Contents

About the Consulting Editor

Anne B. Casto, RHIA, CCS, is the president of Casto Consulting, LLC. Casto Consulting, LLC is a consulting firm that provides services to hospitals and other healthcare stakeholders primarily in the areas of reimbursement and coding. Casto Consulting, LLC specializes in linking coding and billing practices to positive revenue cycle outcomes. Additionally, the firm provides guidance to consulting firms, healthcare organizations and healthcare insurers regarding reimbursement methodologies and Medicare regulations.

Additionally, Ms. Casto is a lecturer in the HIMS department at The Ohio State University, School of Health and Rehabilitation Sciences. Over the past 18 years, Ms. Casto has taught numerous courses in the areas of healthcare reimbursement, coding, healthcare data trending, and coding analytics.

Prior to her current roles, Ms. Casto was the vice president of clinical information for Cleverley & Associates where she worked very closely with APC regulations and guidelines, preparing hospitals for the implementation of the Medicare OPPS. Ms. Casto was also the clinical information product manager for CHIPS/Ingenix. She joined CHIPS/Ingenix in 1998 and spent the majority of her time developing coding compliance products for the inpatient and outpatient settings.

Ms. Casto has been responsible for inpatient and outpatient coding activities in several large hospitals including Mt. Sinai Medical Center (NYC), Beth Israel Medical Center (NYC), and The Ohio State University. She worked extensively with CMI, quality measures, physician documentation, and coding accuracy efforts at these facilities.

Ms. Casto received her degree in Health Information Management at The Ohio State University in 1995. She received her Certified Coding Specialist credential in 1998 from the American Health Information Management Association. In 2009 Ms. Casto received her ICD-10-CM/PCS Trainer certificate from AHIMA. Ms. Casto is the author of an AHIMA-published textbook entitled *Principles of Healthcare Reimbursement*. Additionally, Ms. Casto was a contributing author to the published AHIMA books: *Severity DRGs and Reimbursement; A MS-DRG Primer* and *Effective Management of Coding Services.*

Ms. Casto received the AHIMA Legacy Award, part of the FORE Triumph Awards, in 2007 which honors a significant contribution to the knowledge base of the HIM field through an insightful publication. Additionally, Ms. Casto was honored with the Ohio Health Information Management Association's Distinguished Member Award in 2008 and the Ohio Health Information Management Association's Professional Achievement Award in 2011.

Acknowledgments

Many thanks to my family for their support during this project. Thanks to Dr. Susan White, The Ohio State University; your data manipulation skills are second to none. I thank the reviewers for their thoughtful comments and suggestions. Many thanks to Linda Hyde, RHIA, and Rachael D'Andrea, MS, RHIA, CHTS-TR, CPHQ for their very thorough technical review of the book.

ICD-10-PCS Overview

The *International Classification of Diseases, Tenth Revision, Procedure Coding System* (ICD-10-PCS) was created to accompany the World Health Organization's (WHO) ICD-10 diagnosis classification. This coding system was developed to replace ICD-9-CM procedure codes for reporting inpatient procedures. ICD-10-PCS was designed to enable each code to have a standard structure and be very descriptive, and yet flexible enough to accommodate future needs.

History of ICD-10-PCS

The WHO has maintained the International Classification of Diseases (ICD) for recording cause of death since 1893. It has updated the ICD periodically to reflect new discoveries in epidemiology and changes in medical understanding of disease. The International Classification of Diseases Tenth Revision (ICD-10), published in 1992, is the latest revision of the ICD. The WHO authorized the National Center for Health Statistics (NCHS) to develop a clinical modification of ICD-10 for use in the United States. This version of ICD-10 is called ICD-10-CM, and is intended to replace the previous US clinical modification, ICD-9-CM, that had been in use since 1979. ICD-9-CM contains a procedure classification; ICD-10-CM does not.

The Centers for Medicare and Medicaid Services (CMS), the agency responsible for maintaining the inpatient procedure code set in the United States, contracted with 3M Health Information Systems in 1993 to design and then develop a procedure classification system to replace Volume 3 of ICD-9-CM. ICD-10-PCS is the result. ICD-10-PCS was initially released in 1998. It has been updated annually since that time.

ICD-10-PCS Design

ICD-10-PCS is fundamentally different from previous procedure classification systems in its structure, organization, and capabilities. It was designed and developed to adhere to recommendations made by the National Committee on Vital and Health Statistics (NCVHS). It also incorporates input from a wide range of organizations, individual physicians, healthcare professionals, and researchers. Several structural attributes were recommended for a new procedure coding system. These attributes include a multiaxial structure, completeness, and expandability.

Multiaxial Structure

The key attribute that provides the framework for all other structural attributes is multiaxial code structure. *Multiaxial code structure* makes it possible for the ICD-10-PCS to be complete, expandable, and provide a high degree of flexibility and functionality.

ICD-10-PCS codes are composed of seven characters. Each character represents a category of information that can be specified about the procedure performed. A character defines both the category of information and its physical position in the code. A character's position can be understood as a semi-independent axis of classification that allows different specific values to be inserted into that space, and whose physical position remains stable. Within a defined code range, a character retains the general meaning that it confers on any value in that position.

Completeness

Completeness is considered a key structural attribute for a new procedure coding system. The specific recommendation for completeness included that a unique code be available for each significant procedure, that each code retain its unique definition, and that codes that have been deleted are not reused.

In ICD-10-PCS, a unique code is constructed for every significantly different procedure. Within each section, a character defines a consistent component of a code, and contains all applicable values for that character. The values define individual expressions (Open, Percutaneous) of the character's general meaning (approach) that are then used to construct unique procedure codes. Because all approaches by which a procedure is performed are assigned a separate approach value, every procedure which uses a different approach will have its own unique code. This is true of the other characters as well. The same procedure performed on a different body part has its own unique code; the same procedure performed using a different device has its own unique code, and so on.

Because ICD-10-PCS codes are constructed of individual values rather than lists of fixed codes and text descriptions, the unique, stable definition of a code in the system is retained. New values may be added to the system to represent a specific new approach or device or qualifier, but whole codes by design cannot be given new meanings and reused.

Expandability

Expandability was also recommended as a key structural attribute. The specific recommendation for expandability included that the system be capable of accommodating new procedures and technology and that these new codes could be added to the system without disrupting the existing structure.

ICD-10-PCS is designed to be easily updated as new codes are required for new procedures and new techniques. Changes to ICD-10-PCS can all be made within the existing structure because whole codes are not added. Instead, a new value for a character can be added to the system as needed. Likewise, an existing value for a character can be added to a table(s) in the system.

ICD-10-PCS Additional Characteristics

ICD-10-PCS possesses several additional characteristics in response to government and industry recommendations. These characteristics are

- Standardized terminology within the coding system
- Standardized level of specificity
- No diagnostic information
- No explicit "not otherwise specified" (NOS) code options
- Limited use of "not elsewhere classified" (NEC) code options

Standardized Terminology

Words commonly used in clinical vocabularies may have multiple meanings. This can cause confusion and result in inaccurate data. ICD-10-PCS is standardized and self-contained. Characters and values used in the system are defined in the system. For example, the word *excision* is used to describe a wide variety of surgical procedures. In ICD-10-PCS, the word *excision* describes a single, precise surgical objective, defined as "cutting out or off, without replacement, a portion of a body part."

No Eponyms or Common Procedure Names

The terminology used in ICD-10-PCS is standardized to provide precise and stable definitions of all procedures performed. This standardized terminology is used in all ICD-10-PCS code descriptions. As a result, ICD-10-PCS code descriptions do not include eponyms or common procedure names.

In ICD-10-PCS, physicians' names are not included in a code description, nor are procedures identified by common terms or acronyms such as appendectomy or CABG. Instead, such procedures are coded to the root operation that accurately identifies the objective of the procedure.

ICD-10-PCS assigns procedure codes according to the root operation that matches the objective of the procedure. By relying on the universal objectives defined in root operations rather than eponyms or specific procedure titles that change or become obsolete, ICD-10-PCS preserves the capacity to define past, present, and future procedures accurately using stable terminology in the form of characters and values.

No Combination Codes

With rare exceptions, ICD-10-PCS does not define multiple procedures with one code. This is to preserve standardized terminology and consistency across the system. A procedure that meets the reporting criteria for a separate procedure is coded separately in ICD-10-PCS. This allows the system to respond to changes in technology and medical practice with the maximum degree of stability and flexibility.

Standardized Level of Specificity

ICD-10-PCS provides a standardized level of specificity for each code, so each code represents a single procedure variation. In general, ICD-10-PCS code descriptions are much more specific than previous procedure classification systems but sometimes an ICD-10-PCS code description is actually less specific. ICD-10-PCS provides a standardized level of specificity that can be predicted across the system.

Diagnosis Information Excluded

Another key feature of ICD-10-PCS is that information pertaining to a diagnosis is excluded from the code descriptions. Adding diagnosis information limits the flexibility and functionality of a procedure coding system. It has the effect of placing a code "off limits" because the diagnosis in the medical record does not match the diagnosis in the procedure code description. The code cannot be used even though the procedural part of the code description precisely matches the procedure performed. Diagnosis information is not contained in any ICD-10-PCS code. The diagnosis codes, not the procedure codes, will specify the reason the procedure is performed.

Not Otherwise Specified (NOS) Code Options Restricted

The standardized level of specificity designed into ICD-10-PCS restricts the use of broadly applicable NOS or unspecified code options in the system. A minimal level of specificity is required to construct a valid code.

Limited Not Elsewhere Classified (NEC) Code Options

NEC options are provided in ICD-10-PCS, but only for specific, limited use. In the Medical and Surgical section, two significant NEC options are the root operation value Q, Repair, and the device value Y, Other Device. The root operation Repair is a true NEC value. It is used only when the procedure performed is not one of the other root operations in the Medical and Surgical section. Other Device, on the other hand, is intended to be used to temporarily define new devices that do not have a specific value assigned, until one can be added to the system. No categories of medical or surgical devices are permanently classified to Other Device.

ICD-10-PCS Code Structure

Undergirding ICD-10-PCS is a logical, consistent structure that informs the system as a whole, down to the level of a single code. This means the process of constructing codes in ICD-10-PCS is also logical and consistent: the spaces of the code, called *characters* are filled with individual letters and numbers, called *values*.

Characters

All codes in ICD-10-PCS are seven characters long. Each character in the seven-character code represents an aspect of the procedure. The following are two examples of the code structure: one from the Medical and Surgical section and one from the Ancillary section.

Medical and Surgical Code Structure

Character 1	Character 2	Character 3	Character 4	Character 5	Character 6	Character 7
Section	Body System	Operation	Body Part	Approach	Device	Qualifier

Imaging Section Code Structure

Character 1	Character 2	Character 3	Character 4	Character 5	Character 6	Character 7
Section	Body System	Type	Body Part	Contrast	Qualifier	Qualifier

An ICD-10-PCS code is best understood as the result of a process rather than as an isolated, fixed quantity. The process consists of assigning values from among the valid choices for that part of the system, according to the rules governing the construction of codes.

Values

One of 34 possible values can be assigned to each character in a code: the numbers 0 through 9 and the alphabet (except the letters I and O, because they are easily confused with the numbers 1 and 0). A finished code looks like this: 02103D4.

This code is derived by choosing a specific value for each of the seven characters. Based on details about the procedure performed, values for each character specifying the section, body system, root operation, body part, approach, device, and qualifier are assigned. Because the definition of each character is a function of its physical position in the code, the same value placed in a different position in the code means something different. The value 0 in the first character means something different than 0 in the second character, or 0 in the third character, and so on.

Code Structure Example

The following example defines each character using the code 0LB50ZZ, Excision of right lower arm and wrist tendon, Open approach. This example comes from the Medical and Surgical section of ICD-10-PCS.

Character 1: Section

The first character in the code determines the broad procedure category, or section, where the code is found. In this example, the section is Medical and Surgical. 0 is the value that represents Medical and Surgical in the first character.

Character 1	Character 2	Character 3	Character 4	Character 5	Character 6	Character 7
Section	Body System	Root Operation	Body Part	Approach	Device	Qualifier
0						

Character 2: Body System

The second character defines the body system—the general physiological system or anatomical region involved. Examples of body systems include Lower Arteries, Central Nervous System, and Respiratory System. In this example, the body system is Tendons, represented by the value L.

Character 1	Character 2	Character 3	Character 4	Character 5	Character 6	Character 7
Section	Body System	Root Operation	Body Part	Approach	Device	Qualifier
0	L					

Character 3: Root Operation

The third character defines the root operation, or the objective of the procedure. Some examples of root operations are Bypass, Drainage, and Reattachment. In this example code, the root operation is Excision. When used in the third character of the code, the value B represents Excision.

Character 1	Character 2	Character 3	Character 4	Character 5	Character 6	Character 7
Section	Body System	Root Operation	Body Part	Approach	Device	Qualifier
0	L	B				

Character 4: Body Part

The fourth character defines the body part or specific anatomical site where the procedure was performed. The body system (second character) provides only a general indication of the procedure site. The body part and body system values together provide a precise description of the procedure site. Examples of body parts are Kidney, Tonsils, and Thymus. In this example, the body part value is 5, Lower Arm and Wrist, Right. When the second character is L, the value 5 when used in the fourth character of the code represents the right lower arm and wrist tendon.

Character 1	Character 2	Character 3	Character 4	Character 5	Character 6	Character 7
Section	Body System	Root Operation	Body Part	Approach	Device	Qualifier
0	L	B	5			

Character 5: Approach

The fifth character defines the approach, or the technique used to reach the procedure site. Seven different approach values are used in the Medical and Surgical section to define the approach. Examples of approaches include Open and Percutaneous Endoscopic. In this example code, the approach is Open and is represented by the value 0.

Character 1	Character 2	Character 3	Character 4	Character 5	Character 6	Character 7
Section	Body System	Root Operation	Body Part	Approach	Device	Qualifier
0	L	B	5	0		

Character 6: Device

Depending on the procedure performed, there may be a device left in place at the end of the procedure. The sixth character defines the device. Device values fall into four basic categories:

- Grafts and Prostheses
- Implants
- Simple or Mechanical Appliances
- Electronic Appliances

In this example, there is no device used in the procedure. The value Z is used to represent No Device, as shown here:

Character 1	Character 2	Character 3	Character 4	Character 5	Character 6	Character 7
Section	Body System	Operation	Body Part	Approach	Device	Qualifier
0	L	B	5	0	Z	

Character 7: Qualifier

The seventh character defines a qualifier for the code. A qualifier specifies an additional attribute of the procedure, if applicable. Examples of qualifiers include Diagnostic and Stereotactic. Qualifier choices vary depending on the previous values selected. In this example, there is no specific qualifier applicable to this procedure, so the value is No Qualifier, represented by the letter Z.

Character 1	Character 2	Character 3	Character 4	Character 5	Character 6	Character 7
Section	Body System	Operation	Body Part	Approach	Device	Qualifier
0	L	B	5	0	Z	Z

0LB50ZZ is the complete specification of the procedure "Excision of right lower arm and wrist tendon, open approach."

ICD-10-PCS Organization and Official Conventions

The *ICD-10-PCS Code Book, Professional Edition,* 2021 is based on the official *International Classification of Diseases, Tenth Revision, Procedure Coding System*, issued by the US Department of Health and Human Services (HHS) and CMS. This book is consistent with the content of the government's version of ICD-10-PCS and follows the official conventions.

Index

The Alphabetic Index is provided to assist the user with locating the appropriate table to construct procedure codes. Each table contains all the information required to construct valid procedure codes. Coders should not code from the PCS Index alone; the PCS code tables should always be consulted before assigning a PCS procedure code.

Main Terms

Main terms in the Alphabetic Index reflect the root operations, third character, of procedures. The Index includes not only root operation terms, but also other common procedural terms, anatomical sites, and device terms. The main terms are listed alphabetically. After the coder has located the correct main term and subterm in the Alphabetic Index, he or she is provided with the first three to four digits of the procedure code. The coder should then move to the Tables section of the code book and locate the appropriate table to complete the code construction. Even if the entire seven-digit code is provided in the Index, the coder should still reference the Tables to ensure the correct PCS code has been constructed.

See Reference

Common procedure terms are often listed with the *see* reference. The coder is instructed to follow the reference provided in order to locate the appropriate table to construct the code. For example, the *see* reference is present for the main term Colectomy. The Index excerpt is as follows:

Colectomy

  see Excision, Gastrointestinal System 0DB

  see Resection, Gastrointestinal System 0DT

In this example, the coder should review the definition of the root operations Excision and Resection to determine which is consistent with the medical record documentation. The coder should then proceed to the corresponding table as suggested by the *see* reference.

Use Reference

Anatomical site terms and device terms are often listed with the *use* reference. The coder is instructed to follow the reference provided in order to locate the appropriate main term for the procedure in question. For example, the *use* reference is present for the main term Inferior rectus muscle. The Index excerpt is as follows:

> **Inferior rectus muscle**
>
> > *use* Muscle, Extraocular, Left
> >
> > *use* Muscle, Extraocular, Right

In this example, the coder should identify the root operation for the procedure, and then look for the subterm that identifies the body part indicated in the *use* reference. For example, the procedure is excision of the inferior rectus muscle. The coder would locate the main term Excision. The Index excerpt is as follows:

> **Excision**
>
> > Muscle
> >
> > > Extraocular
> > >
> > > > Left 08BM
> > > >
> > > > Right 08BL

In this example, the coder knows that the Code Table 08B is the correct table because the previous review of the *use* reference identified that the inferior rectus muscle is an extraocular muscle. The coder can now proceed to the 08B Table to finish constructing the PCS code.

In addition to the *use* reference, the coder may also consult appendix D for Body Part Table or appendix E for the Device Table.

Code Tables

ICD-10-PCS contains 17 sections of Code Tables, represented by the numbers 0 through 9 and the letters B through D, F through H, and X. The Tables are organized by general type of procedure. The three main sections of tables include:

1. **Medical and Surgical section**
   - Medical and Surgical (first character 0)

2. **Medical and Surgical Related sections**
   - Obstetrics (first character 1)
   - Placement (first character 2)
   - Administration (first character 3)
   - Measurement and Monitoring (first character 4)
   - Extracorporeal or Systemic Assistance and Performance (first character 5)
   - Extracorporeal or Systemic Therapies (first character 6)
   - Osteopathic (first character 7)
   - Other Procedures (first character 8)
   - Chiropractic (first character 9)

3. **Ancillary sections**
   - Imaging (first character B)
   - Nuclear Medicine (first character C)
   - Radiation Therapy (first character D)
   - Physical Rehabilitation and Diagnostic Audiology (first character F)
   - Mental Health (first character G)
   - Substance Abuse (first character H)
   - New Technology (first character X)

Each code table is defined by the first three characters of the PCS code. Each of these characters is displayed above the table. The table consists of all the options for characters 4 through 7. The root operation or root type, character 3, is present along with its official definition. Table 097 is provided here as an example of the table structure.

0 **Medical and Surgical**

9 **Ear, Nose, Sinus**

7 **Dilation: Expanding an orifice or the lumen of a tubular body part**

Body Part Character 4	Approach Character 5	Device Character 6	Qualifier Character 7
F Eustachian Tube, Right **G** Eustachian Tube, Left	**0** Open **7** Via Natural or Artificial Opening **8** Via Natural or Artificial Opening Endoscopic	**D** Intraluminal Device **Z** No Device	**Z** No Qualifier
F Eustachian Tube, Right **G** Eustachian Tube, Left	**3** Percutaneous **4** Percutaneous Endoscopic	**Z** No Device	**Z** No Qualifier

There can be multiple rows within the table for the first three characters, so the coder must carefully review all the applicable rows. Additionally, a table may cover multiple pages. Therefore, the coder must continue to review the code table options until the end of the table is reached to ensure the correct PCS code has been constructed.

AHA *Coding Clinic* for ICD-10-CM and ICD-10-PCS

The American Hospital Association began publishing coding guidance for ICD-10-CM and ICD-10-PCS in the fourth quarter of 2012. In this code book we identify procedure codes that are discussed in the *Coding Clinic* guidance fourth quarter 2012 through second quarter 2020. In the Medical and Surgical section, after each body system table section, there is an AHA *Coding Clinic* section that lists the references. For all other sections of the code book, the AHA *Coding Clinic* section follows the Tables section. In the AHA *Coding Clinic* section, the PCS codes included in AHA *Coding Clinic* guidance are listed with a sky blue note that alerts the coder to review the AHA *Coding Clinic* prior to assignment of the code to ensure appropriate and accurate reporting. The quarter of publication, year and page number(s) are provided in the note.

AHA CC: 4Q; 2012; pg#-pg#

AHA Coding Clinic Crosswalk for Deleted Codes

Deleted Code	Coding Clinic Reference	Replacement Code
047K3Z6	4Q, 2016, 88-89	047K3ZZ
04CK3Z6	4Q, 2016, 88-89	04CK3ZZ
04V03E6	4Q, 2016, 91-92	04V03EZ
04V03F6	4Q, 2016, 92-94	04V03FZ
0B5S0ZZ	2Q, 2016, 17-18	See 0B5T0ZZ
0BQR0ZZ	2Q, 2016, 22-23	See 0BQT0ZZ
0BQR4ZZ	3Q, 2014, 28	See 0BQT4ZZ
0BQS0ZZ	2Q, 2016, 22-23	See 0BQT0ZZ
0BQS4ZZ	3Q, 2014, 28	See 0BQT4ZZ
0NQS0ZZ	3Q, 2016, 29-30	See 0NQR0ZZ
0NSS04Z	3Q, 2014, 23-24	See 0NSR04Z
0NSS0ZZ	1Q, 2017, 20-21	See 0NSR0ZZ
0NR80JZ	3Q, 2017, 17	See 0NR70JZ

ICD-10-PCS Coding Guidelines

The ICD-10-PCS Coding Guidelines are presented here in the introduction and throughout this manual. Within the manual, the Medical and Surgical Section Guidelines are presented after the Introduction of the Medical and Surgical section. The Obstetric Section Guidelines are presented after the Introduction of the Obstetrics section. Lastly, the New Technology Guidelines are presented after the Introduction of the New Technology section.

ICD-10-PCS Official Guidelines for Coding and Reporting, 2021

The Centers for Medicare and Medicaid Services (CMS) and the National Center for Health Statistics (NCHS), two departments within the US federal government's Department of Health and Human Services (DHHS) provide the following guidelines for coding and reporting using the International Classification of Diseases, 10th Revision, Procedure Coding System (ICD-10-PCS). These guidelines should be used as a companion document to the official version of the ICD-10-PCS as published on the CMS website. The ICD-10-PCS is a procedure classification published by the United States for classifying procedures performed in hospital inpatient health care settings.

These guidelines have been approved by the four organizations that make up the Cooperating Parties for the ICD-10-PCS: the American Hospital Association (AHA), the American Health Information Management Association (AHIMA), CMS, and NCHS.

These guidelines are a set of rules that have been developed to accompany and complement the official conventions and instructions provided within the ICD-10-PCS itself. They are intended to provide direction that is applicable in most circumstances. However, there may be unique circumstances where exceptions are applied. The instructions and conventions of the classification take precedence over guidelines. These guidelines are based on the coding and sequencing instructions in the Tables, Index, and Definitions of ICD-10-PCS, but provide additional instruction. Adherence to these guidelines when assigning ICD-10-PCS procedure codes is required under the Health Insurance Portability and Accountability Act (HIPAA). The procedure codes have been adopted under HIPAA for hospital inpatient healthcare settings. A joint effort between the healthcare provider and the coder is essential to achieve complete and accurate documentation, code assignment, and reporting of diagnoses and procedures. These guidelines have been developed to assist both the healthcare provider and the coder in identifying those procedures that are to be reported. The importance of consistent, complete documentation in the medical record cannot be overemphasized. Without such documentation, accurate coding cannot be achieved.

Conventions

A1. ICD-10-PCS codes are composed of seven characters. Each character is an axis of classification that specifies information about the procedure performed. Within a defined code range, a character specifies the same type of information in that axis of classification.

Example: The fifth axis of classification specifies the approach in sections 0 through 4 and 7 through 9 of the system.

A2. One of 34 possible values can be assigned to each axis of classification in the seven-character code: they are the numbers 0 through 9 and the alphabet (except the letters I and O because they are easily confused with the numbers 1 and 0). The number of unique values used in an axis of classification differs as needed.

Example: Where the fifth axis of classification specifies the approach, seven different approach values are currently used to specify the approach.

A3. The valid values for an axis of classification can be added to as needed.

Example: If a significantly distinct type of device is used in a new procedure, a new device value can be added to the system.

A4. As with words in their context, the meaning of any single value is a combination of its axis of classification and any preceding values on which it may be dependent.

Example: The meaning of a body part value in the Medical and Surgical section is always dependent on the body system value. The body part value 0 in the Central Nervous body system specifies Brain and the body part value 0 in the Peripheral Nervous body system specifies Cervical Plexus.

A5. As the system is expanded to become increasingly detailed, over time more values will depend on preceding values for their meaning.

Example: In the Lower Joints body system, the device value 3 in the root operation Insertion specifies Infusion Device and the device value 3 in the root operation Replacement specifies Ceramic Synthetic Substitute.

A6. The purpose of the Alphabetic Index is to locate the appropriate table that contains all information necessary to construct a procedure code. The PCS Tables should always be consulted to find the most appropriate valid code.

A7. It is not required to consult the Index first before proceeding to the Tables to complete the code. A valid code may be chosen directly from the Tables.

A8. All seven characters must be specified to be a valid code. If the documentation is incomplete for coding purposes, the physician should be queried for the necessary information.

A9. Within a PCS Table, valid codes include all combinations of choices in characters 4 through 7 contained in the same row of the table. In the example below, 0JHT3VZ is a valid code, and 0JHW3VZ is *not* a valid code.

Section:	0	Medical and Surgical
Body System:	J	Subcutaneous Tissue and Fascia
Operation:	H	**Insertion:** Putting in a nonbiological appliance that monitors, assists, performs, or prevents a physiological function but does not physically take the place of a body part

Body Part (4th)	Approach (5th)	Device (6th)	Qualifier (7th)
S Subcutaneous Tissue and Fascia, Head and Neck **V** Subcutaneous Tissue and Fascia, Upper Extremity **W** Subcutaneous Tissue and Fascia, Lower Extremity	**0** Open **3** Percutaneous	**1** Radioactive Element **3** Infusion Device **Y** Other Device	**Z** No Qualifier
T Subcutaneous Tissue and Fascia, Trunk	**0** Open **3** Percutaneous	**1** Radioactive Element **3** Infusion Device **V** Infusion Pump **Y** Other Device	**Z** No Qualifier

A10. "And," when used in a code description, means "and/or," except when used to describe a combination of multiple body parts for which separate values exist for each body part (e.g., Skin and Subcutaneous Tissue used as a qualifier, where there are separate body part values for "Skin" and "Subcutaneous Tissue").

Example: Lower Arm and Wrist Muscle means lower arm and/or wrist muscle.

A11. Many of the terms used to construct PCS codes are defined within the system. It is the coder's responsibility to determine what the documentation in the medical record equates to in the PCS definitions. The physician is not expected to use the terms used in PCS code descriptions, nor is the coder required to query the physician when the correlation between the documentation and the defined PCS terms is clear.

Example: When the physician documents "partial resection" the coder can independently correlate "partial resection" to the root operation Excision without querying the physician for clarification.

Medical and Surgical Section Guidelines (section 0)

B2. Body System
General guidelines
B2.1a

The procedure codes in Anatomical Regions, General, Anatomical Regions, Upper Extremities and Anatomical Regions, Lower Extremities can be used when the procedure is performed on an anatomical region rather than a specific body part, or on the rare occasion when no information is available to support assignment of a code to a specific body part.

Examples: Chest tube drainage of the pleural cavity is coded to the root operation Drainage found in the body system Anatomical Regions, General. Suture repair of the abdominal wall is coded to the root operation Repair in the body system Anatomical Regions, General. Amputation of the foot is coded to the root operation Detachment in the body system Anatomical Regions, Lower Extremities.

B2.1b

Where the general body part values "upper" and "lower" are provided as an option in the Upper Arteries, Lower Arteries, Upper Veins, Lower Veins, Muscles and Tendons body systems, "upper" or "lower "specifies body parts located above or below the diaphragm respectively.

Example: Vein body parts above the diaphragm are found in the Upper Veins body system; vein body parts below the diaphragm are found in the Lower Veins body system.

B3. Root Operation
General guidelines
B3.1a

In order to determine the appropriate root operation, the full definition of the root operation as contained in the PCS Tables must be applied.

B3.1b

Components of a procedure specified in the root operation definition or explanation as integral to that root operation are not coded separately. Procedural steps necessary to reach the operative site and close the operative site, including anastomosis of a tubular body part, are also not coded separately.

Example: Resection of a joint as part of a joint replacement procedure is included in the root operation definition of Replacement and is not coded separately. Laparotomy performed to reach the site of an open liver biopsy is not coded separately. In a resection of sigmoid colon with anastomosis of descending colon to rectum, the anastomosis is not coded separately.

Multiple procedures
B3.2

During the same operative episode, multiple procedures are coded if:

    a.   The same root operation is performed on different body parts as defined by distinct values of the body part character.

        Examples: Diagnostic excision of liver and pancreas are coded separately. Excision of lesion in the ascending colon and excision of lesion in the transverse colon are coded separately.

    b.   The same root operation is repeated in multiple body parts, and those body parts are separate and distinct body parts classified to a single ICD-10-PCS body part value.

        Examples: Excision of the sartorius muscle and excision of the gracilis muscle are both included in the upper leg muscle body part value, and multiple procedures are coded. Extraction of multiple toenails are coded separately.

    c.   Multiple root operations with distinct objectives are performed on the same body part.

        Example: Destruction of sigmoid lesion and bypass of sigmoid colon are coded separately.

    d.   The intended root operation is attempted using one approach but is converted to a different approach.

        Example: Laparoscopic cholecystectomy converted to an open cholecystectomy is coded as percutaneous endoscopic Inspection and open Resection.

Discontinued or incomplete procedures
B3.3

If the intended procedure is discontinued or otherwise not completed, code the procedure to the root operation performed. If a procedure is discontinued before any other root operation is performed, code the root operation Inspection of the body part or anatomical region inspected.

Example: A planned aortic valve replacement procedure is discontinued after the initial thoracotomy and before any incision is made in the heart muscle, when the patient becomes hemodynamically unstable. This procedure is coded as an open Inspection of the mediastinum.

Biopsy procedures
B3.4a

Biopsy procedures are coded using the root operations Excision, Extraction, or Drainage and the qualifier Diagnostic.
Examples: Fine needle aspiration biopsy of fluid in the lung is coded to the root operation Drainage with the qualifier Diagnostic. Biopsy of bone marrow is coded to the root operation Extraction with the qualifier Diagnostic. Lymph node sampling for biopsy is coded to the root operation Excision with the qualifier Diagnostic.

Biopsy followed by more definitive treatment
B3.4b

If a diagnostic Excision, Extraction, or Drainage procedure (biopsy) is followed by a more definitive procedure, such as Destruction, Excision or Resection at the same procedure site, both the biopsy and the more definitive treatment are coded.

Example: Biopsy of breast followed by partial mastectomy at the same procedure site, both the biopsy and the partial mastectomy procedure are coded.

Overlapping body layers
B3.5

If root operations Excision, Extraction, Repair or Inspection are performed on overlapping layers of the musculoskeletal system, the body part specifying the deepest layer is coded.

Example: Excisional debridement that includes skin and subcutaneous tissue and muscle is coded to the muscle body part.

Bypass procedures
B3.6a

Bypass procedures are coded by identifying the body part bypassed "from" and the body part bypassed "to." The fourth character body part specifies the body part bypassed from, and the qualifier specifies the body part bypassed to.

Example: Bypass from stomach to jejunum, stomach is the body part and jejunum is the qualifier.

B3.6b

Coronary artery bypass procedures are coded differently than other bypass procedures as described in the previous guideline. Rather than identifying the body part bypassed from, the body part identifies the number of coronary artery sites bypassed to, and the qualifier specifies the vessel bypassed from.

Example: Aortocoronary artery bypass of the left anterior descending coronary artery and the obtuse marginal coronary artery is classified in the body part axis of classification as two coronary arteries and the qualifier specifies the aorta as the body part bypassed from.

B3.6c

If multiple coronary arteries are bypassed, a separate procedure is coded for each coronary artery that uses a different device and/or qualifier.

Example: Aortocoronary artery bypass and internal mammary coronary artery bypass are coded separately.

Control vs. more definitive root operations
B3.7

The root operation Control is defined as, "Stopping, or attempting to stop, postprocedural or other acute bleeding." If an attempt to stop postprocedural or other acute bleeding is initially unsuccessful, and to stop the bleeding requires performing a more definitive root operation, such as Bypass, Detachment, Excision, Extraction, Reposition, Replacement, or Resection, then the more definitive root operation is coded instead of Control.

Example: Resection of spleen to stop bleeding is coded to Resection instead of Control.

Excision vs. Resection
B3.8

PCS contains specific body parts for anatomical subdivisions of a body part, such as lobes of the lungs or liver and regions of the intestine. Resection of the specific body part is coded whenever all of the body part is cut out or off, rather than coding Excision of a less specific body part.

Example: Left upper lung lobectomy is coded to Resection of Upper Lung Lobe, Left rather than Excision of Lung, Left.

Excision for graft
B3.9

If an autograft is obtained from a different procedure site in order to complete the objective of the procedure, a separate procedure is coded, except when the seventh character qualifier value in the ICD-10-PCS table fully specifies the site from which the autograft was obtained.

Examples: Coronary bypass with excision of saphenous vein graft, excision of saphenous vein is coded separately. Replacement of breast with autologous deep inferior epigastric artery perforator (DIEP) flap, excision of the DIEP flap is not coded separately. The seventh character qualifier value Deep Inferior Epigastric Artery Perforator Flap in the Replacement table fully specifies the site of the autograft harvest.

Fusion procedures of the spine
B3.10a

The body part coded for a spinal vertebral joint(s) rendered immobile by a spinal fusion procedure is classified by the level of the spine (e.g. thoracic). There are distinct body part values for a single vertebral joint and for multiple vertebral joints at each spinal level.

Example: Body part values specify Lumbar Vertebral Joint, Lumbar Vertebral Joints, 2 or More and Lumbosacral Vertebral Joint.

B3.10b

If multiple vertebral joints are fused, a separate procedure is coded for each vertebral joint that uses a different device and/or qualifier.

Example: Fusion of lumbar vertebral joint, posterior approach, anterior column and fusion of lumbar vertebral joint, posterior approach, posterior column are coded separately.

B3.10c

Combinations of devices and materials are often used on a vertebral joint to render the joint immobile. When combinations of devices are used on the same vertebral joint, the device value coded for the procedure is as follows:

- If an interbody fusion device is used to render the joint immobile (containing bone graft or bone graft substitute), the procedure is coded with the device value Interbody Fusion Device
- If bone graft is the *only* device used to render the joint immobile, the procedure is coded with the device value Nonautologous Tissue Substitute or Autologous Tissue Substitute
- If a mixture of autologous and nonautologous bone graft (with or without biological or synthetic extenders or binders) is used to render the joint immobile, code the procedure with the device value Autologous Tissue Substitute

Examples: Fusion of a vertebral joint using a cage style interbody fusion device containing morsellized bone graft is coded to the device Interbody Fusion Device. Fusion of a vertebral joint using a bone dowel interbody fusion device made of cadaver bone and packed with a mixture of local morsellized bone and demineralized bone matrix is coded to the device Interbody Fusion Device. Fusion of a vertebral joint using both autologous bone graft and bone bank bone graft is coded to the device Autologous Tissue Substitute.

Inspection procedures
B3.11a

Inspection of a body part(s) performed in order to achieve the objective of a procedure is not coded separately.

Example: Fiberoptic bronchoscopy performed for irrigation of bronchus, only the irrigation procedure is coded.

B3.11b

If multiple tubular body parts are inspected, the most distal body part (the body part furthest from the starting point of the inspection) is coded. If multiple non-tubular body parts in a region are inspected, the body part that specifies the entire area inspected is coded.

Examples: Cystoureteroscopy with inspection of bladder and ureters is coded to the ureter body part value. Exploratory laparotomy with general inspection of abdominal contents is coded to the peritoneal cavity body part value.

B3.11c

When both an Inspection procedure and another procedure are performed on the same body part during the same episode, if the Inspection procedure is performed using a different approach than the other procedure, the Inspection procedure is coded separately.

Example: Endoscopic Inspection of the duodenum is coded separately when open Excision of the duodenum is performed during the same procedural episode.

Occlusion vs. Restriction for vessel embolization procedures
B3.12

If the objective of an embolization procedure is to completely close a vessel, the root operation Occlusion is coded. If the objective of an embolization procedure is to narrow the lumen of a vessel, the root operation Restriction is coded.

Examples: Tumor embolization is coded to the root operation Occlusion, because the objective of the procedure is to cut off the blood supply to the vessel. Embolization of a cerebral aneurysm is coded to the root operation Restriction, because the objective of the procedure is not to close off the vessel entirely, but to narrow the lumen of the vessel at the site of the aneurysm where it is abnormally wide.

Release procedures
B3.13

In the root operation Release, the body part value coded is the body part being freed and not the tissue being manipulated or cut to free the body part.

Example: Lysis of intestinal adhesions is coded to the specific intestine body part value.

Release vs. Division
B3.14

If the sole objective of the procedure is freeing a body part without cutting the body part, the root operation is Release. If the sole objective of the procedure is separating or transecting a body part, the root operation is Division.

Examples: Freeing a nerve root from surrounding scar tissue to relieve pain is coded to the root operation Release. Severing a nerve root to relieve pain is coded to the root operation Division.

Reposition for fracture treatment
B3.15

Reduction of a displaced fracture is coded to the root operation Reposition and the application of a cast or splint in conjunction with the Reposition procedure is not coded separately. Treatment of a nondisplaced fracture is coded to the procedure performed.

Examples: Casting of a nondisplaced fracture is coded to the root operation Immobilization in the Placement section.

Putting a pin in a nondisplaced fracture is coded to the root operation Insertion.

Transplantation vs. Administration
B3.16

Putting in a mature and functioning living body part taken from another individual or animal is coded to the root operation Transplantation. Putting in autologous or nonautologous cells is coded to the Administration section.

Example: Putting in autologous or nonautologous bone marrow, pancreatic islet cells or stem cells is coded to the Administration section.

Transfer procedures using multiple tissue layers
B3.17

The root operation Transfer contains qualifiers that can be used to specify when a transfer flap is composed of more than one tissue layer, such as a musculocutaneous flap. For procedures involving transfer of multiple tissue layers including skin, subcutaneous tissue, fascia or muscle, the procedure is coded to the body part value that describes the deepest tissue layer in the flap, and the qualifier can be used to describe the other tissue layer(s) in the transfer flap.

Example: A musculocutaneous flap transfer is coded to the appropriate body part value in the body system Muscles, and the qualifier is used to describe the additional tissue layer(s) in the transfer flap.

Excision/Resection followed by replacement
B3.18

If an Excision or Resection of a body part is followed by a Replacement procedure, code both procedures to identify each distinct objective, except when the Excision or Resection is considered integral and preparatory for the Replacement procedure.

Examples: Mastectomy followed by reconstruction, both Resection and Replacement of the breast are coded to fully capture the distinct objectives of the procedures performed. Maxillectomy with obturator reconstruction, both Excision and Replacement of the maxilla are coded to fully capture the distinct objectives of the procedures performed. Excisional debridement of tendon with skin graft, both the Excision of the tendon and the Replacement of the skin with a graft are coded to fully capture the distinct objectives of the procedures performed. Esophagectomy followed by reconstruction with colonic interposition, both the Resection and the Transfer of the large intestine to function as the esophagus are coded to fully capture the distinct objectives of the procedures performed.

Examples: Resection of a joint as part of a joint replacement procedure is considered integral and preparatory for the Replacement of the joint and the Resection is not coded separately. Resection of a valve as part of a valve replacement procedure is considered integral and preparatory for the valve Replacement and the Resection is not coded separately.

B4. Body Part
General guidelines
B4.1a

If a procedure is performed on a portion of a body part that does not have a separate body part value, code the body part value corresponding to the whole body part.

Example: A procedure performed on the alveolar process of the mandible is coded to the mandible body part.

B4.1b

If the prefix "peri" is combined with a body part to identify the site of the procedure, and the site of the procedure is not further specified, then the procedure is coded to the body part named. This guideline applies only when a more specific body part value is not available.

Examples: A procedure site identified as perirenal is coded to the kidney body part when the site of the procedure is not further specified. A procedure site described in the documentation as peri-urethral, and the documentation also indicates that it is the vulvar tissue and not the urethral tissue that is the site of the procedure, then the procedure is coded to the vulva body part. A procedure site documented as involving the periosteum is coded to the corresponding bone body part.

B4.1c

If a procedure is performed on a continuous section of a tubular body part, code the body part value corresponding to the furthest anatomical site from the point of entry.

Example: A procedure performed on a continuous section of artery from the femoral artery to the external iliac artery with the point of entry at the femoral artery is coded to the external iliac body part.

Branches of body parts
B4.2

Where a specific branch of a body part does not have its own body part value in PCS, the body part is typically coded to the closest proximal branch that has a specific body part value. In the cardiovascular body systems, if a general body part is available in the correct root operation table, and coding to a proximal branch would require assigning a code in a different body system, the procedure is coded using the general body part value.

Examples: A procedure performed on the mandibular branch of the trigeminal nerve is coded to the trigeminal nerve body part value. Occlusion of the bronchial artery is coded to the body part value Upper Artery in the body system Upper Arteries, and not to the body part value Thoracic Aorta, Descending in the body system Heart and Great Vessels.

Bilateral body part values
B4.3

Bilateral body part values are available for a limited number of body parts. If the identical procedure is performed on contralateral body parts, and a bilateral body part value exists for that body part, a single procedure is coded using the bilateral body part value. If no bilateral body part value exists, each procedure is coded separately using the appropriate body part value.

Example: The identical procedure performed on both fallopian tubes is coded once using the body part value Fallopian Tube, Bilateral. The identical procedure performed on both knee joints is coded twice using the body part values Knee Joint, Right and Knee Joint, Left.

Coronary arteries
B4.4

The coronary arteries are classified as a single body part that is further specified by number of arteries treated. One procedure code specifying multiple arteries is used when the same procedure is performed, including the same device and qualifier values.

Examples: Angioplasty of two distinct coronary arteries with placement of two stents is coded as Dilation of Coronary Artery, Two Arteries, with Two Intraluminal Devices. Angioplasty of two distinct coronary arteries, one with stent placed and one without, is coded separately as Dilation of Coronary Artery, One Artery with Intraluminal Device, and Dilation of Coronary Artery, One Artery with no device.

Tendons, ligaments, bursae and fascia near a joint
B4.5

Procedures performed on tendons, ligaments, bursae and fascia supporting a joint are coded to the body part in the respective body system that is the focus of the procedure. Procedures performed on joint structures themselves are coded to the body part in the joint body systems.

Example: Repair of the anterior cruciate ligament of the knee is coded to the knee bursa and ligament body part in the Bursae and Ligaments body system. Knee arthroscopy with shaving of articular cartilage is coded to the knee joint body part in the Lower Joints body system.

Skin, subcutaneous tissue and fascia overlying a joint
B4.6

If a procedure is performed on the skin, subcutaneous tissue or fascia overlying a joint, the procedure is coded to the following body part:

- Shoulder is coded to Upper Arm
- Elbow is coded to Lower Arm
- Wrist is coded to Lower Arm
- Hip is coded to Upper Leg
- Knee is coded to Lower Leg
- Ankle is coded to Foot

Fingers and toes
B4.7

If a body system does not contain a separate body part value for fingers, procedures performed on the fingers are coded to the body part value for the hand. If a body system does not contain a separate body part value for toes, procedures performed on the toes are coded to the body part value for the foot.

Example: Excision of finger muscle is coded to one of the hand muscle body part values in the Muscles body system.

Upper and lower intestinal tract
B4.8

In the Gastrointestinal body system, the general body part values Upper Intestinal Tract and Lower Intestinal Tract are provided as an option for the root operations Change, Inspection, Removal and Revision. Upper Intestinal Tract includes the portion of the gastrointestinal tract from the esophagus down to and including the duodenum, and Lower Intestinal Tract includes the portion of the gastrointestinal tract from the jejunum down to and including the rectum and anus.

Example: In the root operation Change table, change of a device in the jejunum is coded using the body part Lower Intestinal Tract.

B5. Approach
Open approach with percutaneous endoscopic assistance
B5.2a

Procedures performed using the open approach with percutaneous endoscopic assistance are coded to the approach Open.

Example: Laparoscopic-assisted sigmoidectomy is coded to the approach Open.

Percutaneous endoscopic approach with extension of incision
B5.2b

Procedures performed using the percutaneous endoscopic approach, with incision or extension of an incision to assist in the removal of all or a portion of a body part or to anastomose a tubular body part to complete the procedure, are coded to the approach value Percutaneous Endoscopic.

Examples: Laparoscopic sigmoid colectomy with extension of stapling port for removal of specimen and direct anastomosis is coded to the approach value Percutaneous Endoscopic. Laparoscopic nephrectomy with midline incision for removing the resected kidney is coded to the approach value Percutaneous Endoscopic. Robotic-assisted laparoscopic prostatectomy with extension of incision for removal of the resected prostate is coded to the approach value Percutaneous Endoscopic.

External approach
B5.3a

Procedures performed within an orifice on structures that are visible without the aid of any instrumentation are coded to the approach External.

Example: Resection of tonsils is coded to the approach External.

B5.3b

Procedures performed indirectly by the application of external force through the intervening body layers are coded to the approach External.

Example: Closed reduction of fracture is coded to the approach External.

Percutaneous procedure via device

B5.4

Procedures performed percutaneously via a device placed for the procedure are coded to the approach Percutaneous.

Example: Fragmentation of kidney stone performed via percutaneous nephrostomy is coded to the approach Percutaneous.

B6. Device
General guidelines

B6.1a

A device is coded only if a device remains after the procedure is completed. If no device remains, the device value No Device is coded. In limited root operations, the classification provides the qualifier values Temporary and Intraoperative, for specific procedures involving clinically significant devices, where the purpose of the device is to be utilized for a brief duration during the procedure or current inpatient stay. If a device that is intended to remain after the procedure is completed requires removal before the end of the operative episode in which it was inserted (for example, the device size is inadequate or a complication occurs), both the insertion and removal of the device should be coded.

B6.1b

Materials such as sutures, ligatures, radiological markers and temporary post-operative wound drains are considered integral to the performance of a procedure and are not coded as devices.

B6.1c

Procedures performed on a device only and not on a body part are specified in the root operations Change, Irrigation, Removal and Revision, and are coded to the procedure performed.

Example: Irrigation of percutaneous nephrostomy tube is coded to the root operation Irrigation of indwelling device in the Administration section.

Drainage device

B6.2

A separate procedure to put in a drainage device is coded to the root operation Drainage with the device value Drainage Device.

Obstetric Section Guidelines (section 1)

C. Obstetrics Section
Products of conception

C1

Procedures performed on the products of conception are coded to the Obstetrics section. Procedures performed on the pregnant female other than the products of conception are coded to the appropriate root operation in the Medical and Surgical section.

Example: Amniocentesis is coded to the products of conception body part in the Obstetrics section. Repair of obstetric urethral laceration is coded to the urethra body part in the Medical and Surgical section.

Procedures following delivery or abortion

C2

Procedures performed following a delivery or abortion for curettage of the endometrium or evacuation of retained products of conception are all coded in the Obstetrics section, to the root operation Extraction and the body part Products of Conception, Retained. Diagnostic or therapeutic dilation and curettage performed during times other than the postpartum or post-abortion period are all coded in the Medical and Surgical section, to the root operation Extraction and the body part Endometrium.

Radiation Therapy Section Guidelines (section D)

D. Radiation Therapy Section
Brachytherapy

D1.a

Brachytherapy is coded to the modality Brachytherapy in the Radiation Therapy section. When a radioactive brachytherapy source is left in the body at the end of the procedure, it is coded separately to the root operation Insertion with the device value Radioactive Element.

Example: Brachytherapy with implantation of a low dose rate brachytherapy source left in the body at the end of the procedure is coded to the applicable treatment site in section D, Radiation Therapy, with the modality Brachytherapy, the modality qualifier value, Low Dose Rate, and the applicable isotope value and qualifier value. The implantation of the brachytherapy source is coded separately to the device value Radioactive Element in the appropriate Insertion table of the Medical and Surgical section. The Radiation Therapy section code identifies the specific modality and isotope of the brachytherapy, and the root operation Insertion code identifies the implantation of the brachytherapy source that remain in the body at the end of the procedure.

Exception: Implantation of Cesium-131 brachytherapy seeds embedded in a collagen matrix to the treatment site after resection of brain tumor is coded to the root operation Insertion with the device value Radioactive Element, Cesium-131 Collagen Implant. The procedure is coded to the root operation Insertion only, because the device value identifies both the implantation of the radioactive element and a specific brachytherapy isotope that is not included in the Radiation Therapy section tables.

D1.b

A separate procedure to place a temporary applicator for delivering the brachytherapy is coded to the root operation Insertion and the device value Other Device.

Examples: Intrauterine brachytherapy applicator placed as a separate procedure from the brachytherapy procedure is coded to Insertion of Other Device, and the brachytherapy is coded separately using the modality Brachytherapy in the Radiation Therapy section. Intrauterine brachytherapy applicator placed concomitantly with delivery of the brachytherapy dose is coded with a single code using the modality Brachytherapy in the Radiation Therapy section.

New Technology Section Guidelines (section X)

E. New Technology Section

General guidelines

E1.a

Section X codes fully represent the specific procedure described in the code title, and do not require any additional codes from other sections of ICD-10-PCS. When section X contains a code title which describes a specific new technology procedure, and it is the only procedure performed, only the section X code is reported for the procedure. There is no need to report an additional code in another section of ICD-10-PCS.

Example: XW04321 Introduction of Ceftazidime-Avibactam Anti-infective into Central Vein, Percutaneous Approach, New Technology Group 1, can be coded to indicate that Ceftazidime-Avibactam Anti-infective was administered via a central vein. A separate code from table 3E0 in the Administration section of ICD-10-PCS is not coded in addition to this code.

E1.b

When multiple procedures are performed, New Technology section X codes are coded following the multiple procedures guideline.

Examples: Dual filter cerebral embolic filtration used during transcatheter aortic valve replacement (TAVR), X2A5312 Cerebral Embolic Filtration, Dual Filter in Innominate Artery and Left Common Carotid Artery, Percutaneous Approach, New Technology Group 2, is coded for the cerebral embolic filtration, along with an ICD-10-PCS code for the TAVR procedure. Magnetically controlled growth rod (MCGR) placed during a spinal fusion procedure, a code from table XNS, Reposition of the Bones is coded for the MCGR, along with an ICD-10-PCS code for the spinal fusion procedure.

F. Selection of Principal Procedure

The following instructions should be applied in the selection of principal procedure and clarification on the importance of the relation to the principal diagnosis when more than one procedure is performed:

1. Procedure performed for definitive treatment of both principal diagnosis and secondary diagnosis

   a. Sequence procedure performed for definitive treatment most related to principal diagnosis as principal procedure.

2. Procedure performed for definitive treatment and diagnostic procedures performed for both principal diagnosis and secondary diagnosis

   a. Sequence procedure performed for definitive treatment most related to principal diagnosis as principal procedure

3. A diagnostic procedure was performed for the principal diagnosis and a procedure is performed for definitive treatment of a secondary diagnosis.

   a. Sequence diagnostic procedure as principal procedure, since the procedure most related to the principal diagnosis takes precedence.

4. No procedures performed that are related to principal diagnosis; procedures performed for definitive treatment and diagnostic procedures were performed for secondary diagnosis

   a. Sequence procedure performed for definitive treatment of secondary diagnosis as principal procedure, since there are no procedures (definitive or nondefinitive treatment) related to principal diagnosis.

Analog radiography
   see Plain Radiography
Anastomosis
   see Bypass
Anatomical snuffbox
   use Muscle, Lower Arm and Wrist, Left
   use Muscle, Lower Arm and Wrist, Right
Andexanet Alfa, Factor Xa Inhibitor Reversal Agent
   use Coagulation Factor Xa, Inactivated
Andexxa
   use Coagulation Factor Xa, Inactivated
AneuRx® AAA Advantage®
   use Intraluminal Device
Angiectomy
   see Excision, Heart and Great Vessels 02B
   see Excision, Upper Arteries 03B
   see Excision, Lower Arteries 04B
   see Excision, Upper Veins 05B
   see Excision, Lower Veins 06B
Angiocardiography
   Combined right and left heart
      see Fluoroscopy, Heart, Right and Left B216
   Left Heart
      see Fluoroscopy, Heart, Left B215
   Right Heart
      see Fluoroscopy, Heart, Right B214
   SPY system intravascular fluorescence
      see Monitoring, Physiological Systems 4A1
Angiography
   see Plain Radiography, Heart B20
   see Fluoroscopy, Heart B21
Angioplasty
   see Dilation, Heart and Great Vessels 027
   see Repair, Heart and Great Vessels 02Q
   see Replacement, Heart and Great Vessels 02R
   see Dilation, Upper Arteries 037
   see Repair, Upper Arteries 03Q
   see Replacement, Upper Arteries 03R
   see Dilation, Lower Arteries 047
   see Repair, Lower Arteries 04Q
   see Replacement, Lower Arteries 04R
   see Supplement, Heart and Great Vessels 02U
   see Supplement, Upper Arteries 03U
   see Supplement, Lower Arteries 04U
Angiorrhaphy
   see Repair, Heart and Great Vessels 02Q
   see Repair, Upper Arteries 03Q
   see Repair, Lower Arteries 04Q
Angioscopy
   02JY4ZZ
   03JY4ZZ
   04JY4ZZ
Angiotensin II
   use Synthetic Human Angiotensin II
Angiotripsy
   see Occlusion, Upper Arteries 03L
   see Occlusion, Lower Arteries 04L
Angular artery
   use Artery, Face
Angular vein
   use Vein, Face, Left
   use Vein, Face, Right
Annular ligament
   use Bursa and Ligament, Elbow, Left
   use Bursa and Ligament, Elbow, Right
Annuloplasty
   see Repair, Heart and Great Vessels 02Q
   see Supplement, Heart and Great Vessels 02U

Annuloplasty ring
   use Synthetic Substitute
Anoplasty
   see Repair, Anus 0DQQ
   see Supplement, Anus 0DUQ
Anorectal junction
   use Rectum
Anoscopy 0DJD8ZZ
Ansa cervicalis
   use Nerve, Cervical Plexus
Antabuse therapy HZ93ZZZ
Antebrachial fascia
   use Subcutaneous Tissue and Fascia, Lower Arm, Left
   use Subcutaneous Tissue and Fascia, Lower Arm, Right
Anterior (pectoral) lymph node
   use Lymphatic, Axillary, Left
   use Lymphatic, Axillary, Right
Anterior cerebral artery
   use Artery, Intracranial
Anterior cerebral vein
   use Vein, Intracranial
Anterior choroidal artery
   use Artery, Intracranial
Anterior circumflex humeral artery
   use Artery, Axillary, Left
   use Artery, Axillary, Right
Anterior communicating artery
   use Artery, Intracranial
Anterior cruciate ligament (ACL)
   use Bursa and Ligament, Knee, Left
   use Bursa and Ligament, Knee, Right
Anterior crural nerve
   use Nerve, Femoral
Anterior facial vein
   use Vein, Face, Left
   use Vein, Face, Right
Anterior intercostal artery
   use Artery, Internal Mammary, Left
   use Artery, Internal Mammary, Right
Anterior interosseous nerve
   use Nerve, Median
Anterior lateral malleolar artery
   use Artery, Anterior Tibial, Left
   use Artery, Anterior Tibial, Right
Anterior lingual gland
   use Gland, Minor Salivary
Anterior medial malleolar artery
   use Artery, Anterior Tibial, Left
   use Artery, Anterior Tibial, Right
Anterior spinal artery
   use Artery, Vertebral, Left
   use Artery, Vertebral, Right
Anterior tibial recurrent artery
   use Artery, Anterior Tibial, Left
   use Artery, Anterior Tibial, Right
Anterior ulnar recurrent artery
   use Artery, Ulnar, Left
   use Artery, Ulnar, Right
Anterior vagal trunk
   use Nerve, Vagus
Anterior vertebral muscle
   use Muscle, Neck, Left
   use Muscle, Neck, Right
Antibacterial Envelope (TYRX) (AIGISRx)
   use Anti-Infective Envelope
Antigen-free air conditioning
   see Atmospheric Control, Physiological Systems 6A0
Antihelix
   use Ear, External, Bilateral
   use Ear, External, Left
   use Ear, External, Right
Antimicrobial envelope
   use Anti-Infective Envelope
Antitragus
   use Ear, External, Bilateral
   use Ear, External, Left
   use Ear, External, Right

Antrostomy
   see Drainage, Ear, Nose, Sinus 099
Antrotomy
   see Drainage, Ear, Nose, Sinus 099
Antrum of Highmore
   use Sinus, Maxillary, Left
   use Sinus, Maxillary, Right
Aortic annulus
   use Valve, Aortic
Aortic arch
   use Thoracic Aorta, Ascending/Arch
Aortic intercostal artery
   use Upper Artery
Aortography
   see Plain Radiography, Upper Arteries B30
   see Fluoroscopy, Upper Arteries B31
   see Plain Radiography, Lower Arteries B40
   see Fluoroscopy, Lower Arteries B41
Aortoplasty
   see Repair, Aorta, Thoracic, Descending 02QW
   see Repair, Aorta, Thoracic, Ascending/Arch 02QX
   see Replacement, Aorta, Thoracic, Descending 02RW
   see Replacement, Aorta, Thoracic, Ascending/Arch 02RX
   see Supplement, Aorta, Thoracic, Descending 02UW
   see Supplement, Aorta, Thoracic, Ascending/Arch 02UX
   see Repair, Aorta, Abdominal 04Q0
   see Replacement, Aorta, Abdominal 04R0
   see Supplement, Aorta, Abdominal 04U0
Apalutamide Antineoplastic XW0DXJ5
Apical (subclavicular) lymph node
   use Lymphatic, Axillary, Left
   use Lymphatic, Axillary, Right
Apneustic center use Pons
Appendectomy
   see Excision, Appendix 0DBJ
   see Resection, Appendix 0DTJ
Appendicolysis
   see Release, Appendix 0DNJ
Appendicotomy
   see Drainage, Appendix 0D9J
Application
   see Introduction of substance in or on
Aquablation therapy, prostate XV508A4
Aquapheresis 6A550Z3
Aqueduct of Sylvius
   use Cerebral Ventricle
Aqueous humour
   use Anterior Chamber, Left
   use Anterior Chamber, Right
Arachnoid mater, intracranial
   use Cerebral Meninges
Arachnoid mater, spinal
   use Spinal Meninges
Arcuate artery
   use Artery, Foot, Left
   use Artery, Foot, Right
Areola
   use Nipple, Left
   use Nipple, Right
AROM (artificial rupture of membranes) 10907ZC
Arterial canal (duct)
   use Artery, Pulmonary, Left
Arterial pulse tracing
   see Measurement, Arterial 4A03
Arteriectomy
   see Excision, Heart and Great Vessels 02B
   see Excision, Upper Arteries 03B
   see Excision, Lower Arteries 04B

Arteriography
   see Plain Radiography, Heart B20
   see Fluoroscopy, Heart B21
   see Plain Radiography, Upper Arteries B30
   see Fluoroscopy, Upper Arteries B31
   see Plain Radiography, Lower Arteries B40
   see Fluoroscopy, Lower Arteries B41
Arterioplasty
   see Repair, Heart and Great Vessels 02Q
   see Replacement, Heart and Great Vessels 02R
   see Repair, Upper Arteries 03Q
   see Replacement, Upper Arteries 03R
   see Repair, Lower Arteries 04Q
   see Replacement, Lower Arteries 04R
   see Supplement, Upper Arteries 03U
   see Supplement, Lower Arteries 04U
   see Supplement, Heart and Great Vessels 02U
Arteriorrhaphy
   see Repair, Heart and Great Vessels 02Q
   see Repair, Upper Arteries 03Q
   see Repair, Lower Arteries 04Q
Arterioscopy
   see Inspection, Artery, Lower 04JY
   see Inspection, Artery, Upper 03JY
   see Inspection, Great Vessel 02JY
Arthrectomy
   see Excision, Upper Joints 0RB
   see Resection, Upper Joints 0RT
   see Excision, Lower Joints 0SB
   see Resection, Lower Joints 0ST
Arthrocentesis
   see Drainage, Upper Joints 0R9
   see Drainage, Lower Joints 0S9
Arthrodesis
   see Fusion, Upper Joints 0RG
   see Fusion, Lower Joints 0SG
Arthrography
   see Plain Radiography, Skull and Facial Bones BN0
   see Plain Radiography, Non-Axial Upper Bones BP0
   see Plain Radiography, Non-Axial Lower Bones BQ0
Arthrolysis
   see Release, Upper Joints 0RN
   see Release, Lower Joints 0SN
Arthropexy
   see Repair, Upper Joints 0RQ
   see Reposition, Upper Joints 0RS
   see Repair, Lower Joints 0SQ
   see Reposition, Lower Joints 0SS
Arthroplasty
   see Repair, Upper Joints 0RQ
   see Replacement, Upper Joints 0RR
   see Repair, Lower Joints 0SQ
   see Replacement, Lower Joints 0SR
   see Supplement, Lower Joints 0SU
   see Supplement, Upper Joints 0RU
Arthroplasty, radial head
   see Replacement, Radius, Left 0PRJ
   see Replacement, Radius, Right 0PRH
Arthroscopy
   see Inspection, Upper Joints 0RJ
   see Inspection, Lower Joints 0SJ
Arthrotomy
   see Drainage, Upper Joints 0R9
   see Drainage, Lower Joints 0S9
Articulating Spacer (Antibiotic)
   use Articulating Spacer in Lower Joints
Artificial anal sphincter (AAS)
   use Artificial Sphincter in Gastrointestinal System
Artificial bowel sphincter (neosphincter)
   use Artificial Sphincter in Gastrointestinal System

Artificial Sphincter
  Insertion of device in
    Anus 0DHQ
    Bladder 0THB
    Bladder Neck 0THC
    Urethra 0THD
  Removal of device from
    Anus 0DPQ
    Bladder 0TPB
    Urethra 0TPD
  Revision of device in
    Anus 0DWQ
    Bladder 0TWB
    Urethra 0TWD
Artificial urinary sphincter (AUS)
  use Artificial Sphincter in Urinary
    System
Aryepiglottic fold
  use Larynx
Arytenoid cartilage
  use Larynx
Arytenoid muscle
  use Muscle, Neck, Left
  use Muscle, Neck, Right
Arytenoidectomy
  see Excision, Larynx 0CBS
Arytenoidopexy
  see Repair, Larynx 0CQS
Ascenda Intrathecal Catheter
  use Infusion Device
Ascending aorta
  use Thoracic Aorta, Ascending/Arch
Ascending palatine artery
  use Artery, Face
Ascending pharyngeal artery
  use Artery, External Carotid, Left
  use Artery, External Carotid, Right
Aspiration, fine needle
  Fluid or gas
    see Drainage
  Tissue biopsy
    see Excision
    see Extraction
Assessment
  Activities of daily living
    see Activities of Daily Living
      Assessment, Rehabilitation
      F02
  Hearing
    see Hearing Assessment,
      Diagnostic Audiology F13
  Hearing aid
    see Hearing Aid Assessment,
      Diagnostic Audiology F14
  Intravascular perfusion, using
    indocyanine green (ICG) dye
    see Monitoring, Physiological
      Systems 4A1
  Motor function
    see Motor Function Assessment,
      Rehabilitation F01
  Nerve function
    see Motor Function Assessment,
      Rehabilitation F01
  Speech
    see Speech Assessment,
      Rehabilitation F00
  Vestibular
    see Vestibular Assessment,
      Diagnostic Audiology F15
  Vocational
    see Activities of Daily Living
      Treatment, Rehabilitation
      F08
Assistance
  Cardiac
    Continuous
      Balloon Pump 5A02210
      Impeller Pump 5A0221D
      Other Pump 5A02216
      Pulsatile Compression
        5A02215

Assistance *(continued)*
  Cardiac *(continued)*
    Intermittent
      Balloon Pump 5A02110
      Impeller Pump 5A0211D
      Other Pump 5A02116
      Pulsatile Compression
        5A02115
  Circulatory
    Continuous
      Hyperbaric 5A05221
      Supersaturated 5A0522C
    Intermittent
      Hyperbaric 5A05121
      Supersaturated 5A0512C
  Respiratory
    24-96 Consecutive Hours
      Continuous Negative Airway
        Pressure 5A09459
      Continuous Positive Airway
        Pressure 5A09457
      High Nasal Flow/Velocity
        5A0945A
      Intermittent Negative Airway
        Pressure 5A0945B
      Intermittent Positive Airway
        Pressure 5A09458
      No Qualifier 5A0945Z
    Continuous, Filtration 5A0920Z
    Greater than 96 Consecutive
      Hours
      Continuous Negative Airway
        Pressure 5A09559
      Continuous Positive Airway
        Pressure 5A09557
      High Nasal Flow/Velocity
        5A0955A
      Intermittent Negative Airway
        Pressure 5A0955B
      Intermittent Positive Airway
        Pressure 5A09558
      No Qualifier 5A0955Z
    Less than 24 Consecutive Hours
      Continuous Negative Airway
        Pressure 5A09359
      Continuous Positive Airway
        Pressure 5A09357
      High Nasal Flow/Velocity
        5A0935A
      Intermittent Negative Airway
        Pressure 5A0935B
      Intermittent Positive Airway
        Pressure 5A09358
      No Qualifier 5A0935Z
Assurant (Cobalt) stent
  use Intraluminal Device
Atezolizumab Antineoplastic XW0
Atherectomy
  see Extirpation, Heart and Great
    Vessels 02C
  see Extirpation, Upper Arteries 03C
  see Extirpation, Lower Arteries 04C
Atlantoaxial joint
  use Joint, Cervical Vertebral
Atmospheric Control 6A0Z
AtriClip LAA Exclusion System
  use Extraluminal Device
Atrioseptoplasty
  see Repair, Heart and Great Vessels
    02Q
  see Replacement, Heart and Great
    Vessels 02R
  see Supplement, Heart and Great
    Vessels 02U
Atrioventricular node
  use Conduction Mechanism
Atrium dextrum cordis
  use Atrium, Right
Atrium pulmonale
  use Atrium, Left
Attain Ability® lead
  use Cardiac Lead, Pacemaker in 02H

Attain Ability® lead *(continued)*
  use Cardiac Lead, Defibrillator in
    02H
Attain StarFix® (OTW) lead
  use Cardiac Lead, Defibrillator in
    02H
  use Cardiac Lead, Pacemaker in 02H
Audiology, diagnostic
  see Hearing Assessment, Diagnostic
    Audiology F13
  see Hearing Aid Assessment,
    Diagnostic Audiology F14
  see Vestibular Assessment,
    Diagnostic Audiology F15
Audiometry
  see Hearing Assessment, Diagnostic
    Audiology F13
Auditory tube
  use Eustachian Tube, Left
  use Eustachian Tube, Right
Auerbach's (myenteric) plexus
  use Nerve, Abdominal Sympathetic
Auricle
  use Ear, External, Bilateral
  use Ear, External, Left
  use Ear, External, Right
Auricularis muscle
  use Muscle, Head
Autograft
  use Autologous Tissue Substitute
Autologous artery graft
  use Autologous Arterial Tissue in
    Heart and Great Vessels
  use Autologous Arterial Tissue in
    Lower Arteries
  use Autologous Arterial Tissue in
    Lower Veins
  use Autologous Arterial Tissue in
    Upper Arteries
  use Autologous Arterial Tissue in
    Upper Veins
Autologous vein graft
  use Autologous Venous Tissue in
    Heart and Great Vessels
  use Autologous Venous Tissue in
    Lower Arteries
  use Autologous Venous Tissue in
    Lower Veins
  use Autologous Venous Tissue in
    Upper Arteries
  use Autologous Venous Tissue in
    Upper Veins
Autotransfusion
  see Transfusion
Autotransplant
  Adrenal tissue
    see Reposition, Endocrine
      System 0GS
  Kidney
    see Reposition, Urinary System
      0TS
  Pancreatic tissue
    see Reposition, Pancreas
      0FSG
  Parathyroid tissue
    see Reposition, Endocrine
      System 0GS
  Thyroid tissue
    see Reposition, Endocrine
      System 0GS
  Tooth
    see Reattachment, Mouth and
      Throat 0CM
Avulsion
  see Extraction
Axial Lumbar Interbody Fusion
  System
  use Interbody Fusion Device in
    Lower Joints
AxiaLIF® System
  use Interbody Fusion Device in
    Lower Joints

Axicabtagene Ciloeucel
  use Engineered Autologous
    Chimeric Antigen Receptor
    T-cell Immunotherapy
Axillary fascia
  use Subcutaneous Tissue and Fascia,
    Upper Arm, Left
  use Subcutaneous Tissue and Fascia,
    Upper Arm, Right
Axillary nerve
  use Nerve, Brachial Plexus
AZEDRA®
  use Iobenguane I-131 Antineoplastic

B

BAK/C® Interbody Cervical Fusion
  System
  use Interbody Fusion Device in
    Upper Joints
BAL (bronchial alveolar lavage),
  diagnostic
  see Drainage, Respiratory System 0B9
Balanoplasty
  see Repair, Penis 0VQS
  see Supplement, Penis 0VUS
Balloon atrial septostomy (BAS)
  02163Z7
Balloon Pump
  Continuous, Output 5A02210
  Intermittent, Output 5A02110
Bandage, Elastic
  see Compression
Banding
  see Occlusion
  see Restriction
Banding, esophageal varices
  see Occlusion, Vein, Esophageal 06L3
Banding, laparoscopic (adjustable)
  gastric
  Initial procedure 0DV64CZ
  Surgical correction
    see Revision of device in,
      Stomach 0DW6
Bard® Composix® (E/X)(LP) mesh
  use Synthetic Substitute
Bard® Composix® Kugel® patch
  use Synthetic Substitute
Bard® Dulex™ mesh
  use Synthetic Substitute
Bard® Ventralex™ hernia patch
  use Synthetic Substitute
Barium swallow
  see Fluoroscopy, Gastrointestinal
    System BD1
Baroreflex Activation Therapy® (BAT®)
  Stimulator Generator in
    Subcutaneous Tissue and Fascia
  use Stimulator Lead in Upper
    Arteries
Barricaid® Annular Closure Device
  (ACD)
  use Synthetic Substitute
Bartholin's (greater vestibular)
  gland
  use Gland, Vestibular
Basal (internal) cerebral vein
  use Vein, Intracranial
Basal metabolic rate (BMR)
  see Measurement, Physiological
    Systems 4A0Z
Basal nuclei
  use Basal Ganglia
Base of Tongue
  use Pharynx
Basilar artery
  use Artery, Intracranial
Basis pontis
  use Pons
Beam Radiation
  Abdomen DW03
    Intraoperative DW033Z0

Beam Radiation (*continued*)
Adrenal Gland DG02
  Intraoperative DG023Z0
Bile Ducts DF02
  Intraoperative DF023Z0
Bladder DT02
  Intraoperative DT023Z0
Bone
  Intraoperative DP0C3Z0
  Other DP0C
Bone Marrow D700
  Intraoperative D7003Z0
Brain D000
  Intraoperative D0003Z0
Brain Stem D001
  Intraoperative D0013Z0
Breast
  Left DM00
    Intraoperative DM003Z0
  Right DM01
    Intraoperative DM013Z0
Bronchus DB01
  Intraoperative DB013Z0
Cervix DU01
  Intraoperative DU013Z0
Chest DW02
  Intraoperative DW023Z0
Chest Wall DB07
  Intraoperative DB073Z0
Colon DD05
  Intraoperative DD053Z0
Diaphragm DB08
  Intraoperative DB083Z0
Duodenum DD02
  Intraoperative DD023Z0
Ear D900
  Intraoperative D9003Z0
Esophagus DD00
  Intraoperative DD003Z0
Eye D800
  Intraoperative D8003Z0
Femur DP09
  Intraoperative DP093Z0
Fibula DP0B
  Intraoperative DP0B3Z0
Gallbladder DF01
  Intraoperative DF013Z0
Gland
  Adrenal DG02
    Intraoperative DG023Z0
  Parathyroid DG04
    Intraoperative DG043Z0
  Pituitary DG00
    Intraoperative DG003Z0
  Thyroid DG05
    Intraoperative DG053Z0
Glands
  Intraoperative D9063Z0
  Salivary D906
Head and Neck DW01
  Intraoperative DW013Z0
Hemibody DW04
  Intraoperative DW043Z0
Humerus DP06
  Intraoperative DP063Z0
Hypopharynx D903
  Intraoperative D9033Z0
Ileum DD04
  Intraoperative DD043Z0
Jejunum DD03
  Intraoperative DD033Z0
Kidney DT00
  Intraoperative DT003Z0
Larynx D90B
  Intraoperative D90B3Z0
Liver DF00
  Intraoperative DF003Z0
Lung DB02
  Intraoperative DB023Z0
Lymphatics
  Abdomen D706
    Intraoperative D7063Z0

Beam Radiation (*continued*)
Lymphatics (*continued*)
  Axillary D704
    Intraoperative D7043Z0
  Inguinal D708
    Intraoperative D7083Z0
  Neck D703
    Intraoperative D7033Z0
  Pelvis D707
    Intraoperative D7073Z0
  Thorax D705
    Intraoperative D7053Z0
Mandible DP03
  Intraoperative DP033Z0
Maxilla DP02
  Intraoperative DP023Z0
Mediastinum DB06
  Intraoperative DB063Z0
Mouth D904
  Intraoperative D9043Z0
Nasopharynx D90D
  Intraoperative D90D3Z0
Neck and Head DW01
  Intraoperative DW013Z0
Nerve
  Intraoperative D0073Z0
  Peripheral D007
Nose D901
  Intraoperative D9013Z0
Oropharynx D90F
  Intraoperative D90F3Z0
Ovary DU00
  Intraoperative DU003Z0
Palate
  Hard D908
    Intraoperative D9083Z0
  Soft D909
    Intraoperative D9093Z0
Pancreas DF03
  Intraoperative DF033Z0
Parathyroid Gland DG04
  Intraoperative DG043Z0
Pelvic Bones DP08
  Intraoperative DP083Z0
Pelvic Region DW06
  Intraoperative DW063Z0
Pineal Body DG01
  Intraoperative DG013Z0
Pituitary Gland DG00
  Intraoperative DG003Z0
Pleura DB05
  Intraoperative DB053Z0
Prostate DV00
  Intraoperative DV003Z0
Radius DP07
  Intraoperative DP073Z0
Rectum DD07
  Intraoperative DD073Z0
Rib DP05
  Intraoperative DP053Z0
Sinuses D907
  Intraoperative D9073Z0
Skin
  Abdomen DH08
    Intraoperative DH083Z0
  Arm DH04
    Intraoperative DH043Z0
  Back DH07
    Intraoperative DH073Z0
  Buttock DH09
    Intraoperative DH093Z0
  Chest DH06
    Intraoperative DH063Z0
  Face DH02
    Intraoperative DH023Z0
  Leg DH0B
    Intraoperative DH0B3Z0
  Neck DH03
    Intraoperative DH033Z0
Skull DP00
  Intraoperative DP003Z0
Spinal Cord D006
  Intraoperative D0063Z0

Beam Radiation (*continued*)
Spleen D702
  Intraoperative D7023Z0
Sternum DP04
  Intraoperative DP043Z0
Stomach DD01
  Intraoperative DD013Z0
Testis DV01
  Intraoperative DV013Z0
Thymus D701
  Intraoperative D7013Z0
Thyroid Gland DG05
  Intraoperative DG053Z0
Tibia DP0B
  Intraoperative DP0B3Z0
Tongue D905
  Intraoperative D9053Z0
Trachea DB00
  Intraoperative DB003Z0
Ulna DP07
  Intraoperative DP073Z0
Ureter DT01
  Intraoperative DT013Z0
Urethra DT03
  Intraoperative DT033Z0
Uterus DU02
  Intraoperative DU023Z0
Whole Body DW05
  Intraoperative DW053Z0
Bedside swallow F00ZJWZ
Berlin Heart Ventricular Assist Device
  use Implantable Heart Assist System
    in Heart and Great Vessels
Bezlotoxumab Monoclonal Antibody
  XW0
Biceps brachii muscle
  use Muscle, Upper Arm, Left
  use Muscle, Upper Arm, Right
Biceps femoris muscle
  use Muscle, Upper Leg, Left
  use Muscle, Upper Leg, Right
Bicipital aponeurosis
  use Subcutaneous Tissue and Fascia,
    Lower Arm, Left
  use Subcutaneous Tissue and Fascia,
    Lower Arm, Right
Bicuspid valve
  use Valve, Mitral
Bili light therapy
  see Phototherapy, Skin 6A60
Bioactive embolization coil(s)
  use Intraluminal Device, Bioactive
    in Upper Arteries
Biofeedback GZC9ZZZ
BioFire® FilmArray® Pneumonia
  Panel XXEBXQ6
Biopsy
  see Drainage with qualifier Diagnostic
  see Excision with qualifier Diagnostic
  see Extraction with qualifier
    Diagnostic
BiPAP
  see Assistance, Respiratory v5A09
Bisection
  see Division
Biventricular external heart assist
  system
  use Short-term External Heart
    Assist System in Heart and Great
    Vessels
Blepharectomy
  see Excision, Eye 08B
  see Resection, Eye 08T
Blepharoplasty
  see Repair, Eye 08Q
  see Replacement, Eye 08R
  see Reposition, Eye 08S
  see Supplement, Eye 08U
Blepharorrhaphy
  see Repair, Eye 08Q
Blepharotomy
  see Drainage, Eye 089

Blinatumomab Antineoplastic
  Immunotherapy XW0
Block, Nerve, anesthetic injection
  3E0T3BZ
Blood glucose monitoring system
  use Monitoring Device
Blood pressure
  see Measurement, Arterial 4A03
BMR (basal metabolic rate)
  see Measurement, Physiological
    Systems 4A0Z
Body of femur
  use Femoral Shaft, Left
  use Femoral Shaft, Right
Body of fibula
  use Fibula, Left
  use Fibula, Right
Bone anchored hearing device
  use Hearing Device, Bone
    Conduction in 09H
  use Hearing Device in Head and Facial
    Bones
Bone bank bone graft
  use Nonautologous Tissue Substitute
Bone Growth Stimulator
  Insertion of device in
    Bone
      Facial 0NHW
      Lower 0QHY
      Nasal 0NHB
      Upper 0PHY
      Skull 0NH0
  Removal of device from
    Bone
      Facial 0NPW
      Lower 0QPY
      Nasal 0NPB
      Upper 0PPY
      Skull 0NP0
  Revision of device in
    Bone
      Facial 0NWW
      Lower 0QWY
      Nasal 0NWB
      Upper 0PWY
      Skull 0NW0
Bone marrow transplant
  see Transfusion, Circulatory 302
Bone morphogenetic protein 2
  (BMP 2)
  use Recombinant Bone
    Morphogenetic Protein
Bone screw (interlocking)(lag)
  (pedicle)(recessed)
  use Internal Fixation Device in Head
    and Facial Bones
  use Internal Fixation Device in
    Lower Bones
  use Internal Fixation Device in Upper
    Bones
Bony labyrinth
  use Ear, Inner, Left
  use Ear, Inner, Right
Bony orbit
  use Orbit, Left
  use Orbit, Right
Bony vestibule
  use Ear, Inner, Left
  use Ear, Inner, Right
Botallo's duct
  use Artery, Pulmonary, Left
Bovine pericardial valve
  use Zooplastic Tissue in Heart and
    Great Vessels
Bovine pericardium graft
  use Zooplastic Tissue in Heart and
    Great Vessels
BP (blood pressure)
  see Measurement, Arterial 4A03
Brachial (lateral) lymph node
  use Lymphatic, Axillary, Left
  use Lymphatic, Axillary, Right

Brachialis muscle
  use Muscle, Upper Arm, Left
  use Muscle, Upper Arm, Right
Brachiocephalic artery
  use Artery, Innominate
Brachiocephalic trunk
  use Artery, Innominate
Brachiocephalic vein
  use Vein, Innominate, Left
  use Vein, Innominate, Right
Brachioradialis muscle
  use Muscle, Lower Arm and Wrist, Left
  use Muscle, Lower Arm and Wrist, Right
Brachytherapy
  Abdomen DW13
  Adrenal Gland DG12
  Back
    Lower DW1L
    Upper DW1K
  Bile Ducts DF12
  Bladder DT12
  Bone Marrow D710
  Brain D010
  Brain Stem D011
  Breast
    Left DM10
    Right DM11
  Bronchus DB11
  Cervix DU11
  Chest DW12
  Chest Wall DB17
  Colon DD15
  Cranial Cavity DW10
  Diaphragm DB18
  Duodenum DD12
  Ear D910
  Esophagus DD10
  Extremity
    Lower DW1Y
    Upper DW1X
  Eye D810
  Gastrointestinal Tract DW1P
  Gallbladder DF11
  Genitourinary Tract DW1R
  Gland
    Adrenal DG12
    Parathyroid DG14
    Pituitary DG10
    Thyroid DG15
  Glands, Salivary D916
  Head and Neck DW11
  Hypopharynx D913
  Ileum DD14
  Jejunum DD13
  Kidney DT10
  Larynx D91B
  Liver DF10
  Lung DB12
  Lymphatics
    Abdomen D716
    Axillary D714
    Inguinal D718
    Neck D713
    Pelvis D717
    Thorax D715
  Mediastinum DB16
  Mouth D914
  Nasopharynx D91D
  Neck and Head DW11
  Nerve, Peripheral D017
  Nose D911
  Oropharynx D91F
  Ovary DU10
  Palate
    Hard D918
    Soft D919
  Pancreas DF13
  Parathyroid Gland DG14
  Pelvic Region DW16

Brachytherapy *(continued)*
  Pineal Body DG11
  Pituitary Gland DG10
  Pleura DB15
  Prostate DV10
  Rectum DD17
  Respiratory Tract DW1Q
  Sinuses D917
  Spinal Cord D016
  Spleen D712
  Stomach DD11
  Testis DV11
  Thymus D711
  Thyroid Gland DG15
  Tongue D915
  Trachea DB10
  Ureter DT11
  Urethra DT13
  Uterus DU12
Brachytherapy, CivaSheet®
  see Brachytherapy with qualifier Unidirectional Source
  see Insertion with device Radioactive Element
Brachytherapy seeds
  use Radioactive Element
Breast procedures, skin only
  use Skin, Chest
Brexanolone XW0
Brexucabtagene Autoleucel
  use Brexucabtagene Autoleucel Immunotherapy
Brexucabtagene Autoleucel Immunotherapy XW2
Broad ligament
  use Uterine Supporting Structure
Bronchial artery
  use Upper Artery
Bronchography
  see Fluoroscopy, Respiratory System BB1
  see Plain Radiography, Respiratory System BB0
Bronchoplasty
  see Repair, Respiratory System 0BQ
  see Supplement, Respiratory System 0BU
Bronchorrhaphy
  see Repair, Respiratory System 0BQ
Bronchoscopy 0BJ08ZZ
Bronchotomy
  see Drainage, Respiratory System 0B9
Bronchus Intermedius
  use Main Bronchus, Right
BRYAN® Cervical Disc System
  use Synthetic Substitute
Buccal gland
  use Buccal Mucosa
Buccinator lymph node
  use Lymphatic, Head
Buccinator muscle
  use Muscle, Facial
Buckling, scleral with implant
  see Supplement, Eye 08U
Bulbospongiosus muscle
  use Muscle, Perineum
Bulbourethral (Cowper's) gland
  use Urethra
Bundle of His
  use Conduction Mechanism
Bundle of Kent
  use Conduction Mechanism
Bunionectomy
  see Excision, Lower Bones 0QB
Bursectomy
  see Excision, Bursae and Ligaments 0MB
  see Resection, Bursae and Ligaments 0MT
Bursocentesis
  see Drainage, Bursae and Ligaments 0M9

Bursography
  see Plain Radiography, Non-Axial Upper Bones BP0
  see Plain Radiography, Non-Axial Lower Bones BQ0
Bursotomy
  see Division, Bursae and Ligaments 0M8
  see Drainage, Bursae and Ligaments 0M9
BVS 5000 Ventricular Assist Device
  use Short-term External Heart Assist System in Heart and Great Vessels
Bypass
  Anterior Chamber
    Left 08133
    Right 08123
  Aorta
    Abdominal 0410
    Thoracic
      Ascending/Arch 021X
      Descending 021W
  Artery
    Anterior Tibial
      Left 041Q
      Right 041P
    Axillary
      Left 03160
      Right 03150
    Brachial
      Left 03180
      Right 03170
    Common Carotid
      Left 031J0
      Right 031H0
    Common Iliac
      Left 041D
      Right 041C
    Coronary
      Four or More Arteries 0213
      One Artery 0210
      Three Arteries 0212
      Two Arteries 0211
    External Carotid
      Left 031N0
      Right 031M0
    External Iliac
      Left 041J
      Right 041H
    Femoral
      Left 041L
      Right 041K
    Foot
      Left 041W
      Right 041V
    Hepatic 0413
    Innominate 03120
    Internal Carotid
      Left 031L0
      Right 031K0
    Internal Iliac
      Left 041F
      Right 041E
    Intracranial 031G0
    Peroneal
      Left 041U
      Right 041T
    Popliteal
      Left 041N
      Right 041M
    Posterior Tibial
      Left 041S
      Right 041R
    Pulmonary
      Left 021R
      Right 021Q
    Pulmonary Trunk 021P
    Radial
      Left 031C
      Right 031B

Bypass *(continued)*
  Artery *(continued)*
    Splenic 0414
    Subclavian
      Left 03140
      Right 03130
    Temporal
      Left 031T0
      Right 031S0
    Ulnar
      Left 031A
      Right 0319
  Atrium
    Left 0217
    Right 0216
  Bladder 0T1B
  Cavity, Cranial 0W110J
  Cecum 0D1H
  Cerebral Ventricle 0016
  Colon
    Ascending 0D1K
    Descending 0D1M
    Sigmoid 0D1N
    Transverse 0D1L
  Duct
    Common Bile 0F19
    Cystic 0F18
    Hepatic
      Common 0F17
      Left 0F16
      Right 0F15
    Lacrimal
      Left 081Y
      Right 081X
    Pancreatic 0F1D
      Accessory 0F1F
  Duodenum 0D19
  Ear
    Left 091E0
    Right 091D0
  Esophagus 0D15
    Lower 0D13
    Middle 0D12
    Upper 0D11
  Fallopian Tube
    Left 0U16
    Right 0U15
  Gallbladder 0F14
  Ileum 0D1B
  Intestine
    Large 0D1E
    Small 0D18
  Jejunum 0D1A
  Kidney Pelvis
    Left 0T14
    Right 0T13
  Pancreas 0F1G
  Pelvic Cavity 0W1J
  Peritoneal Cavity 0W1G
  Pleural Cavity
    Left 0W1B
    Right 0W19
  Spinal Canal 001U
  Stomach 0D16
  Trachea 0B11
  Ureter
    Left 0T17
    Right 0T16
  Ureters, Bilateral 0T18
  Vas Deferens
    Bilateral 0V1Q
    Left 0V1P
    Right 0V1N
  Vein
    Axillary
      Left 0518
      Right 0517
    Azygos 0510
    Basilic
      Left 051C
      Right 051B

Bypass *(continued)*
Vein *(continued)*
Brachial
Left 051A
Right 0519
Cephalic
Left 051F
Right 051D
Colic 0617
Common Iliac
Left 061D
Right 061C
Esophageal 0613
External Iliac
Left 061G
Right 061F
External Jugular
Left 051Q
Right 051P
Face
Left 051V
Right 051T
Femoral
Left 061N
Right 061M
Foot
Left 061V
Right 061T
Gastric 0612
Hand
Left 051H
Right 051G
Hemiazygos 0511
Hepatic 0614
Hypogastric
Left 061J
Right 061H
Inferior Mesenteric 0616
Innominate
Left 0514
Right 0513
Internal Jugular
Left 051N
Right 051M
Intracranial 051L
Portal 0618
Renal
Left 061B
Right 0619
Saphenous
Left 061Q
Right 061P
Splenic 0611
Subclavian
Left 0516
Right 0515
Superior Mesenteric 0615
Vertebral
Left 051S
Right 051R
Vena Cava
Inferior 0610
Superior 021V
Ventricle
Left 021L
Right 021K
Bypass, cardiopulmonary 5A1221Z

C

Caesarean section
see Extraction, Products of Conception 10D0
Calcaneocuboid joint
use Joint, Tarsal, Left
use Joint, Tarsal, Right
Calcaneocuboid ligament
use Bursa and Ligament, Foot, Left
use Bursa and Ligament, Foot, Right
Calcaneofibular ligament
use Bursa and Ligament, Ankle, Left
use Bursa and Ligament, Ankle, Right

Calcaneus
use Tarsal, Left
use Tarsal, Right
Cannulation
see Bypass
see Dilation
see Drainage
see Irrigation
Canthorrhaphy
see Repair, Eye 08Q
Canthotomy
see Release, Eye 08N
Capitate bone
use Carpal, Left
use Carpal, Right
Caplacizumab XW0
Capsulectomy, lens
see Excision, Eye 08B
Capsulorrhaphy, joint
see Repair, Lower Joints 0SQ
see Repair, Upper Joints 0RQ
Cardia
use Esophagogastric Junction
Cardiac contractility modulation lead
use Cardiac Lead in Heart and Great Vessels
Cardiac event recorder
use Monitoring Device
Cardiac Lead
Defibrillator
Atrium
Left 02H7
Right 02H6
Pericardium 02HN
Vein, Coronary 02H4
Ventricle
Left 02HL
Right 02HK
Insertion of device in
Atrium
Left 02H7Z
Right 02H6
Pericardium 02HN
Vein, Coronary 02H4
Ventricle
Left 02HL
Right 02HK
Pacemaker
Atrium
Left 02H7
Right 02H6
Pericardium 02HN
Vein, Coronary 02H4
Ventricle
Left 02HL
Right 02HK
Removal of device from, Heart 02PA
Revision of device in, Heart 02WA
Cardiac plexus
use Nerve, Thoracic Sympathetic
Cardiac Resynchronization Defibrillator Pulse Generator
Abdomen 0JH8
Chest 0JH6
Cardiac Resynchronization Pacemaker Pulse Generator
Abdomen 0JH8
Chest 0JH6
Cardiac resynchronization therapy (CRT) lead
use Cardiac Lead, Defibrillator in 02H
use Cardiac Lead, Pacemaker in 02H
Cardiac Rhythm Related Device
Insertion of device in
Abdomen 0JH8
Chest 0JH6
Removal of device from, Subcutaneous Tissue and Fascia, Trunk 0JPT
Revision of device in, Subcutaneous Tissue and Fascia, Trunk 0JWT

Cardiocentesis
see Drainage, Pericardial Cavity 0W9D
Cardioesophageal junction
use Esophagogastric Junction
Cardiolysis
see Release, Heart and Great Vessels 02N
CardioMEMS® pressure sensor
use Monitoring Device, Pressure Sensor in 02H
Cardiomyotomy
see Division, Esophagogastric Junction 0D84
Cardioplegia
see Introduction of substance in or on, Heart 3E08
Cardiorrhaphy
see Repair, Heart and Great Vessels 02Q
Cardioversion 5A2204Z
Caregiver Training F0FZ
Caroticotympanic artery
use Artery, Internal Carotid, Left
use Artery, Internal Carotid, Right
Carotid (artery) sinus (baroreceptor) lead
use Stimulator Lead in Upper Arteries
Carotid glomus
use Carotid Bodies, Bilateral
use Carotid Body, Left
use Carotid Body, Right
Carotid sinus
use Artery, Internal Carotid, Left
use Artery, Internal Carotid, Right
Carotid sinus nerve
use Nerve, Glossopharyngeal
Carotid WALLSTENT® Monorail® Endoprosthesis
use Intraluminal Device
Carpectomy
see Excision, Upper Bones 0PB
see Resection, Upper Bones 0PT
Carpometacarpal ligament
use Bursa and Ligament, Hand, Left
use Bursa and Ligament, Hand, Right
Casting
see Immobilization
CAT scan
see Computerized Tomography (CT Scan)
Catheterization
see Dilation
see Drainage
Heart
see Measurement, Cardiac 4A02
see Irrigation
see Insertion of device in
Umbilical vein, for infusion 06H033T
Cauda equina
use Spinal Cord, Lumbar
Cauterization
see Destruction
see Repair
Cavernous plexus
use Nerve, Head and Neck Sympathetic
CBMA (Concentrated Bone Marrow Aspirate)
use Concentrated Bone Marrow Aspirate
CBMA (Concentrated Bone Marrow Aspirate) injection, intramuscular XK02303
Cecectomy
see Excision, Cecum 0DBH
see Resection, Cecum 0DTH
Cecocolostomy
see Bypass, Gastrointestinal System 0D1
see Drainage, Gastrointestinal System 0D9

Cecopexy
see Repair, Cecum 0DQH
see Reposition, Cecum 0DSH
Cecoplication
see Restriction, Cecum 0DVH
Cecorrhaphy
see Repair, Cecum 0DQH
Cecostomy
see Bypass, Cecum 0D1H
see Drainage, Cecum 0D9H
Cecotomy
see Drainage, Cecum 0D9H
Cefiderocol Anti-Infective XW0
Ceftazidime-Avibactam Anti-infective XW0
Ceftolozane/Tazobactam Anti-Infective XW0
Celiac (solar) plexus
use Nerve, Abdominal Sympathetic
Celiac ganglion
use Nerve, Abdominal Sympathetic
Celiac lymph node
use Lymphatic, Aortic
Celiac trunk
use Artery, Celiac
Central axillary lymph node
use Lymphatic, Axillary, Left
use Lymphatic, Axillary, Right
Central venous pressure
see Measurement, Venous 4A04
Centrimag® Blood Pump
use Short-term External Heart Assist System in Heart and Great Vessels
Cephalogram BN00ZZZ
Ceramic on ceramic bearing surface
use Synthetic Substitute, Ceramic in 0SR
Cerclage
see Restriction
Cerebral aqueduct (Sylvius)
use Cerebral Ventricle
Cerebral Embolic Filtration
Dual Filter X2A5312
Extracorporeal Flow Reversal Circuit X2A
Single Deflection Filter X2A6325
Cerebrum
use Brain
Cervical esophagus
use Esophagus, Upper
Cervical facet joint
use Joint, Cervical Vertebral
use Joint, Cervical Vertebral, 2 or more
Cervical ganglion
use Nerve, Head and Neck Sympathetic
Cervical interspinous ligament
use Bursa and Ligament, Head and Neck
Cervical intertransverse ligament
use Bursa and Ligament, Head and Neck
Cervical ligamentum flavum
use Bursa and Ligament, Head and Neck
Cervical lymph node
use Lymphatic, Neck, Left
use Lymphatic, Neck, Right
Cervicectomy
see Excision, Cervix 0UBC
see Resection, Cervix 0UTC
Cervicothoracic facet joint
use Joint, Cervicothoracic Vertebral
Cesarean section
see Extraction, Products of Conception 10D0
Cesium-131 Collagen Implant
use Radioactive Element, Cesium-131 Collagen Implant in 00H
Change device in
Abdominal Wall 0W2FX

Back
  Lower 0W2LX
  Upper 0W2KX
Bladder 0T2BX
Bone
  Facial 0N2WX
  Lower 0Q2YX
  Nasal 0N2BX
  Upper 0P2YX
Bone Marrow 072TX
Brain 0020X
Breast
  Left 0H2UX
  Right 0H2TX
Bursa and Ligament
  Lower 0M2YX
  Upper 0M2XX
Cavity, Cranial 0W21X
Chest Wall 0W28X
Cisterna Chyli 072LX
Diaphragm 0B2TX
Duct
  Hepatobiliary 0F2BX
  Pancreatic 0F2DX
Ear
  Left 092JX
  Right 092HX
Epididymis and Spermatic Cord
  0V2MX
Extremity
  Lower
    Left 0Y2BX
    Right 0Y29X
  Upper
    Left 0X27X
    Right 0X26X
Eye
  Left 0821X
  Right 0820X
Face 0W22X
Fallopian Tube 0U28X
Gallbladder 0F24X
Gland
  Adrenal 0G25X
  Endocrine 0G2SX
  Pituitary 0G20X
  Salivary 0C2AX
Head 0W20X
Intestinal Tract
  Lower 0D2DXUZ
  Upper 0D20XUZ
Jaw
  Lower 0W25X
  Upper 0W24X
Joint
  Lower 0S2YX
  Upper 0R2YX
Kidney 0T25X
Larynx 0C2SX
Liver 0F20X
Lung
  Left 0B2LX
  Right 0B2KX
Lymphatic 072NX
  Thoracic Duct 072KX
Mediastinum 0W2CX
Mesentery 0D2VX
Mouth and Throat 0C2YX
Muscle
  Lower 0K2YX
  Upper 0K2XX
Nasal Mucosa and Soft Tissue
  092KX
Neck 0W26X
Nerve
  Cranial 002EX
  Peripheral 012YX
Omentum 0D2UX
Ovary 0U23X
Pancreas 0F2GX
Parathyroid Gland 0G2RX

Pelvic Cavity 0W2JX
Penis 0V2SX
Pericardial Cavity 0W2DX
Perineum
  Female 0W2NX
  Male 0W2MX
Peritoneal Cavity 0W2GX
Peritoneum 0D2WX
Pineal Body 0G21X
Pleura 0B2QX
Pleural Cavity
  Left 0W2BX
  Right 0W29X
Products of Conception 10207
Prostate and Seminal Vesicles
  0V24X
Retroperitoneum 0W2HX
Scrotum and Tunica Vaginalis 0V28X
Sinus 092YX
Skin 0H2PX
Skull 0N20X
Spinal Canal 002UX
Spleen 072PX
Subcutaneous Tissue and Fascia
  Head and Neck 0J2SX
  Lower Extremity 0J2WX
  Trunk 0J2TX
  Upper Extremity 0J2VX
Tendon
  Lower 0L2YX
  Upper 0L2XX
Testis 0V2DX
Thymus 072MX
Thyroid Gland 0G2KX
Trachea 0B21
Tracheobronchial Tree 0B20X
Ureter 0T29X
Urethra 0T2DX
Uterus and Cervix 0U2DXHZ
Vagina and Cul-de-sac 0U2HXGZ
Vas Deferens 0V2RX
Vulva 0U2MX

Change device in or on
Abdominal Wall 2W03X
Anorectal 2Y03X5Z
Arm
  Lower
    Left 2W0DX
    Right 2W0CX
  Upper
    Left 2W0BX
    Right 2W0AX
Back 2W05X
Chest Wall 2W04X
Ear 2Y02X5Z
Extremity
  Lower
    Left 2W0MX
    Right 2W0LX
  Upper
    Left 2W09X
    Right 2W08X
Face 2W01X
Finger
  Left 2W0KX
  Right 2W0JX
Foot
  Left 2W0TX
  Right 2W0SX
Genital Tract, Female 2Y04X5Z
Hand
  Left 2W0FX
  Right 2W0EX
Head 2W00X
Inguinal Region
  Left 2W07X
  Right 2W06X
Leg
  Lower
    Left 2W0RX
    Right 2W0QX

Leg (continued)
  Upper
    Left 2W0PX
    Right 2W0NX
Mouth and Pharynx 2Y00X5Z
Nasal 2Y01X5Z
Neck 2W02X
Thumb
  Left 2W0HX
  Right 2W0GX
Toe
  Left 2W0VX
  Right 2W0UX
Urethra 2Y05X5Z
Chemoembolization
  see Introduction of substance in
    or on
Chemosurgery, Skin 3E00XTZ
Chemothalamectomy
  see Destruction, Thalamus 0059
Chemotherapy, Infusion for cancer
  see Introduction of substance in
    or on
Chest x-ray
  see Plain Radiography, Chest BW03
Chiropractic Manipulation
  Abdomen 9WB9X
  Cervical 9WB1X
  Extremities
    Lower 9WB6X
    Upper 9WB7X
  Head 9WB0X
  Lumbar 9WB3X
  Pelvis 9WB5X
  Rib Cage 9WB8X
  Sacrum 9WB4X
  Thoracic 9WB2X
Choana
  use Nasopharynx
Cholangiogram
  see Plain Radiography,
    Hepatobiliary System and
    Pancreas BF0
  see Fluoroscopy, Hepatobiliary
    System and Pancreas BF1
Cholecystectomy
  see Excision, Gallbladder 0FB4
  see Resection, Gallbladder 0FT4
Cholecystojejunostomy
  see Bypass, Hepatobiliary System
    and Pancreas 0F1
  see Drainage, Hepatobiliary System
    and Pancreas 0F9
Cholecystopexy
  see Repair, Gallbladder 0FQ4
  see Reposition, Gallbladder 0FS4
Cholecystoscopy 0FJ44ZZ
Cholecystostomy
  see Drainage, Gallbladder 0F94
  see Bypass, Gallbladder 0F14
Cholecystotomy
  see Drainage, Gallbladder 0F94
Choledochectomy
  see Excision, Hepatobiliary System
    and Pancreas 0FB
  see Resection, Hepatobiliary System
    and Pancreas 0FT
Choledocholithotomy
  see Extirpation, Duct, Common Bile
    0FC9
Choledochoplasty
  see Repair, Hepatobiliary System
    and Pancreas 0FQ
  see Replacement, Hepatobiliary
    System and Pancreas 0FR
  see Supplement, Hepatobiliary
    System and Pancreas 0FU
Choledochoscopy 0FJB8ZZ
Choledochotomy
  see Drainage, Hepatobiliary System
    and Pancreas 0F9

Cholelithotomy
  see Extirpation, Hepatobiliary
    System and Pancreas 0FC
Chondrectomy
  see Excision, Lower Joints 0SB
  see Excision, Upper Joints 0RB
  Knee
    see Excision, Lower Joints 0SB
  Semilunar cartilage
    see Excision, Lower Joints 0SB
Chondroglossus muscle
  use Muscle, Tongue, Palate, Pharynx
Chorda tympani
  use Nerve, Facial
Chordotomy
  see Division, Central Nervous
    System and Cranial Nerves
    008
Choroid plexus
  use Cerebral Ventricle
Choroidectomy
  see Excision, Eye 08B
  see Resection, Eye 08T
Ciliary body
  use Eye, Left
  use Eye, Right
Ciliary ganglion
  use Nerve, Head and Neck
    Sympathetic
Circle of Willis
  use Artery, Intracranial
Circumcision 0VTTXZZ
Circumflex iliac artery
  use Artery, Femoral, Left
  use Artery, Femoral, Right
CivaSheet®
  use Radioactive Element
CivaSheet® Brachytherapy
  see Brachytherapy with qualifier
    Unidirectional Source
  see Insertion with device
    Radioactive Element
**Clamp and rod internal fixation
    system (CRIF)**
  use Internal Fixation Device in
    Lower Bones
  use Internal Fixation Device in Upper
    Bones
Clamping
  see Occlusion
Claustrum
  use Basal Ganglia
Claviculectomy
  see Excision, Upper Bones 0PB
  see Resection, Upper Bones 0PT
Claviculotomy
  see Division, Upper Bones 0P8
  see Drainage, Upper Bones 0P9
Clipping, aneurysm
  see Occlusion using Extraluminal
    Device
  see Restriction using Extraluminal
    Device
Clitorectomy, clitoridectomy
  see Excision, Clitoris 0UBJ
  see Resection, Clitoris 0UTJ
Clolar
  use Clofarabine
Closure
  see Occlusion
  see Repair
Clysis
  see Introduction of substance in
    or on
Coagulation
  see Destruction
Coagulation Factor Xa, Inactivated
  XW0
**Coagulation Factor Xa,
    (Recombinant) Inactivated**
  use Coagulation Factor Xa,
    Inactivated

COALESCE® radiolucent interbody fusion device
   use Interbody Fusion Device, Radiolucent Porous in New Technology

CoAxia NeuroFlo catheter
   use Intraluminal Device

Cobalt/chromium head and polyethylene socket
   use Synthetic Substitute, Metal on Polyethylene in 0SR

Cobalt/chromium head and socket
   use Synthetic Substitute, Metal in 0SR

Coccygeal body
   use Coccygeal Glomus

Coccygeus muscle
   use Muscle, Trunk, Left
   use Muscle, Trunk, Right

Cochlea
   use Ear, Inner, Left
   use Ear, Inner, Right

Cochlear implant (CI), multiple channel (electrode)
   use Hearing Device, Multiple Channel Cochlear Prosthesis in 09H

Cochlear implant (CI), single channel (electrode)
   use Hearing Device, Single Channel Cochlear Prosthesis in 09H

Cochlear Implant Treatment F0BZ0

Cochlear nerve
   use Nerve, Acoustic

COGNIS® CRT-D
   use Cardiac Resynchronization Defibrillator Pulse Generator in 0JH

COHERE® radiolucent interbody fusion device
   use Interbody Fusion Device, Radiolucent Porous in New Technology

Colectomy
   see Excision, Gastrointestinal System 0DB
   see Resection, Gastrointestinal System 0DT

Collapse
   see Occlusion

Collection from
   Breast, Breast Milk 8E0HX62
   Indwelling Device
     Circulatory System
       Blood 8C02X6K
       Other Fluid 8C02X6L
     Nervous System
       Cerebrospinal Fluid 8C01X6J
       Other Fluid 8C01X6L
   Integumentary System, Breast Milk 8E0HX62
   Reproductive System, Male, Sperm 8E0VX63

Colocentesis
   see Drainage, Gastrointestinal System 0D9

Colofixation
   see Repair, Gastrointestinal System 0DQ
   see Reposition, Gastrointestinal System 0DS

Cololysis
   see Release, Gastrointestinal System 0DN

Colonic Z-Stent®
   use Intraluminal Device

Colonoscopy 0DJD8ZZ

Colopexy
   see Repair, Gastrointestinal System 0DQ
   see Reposition, Gastrointestinal System 0DS

Coloplication
   see Restriction, Gastrointestinal System 0DV

Coloproctectomy
   see Excision, Gastrointestinal System 0DB
   see Resection, Gastrointestinal System 0DT

Coloproctostomy
   see Bypass, Gastrointestinal System 0D1
   see Drainage, Gastrointestinal System 0D9

Colopuncture
   see Drainage, Gastrointestinal System 0D9

Colorrhaphy
   see Repair, Gastrointestinal System 0DQ

Colostomy
   see Bypass, Gastrointestinal System 0D1
   see Drainage, Gastrointestinal System 0D9

Colpectomy
   see Excision, Vagina 0UBG
   see Resection, Vagina 0UTG

Colpocentesis
   see Drainage, Vagina 0U9G

Colpopexy
   see Repair, Vagina 0UQG
   see Reposition, Vagina 0USG

Colpoplasty
   see Repair, Vagina 0UQG
   see Supplement, Vagina 0UUG

Colporrhaphy
   see Repair, Vagina 0UQG

Colposcopy 0UJH8ZZ

Columella
   use Nasal Mucosa and Soft Tissue

Common digital vein
   use Vein, Foot, Left
   use Vein, Foot, Right

Common facial vein
   use Vein, Face, Left
   use Vein, Face, Right

Common fibular nerve
   use Nerve, Peroneal

Common hepatic artery
   use Artery, Hepatic

Common iliac (subaortic) lymph node
   use Lymphatic, Pelvis

Common interosseous artery
   use Artery, Ulnar, Left
   use Artery, Ulnar, Right

Common peroneal nerve
   use Nerve, Peroneal

Complete (SE) stent
   use Intraluminal Device

Compression
   see Restriction
   Abdominal Wall 2W13X
   Arm
     Lower
       Left 2W1DX
       Right 2W1CX
     Upper
       Left 2W1BX
       Right 2W1AX
   Back 2W15X
   Chest Wall 2W14X
   Extremity
     Lower
       Left 2W1MX
       Right 2W1LX
     Upper
       Left 2W19X
       Right 2W18X
   Face 2W11X

Compression *(continued)*
   Finger
     Left 2W1KX
     Right 2W1JX
   Foot
     Left 2W1TX
     Right 2W1SX
   Hand
     Left 2W1FX
     Right 2W1EX
   Head 2W10X
   Inguinal Region
     Left 2W17X
     Right 2W16X
   Leg
     Lower
       Left 2W1RX
       Right 2W1QX
     Upper
       Left 2W1PX
       Right 2W1NX
   Neck 2W12X
   Thumb
     Left 2W1HX
     Right 2W1GX
   Toe
     Left 2W1VX
     Right 2W1UX

Computer Assisted Procedure
   Extremity
     Lower
       No Qualifier 8E0YXBZ
       With Computerized Tomography 8E0YXBG
       With Fluoroscopy 8E0YXBF
       With Magnetic Resonance Imaging 8E0YXBH
     Upper
       No Qualifier 8E0XXBZ
       With Computerized Tomography 8E0XXBG
       With Fluoroscopy 8E0XXBF
       With Magnetic Resonance Imaging 8E0XXBH
   Head and Neck Region
     No Qualifier 8E09XBZ
     With Computerized Tomography 8E09XBG
     With Fluoroscopy 8E09XBF
     With Magnetic Resonance Imaging 8E09XBH
   Trunk Region
     No Qualifier 8E0WXBZ
     With Computerized Tomography 8E0WXBG
     With Fluoroscopy 8E0WXBF
     With Magnetic Resonance Imaging 8E0WXBH

Computerized Tomography (CT Scan)
   Abdomen BW20
     Chest and Pelvis BW25
   Abdomen and Chest BW24
   Abdomen and Pelvis BW21
   Airway, Trachea BB2F
   Ankle
     Left BQ2H
     Right BQ2G
   Aorta
     Abdominal B420
       Intravascular Optical Coherence B420Z2Z
     Thoracic B320
       Intravascular Optical Coherence B320Z2Z
   Arm
     Left BP2F
     Right BP2E

Computerized Tomography (CT Scan) *(continued)*
   Artery
     Celiac B421
       Intravascular Optical Coherence B421Z2Z
     Common Carotid
       Bilateral B325
       Intravascular Optical Coherence B325Z2Z
     Coronary
       Bypass Graft
         Multiple B223
         Intravascular Optical Coherence B223Z2Z
       Multiple B221
         Intravascular Optical Coherence B221Z2Z
     Internal Carotid
       Bilateral B328
       Intravascular Optical Coherence B328Z2Z
     Intracranial B32R
       Intravascular Optical Coherence B32RZ2Z
     Lower Extremity
       Bilateral B42H
       Intravascular Optical Coherence B42HZ2Z
       Left B42G
       Intravascular Optical Coherence B42GZ2Z
       Right B42F
       Intravascular Optical Coherence B42FZ2Z
     Pelvic B42C
       Intravascular Optical Coherence B42CZ2Z
     Pulmonary
       Left B32T
       Intravascular Optical Coherence B32TZ2Z
       Right B32S
       Intravascular Optical Coherence B32SZ2Z
     Renal
       Bilateral B428
       Intravascular Optical Coherence B428Z2Z
       Transplant B42M
       Intravascular Optical Coherence B42MZ2Z
     Superior Mesenteric B424
       Intravascular Optical Coherence B424Z2Z
     Vertebral
       Bilateral B32G
       Intravascular Optical Coherence B32GZ2Z
   Bladder BT20
   Bone
     Facial BN25
     Temporal BN2F
   Brain B020
   Calcaneus
     Left BQ2K
     Right BQ2J
   Cerebral Ventricle B028
   Chest, Abdomen and Pelvis BW25
   Chest and Abdomen BW24
   Cisterna B027
   Clavicle
     Left BP25
     Right BP24
   Coccyx BR2F
   Colon BD24

Computerized Tomography (CT Scan) *(continued)*

Ear B920
Elbow
  Left BP2H
  Right BP2G
Extremity
  Lower
    Left BQ2S
    Right BQ2R
  Upper
    Bilateral BP2V
    Left BP2U
    Right BP2T
Eye
  Bilateral B827
  Left B826
  Right B825
Femur
  Left BQ24
  Right BQ23
Fibula
  Left BQ2C
  Right BQ2B
Finger
  Left BP2S
  Right BP2R
Foot
  Left BQ2M
  Right BQ2L
Forearm
  Left BP2K
  Right BP2J
Gland
  Adrenal, Bilateral BG22
  Parathyroid BG23
  Parotid, Bilateral B926
  Salivary, Bilateral B92D
  Submandibular, Bilateral B929
  Thyroid BG24
Hand
  Left BP2P
  Right BP2N
Hands and Wrists, Bilateral BP2Q
Head BW28
Head and Neck BW29
Heart
  Intravascular Optical Coherence B226Z2Z
  Right and Left B226
Hepatobiliary System, All BF2C
Hip
  Left BQ21
  Right BQ20
Humerus
  Left BP2B
  Right BP2A
Intracranial Sinus B522
  Intravascular Optical Coherence B522Z2Z
Joint
  Acromioclavicular, Bilateral BP23
  Finger
    Left BP2DZZZ
    Right BP2CZZZ
  Foot
    Left BQ2Y
    Right BQ2X
  Hand
    Left BP2DZZZ
    Right BP2CZZZ
  Sacroiliac BR2D
  Sternoclavicular
    Bilateral BP22
    Left BP21
    Right BP20
  Temporomandibular, Bilateral BN29

Computerized Tomography (CT Scan) *(continued)*

Joint *(continued)*
  Toe
    Left BQ2Y
    Right BQ2X
Kidney
  Bilateral BT23
  Left BT22
  Right BT21
  Transplant BT29
Knee
  Left BQ28
  Right BQ27
Larynx B92J
Leg
  Left BQ2F
  Right BQ2D
Liver BF25
Liver and Spleen BF26
Lung, Bilateral BB24
Mandible BN26
Nasopharynx B92F
Neck BW2F
Neck and Head BW29
Orbit, Bilateral BN23
Oropharynx B92F
Pancreas BF27
Patella
  Left BQ2W
  Right BQ2V
Pelvic Region BW2G
Pelvis BR2C
  Chest and Abdomen BW25
Pelvis and Abdomen BW21
Pituitary Gland B029
Prostate BV23
Ribs
  Left BP2Y
  Right BP2X
Sacrum BR2F
Scapula
  Left BP27
  Right BP26
Sella Turcica B029
Shoulder
  Left BP29
  Right BP28
Sinus
  Intracranial B522
    Intravascular Optical Coherence B522Z2Z
  Paranasal B922
Skull BN20
Spinal Cord B02B
Spine
  Cervical BR20
  Lumbar BR29
  Thoracic BR27
Spleen and Liver BF26
Thorax BP2W
Tibia
  Left BQ2C
  Right BQ2B
Toe
  Left BQ2Q
  Right BQ2P
Trachea BB2F
Tracheobronchial Tree
  Bilateral BB29
  Left BB28
  Right BB27
Vein
  Pelvic (Iliac)
    Left B52G
      Intravascular Optical Coherence B52GZ2Z
    Right B52F
      Intravascular Optical Coherence B52FZ2Z

Computerized Tomography (CT Scan) *(continued)*

Vein *(continued)*
  Pelvic (Iliac) Bilateral B52H
    Intravascular Optical Coherence B52HZ2Z
  Portal B52T
    Intravascular Optical Coherence B52TZ2Z
  Pulmonary
    Bilateral B52S
      Intravascular Optical Coherence B52SZ2Z
    Left B52R
      Intravascular Optical Coherence B52RZ2Z
    Right B52Q
      Intravascular Optical Coherence B52QZ2Z
  Renal
    Bilateral B52L
      Intravascular Optical Coherence B52LZ2Z
    Left B52K
      Intravascular Optical Coherence B52KZ2Z
    Right B52J
      Intravascular Optical Coherence B52JZ2Z
  Spanchnic B52T
    Intravascular Optical Coherence B52TZ2Z
  Vena Cava
    Inferior B529
      Intravascular Optical Coherence B529Z2Z
    Superior B528
      Intravascular Optical Coherence B528Z2Z
Ventricle, Cerebral B028
Wrist
  Left BP2M
  Right BP2L

Concentrated Bone Marrow Aspirate (CBMA) injection,
intramuscular XK02303

Concerto II CRT-D
use Cardiac Resynchronization Defibrillator Pulse Generator in 0JH

Condylectomy
see Excision, Head and Facial Bones 0NB
see Excision, Lower Bones 0QB
see Excision, Upper Bones 0PB

Condyloid process
use Mandible, Left
use Mandible, Right

Condylotomy
see Division, Head and Facial Bones 0N8
see Division, Lower Bones 0Q8
see Division, Upper Bones 0P8
see Drainage, Head and Facial Bones 0N9
see Drainage, Lower Bones 0Q9
see Drainage, Upper Bones 0P9

Condylysis
see Release, Head and Facial Bones 0NN
see Release, Lower Bones 0QN
see Release, Upper Bones 0PN

Conization, cervix
see Excision, Cervix 0UBC

Conjunctivoplasty
see Repair, Eye 08Q
see Replacement, Eye 08R

CONSERVE® PLUS Total Resurfacing Hip System
use Resurfacing Device in Lower Joints

Construction

Auricle, ear
  see Bypass, Urinary System 0T1
Ileal conduit
  see Replacement, Ear, Nose, Sinus 09R

Consulta CRT-D
use Cardiac Resynchronization Defibrillator Pulse Generator in 0JH

Consulta CRT-P
use Cardiac Resynchronization Pacemaker Pulse Generator in 0JH

Contact Radiation

Abdomen DWY37ZZ
Adrenal Gland DGY27ZZ
Bile Ducts DFY27ZZ
Bladder DTY27ZZ
Bone, Other DPYC7ZZ
Brain D0Y07ZZ
Brain Stem D0Y17ZZ
Breast
  Left DMY07ZZ
  Right DMY17ZZ
Bronchus DBY17ZZ
Cervix DUY17ZZ
Chest DWY27ZZ
Chest Wall DBY77ZZ
Colon DDY57ZZ
Diaphragm DBY87ZZ
Duodenum DDY27ZZ
Ear D9Y07ZZ
Esophagus DDY07ZZ
Eye D8Y07ZZ
Femur DPY97ZZ
Fibula DPYB7ZZ
Gallbladder DFY17ZZ
Gland
  Adrenal DGY27ZZ
  Parathyroid DGY47ZZ
  Pituitary DGY07ZZ
  Thyroid DGY57ZZ
Glands, Salivary D9Y67ZZ
Head and Neck DWY17ZZ
Hemibody DWY47ZZ
Humerus DPY67ZZ
Hypopharynx D9Y37ZZ
Ileum DDY47ZZ
Jejunum DDY37ZZ
Kidney DTY07ZZ
Larynx D9YB7ZZ
Liver DFY07ZZ
Lung DBY27ZZ
Mandible DPY37ZZ
Maxilla DPY27ZZ
Mediastinum DBY67ZZ
Mouth D9Y47ZZ
Nasopharynx D9YD7ZZ
Neck and Head DWY17ZZ
Nerve, Peripheral D0Y77ZZ
Nose D9Y17ZZ
Oropharynx D9YF7ZZ
Ovary DUY07ZZ
Palate
  Hard D9Y87ZZ
  Soft D9Y97ZZ
Pancreas DFY37ZZ
Parathyroid Gland DGY47ZZ
Pelvic Bones DPY87ZZ
Pelvic Region DWY67ZZ
Pineal Body DGY17ZZ
Pituitary Gland DGY07ZZ
Pleura DBY57ZZ
Prostate DVY07ZZ
Radius DPY77ZZ
Rectum DDY77ZZ
Rib DPY57ZZ
Sinuses D9Y77ZZ

Contact Radiation (continued)
  Skin
    Abdomen DHY87ZZ
    Arm DHY47ZZ
    Back DHY77ZZ
    Buttock DHY97ZZ
    Chest DHY67ZZ
    Face DHY27ZZ
    Leg DHYB7ZZ
    Neck DHY37ZZ
  Skull DPY07ZZ
  Spinal Cord D0Y67ZZ
  Sternum DPY47ZZ
  Stomach DDY17ZZ
  Testis DVY17ZZ
  Thyroid Gland DGY57ZZ
  Tibia DPYB7ZZ
  Tongue D9Y57ZZ
  Trachea DBY07ZZ
  Ulna DPY77ZZ
  Ureter DTY17ZZ
  Urethra DTY37ZZ
  Uterus DUY27ZZ
  Whole Body DWY57ZZ
ContaCT software (Measurement of intracranial arterial flow) 4A03X5D
CONTAK RENEWAL® 3 RF (HE) CRT-D
  use Cardiac Resynchronization Defibrillator Pulse Generator in 0JH
Contegra Pulmonary Valved Conduit
  use Zooplastic Tissue in Heart and Great Vessels
CONTEPO™
  use Fosfomycin Anti-infective
Continuous Glucose Monitoring (CGM) device
  use Monitoring Device
Continuous Negative Airway Pressure
  24-96 Consecutive Hours, Ventilation 5A09459
  Greater than 96 Consecutive Hours, Ventilation 5A09559
  Less than 24 Consecutive Hours, Ventilation 5A09359
Continuous Positive Airway Pressure
  24-96 Consecutive Hours, Ventilation 5A09457
  Greater than 96 Consecutive Hours, Ventilation 5A09557
  Less than 24 Consecutive Hours, Ventilation 5A09357
Continuous renal replacement therapy (CRRT) 5A1D90Z
Contraceptive Device
  Change device in, Uterus and Cervix 0U2DXHZ
  Insertion of device in
    Cervix 0UHC
    Subcutaneous Tissue and Fascia
      Abdomen 0JH8
      Chest 0JH6
      Lower Arm
        Left 0JHH
        Right 0JHG
      Lower Leg
        Left 0JHP
        Right 0JHN
      Upper Arm
        Left 0JHF
        Right 0JHD
      Upper Leg
        Left 0JHM
        Right 0JHL
    Uterus 0UH9
  Removal of device from
    Subcutaneous Tissue and Fascia
      Lower Extremity 0JPW
      Trunk 0JPT
      Upper Extremity 0JPV

Contraceptive Device (continued)
  Removal of device from (continued)
    Uterus and Cervix 0UPD
  Revision of device in
    Subcutaneous Tissue and Fascia
      Lower Extremity 0JWW
      Trunk 0JWT
      Upper Extremity 0JWV
    Uterus and Cervix 0UWD
Contractility Modulation Device
  Abdomen 0JH8
  Chest 0JH6
Control, Epistaxis
  see Control bleeding in, Nasal Mucosa and Soft Tissue 093K
Control bleeding in
  Abdominal Wall 0W3F
  Ankle Region
    Left 0Y3L
    Right 0Y3K
  Arm
    Lower
      Left 0X3F
      Right 0X3D
    Upper
      Left 0X39
      Right 0X38
  Axilla
    Left 0X35
    Right 0X34
  Back
    Lower 0W3L
    Upper 0W3K
  Buttock
    Left 0Y31
    Right 0Y30
  Cavity, Cranial 0W31
  Chest Wall 0W38
  Elbow Region
    Left 0X3C
    Right 0X3B
  Extremity
    Lower
      Left 0Y3B
      Right 0Y39
    Upper
      Left 0X37
      Right 0X36
  Face 0W32
  Femoral Region
    Left 0Y38
    Right 0Y37
  Foot
    Left 0Y3N
    Right 0Y3M
  Gastrointestinal Tract 0W3P
  Genitourinary Tract 0W3R
  Hand
    Left 0X3K
    Right 0X3J
  Head 0W30
  Inguinal Region
    Left 0Y36
    Right 0Y35
  Jaw
    Lower 0W35
    Upper 0W34
  Knee Region
    Left 0Y3G
    Right 0Y3F
  Leg
    Lower
      Left 0Y3J
      Right 0Y3H
    Upper
      Left 0Y3D
      Right 0Y3C
  Mediastinum 0W3C
  Nasal Mucosa and Soft Tissue 093K
  Neck 0W36
  Oral Cavity and Throat 0W33
  Pelvic Cavity 0W3J

Control bleeding in (continued)
  Pericardial Cavity 0W3D
  Perineum
    Female 0W3N
    Male 0W3M
  Peritoneal Cavity 0W3G
  Pleural Cavity
    Left 0W3B
    Right 0W39
  Respiratory Tract 0W3Q
  Retroperitoneum 0W3H
  Shoulder Region
    Left 0X33
    Right 0X32
  Wrist Region
    Left 0X3H
    Right 0X3G
Conus arteriosus
  use Ventricle, Right
Conus medullaris
  use Spinal Cord, Lumbar
Convalescent Plasma (Nonautologous)
  see New Technology, Anatomical Regions XW1
Conversion
  Cardiac rhythm 5A2204Z
  Gastrostomy to jejunostomy feeding device
    see Insertion of device in, Jejunum 0DHA
Cook Biodesign® Fistula Plug(s)
  use Nonautologous Tissue Substitute
Cook Biodesign® Hernia Graft(s)
  use Nonautologous Tissue Substitute
Cook Biodesign® Layered Graft(s)
  use Nonautologous Tissue Substitute
Cook Zenapro™ Layered Graft(s)
  use Nonautologous Tissue Substitute
Cook Zenith AAA Endovascular Graft
  use Intraluminal Device
Cook Zenith® Fenestrated AAA Endovascular Graft
  use Intraluminal Device, Branched or Fenestrated, One or Two Arteries in 04V
  use Intraluminal Device, Branched or Fenestrated, Three or More Arteries in 04V
Coracoacromial ligament
  use Bursa and Ligament, Shoulder, Left
  use Bursa and Ligament, Shoulder, Right
Coracobrachialis muscle
  use Muscle, Upper Arm, Left
  use Muscle, Upper Arm, Right
Coracoclavicular ligament
  use Bursa and Ligament, Shoulder, Left
  use Bursa and Ligament, Shoulder, Right
Coracohumeral ligament
  use Bursa and Ligament, Shoulder, Left
  use Bursa and Ligament, Shoulder, Right
Coracoid process
  use Scapula, Left
  use Scapula, Right
Cordotomy
  see Division, Central Nervous System and Cranial Nerves 008
Core needle biopsy
  see Excision with qualifier Diagnostic
CoreValve transcatheter aortic valve
  use Zooplastic Tissue in Heart and Great Vessels
Cormet Hip Resurfacing System
  use Resurfacing Device in Lower Joints
Corniculate cartilage
  use Larynx

CoRoent® XL
  use Interbody Fusion Device in Lower Joints
Coronary arteriography
  see Fluoroscopy, Heart B21
  see Plain Radiography, Heart B20
Corox (OTW) Bipolar Lead
  use Cardiac Lead, Defibrillator in 02▶
  use Cardiac Lead, Pacemaker in 02▶
Corpus callosum
  use Brain
Corpus cavernosum
  use Penis
Corpus spongiosum
  use Penis
Corpus striatum
  use Basal Ganglia
Corrugator supercilii muscle
  use Muscle, Facial
Cortical strip neurostimulator lead
  use Neurostimulator Lead in Central Nervous System and Cranial Nerves
Corvia IASD®
  use Synthetic Substitute
Costatectomy
  see Excision, Upper Bones 0PB
  see Resection, Upper Bones 0PT
Costectomy
  see Excision, Upper Bones 0PB
  see Resection, Upper Bones 0PT
Costocervical trunk
  use Artery, Subclavian, Left
  use Artery, Subclavian, Right
Costochondrectomy
  see Excision, Upper Bones 0PB
  see Resection, Upper Bones 0PT
Costoclavicular ligament
  use Bursa and Ligament, Shoulder, Left
  use Bursa and Ligament, Shoulder, Right
Costosternoplasty
  see Repair, Upper Bones 0PQ
  see Replacement, Upper Bones 0PR
  see Supplement, Upper Bones 0PU
Costotomy
  see Division, Upper Bones 0P8
  see Drainage, Upper Bones 0P9
Costotransverse joint
  use Joint, Thoracic Vertebral
Costotransverse ligament
  use Rib(s) Bursa and Ligament
Costovertebral joint
  use Joint, Thoracic Vertebral
Costoxiphoid ligament
  use Sternum Bursa and Ligament
Counseling
  Family, for substance abuse, Other Family Counseling HZ63ZZZ
  Group
    12-Step HZ43ZZZ
    Behavioral HZ41ZZZ
    Cognitive HZ40ZZZ
    Cognitive-Behavioral HZ42ZZZ
    Confrontational HZ48ZZZ
    Continuing Care HZ49ZZZ
    Infectious Disease
      Post-Test HZ4CZZZ
      Pre-Test HZ4CZZZ
    Interpersonal HZ44ZZZ
    Motivational Enhancement HZ47ZZZ
    Psychoeducation HZ46ZZZ
    Spiritual HZ4BZZZ
    Vocational HZ45ZZZ
  Individual
    12-Step HZ33ZZZ
    Behavioral HZ31ZZZ
    Cognitive HZ30ZZZ
    Cognitive-Behavioral HZ32ZZZ
    Confrontational HZ38ZZZ

Counseling *(continued)*
  Individual *(continued)*
    Continuing Care HZ39ZZZ
    Infectious Disease
      Post-Test HZ3CZZZ
      Pre-Test HZ3CZZZ
    Interpersonal HZ34ZZZ
    Motivational Enhancement
      HZ37ZZZ
    Psychoeducation HZ36ZZZ
    Spiritual HZ3BZZZ
    Vocational HZ35ZZZ
  Mental Health Services
    Educational GZ60ZZZ
    Other Counseling GZ63ZZZ
    Vocational GZ61ZZZ
Countershock, cardiac 5A2204Z
Cowper's (bulbourethral) gland
  use Urethra
CPAP (continuous positive airway pressure)
  see Assistance, Respiratory 5A09
Craniectomy
  see Excision, Head and Facial Bones 0NB
  see Resection, Head and Facial Bones 0NT
Cranioplasty
  see Repair, Head and Facial Bones 0NQ
  see Replacement, Head and Facial Bones 0NR
  see Supplement, Head and Facial Bones 0NU
Craniotomy
  see Drainage, Central Nervous System and Cranial Nerves 009
  see Division, Head and Facial Bones 0N8
  see Drainage, Head and Facial Bones 0N9
Creation
  Perineum
    Female 0W4N0
    Male 0W4M0
  Valve
    Aortic 024F0
    Mitral 024G0
    Tricuspid 024J0
Cremaster muscle
  use Muscle, Perineum
Cribriform plate
  use Bone, Ethmoid, Left
  use Bone, Ethmoid, Right
Cricoid cartilage
  use Trachea
Cricoidectomy
  see Excision, Larynx 0CBS
Cricothyroid artery
  use Artery, Thyroid, Left
  use Artery, Thyroid, Right
Cricothyroid muscle
  use Muscle, Neck, Left
  use Muscle, Neck, Right
Crisis Intervention GZ2ZZZZ
CRRT (Continuous renal replacement therapy) 5A1D90Z
Crural fascia
  use Subcutaneous Tissue and Fascia, Upper Leg, Left
  use Subcutaneous Tissue and Fascia, Upper Leg, Right
Crushing, nerve
  Cranial
  see Destruction, Central Nervous System and Cranial Nerves 005
  Peripheral
  see Destruction, Peripheral Nervous System 015
Cryoablation
  see Destruction

Cryotherapy
  see Destruction
Cryptorchidectomy
  see Excision, Male Reproductive System 0VB
  see Resection, Male Reproductive System 0VT
Cryptorchiectomy
  see Excision, Male Reproductive System 0VB
  see Resection, Male Reproductive System 0VT
Cryptotomy
  see Division, Gastrointestinal System 0D8
  see Drainage, Gastrointestinal System 0D9
CT scan
  see Computerized Tomography (CT Scan)
CT sialogram
  see Computerized Tomography (CT Scan), Ear, Nose, Mouth and Throat B92
Cubital lymph node
  use Lymphatic, Upper Extremity, Left
  use Lymphatic, Upper Extremity, Right
Cubital nerve
  use Nerve, Ulnar
Cuboid bone
  use Tarsal, Left
  use Tarsal, Right
Cuboideonavicular joint
  use Joint, Tarsal, Left
  use Joint, Tarsal, Right
Culdocentesis
  see Drainage, Cul-de-sac 0U9F
Culdoplasty
  see Repair, Cul-de-sac 0UQF
  see Supplement, Cul-de-sac 0UUF
Culdoscopy 0UJH8ZZ
Culdotomy
  see Drainage, Cul-de-sac 0U9F
Culmen
  use Cerebellum
Cultured epidermal cell autograft
  use Autologous Tissue Substitute
Cuneiform cartilage
  use Larynx
Cuneonavicular joint
  use Joint, Tarsal, Left
  use Joint, Tarsal, Right
Cuneonavicular ligament
  use Bursa and Ligament, Foot, Left
  use Bursa and Ligament, Foot, Right
Curettage
  see Excision
  see Extraction
Cutaneous (transverse) cervical nerve
  use Nerve, Cervical Plexus
CVP (central venous pressure)
  see Measurement, Venous 4A04
Cyclodiathermy
  see Destruction, Eye 085
Cyclophotocoagulation
  see Destruction, Eye 085
CYPHER® Stent
  use Intraluminal Device, Drug-eluting in Heart and Great Vessels
Cystectomy
  see Excision, Bladder 0TBB
  see Resection, Bladder 0TTB
Cystocele repair
  see Repair, Subcutaneous Tissue and Fascia, Pelvic Region 0JQC
Cystography
  see Fluoroscopy, Urinary System BT1
  see Plain Radiography, Urinary System BT0

Cystolithotomy
  see Extirpation, Bladder 0TCB
Cystopexy
  see Repair, Bladder 0TQB
  see Reposition, Bladder 0TSB
Cystoplasty
  see Repair, Bladder 0TQB
  see Replacement, Bladder 0TRB
  see Supplement, Bladder 0TUB
Cystorrhaphy
  see Repair, Bladder 0TQB
Cystoscopy 0TJB8ZZ
Cystostomy
  see Bypass, Bladder 0T1B
Cystostomy tube
  use Drainage Device
Cystotomy
  see Drainage, Bladder 0T9B
Cystourethrography
  see Fluoroscopy, Urinary System BT1
  see Plain Radiography, Urinary System BT0
Cystourethroplasty
  see Repair, Urinary System 0TQ
  see Replacement, Urinary System 0TR
  see Supplement, Urinary System 0TU
Cytarabine and Daunorubicin Liposome Antineoplastic XW0

D

DBS lead
  use Neurostimulator Lead in Central Nervous System and Cranial Nerves
DeBakey Left Ventricular Assist Device
  use Implantable Heart Assist System in Heart and Great Vessels
Debridement
  Excisional
    see Excision
  Non-excisional
    see Extraction
Decompression, Circulatory 6A15
Decortication, lung
  see Extirpation, Respiratory System 0BC
  see Release, Respiratory System 0BN
Deep brain neurostimulator lead
  use Neurostimulator Lead in Central Nervous System and Cranial Nerves
Deep cervical fascia
  use Subcutaneous Tissue and Fascia, Neck, Left
  use Subcutaneous Tissue and Fascia, Neck, Right
Deep cervical vein
  use Vein, Vertebral, Left
  use Vein, Vertebral, Right
Deep circumflex iliac artery
  use Artery, External Iliac, Left
  use Artery, External Iliac, Right
Deep facial vein
  use Vein, Face, Left
  use Vein, Face, Right
Deep femoral (profunda femoris) vein
  use Vein, Femoral, Left
  use Vein, Femoral, Right
Deep femoral artery
  use Artery, Femoral, Left
  use Artery, Femoral, Right
Deep Inferior Epigastric Artery Perforator Flap
  Replacement
    Bilateral 0HRV077
    Left 0HRU077
    Right 0HRT077
  Transfer
    Left 0KXG
    Right 0KXF

Deep palmar arch
  use Artery, Hand, Left
  use Artery, Hand, Right
Deep transverse perineal muscle
  use Muscle, Perineum
Deferential artery
  use Artery, Internal Iliac, Left
  use Artery, Internal Iliac, Right
Defibrillator Generator
  Abdomen 0JH8
  Chest 0JH6
Defibrotide Sodium Anticoagulant XW0
Defitelio
  use Defibrotide Sodium Anticoagulant
Delivery
  Cesarean
    see Extraction, Products of Conception 10D0
  Forceps
    see Extraction, Products of Conception 10D0
  Manually assisted 10E0XZZ
  Products of Conception 10E0XZZ
  Vacuum assisted
    see Extraction, Products of Conception 10D0
Delta frame external fixator
  use External Fixation Device, Hybrid in 0PH
  use External Fixation Device, Hybrid in 0PS
  use External Fixation Device, Hybrid in 0QH
  use External Fixation Device, Hybrid in 0QS
Delta III Reverse shoulder prosthesis
  use Synthetic Substitute, Reverse Ball and Socket in 0RR
Deltoid fascia
  use Subcutaneous Tissue and Fascia, Upper Arm, Left
  use Subcutaneous Tissue and Fascia, Upper Arm, Right
Deltoid ligament
  use Bursa and Ligament, Ankle, Left
  use Bursa and Ligament, Ankle, Right
Deltoid muscle
  use Muscle, Shoulder, Left
  use Muscle, Shoulder, Right
Deltopectoral (infraclavicular) lymph node
  use Lymphatic, Upper Extremity, Left
  use Lymphatic, Upper Extremity, Right
Denervation
  Cranial nerve
    see Destruction, Central Nervous System and Cranial Nerves 005
  Peripheral nerve
    see Destruction, Peripheral Nervous System 015
Dens
  use Cervical Vertebra
Densitometry
  Plain Radiography
    Femur
      Left BQ04ZZ1
      Right BQ03ZZ1
    Hip
      Left BQ01ZZ1
      Right BQ00ZZ1
    Spine
      Cervical BR00ZZ1
      Lumbar BR09ZZ1

Densitometry (continued)
  Plain Radiography (continued)
    Spine (continued)
      Thoracic BR07ZZ1
      Whole BR0GZZ1
  Ultrasonography
    Elbow
      Left BP4HZZ1
      Right BP4GZZ1
    Hand
      Left BP4PZZ1
      Right BP4NZZ1
    Shoulder
      Left BP49ZZ1
      Right BP48ZZ1
    Wrist
      Left BP4MZZ1
      Right BP4LZZ1

Denticulate (dentate) ligament
  use Spinal Meninges
Depressor anguli oris muscle
  use Muscle, Facial
Depressor labii inferioris muscle
  use Muscle, Facial
Depressor septi nasi muscle
  use Muscle, Facial
Depressor supercilii muscle
  use Muscle, Facial
Dermabrasion
  see Extraction, Skin and Breast
    0HD
Dermis
  use Skin
Descending genicular artery
  use Artery, Femoral, Left
  use Artery, Femoral, Right
Destruction
  Acetabulum
    Left 0Q55
    Right 0Q54
  Adenoids 0C5Q
  Ampulla of Vater 0F5C
  Anal Sphincter 0D5R
  Anterior Chamber
    Left 08533ZZ
    Right 08523ZZ
  Anus 0D5Q
  Aorta
    Abdominal 0450
    Thoracic
      Ascending/Arch 025X
      Descending 025W
  Aortic Body 0G5D
  Appendix 0D5J
  Artery
    Anterior Tibial
      Left 045Q
      Right 045P
    Axillary
      Left 0356
      Right 0355
    Brachial
      Left 0358
      Right 0357
    Celiac 0451
    Colic
      Left 0457
      Middle 0458
      Right 0456
    Common Carotid
      Left 035J
      Right 035H
    Common Iliac
      Left 045D
      Right 045C
    External Carotid
      Left 035N
      Right 035M
    External Iliac
      Left 045J
      Right 045H

Destruction (continued)
  Artery (continued)
    Face 035R
    Femoral
      Left 045L
      Right 045K
    Foot
      Left 045W
      Right 045V
    Gastric 0452
    Hand
      Left 035F
      Right 035D
    Hepatic 0453
    Inferior Mesenteric
      045B
    Innominate 0352
    Internal Carotid
      Left 035L
      Right 035K
    Internal Iliac
      Left 045F
      Right 045E
    Internal Mammary
      Left 0351
      Right 0350
    Intracranial 035G
    Lower 045Y
    Peroneal
      Left 045U
      Right 045T
    Popliteal
      Left 045N
      Right 045M
    Posterior Tibial
      Left 045S
      Right 045R
    Pulmonary
      Left 025R
      Right 025Q
    Pulmonary Trunk 025P
    Radial
      Left 035C
      Right 035B
    Renal
      Left 045A
      Right 0459
    Splenic 0454
    Subclavian
      Left 0354
      Right 0353
    Superior Mesenteric
      0455
    Temporal
      Left 035T
      Right 035S
    Thyroid
      Left 035V
      Right 035U
    Ulnar
      Left 035A
      Right 0359
    Upper 035Y
    Vertebral
      Left 035Q
      Right 035P
  Atrium
    Left 0257
    Right 0256
  Auditory Ossicle
    Left 095A
    Right 0959
  Basal Ganglia 0058
  Bladder 0T5B
  Bladder Neck 0T5C
  Bone
    Ethmoid
      Left 0N5G
      Right 0N5F
    Frontal 0N51
    Hyoid 0N5X

Destruction (continued)
  Bone (continued)
    Lacrimal
      Left 0N5J
      Right 0N5H
    Nasal 0N5B
    Occipital 0N57
    Palatine
      Left 0N5L
      Right 0N5K
    Parietal
      Left 0N54
      Right 0N53
    Pelvic
      Left 0Q53
      Right 0Q52
    Sphenoid 0N5C
    Temporal
      Left 0N56
      Right 0N55
    Zygomatic
      Left 0N5N
      Right 0N5M
  Brain 0050
  Breast
    Bilateral 0H5V
    Left 0H5U
    Right 0H5T
  Bronchus
    Lingula 0B59
    Lower Lobe
      Left 0B5B
      Right 0B56
    Main
      Left 0B57
      Right 0B53
    Middle Lobe, Right 0B55
    Upper Lobe
      Left 0B58
      Right 0B54
  Buccal Mucosa 0C54
  Bursa and Ligament
    Abdomen
      Left 0M5J
      Right 0M5H
    Ankle
      Left 0M5R
      Right 0M5Q
    Elbow
      Left 0M54
      Right 0M53
    Foot
      Left 0M5T
      Right 0M5S
    Hand
      Left 0M58
      Right 0M57
    Head and Neck 0M50
    Hip
      Left 0M5M
      Right 0M5L
    Knee
      Left 0M5P
      Right 0M5N
    Lower Extremity
      Left 0M5W
      Right 0M5V
    Rib(s) 0M5G
    Shoulder
      Left 0M52
      Right 0M51
    Spine
      Lower 0M5D
      Upper 0M5C
    Sternum 0M5F
    Upper Extremity
      Left 0M5B
      Right 0M59
    Wrist
      Left 0M56
      Right 0M55

Destruction (continued)
  Carina 0B52
  Carotid Bodies, Bilateral 0G58
  Carotid Body
    Left 0G56
    Right 0G57
  Carpal
    Left 0P5N
    Right 0P5M
  Cecum 0D5H
  Cerebellum 005C
  Cerebral Hemisphere 0057
  Cerebral Meninges 0051
  Cerebral Ventricle 0056
  Cervix 0U5C
  Chordae Tendineae 0259
  Choroid
    Left 085B
    Right 085A
  Cisterna Chyli 075L
  Clavicle
    Left 0P5B
    Right 0P59
  Clitoris 0U5J
  Coccygeal Glomus 0G5B
  Coccyx 0Q5S
  Colon
    Ascending 0D5K
    Descending 0D5M
    Sigmoid 0D5N
    Transverse 0D5L
  Conduction Mechanism 0258
  Conjunctiva
    Left 085TXZZ
    Right 085SXZZ
  Cord
    Bilateral 0V5H
    Left 0V5G
    Right 0V5F
  Cornea
    Left 0859XZZ
    Right 0858XZZ
  Cul-de-sac 0U5F
  Diaphragm 0B5T
  Disc
    Cervical Vertebral 0R53
    Cervicothoracic Vertebral 0R55
    Lumbar Vertebral 0S52
    Lumbosacral 0S54
    Thoracic Vertebral 0R59
    Thoracolumbar Vertebral 0R5B
  Duct
    Common Bile 0F59
    Cystic 0F58
    Hepatic
      Common 0F57
      Left 0F56
      Right 0F55
    Lacrimal
      Left 085Y
      Right 085X
    Pancreatic 0F5D
      Accessory 0F5F
    Parotid
      Left 0C5C
      Right 0C5B
  Duodenum 0D59
  Dura Mater 0052
  Ear
    External
      Left 0951
      Right 0950
    External Auditory Canal
      Left 0954
      Right 0953
    Inner
      Left 095E
      Right 095D
    Middle
      Left 0956
      Right 0955

struction (continued)

Vein (continued)
  Vertebral (continued)
    Right 055R
Vena Cava
  Inferior 0650
  Superior 025V
Ventricle
  Left 025L
  Right 025K
Vertebra
  Cervical 0P53
  Lumbar 0Q50
  Thoracic 0P54
Vesicle
  Bilateral 0V53
  Left 0V52
  Right 0V51
Vitreous
  Left 08553ZZ
  Right 08543ZZ
Vocal Cord
  Left 0C5V
  Right 0C5T
Vulva 0U5M

etachment

Arm
  Lower
    Left 0X6F0Z
    Right 0X6D0Z
  Upper
    Left 0X690Z
    Right 0X680Z
Elbow Region
  Left 0X6C0ZZ
  Right 0X6B0ZZ
Femoral Region
  Left 0Y680ZZ
  Right 0Y670ZZ
Finger
  Index
    Left 0X6P0Z
    Right 0X6N0Z
  Little
    Left 0X6W0Z
    Right 0X6V0Z
  Middle
    Left 0X6R0Z
    Right 0X6Q0Z
  Ring
    Left 0X6T0Z
    Right 0X6S0Z
Foot
  Left 0Y6N0Z
  Right 0Y6M0Z
Forequarter
  Left 0X610ZZ
  Right 0X600ZZ
Hand
  Left 0X6K0Z
  Right 0X6J0Z
Hindquarter
  Bilateral 0Y640ZZ
  Left 0Y630ZZ
  Right 0Y620ZZ
Knee Region
  Left 0Y6G0ZZ
  Right 0Y6F0ZZ
Leg
  Lower
    Left 0Y6J0Z
    Right 0Y6H0Z
  Upper
    Left 0Y6D0Z
    Right 0Y6C0Z
Shoulder Region
  Left 0X630ZZ
  Right 0X620ZZ
Thumb
  Left 0X6M0Z
  Right 0X6L0Z

Detachment (continued)

Toe
  1st
    Left 0Y6Q0Z
    Right 0Y6P0Z
  2nd
    Left 0Y6S0Z
    Right 0Y6R0Z
  3rd
    Left 0Y6U0Z
    Right 0Y6T0Z
  4th
    Left 0Y6W0Z
    Right 0Y6V0Z
  5th
    Left 0Y6Y0Z
    Right 0Y6X0Z

Determination, Mental status GZ14ZZZ

Detorsion
  see Release
  see Reposition

Detoxification Services, for substance abuse HZ2ZZZZ

Device Fitting F0DZ

Diagnostic Audiology
  see Audiology, Diagnostic

Diagnostic imaging
  see Imaging, Diagnostic

Diagnostic radiology
  see Imaging, Diagnostic

Dialysis
  Hemodialysis *see* Performance, Urinary 5A1D
  Peritoneal 3E1M39Z

Diaphragma sellae
  use Dura Mater

Diaphragmatic pacemaker generator
  use Stimulator Generator in Subcutaneous Tissue and Fascia

Diaphragmatic Pacemaker Lead
  Insertion of device in, Diaphragm 0BHT
  Removal of device from, Diaphragm 0BPT
  Revision of device in, Diaphragm 0BWT

Digital radiography, plain
  see Plain Radiography

Dilation

Ampulla of Vater 0F7C
Anus 0D7Q
Aorta
  Abdominal 0470
  Thoracic
    Ascending/Arch 027X
    Descending 027W
Artery
  Anterior Tibial
    Left 047Q
      Sustained Release Drug-eluting Intraluminal Device X27Q385
      Four or More X27Q3C5
      Three X27Q3B5
      Two X27Q395
    Right 047P
      Sustained Release Drug-eluting Intraluminal Device X27P385
      Four or More X27P3C5
      Three X27P3B5
      Two X27P395
  Axillary
    Left 0376
    Right 0375
  Brachial
    Left 0378
    Right 0377
  Celiac 0471

Dilation (continued)

Artery (continued)
  Colic
    Left 0477
    Middle 0478
    Right 0476
  Common Carotid
    Left 037J
    Right 037H
  Common Iliac
    Left 047D
    Right 047C
  Coronary
    Four or More Arteries 0273
    One Artery 0270
    Three Arteries 0272
    Two Arteries 0271
  External Carotid
    Left 037N
    Right 037M
  External Iliac
    Left 047J
    Right 047H
  Face 037R
  Femoral
    Left 047L
      Sustained Release Drug-eluting Intraluminal Device X27J385
      Four or More X27J3C5
      Three X27J3B5
      Two X27J395
    Right 047K
      Sustained Release Drug-eluting Intraluminal Device X27H385
      Four or More X27H3C5
      Three X27H3B5
      Two X27H395
  Foot
    Left 047W
    Right 047V
  Gastric 0472
  Hand
    Left 037F
    Right 037D
  Hepatic 0473
  Inferior Mesenteric 047B
  Innominate 0372
  Internal Carotid
    Left 037L
    Right 037K
  Internal Iliac
    Left 047F
    Right 047E
  Internal Mammary
    Left 0371
    Right 0370
  Intracranial 037G
  Lower 047Y
  Peroneal
    Left 047U
      Sustained Release Drug-eluting Intraluminal Device X27U385
      Four or More X27U3C5
      Three X27U3B5
      Two X27U395
    Right 047T
      Sustained Release Drug-eluting Intraluminal Device X27T385
      Four or More X27T3C5
      Three X27T3B5
      Two X27T395
  Popliteal
    Left 047N

Dilation (continued)

Artery (continued)
  Popliteal (continued)
    Left Distal
      Sustained Release Drug-eluting Intraluminal Device X27N385
      Four or More X27N3C5
      Three X27N3B5
      Two X27N395
    Left Proximal
      Sustained Release Drug-eluting Intraluminal Device X27L385
      Four or More X27L3C5
      Three X27L3B5
      Two X27L395
    Right 047M
    Right Distal
      Sustained Release Drug-eluting Intraluminal Device X27M385
      Four or More X27M3C5
      Three X27M3B5
      Two X27M395
    Right Proximal
      Sustained Release Drug-eluting Intraluminal Device X27K385
      Four or More X27K3C5
      Three X27K3B5
      Two X27K395
  Posterior Tibial
    Left 047S
      Sustained Release Drug-eluting Intraluminal Device X27S385
      Four or More X27S3C5
      Three X27S3B5
      Two X27S395
    Right 047R
      Sustained Release Drug-eluting Intraluminal Device X27R385
      Four or More X27R3C5
      Three X27R3B5
      Two X27R395
  Pulmonary
    Left 027R
    Right 027Q
  Pulmonary Trunk 027P
  Radial
    Left 037C
    Right 037B
  Renal
    Left 047A
    Right 0479
  Splenic 0474
  Subclavian
    Left 0374
    Right 0373
  Superior Mesenteric 0475
  Temporal
    Left 037T
    Right 037S
  Thyroid
    Left 037V
    Right 037U
  Ulnar
    Left 037A
    Right 0379
  Upper 037Y
  Vertebral
    Left 037Q
    Right 037P

Division (continued)

Metatarsal
    Left 0Q8P
    Right 0Q8N
Muscle
    Abdomen
        Left 0K8L
        Right 0K8K
    Facial 0K81
    Foot
        Left 0K8W
        Right 0K8V
    Hand
        Left 0K8D
        Right 0K8C
    Head 0K80
    Hip
        Left 0K8P
        Right 0K8N
    Lower Arm and Wrist
        Left 0K8B
        Right 0K89
    Lower Leg
        Left 0K8T
        Right 0K8S
    Neck
        Left 0K83
        Right 0K82
    Papillary 028D
    Perineum 0K8M
    Shoulder
        Left 0K86
        Right 0K85
    Thorax
        Left 0K8J
        Right 0K8H
    Tongue, Palate, Pharynx 0K84
    Trunk
        Left 0K8G
        Right 0K8F
    Upper Arm
        Left 0K88
        Right 0K87
    Upper Leg
        Left 0K8R
        Right 0K8Q
Nerve
    Abdominal Sympathetic 018M
    Abducens 008L
    Accessory 008R
    Acoustic 008N
    Brachial Plexus 0183
    Cervical 0181
    Cervical Plexus 0180
    Facial 008M
    Femoral 018D
    Glossopharyngeal 008P
    Head and Neck Sympathetic 018K
    Hypoglossal 008S
    Lumbar 018B
    Lumbar Plexus 0189
    Lumbar Sympathetic 018N
    Lumbosacral Plexus 018A
    Median 0185
    Oculomotor 008H
    Olfactory 008F
    Optic 008G
    Peroneal 018H
    Phrenic 0182
    Pudendal 018C
    Radial 0186
    Sacral 018R
    Sacral Plexus 018Q
    Sacral Sympathetic 018P
    Sciatic 018F
    Thoracic 0188
    Thoracic Sympathetic 018L
    Tibial 018G
    Trigeminal 008K
    Trochlear 008J
    Ulnar 0184

Division (continued)

Nerve (continued)
    Vagus 008Q
Orbit
    Left 0N8Q
    Right 0N8P
Ovary
    Bilateral 0U82
    Left 0U81
    Right 0U80
Pancreas 0F8G
Patella
    Left 0Q8F
    Right 0Q8D
Perineum, Female
    0W8NXZZ
Phalanx
    Finger
        Left 0P8V
        Right 0P8T
    Thumb
        Left 0P8S
        Right 0P8R
    Toe
        Left 0Q8R
        Right 0Q8Q
Radius
    Left 0P8J
    Right 0P8H
Ribs
    1 to 2 0P81
    3 or More 0P82
Sacrum 0Q81
Scapula
    Left 0P86
    Right 0P85
Skin
    Abdomen 0H87XZZ
    Back 0H86XZZ
    Buttock 0H88XZZ
    Chest 0H85XZZ
    Ear
        Left 0H83XZZ
        Right 0H82XZZ
    Face 0H81XZZ
    Foot
        Left 0H8NXZZ
        Right 0H8MXZZ
    Hand
        Left 0H8GXZZ
        Right 0H8FXZZ
    Inguinal 0H8AXZZ
    Lower Arm
        Left 0H8EXZZ
        Right 0H8DXZZ
    Lower Leg
        Left 0H8LXZZ
        Right 0H8KXZZ
    Neck 0H84XZZ
    Perineum 0H89XZZ
    Scalp 0H80XZZ
    Upper Arm
        Left 0H8CXZZ
        Right 0H8BXZZ
    Upper Leg
        Left 0H8JXZZ
        Right 0H8HXZZ
Skull 0N80
Spinal Cord
    Cervical 008W
    Lumbar 008Y
    Thoracic 008X
Sternum 0P80
Stomach, Pylorus 0D87
Subcutaneous Tissue and
    Fascia
    Abdomen 0J88
    Back 0J87
    Buttock 0J89
    Chest 0J86
    Face 0J81

Division (continued)

Subcutaneous Tissue and
    Fascia (continued)
    Foot
        Left 0J8R
        Right 0J8Q
    Hand
        Left 0J8K
        Right 0J8J
    Head and Neck 0J8S
    Lower Arm
        Left 0J8H
        Right 0J8G
    Lower Extremity 0J8W
    Lower Leg
        Left 0J8P
        Right 0J8N
    Neck
        Left 0J85
        Right 0J84
    Pelvic Region 0J8C
    Perineum 0J8B
    Scalp 0J80
    Trunk 0J8T
    Upper Arm
        Left 0J8F
        Right 0J8D
    Upper Extremity 0J8V
    Upper Leg
        Left 0J8M
        Right 0J8L
Tarsal
    Left 0Q8M
    Right 0Q8L
Tendon
    Abdomen
        Left 0L8G
        Right 0L8F
    Ankle
        Left 0L8T
        Right 0L8S
    Foot
        Left 0L8W
        Right 0L8V
    Hand
        Left 0L88
        Right 0L87
    Head and Neck 0L80
    Hip
        Left 0L8K
        Right 0L8J
    Knee
        Left 0L8R
        Right 0L8Q
    Lower Arm and Wrist
        Left 0L86
        Right 0L85
    Lower Leg
        Left 0L8P
        Right 0L8N
    Perineum 0L8H
    Shoulder
        Left 0L82
        Right 0L81
    Thorax
        Left 0L8D
        Right 0L8C
    Trunk
        Left 0L8B
        Right 0L89
    Upper Arm
        Left 0L84
        Right 0L83
    Upper Leg
        Left 0L8M
        Right 0L8L
Thyroid Gland Isthmus
    0G8J
Tibia
    Left 0Q8H
    Right 0Q8G

Division (continued)

Turbinate, Nasal 098L
Ulna
    Left 0P8L
    Right 0P8K
Uterine Supporting Structure
    0U84
Vertebra
    Cervical 0P83
    Lumbar 0Q80
    Thoracic 0P84
Doppler study
    see Ultrasonography
Dorsal digital nerve
    use Nerve, Radial
Dorsal metacarpal vein
    use Vein, Hand, Left
    use Vein, Hand, Right
Dorsal metatarsal artery
    use Artery, Foot, Left
    use Artery, Foot, Right
Dorsal metatarsal vein
    use Vein, Foot, Left
    use Vein, Foot, Right
Dorsal scapular artery
    use Artery, Subclavian, Left
    use Artery, Subclavian, Right
Dorsal scapular nerve
    use Nerve, Brachial Plexus
Dorsal venous arch
    use Vein, Foot, Left
    use Vein, Foot, Right
Dorsalis pedis artery
    use Artery, Anterior Tibial, Left
    use Artery, Anterior Tibial, Right
DownStream® System
    5A0512C
    5A0522C
Drainage
    Abdominal Wall 0W9F
    Acetabulum
        Left 0Q95
        Right 0Q94
    Adenoids 0C9Q
    Ampulla of Vater 0F9C
    Anal Sphincter 0D9R
    Ankle Region
        Left 0Y9L
        Right 0Y9K
    Anterior Chamber
        Left 0893
        Right 0892
    Anus 0D9Q
    Aorta, Abdominal 0490
    Aortic Body 0G9D
    Appendix 0D9J
    Arm
        Lower
            Left 0X9F
            Right 0X9D
        Upper
            Left 0X99
            Right 0X98
    Artery
        Anterior Tibial
            Left 049Q
            Right 049P
        Axillary
            Left 0396
            Right 0395
        Brachial
            Left 0398
            Right 0397
        Celiac 0491
        Colic
            Left 0497
            Middle 0498
            Right 0496
        Common Carotid
            Left 039J
            Right 039H

Drainage *(continued)*
  Wrist Region
    Left 0X9H
    Right 0X9G
Dressing
  Abdominal Wall 2W23X4Z
  Arm
    Lower
      Left 2W2DX4Z
      Right 2W2CX4Z
    Upper
      Left 2W2BX4Z
      Right 2W2AX4Z
  Back 2W25X4Z
  Chest Wall 2W24X4Z
  Extremity
    Lower
      Left 2W2MX4Z
      Right 2W2LX4Z
    Upper
      Left 2W29X4Z
      Right 2W28X4Z
  Face 2W21X4Z
  Finger
    Left 2W2KX4Z
    Right 2W2JX4Z
  Foot
    Left 2W2TX4Z
    Right 2W2SX4Z
  Hand
    Left 2W2FX4Z
    Right 2W2EX4Z
  Head 2W20X4Z
  Inguinal Region
    Left 2W27X4Z
    Right 2W26X4Z
  Leg
    Lower
      Left 2W2RX4Z
      Right 2W2QX4Z
    Upper
      Left 2W2PX4Z
      Right 2W2NX4Z
  Neck 2W22X4Z
  Thumb
    Left 2W2HX4Z
    Right 2W2GX4Z
  Toe
    Left 2W2VX4Z
    Right 2W2UX4Z
Driver stent (RX) (OTW)
  use Intraluminal Device
Drotrecogin alfa, infusion
  see Introduction of Recombinant
    Human-activated Protein C
Duct of Santorini
  use Duct, Pancreatic, Accessory
Duct of Wirsung
  use Duct, Pancreatic
Ductogram, mammary
  see Plain Radiography, Skin,
    Subcutaneous Tissue and Breast
    BH0
Ductography, mammary
  see Plain Radiography, Skin,
    Subcutaneous Tissue and Breast
    BH0
Ductus deferens
  use Vas Deferens
  use Vas Deferens, Bilateral
  use Vas Deferens, Left
  use Vas Deferens, Right
Duodenal ampulla
  use Ampulla of Vater
Duodenectomy
  see Excision, Duodenum 0DB9
  see Resection, Duodenum 0DT9
Duodenocholedochotomy
  see Drainage, Gallbladder 0F94
Duodenocystostomy
  see Bypass, Gallbladder 0F14
  see Drainage, Gallbladder 0F94

Duodenoenterostomy
  see Bypass, Gastrointestinal System
    0D1
  see Drainage, Gastrointestinal
    System 0D9
Duodenojejunal flexure
  use Jejunum
Duodenolysis
  see Release, Duodenum 0DN9
Duodenorrhaphy
  see Repair, Duodenum 0DQ9
Duodenostomy
  see Bypass, Duodenum 0D19
  see Drainage, Duodenum 0D99
Duodenotomy
  see Drainage, Duodenum 0D99
DuraGraft® Endothelial Damage
    Inhibitor
  use Endothelial Damage Inhibitor
DuraHeart Left Ventricular Assist
    System
  use Implantable Heart Assist System
    in Heart and Great Vessels
Dural venous sinus
  use Vein, Intracranial
Dura mater, intracranial
  use Dura Mater
Dura mater, spinal
  use Spinal Meninges
Durata® Defibrillation Lead
  use Cardiac Lead, Defibrillator in 02H
Durvalumab Antineoplastic XW0
DynaNail®
  use Internal Fixation Device,
    Sustained Compression in 0RG
  use Internal Fixation Device,
    Sustained Compression in 0SG
DynaNail Mini®
  use Internal Fixation Device,
    Sustained Compression in 0RG
  use Internal Fixation Device,
    Sustained Compression in 0SG
Dynesys® Dynamic Stabilization
    System
  use Spinal Stabilization Device,
    Pedicle-Based in 0RH
  use Spinal Stabilization Device,
    Pedicle-Based in 0SH

E

E-Luminexx™ (Biliary)(Vascular)
    Stent
  use Intraluminal Device
Earlobe
  use Ear, External, Bilateral
  use Ear, External, Left
  use Ear, External, Right
ECCO2R (Extracorporeal Carbon
    Dioxide Removal) 5A0920Z
Echocardiogram
  see Ultrasonography, Heart B24
Echography
  see Ultrasonography
EchoTip® Insight™ Portosystemic
    Pressure Gradient
    Measurement System 4A044B2
ECMO
  see Performance, Circulatory 5A15
ECMO, intraoperative
  see Performance, Circulatory
    5A15A
Eculizumab XW0
EDWARDS INTUITY Elite valve
    system
  use Zooplastic Tissue, Rapid
    Deployment in New Technology
EEG (electroencephalogram)
  see Measurement, Central Nervous
    4A00
EGD (esophagogastroduodenoscopy)
    0DJ08ZZ

Eighth cranial nerve
  use Nerve, Acoustic
Ejaculatory duct
  use Vas Deferens
  use Vas Deferens, Bilateral
  use Vas Deferens, Left
  use Vas Deferens, Right
EKG (electrocardiogram)
  see Measurement, Cardiac 4A02
EKOS™ EkoSonic® Endovascular
    System
  see Fragmentation, Artery
Eladocagene exuparvovec XW0Q316
Electrical bone growth stimulator
    (EBGS)
  use Bone Growth Stimulator in
    Head and Facial Bones
  use Bone Growth Stimulator in
    Lower Bones
  use Bone Growth Stimulator in
    Upper Bones
Electrical muscle stimulation (EMS)
    lead
  use Stimulator Lead in Muscles
Electrocautery
  Destruction
    see Destruction
  Repair
    see Repair
Electroconvulsive Therapy
  Bilateral-Multiple Seizure
    GZB3ZZZ
  Bilateral-Single Seizure GZB2ZZZ
  Electroconvulsive Therapy, Other
    GZB4ZZZ
  Unilateral-Multiple Seizure
    GZB1ZZZ
  Unilateral-Single Seizure GZB0ZZZ
Electroencephalogram (EEG)
  see Measurement, Central Nervous
    4A00
Electromagnetic Therapy
  Central Nervous 6A22
  Urinary 6A21
Electronic muscle stimulator lead
  use Stimulator Lead in Muscles
Electrophysiologic stimulation
    (EPS)
  see Measurement, Cardiac 4A02
Electroshock therapy
  see Electroconvulsive Therapy
Elevation, bone fragments, skull
  see Reposition, Head and Facial
    Bones 0NS
Eleventh cranial nerve
  use Nerve, Accessory
Ellipsys® vascular access system
  Radial Artery, Left 031C
  Radial Artery, Right 031B
  Ulnar Artery, Left 031A
  Ulnar Artery, Right 0319
Eluvia™ Drug-Eluting Vascular Stent
    System
  use Intraluminal Device, Sustained
    Release Drug-eluting in New
    Technology
  use Intraluminal Device, Sustained
    Release Drug-eluting, Two in
    New Technology
  use Intraluminal Device, Sustained
    Release Drug-eluting, Three in
    New Technology
  use Intraluminal Device, Sustained
    Release Drug-eluting, Four or
    More in New Technology
ELZONRIS™
  use Tagraxofusp-erzs Antineoplastic
Embolectomy
  see Extirpation
Embolization
  see Occlusion
  see Restriction

Embolization coil(s)
  use Intraluminal Device
EMG (electromyogram)
  see Measurement, Musculoskeletal
    4A0F
Encephalon
  use Brain
Endarterectomy
  see Extirpation, Lower Arteries 04C
  see Extirpation, Upper Arteries 03C
Endeavor® (III)(IV) (Sprint)
    Zotarolimus-eluting Coronary
    Stent System
  use Intraluminal Device, Drug-
    eluting in Heart and Great Vessels
EndoAVF procedure
  Radial Artery, Left 031C
  Radial Artery, Right 031B
  Ulnar Artery, Left 031A
  Ulnar Artery, Right 0319
Endologix AFX® Endovascular
    AAA System
  use Intraluminal Device
EndoSure® sensor
  use Monitoring Device, Pressure
    Sensor in 02H
Endovascular fistula creation
  Radial Artery, Left 031C
  Radial Artery, Right 031B
  Ulnar Artery, Left 031A
  Ulnar Artery, Right 0319
ENDOTAK RELIANCE® (G)
    Defibrillation Lead
  use Cardiac Lead, Defibrillator in
    02H
Endothelial damage inhibitor, applied
    to vein graft XY0VX83
Endotracheal tube (cuffed)(double-
    lumen)
  use Intraluminal Device, Endotracheal
    Airway in Respiratory System
Endurant® II AAA stent graft system
  use Intraluminal Device
Endurant® Endovascular Stent Graft
  use Intraluminal Device
Engineered Autologous Chimeric
    Antigen Receptor T-cell
    Immunotherapy XW0
Enlargement
  see Dilation
  see Repair
EnRhythm
  use Pacemaker, Dual Chamber in 0JH
ENROUTE® Transcarotid
    Neuroprotection System
  see New Technology,
    Cardiovascular System X2A
Enterorrhaphy
  see Repair, Gastrointestinal System
    0DQ
Enterra gastric neurostimulator
  use Stimulator Generator, Multiple
    Array in 0JH
Enucleation
  Eyeball
    see Resection, Eye 08T
  Eyeball with prosthetic implant
    see Replacement, Eye 08R
Ependyma
  use Cerebral Ventricle
Epicel® cultured epidermal autograft
  use Autologous Tissue Substitute
Epic™ Stented Tissue Valve (aortic)
  use Zooplastic Tissue in Heart and
    Great Vessels
Epidermis
  use Skin
Epididymectomy
  see Excision, Male Reproductive
    System 0VB
  see Resection, Male Reproductive
    System 0VT

Epididymoplasty
 see Repair, Male Reproductive
  System 0VQ
 see Supplement, Male Reproductive
  System 0VU
Epididymorrhaphy
 see Repair, Male Reproductive
  System 0VQ
Epididymotomy
 see Drainage, Male Reproductive
  System 0V9
Epidural space, spinal
 use Spinal Canal
Epiphysiodesis
 see Insertion of device in Lower
  Bones 0QH
 see Insertion of device in Upper
  Bones 0PH
 see Repair, Lower Bones 0QQ
 see Repair, Upper Bones 0PQ
Epiploic foramen
 use Peritoneum
Epiretinal Visual Prosthesis
 Left 08H105Z
 Right 08H005Z
Episiorrhaphy
 see Repair, Perineum, Female 0WQN
Episiotomy
 see Division, Perineum, Female
  0W8N
Epithalamus
 use Thalamus
Epitrochlear lymph node
 use Lymphatic, Upper Extremity,
  Left
 use Lymphatic, Upper Extremity,
  Right
EPS (electrophysiologic stimulation)
 see Measurement, Cardiac 4A02
Eptifibatide, infusion
 see Introduction of Platelet Inhibitor
ERCP (endoscopic retrograde
 cholangiopancreatography)
 see Fluoroscopy, Hepatobiliary
  System and Pancreas BF1
Erdafitinib Antineoplastic XW0DXL5
Erector spinae muscle
 use Muscle, Trunk, Left
 use Muscle, Trunk, Right
ERLEADA™
 use Apalutamide Antineoplastic
Esketamine Hydrochloride
 XW097M5
Esophageal artery
 use Upper Artery
Esophageal obturator airway (EOA)
 use Intraluminal Device, Airway in
  Gastrointestinal System
Esophageal plexus
 use Nerve, Thoracic Sympathetic
Esophagectomy
 see Excision, Gastrointestinal
  System 0DB
 see Resection, Gastrointestinal
  System 0DT
Esophagocoloplasty
 see Repair, Gastrointestinal System
  0DQ
 see Supplement, Gastrointestinal
  System 0DU
Esophagoenterostomy
 see Bypass, Gastrointestinal System
  0D1
 see Drainage, Gastrointestinal
  System 0D9
Esophagoesophagostomy
 see Bypass, Gastrointestinal System
  0D1
 see Drainage, Gastrointestinal
  System 0D9

Esophagogastrectomy
 see Excision, Gastrointestinal
  System 0DB
 see Resection, Gastrointestinal
  System 0DT
Esophagogastroduodenoscopy (EGD)
 0DJ08ZZ
Esophagogastroplasty
 see Repair, Gastrointestinal System
  0DQ
 see Supplement, Gastrointestinal
  System 0DU
Esophagogastroscopy 0DJ68ZZ
Esophagogastrostomy
 see Bypass, Gastrointestinal System
  0D1
 see Drainage, Gastrointestinal
  System 0D9
Esophagojejunoplasty
 see Supplement, Gastrointestinal
  System 0DU
Esophagojejunostomy
 see Bypass, Gastrointestinal System
  0D1
 see Drainage, Gastrointestinal
  System 0D9
Esophagomyotomy
 see Division, Esophagogastric
  Junction 0D84
Esophagoplasty
 see Repair, Gastrointestinal System
  0DQ
 see Replacement, Esophagus 0DR5
 see Supplement, Gastrointestinal
  System 0DU
Esophagoplication
 see Restriction, Gastrointestinal
  System 0DV
Esophagorrhaphy
 see Repair, Gastrointestinal System
  0DQ
Esophagoscopy 0DJ08ZZ
Esophagotomy
 see Drainage, Gastrointestinal
  System 0D9
Esteem® implantable hearing system
 use Hearing Device in Ear, Nose, Sinus
ESWL (extracorporeal shock wave
 lithotripsy)
 see Fragmentation
Ethmoidal air cell
 use Sinus, Ethmoid, Left
 use Sinus, Ethmoid, Right
Ethmoidectomy
 see Excision, Ear, Nose, Sinus 09B
 see Excision, Head and Facial
  Bones 0NB
 see Resection, Ear, Nose, Sinus 09T
 see Resection, Head and Facial
  Bones 0NT
Ethmoidotomy
 see Drainage, Ear, Nose, Sinus 099
Evacuation
 Hematoma
  see Extirpation
 Other Fluid
  see Drainage
Evera (XT)(S)(DR/VR)
 use Defibrillator Generator in 0JH
Everolimus-eluting coronary stent
 use Intraluminal Device, Drug-
  eluting in Heart and Great
  Vessels
Evisceration
 Eyeball
  see Resection, Eye 08T
 Eyeball with prosthetic implant
  see Replacement, Eye 08R
Ex-PRESS™ mini glaucoma shunt
 use Synthetic Substitute

Examination
 see Inspection
Exchange
 see Change device in
Excision
 Abdominal Wall 0WBF
 Acetabulum
  Left 0QB5
  Right 0QB4
 Adenoids 0CBQ
 Ampulla of Vater 0FBC
 Anal Sphincter 0DBR
 Ankle Region
  Left 0YBL
  Right 0YBK
 Anus 0DBQ
 Aorta
  Abdominal 04B0
  Thoracic
   Ascending/Arch 02BX
   Descending 02BW
 Aortic Body 0GBD
 Appendix 0DBJ
 Arm
  Lower
   Left 0XBF
   Right 0XBD
  Upper
   Left 0XB9
   Right 0XB8
 Artery
  Anterior Tibial
   Left 04BQ
   Right 04BP
  Axillary
   Left 03B6
   Right 03B5
  Brachial
   Left 03B8
   Right 03B7
  Celiac 04B1
  Colic
   Left 04B7
   Middle 04B8
   Right 04B6
  Common Carotid
   Left 03BJ
   Right 03BH
  Common Iliac
   Left 04BD
   Right 04BC
  External Carotid
   Left 03BN
   Right 03BM
  External Iliac
   Left 04BJ
   Right 04BH
  Face 03BR
  Femoral
   Left 04BL
   Right 04BK
  Foot
   Left 04BW
   Right 04BV
  Gastric 04B2
  Hand
   Left 03BF
   Right 03BD
  Hepatic 04B3
  Inferior Mesenteric 04BB
  Innominate 03B2
  Internal Carotid
   Left 03BL
   Right 03BK
  Internal Iliac
   Left 04BF
   Right 04BE
  Internal Mammary
   Left 03B1
   Right 03B0

Excision *(continued)*
 Artery *(continued)*
  Intracranial 03BG
  Lower 04BY
  Peroneal
   Left 04BU
   Right 04BT
  Popliteal
   Left 04BN
   Right 04BM
  Posterior Tibial
   Left 04BS
   Right 04BR
  Pulmonary
   Left 02BR
   Right 02BQ
  Pulmonary Trunk 02BP
  Radial
   Left 03BC
   Right 03BB
  Renal
   Left 04BA
   Right 04B9
  Splenic 04B4
  Subclavian
   Left 03B4
   Right 03B3
  Superior Mesenteric 04B5
  Temporal
   Left 03BT
   Right 03BS
  Thyroid
   Left 03BV
   Right 03BU
  Ulnar
   Left 03BA
   Right 03B9
  Upper 03BY
  Vertebral
   Left 03BQ
   Right 03BP
 Atrium
  Left 02B7
  Right 02B6
 Auditory Ossicle
  Left 09BA
  Right 09B9
 Axilla
  Left 0XB5
  Right 0XB4
 Back
  Lower 0WBL
  Upper 0WBK
 Basal Ganglia 00B8
 Bladder 0TBB
 Bladder Neck 0TBC
 Bone
  Ethmoid
   Left 0NBG
   Right 0NBF
  Frontal 0NB1
  Hyoid 0NBX
  Lacrimal
   Left 0NBJ
   Right 0NBH
  Nasal 0NBB
  Occipital 0NB7
  Palatine
   Left 0NBL
   Right 0NBK
  Parietal
   Left 0NB4
   Right 0NB3
  Pelvic
   Left 0QB3
   Right 0QB2
  Sphenoid 0NBC
  Temporal
   Left 0NB6
   Right 0NB5

Excision *(continued)*

Joint *(continued)*
  Sternoclavicular
    Left 0RBF
    Right 0RBE
  Tarsal
    Left 0SBJ
    Right 0SBH
  Tarsometatarsal
    Left 0SBL
    Right 0SBK
  Temporomandibular
    Left 0RBD
    Right 0RBC
  Thoracic Vertebral 0RB6
  Thoracolumbar Vertebral
    0RBA
  Toe Phalangeal
    Left 0SBQ
    Right 0SBP
  Wrist
    Left 0RBP
    Right 0RBN
Kidney
  Left 0TB1
  Right 0TB0
Kidney Pelvis
  Left 0TB4
  Right 0TB3
Knee Region
  Left 0YBG
  Right 0YBF
Larynx 0CBS
Leg
  Lower
    Left 0YBJ
    Right 0YBH
  Upper
    Left 0YBD
    Right 0YBC
Lens
  Left 08BK3Z
  Right 08BJ3Z
Lip
  Lower 0CB1
  Upper 0CB0
Liver 0FB0
  Left Lobe 0FB2
  Right Lobe 0FB1
Lung
  Bilateral 0BBM
  Left 0BBL
  Lower Lobe
    Left 0BBJ
    Right 0BBF
  Middle Lobe, Right 0BBD
  Right 0BBK
  Upper Lobe
    Left 0BBG
    Right 0BBC
Lung Lingula 0BBH
Lymphatic
  Aortic 07BD
  Axillary
    Left 07B6
    Right 07B5
  Head 07B0
  Inguinal
    Left 07BJ
    Right 07BH
  Internal Mammary
    Left 07B9
    Right 07B8
  Lower Extremity
    Left 07BG
    Right 07BF
  Mesenteric 07BB
  Neck
    Left 07B2
    Right 07B1

Excision *(continued)*

Lymphatic *(continued)*
  Pelvis 07BC
  Thoracic Duct 07BK
  Thorax 07B7
  Upper Extremity
    Left 07B4
    Right 07B3
Mandible
  Left 0NBV
  Right 0NBT
Maxilla 0NBR
Mediastinum 0WBC
Medulla Oblongata 00BD
Mesentery 0DBV
Metacarpal
  Left 0PBQ
  Right 0PBP
Metatarsal
  Left 0QBP
  Right 0QBN
Muscle
  Abdomen
    Left 0KBL
    Right 0KBK
  Extraocular
    Left 08BM
    Right 08BL
  Facial 0KB1
  Foot
    Left 0KBW
    Right 0KBV
  Hand
    Left 0KBD
    Right 0KBC
  Head 0KB0
  Hip
    Left 0KBP
    Right 0KBN
  Lower Arm and Wrist
    Left 0KBB
    Right 0KB9
  Lower Leg
    Left 0KBT
    Right 0KBS
  Neck
    Left 0KB3
    Right 0KB2
  Papillary 02BD
  Perineum 0KBM
  Shoulder
    Left 0KB6
    Right 0KB5
  Thorax
    Left 0KBJ
    Right 0KBH
  Tongue, Palate, Pharynx 0KB4
  Trunk
    Left 0KBG
    Right 0KBF
  Upper Arm
    Left 0KB8
    Right 0KB7
  Upper Leg
    Left 0KBR
    Right 0KBQ
Nasal Mucosa and Soft Tissue
  09BK
Nasopharynx 09BN
Neck 0WB6
Nerve
  Abdominal Sympathetic
    01BM
  Abducens 00BL
  Accessory 00BR
  Acoustic 00BN
  Brachial Plexus 01B3
  Cervical 01B1
  Cervical Plexus 01B0
  Facial 00BM

Excision *(continued)*

Nerve *(continued)*
  Femoral 01BD
  Glossopharyngeal 00BP
  Head and Neck Sympathetic
    01BK
  Hypoglossal 00BS
  Lumbar 01BB
  Lumbar Plexus 01B9
  Lumbar Sympathetic 01BN
  Lumbosacral Plexus 01BA
  Median 01B5
  Oculomotor 00BH
  Olfactory 00BF
  Optic 00BG
  Peroneal 01BH
  Phrenic 01B2
  Pudendal 01BC
  Radial 01B6
  Sacral 01BR
  Sacral Plexus 01BQ
  Sacral Sympathetic 01BP
  Sciatic 01BF
  Thoracic 01B8
  Thoracic Sympathetic 01BL
  Tibial 01BG
  Trigeminal 00BK
  Trochlear 00BJ
  Ulnar 01B4
  Vagus 00BQ
Nipple
  Left 0HBX
  Right 0HBW
Omentum 0DBU
Oral Cavity and Throat 0WB3
Orbit
  Left 0NBQ
  Right 0NBP
Ovary
  Bilateral 0UB2
  Left 0UB1
  Right 0UB0
Palate
  Hard 0CB2
  Soft 0CB3
Pancreas 0FBG
Para-aortic Body 0GB9
Paraganglion Extremity 0GBF
Parathyroid Gland 0GBR
  Inferior
    Left 0GBP
    Right 0GBN
  Multiple 0GBQ
  Superior
    Left 0GBM
    Right 0GBL
Patella
  Left 0QBF
  Right 0QBD
Penis 0VBS
Pericardium 02BN
Perineum
  Female 0WBN
  Male 0WBM
Peritoneum 0DBW
Phalanx
  Finger
    Left 0PBV
    Right 0PBT
  Thumb
    Left 0PBS
    Right 0PBR
  Toe
    Left 0QBR
    Right 0QBQ
Pharynx 0CBM
Pineal Body 0GB1
Pleura
  Left 0BBP
  Right 0BBN

Excision *(continued)*

Pons 00BB
Prepuce 0VBT
Prostate 0VB0
Radius
  Left 0PBJ
  Right 0PBH
Rectum 0DBP
Retina
  Left 08BF3Z
  Right 08BE3Z
Retroperitoneum
  0WBH
Ribs
  1 to 2 0PB1
  3 or More 0PB2
Sacrum 0QB1
Scapula
  Left 0PB6
  Right 0PB5
Sclera
  Left 08B7XZ
  Right 08B6XZ
Scrotum 0VB5
Septum
  Atrial 02B5
  Nasal 09BM
  Ventricular 02BM
Shoulder Region
  Left 0XB3
  Right 0XB2
Sinus
  Accessory 09BP
  Ethmoid
    Left 09BV
    Right 09BU
  Frontal
    Left 09BT
    Right 09BS
  Mastoid
    Left 09BC
    Right 09BB
  Maxillary
    Left 09BR
    Right 09BQ
  Sphenoid
    Left 09BX
    Right 09BW
Skin
  Abdomen 0HB7XZ
  Back 0HB6XZ
  Buttock 0HB8XZ
  Chest 0HB5XZ
  Ear
    Left 0HB3XZ
    Right 0HB2XZ
  Face 0HB1XZ
  Foot
    Left 0HBNXZ
    Right 0HBMXZ
  Hand
    Left 0HBGXZ
    Right 0HBFXZ
  Inguinal 0HBAXZ
  Lower Arm
    Left 0HBEXZ
    Right 0HBDXZ
  Lower Leg
    Left 0HBLXZ
    Right 0HBKXZ
  Neck 0HB4XZ
  Perineum 0HB9XZ
  Scalp 0HB0XZ
  Upper Arm
    Left 0HBCXZ
    Right 0HBBXZ
  Upper Leg
    Left 0HBJXZ
    Right 0HBHXZ
Skull 0NB0

Excision (continued)

Spinal Cord
    Cervical 00BW
    Lumbar 00BY
    Thoracic 00BX
Spinal Meninges 00BT
Spleen 07BP
Sternum 0PB0
Stomach 0DB6
    Pylorus 0DB7
Subcutaneous Tissue and Fascia
    Abdomen 0JB8
    Back 0JB7
    Buttock 0JB9
    Chest 0JB6
    Face 0JB1
    Foot
        Left 0JBR
        Right 0JBQ
    Hand
        Left 0JBK
        Right 0JBJ
    Lower Arm
        Left 0JBH
        Right 0JBG
    Lower Leg
        Left 0JBP
        Right 0JBN
    Neck
        Left 0JB5
        Right 0JB4
    Pelvic Region 0JBC
    Perineum 0JBB
    Scalp 0JB0
    Upper Arm
        Left 0JBF
        Right 0JBD
    Upper Leg
        Left 0JBM
        Right 0JBL
Tarsal
    Left 0QBM
    Right 0QBL
Tendon
    Abdomen
        Left 0LBG
        Right 0LBF
    Ankle
        Left 0LBT
        Right 0LBS
    Foot
        Left 0LBW
        Right 0LBV
    Hand
        Left 0LB8
        Right 0LB7
    Head and Neck
        0LB0
    Hip
        Left 0LBK
        Right 0LBJ
    Knee
        Left 0LBR
        Right 0LBQ
    Lower Arm and Wrist
        Left 0LB6
        Right 0LB5
    Lower Leg
        Left 0LBP
        Right 0LBN
    Perineum 0LBH
    Shoulder
        Left 0LB2
        Right 0LB1
    Thorax
        Left 0LBD
        Right 0LBC
    Trunk
        Left 0LBB
        Right 0LB9

Excision (continued)

Tendon (continued)
    Upper Arm
        Left 0LB4
        Right 0LB3
    Upper Leg
        Left 0LBM
        Right 0LBL
Testis
    Bilateral 0VBC
    Left 0VBB
    Right 0VB9
Thalamus 00B9
Thymus 07BM
Thyroid Gland
    Left Lobe 0GBG
    Right Lobe 0GBH
Thyroid Gland Isthmus
    0GBJ
Tibia
    Left 0QBH
    Right 0QBG
Toe Nail 0HBRXZ
Tongue 0CB7
Tonsils 0CBP
Tooth
    Lower 0CBX
    Upper 0CBW
Trachea 0BB1
Tunica Vaginalis
    Left 0VB7
    Right 0VB6
Turbinate, Nasal 09BL
Tympanic Membrane
    Left 09B8
    Right 09B7
Ulna
    Left 0PBL
    Right 0PBK
Ureter
    Left 0TB7
    Right 0TB6
Urethra 0TBD
Uterine Supporting Structure
    0UB4
Uterus 0UB9
Uvula 0CBN
Vagina 0UBG
Valve
    Aortic 02BF
    Mitral 02BG
    Pulmonary 02BH
    Tricuspid 02BJ
Vas Deferens
    Bilateral 0VBQ
    Left 0VBP
    Right 0VBN
Vein
    Axillary
        Left 05B8
        Right 05B7
    Azygos 05B0
    Basilic
        Left 05BC
        Right 05BB
    Brachial
        Left 05BA
        Right 05B9
    Cephalic
        Left 05BF
        Right 05BD
    Colic 06B7
    Common Iliac
        Left 06BD
        Right 06BC
    Coronary 02B4
    Esophageal 06B3
    External Iliac
        Left 06BG
        Right 06BF

Excision (continued)

Vein (continued)
    External Jugular
        Left 05BQ
        Right 05BP
    Face
        Left 05BV
        Right 05BT
    Femoral
        Left 06BN
        Right 06BM
    Foot
        Left 06BV
        Right 06BT
    Gastric 06B2
    Hand
        Left 05BH
        Right 05BG
    Hemiazygos 05B1
    Hepatic 06B4
    Hypogastric
        Left 06BJ
        Right 06BH
    Inferior Mesenteric 06B6
    Innominate
        Left 05B4
        Right 05B3
    Internal Jugular
        Left 05BN
        Right 05BM
    Intracranial 05BL
    Lower 06BY
    Portal 06B8
    Pulmonary
        Left 02BT
        Right 02BS
    Renal
        Left 06BB
        Right 06B9
    Saphenous
        Left 06BQ
        Right 06BP
    Splenic 06B1
    Subclavian
        Left 05B6
        Right 05B5
    Superior Mesenteric 06B5
    Upper 05BY
    Vertebral
        Left 05BS
        Right 05BR
Vena Cava
    Inferior 06B0
    Superior 02BV
Ventricle
    Left 02BL
    Right 02BK
Vertebra
    Cervical 0PB3
    Lumbar 0QB0
    Thoracic 0PB4
Vesicle
    Bilateral 0VB3
    Left 0VB2
    Right 0VB1
Vitreous
    Left 08B53Z
    Right 08B43Z
Vocal Cord
    Left 0CBV
    Right 0CBT
Vulva 0UBM
Wrist Region
    Left 0XBH
    Right 0XBG

EXCLUDER® AAA Endoprosthesis
    use Intraluminal Device
    use Intraluminal Device, Branched
        or Fenestrated, One or Two
        Arteries in 04V

EXCLUDER® AAA Endoprosthesis
    (continued)
    use Intraluminal Device, Branched
        or Fenestrated, Three or More
        Arteries in 04V
EXCLUDER® IBE Endoprosthesis
    use Intraluminal Device, Branched
        or Fenestrated, One or Two
        Arteries in 04V
Exclusion, Left atrial appendage
    (LAA)
    see Occlusion, Atrium, Left
        02L7
Exercise, rehabilitation
    see Motor Treatment, Rehabilitation
        F07
Exploration
    see Inspection
Express® (LD) Premounted Stent
    System
    use Intraluminal Device
Express® Biliary SD Monorail®
    Premounted Stent System
    use Intraluminal Device
Express® SD Renal Monorail®
    Premounted Stent System
    use Intraluminal Device
Extensor carpi radialis muscle
    use Muscle, Lower Arm and Wrist,
        Left
Extensor carpi radialis muscle
    use Muscle, Lower Arm and Wrist,
        Right
Extensor carpi ulnaris muscle
    use Muscle, Lower Arm and Wrist,
        Left
    use Muscle, Lower Arm and Wrist,
        Right
Extensor digitorum brevis muscle
    use Muscle, Foot, Left
    use Muscle, Foot, Right
Extensor digitorum longus muscle
    use Muscle, Lower Leg, Left
    use Muscle, Lower Leg, Right
Extensor hallucis brevis muscle
    use Muscle, Foot, Left
    use Muscle, Foot, Right
Extensor hallucis longus muscle
    use Muscle, Lower Leg, Left
    use Muscle, Lower Leg, Right
External anal sphincter
    use Anal Sphincter
External auditory meatus
    use Ear, External Auditory Canal,
        Left
    use Ear, External Auditory Canal,
        Right
External fixator
    use External Fixation Device in
        Head and Facial Bones
    use External Fixation Device in
        Lower Bones
    use External Fixation Device in
        Lower Joints
    use External Fixation Device in
        Upper Bones
    use External Fixation Device in
        Upper Joints
External maxillary artery
    use Artery, Face
External naris
    use Nasal Mucosa and Soft Tissue
External oblique aponeurosis
    use Subcutaneous Tissue and Fascia,
        Trunk
External oblique muscle
    use Muscle, Abdomen, Left
    use Muscle, Abdomen, Right
External popliteal nerve
    use Nerve, Peroneal

External pudendal artery
use Artery, Femoral, Left
use Artery, Femoral, Right
External pudendal vein
use Vein, Saphenous, Left
use Vein, Saphenous, Right
External urethral sphincter
use Urethra
Extirpation
Acetabulum
    Left 0QC5
    Right 0QC4
Adenoids 0CCQ
Ampulla of Vater 0FCC
Anal Sphincter 0DCR
Anterior Chamber
    Left 08C3
    Right 08C2
Anus 0DCQ
Aorta
    Abdominal 04C0
    Thoracic
        Ascending/Arch 02CX
        Descending 02CW
Aortic Body 0GCD
Appendix 0DCJ
Artery
    Anterior Tibial
        Left 04CQ
        Right 04CP
    Axillary
        Left 03C6
        Right 03C5
    Brachial
        Left 03C8
        Right 03C7
    Celiac 04C1
    Colic
        Left 04C7
        Middle 04C8
        Right 04C6
    Common Carotid
        Left 03CJ
        Right 03CH
    Common Iliac
        Left 04CD
        Right 04CC
    Coronary
        Four or More Arteries 02C3
        One Artery 02C0
        Three Arteries 02C2
        Two Arteries 02C1
    External Carotid
        Left 03CN
        Right 03CM
    External Iliac
        Left 04CJ
        Right 04CH
    Face 03CR
    Femoral
        Left 04CL
        Right 04CK
    Foot
        Left 04CW
        Right 04CV
    Gastric 04C2
    Hand
        Left 03CF
        Right 03CD
    Hepatic 04C3
    Inferior Mesenteric 04CB
    Innominate 03C2
    Internal Carotid
        Left 03CL
        Right 03CK
    Internal Iliac
        Left 04CF
        Right 04CE
    Internal Mammary
        Left 03C1
        Right 03C0

Extirpation *(continued)*
Artery *(continued)*
    Intracranial 03CG
    Lower 04CY
    Peroneal
        Left 04CU
        Right 04CT
    Popliteal
        Left 04CN
        Right 04CM
    Posterior Tibial
        Left 04CS
        Right 04CR
    Pulmonary
        Left 02CR
        Right 02CQ
    Pulmonary Trunk
        02CP
    Radial
        Left 03CC
        Right 03CB
    Renal
        Left 04CA
        Right 04C9
    Splenic 04C4
    Subclavian
        Left 03C4
        Right 03C3
    Superior Mesenteric
        04C5
    Temporal
        Left 03CT
        Right 03CS
    Thyroid
        Left 03CV
        Right 03CU
    Ulnar
        Left 03CA
        Right 03C9
    Upper 03CY
    Vertebral
        Left 03CQ
        Right 03CP
Atrium
    Left 02C7
    Right 02C6
Auditory Ossicle
    Left 09CA
    Right 09C9
Basal Ganglia 00C8
Bladder 0TCB
Bladder Neck
    0TCC
Bone
    Ethmoid
        Left 0NCG
        Right 0NCF
    Frontal 0NC1
    Hyoid 0NCX
    Lacrimal
        Left 0NCJ
        Right 0NCH
    Nasal 0NCB
    Occipital 0NC7
    Palatine
        Left 0NCL
        Right 0NCK
    Parietal
        Left 0NC4
        Right 0NC3
    Pelvic
        Left 0QC3
        Right 0QC2
    Sphenoid 0NCC
    Temporal
        Left 0NC6
        Right 0NC5
    Zygomatic
        Left 0NCN
        Right 0NCM
Brain 00C0

Extirpation *(continued)*
Breast
    Bilateral 0HCV
    Left 0HCU
    Right 0HCT
Bronchus
    Lingula 0BC9
    Lower Lobe
        Left 0BCB
        Right 0BC6
    Main
        Left 0BC7
        Right 0BC3
    Middle Lobe, Right
        0BC5
    Upper Lobe
        Left 0BC8
        Right 0BC4
Buccal Mucosa 0CC4
Bursa and Ligament
    Abdomen
        Left 0MCJ
        Right 0MCH
    Ankle
        Left 0MCR
        Right 0MCQ
    Elbow
        Left 0MC4
        Right 0MC3
    Foot
        Left 0MCT
        Right 0MCS
    Hand
        Left 0MC8
        Right 0MC7
    Head and Neck 0MC0
    Hip
        Left 0MCM
        Right 0MCL
    Knee
        Left 0MCP
        Right 0MCN
    Lower Extremity
        Left 0MCW
        Right 0MCV
    Perineum 0MCK
    Rib(s) 0MCG
    Shoulder
        Left 0MC2
        Right 0MC1
    Spine
        Lower 0MCD
        Upper 0MCC
    Sternum 0MCF
    Upper Extremity
        Left 0MCB
        Right 0MC9
    Wrist
        Left 0MC6
        Right 0MC5
Carina 0BC2
Carotid Bodies, Bilateral
    0GC8
Carotid Body
    Left 0GC6
    Right 0GC7
Carpal
    Left 0PCN
    Right 0PCM
Cavity, Cranial 0WC1
Cecum 0DCH
Cerebellum 00CC
Cerebral Hemisphere 00C7
Cerebral Meninges 00C1
Cerebral Ventricle 00C6
Cervix 0UCC
Chordae Tendineae 02C9
Choroid
    Left 08CB
    Right 08CA
Cisterna Chyli 07CL

Extirpation *(continued)*
Clavicle
    Left 0PCB
    Right 0PC9
Clitoris 0UCJ
Coccygeal Glomus 0GCB
Coccyx 0QCS
Colon
    Ascending 0DCK
    Descending 0DCM
    Sigmoid 0DCN
    Transverse 0DCL
Conduction Mechanism 02C8
Conjunctiva
    Left 08CTXZZ
    Right 08CSXZZ
Cord
    Bilateral 0VCH
    Left 0VCG
    Right 0VCF
Cornea
    Left 08C9XZZ
    Right 08C8XZZ
Cul-de-sac 0UCF
Diaphragm 0BCT
Disc
    Cervical Vertebral 0RC3
    Cervicothoracic Vertebral 0RC5
    Lumbar Vertebral 0SC2
    Lumbosacral 0SC4
    Thoracic Vertebral 0RC9
    Thoracolumbar Vertebral
        0RCB
Duct
    Common Bile 0FC9
    Cystic 0FC8
    Hepatic
        Common 0FC7
        Left 0FC6
        Right 0FC5
    Lacrimal
        Left 08CY
        Right 08CX
    Pancreatic 0FCD
        Accessory 0FCF
    Parotid
        Left 0CCC
        Right 0CCB
Duodenum 0DC9
Dura Mater 00C2
Ear
    External
        Left 09C1
        Right 09C0
    External Auditory Canal
        Left 09C4
        Right 09C3
    Inner
        Left 09CE
        Right 09CD
    Middle
        Left 09C6
        Right 09C5
Endometrium 0UCB
Epididymis
    Bilateral 0VCL
    Left 0VCK
    Right 0VCJ
Epidural Space, Intracranial 00C3
Epiglottis 0CCR
Esophagogastric Junction 0DC4
Esophagus 0DC5
    Lower 0DC3
    Middle 0DC2
    Upper 0DC1
Eustachian Tube
    Left 09CG
    Right 09CF
Eye
    Left 08C1XZZ
    Right 08C0XZZ

Feeding Device *(continued)*
  Removal of device from
    Esophagus 0DP5
    Intestinal Tract
      Lower 0DPD
      Upper 0DP0
    Stomach 0DP6
  Revision of device in
    Intestinal Tract
      Lower 0DWD
      Upper 0DW0
    Stomach 0DW6

Femoral head
  use Femur, Upper, Left
  use Femur, Upper, Right

Femoral lymph node
  use Lymphatic, Lower Extremity, Left
  use Lymphatic, Lower Extremity, Right

Femoropatellar joint
  use Joint, Knee, Left
  use Joint, Knee, Left, Femoral Surface
  use Joint, Knee, Right
  use Joint, Knee, Right, Femoral Surface

Femorotibial joint
  use Joint, Knee, Left
  use Joint, Knee, Left, Tibial Surface
  use Joint, Knee, Right
  use Joint, Knee, Right, Tibial Surface

FETROJA®
  use Cefiderocol Anti-infective

FGS (fluorescence-guided surgery)
  see Fluorescence Guided Procedure

Fibular artery
  use Artery, Peroneal, Left
  use Artery, Peroneal, Right

Fibularis brevis muscle
  use Muscle, Lower Leg, Left
  use Muscle, Lower Leg, Right

Fibularis longus muscle
  use Muscle, Lower Leg, Left
  use Muscle, Lower Leg, Right

Fifth cranial nerve
  use Nerve, Trigeminal

Filum terminale
  use Spinal Meninges

Fimbriectomy
  see Excision, Female Reproductive System 0UB
  see Resection, Female Reproductive System 0UT

Fine needle aspiration
  Fluid or gas
    see Drainage
  Tissue biopsy
    see Excision
    see Extraction

First cranial nerve
  use Nerve, Olfactory

First intercostal nerve
  use Nerve, Brachial Plexus

Fistulization
  see Bypass
  see Drainage
  see Repair

Fitting
  Arch bars, for fracture reduction
    see Reposition, Mouth and Throat 0CS
  Arch bars, for immobilization
    see Immobilization, Face 2W31
  Artificial limb
    see Device Fitting, Rehabilitation F0D
  Hearing aid
    see Device Fitting, Rehabilitation F0D
  Ocular prosthesis F0DZ8UZ

Fitting *(continued)*
  Prosthesis, limb
    see Device Fitting, Rehabilitation F0D
  Prosthesis, ocular F0DZ8UZ

Fixation, bone
  External, with fracture reduction
    see Reposition
  External, without fracture reduction
    see Insertion
  Internal, with fracture reduction
    see Reposition
  Internal, without fracture reduction
    see Insertion

FLAIR® Endovascular Stent Graft
  use Intraluminal Device

Flexible Composite Mesh
  use Synthetic Substitute

Flexor carpi radialis muscle
  use Muscle, Lower Arm and Wrist, Left
  use Muscle, Lower Arm and Wrist, Right

Flexor carpi ulnaris muscle
  use Muscle, Lower Arm and Wrist, Left
  use Muscle, Lower Arm and Wrist, Right

Flexor digitorum brevis muscle
  use Muscle, Foot, Left
  use Muscle, Foot, Right

Flexor digitorum longus muscle
  use Muscle, Lower Leg, Left
  use Muscle, Lower Leg, Right

Flexor hallucis brevis muscle
  use Muscle, Foot, Left
  use Muscle, Foot, Right

Flexor hallucis longus muscle
  use Muscle, Lower Leg, Left
  use Muscle, Lower Leg, Right

Flexor pollicis longus muscle
  use Muscle, Lower Arm and Wrist, Left
  use Muscle, Lower Arm and Wrist, Right

Flow Diverter embolization device
  use Intraluminal Device, Flow Diverter in 03V

Fluorescence Guided Procedure
  Extremity
    Lower 8E0Y
    Upper 8E0X
  Head and Neck Region 8E09
    Aminolevulinic Acid 8E09
    No Qualifier 8E09
  Trunk Region 8E0W

Fluorescent Pyrazine, Kidney
  XT25XE5

Fluoroscopy
  Abdomen and Pelvis BW11
  Airway, Upper BB1DZZZ
  Ankle
    Left BQ1
    Right BQ1G
  Aorta
    Abdominal B410
      Laser, Intraoperative B410
    Thoracic B310
      Laser, Intraoperative B310
    Thoraco-Abdominal B31P
      Laser, Intraoperative B31P
  Aorta and Bilateral Lower Extremity Arteries B41D
    Laser, Intraoperative B41D
  Arm
    Left BP1FZZZ
    Right BP1EZZZ
  Artery
    Brachiocephalic-Subclavian
      Right B311
      Laser, Intraoperative B311

Fluoroscopy *(continued)*
  Artery *(continued)*
    Bronchial B31L
      Laser, Intraoperative B31L
    Bypass Graft, Other B21F
    Cervico-Cerebral Arch B31Q
      Laser, Intraoperative B31Q
    Common Carotid
      Bilateral B315
        Laser, Intraoperative B315
      Left B314
        Laser, Intraoperative B314
      Right B313
        Laser, Intraoperative B313
    Coronary
      Bypass Graft
        Multiple B213
          Laser, Intraoperative B213
        Single B212
          Laser, Intraoperative B212
      Multiple B211
        Laser, Intraoperative B211
      Single B210
        Laser, Intraoperative B210
    External Carotid
      Bilateral B31C
        Laser, Intraoperative B31C
      Left B31B
        Laser, Intraoperative B31B
      Right B319
        Laser, Intraoperative B319
    Hepatic B412
      Laser, Intraoperative B412
    Inferior Mesenteric B415
      Laser, Intraoperative B415
    Intercostal B31L
      Laser, Intraoperative B31L
    Internal Carotid
      Bilateral B318
        Laser, Intraoperative B318
      Left B317
        Laser, Intraoperative B317
      Right B316
        Laser, Intraoperative B316
    Internal Mammary Bypass Graft
      Left B218
      Right B217
    Intra-Abdominal
      Laser, Intraoperative B41B
      Other B41B
    Intracranial B31R
      Laser, Intraoperative B31R
    Lower
      Laser, Intraoperative B41J
      Other B41J
    Lower Extremity
      Bilateral and Aorta B41D
        Laser, Intraoperative B41D
      Left B41G
        Laser, Intraoperative B41G
      Right B41F
        Laser, Intraoperative B41F
    Lumbar B419
      Laser, Intraoperative B419
    Pelvic B41C
      Laser, Intraoperative B41C

Fluoroscopy *(continued)*
  Artery *(continued)*
    Pulmonary
      Left B31T
        Laser, Intraoperative B31T
      Right B31S
        Laser, Intraoperative B31S
    Pulmonary Trunk B31U
      Laser, Intraoperative B31U
    Renal
      Bilateral B418
        Laser, Intraoperative B418
      Left B417
        Laser, Intraoperative B417
      Right B416
        Laser, Intraoperative B416
    Spinal B31M
      Laser, Intraoperative B31M
    Splenic B413
      Laser, Intraoperative B413
    Subclavian
      Laser, Intraoperative B312
      Left B312
    Superior Mesenteric B414
      Laser, Intraoperative B414
    Upper
      Laser, Intraoperative B31N
      Other B31N
    Upper Extremity
      Bilateral B31K
        Laser, Intraoperative B31K
      Left B31J
        Laser, Intraoperative B31J
      Right B31H
        Laser, Intraoperative B31H
    Vertebral
      Bilateral B31G
        Laser, Intraoperative B31G
      Left B31F
        Laser, Intraoperative B31F
      Right B31D
        Laser, Intraoperative B31D
  Bile Duct BF10
    Pancreatic Duct and Gallbladder BF14
  Bile Duct and Gallbladder BF13
  Biliary Duct BF11
  Bladder BT10
    Kidney and Ureter BT14
    Left BT1F
    Right BT1D
  Bladder and Urethra BT1B
  Bowel, Small BD1
  Calcaneus
    Left BQ1KZZZ
    Right BQ1JZZZ
  Clavicle
    Left BP15ZZZ
    Right BP14ZZZ
  Coccyx BR1F
  Colon BD14
  Corpora Cavernosa BV10
  Dialysis Fistula B51W
  Dialysis Shunt B51W
  Diaphragm BB16ZZZ
  Disc
    Cervical BR11
    Lumbar BR13
    Thoracic BR12

Fragmentation *(continued)*
   Fallopian Tubes, Bilateral 0UF7
   Gallbladder 0FF4
   Gastrointestinal Tract 0WFP
   Genitourinary Tract 0WFR
   Ileum 0DFB
   Intestine
      Large 0DFE
         Left 0DFG
         Right 0DFF
      Small 0DF8
   Jejunum 0DFA
   Kidney Pelvis
      Left 0TF4
      Right 0TF3
   Mediastinum 0WFC
   Oral Cavity and Throat 0WF3
   Pelvic Cavity 0WFJ
   Pericardial Cavity 0WFD
   Pericardium 02FN
   Peritoneal Cavity 0WFG
   Pleural Cavity
      Left 0WFB
      Right 0WF9
   Rectum 0DFP
   Respiratory Tract 0WFQ
   Spinal Canal 00FU
   Stomach 0DF6
   Subarachnoid Space, Intracranial 00F5
   Subdural Space, Intracranial 00F4
   Trachea 0BF1
   Ureter
      Left 0TF7
      Right 0TF6
   Urethra 0TFD
   Uterus 0UF9
   Vein
      Axillary
         Left 05F83Z
         Right 05F73Z
      Basilic
         Left 05FC3Z
         Right 05FB3Z
      Brachial
         Left 05FA3Z
         Right 05F93Z
      Cephalic
         Left 05FF3Z
         Right 05FD3Z
      Common Iliac
         Left 06FD3Z
         Right 06FC3Z
      External Iliac
         Left 06FG3Z
         Right 06FF3Z
      Femoral
         Left 06FN3Z
         Right 06FM3Z
      Hypogastric
         Left 06FJ3Z
         Right 06FH3Z
      Innominate
         Left 05F43Z
         Right 05F33Z
      Lower 06FY3Z
      Pulmonary
         Left 02FT3Z
         Right 02FS3Z
      Saphenous
         Left 06FQ3Z
         Right 06FP3Z
      Subclavian
         Left 05F63Z
         Right 05F53Z
      Upper 05FY3Z
   Vitreous
      Left 08F5
      Right 08F4
Fragmentation, Ultrasonic
   see Fragmentation, Artery

Freestyle (Stentless) Aortic Root Bioprosthesis
   use Zooplastic Tissue in Heart and Great Vessels
Frenectomy
   see Excision, Mouth and Throat 0CB
   see Resection, Mouth and Throat 0CT
Frenoplasty, frenuloplasty
   see Repair, Mouth and Throat 0CQ
   see Replacement, Mouth and Throat 0CR
   see Supplement, Mouth and Throat 0CU
Frenotomy
   see Drainage, Mouth and Throat 0C9
   see Release, Mouth and Throat 0CN
Frenulotomy
   see Drainage, Mouth and Throat 0C9
   see Release, Mouth and Throat 0CN
Frenulum labii inferioris
   use Lip, Lower
Frenulum labii superioris
   use Lip, Upper
Frenulum linguae
   use Tongue
Frenulumectomy
   see Excision, Mouth and Throat 0CB
   see Resection, Mouth and Throat 0CT
Frontal lobe
   use Cerebral Hemisphere
Frontal vein
   use Vein, Face, Left
   use Vein, Face, Right
Fulguration
   see Destruction
Fundoplication, gastroesophageal
   see Restriction, Esophagogastric Junction 0DV4
Fundus uteri
   use Uterus
Fusion
   Acromioclavicular
      Left 0RGH
      Right 0RGG
   Ankle
      Left 0SGG
      Right 0SGF
   Carpal
      Left 0RGR
      Right 0RGQ
   Carpometacarpal
      Left 0RGT
      Right 0RGS
   Cervical Vertebral 0RG1
      2 or more 0RG2
         Interbody Fusion Device
            Nanotextured Surface XRG2092
            Radiolucent Porous XRG20F3
      Interbody Fusion Device, Nanotextured Surface XRG1092
         Radiolucent Porous XRG10F3
   Cervicothoracic Vertebral 0RG4
      Interbody Fusion Device
         Nanotextured Surface XRG4092
         Radiolucent Porous XRG40F3
   Coccygeal 0SG6

Fusion *(continued)*
   Elbow
      Left 0RGM
      Right 0RGL
   Finger Phalangeal
      Left 0RGX
      Right 0RGW
   Hip
      Left 0SGB
      Right 0SG9
   Knee
      Left 0SGD
      Right 0SGC
   Lumbar Vertebral 0SG0
      2 or more 0SG1
         Interbody Fusion Device
            Nanotextured Surface XRGC092
            Radiolucent Porous XRGC0F3
      Interbody Fusion Device
         Nanotextured Surface XRGB092
         Radiolucent Porous XRGB0F3
   Lumbosacral 0SG3
      Interbody Fusion Device
         Nanotextured Surface XRGD092
         Radiolucent Porous XRGD0F3
   Metacarpophalangeal
      Left 0RGV
      Right 0RGU
   Metatarsal-Phalangeal
      Left 0SGN
      Right 0SGM
   Occipital-cervical 0RG0
      Interbody Fusion Device
         Nanotextured Surface XRG0092
         Radiolucent Porous XRG00F3
   Sacrococcygeal 0SG5
   Sacroiliac
      Left 0SG8
      Right 0SG7
   Shoulder
      Left 0RGK
      Right 0RGJ
   Sternoclavicular
      Left 0RGF
      Right 0RGE
   Tarsal
      Left 0SGJ
      Right 0SGH
   Tarsometatarsal
      Left 0SGL
      Right 0SGK
   Temporomandibular
      Left 0RGD
      Right 0RGC
   Thoracic Vertebral 0RG6
      2 to 7 0RG7
         Interbody Fusion Device Nanotextured Surface XRG7092
         Radiolucent Porous XRG70F3
      8 or more 0RG8
         Interbody Fusion Device
            Nanotextured Surface XRG8092
            Radiolucent Porous XRG80F3
      Interbody Fusion Device
         Nanotextured Surface XRG6092
         Radiolucent Porous XRG60F3

Fusion *(continued)*
      Thoracolumbar Vertebral 0RGA
      Interbody Fusion Device
         Nanotextured Surface XRGA092
         Radiolucent Porous XRGA0F3
   Toe Phalangeal
      Left 0SGQ
      Right 0SGP
   Wrist
      Left 0RGP
      Right 0RGN
Fusion screw (compression)(lag) (locking)
   use Internal Fixation Device in Lower Joints
   use Internal Fixation Device in Upper Joints

G

Gait training
   see Motor Treatment, Rehabilitation F07
Galea aponeurotica
   use Subcutaneous Tissue and Fascia, Scalp
GammaTile™
   use Radioactive Element, Cesium-131 Collagen Implant in 00H
Ganglion impar (ganglion of Walther)
   use Nerve, Sacral Sympathetic
Ganglionectomy
   Destruction of lesion
      see Destruction
   Excision of lesion
      see Excision
Gasserian ganglion
   use Nerve, Trigeminal
Gastrectomy
   Partial
      see Excision, Stomach 0DB6
   Total
      see Resection, Stomach 0DT6
   Vertical (sleeve)
      see Excision, Stomach 0DB6
Gastric electrical stimulation (GES) lead
   use Stimulator Lead in Gastrointestinal System
Gastric lymph node
   use Lymphatic, Aortic
Gastric pacemaker lead
   use Stimulator Lead in Gastrointestinal System
Gastric plexus
   use Nerve, Abdominal Sympathetic
Gastrocnemius muscle
   use Muscle, Lower Leg, Left
   use Muscle, Lower Leg, Right
Gastrocolic ligament
   use Omentum
Gastrocolic omentum
   use Omentum
Gastrocolostomy
   see Bypass, Gastrointestinal System 0D1
   see Drainage, Gastrointestinal System 0D9
Gastroduodenal artery
   use Artery, Hepatic
Gastroduodenectomy
   see Excision, Gastrointestinal System 0DB
   see Resection, Gastrointestinal System 0DT
Gastroduodenoscopy 0DJ08ZZ

Gastroenteroplasty
  see Repair, Gastrointestinal System 0DQ
  see Supplement, Gastrointestinal System 0DU
Gastroenterostomy
  see Bypass, Gastrointestinal System 0D1
  see Drainage, Gastrointestinal System 0D9
Gastroesophageal (GE) junction
  use Esophagogastric Junction
Gastrogastrostomy
  see Bypass, Stomach 0D16
  see Drainage, Stomach 0D96
Gastrohepatic omentum
  use Omentum
Gastrojejunostomy
  see Bypass, Stomach 0D16
  see Drainage, Stomach 0D96
Gastrolysis
  see Release, Stomach 0DN6
Gastropexy
  see Repair, Stomach 0DQ6
  see Reposition, Stomach 0DS6
Gastrophrenic ligament
  use Omentum
Gastroplasty
  see Repair, Stomach 0DQ6
  see Supplement, Stomach 0DU6
Gastroplication
  see Restriction, Stomach 0DV6
Gastropylorectomy
  see Excision, Gastrointestinal System 0DB
Gastrorrhaphy
  see Repair, Stomach 0DQ6
Gastroscopy 0DJ68ZZ
Gastrosplenic ligament
  use Omentum
Gastrostomy
  see Bypass, Stomach 0D16
  see Drainage, Stomach 0D96
Gastrotomy
  see Drainage, Stomach 0D96
Gemellus muscle
  use Muscle, Hip, Left
  use Muscle, Hip, Right
Geniculate ganglion
  use Nerve, Facial
Geniculate nucleus
  use Thalamus
Genioglossus muscle
  use Muscle, Tongue, Palate, Pharynx
Genioplasty
  see Alteration, Jaw, Lower 0W05
Genitofemoral nerve
  use Nerve, Lumbar Plexus
GIAPREZA™
  use Synthetic Human Angiotensin II
Gilteritinib Antineoplastic XW0DXV5
Gingivectomy
  see Excision, Mouth and Throat 0CB
Gingivoplasty
  see Repair, Mouth and Throat 0CQ
  see Replacement, Mouth and Throat 0CR
  see Supplement, Mouth and Throat 0CU
Glans penis
  use Prepuce
Glenohumeral joint
  use Joint, Shoulder, Left
  use Joint, Shoulder, Right
Glenohumeral ligament
  use Bursa and Ligament, Shoulder, Left
  use Bursa and Ligament, Shoulder, Right
Glenoid fossa (of scapula)
  use Glenoid Cavity, Left
  use Glenoid Cavity, Right

Glenoid ligament (labrum)
  use Shoulder Joint, Left
  use Shoulder Joint, Right
Globus pallidus
  use Basal Ganglia
Glomectomy
  see Excision, Endocrine System 0GB
  see Resection, Endocrine System 0GT
Glossectomy
  see Excision, Tongue 0CB7
  see Resection, Tongue 0CT7
Glossoepiglottic fold
  use Epiglottis
Glossopexy
  see Repair, Tongue 0CQ7
  see Reposition, Tongue 0CS7
Glossoplasty
  see Repair, Tongue 0CQ7
  see Replacement, Tongue 0CR7
  see Supplement, Tongue 0CU7
Glossorrhaphy
  see Repair, Tongue 0CQ7
Glossotomy
  see Drainage, Tongue 0C97
Glottis
  use Larynx
Gluteal Artery Perforator Flap
  Replacement
    Bilateral 0HRV079
    Left 0HRU079
    Right 0HRT079
  Transfer
    Left 0KXG
    Right 0KXF
Gluteal lymph node
  use Lymphatic, Pelvis
Gluteal vein
  use Vein, Hypogastric, Left
  use Vein, Hypogastric, Right
Gluteus maximus muscle
  use Muscle, Hip, Left
  use Muscle, Hip, Right
Gluteus medius muscle
  use Muscle, Hip, Left
  use Muscle, Hip, Right
Gluteus minimus muscle
  use Muscle, Hip, Left
  use Muscle, Hip, Right
GORE® DUALMESH®
  use Synthetic Substitute
GORE EXCLUDER® AAA Endoprosthesis
  use Intraluminal Device
  use Intraluminal Device, Branched or Fenestrated, One or Two Arteries in 04V
  use Intraluminal Device, Branched or Fenestrated, Three or More Arteries in 04V
GORE EXCLUDER® IBE Endoprosthesis
  use Intraluminal Device, Branched or Fenestrated, One or Two Arteries in 04V
GORE TAG® Thoracic Endoprosthesis
  use Intraluminal Device
Gracilis muscle
  use Muscle, Upper Leg, Left
  use Muscle, Upper Leg, Right
Graft
  see Replacement
  see Supplement
Great auricular nerve
  use Nerve, Cervical Plexus
Great cerebral vein
  use Vein, Intracranial
Great(er) saphenous vein
  use Vein, Saphenous, Left
  use Vein, Saphenous, Right

Greater alar cartilage
  use Nasal Mucosa and Soft Tissue
Greater occipital nerve
  use Nerve, Cervical
Greater Omentum
  use Omentum
Greater splanchnic nerve
  use Nerve, Thoracic Sympathetic
Greater superficial petrosal nerve
  use Nerve, Facial
Greater trochanter
  use Femur, Upper, Left
  use Femur, Upper, Right
Greater tuberosity
  use Humeral Head, Left
  use Humeral Head, Right
Greater vestibular (Bartholin's) gland
  use Gland, Vestibular
Greater wing
  use Bone, Sphenoid
GS-5734 *use* Remdesivir Anti-infective
Guedel airway
  use Intraluminal Device, Airway in Mouth and Throat
Guidance, catheter placement
  EKG
    see Measurement, Physiological Systems 4A0
  Fluoroscopy
    see Fluoroscopy, Veins B51
  Ultrasound
    see Ultrasonography, Veins B54

H

Hallux
  use Toe, 1st, Left
  use Toe, 1st, Right
Hamate bone
  use Carpal, Left
  use Carpal, Right
Hancock Bioprosthesis (aortic) (mitral) valve
  use Zooplastic Tissue in Heart and Great Vessels
Hancock Bioprosthetic Valved Conduit
  use Zooplastic Tissue in Heart and Great Vessels
Harvesting, stem cells
  see Pheresis, Circulatory 6A55
Head of fibula
  use Fibula, Left
  use Fibula, Right
Hearing Aid Assessment F14Z
Hearing Assessment F13Z
Hearing Device
  Bone Conduction
    Left 09HE
    Right 09HD
  Insertion of device in
    Left 0NH6
    Right 0NH5
  Multiple Channel Cochlear Prosthesis
    Left 09HE
    Right 09HD
  Removal of device from, Skull 0NP0
  Revision of device in, Skull 0NW0
  Single Channel Cochlear Prosthesis
    Left 09HE
    Right 09HD
Hearing Treatment F09Z
Heart Assist System
  Implantable
    Insertion of device in, Heart 02HA
    Removal of device from, Heart 02PA
    Revision of device in, Heart 02WA
  Short-term External
    Insertion of device in, Heart 02HA

Heart Assist System *(continued)*
  Short-term External *(continued)*
    Removal of device from, Heart 02PA
    Revision of device in, Heart 02WA
HeartMate II® Left Ventricular Assist Device (LVAD)
  use Implantable Heart Assist System in Heart and Great Vessels
HeartMate 3™ LVAS
  use Implantable Heart Assist System in Heart and Great Vessels
HeartMate XVE® Left Ventricular Assist Device (LVAD)
  use Implantable Heart Assist System in Heart and Great Vessels
HeartMate® implantable heart assist system
  see Insertion of device in, Heart 02H
Helix
  use Ear, External, Bilateral
  use Ear, External, Left
  use Ear, External, Right
Hematopoietic cell transplant (HCT)
  see Transfusion, Circulatory 302
Hemicolectomy
  see Resection, Gastrointestinal System 0DT
Hemicystectomy
  see Excision, Urinary System 0TB
Hemigastrectomy
  see Excision, Gastrointestinal System 0DB
Hemiglossectomy
  see Excision, Mouth and Throat 0C
Hemilaminectomy
  see Excision, Lower Bones 0QB
  see Excision, Upper Bones 0PB
Hemilaminotomy
  see Drainage, Lower Bones 0Q9
  see Drainage, Upper Bones 0P9
  see Excision, Lower Bones 0QB
  see Excision, Upper Bones 0PB
  see Release, Central Nervous System and Cranial Nerves 00
  see Release, Lower Bones 0QN
  see Release, Peripheral Nervous System 01N
  see Release, Upper Bones 0PN
Hemilaryngectomy
  see Excision, Larynx 0CBS
Hemimandibulectomy
  see Excision, Head and Facial Bones 0NB
Hemimaxillectomy
  see Excision, Head and Facial Bones 0NB
Hemipylorectomy
  see Excision, Gastrointestinal System 0DB
Hemispherectomy
  see Excision, Central Nervous System and Cranial Nerves 00
  see Resection, Central Nervous System and Cranial Nerves 00
Hemithyroidectomy
  see Excision, Endocrine System 0C
  see Excision, Endocrine System 0C
Hemodialysis
  see Performance, Urinary 5A1D
Hemolung® Respiratory Assist System (RAS) 5A0920Z
Hemospray® Endoscopic Hemostat
  use Mineral-based Topical Hemostatic Agent
Hepatectomy
  see Excision, Hepatobiliary System and Pancreas 0FB
  see Resection, Hepatobiliary System and Pancreas 0FT

Hepatic artery proper
  use Artery, Hepatic
Hepatic flexure
  use Colon, Transverse
Hepatic lymph node
  use Lymphatic, Aortic
Hepatic plexus
  use Nerve, Abdominal Sympathetic
Hepatic portal vein
  use Vein, Portal
Hepaticoduodenostomy
  see Bypass, Hepatobiliary System
    and Pancreas 0F1
  see Drainage, Hepatobiliary System
    and Pancreas 0F9
Hepaticotomy
  see Drainage, Hepatobiliary System
    and Pancreas 0F9
Hepatocholedochostomy
  see Drainage, Duct, Common Bile
    0F99
Hepatogastric ligament
  use Omentum
Hepatopancreatic ampulla
  use Ampulla of Vater
Hepatopexy
  see Repair, Hepatobiliary System
    and Pancreas 0FQ
  see Reposition, Hepatobiliary
    System and Pancreas 0FS
Hepatorrhaphy
  see Repair, Hepatobiliary System
    and Pancreas 0FQ
Hepatotomy
  see Drainage, Hepatobiliary System
    and Pancreas 0F9
Herculink (RX) Elite Renal Stent
  System
  use Intraluminal Device
Herniorrhaphy
  see Repair, Anatomical Regions,
    General 0WQ
  see Repair, Anatomical Regions,
    Lower Extremities 0YQ
  With synthetic substitute
    see Supplement, Anatomical
      Regions, General 0WU
    see Supplement, Anatomical
      Regions, Lower Extremities
      0YU
Hip (joint) liner
  use Liner in Lower Joints
HIPEC (hyperthermic
  intraperitoneal
  chemotherapy) 3E0M30Y
Holter monitoring 4A12X45
Holter valve ventricular shunt
  use Synthetic Substitute
Human angiotensin II, synthetic
  use Synthetic Human Angiotensin II
Humeroradial joint
  use Joint, Elbow, Left
  use Joint, Elbow, Right
Humeroulnar joint
  use Joint, Elbow, Left
  use Joint, Elbow, Right
Humerus, distal
  use Humeral Shaft, Left
  use Humeral Shaft, Right
Hydrocelectomy
  see Excision, Male Reproductive
    System 0VB
Hydrotherapy
  Assisted exercise in pool
    see Motor Treatment,
      Rehabilitation F07
  Whirlpool
    see Activities of Daily Living
      Treatment, Rehabilitation F08
Hymenectomy
  see Excision, Hymen 0UBK
  see Resection, Hymen 0UTK

Hymenoplasty
  see Repair, Hymen 0UQK
  see Supplement, Hymen 0UUK
Hymenorrhaphy
  see Repair, Hymen 0UQK
Hymenotomy
  see Division, Hymen 0U8K
  see Drainage, Hymen 0U9K
Hyoglossus muscle
  use Muscle, Tongue, Palate, Pharynx
Hyoid artery
  use Artery, Thyroid, Left
  use Artery, Thyroid, Right
Hyperalimentation
  see Introduction of substance in or on
Hyperbaric oxygenation
  Decompression sickness
    treatment
    see Decompression, Circulatory
      6A15
  Wound treatment
    see Assistance, Circulatory
      5A05
Hyperthermia
  Radiation Therapy
    Abdomen DWY38ZZ
    Adrenal Gland DGY28ZZ
    Bile Ducts DFY28ZZ
    Bladder DTY28ZZ
    Bone, Other DPYC8ZZ
    Bone Marrow D7Y08ZZ
    Brain D0Y08ZZ
    Brain Stem D0Y18ZZ
    Breast
      Left DMY08ZZ
      Right DMY18ZZ
    Bronchus DBY18ZZ
    Cervix DUY18ZZ
    Chest DWY28ZZ
    Chest Wall DBY78ZZ
    Colon DDY58ZZ
    Diaphragm DBY88ZZ
    Duodenum DDY28ZZ
    Ear D9Y08ZZ
    Esophagus DDY08ZZ
    Eye D8Y08ZZ
    Femur DPY98ZZ
    Fibula DPYB8ZZ
    Gallbladder DFY18ZZ
    Gland
      Adrenal DGY28ZZ
      Parathyroid DGY48ZZ
      Pituitary DGY08ZZ
      Thyroid DGY58ZZ
    Glands, Salivary D9Y68ZZ
    Head and Neck DWY18ZZ
    Hemibody DWY48ZZ
    Humerus DPY68ZZ
    Hypopharynx D9Y38ZZ
    Ileum DDY48ZZ
    Jejunum DDY38ZZ
    Kidney DTY08ZZ
    Larynx D9YB8ZZ
    Liver DFY08ZZ
    Lung DBY28ZZ
    Lymphatics
      Abdomen D7Y68ZZ
      Axillary D7Y48ZZ
      Inguinal D7Y88ZZ
      Neck D7Y38ZZ
      Pelvis D7Y78ZZ
      Thorax D7Y58ZZ
    Mandible DPY38ZZ
    Maxilla DPY28ZZ
    Mediastinum DBY68ZZ
    Mouth D9Y48ZZ
    Nasopharynx D9YD8ZZ
    Neck and Head DWY18ZZ
    Nerve, Peripheral D0Y78ZZ
    Nose D9Y18ZZ
    Oropharynx D9YF8ZZ
    Ovary DUY08ZZ

Hyperthermia *(continued)*
  Radiation Therapy *(continued)*
    Palate
      Hard D9Y88ZZ
      Soft D9Y98ZZ
    Pancreas DFY38ZZ
    Parathyroid Gland DGY48ZZ
    Pelvic Bones DPY88ZZ
    Pelvic Region DWY68ZZ
    Pineal Body DGY18ZZ
    Pituitary Gland DGY08ZZ
    Pleura DBY58ZZ
    Prostate DVY08ZZ
    Radius DPY78ZZ
    Rectum DDY78ZZ
    Rib DPY58ZZ
    Sinuses D9Y78ZZ
    Skin
      Abdomen DHY88ZZ
      Arm DHY48ZZ
      Back DHY78ZZ
      Buttock DHY98ZZ
      Chest DHY68ZZ
      Face DHY28ZZ
      Leg DHYB8ZZ
      Neck DHY38ZZ
    Skull DPY08ZZ
    Spinal Cord D0Y68ZZ
    Spleen D7Y28ZZ
    Sternum DPY48ZZ
    Stomach DDY18ZZ
    Testis DVY18ZZ
    Thymus D7Y18ZZ
    Thyroid Gland DGY58ZZ
    Tibia DPYB8ZZ
    Tongue D9Y58ZZ
    Trachea DBY08ZZ
    Ulna DPY78ZZ
    Ureter DTY18ZZ
    Urethra DTY38ZZ
    Uterus DUY28ZZ
    Whole Body DWY58ZZ
  Whole Body 6A3Z
Hyperthermic intraperitoneal
  chemotherapy (HIPEC)
  3E0M30Y
Hypnosis GZFZZZZ
Hypogastric artery
  use Artery, Internal Iliac, Left
  use Artery, Internal Iliac, Right
Hypopharynx
  use Pharynx
Hypophysectomy
  see Excision, Gland, Pituitary
    0GB0
  see Resection, Gland, Pituitary
    0GT0
Hypophysis
  use Gland, Pituitary
Hypothalamotomy
  see Destruction, Thalamus 0059
Hypothenar muscle
  use Muscle, Hand, Left
  use Muscle, Hand, Right
Hypothermia, Whole Body 6A4Z
Hysterectomy
  Supracervical
    see Resection, Uterus 0UT9
  Total
    see Resection, Uterus 0UT9
Hysterolysis
  see Release, Uterus 0UN9
Hysteropexy
  see Repair, Uterus 0UQ9
  see Reposition, Uterus 0US9
Hysteroplasty
  see Repair, Uterus 0UQ9
Hysterorrhaphy
  see Repair, Uterus 0UQ9
Hysteroscopy 0UJD8ZZ
Hysterotomy
  see Drainage, Uterus 0U99

Hysterotrachelectomy
  see Resection, Cervix 0UTC
  see Resection, Uterus 0UT9
Hysterotracheloplasty
  see Repair, Uterus 0UQ9
Hysterotrachelorrhaphy
  see Repair, Uterus 0UQ9

I

IABP (Intra-aortic balloon pump)
  see Assistance, Cardiac 5A02
IAEMT (Intraoperative anesthetic
  effect monitoring and
  titration)
  see Monitoring, Central Nervous
    4A10
IASD® (InterAtrial Shunt Device),
  Corvia
  use Synthetic Substitute
Idarucizumab, Dabigatran Reversal
  Agent XW0
IHD (Intermittent hemodialysis)
  5A1D70Z
Ileal artery
  use Artery, Superior Mesenteric
Ileectomy
  see Excision, Ileum 0DBB
  see Resection, Ileum 0DTB
Ileocolic artery
  use Artery, Superior Mesenteric
Ileocolic vein
  use Vein, Colic
Ileopexy
  see Repair, Ileum 0DQB
  see Reposition, Ileum 0DSB
Ileorrhaphy
  see Repair, Ileum 0DQB
Ileoscopy 0DJD8ZZ
Ileostomy
  see Bypass, Ileum 0D1B
  see Drainage, Ileum 0D9B
Ileotomy
  see Drainage, Ileum 0D9B
Ileoureterostomy
  see Bypass, Urinary System 0T1
Iliac crest
  use Bone, Pelvic, Left
  use Bone, Pelvic, Right
Iliac fascia
  use Subcutaneous Tissue and Fascia,
    Upper Leg, Left
  use Subcutaneous Tissue and Fascia,
    Upper Leg, Right
Iliac lymph node
  use Lymphatic, Pelvis
Iliacus muscle
  use Muscle, Hip, Left
  use Muscle, Hip, Right
Iliofemoral ligament
  use Bursa and Ligament, Hip,
    Left
  use Bursa and Ligament, Hip,
    Right
Iliohypogastric nerve
  use Nerve, Lumbar Plexus
Ilioinguinal nerve
  use Nerve, Lumbar Plexus
Iliolumbar artery
  use Artery, Internal Iliac, Left
  use Artery, Internal Iliac, Right
Iliolumbar ligament
  use Bursa and Ligament, Lower
    Spine
Iliotibial tract (band)
  use Subcutaneous Tissue and Fascia,
    Upper Leg, Left
  use Subcutaneous Tissue and Fascia,
    Upper Leg, Right
Ilium
  use Bone, Pelvic, Left
  use Bone, Pelvic, Right

Ilizarov external fixator
- *use* External Fixation Device, Ring in 0PH
- *use* External Fixation Device, Ring in 0PS
- *use* External Fixation Device, Ring in 0QH
- *use* External Fixation Device, Ring in 0QS

Ilizarov-Vecklich device
- *use* External Fixation Device, Limb Lengthening in 0QH
- *use* External Fixation Device, Limb Lengthening in 0PH

Imaging, diagnostic
- *see* Computerized Tomography (CT Scan)
- *see* Fluoroscopy
- *see* Magnetic Resonance Imaging (MRI)
- *see* Plain Radiography
- *see* Ultrasonography

IMFINZI®
- *use* Durvalumab Antineoplastic

IMI/REL
- *use* Imipenem-cilastatin-relebactam Anti-infective

Imipenem-cilastatin-relebactam Anti-infective XW0

Immobilization
- Abdominal Wall 2W33X
- Arm
  - Lower
    - Left 2W3DX
    - Right 2W3CX
  - Upper
    - Left 2W3BX
    - Right 2W3AX
- Back 2W35X
- Chest Wall 2W34X
- Extremity
  - Lower
    - Left 2W3MX
    - Right 2W3LX
  - Upper
    - Left 2W39X
    - Right 2W38X
- Face 2W31X
- Finger
  - Left 2W3KX
  - Right 2W3JX
- Foot
  - Left 2W3TX
  - Right 2W3SX
- Hand
  - Left 2W3FX
  - Right 2W3EX
- Head 2W30X
- Inguinal Region
  - Left 2W37X
  - Right 2W36X
- Leg
  - Lower
    - Left 2W3RX
    - Right 2W3QX
  - Upper
    - Left 2W3PX
    - Right 2W3NX
- Neck 2W32X
- Thumb
  - Left 2W3H
  - Right 2W3GX
- Toe
  - Left 2W3VX
  - Right 2W3UX

Immunization
- *see* Introduction of Serum, Toxoid, and Vaccine

Immunotherapy
- *see* Introduction of Immunotherapeutic Substance

Immunotherapy, antineoplastic
- Interferon
  - *see* Introduction of Low-dose Interleukin-2
- Interleukin-2, high-dose
  - *see* Introduction of High-dose Interleukin-2
- Interleukin-2, low-dose
  - *see* Introduction of Low-dose Interleukin-2
- Monoclonal antibody
  - *see* Introduction of Monoclonal Antibody
- Proleukin, high-dose
  - *see* Introduction of High-dose Interleukin-2
- Proleukin, low-dose
  - *see* Introduction of Low-dose Interleukin-2

Impella® heart pump
- *use* Short-term External Heart Assist System in Heart and Great Vessels

Impeller Pump
- Continuous, Output 5A0221D
- Intermittent, Output 5A0211D

Implantable cardioverter-defibrillator (ICD)
- *use* Defibrillator Generator in 0JH

Implantable drug infusion pump (anti-spasmodic) (chemotherapy)(pain)
- *use* Infusion Device, Pump in Subcutaneous Tissue and Fascia

Implantable glucose monitoring device
- *use* Monitoring Device

Implantable hemodynamic monitor (IHM)
- *use* Monitoring Device, Hemodynamic in 0JH

Implantable hemodynamic monitoring system (IHMS)
- *use* Monitoring Device, Hemodynamic in 0JH

Implantable Miniature Telescope™ (IMT)
- *use* Synthetic Substitute, Intraocular Telescope in 08R

Implantation
- *see* Insertion
- *see* Replacement

Implanted (venous)(access) port
- *use* Vascular Access Device, Totally Implantable in Subcutaneous Tissue and Fascia

IMV (intermittent mandatory ventilation)
- *see* Assistance, Respiratory 5A09

In Vitro Fertilization 8E0ZXY1

Incision, abscess
- *see* Drainage

Incudectomy
- *see* Excision, Ear, Nose, Sinus 09B
- *see* Resection, Ear, Nose, Sinus 09T

Incudopexy
- *see* Reposition, Ear, Nose, Sinus 09S
- *see* Repair, Ear, Nose, Sinus 09Q

Incus
- *use* Auditory Ossicle, Left
- *use* Auditory Ossicle, Right

Induction of labor
- Artificial rupture of membranes
  - *see* Drainage, Pregnancy 109
- Oxytocin
  - *see* Introduction of Hormone

InDura, intrathecal catheter (1P) (spinal)
- *use* Infusion Device

Inferior cardiac nerve
- *use* Nerve, Thoracic Sympathetic

Inferior cerebellar vein
- *use* Vein, Intracranial

Inferior cerebral vein
- *use* Vein, Intracranial

Inferior epigastric artery
- *use* Artery, External Iliac, Left
- *use* Artery, External Iliac, Right

Inferior epigastric lymph node
- *use* Lymphatic, Pelvis

Inferior genicular artery
- *use* Artery, Popliteal, Left
- *use* Artery, Popliteal, Right

Inferior gluteal artery
- *use* Artery, Internal Iliac, Left
- *use* Artery, Internal Iliac, Right

Inferior gluteal nerve
- *use* Nerve, Sacral Plexus

Inferior hypogastric plexus
- *use* Nerve, Abdominal Sympathetic

Inferior labial artery
- *use* Artery, Face

Inferior longitudinal muscle
- *use* Muscle, Tongue, Palate, Pharynx

Inferior mesenteric ganglion
- *use* Nerve, Abdominal Sympathetic

Inferior mesenteric lymph node
- *use* Lymphatic, Mesenteric

Inferior mesenteric plexus
- *use* Nerve, Abdominal Sympathetic

Inferior oblique muscle
- *use* Muscle, Extraocular, Left
- *use* Muscle, Extraocular, Right

Inferior pancreaticoduodenal artery
- *use* Artery, Superior Mesenteric

Inferior phrenic artery
- *use* Aorta, Abdominal

Inferior rectus muscle
- *use* Muscle, Extraocular, Left
- *use* Muscle, Extraocular, Right

Inferior suprarenal artery
- *use* Artery, Renal, Left
- *use* Artery, Renal, Right

Inferior tarsal plate
- *use* Eyelid, Lower, Left
- *use* Eyelid, Lower, Right

Inferior thyroid vein
- *use* Vein, Innominate, Left
- *use* Vein, Innominate, Right

Inferior tibiofibular joint
- *use* Joint, Ankle, Left
- *use* Joint, Ankle, Right

Inferior turbinate
- *use* Turbinate, Nasal

Inferior ulnar collateral artery
- *use* Artery, Brachial, Left
- *use* Artery, Brachial, Right

Inferior vesical artery
- *use* Artery, Internal Iliac, Left
- *use* Artery, Internal Iliac, Right

Infraauricular lymph node
- *use* Lymphatic, Head

Infraclavicular (deltopectoral) lymph node
- *use* Lymphatic, Upper Extremity, Left
- *use* Lymphatic, Upper Extremity, Right

Infrahyoid muscle
- *use* Muscle, Neck, Left
- *use* Muscle, Neck, Right

Infraparotid lymph node
- *use* Lymphatic, Head

Infraspinatus fascia
- *use* Subcutaneous Tissue and Fascia, Upper Arm, Left
- *use* Subcutaneous Tissue and Fascia, Upper Arm, Right

Infraspinatus muscle
- *use* Muscle, Shoulder, Left
- *use* Muscle, Shoulder, Right

Infundibulopelvic ligament
- *use* Uterine Supporting Structure

Infusion
- *see* Introduction of substance in or on

Infusion Device, Pump
- Insertion of device in
  - Abdomen 0JH8
  - Back 0JH7
  - Chest 0JH6
  - Lower Arm
    - Left 0JHH
    - Right 0JHG
  - Lower Leg
    - Left 0JHP
    - Right 0JHN
  - Trunk 0JHT
  - Upper Arm
    - Left 0JHF
    - Right 0JHD
  - Upper Leg
    - Left 0JHM
    - Right 0JHL
- Removal of device from
  - Lower Extremity 0JPW
  - Trunk 0JPT
  - Upper Extremity 0JPV
- Revision of device in
  - Lower Extremity 0JWW
  - Trunk 0JWT
  - Upper Extremity 0JWV

Infusion, glucarpidase
- Central vein 3E043GQ
- Peripheral vein 3E033GQ

Inguinal canal
- *use* Inguinal Region, Bilateral
- *use* Inguinal Region, Left
- *use* Inguinal Region, Right

Inguinal triangle
- *use* Inguinal Region, Bilateral
- *use* Inguinal Region, Left
- *use* Inguinal Region, Right

Injection
- *see* Introduction of substance in or on

Injection, Concentrated Bone Marrow Aspirate (CBMA), intramuscular XK02303

Injection reservoir, port
- *use* Vascular Access Device, Totally Implantable in Subcutaneous Tissue and Fascia

Injection reservoir, pump
- *use* Infusion Device, Pump in Subcutaneous Tissue and Fascia

Insemination, artificial 3E0P7LZ

Insertion
- Antimicrobial envelope
  - *see* Introduction of Anti-infective
- Aqueous drainage shunt
  - *see* Bypass, Eye 081
  - *see* Drainage, Eye 089
- Products of Conception 10H0
- Spinal Stabilization Device
  - *see* Insertion of device in, Upper Joints 0RH
  - *see* Insertion of device in, Lower Joints 0SH

Insertion of device in
- Abdominal Wall 0WHF
- Acetabulum
  - Left 0QH5
  - Right 0QH4
- Anal Sphincter 0DHR
- Ankle Region
  - Left 0YHL
  - Right 0YHK
- Anus 0DHQ
- Aorta
  - Abdominal 04H0
  - Thoracic
    - Ascending/Arch 02HX
    - Descending 02HW

Arm
  Lower
    Left 0XHF
    Right 0XHD
  Upper
    Left 0XH9
    Right 0XH8
Artery
  Anterior Tibial
    Left 04HQ
    Right 04HP
  Axillary
    Left 03H6
    Right 03H5
  Brachial
    Left 03H8
    Right 03H7
  Celiac 04H1
  Colic
    Left 04H7
    Middle 04H8
    Right 04H6
  Common Carotid
    Left 03HJ
    Right 03HH
  Common Iliac
    Left 04HD
    Right 04HC
  Coronary
    Four or More Arteries
      02H3
    One Artery 02H0
    Three Arteries 02H2
    Two Arteries 02H1
  External Carotid
    Left 03HN
    Right 03HM
  External Iliac
    Left 04HJ
    Right 04HH
  Face 03HR
  Femoral
    Left 04HL
    Right 04HK
  Foot
    Left 04HW
    Right 04HV
  Gastric 04H2
  Hand
    Left 03HF
    Right 03HD
  Hepatic 04H3
  Inferior Mesenteric 04HB
  Innominate 03H2
  Internal Carotid
    Left 03HL
    Right 03HK
  Internal Iliac
    Left 04HF
    Right 04HE
  Internal Mammary
    Left 03H1
    Right 03H0
  Intracranial 03HG
  Lower 04HY
  Peroneal
    Left 04HU
    Right 04HT
  Popliteal
    Left 04HN
    Right 04HM
  Posterior Tibial
    Left 04HS
    Right 04HR
  Pulmonary
    Left 02HR
    Right 02HQ
  Pulmonary Trunk 02HP
  Radial
    Left 03HC
    Right 03HB

Artery *(continued)*
  Renal
    Left 04HA
    Right 04H9
  Splenic 04H4
  Subclavian
    Left 03H4
    Right 03H3
  Superior Mesenteric 04H5
  Temporal
    Left 03HT
    Right 03HS
  Thyroid
    Left 03HV
    Right 03HU
  Ulnar
    Left 03HA
    Right 03H9
  Upper 03HY
  Vertebral
    Left 03HQ
    Right 03HP
Atrium
  Left 02H7
  Right 02H6
Axilla
  Left 0XH5
  Right 0XH4
Back
  Lower 0WHL
  Upper 0WHK
Bladder 0THB
Bladder Neck 0THC
Bone
  Ethmoid
    Left 0NHG
    Right 0NHF
  Facial 0NHW
  Frontal 0NH1
  Hyoid 0NHX
  Lacrimal
    Left 0NHJ
    Right 0NHH
  Lower 0QHY
  Nasal 0NHB
  Occipital 0NH7
  Palatine
    Left 0NHL
    Right 0NHK
  Parietal
    Left 0NH4
    Right 0NH3
  Pelvic
    Left 0QH3
    Right 0QH2
  Sphenoid 0NHC
  Temporal
    Left 0NH6
    Right 0NH5
  Upper 0PHY
  Zygomatic
    Left 0NHN
    Right 0NHM
Bone Marrow 07HT
Brain 00H0
Breast
  Bilateral 0HHV
  Left 0HHU
  Right 0HHT
Bronchus
  Lingula 0BH9
  Lower Lobe
    Left 0BHB
    Right 0BH6
  Main
    Left 0BH7
    Right 0BH3
  Middle Lobe, Right 0BH5
  Upper Lobe
    Left 0BH8
    Right 0BH4

Bursa and Ligament
  Lower 0MHY
  Upper 0MHX
Buttock
  Left 0YH1
  Right 0YH0
Carpal
  Left 0PHN
  Right 0PHM
Cavity, Cranial 0WH1
Cerebral Ventricle 00H6
Cervix 0UHC
Chest Wall 0WH8
Cisterna Chyli 07HL
Clavicle
  Left 0PHB
  Right 0PH9
Coccyx 0QHS
Cul-de-sac 0UHF
Diaphragm 0BHT
Disc
  Cervical Vertebral 0RH3
  Cervicothoracic Vertebral
    0RH5
  Lumbar Vertebral 0SH2
  Lumbosacral 0SH4
  Thoracic Vertebral 0RH9
  Thoracolumbar Vertebral 0RHB
Duct
  Hepatobiliary 0FHB
  Pancreatic 0FHD
Duodenum 0DH9
Ear
  Inner
    Left 09HE
    Right 09HD
  Left 09HJ
  Right 09HH
Elbow Region
  Left 0XHC
  Right 0XHB
Epididymis and Spermatic Cord
  0VHM
Esophagus 0DH5
Extremity
  Lower
    Left 0YHB
    Right 0YH9
  Upper
    Left 0XH7
    Right 0XH6
Eye
  Left 08H1
  Right 08H0
Face 0WH2
Fallopian Tube 0UH8
Femoral Region
  Left 0YH8
  Right 0YH7
Femoral Shaft
  Left 0QH9
  Right 0QH8
Femur
  Lower
    Left 0QHC
    Right 0QHB
  Upper
    Left 0QH7
    Right 0QH6
Fibula
  Left 0QHK
  Right 0QHJ
Foot
  Left 0YHN
  Right 0YHM
Gallbladder 0FH4
Gastrointestinal Tract 0WHP
Genitourinary Tract 0WHR
Gland
  Endocrine 0GHS
  Salivary 0CHA

Glenoid Cavity
  Left 0PH8
  Right 0PH7
Hand
  Left 0XHK
  Right 0XHJ
Head 0WH0
Heart 02HA
Humeral Head
  Left 0PHD
  Right 0PHC
Humeral Shaft
  Left 0PHG
  Right 0PHF
Ileum 0DHB
Inguinal Region
  Left 0YH6
  Right 0YH5
Intestinal Tract
  Lower 0DHD
  Upper 0DH0
Intestine
  Large 0DHE
  Small 0DH8
Jaw
  Lower 0WH5
  Upper 0WH4
Jejunum 0DHA
Joint
  Acromioclavicular
    Left 0RHH
    Right 0RHG
  Ankle
    Left 0SHG
    Right 0SHF
  Carpal
    Left 0RHR
    Right 0RHQ
  Carpometacarpal
    Left 0RHT
    Right 0RHS
  Cervical Vertebral 0RH1
  Cervicothoracic Vertebral 0RH4
  Coccygeal 0SH6
  Elbow
    Left 0RHM
    Right 0RHL
  Finger Phalangeal
    Left 0RHX
    Right 0RHW
  Hip
    Left 0SHB
    Right 0SH9
  Knee
    Left 0SHD
    Right 0SHC
  Lumbar Vertebral 0SH0
  Lumbosacral 0SH3
  Metacarpophalangeal
    Left 0RHV
    Right 0RHU
  Metatarsal-Phalangeal
    Left 0SHN
    Right 0SHM
  Occipital-cervical 0RH0
  Sacrococcygeal 0SH5
  Sacroiliac
    Left 0SH8
    Right 0SH7
  Shoulder
    Left 0RHK
    Right 0RHJ
  Sternoclavicular
    Left 0RHF
    Right 0RHE
  Tarsal
    Left 0SHJ
    Right 0SHH
  Tarsometatarsal
    Left 0SHL
    Right 0SHK

Internal carotid artery, intracranial portion
  use Intracranial Artery
Internal carotid plexus
  use Nerve, Head and Neck Sympathetic
Internal iliac vein
  use Vein, Hypogastric, Left
  use Vein, Hypogastric, Right
Internal maxillary artery
  use Artery, External Carotid, Left
  use Artery, External Carotid, Right
Internal naris
  use Nasal Mucosa and Soft Tissue
Internal oblique muscle
  use Muscle, Abdomen, Left
  use Muscle, Abdomen, Right
Internal pudendal artery
  use Artery, Internal Iliac, Left
  use Artery, Internal Iliac, Right
Internal pudendal vein
  use Vein, Hypogastric, Left
  use Vein, Hypogastric, Right
Internal thoracic artery
  use Artery, Internal Mammary, Left
  use Artery, Internal Mammary, Right
  use Artery, Subclavian, Left
  use Artery, Subclavian, Right
Internal urethral sphincter
  use Urethra
Interphalangeal (IP) joint
  use Joint, Finger Phalangeal, Left
  use Joint, Finger Phalangeal, Right
  use Joint, Toe Phalangeal, Left
  use Joint, Toe Phalangeal, Right
Interphalangeal ligament
  use Bursa and Ligament, Foot, Left
  use Bursa and Ligament, Foot, Right
  use Bursa and Ligament, Hand, Left
  use Bursa and Ligament, Hand, Right
Interrogation, cardiac rhythm related device
  Interrogation only
    see Measurement, Cardiac 4B02
  With cardiac function testing
    see Measurement, Cardiac 4A02
Interruption
  see Occlusion
Interspinalis muscle
  use Muscle, Trunk, Left
  use Muscle, Trunk, Right
Interspinous ligament, cervical
  use Head and Neck Bursa and Ligament
Interspinous ligament, lumbar
  use Lower Spine Bursa and Ligament
Interspinous ligament, thoracic
  use Upper Spine Bursa and Ligament
Interspinous process spinal stabilization device
  use Spinal Stabilization Device, Interspinous Process in 0RH
  use Spinal Stabilization Device, Interspinous Process in 0SH
InterStim® Therapy lead
  use Neurostimulator Lead in Peripheral Nervous System
InterStim® Therapy neurostimulator
  use Stimulator Generator, Single Array in 0JH
Intertransversarius muscle
  use Muscle, Trunk, Left
  use Muscle, Trunk, Right
Intertransverse ligament, cervical
  use Head and Neck Bursa and Ligament
Intertransverse ligament, lumbar
  use Lower Spine Bursa and Ligament

Intertransverse ligament, thoracic
  use Upper Spine Bursa and Ligament
Interventricular foramen (Monro)
  use Cerebral Ventricle
Interventricular septum
  use Septum, Ventricular
Intestinal lymphatic trunk
  use Cisterna Chyli
Intraluminal Device
  Airway
    Esophagus 0DH5
    Mouth and Throat 0CHY
    Nasopharynx 09HN
  Bioactive
    Occlusion
      Common Carotid
        Left 03LJ
        Right 03LH
      External Carotid
        Left 03LN
        Right 03LM
      Internal Carotid
        Left 03LL
        Right 03LK
      Intracranial 03LG
      Vertebral
        Left 03LQ
        Right 03LP
    Restriction
      Common Carotid
        Left 03VJ
        Right 03VH
      External Carotid
        Left 03VN
        Right 03VM
      Internal Carotid
        Left 03VL
        Right 03VK
      Intracranial 03VG
      Vertebral
        Left 03VQ
        Right 03VP
  Endobronchial Valve
    Lingula 0BH9
    Lower Lobe
      Left 0BHB
      Right 0BH6
    Main
      Left 0BH7
      Right 0BH3
    Middle Lobe, Right 0BH5
    Upper Lobe
      Left 0BH8
      Right 0BH4
  Endotracheal Airway
    Change device in, Trachea 0B21XEZ
    Insertion of device in, Trachea 0BH1
  Pessary
    Change device in, Vagina and Cul-de-sac 0U2HXGZ
    Insertion of device in Cul-de-sac 0UHF
    Vagina 0UHG
Intramedullary (IM) rod (nail)
  use Internal Fixation Device, Intramedullary in Lower Bones
  use Internal Fixation Device, Intramedullary in Upper Bones
Intramedullary skeletal kinetic distractor (ISKD)
  use Internal Fixation Device, Intramedullary in Lower Bones
  use Internal Fixation Device, Intramedullary in Upper Bones
Intraocular Telescope
  Left 08RK30Z
  Right 08RJ30Z

Intra.OX 8E02XDZ
Intraoperative Knee Replacement Sensor XR2
Intraoperative Radiation Therapy (IORT)
  Anus DDY8CZZ
  Bile Ducts DFY2CZZ
  Bladder DTY2CZZ
  Brain D0Y0CZZ
  Brain Stem D0Y1CZZ
  Cervix DUY1CZZ
  Colon DDY5CZZ
  Duodenum DDY2CZZ
  Gallbladder DFY1CZZ
  Ileum DDY4CZZ
  Jejunum DDY3CZZ
  Kidney DTY0CZZ
  Larynx D9YBCZZ
  Liver DFY0CZZ
  Mouth D9Y4CZZ
  Nasopharynx D9YDCZZ
  Nerve, Peripheral D0Y7CZZ
  Ovary DUY0CZZ
  Pancreas DFY3CZZ
  Pharynx D9YCCZZ
  Prostate DVY0CZZ
  Rectum DDY7CZZ
  Spinal Cord D0Y6CZZ
  Stomach DDY1CZZ
  Ureter DTY1CZZ
  Urethra DTY3CZZ
  Uterus DUY2CZZ
Intrauterine device (IUD)
  use Contraceptive Device in Female Reproductive System
Intravascular fluorescence angiography (IFA)
  see Monitoring, Physiological Systems 4A1
Intravascular Lithotripsy (IVL)
  see Fragmentation
Intravascular ultrasound assisted thrombolysis
  see Fragmentation, Artery
Introduction of substance in or on
  Artery
    Central 3E06
      Analgesics 3E06
      Anesthetic, Intracirculatory 3E06
      Anti-infective 3E06
      Anti-inflammatory 3E06
      Antiarrhythmic 3E06
      Antineoplastic 3E06
      Destructive Agent 3E06
      Diagnostic Substance, Other 3E06
      Electrolytic Substance 3E06
      Hormone 3E06
      Hypnotics 3E06
      Immunotherapeutic 3E06
      Nutritional Substance 3E06
      Platelet Inhibitor 3E06
      Radioactive Substance 3E06
      Sedatives 3E06
      Serum 3E06
      Thrombolytic 3E06
      Toxoid 3E06
      Vaccine 3E06
      Vasopressor 3E06
      Water Balance Substance 3E06
    Coronary 3E07
      Diagnostic Substance, Other 3E07

Introduction of substance in or on *(continued)*
  Artery *(continued)*
    Coronary *(continued)*
      Platelet Inhibitor 3E07
      Thrombolytic 3E07
    Peripheral 3E05
      Analgesics 3E05
      Anesthetic, Intracirculatory 3E05
      Anti-infective 3E052
      Anti-inflammatory 3E05
      Antiarrhythmic 3E05
      Antineoplastic 3E05
      Destructive Agent 3E05
      Diagnostic Substance, Other 3E05
      Electrolytic Substance 3E05
      Hormone 3E05
      Hypnotics 3E05
      Immunotherapeutic 3E05
      Nutritional Substance 3E05
      Platelet Inhibitor 3E05
      Radioactive Substance 3E05
      Sedatives 3E05
      Serum 3E05
      Thrombolytic 3E05
      Toxoid 3E05
      Vaccine 3E05
      Vasopressor 3E05
      Water Balance Substance 3E05
  Biliary Tract 3E0J
    Analgesics 3E0J
    Anesthetic, Agent 3E0J
    Anti-infective 3E0J
    Anti-inflammatory 3E0J
    Antineoplastic 3E0J
    Destructive Agent 3E0J
    Diagnostic Substance, Other 3E0J
    Electrolytic Substance 3E0J
    Gas 3E0J
    Hypnotics 3E0J
    Islet Cells, Pancreatic 3E0J
    Nutritional Substance 3E0J
    Radioactive Substance 3E0J
    Sedatives 3E0J
    Water Balance Substance 3E0J
  Bone 3E0V
    Analgesics 3E0V3NZ
    Anesthetic, Agent 3E0V3BZ
    Anti-infective 3E0V32
    Anti-inflammatory 3E0V33Z
    Antineoplastic 3E0V30
    Destructive Agent 3E0V3TZ
    Diagnostic Substance, Other 3E0V3KZ
    Electrolytic Substance 3E0V37Z
    Hypnotics 3E0V3NZ
    Nutritional Substance 3E0V36Z
    Radioactive Substance 3E0V3HZ
    Sedatives 3E0V3NZ
    Water Balance Substance 3E0V37Z
  Bone Marrow 3E0A3GC
    Antineoplastic 3E0A30
  Brain 3E0Q
    Analgesics 3E0Q
    Anesthetic, Agent 3E0Q
    Anti-infective 3E0Q
    Anti-inflammatory 3E0Q
    Antineoplastic 3E0Q
    Destructive Agent 3E0Q
    Diagnostic Substance, Other 3E0Q
    Electrolytic Substance 3E0Q

Brain *(continued)*
Gas 3E0Q
Hypnotics 3E0Q
Nutritional Substance
3E0Q
Radioactive Substance
3E0Q
Sedatives 3E0Q
Stem Cells
Embryonic 3E0Q
Somatic 3E0Q
Water Balance Substance
3E0Q
Cranial Cavity 3E0Q
Analgesics 3E0Q
Anesthetic Agent 3E0Q
Anti-infective 3E0Q
Anti-inflammatory 3E0Q
Antineoplastic 3E0Q
Destructive Agent 3E0Q
Diagnostic Substance, Other
3E0Q
Electrolytic Substance 3E0Q
Gas 3E0Q
Hypnotics 3E0Q
Nutritional Substance
3E0Q
Radioactive Substance 3E0Q
Sedatives 3E0Q
Stem Cells
Embryonic 3E0Q
Somatic 3E0Q
Water Balance Substance
3E0Q
Ear 3E0B
Analgesics 3E0B
Anesthetic Agentl 3E0B
Anti-infective 3E0B
Anti-inflammatory 3E0B
Antineoplastic 3E0B
Destructive Agent 3E0B
Diagnostic Substance, Other
3E0B
Hypnotics 3E0B
Radioactive Substance 3E0B
Sedatives 3E0B
Epidural Space 3E0S3GC
Analgesics 3E0S3NZ
Anesthetic Agent 3E0S3BZ
Anti-infective 3E0S32
Anti-inflammatory 3E0S33Z
Antineoplastic 3E0S30
Destructive Agent 3E0S3TZ
Diagnostic Substance, Other
3E0S3KZ
Electrolytic Substance 3E0S37Z
Gas 3E0S
Hypnotics 3E0S3NZ
Nutritional Substance 3E0S36Z
Radioactive Substance
3E0S3HZ
Sedatives 3E0S3NZ
Water Balance Substance
3E0S37Z
Eye 3E0C
Analgesics 3E0C
Anesthetic Agent 3E0C
Anti-infective 3E0C
Anti-inflammatory 3E0C
Antineoplastic 3E0C
Destructive Agent 3E0C
Diagnostic Substance, Other
3E0C
Gas 3E0C
Hypnotics 3E0C
Pigment 3E0C
Radioactive Substance
3E0C
Sedatives 3E0C

Gastrointestinal Tract
Lower 3E0H
Analgesics 3E0H
Anesthetic Agent 3E0H
Anti-infective 3E0H
Anti-inflammatory 3E0H
Antineoplastic 3E0H
Destructive Agent 3E0H
Diagnostic Substance, Other
3E0H
Electrolytic Substance 3E0H
Gas 3E0H
Hypnotics 3E0H
Nutritional Substance 3E0H
Radioactive Substance
3E0H
Sedatives 3E0H
Water Balance Substance
3E0H
Upper 3E0G
Analgesics 3E0G
Anesthetic Agent 3E0G
Anti-infective 3E0G
Anti-inflammatory 3E0G
Antineoplastic 3E0G
Destructive Agent 3E0G
Diagnostic Substance, Other
3E0G
Electrolytic Substance
3E0G
Gas 3E0G
Hypnotics 3E0G
Nutritional Substance
3E0G
Radioactive Substance
3E0G
Sedatives 3E0G
Water Balance Substance
3E0G
Genitourinary Tract 3E0K
Analgesics 3E0K
Anesthetic Agent 3E0K
Anti-infective 3E0K
Anti-inflammatory 3E0K
Antineoplastic 3E0K
Destructive Agent 3E0K
Diagnostic Substance, Other
3E0K
Electrolytic Substance 3E0K
Gas 3E0K
Hypnotics 3E0K
Nutritional Substance 3E0K
Radioactive Substance 3E0K
Sedatives 3E0K
Water Balance Substance 3E0K
Heart 3E08
Diagnostic Substance, Other
3E08
Platelet Inhibitor 3E08
Thrombolytic 3E08
Joint 3E0U
Analgesics 3E0U3NZ
Anesthetic Agent 3E0U3BZ
Anti-infective 3E0U
Anti-inflammatory 3E0U33Z
Antineoplastic 3E0U30
Destructive Agent 3E0U3TZ
Diagnostic Substance, Other
3E0U3KZ
Electrolytic Substance
3E0U37Z
Gas 3E0U3SF
Hypnotics 3E0U3NZ
Nutritional Substance 3E0U36Z
Radioactive Substance
3E0U3HZ
Sedatives 3E0U3NZ
Water Balance Substance
3E0U37Z

Lymphatic 3E0W3GC
Analgesics 3E0W3NZ
Anesthetic Agent 3E0W3BZ
Anti-infective 3E0W32
Anti-inflammatory 3E0W33Z
Antineoplastic 3E0W30
Destructive Agent 3E0W3TZ
Diagnostic Substance, Other
3E0W3KZ
Electrolytic Substance
3E0W37Z
Hypnotics 3E0W3NZ
Nutritional Substance 3E0W36Z
Radioactive Substance
3E0W3HZ
Sedatives 3E0W3NZ
Water Balance Substance
3E0W37Z
Mouth 3E0D
Analgesics 3E0D
Anesthetic Agent 3E0D
Anti-infective 3E0D
Anti-inflammatory 3E0D
Antiarrhythmic 3E0D
Antineoplastic 3E0D
Destructive Agent 3E0D
Diagnostic Substance, Other
3E0D
Electrolytic Substance 3E0D
Hypnotics 3E0D
Nutritional Substance 3E0D
Radioactive Substance 3E0D
Sedatives 3E0D
Serum 3E0D
Toxoid 3E0D
Vaccine 3E0D
Water Balance Substance
3E0D
Mucous Membrane 3E00XGC
Analgesics 3E00XNZ
Anesthetic Agent 3E00XBZ
Anti-infective 3E00X2
Anti-inflammatory 3E00X3Z
Antineoplastic 3E00X0
Destructive Agent 3E00XTZ
Diagnostic Substance, Other
3E00XKZ
Hypnotics 3E00XNZ
Pigment 3E00XMZ
Sedatives 3E00XNZ
Serum 3E00X4Z
Toxoid 3E00X4Z
Vaccine 3E00X4Z
Muscle 3E023GC
Analgesics 3E023NZ
Anesthetic Agent 3E023BZ
Anti-infective 3E0232
Anti-inflammatory 3E0233Z
Antineoplastic 3E0230
Destructive Agent 3E023TZ
Diagnostic Substance, Other
3E023KZ
Electrolytic Substance 3E0237Z
Hypnotics 3E023NZ
Nutritional Substance 3E0236Z
Radioactive Substance
3E023HZ
Sedatives 3E023NZ
Serum 3E0234Z
Toxoid 3E0234Z
Vaccine 3E0234Z
Water Balance Substance
3E0237Z
Nerve
Cranial 3E0X3GC
Anesthetic Agent 3E0X3BZ
Anti-inflammatory
3E0X33Z
Destructive Agent 3E0X3TZ

Nerve *(continued)*
Peripheral 3E0T3GC
Anesthetic Agent 3E0T3BZ
Anti-inflammatory 3E0T33Z
Destructive Agent 3E0T3TZ
Plexus 3E0T3GC Agent
3E0T3BZ
Anti-inflammatory 3E0T33Z
Destructive Agent 3E0T3TZ
Nose 3E09
Analgesics 3E09
Anesthetic Agent 3E09
Anti-infective 3E09
Anti-inflammatory 3E09
Antineoplastic 3E09
Destructive Agent 3E09
Diagnostic Substance, Other
3E09
Hypnotics 3E09
Radioactive Substance 3E09
Sedatives 3E09
Serum 3E09
Toxoid 3E09
Vaccine 3E09
Pancreatic Tract 3E0J
Analgesics 3E0J
Anesthetic Agent 3E0J
Anti-infective 3E0J
Anti-inflammatory 3E0J
Antineoplastic 3E0J0
Destructive Agent 3E0J
Diagnostic Substance, Other
3E0J
Electrolytic Substance 3E0J
Gas 3E0J
Hypnotics 3E0J
Islet Cells, Pancreatic 3E0JU
Nutritional Substance 3E0J
Radioactive Substance 3E0J
Sedatives 3E0J
Water Balance Substance 3E0J
Pericardial Cavity 3E0Y
Analgesics 3E0Y3NZ
Anesthetic Agent 3E0Y3BZ
Anti-infective 3E0Y32
Anti-inflammatory 3E0Y33Z
Antineoplastic 3E0Y
Destructive Agent 3E0Y3TZ
Diagnostic Substance, Other
3E0Y3KZ
Electrolytic Substance 3E0Y37Z
Gas 3E0Y
Hypnotics 3E0Y3NZ
Nutritional Substance 3E0Y36Z
Radioactive Substance
3E0Y3HZ
Sedatives 3E0Y3NZ
Water Balance Substance
3E0Y37Z
Peritoneal Cavity 3E0M
Adhesion Barrier 3E0M
Analgesics 3E0M3NZ
Anesthetic Agent 3E0M3BZ
Anti-infective 3E0M32
Anti-inflammatory 3E0M33Z
Antineoplastic 3E0M
Destructive Agent 3E0M3TZ
Diagnostic Substance, Other
3E0M3KZ
Electrolytic Substance
3E0M37Z
Gas 3E0M
Hypnotics 3E0M3NZ
Nutritional Substance 3E0M36Z
Radioactive Substance
3E0M3HZ
Sedatives 3E0M3NZ
Water Balance Substance
3E0M37Z

Isolation 8E0ZXY6
Isotope Administration, Whole Body
DWY5G
Itrel (3)(4) neurostimulator
use Stimulator Generator, Single
Array in 0JH

J

Jakafi®
use Ruxolitinib
Jejunal artery
use Artery, Superior Mesenteric
Jejunectomy
see Excision, Jejunum 0DBA
see Resection, Jejunum 0DTA
Jejunocolostomy
see Bypass, Gastrointestinal System
0D1
see Drainage, Gastrointestinal
System 0D9
Jejunopexy
see Repair, Jejunum 0DQA
see Reposition, Jejunum 0DSA
Jejunostomy
see Bypass, Jejunum 0D1A
see Drainage, Jejunum 0D9A
Jejunotomy
see Drainage, Jejunum 0D9A
Joint fixation plate
use Internal Fixation Device in
Lower Joints
use Internal Fixation Device in
Upper Joints
Joint liner (insert)
use Liner in Lower Joints
Joint spacer (antibiotic)
use Spacer in Lower Joints
use Spacer in Upper Joints
Jugular body
use Glomus Jugulare
Jugular lymph node
use Lymphatic, Neck, Left
use Lymphatic, Neck, Right

K

Kappa
use Pacemaker, Dual Chamber in 0JH
Kcentra
use 4-Factor Prothrombin Complex
Concentrate
Keratectomy, kerectomy
see Excision, Eye 08B
see Resection, Eye 08T
Keratocentesis
see Drainage, Eye 089
Keratoplasty
see Repair, Eye 08Q
see Replacement, Eye 08R
see Supplement, Eye 08U
Keratotomy
see Drainage, Eye 089
see Repair, Eye 08Q
KEVZARA® *use* Sarilumab
**Keystone Heart TriGuard 3™ CEPD
(cerebral embolic protection
device)** X2A6325
Kirschner wire (K-wire)
use Internal Fixation Device in
Head and Facial Bones
use Internal Fixation Device in
Lower Bones
use Internal Fixation Device in
Lower Joints
use Internal Fixation Device in
Upper Bones
use Internal Fixation Device in
Upper Joints
Knee (implant) insert
use Liner in Lower Joints

KUB x-ray
see Plain Radiography, Kidney,
Ureter and Bladder BT04
Kuntscher nail
use Internal Fixation Device,
Intramedullary in Lower Bones
use Internal Fixation Device,
Intramedullary in Upper Bones
KYMRIAH
use Engineered Autologous
Chimeric Antigen Receptor
T-cell Immunotherapy

L

Labia majora
use Vulva
Labia minora
use Vulva
Labial gland
use Lip, Lower
use Lip, Upper
Labiectomy
see Excision, Female Reproductive
System 0UB
see Resection, Female Reproductive
System 0UT
see Release, Central Nervous
System 00N
see Release, Peripheral Nervous
System 01N
Lacrimal canaliculus
use Duct, Lacrimal, Left
use Duct, Lacrimal, Right
Lacrimal punctum
use Duct, Lacrimal, Left
use Duct, Lacrimal, Right
Lacrimal sac
use Duct, Lacrimal, Left
use Duct, Lacrimal, Right
**LAGB (laparoscopic adjustable
gastric banding)**
Initial procedure 0DV64CZ
Surgical correction
see Revision of device in,
Stomach 0DW6
Laminectomy
see Excision, Lower Bones 0QB
see Excision, Upper Bones 0PB
see Release, Central Nervous
System and Cranial Nerves 00N
see Release, Peripheral Nervous
System 01N
Laminotomy
see Drainage, Lower Bones 0Q9
see Drainage, Upper Bones 0P9
see Excision, Lower Bones 0QB
see Excision, Upper Bones 0PB
see Release, Central Nervous
System and Cranial Nerves 00N
see Release, Lower Bones 0QN
see Release, Peripheral Nervous
System 01N
see Release, Upper Bones 0PN
**LAP-BAND® adjustable gastric
banding system**
use Extraluminal Device
**Laparoscopic-assisted transanal
pull-through**
see Excision, Gastrointestinal
System 0DB
see Resection, Gastrointestinal
System 0DT
Laparoscopy
see Inspection
Laparotomy
Drainage
see Drainage, Peritoneal Cavity 0W9G
Exploratory
see Inspection, Peritoneal Cavity
0WJG

Laryngectomy
see Excision, Larynx 0CBS
see Resection, Larynx 0CTS
Laryngocentesis
see Drainage, Larynx 0C9S
Laryngogram
see Fluoroscopy, Larynx B91J
Laryngopexy
see Repair, Larynx 0CQS
Laryngopharynx
use Pharynx
Laryngoplasty
see Repair, Larynx 0CQS
see Replacement, Larynx 0CRS
see Supplement, Larynx 0CUS
Laryngorrhaphy
see Repair, Larynx 0CQS
Laryngoscopy 0CJS8ZZ
Laryngotomy
see Drainage, Larynx 0C9S
Laser Interstitial Thermal Therapy
Adrenal Gland DGY2KZZ
Anus DDY8KZZ
Bile Ducts DFY2KZZ
Brain D0Y0KZZ
Brain Stem D0Y1KZZ
Breast
Left DMY0KZZ
Right DMY1KZZ
Bronchus DBY1KZZ
Chest Wall DBY7KZZ
Colon DDY5KZZ
Diaphragm DBY8KZZ
Duodenum DDY2KZZ
Esophagus DDY0KZZ
Gallbladder DFY1KZZ
Gland
Adrenal DGY2KZZ
Parathyroid DGY4KZZ
Pituitary DGY0KZZ
Thyroid DGY5KZZ
Ileum DDY4KZZ
Jejunum DDY3KZZ
Liver DFY0KZZ
Lung DBY2KZZ
Mediastinum DBY6KZZ
Nerve, Peripheral D0Y7KZZ
Pancreas DFY3KZZ
Parathyroid Gland DGY4KZZ
Pineal Body DGY1KZZ
Pituitary Gland DGY0KZZ
Pleura DBY5KZZ
Prostate DVY0KZZ
Rectum DDY7KZZ
Spinal Cord D0Y6KZZ
Stomach DDY1KZZ
Thyroid Gland DGY5KZZ
Trachea DBY0KZZ
Lateral (brachial) lymph node
use Lymphatic, Axillary, Left
use Lymphatic, Axillary, Right
Lateral canthus
use Eyelid, Upper, Left
use Eyelid, Upper, Right
Lateral collateral ligament (LCL)
use Bursa and Ligament, Knee,
Left
use Bursa and Ligament, Knee,
Right
Lateral condyle of femur
use Femur, Lower, Left
use Femur, Lower, Right
Lateral condyle of tibia
use Tibia, Left
use Tibia, Right
Lateral cuneiform bone
use Tarsal, Left
use Tarsal, Right
Lateral epicondyle of femur
use Femur, Lower, Left
use Femur, Lower, Right

Lateral epicondyle of humerus
use Humeral Shaft, Left
use Humeral Shaft, Right
Lateral femoral cutaneous nerve
use Nerve, Lumbar Plexus
Lateral malleolus
use Fibula, Left
use Fibula, Right
Lateral meniscus
use Joint, Knee, Left
use Joint, Knee, Right
Lateral nasal cartilage
use Nasal Mucosa and Soft Tissue
Lateral plantar artery
use Artery, Foot, Left
use Artery, Foot, Right
Lateral plantar nerve
use Nerve, Tibial
Lateral rectus muscle
use Muscle, Extraocular, Left
use Muscle, Extraocular, Right
Lateral sacral artery
use Artery, Internal Iliac, Left
use Artery, Internal Iliac, Right
Lateral sacral vein
use Vein, Hypogastric, Left
use Vein, Hypogastric, Right
Lateral sural cutaneous nerve
use Nerve, Peroneal
Lateral tarsal artery
use Artery, Foot, Left
use Artery, Foot, Right
Lateral temporomandibular ligament
use Bursa and Ligament, Head and
Neck
Lateral thoracic artery
use Artery, Axillary, Left
use Artery, Axillary, Right
Latissimus dorsi muscle
use Muscle, Trunk, Left
use Muscle, Trunk, Right
Latissimus Dorsi Myocutaneous Flap
Replacement
Bilateral 0HRV075
Left 0HRU075
Right 0HRT075
Transfer
Left 0KXG
Right 0KXF
Lavage
see Irrigation
Bronchial alveolar, diagnostic
see Drainage, Respiratory
System 0B9
Least splanchnic nerve
use Nerve, Thoracic Sympathetic
Lefamulin Anti-infective XW0
Left ascending lumbar vein
use Vein, Hemiazygos
Left atrioventricular valve
use Valve, Mitral
Left auricular appendix
use Atrium, Left
Left colic vein
use Vein, Colic
Left coronary sulcus
use Heart, Left
Left gastric artery
use Artery, Gastric
Left gastroepiploic artery
use Artery, Splenic
Left gastroepiploic vein
use Vein, Splenic
Left inferior phrenic vein
use Vein, Renal, Left
Left inferior pulmonary vein
use Vein, Pulmonary, Left
Left jugular trunk
use Lymphatic, Thoracic Duct
Left lateral ventricle
use Cerebral Ventricle

Left ovarian vein
  use Vein, Renal, Left
Left second lumbar vein
  use Vein, Renal, Left
Left subclavian trunk
  use Lymphatic, Thoracic Duct
Left subcostal vein
  use Vein, Hemiazygos
Left superior pulmonary vein
  use Vein, Pulmonary, Left
Left suprarenal vein
  use Vein, Renal, Left
Left testicular vein
  use Vein, Renal, Left
Lengthening
  Bone, with device
    see Insertion of Limb
      Lengthening Device
  Muscle, by incision
    see Division, Muscles 0K8
  Tendon, by incision
    see Division, Tendons 0L8
Leptomeninges, intracranial
  use Cerebral Meninges
Leptomeninges, spinal
  use Spinal Meninges
Lesser alar cartilage
  use Nasal Mucosa and Soft Tissue
Lesser occipital nerve
  use Nerve, Cervical Plexus
Lesser Omentum
  use Omentum
Lesser saphenous vein
  use Saphenous Vein, Left
  use Saphenous Vein, Right
Lesser splanchnic nerve
  use Nerve, Thoracic
    Sympathetic
Lesser trochanter
  use Femur, Upper, Left
  use Femur, Upper, Right
Lesser tuberosity
  use Humeral Head, Left
  use Humeral Head, Right
Lesser wing
  use Bone, Sphenoid
Leukopheresis, therapeutic
  see Pheresis, Circulatory 6A55
Levator anguli oris muscle
  use Muscle, Facial
Levator ani muscle
  use Perineum Muscle
Levator labii superioris alaeque nasi muscle
  use Muscle, Facial
Levator labii superioris muscle
  use Muscle, Facial
Levator palpebrae superioris muscle
  use Eyelid, Upper, Left
  use Eyelid, Upper, Right
Levator scapulae muscle
  use Muscle, Neck, Left
  use Muscle, Neck, Right
Levator veli palatini muscle
  use Muscle, Tongue, Palate, Pharynx
Levatores costarum muscle
  use Muscle, Thorax, Left
  use Muscle, Thorax, Right
LifeStent® (Flexstar)(XL) Vascular Stent System
  use Intraluminal Device
Ligament of head of fibula
  use Bursa and Ligament, Knee, Left
  use Bursa and Ligament, Knee, Right
Ligament of the lateral malleolus
  use Bursa and Ligament, Ankle, Left
  use Bursa and Ligament, Ankle, Right
Ligamentum flavum, cervical
  use Head and Neck Bursa and Ligament

Ligamentum flavum, lumbar
  use Lower Spine Bursa and Ligament
Ligamentum flavum, thoracic
  use Upper Spine Bursa and Ligament
Ligation
  see Occlusion
Ligation, hemorrhoid
  see Occlusion, Lower Veins, Hemorrhoidal Plexus
Light Therapy GZJZZZZ
Liner
  Removal of device from
    Hip
      Left 0SPB09Z
      Right 0SP909Z
    Knee
      Left 0SPD09Z
      Right 0SPC09Z
  Revision of device in
    Hip
      Left 0SWB09Z
      Right 0SW909Z
    Knee
      Left 0SWD09Z
      Right 0SWC09Z
  Supplement
    Hip
      Left 0SUB09Z
        Acetabular Surface 0SUE09Z
        Femoral Surface 0SUS09Z
      Right 0SU909Z
        Acetabular Surface 0SUA09Z
        Femoral Surface 0SUR09Z
    Knee
      Left 0SUD09
        Femoral Surface 0SUU09Z
        Tibial Surface 0SUW09Z
      Right 0SUC09
        Femoral Surface 0SUT09Z
        Tibial Surface 0SUV09Z
Lingual artery
  use Artery, External Carotid, Left
  use Artery, External Carotid, Right
Lingual tonsil
  use Pharynx
Lingulectomy, lung
  see Excision, Lung Lingula 0BBH
  see Resection, Lung Lingula 0BTH
Lisocabtagene Maraleucel
  use Lisocabtagene Maraleucel Immunotherapy
Lisocabtagene Maraleucel Immunotherapy XW2
Lithoplasty
  see Fragmentation
Lithotripsy
  see Fragmentation
  With removal of fragments
    see Extirpation
LITT (laser interstitial thermal therapy)
  see Laser Interstitial Thermal Therapy
LIVIAN™ CRT-D
  use Cardiac Resynchronization Defibrillator Pulse Generator in 0JH
Lobectomy
  see Excision, Central Nervous System and Cranial Nerves 00B
  see Excision, Endocrine System 0GB
  see Excision, Hepatobiliary System and Pancreas 0FB
  see Excision, Respiratory System 0BB
  see Resection, Endocrine System 0GT

Lobectomy *(continued)*
  see Resection, Hepatobiliary System and Pancreas 0FT
  see Resection, Respiratory System 0BT
Lobotomy
  see Division, Brain 0080
Localization
  see Map
  see Imaging
Locus ceruleus
  use Pons
Long thoracic nerve
  use Nerve, Brachial Plexus
Loop ileostomy
  see Bypass, Ileum 0D1B
Loop recorder, implantable
  use Monitoring Device
Lower GI series
  see Fluoroscopy, Colon BD14
Lower Respiratory Fluid Nucleic Acid-base Microbial Detection XXEBXQ6
Lumbar artery
  use Aorta, Abdominal
Lumbar facet joint
  use Joint, Lumbar Vertebral
Lumbar ganglion
  use Nerve, Lumbar Sympathetic
Lumbar lymph node
  use Lymphatic, Aortic
Lumbar lymphatic trunk
  use Cisterna Chyli
Lumbar splanchnic nerve
  use Nerve, Lumbar Sympathetic
Lumbosacral facet joint
  use Joint, Lumbosacral
Lumbosacral trunk
  use Nerve, Lumbar
Lumpectomy
  see Excision
Lunate bone
  use Carpal, Left
  use Carpal, Right
Lunotriquetral ligament
  use Bursa and Ligament, Hand, Left
  use Bursa and Ligament, Hand, Right
Lymphadenectomy
  see Excision, Lymphatic and Hemic Systems 07B
  see Resection, Lymphatic and Hemic Systems 07T
Lymphadenotomy
  see Drainage, Lymphatic and Hemic Systems 079
Lymphangiectomy
  see Excision, Lymphatic and Hemic Systems 07B
  see Resection, Lymphatic and Hemic Systems 07T
Lymphangiogram
  see Plain Radiography, Lymphatic System B70
Lymphangioplasty
  see Repair, Lymphatic and Hemic Systems 07Q
  see Supplement, Lymphatic and Hemic Systems 07U
Lymphangiorrhaphy
  see Repair, Lymphatic and Hemic Systems 07Q
Lymphangiotomy
  see Drainage, Lymphatic and Hemic Systems 079
Lysis
  see Release

M

Macula
  use Retina, Left
  use Retina, Right

MAGEC® Spinal Bracing and Distraction System
  use Magnetically Controlled Growth Rod(s) in New Technology
Magnet extraction, ocular foreign body
  see Extirpation, Eye 08C
Magnetic-guided radiofrequency endovascular fistula
  Radial Artery, Left 031C
  Radial Artery, Right 031B
  Ulnar Artery, Left 031A
  Ulnar Artery, Right 0319
Magnetic Resonance Imaging (MRI)
  Abdomen BW30
  Ankle
    Left BQ3H
    Right BQ3G
  Aorta
    Abdominal B430
    Thoracic B330
  Arm
    Left BP3F
    Right BP3E
  Artery
    Celiac B431
    Cervico-Cerebral Arch B33Q
    Common Carotid, Bilateral B335
    Coronary
      Bypass Graft, Multiple B233
      Multiple B231
    Internal Carotid, Bilateral B338
    Intracranial B33R
    Lower Extremity
      Bilateral B43H
      Left B43G
      Right B43F
    Pelvic B43C
    Renal, Bilateral B438
    Spinal B33M
    Superior Mesenteric B434
    Upper Extremity
      Bilateral B33K
      Left B33J
      Right B33H
    Vertebral, Bilateral B33G
  Bladder BT30
  Brachial Plexus BW3P
  Brain B030
  Breast
    Bilateral BH32
    Left BH31
    Right BH30
  Calcaneus
    Left BQ3K
    Right BQ3J
  Chest BW33Y
  Coccyx BR3F
  Connective Tissue
    Lower Extremity BL31
    Upper Extremity BL30
  Corpora Cavernosa BV30
  Disc
    Cervical BR31
    Lumbar BR33
    Thoracic BR32
  Ear B930
  Elbow
    Left BP3H
    Right BP3G
  Eye
    Bilateral B837
    Left B836
    Right B835
  Femur
    Left BQ34
    Right BQ33
  Fetal Abdomen BY33
  Fetal Extremity BY35

Magnetic Resonance Imaging (MRI) *(continued)*

Fetal Head BY30
Fetal Heart BY31
Fetal Spine BY34
Fetal Thorax BY32
Fetus, Whole BY36
Foot
   Left BQ3M
   Right BQ3L
Forearm
   Left BP3K
   Right BP3J
Gland
   Adrenal, Bilateral BG32
   Parathyroid BG33
   Parotid, Bilateral B936
   Salivary, Bilateral B93D
   Submandibular, Bilateral
      B939
   Thyroid BG34
Head BW38
Heart, Right and Left B236
Hip
   Left BQ31
   Right BQ30
Intracranial Sinus B532
Joint
   Finger
      Left BP3D
      Right BP3C
   Hand
      Left BP3D
      Right BP3C
   Temporomandibular, Bilateral
      BN39
Kidney
   Bilateral BT33
   Left BT32
   Right BT31
   Transplant BT39
Knee
   Left BQ38
   Right BQ37
Larynx B93J
Leg
   Left BQ3F
   Right BQ3D
Liver BF35
Liver and Spleen BF36
Lung Apices BB3G
Nasopharynx B93F
Neck BW3F
Nerve
   Acoustic B03C
   Brachial Plexus BW3P
Oropharynx B93F
Ovary
   Bilateral BU35
   Left BU34
   Right BU33
Ovary and Uterus BU3C
Pancreas BF37
Patella
   Left BQ3W
   Right BQ3V
Pelvic Region BW3G
Pelvis BR3C
Pituitary Gland B039
Plexus, Brachial BW3P
Prostate BV33
Retroperitoneum BW3H
Sacrum BR3F
Scrotum BV34
Sella Turcica B039
Shoulder
   Left BP39
   Right BP38
Sinus
   Intracranial B532
   Paranasal B932
Spinal Cord B03B

Magnetic Resonance Imaging (MRI) *(continued)*

Spine
   Cervical BR30
   Lumbar BR39
   Thoracic BR37
Spleen and Liver BF36
Subcutaneous Tissue
   Abdomen BH3H
   Extremity
      Lower BH3J
      Upper BH3F
   Head BH3D
   Neck BH3D
   Pelvis BH3H
   Thorax BH3G
Tendon
   Lower Extremity BL33
   Upper Extremity BL32
Testicle
   Bilateral BV37
   Left BV36
   Right BV35
Toe
   Left BQ3Q
   Right BQ3P
Uterus BU36
   Pregnant BU3B
Uterus and Ovary BU3C
Vagina BU39
Vein
   Cerebellar B531
   Cerebral B531
   Jugular, Bilateral B535
   Lower Extremity
      Bilateral B53D
      Left B53C
      Right B53B
   Other B53V
   Pelvic (Iliac) Bilateral B53H
   Portal B53T
   Pulmonary, Bilateral B53S
   Renal, Bilateral B53L
   Spanchnic B53T
   Upper Extremity
      Bilateral B53P
      Left B53N
      Right B53M
Vena Cava
   Inferior B539
   Superior B538
Wrist
   Left BP3M
   Right BP3L

Magnetically Controlled Growth Rod(s)

Cervical XNS3
Lumbar XNS0
Thoracic XNS4

Malleotomy

see Drainage, Ear, Nose, Sinus 099

Malleus

use Auditory Ossicle, Left
use Auditory Ossicle, Right

Mammaplasty, mammoplasty

see Alteration, Skin and Breast
    0H0
see Repair, Skin and Breast 0HQ
see Replacement, Skin and Breast
    0HR
see Supplement, Skin and Breast 0HU

Mammary duct

use Breast, Bilateral
use Breast, Left
use Breast, Right

Mammary gland

use Breast, Bilateral
use Breast, Left
use Breast, Right

Mammectomy

see Excision, Skin and Breast 0HB
see Resection, Skin and Breast 0HT

Mammillary body

use Hypothalamus

Mammography

see Plain Radiography, Skin,
    Subcutaneous Tissue and Breast
    BH0

Mammotomy

see Drainage, Skin and Breast 0H9

Mandibular nerve

use Nerve, Trigeminal

Mandibular notch

use Mandible, Left
use Mandible, Right

Mandibulectomy

see Excision, Head and Facial
    Bones 0NB
see Resection, Head and Facial
    Bones 0NT

Manipulation

Adhesions
   see Release
Chiropractic
   see Chiropractic Manipulation

Manual removal, retained placenta

see Extraction, Products of
    Conception, Retained 10D1

Manubrium

use Sternum

Map

Basal Ganglia 00K8
Brain 00K0
Cerebellum 00KC
Cerebral Hemisphere 00K7
Conduction Mechanism 02K8
Hypothalamus 00KA
Medulla Oblongata 00KD
Pons 00KB
Thalamus 00K9

Mapping

Doppler ultrasound
   see Ultrasonography
Electrocardiogram only
   see Measurement, Cardiac 4A02

Mark IV Breathing Pacemaker System

use Stimulator Generator in
    Subcutaneous Tissue and Fascia

Marsupialization

see Drainage
see Excision

Massage, cardiac

External 5A12012
Open 02QA0ZZ

Masseter muscle

use Muscle, Head

Masseteric fascia

use Subcutaneous Tissue and Fascia,
    Face

Mastectomy

see Excision, Skin and Breast 0HB
see Resection, Skin and Breast 0HT

Mastoid (postauricular) lymph node

use Lymphatic, Neck, Left
use Lymphatic, Neck, Right

Mastoid air cells

use Sinus, Mastoid, Left
use Sinus, Mastoid, Right

Mastoid process

use Bone, Temporal, Left
use Bone, Temporal, Right

Mastoidectomy

see Excision, Ear, Nose, Sinus 09B
see Resection, Ear, Nose, Sinus
    09T

Mastoidotomy

see Drainage, Ear, Nose, Sinus 099

Mastopexy

see Repair, Skin and Breast 0HQ
see Reposition, Skin and Breast
    0HS

Mastorrhaphy

see Repair, Skin and Breast 0HQ

Mastotomy

see Drainage, Skin and Breast
    0H9

Maxillary artery

use Artery, External Carotid, Left
use Artery, External Carotid, Right

Maxillary nerve

use Nerve, Trigeminal

Maximo II DR (VR)

use Defibrillator Generator in 0JH

Maximo II DR CRT-D

use Cardiac Resynchronization
    Defibrillator Pulse Generator
    in 0JH

Measurement

Arterial
   Flow
      Coronary 4A03
      Intracranial 4A03X5D
      Peripheral 4A03
      Pulmonary 4A03
   Pressure
      Coronary 4A03
      Peripheral 4A03
      Pulmonary 4A03
      Thoracic, Other 4A03
   Pulse
      Coronary 4A03
      Peripheral 4A03
      Pulmonary 4A03
   Saturation, Peripheral 4A03
   Sound, Peripheral 4A03
Biliary
   Flow 4A0C
   Pressure 4A0C
Cardiac
   Action Currents 4A02
   Defibrillator 4B02XTZ
   Electrical Activity 4A02
      Guidance 4A02X4A
      No Qualifier 4A02X4Z
   Output 4A02
   Pacemaker 4B02XSZ
   Rate 4A02
   Rhythm 4A02
   Sampling and Pressure
      Bilateral 4A02
      Left Heart 4A02
      Right Heart 4A02
   Sound 4A02
   Total Activity, Stress 4A02XM4
Central Nervous
   Conductivity 4A00
   Electrical Activity 4A00
   Pressure 4A000BZ
      Intracranial 4A00
   Saturation, Intracranial 4A00
   Stimulator 4B00XVZ
   Temperature, Intracranial 4A00
Circulatory, Volume 4A05XLZ
Gastrointestinal
   Motility 4A0B
   Pressure 4A0B
   Secretion 4A0B
Lower Respiratory Fluid Nucleic
   Acid-base Microbial Detection
   XXEBXQ6
Lymphatic
   Flow 4A06
   Pressure 4A06
Metabolism 4A0Z
Musculoskeletal
   Contractility 4A0F
   Pressure 4A0F3BE
   Stimulator 4B0FXVZ
Olfactory, Acuity 4A08X0Z
Peripheral Nervous
   Conductivity
      Motor 4A01
      Sensory 4A01
   Electrical Activity 4A01
   Stimulator 4B01XVZ

Measurement (*continued*)
Positive Blood Culture Fluorescence
Hybridization for Organism
Identification, Concentration and
Susceptibility XXE5XN6
Products of Conception
Cardiac
Electrical Activity 4A0H
Rate 4A0H
Rhythm 4A0H
Sound 4A0HH
Nervous
Conductivity 4A0J
Electrical Activity 4A0J
Pressure 4A0J
Respiratory
Capacity 4A09
Flow 4A09
Pacemaker 4B09X
Rate 4A09
Resistance 4A09
Total Activity 4A09
Volume 4A09
Sleep 4A0ZXQZ
Temperature 4A0Z
Urinary
Contractility 4A0D
Flow 4A0D
Pressure 4A0D
Resistance 4A0D
Volume 4A0D
Venous
Flow
Central 4A04
Peripheral 4A04
Portal 4A04
Pulmonary 4A04
Pressure
Central 4A04
Peripheral 4A04
Portal 4A04
Pulmonary 4A04
Pulse
Central 4A04
Peripheral 4A04
Portal 4A04
Pulmonary 4A04
Saturation, Peripheral 4A04
Visual
Acuity 4A07X0Z
Mobility 4A07X7Z
Pressure 4A07XBZ
Whole Blood Nucleic Acid-
base Microbial Detection
XXE5XM5
Meatoplasty, urethra
see Repair, Urethra 0TQD
Meatotomy
see Drainage, Urinary System 0T9
Mechanical ventilation
see Performance, Respiratory 5A19
Medial canthus
use Eyelid, Lower, Left
use Eyelid, Lower, Right
Medial collateral ligament (MCL)
use Bursa and Ligament, Knee, Left
use Bursa and Ligament, Knee, Right
Medial condyle of femur
use Femur, Lower, Left
use Femur, Lower, Right
Medial condyle of tibia
use Tibia, Left
use Tibia, Right
Medial cuneiform bone
use Tarsal, Left
use Tarsal, Right
Medial epicondyle of femur
use Femur, Lower, Left
use Femur, Lower, Right
Medial epicondyle of humerus
use Humeral Shaft, Left
use Humeral Shaft, Right

Medial malleolus
use Tibia, Left
use Tibia, Right
Medial meniscus
use Joint, Knee, Left
use Joint, Knee, Right
Medial plantar artery
use Artery, Foot, Left
use Artery, Foot, Right
Medial plantar nerve
use Nerve, Tibial
Medial popliteal nerve
use Nerve, Tibial
Medial rectus muscle
use Muscle, Extraocular, Left
use Muscle, Extraocular, Right
Medial sural cutaneous nerve
use Nerve, Tibial
Median antebrachial vein
use Vein, Basilic, Left
use Vein, Basilic, Right
Median cubital vein
use Vein, Basilic, Left
use Vein, Basilic, Right
Median sacral artery
use Aorta, Abdominal
Mediastinal cavity
use Mediastinum
Mediastinal lymph node
use Lymphatic, Thorax
Mediastinal space
use Mediastinum
Mediastinoscopy 0WJC4ZZ
Medication Management GZ3ZZZZ
for substance abuse
Antabuse HZ83ZZZ
Bupropion HZ87ZZZ
Clonidine HZ86ZZZ
Levo-alpha-acetyl-methadol
(LAAM) HZ82ZZZ
Methadone Maintenance
HZ81ZZZ
Naloxone HZ85ZZZ
Naltrexone HZ84ZZZ
Nicotine Replacement
HZ80ZZZ
Other Replacement Medication
HZ89ZZZ
Psychiatric Medication
HZ88ZZZ
Meditation 8E0ZXY5
**Medtronic Endurant® II AAA stent
graft system**
use Intraluminal Device
Meissner's (submucous) plexus
use Nerve, Abdominal Sympathetic
**Melody® transcatheter pulmonary
valve**
use Zooplastic Tissue in Heart and
Great Vessels
Membranous urethra
use Urethra
Meningeorrhaphy
see Repair, Cerebral Meninges
00Q1
see Repair, Spinal Meninges 00QT
Meniscectomy, knee
see Excision, Joint, Knee, Left
0SBD
see Excision, Joint, Knee, Right
0SBC
Mental foramen
use Mandible, Left
use Mandible, Right
Mentalis muscle
use Muscle, Facial
Mentoplasty
see Alteration, Jaw, Lower 0W05
**Meropenem-vaborbactam Anti-
infective** XW0
Mesenterectomy
see Excision, Mesentery 0DBV

**Mesenteriorrhaphy,
mesenterorrhaphy**
see Repair, Mesentery 0DQV
Mesenteriplication
see Repair, Mesentery 0DQV
Mesoappendix
use Mesentery
Mesocolon
use Mesentery
Metacarpal ligament
use Bursa and Ligament, Hand, Left
use Bursa and Ligament, Hand,
Right
Metacarpophalangeal ligament
use Bursa and Ligament, Hand, Left
use Bursa and Ligament, Hand,
Right
Metal on metal bearing surface
use Synthetic Substitute, Metal in
0SR
Metatarsal ligament
use Bursa and Ligament, Foot, Left
use Bursa and Ligament, Foot, Right
Metatarsectomy
see Excision, Lower Bones 0QB
see Resection, Lower Bones 0QT
Metatarsophalangeal (MTP) joint
use Joint, Metatarsal-Phalangeal,
Left
use Joint, Metatarsal-Phalangeal,
Right
Metatarsophalangeal ligament
use Bursa and Ligament, Foot, Left
use Bursa and Ligament, Foot, Right
Metathalamus
use Thalamus
Micro-Driver stent (RX) (OTW)
use Intraluminal Device
MicroMed HeartAssist
use Implantable Heart Assist
System in Heart and Great
Vessels
Micrus CERECYTE microcoil
use Intraluminal Device, Bioactive
in Upper Arteries
Midcarpal joint
use Joint, Carpal, Left
use Joint, Carpal, Right
Middle cardiac nerve
use Nerve, Thoracic Sympathetic
Middle cerebral artery
use Artery, Intracranial
Middle cerebral vein
use Vein, Intracranial
Middle colic vein
use Vein, Colic
Middle genicular artery
use Artery, Popliteal, Left
use Artery, Popliteal, Right
Middle hemorrhoidal vein
use Vein, Hypogastric, Left
use Vein, Hypogastric, Right
Middle rectal artery
use Artery, Internal Iliac, Left
use Artery, Internal Iliac, Right
Middle suprarenal artery
use Aorta, Abdominal
Middle temporal artery
use Artery, Temporal, Left
use Artery, Temporal, Right
Middle turbinate
use Turbinate, Nasal
**Mineral-based Topical Hemostatic
Agent** XW0
**MIRODERM™ Biologic Wound
Matrix**
use Skin Substitute, Porcine Liver
Derived in New Technology
MitraClip valve repair system
use Synthetic Substitute
Mitral annulus
use Valve, Mitral

**Mitroflow® Aortic Pericardial Heart
Valve**
use Zooplastic Tissue in Heart and
Great Vessels
Mobilization, adhesions
see Release
Molar gland
use Buccal Mucosa
MolecuLight i:X® wound imaging
see Other Imaging, Anatomical
Regions BW5
Monitoring
Arterial
Flow
Coronary 4A13
Peripheral 4A13
Pulmonary 4A13
Pressure
Coronary 4A13
Peripheral 4A13
Pulmonary 4A13
Pulse
Coronary 4A13
Peripheral 4A13
Pulmonary 4A13
Saturation, Peripheral 4A13
Sound, Peripheral 4A13
Cardiac
Electrical Activity 4A12
Ambulatory 4A12X45
No Qualifier 4A12X4Z
Output 4A12
Rate 4A12
Rhythm 4A12
Sound 4A12
Total Activity, Stress
4A12XM4
Vascular Perfusion, Indocyanine
Green Dye 4A12XSH
Central Nervous
Conductivity 4A10
Electrical Activity
Intraoperative 4A10
No Qualifier 4A10
Pressure 4A100BZ
Intracranial 4A10
Saturation, Intracranial 4A10
Temperature, Intracranial
4A10
Gastrointestinal
Motility 4A1B
Pressure 4A1B
Secretion 4A1B
Vascular Perfusion, Indocyanin
Green Dye 4A1BXSH
Intraoperative Knee Replacement
Sensor XR2
Kidney, Fluorescent Pyrazine
XT25XE5
Lymphatic
Flow
Indocyanine Green Dye
4A16
No Qualifier A416
Pressure 4A16
Peripheral Nervous
Conductivity
Motor 4A11
Sensory 4A11
Electrical Activity
Intraoperative 4A11
No Qualifier 4A11
Products of Conception
Cardiac
Electrical Activity 4A1H
Rate 4A1H
Rhythm 4A1H
Sound 4A1H
Nervous
Conductivity 4A1J
Electrical Activity 4A1J
Pressure 4A1J

Monitoring (continued)
- Respiratory
  - Capacity 4A19
  - Flow 4A19
  - Rate 4A19
  - Resistance 4A19
  - Volume 4A19
- Skin and Breast
  - Vascular Perfusion,
    - Indocyanine Green Dye 4A1GXSH
- Sleep 4A1ZXQZ
- Temperature 4A1Z
- Urinary
  - Contractility 4A1D
  - Flow 4A1D
  - Pressure 4A1D
  - Resistance 4A1D
  - Volume 4A1D
- Venous
  - Flow
    - Central 4A14
    - Peripheral 4A14
    - Portal 4A14
    - Pulmonary 4A14
  - Pressure
    - Central 4A14
    - Peripheral 4A14
    - Portal 4A14
    - Pulmonary 4A14
  - Pulse
    - Central 4A14
    - Peripheral 4A14
    - Portal 4A14
    - Pulmonary 4A14
  - Saturation
    - Central 4A14
    - Portal 4A14
    - Pulmonary 4A14

Monitoring Device, Hemodynamic
- Abdomen 0JH8
- Chest 0JH6

Mosaic Bioprosthesis (aortic) (mitral) valve
- *use* Zooplastic Tissue in Heart and Great Vessels

Motor Function Assessment F01
Motor Treatment F07
MR Angiography
- *see* Magnetic Resonance Imaging (MRI), Heart B23
- *see* Magnetic Resonance Imaging (MRI), Lower Arteries B43
- *see* Magnetic Resonance Imaging (MRI), Upper Arteries B33

MULTI-LINK (VISION)(MINI-VISION)(ULTRA) Coronary Stent System
- *use* Intraluminal Device

Multiple sleep latency test 4A0ZXQZ

Musculocutaneous nerve
- *use* Nerve, Brachial Plexus

Musculopexy
- *see* Repair, Muscles 0KQ
- *see* Reposition, Muscles 0KS

Musculophrenic artery
- *use* Artery, Internal Mammary, Left
- *use* Artery, Internal Mammary, Right

Musculoplasty
- *see* Repair, Muscles 0KQ
- *see* Supplement, Muscles 0KU

Musculorrhaphy
- *see* Repair, Muscles 0KQ

Musculospiral nerve
- *use* Nerve, Radial

Myectomy
- *see* Excision, Muscles 0KB
- *see* Resection, Muscles 0KT

Myelencephalon
- *use* Medulla Oblongata

Myelogram
- CT
  - *see* Computerized Tomography (CT Scan), Central Nervous System B02
- MRI
  - *see* Magnetic Resonance Imaging (MRI), Central Nervous System B03

Myenteric (Auerbach's) plexus
- *use* Nerve, Abdominal Sympathetic

Myocardial Bridge Release
- *see* Release, Artery, Coronary

Myomectomy
- *see* Excision, Female Reproductive System 0UB

Myometrium
- *use* Uterus

Myopexy
- *see* Repair, Muscles 0KQ
- *see* Reposition, Muscles 0KS

Myoplasty
- *see* Repair, Muscles 0KQ
- *see* Supplement, Muscles 0KU

Myorrhaphy
- *see* Repair, Muscles 0KQ

Myoscopy
- *see* Inspection, Muscles 0KJ

Myotomy
- *see* Division, Muscles 0K8
- *see* Drainage, Muscles 0K9

Myringectomy
- *see* Excision, Ear, Nose, Sinus 09B
- *see* Resection, Ear, Nose, Sinus 09T

Myringoplasty
- *see* Repair, Ear, Nose, Sinus 09Q
- *see* Replacement, Ear, Nose, Sinus 09R
- *see* Supplement, Ear, Nose, Sinus 09U

Myringostomy
- *see* Drainage, Ear, Nose, Sinus 099

Myringotomy
- *see* Drainage, Ear, Nose, Sinus 099

N

NA-1 (Nerinitide)
- *use* Nerinitide

Nail bed
- *use* Finger Nail
- *use* Toe Nail

Nail plate
- *use* Finger Nail
- *use* Toe Nail

nanoLOCK™ interbody fusion device
- *use* Interbody Fusion Device, Nanotextured Surface in New Technology

Narcosynthesis GZGZZZZ

Nasal cavity
- *use* Nasal Mucosa and Soft Tissue

Nasal concha
- *use* Turbinate, Nasal

Nasalis muscle
- *use* Muscle, Facial

Nasolacrimal duct
- *use* Duct, Lacrimal, Left
- *use* Duct, Lacrimal, Right

Nasopharyngeal airway (NPA)
- *use* Intraluminal Device, Airway in Ear, Nose, Sinus

Navicular bone
- *use* Tarsal, Left
- *use* Tarsal, Right

Near Infrared Spectroscopy, Circulatory System 8E02

Neck of femur
- *use* Femur, Upper, Left
- *use* Femur, Upper, Right

Neck of humerus (anatomical) (surgical)
- *use* Humeral Head, Left
- *use* Humeral Head, Right

Nephrectomy
- *see* Excision, Urinary System 0TB
- *see* Resection, Urinary System 0TT

Nephrolithotomy
- *see* Extirpation, Urinary System 0TC

Nephrolysis
- *see* Release, Urinary System 0TN

Nephropexy
- *see* Repair, Urinary System 0TQ
- *see* Reposition, Urinary System 0TS

Nephroplasty
- *see* Repair, Urinary System 0TQ
- *see* Supplement, Urinary System 0TU

Nephropyeloureterostomy
- *see* Bypass, Urinary System 0T1
- *see* Drainage, Urinary System 0T9

Nephrorrhaphy
- *see* Repair, Urinary System 0TQ

Nephroscopy, transurethral 0TJ58ZZ

Nephrostomy
- *see* Bypass, Urinary System 0T1
- *see* Drainage, Urinary System 0T9

Nephrotomography
- *see* Fluoroscopy, Urinary System BT1
- *see* Plain Radiography, Urinary System BT0

Nephrotomy
- *see* Division, Urinary System 0T8
- *see* Drainage, Urinary System 0T9

Nerinitide XW0

Nerve conduction study
- *see* Measurement, Central Nervous 4A00
- *see* Measurement, Peripheral Nervous 4A01

Nerve Function Assessment F01
Nerve to the stapedius
- *use* Nerve, Facial

Nesiritide
- *use* Human B-type Natriuretic Peptide

Neurectomy
- *see* Excision, Central Nervous System and Cranial Nerves 00B
- *see* Excision, Peripheral Nervous System 01B

Neurexeresis
- *see* Extraction, Central Nervous System and Cranial Nerves 00D
- *see* Extraction, Peripheral Nervous System 01D

Neurohypophysis
- *use* Gland, Pituitary

Neurolysis
- *see* Release, Central Nervous System and Cranial Nerves 00N
- *see* Release, Peripheral Nervous System 01N

Neuromuscular electrical stimulation (NEMS) lead
- *use* Stimulator Lead in Muscles

Neurophysiologic monitoring
- *see* Monitoring, Central Nervous 4A10

Neuroplasty
- *see* Repair, Central Nervous System and Cranial Nerves 00Q
- *see* Repair, Peripheral Nervous System 01Q
- *see* Supplement, Central Nervous System and Cranial Nerves 00U
- *see* Supplement, Peripheral Nervous System 01U

Neurorrhaphy
- *see* Repair, Central Nervous System and Cranial Nerves 00Q
- *see* Repair, Peripheral Nervous System 01Q

Neurostimulator Generator
- Insertion of device in, Skull 0NH00NZ
- Removal of device from, Skull 0NP00NZ
- Revision of device in, Skull 0NW00NZ

Neurostimulator generator, multiple channel
- *use* Stimulator Generator, Multiple Array in 0JH

Neurostimulator generator, multiple channel rechargeable
- *use* Stimulator Generator, Multiple Array Rechargeable in 0JH

Neurostimulator generator, single channel
- *use* Stimulator Generator, Single Array in 0JH

Neurostimulator generator, single channel rechargeable
- *use* Stimulator Generator, Single Array Rechargeable in 0JH

Neurostimulator Lead
- Insertion of device in
  - Brain 00H0
  - Cerebral Ventricle 00H6
  - Nerve
    - Cranial 00HE
    - Peripheral 01HY
  - Spinal Canal 00HU
  - Spinal Cord 00HV
  - Vein
    - Azygos 05H0
    - Innominate
      - Left 05H4
      - Right 05H3
- Removal of device from
  - Brain 00P0
  - Cerebral Ventricle 00P6
  - Nerve
    - Cranial 00PE
    - Peripheral 01PY
  - Spinal Canal 00PU
  - Spinal Cord 00PV
  - Vein
    - Azygos 05P0
    - Innominate
      - Left 05P4
      - Right 05HP3
- Revision of device in
  - Brain 00W0
  - Cerebral Ventricle 00W6
  - Nerve
    - Cranial 00WE
    - Peripheral 01WY
  - Spinal Canal 00WU
  - Spinal Cord 00WV
  - Vein
    - Azygos 05W0
    - Innominate
      - Left 05W4
      - Right 05HW3

Neurotomy
- *see* Division, Central Nervous System and Cranial Nerves 008
- *see* Division, Peripheral Nervous System and Cranial Nerves 018

Neurotripsy
see Destruction, Central Nervous
System and Cranial Nerves 005
see Destruction, Peripheral Nervous
System 015
Neutralization plate
use Internal Fixation Device in Head
and Facial Bones
use Internal Fixation Device in
Lower Bones
use Internal Fixation Device in
Upper Bones
New Technology
Apalutamide Antineoplstic XW0DJX5
Atezolizumab Antineoplastic XW0
Bezlotoxumab Monoclonal
Antibody XW0
Blinatumomab Antineoplastic
Immunotherapy XW0
Brexanolone XW0
Brexucabtagene Autoleucel
Immunotherapy XW2
Caplacizumab XW0
Cefiderocol Anti-infective XW0
Ceftazidime-Avibactam Anti-
infective XW0
Ceftolozane/Tazobactam Anti-
infective XW0
Cerebral Embolic Filtration
Dual Filter X2A5312
Extracorporeal Flow Reversal
Circuit X2A
Single Deflection Filter X2A6325
Coagulation Factor Xa, Inactivated
XW0
Concentrated Bone Marrow Aspirate
XK02303
Cytarabine and Daunorubicin
Liposome Antineoplastic XW0
Defibrotide Sodium Anticoagulant
XW0
Destruction, Prostate, Robotic
Waterjet Ablation XV508A4
Dilation
Anterior Tibial
Left
Sustained Release Drug-
eluting Intraluminal
Device X27Q385
Four or More X27Q3C5
Three X27Q3B5
Two X27Q395
Right
Sustained Release Drug-
eluting Intraluminal
Device X27P385
Four or More X27P3C5
Three X27P3B5
Two X27P395
Femoral
Left
Sustained Release Drug-
eluting Intraluminal
Device X27J385
Four or More X27J3C5
Three X27J3B5
Two X27J395
Right
Sustained Release Drug-
eluting Intraluminal
Device X27H385
Four or More X27H3C5
Three X27H3B5
Two X27H395
Peroneal
Left
Sustained Release Drug-
eluting Intraluminal
Device X27U385
Four or More X27U3C5
Three X27U3B5
Two X27U395

New Technology *(continued)*
Dilation *(continued)*
Peroneal *(continued)*
Right
Sustained Release Drug-
eluting Intraluminal
Device X27T385
Four or More X27T3C5
Three X27T3B5
Two X27T395
Popliteal
Left Distal
Sustained Release Drug-
eluting Intraluminal
Device X27N385
Four or More X27N3C5
Three X27N3B5
Two X27N395
Left Proximal
Sustained Release Drug-
eluting Intraluminal
Device X27L385
Four or More X27L3C5
Three X27L3B5
Two X27L395
Right Distal
Sustained Release Drug-
eluting Intraluminal
Device X27M385
Four or More X27M3C5
Three X27M3B5
Two X27M395
Right Proximal
Sustained Release Drug-
eluting Intraluminal
Device X27K385
Four or More X27K3C5
Three X27QK3B5
Two X27K395
Posterior Tibial
Left
Sustained Release Drug-
eluting Intraluminal
Device X27S385
Four or More X27S3C5
Three X27S3B5
Two X27S395
Right
Sustained Release Drug-
eluting Intraluminal
Device X27R385
Four or More X27R3C5
Three X27R3B5
Two X27R395
Durvalumab Antineoplastic XW0
Eculizumab XW0
Eladocagene exuparvovec XW0Q316
Endothelial Damage Inhibitor
XY0VX83
Engineered Autologous Chimeric
Antigen Receptor T-cell
Immunotherapy XW0
Erdafitinib Antineoplastic XW0DXL5
Esketamine Hydrochloride
XW097M5
Fosfomycin Anti-infective XW0
Fusion
Cervical Vertebral
2 or more
Nanotextured Surface
XRG2092
Radiolucent Porous
XRG20F3
Interbody Fusion Device
Nanotextured Surface
XRG1092
Radiolucent Porous
XRG10F3
Cervicothoracic Vertebral
Nanotextured Surface
XRG4092
Radiolucent Porous XRG40F3

New Technology *(continued)*
Fusion *(continued)*
Lumbar Vertebral
2 or more
Nanotextured Surface
XRGC092
Radiolucent Porous
XRGC0F3
Interbody Fusion Device
Nanotextured Surface
XRGB092
Radiolucent Porous
XRGB0F3
Lumbosacral
Nanotextured Surface
XRGD092
Radiolucent Porous
XRGD0F3
Occipital-cervical
Nanotextured Surface
XRG0092
Radiolucent Porous
XRG00F3
Thoracic Vertebral
2 to 7
Nanotextured Surface
XRG7092
Radiolucent Porous
XRG70F3
8 or more
Nanotextured Surface
XRG8092
Radiolucent Porous
XRG80F3
Interbody Fusion Device
Nanotextured Surface
XRG6092
Radiolucent Porous
XRG60F3
Thoracolumbar Vertebral
Nanotextured Surface
XRGA092
Radiolucent Porous
XRGA0F3
Gilteritinib Antineoplastic
XW0DXV5
Idarucizumab, Dabigatran Reversal
Agent XW0
Imipenem-cilastatin-relebactam
Anti-infective XW0
Intraoperative Knee Replacement
Sensor XR2
Iobenguane I-131 Antineoplastic XW0
Isavuconazole Anti-infective XW0
Kidney, Fluorescent Pyrazine
XT25XE5
Lefamulin Anti-infective XW0
Lisocabtagene Maraleucel
Immunotherapy XW2
Lower Respiratory Fluid Nucleic
Acid-base Microbial Detection
XXEBXQ6
Meropenem-vaborbactam Anti-
infective XW0
Mineral-based Topical Hemostatic
Agent XW0
Nerinitide XW0
Omadacycline Anti-infective XW0
Orbital Atherectomy Technology X2C
Other New Technology Therapeutic
Substance XW0
Plasma, Convalescent
(Nonautologous) XW1
Plazomicin Anti-infective XW0
Positive Blood Culture Fluorescence
Hybridization for Organism
Identification, Concentration and
Susceptibility XXE5XN6
Remdesivir Anti-infective XW0
Replacement
Skin Substitute, Porcine Liver
Derived XHRPXL2

New Technology *(continued)*
Replacement *(continued)*
Zooplastic Tissue, Rapid
Deployment Technique X2RF
Reposition
Cervical, Magnetically Controlled
Growth Rod(s) XNS3
Lumbar, Magnetically Controlled
Growth Rod(s) XNS0
Thoracic, Magnetically Controlled
Growth Rod(s) XNS4
Ruxolitinib XW0DXT5
Sarilumab XW0
Supplement
Lumbar, Mechanically
Expandable (Paired)
Synthetic Substitute
XNU0356
Thoracic, Mechanically
Expandable (Paired)
Synthetic Substitute
XNU4356
Synthetic Human Angiotensin II
XW0
Tagraxofusp-erzs Antineoplastic
XW0
Tocilizumab XW0
Uridine Triacetate XW0DX82
Venetoclax Antineoplastic
XW0DXR5
Whole Blood Nucleic Acid-base
Microbial Detection XXE5XM5
Ninth cranial nerve
use Nerve, Glossopharyngeal
NIRS (Near Infrared Spectroscopy)
see Physiological Systems and
Anatomical Regions 8E0
Nitinol framed polymer mesh
use Synthetic Substitute
Non-tunneled central venous catheter
use Infusion Device
Nonimaging Nuclear Medicine Assay
Bladder, Kidneys and Ureters CT63
Blood C763
Kidneys, Ureters and Bladder CT63
Lymphatics and Hematologic
System C76YYZZ
Ureters, Kidneys and Bladder CT63
Urinary System CT6YYZZ
Nonimaging Nuclear Medicine Probe
Abdomen CW50
Abdomen and Chest CW54
Abdomen and Pelvis CW51
Brain C050
Central Nervous System C05YYZZ
Chest CW53ZZ
Chest and Abdomen CW54
Chest and Neck CW56
Extremity
Lower CP5PZZZ
Upper CP5NZZZ
Head and Neck CW5B
Heart C25YYZZ
Right and Left C256
Lymphatics
Head C75J
Head and Neck C755
Lower Extremity C75P
Neck C75K
Pelvic C75D
Trunk C75M
Upper Chest C75L
Upper Extremity C75N
Lymphatics and Hematologic
System C75YYZZ
Musculoskeletal System, Other
CP5YYZZ
Neck and Chest CW56
Neck and Head CW5B
Pelvic Region CW5J
Pelvis and Abdomen CW51
Spine CP55ZZZ

Occlusion (*continued*)
  Vein (*continued*)
    Intracranial 05LL
    Lower 06LY
    Portal 06L8
    Pulmonary
      Left 02LT
      Right 02LS
    Renal
      Left 06LB
      Right 06L9
    Saphenous
      Left 06LQ
      Right 06LP
    Splenic 06L1
    Subclavian
      Left 05L6
      Right 05L5
    Superior Mesenteric 06L5
    Upper 05LY
    Vertebral
      Left 05LS
      Right 05LR
  Vena Cava
    Inferior 06L0
    Superior 02LV
Occlusion, REBOA (resuscitative endovascular balloon occlusion of the aorta)
  02LW3DJ
  04L03DJ
Occupational therapy
  see Activities of Daily Living Treatment, Rehabilitation F08
Odentectomy
  see Excision, Mouth and Throat 0CB
  see Resection, Mouth and Throat 0CT
Odontoid process
  use Cervical Vertebra
Olecranon bursa
  use Bursa and Ligament, Elbow, Left
  use Bursa and Ligament, Elbow, Right
Olecranon process
  use Ulna, Left
  use Ulna, Right
Olfactory bulb
  use Nerve, Olfactory
Omadacycline Anti-infective XW0
Omentectomy, omentumectomy
  see Excision, Gastrointestinal System 0DB
  see Resection, Gastrointestinal System 0DT
Omentofixation
  see Repair, Gastrointestinal System 0DQ
Omentoplasty
  see Repair, Gastrointestinal System 0DQ
  see Replacement, Gastrointestinal System 0DR
  see Supplement, Gastrointestinal System 0DU
Omentorrhaphy
  see Repair, Gastrointestinal System 0DQ
Omentotomy
  see Drainage, Gastrointestinal System 0D9
Omnilink Elite Vascular Balloon Expandable Stent System
  use Intraluminal Device
Onychectomy
  see Excision, Skin and Breast 0HB
  see Resection, Skin and Breast 0HT
Onychoplasty
  see Repair, Skin and Breast 0HQ
  see Replacement, Skin and Breast 0HR
Onychotomy
  see Drainage, Skin and Breast 0H9

Oophorectomy
  see Excision, Female Reproductive System 0UB
  see Resection, Female Reproductive System 0UT
Oophoropexy
  see Repair, Female Reproductive System 0UQ
  see Reposition, Female Reproductive System 0US
Oophoroplasty
  see Repair, Female Reproductive System 0UQ
  see Supplement, Female Reproductive System 0UU
Oophororrhaphy
  see Repair, Female Reproductive System 0UQ
Oophorostomy
  see Drainage, Female Reproductive System 0U9
Oophorotomy
  see Drainage, Female Reproductive System 0U9
  see Division, Female Reproductive System 0U8
Oophorrhaphy
  see Repair, Female Reproductive System 0UQ
Open Pivot (mechanical) valve
  use Synthetic Substitute
Open Pivot Aortic Valve Graft (AVG)
  use Synthetic Substitute
Ophthalmic artery
  use Intracranial Artery
Ophthalmic nerve
  use Nerve, Trigeminal
Ophthalmic vein
  use Vein, Intracranial
Opponensplasty
  Tendon replacement
    see Replacement, Tendons 0LR
  Tendon transfer
    see Transfer, Tendons 0LX
Optic chiasma
  use Nerve, Optic
Optic disc
  use Retina, Left
  use Retina, Right
Optic foramen
  use Bone, Sphenoid
Optical coherence tomography, intravascular
  see Computerized Tomography (CT Scan)
Optimizer™ III implantable pulse generator
  use Contractility Modulation Device in 0JH
Orbicularis oculi muscle
  use Eyelid, Upper, Left
  use Eyelid, Upper, Right
Orbicularis oris muscle
  use Muscle, Facial
Orbital Atherectomy Technology X2C
Orbital fascia
  use Subcutaneous Tissue and Fascia, Face
Orbital portion of ethmoid bone
  use Orbit, Left
  use Orbit, Right
Orbital portion of frontal bone
  use Orbit, Left
  use Orbit, Right
Orbital portion of lacrimal bone
  use Orbit, Left
  use Orbit, Right

Orbital portion of maxilla
  use Orbit, Left
  use Orbit, Right
Orbital portion of palatine bone
  use Orbit, Left
  use Orbit, Right
Orbital portion of sphenoid bone
  use Orbit, Left
  use Orbit, Right
Orbital portion of zygomatic bone
  use Orbit, Left
  use Orbit, Right
Orchectomy, orchidectomy, orchiectomy
  see Excision, Male Reproductive System 0VB
  see Resection, Male Reproductive System 0VT
Orchidoplasty, orchioplasty
  see Repair, Male Reproductive System 0VQ
  see Replacement, Male Reproductive System 0VR
  see Supplement, Male Reproductive System 0VU
Orchidorrhaphy, orchiorrhaphy
  see Repair, Male Reproductive System 0VQ
Orchidotomy, orchiotomy, orchotomy
  see Drainage, Male Reproductive System 0V9
Orchiopexy
  see Repair, Male Reproductive System 0VQ
  see Reposition, Male Reproductive System 0VS
Oropharyngeal airway (OPA)
  use Intraluminal Device, Airway in Mouth and Throat
Oropharynx
  use Pharynx
Ossiculectomy
  see Excision, Ear, Nose, Sinus 09B
  see Resection, Ear, Nose, Sinus 09T
Ossiculotomy
  see Drainage, Ear, Nose, Sinus 099
Ostectomy
  see Excision, Head and Facial Bones 0NB
  see Excision, Lower Bones 0QB
  see Excision, Upper Bones 0PB
  see Resection, Head and Facial Bones 0NT
  see Resection, Lower Bones 0QT
  see Resection, Upper Bones 0PT
Osteoclasis
  see Division, Head and Facial Bones 0N8
  see Division, Lower Bones 0Q8
  see Division, Upper Bones 0P8
Osteolysis
  see Release, Head and Facial Bones 0NN
  see Release, Lower Bones 0QN
  see Release, Upper Bones 0PN
Osteopathic Treatment
  Abdomen 7W09X
  Cervical 7W01X
  Extremity
    Lower 7W06X
    Upper 7W07X
  Head 7W00X
  Lumbar 7W03X
  Pelvis 7W05X
  Rib Cage 7W08X
  Sacrum 7W04X
  Thoracic 7W02X

Osteopexy
  see Repair, Head and Facial Bones 0NQ
  see Repair, Lower Bones 0QQ
  see Repair, Upper Bones 0PQ
  see Reposition, Head and Facial Bones 0NS
  see Reposition, Lower Bones 0QS
  see Reposition, Upper Bones 0PS
Osteoplasty
  see Repair, Head and Facial Bones 0NQ
  see Repair, Lower Bones 0QQ
  see Repair, Upper Bones 0PQ
  see Replacement, Head and Facial Bones 0NR
  see Replacement, Lower Bones 0QR
  see Replacement, Upper Bones 0PR
  see Supplement, Head and Facial Bones 0NU
  see Supplement, Lower Bones 0QU
  see Supplement, Upper Bones 0PU
Osteorrhaphy
  see Repair, Head and Facial Bones 0NQ
  see Repair, Lower Bones 0QQ
  see Repair, Upper Bones 0PQ
Osteotomy, ostotomy
  see Division, Head and Facial Bones 0N8
  see Division, Lower Bones 0Q8
  see Division, Upper Bones 0P8
  see Drainage, Head and Facial Bones 0N9
  see Drainage, Lower Bones 0Q9
  see Drainage, Upper Bones 0P9
Other Imaging
  Bile Duct, Indocyanine Green Dye, Intraoperative BF50200
  Bile Duct and Gallbladder, Indocyanine Green Dye, Intraoperative BF53200
  Extremity
    Lower BW5CZ1Z
    Upper BW5JZ1Z
  Gallbladder, Indocyanine Green Dye, Intraoperative BF52200
  Gallbladder and Bile Duct, Indocyanine Green Dye, Intraoperative BF53200
  Head and Neck BW59Z1Z
  Hepatobiliary System, All, Indocyanine Green Dye, Intraoperative BF5C200
  Liver, Indocyanine Green Dye, Intraoperative BF55200
  Liver and Spleen, Indocyanine Green Dye, Intraoperative BF56200
  Neck and Head BW59Z1Z
  Pancreas, Indocyanine Green Dye, Intraoperative BF57200
  Spleen and Liver, Indocyanine Green Dye, Intraoperative BF56200
  Trunk BW52Z1Z
Other New Technology Therapeutic Substance XW0
Otic ganglion
  use Nerve, Head and Neck Sympathetic
OTL-101
  use Hematopoietic Stem/Progenitor Cells, Genetically Modified
Otoplasty
  see Repair, Ear, Nose, Sinus 09Q
  see Replacement, Ear, Nose, Sinus 09R
  see Supplement, Ear, Nose, Sinus 09U

Otoscopy
  see Inspection, Ear, Nose, Sinus 09J

Oval window
  use Ear, Middle, Left
  use Ear, Middle, Right

Ovarian artery
  use Aorta, Abdominal

Ovarian ligament
  use Uterine Supporting Structure

Ovariectomy
  see Excision, Female Reproductive System 0UB
  see Resection, Female Reproductive System 0UT

Ovariocentesis
  see Drainage, Female Reproductive System 0U9

Ovariopexy
  see Repair, Female Reproductive System 0UQ
  see Reposition, Female Reproductive System 0US

Ovariotomy
  see Division, Female Reproductive System 0U8
  see Drainage, Female Reproductive System 0U9

Ovatio™ CRT-D
  use Cardiac Resynchronization Defibrillator Pulse Generator in 0JH

Oversewing
  Gastrointestinal ulcer
    see Repair, Gastrointestinal System 0DQ
  Pleural bleb
    see Repair, Respiratory System 0BQ

Oviduct
  use Fallopian Tube, Left
  use Fallopian Tube, Right

Oximetry, Fetal pulse 10H073Z

OXINIUM
  use Synthetic Substitute, Oxidized Zirconium on Polyethylene in 0SR

Oxygenation
  Extracorporeal membrane (ECMO)
    see Performance, Circulatory 5A15
  Hyperbaric
    see Assistance, Circulatory 5A05
  Supersaturated
    see Assistance, Circulatory 5A05

P

Pacemaker
  Dual Chamber
    Abdomen 0JH8
    Chest 0JH6
  Intracardiac
    Insertion of device in
      Atrium
        Left 02H7
        Right 02H6
      Vein, Coronary 02H4
      Ventricle
        Left 02HL
        Right 02HK
    Removal of device from
      Heart 02PA
    Revision of device in
      Heart 02WA
  Single Chamber
    Abdomen 0JH8
    Chest 0JH6
  Single Chamber Rate Responsive
    Abdomen 0JH8
    Chest 0JH6

Packing
  Abdominal Wall 2W43X5Z
  Anorectal 2Y43X5Z
  Arm
    Lower
      Left 2W4DX5Z
      Right 2W4CX5Z
    Upper
      Left 2W4BX5Z
      Right 2W4AX5Z
  Back 2W45X5Z
  Chest Wall 2W44X5Z
  Ear 2Y42X5Z
  Extremity
    Lower
      Left 2W4MX5Z
      Right 2W4LX5Z
    Upper
      Left 2W49X5Z
      Right 2W48X5Z
  Face 2W41X5Z
  Finger
    Left 2W4KX5Z
    Right 2W4JX5Z
  Foot
    Left 2W4TX5Z
    Right 2W4SX5Z
  Genital Tract, Female 2Y44X5Z
  Hand
    Left 2W4FX5Z
    Right 2W4EX5Z
  Head 2W40X5Z
  Inguinal Region
    Left 2W47X5Z
    Right 2W46X5Z
  Leg
    Lower
      Left 2W4RX5Z
      Right 2W4QX5Z
    Upper
      Left 2W4PX5Z
      Right 2W4NX5Z
  Mouth and Pharynx 2Y40X5Z
  Nasal 2Y41X5Z
  Neck 2W42X5Z
  Thumb
    Left 2W4HX5Z
    Right 2W4GX5Z
  Toe
    Left 2W4VX5Z
    Right 2W4UX5Z
  Urethra 2Y45X5Z

Paclitaxel-eluting coronary stent
  use Intraluminal Device, Drug-eluting in Heart and Great Vessels

Paclitaxel-eluting peripheral stent
  use Intraluminal Device, Drug-eluting in Lower Arteries
  use Intraluminal Device, Drug-eluting in Upper Arteries

Palatine gland
  use Buccal Mucosa

Palatine tonsil
  use Tonsils

Palatine uvula
  use Uvula

Palatoglossal muscle
  use Muscle, Tongue, Palate, Pharynx

Palatopharyngeal muscle
  use Muscle, Tongue, Palate, Pharynx

Palatoplasty
  see Repair, Mouth and Throat 0CQ
  see Replacement, Mouth and Throat 0CR
  see Supplement, Mouth and Throat 0CU

Palatorrhaphy
  see Repair, Mouth and Throat 0CQ

Palmar (volar) digital vein
  use Vein, Hand, Left
  use Vein, Hand, Right

Palmar (volar) metacarpal vein
  use Vein, Hand, Left
  use Vein, Hand, Right

Palmar cutaneous nerve
  use Nerve, Median
  use Nerve, Radial

Palmar fascia (aponeurosis)
  use Subcutaneous Tissue and Fascia, Hand, Left
  use Subcutaneous Tissue and Fascia, Hand, Right

Palmar interosseous muscle
  use Muscle, Hand, Left
  use Muscle, Hand, Right

Palmar ulnocarpal ligament
  use Bursa and Ligament, Wrist, Left
  use Bursa and Ligament, Wrist, Right

Palmaris longus muscle
  use Muscle, Lower Arm and Wrist, Left
  use Muscle, Lower Arm and Wrist, Right

Pancreatectomy
  see Excision, Pancreas 0FBG
  see Resection, Pancreas 0FTG

Pancreatic artery
  use Artery, Splenic

Pancreatic plexus
  use Nerve, Abdominal Sympathetic

Pancreatic vein
  use Vein, Splenic

Pancreaticoduodenostomy
  see Bypass, Hepatobiliary System and Pancreas 0F1

Pancreaticosplenic lymph node
  use Lymphatic, Aortic

Pancreatogram, endoscopic retrograde
  see Fluoroscopy, Pancreatic Duct BF18

Pancreatolithotomy
  see Extirpation, Pancreas 0FCG

Pancreatotomy
  see Division, Pancreas 0F8G
  see Drainage, Pancreas 0F9G

Panniculectomy
  see Excision, Skin, Abdomen 0HB7
  see Excision, Subcutaneous Tissue and Fascia, Abdomen 0JB8

Paraaortic lymph node
  use Lymphatic, Aortic

Paracentesis
  Eye
    see Drainage, Eye 089
  Peritoneal Cavity
    see Drainage, Peritoneal Cavity 0W9G
  Tympanum
    see Drainage, Ear, Nose, Sinus 099

Pararectal lymph node
  use Lymphatic, Mesenteric

Parasternal lymph node
  use Lymphatic, Thorax

Parathyroidectomy
  see Excision, Endocrine System 0GB
  see Resection, Endocrine System 0GT

Paratracheal lymph node
  use Lymphatic, Thorax

Paraurethral (Skene's) gland
  use Gland, Vestibular

Parenteral nutrition, total
  see Introduction of Nutritional Substance

Parietal lobe
  use Cerebral Hemisphere

Parotid lymph node
  use Lymphatic, Head

Parotid plexus
  use Nerve, Facial

Parotidectomy
  see Excision, Mouth and Throat 0CB
  see Resection, Mouth and Throat 0CT

Pars flaccida
  use Tympanic Membrane, Left
  use Tympanic Membrane, Right

Partial joint replacement
  Hip
    see Replacement, Lower Joints 0SR
  Knee
    see Replacement, Lower Joints 0SR
  Shoulder
    see Replacement, Upper Joints 0RR

Partially absorbable mesh
  use Synthetic Substitute

Patch, blood, spinal 3E0R3GC

Patellapexy
  see Repair, Lower Bones 0QQ
  see Reposition, Lower Bones 0QS

Patellaplasty
  see Repair, Lower Bones 0QQ
  see Replacement, Lower Bones 0QR
  see Supplement, Lower Bones 0QU

Patellar ligament
  use Bursa and Ligament, Knee, Left
  use Bursa and Ligament, Knee, Right

Patellar tendon
  use Tendon, Knee, Left
  use Tendon, Knee, Right

Patellectomy
  see Excision, Lower Bones 0QB
  see Resection, Lower Bones 0QT

Patellofemoral joint
  use Joint, Knee, Left
  use Joint, Knee, Left, Femoral Surface
  use Joint, Knee, Right
  use Joint, Knee, Right, Femoral Surface

Pectineus muscle
  use Muscle, Upper Leg, Left
  use Muscle, Upper Leg, Right

Pectoral (anterior) lymph node
  use Lymphatic, Axillary, Left
  use Lymphatic, Axillary, Right

Pectoral fascia
  use Subcutaneous Tissue and Fascia, Chest

Pectoralis major muscle
  use Muscle, Thorax, Left
  use Muscle, Thorax, Right

Pectoralis minor muscle
  use Muscle, Thorax, Left
  use Muscle, Thorax, Right

Pedicle-based dynamic stabilization device
  use Spinal Stabilization Device, Pedicle-Based in 0RH
  use Spinal Stabilization Device, Pedicle-Based in 0SH

PEEP (positive end expiratory pressure)
  see Assistance, Respiratory 5A09

PEG (percutaneous endoscopic gastrostomy) 0DH63UZ

PEJ (percutaneous endoscopic jejunostomy) 0DHA3UZ

Pelvic splanchnic nerve
use Nerve, Abdominal Sympathetic
use Nerve, Sacral Sympathetic
Penectomy
see Excision, Male Reproductive System 0VB
see Resection, Male Reproductive System 0VT
Penile urethra
use Urethra
Perceval sutureless valve
use Zooplastic Tissue, Rapid Deployment Technique in New Technology
Percutaneous endoscopic gastrojejunostomy (PEG/J) tube
use Feeding Device in Gastrointestinal System
Percutaneous endoscopic gastrostomy (PEG) tube
use Feeding Device in Gastrointestinal System
Percutaneous nephrostomy catheter
use Drainage Device
Percutaneous transluminal coronary angioplasty (PTCA)
see Dilation, Heart and Great Vessels 027
Performance
Biliary
Multiple, Filtration 5A1C60Z
Single, Filtration 5A1C00Z
Cardiac
Continuous
Output 5A1221Z
Pacing 5A1223Z
Intermittent, Pacing 5A1213Z
Single, Output, Manual 5A12012
Circulatory
Continuous
Central Membrane 5A1522F
Peripheral Veno-arterial Membrane 5A1522G
Peripheral Veno-venous Membrane 5A1522H
Intraoperative
Central Membrane 5A15A2F
Peripheral Veno-arterial Membrane 5A15A2G
Peripheral Veno-venous Membrane 5A15A2H
Respiratory
24-96 Consecutive Hours, Ventilation 5A1945Z
Greater than 96 Consecutive Hours, Ventilation 5A1955Z
Less than 24 Consecutive Hours, Ventilation 5A1935Z
Single, Ventilation, Nonmechanical 5A19054
Urinary
Continuous, Greater than 18 hours per day, Filtration 5A1D90Z
Intermittent, Less than 6 hours per day, Filtration 5A1D70Z
Prolonged Intermittent, 6-18 hours per day, Filtration 5A1D80Z
Perfusion
see Introduction of substance in or on
Perfusion, donor organ
Heart 6AB50BZ
Kidney(s) 6ABT0BZ
Liver 6ABF0BZ
Lung(s) 6ABB0BZ

Pericardiectomy
see Excision, Pericardium 02BN
see Resection, Pericardium 02TN
Pericardiocentesis
see Drainage, Pericardial Cavity 0W9D
Pericardiolysis
see Release, Pericardium 02NN
Pericardiophrenic artery
use Artery, Internal Mammary, Left
use Artery, Internal Mammary, Right
Pericardioplasty
see Repair, Pericardium 02QN
see Replacement, Pericardium 02RN
see Supplement, Pericardium 02UN
Pericardiorrhaphy
see Repair, Pericardium 02QN
Pericardiostomy
see Drainage, Pericardial Cavity 0W9D
Pericardiotomy
see Drainage, Pericardial Cavity 0W9D
Perimetrium
use Uterus
Peripheral Intravascular Lithotripsy (Peripheral IVL)
see Fragmentation
Peripheral parenteral nutrition
see Introduction of Nutritional Substance
Peripherally inserted central catheter (PICC)
use Infusion Device
Peritoneal dialysis 3E1M39Z
Peritoneocentesis
see Drainage, Peritoneal Cavity 0W9G
see Drainage, Peritoneum 0D9W
Peritoneoplasty
see Repair, Peritoneum 0DQW
see Replacement, Peritoneum 0DRW
see Supplement, Peritoneum 0DUW
Peritoneoscopy 0DJW4ZZ
Peritoneotomy
see Drainage, Peritoneum 0D9W
Peritoneumectomy
see Excision, Peritoneum 0DBW
Peroneus brevis muscle
use Muscle, Lower Leg, Left
use Muscle, Lower Leg, Right
Peroneus longus muscle
use Muscle, Lower Leg, Left
use Muscle, Lower Leg, Right
Pessary ring
use Intraluminal Device, Pessary in Female Reproductive System
PET scan
see Positron Emission Tomographic (PET) Imaging
Petrous part of temporal bone
use Bone, Temporal, Left
use Bone, Temporal, Right
Phacoemulsification, lens
With IOL implant
see Replacement, Eye 08R
Without IOL implant
see Extraction, Eye 08D
Phalangectomy
see Excision, Lower Bones 0QB
see Excision, Upper Bones 0PB
see Resection, Lower Bones 0QT
see Resection, Upper Bones 0PT

Phallectomy
see Excision, Penis 0VBS
see Resection, Penis 0VTS
Phalloplasty
see Repair, Penis 0VQS
see Supplement, Penis 0VUS
Phallotomy
see Drainage, Penis 0V9S
Pharmacotherapy, for substance abuse
Antabuse HZ93ZZZ
Bupropion HZ97ZZZ
Clonidine HZ96ZZZ
Levo-alpha-acetyl-methadol (LAAM) HZ92ZZZ
Methadone Maintenance HZ91ZZZ
Naloxone HZ95ZZZ
Naltrexone HZ94ZZZ
Nicotine Replacement HZ90ZZZ
Psychiatric Medication HZ98ZZZ
Replacement Medication, Other HZ99ZZZ
Pharyngeal constrictor muscle
use Muscle, Tongue, Palate, Pharynx
Pharyngeal plexus
use Nerve, Vagus
Pharyngeal recess
use Nasopharynx
Pharyngeal tonsil
use Adenoids
Pharyngogram
see Fluoroscopy, Pharynix B91G
Pharyngoplasty
see Repair, Mouth and Throat 0CQ
see Replacement, Mouth and Throat 0CR
see Supplement, Mouth and Throat 0CU
Pharyngorrhaphy
see Repair, Mouth and Throat 0CQ
Pharyngotomy
see Drainage, Mouth and Throat 0C9
Pharyngotympanic tube
use Eustachian Tube, Left
use Eustachian Tube, Right
Pheresis
Erythrocytes 6A55
Leukocytes 6A55
Plasma 6A55
Platelets 6A55
Stem Cells
Cord Blood 6A55
Hematopoietic 6A55
Phlebectomy
see Excision, Lower Veins 06B
see Excision, Upper Veins 05B
see Extraction, Lower Veins 06D
see Extraction, Upper Veins 05D
Phlebography
see Plain Radiography, Veins B50
Impedance 4A04X51
Phleborrhaphy
see Repair, Lower Veins 06Q
see Repair, Upper Veins 05Q
Phlebotomy
see Drainage, Lower Veins 069
see Drainage, Upper Veins 059
Photocoagulation
For Destruction
see Destruction
For Repair
see Repair
Photopheresis, therapeutic
see Phototherapy, Circulatory 6A65
Phototherapy
Circulatory 6A65
Skin 6A60
Ultraviolet light
see Ultraviolet Light Therapy, Physiological Systems 6A8

Phrenectomy, phrenoneurectomy
see Excision, Nerve, Phrenic 01B2
Phrenemphraxis
see Destruction, Nerve, Phrenic 0152
Phrenic nerve stimulator generator
use Stimulator Generator in Subcutaneous Tissue and Fascia
Phrenic nerve stimulator lead
use Diaphragmatic Pacemaker Lead in Respiratory System
Phreniclasis
see Destruction, Nerve, Phrenic 0152
Phrenicoexeresis
see Extraction, Nerve, Phrenic 01D2
Phrenicotomy
see Division, Nerve, Phrenic 0182
Phrenicotripsy
see Destruction, Nerve, Phrenic 0152
Phrenoplasty
see Repair, Respiratory System 0BQ
see Supplement, Respiratory System 0BU
Phrenotomy
see Drainage, Respiratory System 0B9
Physiatry
see Motor Treatment, Rehabilitation F07
Physical medicine
see Motor Treatment, Rehabilitation F07
Physical therapy
see Motor Treatment, Rehabilitation F07
PHYSIOMESH™ Flexible Composite Mesh
use Synthetic Substitute
Pia mater, intracranial
use Cerebral Meninges
Pia mater, spinal
use Spinal Meninges
Pinealectomy
see Excision, Pineal Body 0GB1
see Resection, Pineal Body 0GT1
Pinealoscopy 0GJ14ZZ
Pinealotomy
see Drainage, Pineal Body 0G91
Pinna
use Ear, External, Bilateral
use Ear, External, Left
use Ear, External, Right
Pipeline™ (Flex) embolization device
use Intraluminal Device, Flow Diverter in 03V
Piriform recess (sinus)
use Pharynx
Piriformis muscle
use Muscle, Hip, Right
use Muscle, Hip, Left
PIRRT (Prolonged intermittent renal replacement therapy) 5A1D80Z
Pisiform bone
use Carpal, Left
use Carpal, Right
Pisohamate ligament
use Bursa and Ligament, Hand, Left
use Bursa and Ligament, Hand, Right
Pisometacarpal ligament
use Bursa and Ligament, Hand, Left
use Bursa and Ligament, Hand, Right
Pituitectomy
see Excision, Gland, Pituitary 0GB0
see Resection, Gland, Pituitary 0GT0

Plain film radiology
see Plain Radiography
Plain Radiography
Abdomen BW00ZZZ
Abdomen and Pelvis BW01ZZZ
Abdominal Lymphatic
   Bilateral B701
   Unilateral B700
Airway, Upper BB0DZZZ
Ankle
   Left BQ0H
   Right BQ0G
Aorta
   Abdominal B400
   Thoracic B300
   Thoraco-Abdominal B30P
Aorta and Bilateral Lower Extremity
   Arteries B40D
Arch
   Bilateral BN0DZZZ
   Left BN0CZZZ
   Right BN0BZZZ
Arm
   Left BP0FZZZ
   Right BP0EZZZ
Artery
   Brachiocephalic-Subclavian,
      Right B301
   Bronchial B30L
   Bypass Graft, Other B20F
   Cervico-Cerebral Arch B30Q
   Common Carotid
      Bilateral B305
      Left B304
      Right B303
   Coronary
      Bypass Graft
         Multiple B203
         Single B202
      Multiple B201
      Single B200
   External Carotid
      Bilateral B30C
      Left B30B
      Right B309
   Hepatic B402
   Inferior Mesenteric B405
   Intercostal B30L
   Internal Carotid
      Bilateral B308
      Left B307
      Right B306
   Internal Mammary Bypass Graft
      Left B208
      Right B207
   Intra-Abdominal, Other B40B
   Intracranial B30R
   Lower, Other B40J
   Lower Extremity
      Bilateral and Aorta
         B40D
      Left B40G
      Right B40F
   Lumbar B409
   Pelvic B40C
   Pulmonary
      Left B30T
      Right B30S
   Renal
      Bilateral B408
      Left B407
      Right B406
      Transplant B40M
   Spinal B30M
   Splenic B403
   Subclavian, Left B302
   Superior Mesenteric B404
   Upper, Other B30N
   Upper Extremity
      Bilateral B30K
      Left B30J
      Right B30H

Artery *(continued)*
   Vertebral
      Bilateral B30G
      Left B30F
      Right B30D
Bile Duct BF00
Bile Duct and Gallbladder BF03
Bladder BT00
   Kidney and Ureter BT04
Bladder and Urethra BT0B
Bone
   Facial BN05ZZZ
   Nasal BN04ZZZ
Bones, Long, All BW0BZZZ
Breast
   Bilateral BH02ZZZ
   Left BH01ZZZ
   Right BH00ZZZ
Calcaneus
   Left BQ0KZZZ
   Right BQ0JZZZ
Chest BW03ZZZ
Clavicle
   Left BP05ZZZ
   Right BP04ZZZ
Coccyx BR0FZZZ
Corpora Cavernosa BV00
Dialysis Fistula B50W
Dialysis Shunt B50W
Disc
   Cervical BR01
   Lumbar BR03
   Thoracic BR02
Duct
   Lacrimal
      Bilateral B802
      Left B801
      Right B800
   Mammary
      Multiple
         Left BH06
         Right BH05
      Single
         Left BH04
         Right BH03
Elbow
   Left BP0H
   Right BP0G
Epididymis
   Left BV02
   Right BV01
Extremity
   Lower BW0CZZZ
   Upper BW0JZZZ
Eye
   Bilateral B807ZZZ
   Left B806ZZZ
   Right B805ZZZ
Facet Joint
   Cervical BR04
   Lumbar BR06
   Thoracic BR05
Fallopian Tube
   Bilateral BU02
   Left BU01
   Right BU00
Fallopian Tube and Uterus
   BU08
Femur
   Left, Densitometry BQ04ZZ1
   Right, Densitometry BQ03ZZ1
Finger
   Left BP0SZZZ
   Right BP0RZZZ
Foot
   Left BQ0MZZZ
   Right BQ0LZZZ
Forearm
   Left BP0KZZZ
   Right BP0JZZZ
Gallbladder and Bile Duct BF03

Gland
   Parotid
      Bilateral B906
      Left B905
      Right B904
   Salivary
      Bilateral B90D
      Left B90C
      Right B90B
   Submandibular
      Bilateral B909
      Left B908
      Right B907
Hand
   Left BP0PZZZ
   Right BP0NZZZ
Heart
   Left B205
   Right B204
   Right and Left B206
Hepatobiliary System, All
   BF0C
Hip
   Left BQ01
      Densitometry BQ01ZZ1
   Right BQ00
      Densitometry BQ00ZZ1
Humerus
   Left BP0BZZZ
   Right BP0AZZZ
Ileal Diversion Loop BT0C
Intracranial Sinus B502
Joint
   Acromioclavicular, Bilateral
      BP03ZZZ
   Finger
      Left BP0D
      Right BP0C
   Foot
      Left BQ0Y
      Right BQ0X
   Hand
      Left BP0D
      Right BP0C
   Lumbosacral BR0BZZZ
   Sacroiliac BR0D
   Sternoclavicular
      Bilateral BP02ZZZ
      Left BP01ZZZ
      Right BP00ZZZ
   Temporomandibular
      Bilateral BN09
      Left BN08
      Right BN07
   Thoracolumbar BR08ZZZ
   Toe
      Left BQ0Y
      Right BQ0X
Kidney
   Bilateral BT03
   Left BT02
   Right BT01
   Ureter and Bladder BT04
Knee
   Left BQ08
   Right BQ07
Leg
   Left BQ0FZZZ
   Right BQ0DZZZ
Lymphatic
   Head B704
   Lower Extremity
      Bilateral B70B
      Left B709
      Right B708
   Neck B704
   Pelvic B70C
   Upper Extremity
      Bilateral B707
      Left B706
      Right B705

Mandible BN06ZZZ
Mastoid B90HZZZ
Nasopharynx B90FZZZ
Optic Foramina
   Left B804ZZZ
   Right B803ZZZ
Orbit
   Bilateral BN03ZZZ
   Left BN02ZZZ
   Right BN01ZZZ
Oropharynx B90FZZZ
Patella
   Left BQ0WZZZ
   Right BQ0VZZZ
Pelvis BR0CZZZ
Pelvis and Abdomen BW01ZZZ
Prostate BV03
Retroperitoneal Lymphatic
   Bilateral B701
   Unilateral B700
Ribs
   Left BP0YZZZ
   Right BP0XZZZ
Sacrum BR0FZZZ
Scapula
   Left BP07ZZZ
   Right BP06ZZZ
Shoulder
   Left BP09
   Right BP08
Sinus
   Intracranial B502
   Paranasal B902ZZZ
Skull BN00ZZZ
Spinal Cord B00B
Spine
   Cervical, Densitometry
      BR00ZZ1
   Lumbar, Densitometry
      BR09ZZ1
   Thoracic, Densitometry
      BR07ZZ1
   Whole, Densitometry BR0GZZ1
Sternum BR0HZZZ
Teeth
   All BN0JZZZ
   Multiple BN0HZZZ
Testicle
   Left BV06
   Right BV05
Toe
   Left BQ0QZZZ
   Right BQ0PZZZ
Tooth, Single BN0GZZZ
Tracheobronchial Tree
   Bilateral BB09YZZ
   Left BB08Y
   Right BB07Y
Ureter
   Bilateral BT08
   Kidney and Bladder BT04
   Left BT07
   Right BT06
Urethra BT05
Urethra and Bladder BT0B
Uterus BU06
Uterus and Fallopian Tube BU08
Vagina BU09
Vasa Vasorum BV08
Vein
   Cerebellar B501
   Cerebral B501
   Epidural B500
   Jugular
      Bilateral B505
      Left B504
      Right B503
   Lower Extremity
      Bilateral B50D
      Left B50C
      Right B50B

Plain Radiography (continued)

Vein (continued)
  Other B50V
  Pelvic (Iliac)
    Left B50G
    Right B50F
  Pelvic (Iliac) Bilateral B50H
  Portal B50T
  Pulmonary
    Bilateral B50S
    Left B50R
    Right B50Q
  Renal
    Bilateral B50L
    Left B50K
    Right B50J
  Spanchnic B50T
  Subclavian
    Left B507
    Right B506
  Upper Extremity
    Bilateral B50P
    Left B50N
    Right B50M
Vena Cava
  Inferior B509
  Superior B508
Whole Body BW0KZZZ
  Infant BW0MZZZ
Whole Skeleton BW0LZZZ
Wrist
  Left BP0M
  Right BP0L

Planar Nuclear Medicine Imaging

Abdomen CW10
Abdomen and Chest CW14
Abdomen and Pelvis CW11
Anatomical Regions, Multiple CW1YYZZ
Anatomical Region, Other CW1ZZZZ
Bladder, Kidneys and Ureters CT13
Bladder and Ureters CT1H
Blood C713
Bone Marrow C710
Brain C010
Breast CH1YYZZ
  Bilateral CH12
  Left CH11
  Right CH10
Bronchi and Lungs CB12
Central Nervous System C01YYZZ
Cerebrospinal Fluid C015
Chest CW13
Chest and Abdomen CW14
Chest and Neck CW16
Digestive System CD1YYZZ
Ducts, Lacrimal, Bilateral C819
Ear, Nose, Mouth and Throat C91YYZZ
Endocrine System CG1YYZZ
Extremity
  Lower CW1D
    Bilateral CP1F
    Left CP1D
    Right CP1C
  Upper CW1M
    Bilateral CP1B
    Left CP19
    Right CP18
Eye C81YYZZ
Gallbladder CF14
Gastrointestinal Tract CD17
  Upper CD15
Gland
  Adrenal, Bilateral CG14
  Parathyroid CG11
  Thyroid CG12
Glands, Salivary, Bilateral C91B
Head and Neck CW1B
Heart C21YYZZ
  Right and Left C216

Planar Nuclear Medicine Imaging (continued)

Hepatobiliary System, All CF1C
Hepatobiliary System and Pancreas CF1YYZZ
Kidneys, Ureters and Bladder CT13
Liver CF15
Liver and Spleen CF16
Lungs and Bronchi CB12
Lymphatics
  Head C71J
  Head and Neck C715
  Lower Extremity C71P
  Neck C71K
  Pelvic C71D
  Trunk C71M
  Upper Chest C71L
  Upper Extremity C71N
Lymphatics and Hematologic System C71YYZZ
Musculoskeletal System
  All CP1Z
  Other CP1YYZZ
Myocardium C21G
Neck and Chest CW16
Neck and Head CW1B
Pancreas and Hepatobiliary System CF1YYZZ
Pelvic Region CW1J
Pelvis CP16
Pelvis and Abdomen CW11
Pelvis and Spine CP17
Reproductive System, Male CV1YYZZ
Respiratory System CB1YYZZ
Skin CH1YYZZ
Skull CP11
Spine CP15
Spine and Pelvis CP17
Spleen C712
Spleen and Liver CF16
Subcutaneous Tissue CH1YYZZ
Testicles, Bilateral CV19
Thorax CP14
Ureters, Kidneys and Bladder CT13
Ureters and Bladder CT1H
Urinary System CT1YYZZ
Veins C51YYZZ
  Central C51R
  Lower Extremity
    Bilateral C51D
    Left C51C
    Right C51B
  Upper Extremity
    Bilateral C51Q
    Left C51P
    Right C51N
Whole Body CW1N

Plantar digital vein
  use Vein, Foot, Left
  use Vein, Foot, Right
Plantar fascia (aponeurosis)
  use Subcutaneous Tissue and Fascia, Foot, Left
  use Subcutaneous Tissue and Fascia, Foot, Right
Plantar metatarsal vein
  use Vein, Foot, Left
  use Vein, Foot, Right
Plantar venous arch
  use Vein, Foot, Left
  use Vein, Foot, Right
Plaque Radiation
  Abdomen DWY3FZZ
  Adrenal Gland DGY2FZZ
  Anus DDY8FZZ
  Bile Ducts DFY2FZZ
  Bladder DTY2FZZ
  Bone, Other DPYCFZZ
  Bone Marrow D7Y0FZZ

Plaque Radiation (continued)

Brain D0Y0FZZ
Brain Stem D0Y1FZZ
Breast
  Left DMY0FZZ
  Right DMY1FZZ
Bronchus DBY1FZZ
Cervix DUY1FZZ
Chest DWY2FZZ
Chest Wall DBY7FZZ
Colon DDY5FZZ
Diaphragm DBY8FZZ
Duodenum DDY2FZZ
Ear D9Y0FZZ
Esophagus DDY0FZZ
Eye D8Y0FZZ
Femur DPY9FZZ
Fibula DPYBFZZ
Gallbladder DFY1FZZ
Gland
  Adrenal DGY2FZZ
  Parathyroid DGY4FZZ
  Pituitary DGY0FZZ
  Thyroid DGY5FZZ
Glands, Salivary D9Y6FZZ
Head and Neck DWY1FZZ
Hemibody DWY4FZZ
Humerus DPY6FZZ
Ileum DDY4FZZ
Jejunum DDY3FZZ
Kidney DTY0FZZ
Larynx D9YBFZZ
Liver DFY0FZZ
Lung DBY2FZZ
Lymphatics
  Abdomen D7Y6FZZ
  Axillary D7Y4FZZ
  Inguinal D7Y8FZZ
  Neck D7Y3FZZ
  Pelvis D7Y7FZZ
  Thorax D7Y5FZZ
Mandible DPY3FZZ
Maxilla DPY2FZZ
Mediastinum DBY6FZZ
Mouth D9Y4FZZ
Nasopharynx D9YDFZZ
Neck and Head DWY1FZZ
Nerve, Peripheral D0Y7FZZ
Nose D9Y1FZZ
Ovary DUY0FZZ
Palate
  Hard D9Y8FZZ
  Soft D9Y9FZZ
Pancreas DFY3FZZ
Parathyroid Gland DGY4FZZ
Pelvic Bones DPY8FZZ
Pelvic Region DWY6FZZ
Pharynx D9YCFZZ
Pineal Body DGY1FZZ
Pituitary Gland DGY0FZZ
Pleura DBY5FZZ
Prostate DVY0FZZ
Radius DPY7FZZ
Rectum DDY7FZZ
Rib DPY5FZZ
Sinuses D9Y7FZZ
Skin
  Abdomen DHY8FZZ
  Arm DHY4FZZ
  Back DHY7FZZ
  Buttock DHY9FZZ
  Chest DHY6FZZ
  Face DHY2FZZ
  Foot DHYCFZZ
  Hand DHY5FZZ
  Leg DHYBFZZ
  Neck DHY3FZZ
Skull DPY0FZZ
Spinal Cord D0Y6FZZ
Spleen D7Y2FZZ
Sternum DPY4FZZ
Stomach DDY1FZZ

Plaque Radiation (continued)

Testis DVY1FZZ
Thymus D7Y1FZZ
Thyroid Gland DGY5FZZ
Tibia DPYBFZZ
Tongue D9Y5FZZ
Trachea DBY0FZZ
Ulna DPY7FZZ
Ureter DTY1FZZ
Urethra DTY3FZZ
Uterus DUY2FZZ
Whole Body DWY5FZZ
Plasma, Convalescent (Nonautologous) XW1
Plasmapheresis, therapeutic
  see Pheresis, Physiological Systems 6A5
Plateletpheresis, therapeutic
  see Pheresis, Physiological Systems 6A5
Platysma muscle
  use Muscle, Neck, Left
  use Muscle, Neck, Right
Plazomicin Anti-infective XW0
Pleurectomy
  see Excision, Respiratory System 0BB
  see Resection, Respiratory System 0BT
Pleurocentesis
  see Drainage, Anatomical Regions, General 0W9
Pleurodesis, pleurosclerosis
  Chemical injection
    see Introduction of substance in or on, Pleural Cavity 3E0L
  Surgical
    see Destruction, Respiratory System 0B5
Pleurolysis
  see Release, Respiratory System 0BN
Pleuroscopy 0BJQ4ZZ
Pleurotomy
  see Drainage, Respiratory System 0B9
Plica semilunaris
  use Conjunctiva, Left
  use Conjunctiva, Right
Plication
  see Restriction
Pneumectomy
  see Excision, Respiratory System 0BB
  see Resection, Respiratory System 0BT
Pneumocentesis
  see Drainage, Respiratory System 0B9
Pneumogastric nerve
  use Nerve, Vagus
Pneumolysis
  see Release, Respiratory System 0BN
Pneumonectomy
  see Resection, Respiratory System 0BT
Pneumonolysis
  see Release, Respiratory System 0BN
Pneumonopexy
  see Repair, Respiratory System 0BQ
  see Reposition, Respiratory System 0BS
Pneumonorrhaphy
  see Repair, Respiratory System 0BQ
Pneumonotomy
  see Drainage, Respiratory System 0B9
Pneumotaxic center
  use Pons
Pneumotomy
  see Drainage, Respiratory System 0B9

Pollicization
    see Transfer, Anatomical Regions, Upper Extremities 0XX

Polyethylene socket
    use Synthetic Substitute, Polyethylene in 0SR

Polymethylmethacrylate (PMMA)
    use Synthetic Substitute

Polypectomy, gastrointestinal
    see Excision, Gastrointestinal System 0DB

Polypropylene mesh
    use Synthetic Substitute

Polysomnogram 4A1ZXQZ

Pontine tegmentum
    use Pons

Popliteal ligament
    use Bursa and Ligament, Knee, Left
    use Bursa and Ligament, Knee, Right

Popliteal lymph node
    use Lymphatic, Lower Extremity, Left
    use Lymphatic, Lower Extremity, Right

Popliteal vein
    use Vein, Femoral, Left
    use Vein, Femoral, Right

Popliteus muscle
    use Muscle, Lower Leg, Left
    use Muscle, Lower Leg, Right

Porcine (bioprosthetic) valve
    use Zooplastic Tissue in Heart and Great Vessels

Positive Blood Culture Fluorescence Hybridization for Organism Identification, Concentration and Susceptibility XXE5XN6

Positive end expiratory pressure
    see Performance, Respiratory 5A19

Positron Emission Tomographic (PET) Imaging
    Brain C030
    Bronchi and Lungs CB32
    Central Nervous System C03YYZZ
    Heart C23YYZZ
    Lungs and Bronchi CB32
    Myocardium C23G
    Respiratory System CB3YYZZ
    Whole Body CW3NYZZ

Positron emission tomography
    see Positron Emission Tomographic (PET) Imaging

Postauricular (mastoid) lymph node
    use Lymphatic, Neck, Left
    use Lymphatic, Neck, Right

Postcava
    use Vena Cava, Inferior

Posterior (subscapular) lymph node
    use Lymphatic, Axillary, Left
    use Lymphatic, Axillary, Right

Posterior auricular artery
    use Artery, External Carotid, Left
    use Artery, External Carotid, Right

Posterior auricular nerve
    use Nerve, Facial

Posterior auricular vein
    use Vein, External Jugular, Left
    use Vein, External Jugular, Right

Posterior cerebral artery
    use Artery, Intracranial

Posterior chamber
    use Eye, Left
    use Eye, Right

Posterior circumflex humeral artery
    use Artery, Axillary, Left
    use Artery, Axillary, Right

Posterior communicating artery
    use Artery, Intracranial

Posterior cruciate ligament (PCL)
    use Bursa and Ligament, Knee, Left
    use Bursa and Ligament, Knee, Right

Posterior facial (retromandibular) vein
    use Vein, Face, Left
    use Vein, Face, Right

Posterior femoral cutaneous nerve
    use Nerve, Sacral Plexus

Posterior inferior cerebellar artery (PICA)
    use Artery, Intracranial

Posterior interosseous nerve
    use Nerve, Radial

Posterior labial nerve
    use Nerve, Pudendal

Posterior scrotal nerve
    use Nerve, Pudendal

Posterior spinal artery
    use Artery, Vertebral, Left
    use Artery, Vertebral, Right

Posterior tibial recurrent artery
    use Artery, Anterior Tibial, Left
    use Artery, Anterior Tibial, Right

Posterior ulnar recurrent artery
    use Artery, Ulnar, Left
    use Artery, Ulnar, Right

Posterior vagal trunk
    use Nerve, Vagus

PPN (peripheral parenteral nutrition)
    see Introduction of Nutritional Substance

Preauricular lymph node
    use Lymphatic, Head

Precava
    use Vena Cava, Superior

PRECICE intramedullary limb lengthening system
    use Internal Fixation Device, Intramedullary Limb Lengthening in 0PH
    use Internal Fixation Device, Intramedullary Limb Lengthening in 0QH

Prepatellar bursa
    use Bursa and Ligament, Knee, Left
    use Bursa and Ligament, Knee, Right

Preputiotomy
    see Drainage, Male Reproductive System 0V9

Pressure support ventilation
    see Performance, Respiratory 5A19

PRESTIGE® Cervical Disc
    use Synthetic Substitute

Pretracheal fascia
    use Subcutaneous Tissue and Fascia, Neck, Left
    use Subcutaneous Tissue and Fascia, Neck, Right

Prevertebral fascia
    use Subcutaneous Tissue and Fascia, Neck, Left
    use Subcutaneous Tissue and Fascia, Neck, Right

PrimeAdvanced neurostimulator (SureScan)(MRI Safe)
    use Stimulator Generator, Multiple Array in 0JH

Princeps pollicis artery
    use Artery, Hand, Left
    use Artery, Hand, Right

Probing, duct
    Diagnostic
        see Inspection
    Dilation
        see Dilation

PROCEED™ Ventral Patch
    use Synthetic Substitute

Procerus muscle
    use Muscle, Facial

Proctectomy
    see Excision, Rectum 0DBP
    see Resection, Rectum 0DTP

Proctoclysis
    see Introduction of substance in or on, Gastrointestinal Tract, Lower 3E0H

Proctocolectomy
    see Excision, Gastrointestinal System 0DB
    see Resection, Gastrointestinal System 0DT

Proctocolpoplasty
    see Repair, Gastrointestinal System 0DQ
    see Supplement, Gastrointestinal System 0DU

Proctoperineoplasty
    see Repair, Gastrointestinal System 0DQ
    see Supplement, Gastrointestinal System 0DU

Proctoperineorrhaphy
    see Repair, Gastrointestinal System 0DQ

Proctopexy
    see Repair, Rectum 0DQP
    see Reposition, Rectum 0DSP

Proctoplasty
    see Repair, Rectum 0DQP
    see Supplement, Rectum 0DUP

Proctorrhaphy
    see Repair, Rectum 0DQP

Proctoscopy 0DJD8ZZ

Proctosigmoidectomy
    see Excision, Gastrointestinal System 0DB
    see Resection, Gastrointestinal System 0DT

Proctosigmoidoscopy 0DJD8ZZ

Proctostomy
    see Drainage, Rectum 0D9P

Proctotomy
    see Drainage, Rectum 0D9P

Prodisc-C
    use Synthetic Substitute

Prodisc-L
    use Synthetic Substitute

Production, atrial septal defect
    see Excision, Septum, Atrial 02B5

Profunda brachii
    use Artery, Brachial, Left
    use Artery, Brachial, Right

Profunda femoris (deep femoral) vein
    use Vein, Femoral, Left
    use Vein, Femoral, Right

PROLENE Polypropylene Hernia System (PHS)
    use Synthetic Substitute

Prolonged intermittent renal replacement therapy (PIRRT) 5A1D80Z

Pronator quadratus muscle
    use Muscle, Lower Arm and Wrist, Left
    use Muscle, Lower Arm and Wrist, Right

Pronator teres muscle
    use Muscle, Lower Arm and Wrist, Left
    use Muscle, Lower Arm and Wrist, Right

Prostatectomy
    see Excision, Prostate 0VB0
    see Resection, Prostate 0VT0

Prostatic urethra
    use Urethra

Prostatomy, prostatotomy
    see Drainage, Prostate 0V90

Protecta XT CRT-D
    use Cardiac Resynchronization Defibrillator Pulse Generator in 0JH

Protecta XT DR (XT VR)
    use Defibrillator Generator in 0JH

Protégé® RX Carotid Stent System
    use Intraluminal Device

Proximal radioulnar joint
    use Joint, Elbow, Left
    use Joint, Elbow, Right

Psoas muscle
    use Muscle, Hip, Left
    use Muscle, Hip, Right

PSV (pressure support ventilation)
    see Performance, Respiratory 5A19

Psychoanalysis GZ54ZZZ

Psychological Tests
    Cognitive Status GZ14ZZZ
    Developmental GZ10ZZZ
    Intellectual and Psychoeducational GZ12ZZZ
    Neurobehavioral Status GZ14ZZZ
    Neuropsychological GZ13ZZZ
    Personality and Behavioral GZ11ZZZ

Psychotherapy
    Family, Mental Health Services GZ72ZZZ
    Group
        GZHZZZZ
        Mental Health Services GZHZZZZ
    Individual
        see Psychotherapy, Individual, Mental Health Services
        for substance abuse
        12-Step HZ53ZZZ
        Behavioral HZ51ZZZ
        Cognitive HZ50ZZZ
        Cognitive-Behavioral HZ52ZZZ
        Confrontational HZ58ZZZ
        Interactive HZ55ZZZ
        Interpersonal HZ54ZZZ
        Motivational Enhancement HZ57ZZZ
        Psychoanalysis HZ5BZZZ
        Psychodynamic HZ5CZZZ
        Psychoeducation HZ56ZZZ
        Psychophysiological HZ5DZZZ
        Supportive HZ59ZZZ
        Mental Health Services
            Behavioral GZ51ZZZ
            Cognitive GZ52ZZZ
            Cognitive-Behavioral GZ58ZZZ
            Interactive GZ50ZZZ
            Interpersonal GZ53ZZZ
            Psychoanalysis GZ54ZZZ
            Psychodynamic GZ55ZZZ
            Psychophysiological GZ59ZZZ
            Supportive GZ56ZZZ

PTCA (percutaneous transluminal coronary angioplasty)
    see Dilation, Heart and Great Vessels 027

Pterygoid muscle
    use Muscle, Head

Pterygoid process
    use Bone, Sphenoid

Pterygopalatine (sphenopalatine) ganglion
    use Nerve, Head and Neck Sympathetic

Pubis
use Bone, Pelvic, Left
use Bone, Pelvic, Right
Pubofemoral ligament
use Bursa and Ligament, Hip, Left
use Bursa and Ligament, Hip, Right
Pudendal nerve
use Nerve, Sacral Plexus
Pull-through, laparoscopic-assisted transanal
see Excision, Gastrointestinal System 0DB
see Resection, Gastrointestinal System 0DT
Pull-through, rectal
see Resection, Rectum 0DTP
Pulmoaortic canal
use Artery, Pulmonary, Left
Pulmonary annulus
use Valve, Pulmonary
Pulmonary artery wedge monitoring
see Monitoring, Arterial 4A13
Pulmonary plexus
use Nerve, Thoracic Sympathetic
use Nerve, Vagus
Pulmonic valve
use Valve, Pulmonary
Pulpectomy
see Excision, Mouth and Throat 0CB
Pulverization
see Fragmentation
Pulvinar
use Thalamus
Pump reservoir
use Infusion Device, Pump in Subcutaneous Tissue and Fascia
Punch biopsy
see Excision with qualifier Diagnostic
Puncture
see Drainage
Puncture, lumbar
see Drainage, Spinal Canal 009U
Pyelography
see Fluoroscopy, Urinary System BT1
see Plain Radiography, Urinary System BT0
Pyeloileostomy, urinary diversion
see Bypass, Urinary System 0T1
Pyeloplasty
see Repair, Urinary System 0TQ
see Replacement, Urinary System 0TR
see Supplement, Urinary System 0TU
Pyeloplasty, dismembered
see Repair, Kidney Pelvis
Pyelorrhaphy
see Repair, Urinary System 0TQ
Pyeloscopy 0TJ58ZZ
Pyelostomy
see Drainage, Urinary System 0T9
see Bypass, Urinary System 0T1
Pyelotomy
see Drainage, Urinary System 0T9
Pylorectomy
see Excision, Stomach, Pylorus 0DB7
see Resection, Stomach, Pylorus 0DT7
Pyloric antrum
use Stomach, Pylorus
Pyloric canal
use Stomach, Pylorus
Pyloric sphincter
use Stomach, Pylorus
Pylorodiosis
see Dilation, Stomach, Pylorus 0D77

Pylorogastrectomy
see Excision, Gastrointestinal System 0DB
see Resection, Gastrointestinal System 0DT
Pyloroplasty
see Repair, Stomach, Pylorus 0DQ7
see Supplement, Stomach, Pylorus 0DU7
Pyloroscopy 0DJ68ZZ
Pylorotomy
see Drainage, Stomach, Pylorus 0D97
Pyramidalis muscle
use Muscle, Abdomen, Left
use Muscle, Abdomen, Right

Q

Quadrangular cartilage
use Septum, Nasal
Quadrant resection of breast
see Excision, Skin and Breast 0HB
Quadrate lobe
use Liver
Quadrate femoris muscle
use Muscle, Hip, Left
use Muscle, Hip, Right
Quadratus lumborum muscle
use Muscle, Trunk, Left
use Muscle, Trunk, Right
Quadratus plantae muscle
use Muscle, Foot, Left
use Muscle, Foot, Right
Quadriceps (femoris)
use Muscle, Upper Leg, Left
use Muscle, Upper Leg, Right
Quarantine 8E0ZXY6

R

Radial collateral carpal ligament
use Bursa and Ligament, Wrist, Left
use Bursa and Ligament, Wrist, Right
Radial collateral ligament
use Bursa and Ligament, Elbow, Left
use Bursa and Ligament, Elbow, Right
Radial notch
use Ulna, Left
use Ulna, Right
Radial recurrent artery
use Artery, Radial, Left
use Artery, Radial, Right
Radial vein
use Vein, Brachial, Left
use Vein, Brachial, Right
Radialis indicis
use Artery, Hand, Left
use Artery, Hand, Right
Radiation Therapy
see Beam Radiation
see Brachytherapy
see Stereotactic Radiosurgery
Radiation treatment
see Radiation Therapy
Radiocarpal joint
use Joint, Wrist, Left
use Joint, Wrist, Right
Radiocarpal ligament
use Bursa and Ligament, Wrist, Left
use Bursa and Ligament, Wrist, Right
Radiography
see Plain Radiography

Radiology, analog
see Plain Radiography
Radiology, diagnostic
see Imaging, Diagnostic
Radioulnar ligament
use Bursa and Ligament, Wrist, Left
use Bursa and Ligament, Wrist, Right
Range of motion testing
see Motor Function Assessment, Rehabilitation F01
REALIZE® Adjustable Gastric Band
use Extraluminal Device
Reattachment
Abdominal Wall 0WMF0ZZ
Ampulla of Vater 0FMC
Ankle Region
    Left 0YML0ZZ
    Right 0YMK0ZZ
Arm
    Lower
        Left 0XMF0ZZ
        Right 0XMD0ZZ
    Upper
        Left 0XM90ZZ
        Right 0XM80ZZ
Axilla
    Left 0XM50ZZ
    Right 0XM40ZZ
Back
    Lower 0WML0ZZ
    Upper 0WMK0ZZ
Bladder 0TMB
Bladder Neck 0TMC
Breast
    Bilateral 0HMVXZZ
    Left 0HMUXZZ
    Right 0HMTXZZ
Bronchus
    Lingula 0BM90ZZ
    Lower Lobe
        Left 0BMB0ZZ
        Right 0BM60ZZ
    Main
        Left 0BM70ZZ
        Right 0BM30ZZ
    Middle Lobe, Right 0BM50ZZ
    Upper Lobe
        Left 0BM80ZZ
        Right 0BM40ZZ
Bursa and Ligament
    Abdomen
        Left 0MMJ
        Right 0MMH
    Ankle
        Left 0MMR
        Right 0MMQ
    Elbow
        Left 0MM4
        Right 0MM3
    Foot
        Left 0MMT
        Right 0MMS
    Hand
        Left 0MM8
        Right 0MM7
    Head and Neck 0MM0
    Hip
        Left 0MMM
        Right 0MML
    Knee
        Left 0MMP
        Right 0MMN
    Lower Extremity
        Left 0MMW
        Right 0MMV
    Perineum 0MMK
    Rib(s) 0MMG

Reattachment *(continued)*
Bursa and Ligament *(continued)*
    Shoulder
        Left 0MM2
        Right 0MM1
    Spine
        Lower 0MMD
        Upper 0MMC
    Sternum 0MMF
    Upper Extremity
        Left 0MMB
        Right 0MM9
    Wrist
        Left 0MM6
        Right 0MM5
Buttock
    Left 0YM10ZZ
    Right 0YM00ZZ
Carina 0BM20ZZ
Cecum 0DMH
Cervix 0UMC
Chest Wall 0WM80ZZ
Clitoris 0UMJXZZ
Colon
    Ascending 0DMK
    Descending 0DMM
    Sigmoid 0DMN
    Transverse 0DML
Cord
    Bilateral 0VMH
    Left 0VMG
    Right 0VMF
Cul-de-sac 0UMF
Diaphragm 0BMT0ZZ
Duct
    Common Bile 0FM9
    Cystic 0FM8
    Hepatic
        Common 0FM7
        Left 0FM6
        Right 0FM5
    Pancreatic 0FMD
        Accessory 0FMF
Duodenum 0DM9
Ear
    Left 09M1XZZ
    Right 09M0XZZ
Elbow Region
    Left 0XMC0ZZ
    Right 0XMB0ZZ
Esophagus 0DM5
Extremity
    Lower
        Left 0YMB0ZZ
        Right 0YM90ZZ
    Upper
        Left 0XM70ZZ
        Right 0XM60ZZ
Eyelid
    Lower
        Left 08MRXZZ
        Right 08MQXZZ
    Upper
        Left 08MPXZZ
        Right 08MNXZZ
Face 0WM20ZZ
Fallopian Tube
    Left 0UM6
    Right 0UM5
Fallopian Tubes, Bilateral 0UM7
Femoral Region
    Left 0YM80ZZ
    Right 0YM70ZZ
Finger
    Index
        Left 0XMP0ZZ
        Right 0XMN0ZZ
    Little
        Left 0XMW0ZZ
        Right 0XMV0ZZ

Reattachment *(continued)*
Finger *(continued)*
  Middle
    Left 0XMR0ZZ
    Right 0XMQ0ZZ
  Ring
    Left 0XMT0ZZ
    Right 0XMS0ZZ
Foot
  Left 0YMN0ZZ
  Right 0YMM0ZZ
Forequarter
  Left 0XM10ZZ
  Right 0XM00ZZ
Gallbladder 0FM4
Gland
  Left 0GM2
  Right 0GM3
Hand
  Left 0XMK0ZZ
  Right 0XMJ0ZZ
Hindquarter
  Bilateral 0YM40ZZ
  Left 0YM30ZZ
  Right 0YM20ZZ
Hymen 0UMK
Ileum 0DMB
Inguinal Region
  Left 0YM60ZZ
  Right 0YM50ZZ
Intestine
  Large 0DME
    Left 0DMG
    Right 0DMF
  Small 0DM8
Jaw
  Lower 0WM50ZZ
  Upper 0WM40ZZ
Jejunum 0DMA
Kidney
  Left 0TM1
  Right 0TM0
Kidney Pelvis
  Left 0TM4
  Right 0TM3
Kidneys, Bilateral
  0TM2
Knee Region
  Left 0YMG0ZZ
  Right 0YMF0ZZ
Leg
  Lower
    Left 0YMJ0ZZ
    Right 0YMH0ZZ
  Upper
    Left 0YMD0ZZ
    Right 0YMC0ZZ
Lip
  Lower 0CM10ZZ
  Upper 0CM00ZZ
Liver 0FM0
  Left Lobe 0FM2
  Right Lobe 0FM1
Lung
  Left 0BML0ZZ
  Lower Lobe
    Left 0BMJ0ZZ
    Right 0BMF0ZZ
  Middle Lobe, Right
    0BMD0ZZ
  Right 0BMK0ZZ
  Upper Lobe
    Left 0BMG0ZZ
    Right 0BMC0ZZ
Lung Lingula 0BMH0ZZ
Muscle
  Abdomen
    Left 0KML
    Right 0KMK
  Facial 0KM1

Reattachment *(continued)*
Muscle *(continued)*
  Foot
    Left 0KMW
    Right 0KMV
  Hand
    Left 0KMD
    Right 0KMC
  Head 0KM0
  Hip
    Left 0KMP
    Right 0KMN
  Lower Arm and Wrist
    Left 0KMB
    Right 0KM9
  Lower Leg
    Left 0KMT
    Right 0KMS
  Neck
    Left 0KM3
    Right 0KM2
  Perineum 0KMM
  Shoulder
    Left 0KM6
    Right 0KM5
  Thorax
    Left 0KMJ
    Right 0KMH
  Tongue, Palate, Pharynx 0KM4
  Trunk
    Left 0KMG
    Right 0KMF
  Upper Arm
    Left 0KM8
    Right 0KM7
  Upper Leg
    Left 0KMR
    Right 0KMQ
Nasal Mucosa and Soft Tissue
  09MKXZZ
Neck 0WM60ZZ
Nipple
  Left 0HMXXZZ
  Right 0HMWXZZ
Ovary
  Bilateral 0UM2
  Left 0UM1
  Right 0UM0
Palate, Soft 0CM30ZZ
Pancreas 0FMG
Parathyroid Gland
  0GMR
  Inferior
    Left 0GMP
    Right 0GMN
  Multiple 0GMQ
  Superior
    Left 0GMM
    Right 0GML
Penis 0VMSXZZ
Perineum
  Female 0WMN0ZZ
  Male 0WMM0ZZ
Rectum 0DMP
Scrotum 0VM5XZZ
Shoulder Region
  Left 0XM30ZZ
  Right 0XM20ZZ
Skin
  Abdomen 0HM7XZZ
  Back 0HM6XZZ
  Buttock 0HM8XZZ
  Chest 0HM5XZZ
  Ear
    Left 0HM3XZZ
    Right 0HM2XZZ
  Face 0HM1XZZ
  Foot
    Left 0HMNXZZ
    Right 0HMMXZZ

Reattachment *(continued)*
Skin *(continued)*
  Hand
    Left 0HMGXZZ
    Right 0HMFXZZ
  Inguinal 0HMAXZZ
  Lower Arm
    Left 0HMEXZZ
    Right 0HMDXZZ
  Lower Leg
    Left 0HMLXZZ
    Right 0HMKXZZ
  Neck 0HM4XZZ
  Perineum 0HM9XZZ
  Scalp 0HM0XZZ
  Upper Arm
    Left 0HMCXZZ
    Right 0HMBXZZ
  Upper Leg
    Left 0HMJXZZ
    Right 0HMHXZZ
Stomach 0DM6
Tendon
  Abdomen
    Left 0LMG
    Right 0LMF
  Ankle
    Left 0LMT
    Right 0LMS
  Foot
    Left 0LMW
    Right 0LMV
  Hand
    Left 0LM8
    Right 0LM7
  Head and Neck
    0LM0
  Hip
    Left 0LMK
    Right 0LMJ
  Knee
    Left 0LMR
    Right 0LMQ
  Lower Arm and
  Wrist
    Left 0LM6
    Right 0LM5
  Lower Leg
    Left 0LMP
    Right 0LMN
  Perineum 0LMH
  Shoulder
    Left 0LM2
    Right 0LM1
  Thorax
    Left 0LMD
    Right 0LMC
  Trunk
    Left 0LMB
    Right 0LM9
  Upper Arm
    Left 0LM4
    Right 0LM3
  Upper Leg
    Left 0LMM
    Right 0LML
Testis
  Bilateral 0VMC
  Left 0VMB
  Right 0VM9
Thumb
  Left 0XMM0ZZ
  Right 0XML0ZZ
Thyroid Gland
  Left Lobe 0GMG
  Right Lobe 0GMH
Toe
  1st
    Left 0YMQ0ZZ
    Right 0YMP0ZZ

Reattachment *(continued)*
Toe *(continued)*
  2nd
    Left 0YMS0ZZ
    Right 0YMR0ZZ
  3rd
    Left 0YMU0ZZ
    Right 0YMT0ZZ
  4th
    Left 0YMW0ZZ
    Right 0YMV0ZZ
  5th
    Left 0YMY0ZZ
    Right 0YMX0ZZ
Tongue 0CM70ZZ
Tooth
  Lower 0CMX
  Upper 0CMW
Trachea 0BM10ZZ
Tunica Vaginalis
  Left 0VM7
  Right 0VM6
Ureter
  Left 0TM7
  Right 0TM6
Ureters, Bilateral 0TM8
Urethra 0TMD
Uterine Supporting Structure
  0UM4
Uterus 0UM9
Uvula 0CMN0ZZ
Vagina 0UMG
Vulva 0UMMXZZ
Wrist Region
  Left 0XMH0ZZ
  Right 0XMG0ZZ
REBOA (resuscitative
  endovascular balloon
  occlusion of the aorta)
  02LW3DJ
  04L03DJ
Rebound HRD® (Hernia Repair
  Device)
  use Synthetic Substitute
RECELL® cell suspension
  autograft
  see Replacement, Skin and Breast
  0HR
Recession
  see Repair
  see Reposition
Reclosure, disrupted abdominal wall
  0WQFXZZ
Reconstruction
  see Repair
  see Replacement
  see Supplement
Rectectomy
  see Excision, Rectum 0DBP
  see Resection, Rectum 0DTP
Rectocele repair
  see Repair, Subcutaneous Tissue
  and Fascia, Pelvic Region
  0JQC
Rectopexy
  see Repair, Gastrointestinal System
  0DQ
  see Reposition, Gastrointestinal
  System 0DS
Rectoplasty
  see Repair, Gastrointestinal System
  0DQ
  see Supplement, Gastrointestinal
  System 0DU
Rectorrhaphy
  see Repair, Gastrointestinal System
  0DQ
Rectoscopy 0DJD8ZZ
Rectosigmoid junction
  use Colon, Sigmoid

Rectosigmoidectomy
  see Excision, Gastrointestinal
    System 0DB
  see Resection, Gastrointestinal
    System 0DT
Rectostomy
  see Drainage, Rectum 0D9P
Rectotomy
  see Drainage, Rectum 0D9P
Rectus abdominis muscle
  use Muscle, Abdomen, Left
  use Muscle, Abdomen, Right
Rectus femoris muscle
  use Muscle, Upper Leg,
    Left
  use Muscle, Upper Leg,
    Right
Recurrent laryngeal nerve
  use Nerve, Vagus
Reduction
  Dislocation
    see Reposition
  Fracture
    see Reposition
  Intussusception, intestinal
    see Reposition, Gastrointestinal
      System 0DS
  Mammoplasty
    see Excision, Skin and Breast
      0HB
  Prolapse
    see Reposition
  Torsion
    see Reposition
  Volvulus, gastrointestinal
    see Reposition, Gastrointestinal
      System 0DS
Refusion
  see Fusion
Rehabilitation
  see Activities of Daily Living
    Assessment, Rehabilitation
    F02
  see Activities of Daily Living
    Treatment, Rehabilitation
    F08
  see Caregiver Training,
    Rehabilitation F0F
  see Cochlear Implant Treatment,
    Rehabilitation F0B
  see Device Fitting, Rehabilitation
    F0D
  see Hearing Treatment,
    Rehabilitation F09
  see Motor Function Assessment,
    Rehabilitation F01
  see Motor Treatment, Rehabilitation
    F07
  see Speech Assessment,
    Rehabilitation F00
  see Speech Treatment,
    Rehabilitation F06
  see Vestibular Treatment,
    Rehabilitation F0C
Reimplantation
  see Reattachment
  see Reposition
  see Transfer
Reinforcement
  see Repair
  see Supplement
Relaxation, scar tissue
  see Release
Release
  Acetabulum
    Left 0QN5
    Right 0QN4
  Adenoids 0CNQ
  Ampulla of Vater 0FNC
  Anal Sphincter 0DNR

Release *(continued)*
  Anterior Chamber
    Left 08N33ZZ
    Right 08N23ZZ
  Anus 0DNQ
  Aorta
    Abdominal 04N0
    Thoracic
      Ascending/Arch
      02NX
      Descending 02NW
  Aortic Body 0GND
  Appendix 0DNJ
  Artery
    Anterior Tibial
      Left 04NQ
      Right 04NP
    Axillary
      Left 03N6
      Right 03N5
    Brachial
      Left 03N8
      Right 03N7
    Celiac 04N1
    Colic
      Left 04N7
      Middle 04N8
      Right 04N6
    Common Carotid
      Left 03NJ
      Right 03NH
    Common Iliac
      Left 04ND
      Right 04NC
    Coronary
      Four or More Arteries 02N3
      One Artery 02N0
      Three Arteries 02N2
      Two Arteries 02N1
    External Carotid
      Left 03NN
      Right 03NM
    External Iliac
      Left 04NJ
      Right 04NH
    Face 03NR
    Femoral
      Left 04NL
      Right 04NK
    Foot
      Left 04NW
      Right 04NV
    Gastric 04N2
    Hand
      Left 03NF
      Right 03ND
    Hepatic 04N3
    Inferior Mesenteric
      04NB
    Innominate 03N2
    Internal Carotid
      Left 03NL
      Right 03NK
    Internal Iliac
      Left 04NF
      Right 04NE
    Internal Mammary
      Left 03N1
      Right 03N0
    Intracranial 03NG
    Lower 04NY
    Peroneal
      Left 04NU
      Right 04NT
    Popliteal
      Left 04NN
      Right 04NM
    Posterior Tibial
      Left 04NS
      Right 04NR

Release *(continued)*
  Artery *(continued)*
    Pulmonary
      Left 02NR
      Right 02NQ
    Pulmonary Trunk
      02NP
    Radial
      Left 03NC
      Right 03NB
    Renal
      Left 04NA
      Right 04N9
    Splenic 04N4
    Subclavian
      Left 03N4
      Right 03N3
    Superior Mesenteric 04N5
    Temporal
      Left 03NT
      Right 03NS
    Thyroid
      Left 03NV
      Right 03NU
    Ulnar
      Left 03NA
      Right 03N9
    Upper 03NY
    Vertebral
      Left 03NQ
      Right 03NP
  Atrium
    Left 02N7
    Right 02N6
  Auditory Ossicle
    Left 09NA
    Right 09N9
  Basal Ganglia 00N8
  Bladder 0TNB
  Bladder Neck 0TNC
  Bone
    Ethmoid
      Left 0NNG
      Right 0NNF
    Frontal 0NN1
    Hyoid 0NNX
    Lacrimal
      Left 0NNJ
      Right 0NNH
    Nasal 0NNB
    Occipital 0NN7
    Palatine
      Left 0NNL
      Right 0NNK
    Parietal
      Left 0NN4
      Right 0NN3
    Pelvic
      Left 0QN3
      Right 0QN2
    Sphenoid 0NNC
    Temporal
      Left 0NN6
      Right 0NN5
    Zygomatic
      Left 0NNN
      Right 0NNM
  Brain 00N0
  Breast
    Bilateral 0HNV
    Left 0HNU
    Right 0HNT
  Bronchus
    Lingula 0BN9
    Lower Lobe
      Left 0BNB
      Right 0BN6
    Main
      Left 0BN7
      Right 0BN3

Release *(continued)*
  Bronchus *(continued)*
    Middle Lobe, Right
      0BN5
    Upper Lobe
      Left 0BN8
      Right 0BN4
  Buccal Mucosa 0CN4
  Bursa and Ligament
    Abdomen
      Left 0MNJ
      Right 0MNH
    Ankle
      Left 0MNR
      Right 0MNQ
    Elbow
      Left 0MN4
      Right 0MN3
    Foot
      Left 0MNT
      Right 0MNS
    Hand
      Left 0MN8
      Right 0MN7
    Head and Neck 0MN0
    Hip
      Left 0MNM
      Right 0MNL
    Knee
      Left 0MNP
      Right 0MNN
    Lower Extremity
      Left 0MNW
      Right 0MNV
    Perineum 0MNK
    Rib(s) 0MNG
    Shoulder
      Left 0MN2
      Right 0MN1
    Spine
      Lower 0MND
      Upper 0MNC
    Sternum 0MNF
    Upper Extremity
      Left 0MNB
      Right 0MN9
    Wrist
      Left 0MN6
      Right 0MN5
  Carina 0BN2
  Carotid Bodies, Bilateral 0GN8
  Carotid Body
    Left 0GN6
    Right 0GN7
  Carpal
    Left 0PNN
    Right 0PNM
  Cecum 0DNH
  Cerebellum 00NC
  Cerebral Hemisphere 00N7
  Cerebral Meninges 00N1
  Cerebral Ventricle 00N6
  Cervix 0UNC
  Chordae Tendineae 02N9
  Choroid
    Left 08NB
    Right 08NA
  Cisterna Chyli 07NL
  Clavicle
    Left 0PNB
    Right 0PN9
  Clitoris 0UNJ
  Coccygeal Glomus 0GNB
  Coccyx 0QNS
  Colon
    Ascending 0DNK
    Descending 0DNM
    Sigmoid 0DNN
    Transverse 0DNL
  Conduction Mechanism 02N8

Muscle (continued)
Upper Arm
Left 0KN8
Right 0KN7
Upper Leg
Left 0KNR
Right 0KNQ
Myocardial Bridge
see Release, Artery,
Coronary
Nasal Mucosa and Soft Tissue
09NK
Nasopharynx 09NN
Nerve
Abdominal Sympathetic
01NM
Abducens 00NL
Accessory 00NR
Acoustic 00NN
Brachial Plexus 01N3
Cervical 01N1
Cervical Plexus 01N0
Facial 00NM
Femoral 01ND
Glossopharyngeal 00NP
Head and Neck Sympathetic
01NK
Hypoglossal 00NS
Lumbar 01NB
Lumbar Plexus 01N9
Lumbar Sympathetic 01NN
Lumbosacral Plexus 01NA
Median 01N5
Oculomotor 00NH
Olfactory 00NF
Optic 00NG
Peroneal 01NH
Phrenic 01N2
Pudendal 01NC
Radial 01N6
Sacral 01NR
Sacral Plexus 01NQ
Sacral Sympathetic 01NP
Sciatic 01NF
Thoracic 01N8
Thoracic Sympathetic
01NL
Tibial 01NG
Trigeminal 00NK
Trochlear 00NJ
Ulnar 01N4
Vagus 00NQ
Nipple
Left 0HNX
Right 0HNW
Nose 09NKZZ
Omentum 0DNU
Orbit
Left 0NNQ
Right 0NNP
Ovary
Bilateral 0UN2
Left 0UN1
Right 0UN0
Palate
Hard 0CN2
Soft 0CN3
Pancreas 0FNG
Para-aortic Body 0GN9
Paraganglion Extremity 0GNF
Parathyroid Gland 0GNR
Inferior
Left 0GNP
Right 0GNN
Multiple 0GNQ
Superior
Left 0GNM
Right 0GNL

Patella
Left 0QNF
Right 0QND
Penis 0VNSZZ
Pericardium 02NN
Peritoneum 0DNW
Phalanx
Finger
Left 0PNV
Right 0PNT
Thumb
Left 0PNS
Right 0PNR
Toe
Left 0QNR
Right 0QNQ
Pharynx 0CNM
Pineal Body 0GN1
Pleura
Left 0BNP
Right 0BNN
Pons 00NB
Prepuce 0VNT
Prostate 0VN0
Radius
Left 0PNJ
Right 0PNH
Rectum 0DNP
Retina
Left 08NF3ZZ
Right 08NE3ZZ
Retinal Vessel
Left 08NH3ZZ
Right 08NG3ZZ
Ribs
1 to 2 0PN1
3 or More 0PN2
Sacrum 0QN1
Scapula
Left 0PN6
Right 0PN5
Sclera
Left 08N7XZZ
Right 08N6XZZ
Scrotum 0VN5
Septum
Atrial 02N5
Nasal 09NM
Ventricular 02NM
Sinus
Accessory 09NP
Ethmoid
Left 09NV
Right 09NU
Frontal
Left 09NT
Right 09NS
Mastoid
Left 09NC
Right 09NB
Maxillary
Left 09NR
Right 09NQ
Sphenoid
Left 09NX
Right 09NW
Skin
Abdomen 0HN7XZZ
Back 0HN6XZZ
Buttock 0HN8XZZ
Chest 0HN5XZZ
Ear
Left 0HN3XZZ
Right 0HN2XZZ
Face 0HN1XZZ
Foot
Left 0HNNXZZ
Right 0HNMXZZ

Skin (continued)
Hand
Left 0HNGXZZ
Right 0HNFXZZ
Inguinal 0HNAXZZ
Lower Arm
Left 0HNEXZZ
Right 0HNDXZZ
Lower Leg
Left 0HNLXZZ
Right 0HNKXZZ
Neck 0HN4XZZ
Perineum 0HN9XZZ
Scalp 0HN0XZZ
Upper Arm
Left 0HNCXZZ
Right 0HNBXZZ
Upper Leg
Left 0HNJXZZ
Right 0HNHXZZ
Spinal Cord
Cervical 00NW
Lumbar 00NY
Thoracic 00NX
Spinal Meninges 00NT
Spleen 07NP
Sternum 0PN0
Stomach 0DN6
Pylorus 0DN7
Subcutaneous Tissue and
Fascia
Abdomen 0JN8
Back 0JN7
Buttock 0JN9
Chest 0JN6
Face 0JN1
Foot
Left 0JNR
Right 0JNQ
Hand
Left 0JNK
Right 0JNJ
Lower Arm
Left 0JNH
Right 0JNG
Lower Leg
Left 0JNP
Right 0JNN
Neck
Left 0JN5
Right 0JN4
Pelvic Region
0JNC
Perineum 0JNB
Scalp 0JN0
Upper Arm
Left 0JNF
Right 0JND
Upper Leg
Left 0JNM
Right 0JNL
Tarsal
Left 0QNM
Right 0QNL
Tendon
Abdomen
Left 0LNG
Right 0LNF
Ankle
Left 0LNT
Right 0LNS
Foot
Left 0LNW
Right 0LNV
Hand
Left 0LN8
Right 0LN7
Head and Neck 0LN0

Tendon (continued)
Hip
Left 0LNK
Right 0LNJ
Knee
Left 0LNR
Right 0LNQ
Lower Arm and
Wrist
Left 0LN6
Right 0LN5
Lower Leg
Left 0LNP
Right 0LNN
Perineum 0LNH
Shoulder
Left 0LN2
Right 0LN1
Thorax
Left 0LND
Right 0LNC
Trunk
Left 0LNB
Right 0LN9
Upper Arm
Left 0LN4
Right 0LN3
Upper Leg
Left 0LNM
Right 0LNL
Testis
Bilateral 0VNC
Left 0VNB
Right 0VN9
Thalamus 00N9
Thymus 07NM
Thyroid Gland
0GNK
Left Lobe 0GNG
Right Lobe
0GNH
Tibia
Left 0QNH
Right 0QNG
Toe Nail 0HNRXZZ
Tongue 0CN7
Tonsils 0CNP
Tooth
Lower 0CNX
Upper 0CNW
Trachea 0BN1
Tunica Vaginalis
Left 0VN7
Right 0VN6
Turbinate, Nasal 09NL
Tympanic Membrane
Left 09N8
Right 09N7
Ulna
Left 0PNL
Right 0PNK
Ureter
Left 0TN7
Right 0TN6
Urethra 0TND
Uterine Supporting Structure 0UN4
Uterus 0UN9
Uvula 0CNN
Vagina 0UNG
Valve
Aortic 02NF
Mitral 02NG
Pulmonary 02NH
Tricuspid 02NJ
Vas Deferens
Bilateral 0VNQ
Left 0VNP
Right 0VNN

Release *(continued)*

Vein
Axillary
Left 05N8
Right 05N7
Azygos 05N0
Basilic
Left 05NC
Right 05NB
Brachial
Left 05NA
Right 05N9
Cephalic
Left 05NF
Right 05ND
Colic 06N7
Common Iliac
Left 06ND
Right 06NC
Coronary 02N4
Esophageal 06N3
External Iliac
Left 06NG
Right 06NF
External Jugular
Left 05NQ
Right 05NP
Face
Left 05NV
Right 05NT
Femoral
Left 06NN
Right 06NM
Foot
Left 06NV
Right 06NT
Gastric 06N2
Hand
Left 05NH
Right 05NG
Hemiazygos 05N1
Hepatic 06N4
Hypogastric
Left 06NJ
Right 06NH
Inferior Mesenteric 06N6
Innominate
Left 05N4
Right 05N3
Internal Jugular
Left 05NN
Right 05NM
Intracranial 05NL
Lower 06NY
Portal 06N8
Pulmonary
Left 02NT
Right 02NS
Renal
Left 06NB
Right 06N9
Saphenous
Left 06NQ
Right 06NP
Splenic 06N1
Subclavian
Left 05N6
Right 05N5
Superior Mesenteric 06N5
Upper 05NY
Vertebral
Left 05NS
Right 05NR
Vena Cava
Inferior 06N0
Superior 02NV
Ventricle
Left 02NL
Right 02NK

Release *(continued)*

Vertebra
Cervical 0PN3
Lumbar 0QN0
Thoracic 0PN4
Vesicle
Bilateral 0VN3
Left 0VN2
Right 0VN1
Vitreous
Left 08N53ZZ
Right 08N43ZZ
Vocal Cord
Left 0CNV
Right 0CNT
Vulva 0UNM

Relocation
see Reposition

Remdesivir Anti-infective XW0

Removal
Abdominal Wall 2W53X
Anorectal 2Y53X5
Arm
Lower
Left 2W5DX
Right 2W5CX
Upper
Left 2W5BX
Right 2W5AX
Back 2W55X
Chest Wall 2W54X
Ear 2Y52X5Z
Extremity
Lower
Left 2W5MX
Right 2W5LX
Upper
Left 2W59X
Right 2W58X
Face 2W51X
Finger
Left 2W5KX
Right 2W5JX
Foot
Left 2W5TX
Right 2W5SX
Genital Tract, Female
2Y54X5Z
Hand
Left 2W5FX
Right 2W5EX
Head 2W50X
Inguinal Region
Left 2W57X
Right 2W56X
Leg
Lower
Left 2W5RX
Right 2W5QX
Upper
Left 2W5PX
Right 2W5NX
Mouth and Pharynx 2Y50X5Z
Nasal 2Y51X5Z
Neck 2W52X
Thumb
Left 2W5HX
Right 2W5GX
Toe
Left 2W5VX
Right 2W5UX
Urethra 2Y55X5Z

Removal of device from
Abdominal Wall 0WPF
Acetabulum
Left 0QP5
Right 0QP4
Anal Sphincter 0DPR
Anus 0DPQ

Removal of device from *(continued)*

Artery
Lower 04PY
Upper 03PY
Back
Lower 0WPL
Upper 0WPK
Bladder 0TPB
Bone
Facial 0NPW
Lower 0QPY
Nasal 0NPB
Pelvic
Left 0QP3
Right 0QP2
Upper 0PPY
Bone Marrow 07PT
Brain 00P0
Breast
Left 0HPU
Right 0HPT
Bursa and Ligament
Lower 0MPY
Upper 0MPX
Carpal
Left 0PPN
Right 0PPM
Cavity, Cranial 0WP1
Cerebral Ventricle 00P6
Chest Wall 0WP8
Cisterna Chyli 07PL
Clavicle
Left 0PPB
Right 0PP9
Coccyx 0QPS
Diaphragm 0BPT
Disc
Cervical Vertebral
0RP3
Cervicothoracic Vertebral
0RP5
Lumbar Vertebral 0SP2
Lumbosacral 0SP4
Thoracic Vertebral 0RP9
Thoracolumbar Vertebral 0RPB
Duct
Hepatobiliary 0FPB
Pancreatic 0FPD
Ear
Inner
Left 09PE
Right 09PD
Left 09PJ
Right 09PH
Epididymis and Spermatic Cord
0VPM
Esophagus 0DP5
Extremity
Lower
Left 0YPB
Right 0YP9
Upper
Left 0XP7
Right 0XP6
Eye
Left 08P1
Right 08P0
Face 0WP2
Fallopian Tube 0UP8
Femoral Shaft
Left 0QP9
Right 0QP8
Femur
Lower
Left 0QPC
Right 0QPB
Upper
Left 0QP7
Right 0QP6

Removal of device from *(continued)*

Fibula
Left 0QPK
Right 0QPJ
Finger Nail 0HPQX
Gallbladder 0FP4
Gastrointestinal Tract 0WPP
Genitourinary Tract 0WPR
Gland
Adrenal 0GP5
Endocrine 0GPS
Pituitary 0GP0
Salivary 0CPA
Glenoid Cavity
Left 0PP8
Right 0PP7
Great Vessel 02PY
Hair 0HPSX
Head 0WP0
Heart 02PA
Humeral Head
Left 0PPD
Right 0PPC
Humeral Shaft
Left 0PPG
Right 0PPF
Intestinal Tract
Lower 0DPD
Upper 0DP0
Jaw
Lower 0WP5
Upper 0WP4
Joint
Acromioclavicular
Left 0RPH
Right 0RPG
Ankle
Left 0SPG
Right 0SPF
Carpal
Left 0RPR
Right 0RPQ
Carpometacarpal
Left 0RPT
Right 0RPS
Cervical Vertebral 0RP1
Cervicothoracic Vertebral 0RP4
Coccygeal 0SP6
Elbow
Left 0RPM
Right 0RPL
Finger Phalangeal
Left 0RPX
Right 0RPW
Hip
Left 0SPB
Acetabular Surface 0SPE
Femoral Surface 0SPS
Right 0SP9
Acetabular Surface
0SPA
Femoral Surface 0SPR
Knee
Left 0SPD
Femoral Surface 0SPU
Tibial Surface 0SPW
Right 0SPC
Femoral Surface 0SPT
Tibial Surface 0SPV
Lumbar Vertebral 0SP0
Lumbosacral 0SP3
Metacarpophalangeal
Left 0RPV
Right 0RPU
Metatarsal-Phalangeal
Left 0SPN
Right 0SPM
Occipital-cervical 0RP0
Sacrococcygeal 0SP5

Removal of device from (continued)
Joint (continued)
  Sacroiliac
    Left 0SP8
    Right 0SP7
  Shoulder
    Left 0RPK
    Right 0RPJ
  Sternoclavicular
    Left 0RPF
    Right 0RPE
  Tarsal
    Left 0SPJ
    Right 0SPH
  Tarsometatarsal
    Left 0SPL
    Right 0SPK
  Temporomandibular
    Left 0RPD
    Right 0RPC
  Thoracic Vertebral 0RP6
  Thoracolumbar Vertebral
    0RPA
  Toe Phalangeal
    Left 0SPQ
    Right 0SPP
  Wrist
    Left 0RPP
    Right 0RPN
Kidney 0TP5
Larynx 0CPS
Lens
  Left 08PK3
  Right 08PJ3
Liver 0FP0
Lung
  Left 0BPL
  Right 0BPK
Lymphatic 07PN
  Thoracic Duct 07PK
Mediastinum 0WPC
Mesentery 0DPV
Metacarpal
  Left 0PPQ
  Right 0PPP
Metatarsal
  Left 0QPP
  Right 0QPN
Mouth and Throat 0CPY
Muscle
  Extraocular
    Left 08PM
    Right 08PL
  Lower 0KPY
  Upper 0KPX
Nasal Mucosa and Soft Tissue
  09PK
Neck 0WP6
Nerve
  Cranial 00PE
  Peripheral 01PY
Omentum 0DPU
Ovary 0UP3
Pancreas 0FPGZ
Parathyroid Gland 0GPR0
Patella
  Left 0QPF
  Right 0QPD
Pelvic Cavity 0WPJ
Penis 0VPS
Pericardial Cavity 0WPD
Perineum
  Female 0WPN
  Male 0WPM
Peritoneal Cavity 0WPG
Peritoneum 0DPW
Phalanx
  Finger
    Left 0PPV
    Right 0PPT

Removal of device from (continued)
Phalanx (continued)
  Thumb
    Left 0PPS
    Right 0PPR
  Toe
    Left 0QPR
    Right 0QPQ
Pineal Body 0GP10
Pleura 0BPQ
Pleural Cavity
  Left 0WPB
  Right 0WP9
Products of Conception 10P0
Prostate and Seminal Vesicles
  0VP4
Radius
  Left 0PPJ
  Right 0PPH
Rectum 0DPP1
Respiratory Tract 0WPQZ
Retroperitoneum 0WPH
Ribs
  1 to 2 0PP1
  3 or More 0PP2
Sacrum 0QP1
Scapula
  Left 0PP6
  Right 0PP5
Scrotum and Tunica Vaginalis
  0VP8
Sinus 09PY0
Skin 0HPPX
Skull 0NP0
Spinal Canal 00PU
Spinal Cord 00PV
Spleen 07PP
Sternum 0PP0
Stomach 0DP6
Subcutaneous Tissue and
  Fascia
    Head and Neck 0JPS
    Lower Extremity 0JPW
    Trunk 0JPT
    Upper Extremity 0JPV
Tarsal
  Left 0QPM
  Right 0QPL
Tendon
  Lower 0LPY
  Upper 0LPX
Testis 0VPD
Thymus 07PM
Thyroid Gland 0GPK0
Tibia
  Left 0QPH
  Right 0QPG
Toe Nail 0HPRXZ
Trachea 0BP1
Tracheobronchial Tree 0BP0
Tympanic Membrane
  Left 09P80
  Right 09P70
Ulna
  Left 0PPL
  Right 0PPK
Ureter 0TP9
Urethra 0TPD
Uterus and Cervix
  0UPD
Vagina and Cul-de-sac
  0UPH
Vas Deferens 0VPR
Vein
  Azygos 05P0
  Innominate
    Left 05P4
    Right 05P3
  Lower 06PY
  Upper 05PY

Removal of device from (continued)
Vertebra
  Cervical 0PP3
  Lumbar 0QP0
  Thoracic 0PP4
Vulva 0UPM
Renal calyx
  use Kidney
  use Kidneys, Bilateral
  use Kidney, Left
  use Kidney, Right
Renal capsule
  use Kidney
  use Kidneys, Bilateral
  use Kidney, Left
  use Kidney, Right
Renal cortex
  use Kidney
  use Kidneys, Bilateral
  use Kidney, Left
  use Kidney, Right
Renal dialysis
  see Performance, Urinary 5A1D
Renal nerve
  use Abdominal Sympathetic Nerve
Renal plexus
  use Nerve, Abdominal Sympathetic
Renal segment
  use Kidney
  use Kidneys, Bilateral
  use Kidney, Left
  use Kidney, Right
Renal segmental artery
  use Artery, Renal, Left
  use Artery, Renal, Right
Reopening, operative site
  Control of bleeding
    see Control bleeding in
  Inspection only
    see Inspection
Repair
  Abdominal Wall 0WQF
  Acetabulum
    Left 0QQ5
    Right 0QQ4
  Adenoids 0CQQ
  Ampulla of Vater 0FQC
  Anal Sphincter 0DQR
  Ankle Region
    Left 0YQL
    Right 0YQK
  Anterior Chamber
    Left 08Q33
    Right 08Q23
  Anus 0DQQ
  Aorta
    Abdominal 04Q0
    Thoracic
      Ascending/Arch 02QX
      Descending 02QW
  Aortic Body 0GQD
  Appendix 0DQJ
  Arm
    Lower
      Left 0XQF
      Right 0XQD
    Upper
      Left 0XQ9
      Right 0XQ8
  Artery
    Anterior Tibial
      Left 04QQ
      Right 04QP
    Axillary
      Left 03Q6
      Right 03Q5
    Brachial
      Left 03Q8
      Right 03Q7
    Celiac 04Q1

Repair (continued)
Artery (continued)
  Colic
    Left 04Q7
    Middle 04Q8
    Right 04Q6
  Common Carotid
    Left 03QJ
    Right 03QH
  Common Iliac
    Left 04QD
    Right 04QC
  Coronary
    Four or More Arteries
      02Q3
    One Artery 02Q0
    Three Arteries
      02Q2
    Two Arteries 02Q1
  External Carotid
    Left 03QN
    Right 03QM
  External Iliac
    Left 04QJ
    Right 04QH
  Face 03QR
  Femoral
    Left 04QL
    Right 04QK
  Foot
    Left 04QW
    Right 04QV
  Gastric 04Q2
  Hand
    Left 03QF
    Right 03QD
  Hepatic 04Q3
  Inferior Mesenteric
    04QB
  Innominate 03Q2
  Internal Carotid
    Left 03QL
    Right 03QK
  Internal Iliac
    Left 04QF
    Right 04QE
  Internal Mammary
    Left 03Q1
    Right 03Q0
  Intracranial 03QG
  Lower 04QY
  Peroneal
    Left 04QU
    Right 04QT
  Popliteal
    Left 04QN
    Right 04QM
  Posterior Tibial
    Left 04QS
    Right 04QR
  Pulmonary
    Left 02QR
    Right 02QQ
  Pulmonary Trunk
    02QP
  Radial
    Left 03QC
    Right 03QB
  Renal
    Left 04QA
    Right 04Q9
  Splenic 04Q4
  Subclavian
    Left 03Q4
    Right 03Q3
  Superior Mesenteric
    04Q5
  Temporal
    Left 03QT
    Right 03QS

Hand
   Left 0XQK
   Right 0XQJ
Head 0WQ0
Heart 02QA
   Left 02QC
   Right 02QB
Humeral Head
   Left 0PQD
   Right 0PQC
Humeral Shaft
   Left 0PQG
   Right 0PQF
Hymen 0UQK
Hypothalamus 00QA
Ileocecal Valve 0DQC
Ileum 0DQB
Inguinal Region
   Bilateral 0YQA
   Left 0YQ6
   Right 0YQ5
Intestine
   Large 0DQE
     Left 0DQG
     Right 0DQF
   Small 0DQ8
Iris
   Left 08QD3ZZ
   Right 08QC3ZZ
Jaw
   Lower 0WQ5
   Upper 0WQ4
Jejunum 0DQA
Joint
   Acromioclavicular
     Left 0RQH
     Right 0RQG
   Ankle
     Left 0SQG
     Right 0SQF
   Carpal
     Left 0RQR
     Right 0RQQ
   Carpometacarpal
     Left 0RQT
     Right 0RQS
   Cervical Vertebral 0RQ1
   Cervicothoracic Vertebral
     0RQ4
   Coccygeal 0SQ6
   Elbow
     Left 0RQM
     Right 0RQL
   Finger Phalangeal
     Left 0RQX
     Right 0RQW
   Hip
     Left 0SQB
     Right 0SQ9
   Knee
     Left 0SQD
     Right 0SQC
   Lumbar Vertebral 0SQ0
   Lumbosacral 0SQ3
   Metacarpophalangeal
     Left 0RQV
     Right 0RQU
   Metatarsal-Phalangeal
     Left 0SQN
     Right 0SQM
   Occipital-cervical
     0RQ0
   Sacrococcygeal 0SQ5
   Sacroiliac
     Left 0SQ8
     Right 0SQ7
   Shoulder
     Left 0RQK
     Right 0RQJ

Joint *(continued)*
   Sternoclavicular
     Left 0RQF
     Right 0RQE
   Tarsal
     Left 0SQJ
     Right 0SQH
   Tarsometatarsal
     Left 0SQL
     Right 0SQK
   Temporomandibular
     Left 0RQD
     Right 0RQC
   Thoracic Vertebral 0RQ6
   Thoracolumbar Vertebral 0RQA
   Toe Phalangeal
     Left 0SQQ
     Right 0SQP
   Wrist
     Left 0RQP
     Right 0RQN
Kidney
   Left 0TQ1
   Right 0TQ0
Kidney Pelvis
   Left 0TQ4
   Right 0TQ3
Knee Region
   Left 0YQG
   Right 0YQF
Larynx 0CQS
Leg
   Lower
     Left 0YQJ
     Right 0YQH
   Upper
     Left 0YQD
     Right 0YQC
Lens
   Left 08QK3ZZ
   Right 08QJ3ZZ
Lip
   Lower 0CQ1
   Upper 0CQ0
Liver 0FQ0
   Left Lobe 0FQ2
   Right Lobe 0FQ1
Lung
   Bilateral 0BQM
   Left 0BQL
   Lower Lobe
     Left 0BQJ
     Right 0BQF
   Middle Lobe, Right 0BQD
   Right 0BQK
   Upper Lobe
     Left 0BQG
     Right 0BQC
Lung Lingula 0BQH
Lymphatic
   Aortic 07QD
   Axillary
     Left 07Q6
     Right 07Q5
   Head 07Q0
   Inguinal
     Left 07QJ
     Right 07QH
   Internal Mammary
     Left 07Q9
     Right 07Q8
   Lower Extremity
     Left 07QG
     Right 07QF
   Mesenteric 07QB
   Neck
     Left 07Q2
     Right 07Q1
   Pelvis 07QC

Lymphatic *(continued)*
   Thoracic Duct 07QK
   Thorax 07Q7
   Upper Extremity
     Left 07Q4
     Right 07Q3
Mandible
   Left 0NQV
   Right 0NQT
Maxilla 0NQR
Mediastinum 0WQC
Medulla Oblongata 00QD
Mesentery 0DQV
Metacarpal
   Left 0PQQ
   Right 0PQP
Metatarsal
   Left 0QQP
   Right 0QQN
Muscle
   Abdomen
     Left 0KQL
     Right 0KQK
   Extraocular
     Left 08QM
     Right 08QL
   Facial 0KQ1
   Foot
     Left 0KQW
     Right 0KQV
   Hand
     Left 0KQD
     Right 0KQC
   Head 0KQ0
   Hip
     Left 0KQP
     Right 0KQN
   Lower Arm and Wrist
     Left 0KQB
     Right 0KQ9
   Lower Leg
     Left 0KQT
     Right 0KQS
   Neck
     Left 0KQ3
     Right 0KQ2
   Papillary 02QD
   Perineum 0KQM
   Shoulder
     Left 0KQ6
     Right 0KQ5
   Thorax
     Left 0KQJ
     Right 0KQH
   Tongue, Palate, Pharynx
     0KQ4
   Trunk
     Left 0KQG
     Right 0KQF
   Upper Arm
     Left 0KQ8
     Right 0KQ7
   Upper Leg
     Left 0KQR
     Right 0KQQ
Nasal Mucosa and Soft Tissue
   09QK
Nasopharynx 09QN
Neck 0WQ6
Nerve
   Abdominal Sympathetic
     01QM
   Abducens 00QL
   Accessory 00QR
   Acoustic 00QN
   Brachial Plexus 01Q3
   Cervical 01Q1
   Cervical Plexus 01Q0
   Facial 00QM

Nerve *(continued)*
   Femoral 01QD
   Glossopharyngeal 00QP
   Head and Neck Sympathetic
     01QK
   Hypoglossal 00QS
   Lumbar 01QB
   Lumbar Plexus 01Q9
   Lumbar Sympathetic 01QN
   Lumbosacral Plexus 01QA
   Median 01Q5
   Oculomotor 00QH
   Olfactory 00QF
   Optic 00QG
   Peroneal 01QH
   Phrenic 01Q2
   Pudendal 01QC
   Radial 01Q6
   Sacral 01QR
   Sacral Plexus 01QQ
   Sacral Sympathetic 01QP
   Sciatic 01QF
   Thoracic 01Q8
   Thoracic Sympathetic
     01QL
   Tibial 01QG
   Trigeminal 00QK
   Trochlear 00QJ
   Ulnar 01Q4
   Vagus 00QQ
Nipple
   Left 0HQX
   Right 0HQW
Omentum 0DQU
Oral Cavity and Throat
   0WQ3
Orbit
   Left 0NQQ
   Right 0NQP
Ovary
   Bilateral 0UQ2
   Left 0UQ1
   Right 0UQ0
Palate
   Hard 0CQ2
   Soft 0CQ3
Pancreas 0FQG
Para-aortic Body 0GQ9
Paraganglion Extremity
   0GQF
Parathyroid Gland 0GQR
   Inferior
     Left 0GQP
     Right 0GQN
   Multiple 0GQQ
   Superior
     Left 0GQM
     Right 0GQL
Patella
   Left 0QQF
   Right 0QQD
Penis 0VQS
Pericardium 02QN
Perineum
   Female 0WQN
   Male 0WQM
Peritoneum 0DQW
Phalanx
   Finger
     Left 0PQV
     Right 0PQT
   Thumb
     Left 0PQS
     Right 0PQR
   Toe
     Left 0QQR
     Right 0QQQ
Pharynx 0CQM
Pineal Body 0GQ1

Repair *(continued)*

Pleura
  Left 0BQP
  Right 0BQN
Pons 00QB
Prepuce 0VQT
Products of Conception
  10Q0
Prostate 0VQ0
Radius
  Left 0PQJ
  Right 0PQH
Rectum 0DQP
Retina
  Left 08QF3ZZ
  Right 08QE3ZZ
Retinal Vessel
  Left 08QH3ZZ
  Right 08QG3ZZ
Ribs
  1 to 2 0PQ1
  3 or More 0PQ2
Sacrum 0QQ1
Scapula
  Left 0PQ6
  Right 0PQ5
Sclera
  Left 08Q7XZZ
  Right 08Q6XZZ
Scrotum 0VQ5
Septum
  Atrial 02Q5
  Nasal 09QM
  Ventricular 02QM
Shoulder Region
  Left 0XQ3
  Right 0XQ2
Sinus
  Accessory 09QP
  Ethmoid
    Left 09QV
    Right 09QU
  Frontal
    Left 09QT
    Right 09QS
  Mastoid
    Left 09QC
    Right 09QB
  Maxillary
    Left 09QR
    Right 09QQ
  Sphenoid
    Left 09QX
    Right 09QW
Skin
  Abdomen 0HQ7XZZ
  Back 0HQ6XZZ
  Buttock 0HQ8XZZ
  Chest 0HQ5XZZ
  Ear
    Left 0HQ3XZZ
    Right 0HQ2XZZ
  Face 0HQ1XZZ
  Foot
    Left 0HQNXZZ
    Right 0HQMXZZ
  Hand
    Left 0HQGXZZ
    Right 0HQFXZZ
  Inguinal 0HQAXZZ
  Lower Arm
    Left 0HQEXZZ
    Right 0HQDXZZ
  Lower Leg
    Left 0HQLXZZ
    Right 0HQKXZZ
  Neck 0HQ4XZZ
  Perineum 0HQ9XZZ
  Scalp 0HQ0XZZ

Repair *(continued)*

Skin *(continued)*
  Upper Arm
    Left 0HQCXZZ
    Right 0HQBXZZ
  Upper Leg
    Left 0HQJXZZ
    Right 0HQHXZZ
Skull 0NQ0
Spinal Cord
  Cervical 00QW
  Lumbar 00QY
  Thoracic 00QX
Spinal Meninges 00QT
Spleen 07QP
Sternum 0PQ0
Stomach 0DQ6
  Pylorus 0DQ7
Subcutaneous Tissue and
  Fascia
  Abdomen 0JQ8
  Back 0JQ7
  Buttock 0JQ9
  Chest 0JQ6
  Face 0JQ1
  Foot
    Left 0JQR
    Right 0JQQ
  Hand
    Left 0JQK
    Right 0JQJ
  Lower Arm
    Left 0JQH
    Right 0JQG
  Lower Leg
    Left 0JQP
    Right 0JQN
  Neck
    Left 0JQ5
    Right 0JQ4
  Pelvic Region 0JQC
  Perineum 0JQB
  Scalp 0JQ0
  Upper Arm
    Left 0JQF
    Right 0JQD
  Upper Leg
    Left 0JQM
    Right 0JQL
Tarsal
  Left 0QQM
  Right 0QQL
Tendon
  Abdomen
    Left 0LQG
    Right 0LQF
  Ankle
    Left 0LQT
    Right 0LQS
  Foot
    Left 0LQW
    Right 0LQV
  Hand
    Left 0LQ8
    Right 0LQ7
  Head and Neck
    0LQ0
  Hip
    Left 0LQK
    Right 0LQJ
  Knee
    Left 0LQR
    Right 0LQQ
  Lower Arm and Wrist
    Left 0LQ6
    Right 0LQ5
  Lower Leg
    Left 0LQP
    Right 0LQN
  Perineum 0LQH

Repair *(continued)*

Tendon *(continued)*
  Shoulder
    Left 0LQ2
    Right 0LQ1
  Thorax
    Left 0LQD
    Right 0LQC
  Trunk
    Left 0LQB
    Right 0LQ9
  Upper Arm
    Left 0LQ4
    Right 0LQ3
  Upper Leg
    Left 0LQM
    Right 0LQL
Testis
  Bilateral 0VQC
  Left 0VQB
  Right 0VQ9
Thalamus 00Q9
Thumb
  Left 0XQM
  Right 0XQL
Thymus 07QM
Thyroid Gland 0GQK
  Left Lobe 0GQG
  Right Lobe 0GQH
Thyroid Gland Isthmus
  0GQJ
Tibia
  Left 0QQH
  Right 0QQG
Toe
  1st
    Left 0YQQ
    Right 0YQP
  2nd
    Left 0YQS
    Right 0YQR
  3rd
    Left 0YQU
    Right 0YQT
  4th
    Left 0YQW
    Right 0YQV
  5th
    Left 0YQY
    Right 0YQX
Toe Nail 0HQRXZZ
Tongue 0CQ7
Tonsils 0CQP
Tooth
  Lower 0CQX
  Upper 0CQW
Trachea 0BQ1
Tunica Vaginalis
  Left 0VQ7
  Right 0VQ6
  Turbinate, Nasal
    09QL
Tympanic Membrane
  Left 09Q8
  Right 09Q7
Ulna
  Left 0PQL
  Right 0PQK
Ureter
  Left 0TQ7
  Right 0TQ6
Urethra 0TQD
Uterine Supporting Structure
  0UQ4
Uterus 0UQ9
Uvula 0CQN
Vagina 0UQG
Valve
  Aortic 02QF
  Mitral 02QG

Repair *(continued)*

Valve *(continued)*
  Pulmonary 02QH
  Tricuspid 02QJ
Vas Deferens
  Bilateral 0VQQ
  Left 0VQP
  Right 0VQN
Vein
  Axillary
    Left 05Q8
    Right 05Q7
  Azygos 05Q0
  Basilic
    Left 05QC
    Right 05QB
  Brachial
    Left 05QA
    Right 05Q9
  Cephalic
    Left 05QF
    Right 05QD
  Colic 06Q7
  Common Iliac
    Left 06QD
    Right 06QC
  Coronary 02Q4
  Esophageal 06Q3
  External Iliac
    Left 06QG
    Right 06QF
  External Jugular
    Left 05QQ
    Right 05QP
  Face
    Left 05QV
    Right 05QT
  Femoral
    Left 06QN
    Right 06QM
  Foot
    Left 06QV
    Right 06QT
  Gastric 06Q2
  Hand
    Left 05QH
    Right 05QG
  Hemiazygos 05Q1
  Hepatic 06Q4
  Hypogastric
    Left 06QJ
    Right 06QH
  Inferior Mesenteric
    06Q6
  Innominate
    Left 05Q4
    Right 05Q3
  Internal Jugular
    Left 05QN
    Right 05QM
  Intracranial 05QL
  Lower 06QY
  Portal 06Q8
  Pulmonary
    Left 02QT
    Right 02QS
  Renal
    Left 06QB
    Right 06Q9
  Saphenous
    Left 06QQ
    Right 06QP
  Splenic 06Q1
  Subclavian
    Left 05Q6
    Right 05Q5
  Superior Mesenteric 06Q5
  Upper 05QY
  Vertebral
    Left 05QS

Repair (continued)

Vein (continued)

Vertebral (continued)

Right 05QR

Vena Cava

Inferior 06Q0

Superior 02QV

Ventricle

Left 02QL

Right 02QK

Vertebra

Cervical 0PQ3

Lumbar 0QQ0

Thoracic 0PQ4

Vesicle

Bilateral 0VQ3

Left 0VQ2

Right 0VQ1

Vitreous

Left 08Q53ZZ

Right 08Q43ZZ

Vocal Cord

Left 0CQV

Right 0CQT

Vulva 0UQM

Wrist Region

Left 0XQH

Right 0XQG

Repair, obstetric laceration, periurethral

0UQMXZZ

Replacement

Acetabulum

Left 0QR5

Right 0QR4

Ampulla of Vater 0FRC

Anal Sphincter 0DRR

Aorta

Abdominal 04R0

Thoracic

Ascending/Arch 02RX

Descending 02RW

Artery

Anterior Tibial

Left 04RQ

Right 04RP

Axillary

Left 03R6

Right 03R5

Brachial

Left 03R8

Right 03R7

Celiac 04R1

Colic

Left 04R7

Middle 04R8

Right 04R6

Common Carotid

Left 03RJ

Right 03RH

Common Iliac

Left 04RD

Right 04RC

External Carotid

Left 03RN

Right 03RM

External Iliac

Left 04RJ

Right 04RH

Face 03RR

Femoral

Left 04RL

Right 04RK

Foot

Left 04RW

Right 04RV

Gastric 04R2

Replacement (continued)

Artery (continued)

Hand

Left 03RF

Right 03RD

Hepatic 04R3

Inferior Mesenteric 04R B

Innominate 03R2

Internal Carotid

Left 03RL

Right 03RK

Internal Iliac

Left 04RF

Right 04RE

Internal Mammary

Left 03R1

Right 03R0

Intracranial 03RG

Lower 04RY

Peroneal

Left 04RU

Right 04RT

Popliteal

Left 04RN

Right 04RM

Posterior Tibial

Left 04RS

Right 04RR

Pulmonary

Left 02RR

Right 02RQ

Pulmonary Trunk 02RP

Radial

Left 03RC

Right 03RB

Renal

Left 04RA

Right 04R9

Splenic 04R4

Subclavian

Left 03R4

Right 03R3

Superior Mesenteric 04R5

Temporal

Left 03RT

Right 03RS

Thyroid

Left 03RV

Right 03RU

Ulnar

Left 03RA

Right 03R9

Upper 03RY

Vertebral

Left 03RQ

Right 03RP

Atrium

Left 02R

Right 02R6

Auditory Ossicle

Left 09RA0

Right 09R90

Bladder 0TRB

Bladder Neck 0TRC

Bone

Ethmoid

Left 0NRG

Right 0NRF

Frontal 0NR1

Hyoid 0NRX

Lacrimal

Left 0NRJ

Right 0NRH

Nasal 0NRB

Occipital 0NR7

Palatine

Left 0NRL

Right 0NRK

Replacement (continued)

Bone (continued)

Parietal

Left 0NR4

Right 0NR3

Pelvic

Left 0QR3

Right 0QR2

Sphenoid 0NRC

Temporal

Left 0NR6

Right 0NR5

Zygomatic

Left 0NRN

Right 0NRM

Breast

Bilateral 0HRV

Left 0HRU

Right 0HRT

Bronchus

Lingula 0BR9

Lower Lobe

Left 0BRB

Right 0BR6

Main

Left 0BR7

Right 0BR3

Middle Lobe, Right 0BR5

Upper Lobe

Left 0BR8

Right 0BR4

Buccal Mucosa 0CR4

Bursa and Ligament

Abdomen

Left 0MRJ

Right 0MRH

Ankle

Left 0MRR

Right 0MRQ

Elbow

Left 0MR4

Right 0MR3

Foot

Left 0MRT

Right 0MRS

Hand

Left 0MR8

Right 0MR7

Head and Neck 0MR0

Hip

Left 0MRM

Right 0MRL

Knee

Left 0MRP

Right 0MRN

Lower Extremity

Left 0MRW

Right 0MRV

Perineum 0MRK

Rib(s) 0MRG

Shoulder

Left 0MR2

Right 0MR1

Spine

Lower 0MRD

Upper 0MRC

Sternum 0MRF

Upper Extremity

Left 0MRB

Right 0MR9

Wrist

Left 0MR6

Right 0MR5

Carina 0BR2

Carpal

Left 0PRN

Right 0PRM

Cerebral Meninges 00R1

Cerebral Ventricle 00R6

Replacement (continued)

Chordae Tendineae 02R9

Choroid

Left 08RB

Right 08RA

Clavicle

Left 0PRB

Right 0PR9

Coccyx 0QRS

Conjunctiva

Left 08RTX

Right 08RSX

Cornea

Left 08R9

Right 08R8

Diaphragm 0BRT

Disc

Cervical Vertebral 0RR30

Cervicothoracic Vertebral 0RR50

Lumbar Vertebral 0SR20

Lumbosacral 0SR40

Thoracic Vertebral 0RR90

Thoracolumbar Vertebral 0RRB0

Duct

Common Bile 0FR9

Cystic 0FR8

Hepatic

Common 0FR7

Left 0FR6

Right 0FR5

Lacrimal

Left 08RY

Right 08RX

Pancreatic 0FRD

Accessory 0FRF

Parotid

Left 0CRC

Right 0CRB

Dura Mater 00R2

Ear

External

Bilateral 09R2

Left 09R1

Right 09R0

Inner

Left 09RE0

Right 09RD0

Middle

Left 09R60

Right 09R50

Epiglottis 0CRR

Esophagus 0DR5

Eye

Left 08R1

Right 08R0

Eyelid

Lower

Left 08RR

Right 08RQ

Upper

Left 08RP

Right 08RN

Femoral Shaft

Left 0QR9

Right 0QR8

Femur

Lower

Left 0QRC

Right 0QRB

Upper

Left 0QR7

Right 0QR6

Fibula

Left 0QRK

Right 0QRJ

Finger Nail 0HRQX

Gingiva

Lower 0CR6

Upper 0CR5

Revision of device in (*continued*)
Vertebra
Cervical 0PW3
Lumbar 0QW0
Thoracic 0PW4
Vulva 0UWM
Revo MRI™ SureScan® pacemaker
use Pacemaker, Dual Chamber in 0JH
rhBMP-2
use Recombinant Bone Morphogenetic Protein
Rheos® System device
use Stimulator Generator in Subcutaneous Tissue and Fascia
Rheos® System lead
use Stimulator Lead in Upper Arteries
Rhinopharynx
use Nasopharynx
Rhinoplasty
see Alteration, Nasal Mucosa and Soft Tissue 090K
see Repair, Nasal Mucosa and Soft Tissue 09QK
see Replacement, Nasal Mucosa and Soft Tissue 09RK
see Supplement, Nasal Mucosa and Soft Tissue 09UK
Rhinorrhaphy
see Repair, Nasal Mucosa and Soft Tissue 09QK
Rhinoscopy 09JKXZZ
Rhizotomy
see Division, Central Nervous System and Cranial Nerves 008
see Division, Peripheral Nervous System 018
Rhomboid major muscle
use Muscle, Trunk, Left
use Muscle, Trunk, Right
Rhomboid minor muscle
use Muscle, Trunk, Left
use Muscle, Trunk, Right
Rhythm electrocardiogram
see Measurement, Cardiac 4A02
Rhytidectomy
see Alteration, Face 0W02
Right ascending lumbar vein
use Vein, Azygos
Right atrioventricular valve
use Valve, Tricuspid
Right auricular appendix
use Atrium, Right
Right colic vein
use Vein, Colic
Right coronary sulcus
use Heart, Right
Right gastric artery
use Artery, Gastric
Right gastroepiploic vein
use Vein, Superior Mesenteric
Right inferior phrenic vein
use Vena Cava, Inferior
Right inferior pulmonary vein
use Vein, Pulmonary, Right
Right jugular trunk
use Lymphatic, Neck, Right
Right lateral ventricle
use Cerebral Ventricle
Right lymphatic duct
use Lymphatic, Neck, Right
Right ovarian vein
use Vena Cava, Inferior
Right second lumbar vein
use Vena Cava, Inferior
Right subclavian trunk
use Lymphatic, Neck, Right
Right subcostal vein
use Vein, Azygos

Right superior pulmonary vein
use Vein, Pulmonary, Right
Right suprarenal vein
use Vena Cava, Inferior
Right testicular vein
use Vena Cava, Inferior
Rima glottidis
use Larynx
Risorius muscle
use Muscle, Facial
RNS System lead
use Neurostimulator Lead in Central Nervous System and Cranial Nerves
RNS system neurostimulator generator
use Neurostimulator Generator in Head and Facial Bones
Robotic Assisted Procedure
Extremity
Lower 8E0Y
Upper 8E0X
Head and Neck Region 8E09
Trunk Region 8E0W
Robotic Waterjet Ablation, Destruction, Prostate XV508A4
Rotation of fetal head
Forceps 10S07ZZ
Manual 10S0XZZ
Round ligament of uterus
use Uterine Supporting Structure
Round window
use Ear, Inner, Left
use Ear, Inner, Right
Roux-en-Y operation
see Bypass, Gastrointestinal System 0D1
see Bypass, Hepatobiliary System and Pancreas 0F1
Rupture
Adhesions
see Release
Fluid collection
see Drainage
Ruxolitinib XW0DXT5

S

S-ICD™ lead
use SubcutaneousDifibrillator Lead in Subcutaneous Tissue and Fascia
Sacral ganglion
use Nerve, Sacral Sympathetic
Sacral lymph node
use Lymphatic, Pelvis
Sacral nerve modulation (SNM) lead
use Stimulator Lead in Urinary System
Sacral neuromodulation lead
use Stimulator Lead in Urinary System
Sacral splanchnic nerve
use Nerve, Sacral Sympathetic
Sacrectomy
see Excision, Lower Bones 0QB
Sacrococcygeal ligament
use Bursa and Ligament, Lower Spine
Sacrococcygeal symphysis
use Joint, Sacrococcygeal
Sacroiliac ligament
use Bursa and Ligament, Lower Spine
Sacrospinous ligament
use Bursa and Ligament, Lower Spine

Sacrotuberous ligament
use Bursa and Ligament, Lower Spine
Salpingectomy
see Excision, Female Reproductive System 0UB
see Resection, Female Reproductive System 0UT
Salpingolysis
see Release, Female Reproductive System 0UN
Salpingopexy
see Repair, Female Reproductive System 0UQ
see Reposition, Female Reproductive System 0US
Salpingopharyngeus muscle
use Muscle, Tongue, Palate, Pharynx
Salpingoplasty
see Repair, Female Reproductive System 0UQ
see Supplement, Female Reproductive System 0UU
Salpingorrhaphy
see Repair, Female Reproductive System 0UQ
Salpingoscopy 0UJ88ZZ
Salpingostomy
see Drainage, Female Reproductive System 0U9
Salpingotomy
see Drainage, Female Reproductive System 0U9
Salpinx
use Fallopian Tube, Left
use Fallopian Tube, Right
Saphenous nerve
use Nerve, Femoral
SAPIEN transcatheter aortic valve
use Zooplastic Tissue in Heart and Great Vessels
Sarilumab XW0
Sartorius muscle
use Muscle, Upper Leg, Left
use Muscle, Upper Leg, Right
SAVAL below-the-knee (BTK) drug-eluting stent system
use Intraluminal Device, Sustained Release Drug-eluting in New Technology
use Intraluminal Device, Sustained Release Drug-eluting, Four or More in New Technology
use Intraluminal Device, Sustained Release Drug-eluting, Three in New Technology
use Intraluminal Device, Sustained Release Drug-eluting, Two in New Technology
Scalene muscle
use Muscle, Neck, Left
use Muscle, Neck, Right
Scan
Computerized Tomography (CT)
see Computerized Tomography (CT Scan)
Radioisotope
see Planar Nuclear Medicine Imaging
Scaphoid bone
use Carpal, Left
use Carpal, Right
Scapholunate ligament
use Bursa and Ligament, Wrist, Left
use Bursa and Ligament, Wrist, Right
Scaphotrapezium ligament
use Bursa and Ligament, Hand, Left
use Bursa and Ligament, Hand, Right

Scapulectomy
see Excision, Upper Bones 0PB
see Resection, Upper Bones 0PT
Scapulopexy
see Repair, Upper Bones 0PQ
see Reposition, Upper Bones 0PS
Scarpa's (vestibular) ganglion
use Nerve, Acoustic
Sclerectomy
see Excision, Eye 08B
Sclerotherapy, mechanical
see Destruction
Sclerotherapy, via injection of sclerosing agent
see Introduction, Destructive Agent
Sclerotomy
see Drainage, Eye 089
Scrotectomy
see Excision, Male Reproductive System 0VB
see Resection, Male Reproductive System 0VT
Scrotoplasty
see Repair, Male Reproductive System 0VQ
see Supplement, Male Reproductive System 0VU
Scrotorrhaphy
see Repair, Male Reproductive System 0VQ
Scrototomy
see Drainage, Male Reproductive System 0V9
Sebaceous gland
use Skin
Second cranial nerve
use Nerve, Optic
Section, cesarean
see Extraction, Pregnancy 10D
Secura (DR) (VR)
use Defibrillator Generator in 0JH
Sella Turcica
use Bone, Sphenoid
Semicircular canal
use Ear, Inner, Left
use Ear, Inner, Right
Semimembranosus muscle
use Muscle, Upper Leg, Left
use Muscle, Upper Leg, Right
Semitendinosus muscle
use Muscle, Upper Leg, Left
use Muscle, Upper Leg, Right
Sentinel™ Cerebral Protection System (CPS) X2A5312
Seprafilm
use Adhesion Barrier
Septal cartilage
use Septum, Nasal
Septectomy
see Excision, Ear, Nose, Sinus 09B
see Excision, Heart and Great Vessels 02B
see Resection, Ear, Nose, Sinus 09T
see Resection, Heart and Great Vessels 02T
Septoplasty
see Repair, Ear, Nose, Sinus 09Q
see Repair, Heart and Great Vessels 02Q
see Replacement, Ear, Nose, Sinus 09R
see Replacement, Heart and Great Vessels 02R
see Reposition, Ear, Nose, Sinus 09S
see Supplement, Ear, Nose, Sinus 09U
see Supplement, Heart and Great Vessels 02U

Septostomy, balloon atrial 02163Z7
Septotomy
see Drainage, Ear, Nose, Sinus
099
Sequestrectomy, bone
see Extirpation
Serratus anterior muscle
use Muscle, Thorax, Left
use Muscle, Thorax, Right
Serratus posterior muscle
use Muscle, Trunk, Left
use Muscle, Trunk, Right
Seventh cranial nerve
use Nerve, Facial
Sheffield hybrid external fixator
use External Fixation Device,
Hybrid in 0PH
use External Fixation Device,
Hybrid in 0PS
use External Fixation Device,
Hybrid in 0QH
use External Fixation Device,
Hybrid in 0QS
Sheffield ring external fixator
use External Fixation Device, Ring
in 0PH
use External Fixation Device, Ring
in 0PS
use External Fixation Device, Ring
in 0QH
use External Fixation Device, Ring
in 0QS
Shirodkar cervical cerclage 0UVC7ZZ
**Shockwave Intravascular Lithotripsy
(Shockwave IVL)**
see Fragmentation
**Shock Wave Therapy,
Musculoskeletal** 6A93
Short gastric artery
use Artery, Splenic
Shortening
see Excision
see Repair
see Reposition
Shunt creation
see Bypass
Sialoadenectomy
Complete
see Resection, Mouth and
Throat 0CT
Partial
see Excision, Mouth and Throat
0CB
Sialodochoplasty
see Repair, Mouth and Throat 0CQ
see Replacement, Mouth and Throat
0CR
see Supplement, Mouth and Throat
0CU
Sialoectomy
see Excision, Mouth and Throat
0CB
see Resection, Mouth and Throat
0CT
Sialography
see Plain Radiography, Ear, Nose,
Mouth and Throat B90
Sialolithotomy
see Extirpation, Mouth and Throat
0CC
Sigmoid artery
use Artery, Inferior Mesenteric
Sigmoid flexure
use Colon, Sigmoid
Sigmoid vein
use Vein, Inferior Mesenteric
Sigmoidectomy
see Excision, Gastrointestinal
System 0DB
see Resection, Gastrointestinal
System 0DT

Sigmoidorrhaphy
see Repair, Gastrointestinal System
0DQ
Sigmoidoscopy 0DJD8ZZ
Sigmoidotomy
see Drainage, Gastrointestinal
System 0D9
**Single lead pacemaker (atrium)
(ventricle)**
use Pacemaker, Single Chamber
in 0JH
**Single lead rate responsive pacemaker
(atrium)(ventricle)**
use Pacemaker, Single Chamber
Rate Responsive in 0JH
Sinoatrial node
use Conduction Mechanism
Sinogram
Abdominal Wall
see Fluoroscopy, Abdomen and
Pelvis BW11
Chest Wall
see Plain Radiography, Chest
BW03
Retroperitoneum
see Fluoroscopy, Abdomen and
Pelvis BW11
Sinusectomy
see Excision, Ear, Nose, Sinus
09B
see Resection, Ear, Nose, Sinus
09T
Sinusoscopy 09JY4ZZ
Sinusotomy
see Drainage, Ear, Nose, Sinus 099
Sinus venosus
use Atrium, Right
Sirolimus-eluting coronary stent
use Intraluminal Device, Drug-
eluting in Heart and Great
Vessels
Sixth cranial nerve
use Nerve, Abducens
Size reduction, breast
see Excision, Skin and Breast
0HB
SJM Biocor® Stented Valve System
use Zooplastic Tissue in Heart and
Great Vessels
Skene's (paraurethral) gland
use Gland, Vestibular
**Skin Substitute, Porcine Liver
Derived, Replacement**
XHRPXL2
Sling
Fascial, orbicularis muscle
(mouth)
see Supplement, Muscle, Facial
0KU1
Levator muscle, for urethral
suspension
see Reposition, Bladder Neck
0TSC
Pubococcygeal, for urethral
suspension
see Reposition, Bladder Neck
0TSC
Rectum
see Reposition, Rectum 0DSP
Small bowel series
see Fluoroscopy, Bowel, Small
BD13
Small saphenous vein
use Vein, Saphenous, Left
use Vein, Saphenous, Right
Snapshot_NIR 8E02XDZ
Snaring, polyp, colon
see Excision, Gastrointestinal
System 0DB
Solar (celiac) plexus
use Nerve, Abdominal Sympathetic

Soleus muscle
use Muscle, Lower Leg, Left
use Muscle, Lower Leg, Right
Soliris®
see Eculizumab
Spacer
Insertion of device in
Disc
Lumbar Vertebral
0SH2
Lumbosacral 0SH4
Joint
Acromioclavicular
Left 0RHH
Right 0RHG
Ankle
Left 0SHG
Right 0SHF
Carpal
Left 0RHR
Right 0RHQ
Carpometacarpal
Left 0RHT
Right 0RHS
Cervical Vertebral 0RH1
Cervicothoracic Vertebral
0RH4
Coccygeal 0SH6
Elbow
Left 0RHM
Right 0RHL
Finger Phalangeal
Left 0RHX
Right 0RHW
Hip
Left 0SHB
Right 0SH9
Knee
Left 0SHD
Right 0SHC
Lumbar Vertebral 0SH0
Lumbosacral 0SH3
Metacarpophalangeal
Left 0RHV
Right 0RHU
Metatarsal-Phalangeal
Left 0SHN
Right 0SHM
Occipital-cervical 0RH0
Sacrococcygeal 0SH5
Sacroiliac
Left 0SH8
Right 0SH7
Shoulder
Left 0RHK
Right 0RHJ
Sternoclavicular
Left 0RHF
Right 0RHE
Tarsal
Left 0SHJ
Right 0SHH
Tarsometatarsal
Left 0SHL
Right 0SHK
Temporomandibular
Left 0RHD
Right 0RHC
Thoracic Vertebral 0RH6
Thoracolumbar Vertebral
0RHA
Toe Phalangeal
Left 0SHQ
Right 0SHP
Wrist
Left 0RHP
Right 0RHN
Removal of device from
Acromioclavicular
Left 0RPH
Right 0RPG

Spacer *(continued)*
Removal of device from *(continued)*
Ankle
Left 0SPG
Right 0SPF
Carpal
Left 0RPR
Right 0RPQ
Carpometacarpal
Left 0RPT
Right 0RPS
Cervical Vertebral 0RP1
Cervicothoracic Vertebral
0RP4
Coccygeal 0SP6
Elbow
Left 0RPM
Right 0RPL
Finger Phalangeal
Left 0RPX
Right 0RPW
Hip
Left 0SPB
Right 0SP9
Knee
Left 0SPD
Right 0SPC
Lumbar Vertebral 0SP0
Lumbosacral 0SP3
Metacarpophalangeal
Left 0RPV
Right 0RPU
Metatarsal-Phalangeal
Left 0SPN
Right 0SPM
Occipital-cervical 0RP0
Sacrococcygeal 0SP5
Sacroiliac
Left 0SP8
Right 0SP7
Shoulder
Left 0RPK
Right 0RPJ
Sternoclavicular
Left 0RPF
Right 0RPE
Tarsal
Left 0SPJ
Right 0SPH
Tarsometatarsal
Left 0SPL
Right 0SPK
Temporomandibular
Left 0RPD
Right 0RPC
Thoracic Vertebral 0RP6
Thoracolumbar Vertebral
0RPA
Toe Phalangeal
Left 0SPQ
Right 0SPP
Wrist
Left 0RPP
Right 0RPN
Revision of device in
Acromioclavicular
Left 0RWH
Right 0RWG
Ankle
Left 0SWG
Right 0SWF
Carpal
Left 0RWR
Right 0RWQ
Carpometacarpal
Left 0RWT
Right 0RWS
Cervical Vertebral 0RW1
Cervicothoracic Vertebral
0RW4
Coccygeal 0SW6

Spacer *(continued)*
  Revision of device in *(continued)*
    Elbow
      Left 0RWM
      Right 0RWL
    Finger Phalangeal
      Left 0RWX
      Right 0RWW
    Hip
      Left 0SWB
      Right 0SW9
    Knee
      Left 0SWD
      Right 0SWC
    Lumbar Vertebral 0SW0
    Lumbosacral 0SW3
    Metacarpophalangeal
      Left 0RWV
      Right 0RWU
    Metatarsal-Phalangeal
      Left 0SWN
      Right 0SWM
    Occipital-cervical 0RW0
    Sacrococcygeal 0SW5
    Sacroiliac
      Left 0SW8
      Right 0SW7
    Shoulder
      Left 0RWK
      Right 0RWJ
    Sternoclavicular
      Left 0RWF
      Right 0RWE
    Tarsal
      Left 0SWJ
      Right 0SWH
    Tarsometatarsal
      Left 0SWL
      Right 0SWK
    Temporomandibular
      Left 0RWD
      Right 0RWC
    Thoracic Vertebral 0RW6
    Thoracolumbar Vertebral 0RWA
    Toe Phalangeal
      Left 0SWQ
      Right 0SWP
    Wrist
      Left 0RWP
      Right 0RWN
Spacer, Articulating (Antibiotic)
  use Articulating Spacer in Lower
    Joints
Spacer, Static (Antibiotic)
  use Spacer in Lower Joints
Spectroscopy
  Intravascular Near Infrared 8E023DZ
  Near Infrared
    see Physiological Systems and
      Anatomical Regions 8E0
Speech Assessment F00
Speech therapy
  see Speech Treatment,
    Rehabilitation F06
Speech Treatment F06
Sphenoidectomy
  see Excision, Ear, Nose, Sinus 09B
  see Excision, Head and Facial
    Bones 0NB
  see Resection, Ear, Nose, Sinus 09T
  see Resection, Head and Facial
    Bones 0NT
Sphenoidotomy
  see Drainage, Ear, Nose, Sinus 099
Sphenomandibular ligament
  use Bursa and Ligament, Head and
    Neck
**Sphenopalatine (pterygopalatine)
  ganglion**
  use Nerve, Head and Neck
    Sympathetic

Sphincterorrhaphy, anal
  see Repair, Anal Sphincter 0DQR
Sphincterotomy, anal
  see Division, Anal Sphincter 0D8R
  see Drainage, Anal Sphincter 0D9R
Spinal cord neurostimulator lead
  use Neurostimulator Lead in Central
    Nervous System and Cranial
    Nerves
**Spinal growth rod(s), magnetically
  controlled**
  use Magnetically Controlled Growth
    Rod(s) in New Technology
Spinal nerve, cervical
  use Nerve, Cervical
Spinal nerve, lumbar
  use Nerve, Lumbar
Spinal nerve, sacral
  use Nerve, Sacral
Spinal nerve, thoracic
  use Nerve, Thoracic
Spinal Stabilization Device
  Facet Replacement
    Cervical Vertebral 0RH1
    Cervicothoracic Vertebral 0RH4
    Lumbar Vertebral 0SH0
    Lumbosacral 0SH3
    Occipital-cervical 0RH0
    Thoracic Vertebral 0RH6
    Thoracolumbar Vertebral 0RHA
  Interspinous Process
    Cervical Vertebral 0RH1
    Cervicothoracic Vertebral
      0RH4
    Lumbar Vertebral 0SH0
    Lumbosacral 0SH3
    Occipital-cervical 0RH0
    Thoracic Vertebral 0RH6
    Thoracolumbar Vertebral
      0RHA
  Pedicle-Based
    Cervical Vertebral 0RH1
    Cervicothoracic Vertebral
      0RH4
    Lumbar Vertebral 0SH0
    Lumbosacral 0SH3
    Occipital-cervical 0RH0
    Thoracic Vertebral 0RH6
    Thoracolumbar Vertebral
      0RHA
SpineJack® system
  use Synthetic Substitute,
    Mechanically Expandable
    (Paired) in New Technology
Spinous process
  use Vertebra, Cervical
  use Vertebra, Lumbar
  use Vertebra, Thoracic
Spiral ganglion
  use Nerve, Acoustic
Spiration IBV™ Valve System
  use Intraluminal Device,
    Endobronchial Valve in
    Respiratory System
Splenectomy
  see Excision, Lymphatic and Hemic
    Systems 07B
  see Resection, Lymphatic and
    Hemic Systems 07T
Splenic flexure
  use Colon, Transverse
Splenic plexus
  use Nerve, Abdominal Sympathetic
Splenius capitis muscle
  use Muscle, Head
Splenius cervicis muscle
  use Muscle, Neck, Left
  use Muscle, Neck, Right
Splenolysis
  see Release, Lymphatic and Hemic
    Systems 07N

Splenopexy
  see Repair, Lymphatic and Hemic
    Systems 07Q
  see Reposition, Lymphatic and
    Hemic Systems 07S
Splenoplasty
  see Repair, Lymphatic and Hemic
    Systems 07Q
Splenorrhaphy
  see Repair, Lymphatic and Hemic
    Systems 07Q
Splenotomy
  see Drainage, Lymphatic and Hemic
    Systems 079
Splinting, musculoskeletal
  see Immobilization, Anatomical
    Regions 2W3
SPRAVATO™
  use Esketamine Hydrochloride
**SPY system intravascular
  fluorescence angiography**
  see Monitoring, Physiological
    Systems 4A1
**SPY PINPOINT fluorescence
  imaging system**
  see Monitoring, Physiological
    Systems 4A1
  see Other Imaging, Hepatobiliary
    System and Pancreas BF5
**SPY system intraoperative
  fluorescence cholangiography**
  see Other Imaging, Hepatobiliary
    System and Pancreas BF5
Stapedectomy
  see Excision, Ear, Nose, Sinus 09B
  see Resection, Ear, Nose, Sinus 09T
Stapediolysis
  see Release, Ear, Nose, Sinus 09N
Stapedioplasty
  see Repair, Ear, Nose, Sinus 09Q
  see Replacement, Ear, Nose, Sinus
    09R
  see Supplement, Ear, Nose, Sinus 09U
Stapedotomy
  see Drainage, Ear, Nose, Sinus 099
Stapes
  use Auditory Ossicle, Left
  use Auditory Ossicle, Right
Static Spacer (Antibiotic)
  use Spacer in Lower Joints
STELARA®
  use Other New Technology
    Therapeutic Substance
Stellate ganglion
  use Nerve, Head and Neck
    Sympathetic
Stem cell transplant
  see Transfusion, Circulatory 302
Stensen's duct
  use Duct, Parotid, Left
  use Duct, Parotid, Right
Stent retriever thrombectomy
  see Extirpation, Upper Arteries 03C
**Stent, intraluminal (cardiovascular)
  (gastrointestinal)
  (hepatobiliary)(urinary)**
  use Intraluminal Device
Stented tissue valve
  use Zooplastic Tissue in Heart and
    Great Vessels
Stereotactic Radiosurgery
  Abdomen DW23
  Adrenal Gland DG22
  Bile Ducts DF22
  Bladder DT22
  Bone Marrow D720
  Brain D020
  Brain Stem D021
  Breast
    Left DM20
    Right DM21

Stereotactic Radiosurgery *(continued)*
  Bronchus DB21
  Cervix DU21
  Chest DW22
  Chest Wall DB27
  Colon DD25
  Diaphragm DB28
  Duodenum DD22
  Ear D920
  Esophagus DD20
  Eye D820
  Gallbladder DF21
  Gamma Beam
    Abdomen DW23JZZ
    Adrenal Gland DG22JZZ
    Bile Ducts DF22JZZ
    Bladder DT22JZZ
    Bone Marrow D720JZZ
    Brain D020JZZ
    Brain Stem D021JZZ
    Breast
      Left DM20JZZ
      Right DM21JZZ
    Bronchus DB21JZZ
    Cervix DU21JZZ
    Chest DW22JZZ
    Chest Wall DB27JZZ
    Colon DD25JZZ
    Diaphragm DB28JZZ
    Duodenum DD22JZZ
    Ear D920JZZ
    Esophagus DD20JZZ
    Eye D820JZZ
    Gallbladder DF21JZZ
    Gland
      Adrenal DG22JZZ
      Parathyroid DG24JZZ
      Pituitary DG20JZZ
      Thyroid DG25JZZ
    Glands, Salivary D926JZZ
    Head and Neck DW21JZZ
    Ileum DD24JZZ
    Jejunum DD23JZZ
    Kidney DT20JZZ
    Larynx D92BJZZ
    Liver DF20JZZ
    Lung DB22JZZ
    Lymphatics
      Abdomen D726JZZ
      Axillary D724JZZ
      Inguinal D728JZZ
      Neck D723JZZ
      Pelvis D727JZZ
      Thorax D725JZZ
    Mediastinum DB26JZZ
    Mouth D924JZZ
    Nasopharynx D92DJZZ
    Neck and Head DW21JZZ
    Nerve, Peripheral D027JZZ
    Nose D921JZZ
    Ovary DU20JZZ
    Palate
      Hard D928JZZ
      Soft D929JZZ
    Pancreas DF23JZZ
    Parathyroid Gland DG24JZZ
    Pelvic Region DW26JZZ
    Pharynx D92CJZZ
    Pineal Body DG21JZZ
    Pituitary Gland DG20JZZ
    Pleura DB25JZZ
    Prostate DV20JZZ
    Rectum DD27JZZ
    Sinuses D927JZZ
    Spinal Cord D026JZZ
    Spleen D722JZZ
    Stomach DD21JZZ
    Testis DV21JZZ
    Thymus D721JZZ
    Thyroid Gland DG25JZZ
    Tongue D925JZZ

Stereotactic Radiosurgery (continued)

Gamma Beam (continued)

Trachea DB20JZZ
Ureter DT21JZZ
Urethra DT23JZZ
Uterus DU22JZZ

Gland

Adrenal DG22
Parathyroid DG24
Pituitary DG20
Thyroid DG25

Glands, Salivary D926
Head and Neck DW21
Ileum DD24
Jejunum DD23
Kidney DT20
Larynx D92B
Liver DF20
Lung DB22

Lymphatics

Abdomen D726
Axillary D724
Inguinal D728
Neck D723
Pelvis D727
Thorax D725

Mediastinum DB26
Mouth D924
Nasopharynx D92D
Neck and Head DW21
Nerve, Peripheral D027
Nose D921

Other Photon

Abdomen DW23DZZ
Adrenal Gland DG22DZZ
Bile Ducts DF22DZZ
Bladder DT22DZZ
Bone Marrow D720DZZ
Brain D020DZZ
Brain Stem D021DZZ

Breast

Left DM20DZZ
Right DM21DZZ

Bronchus DB21DZZ
Cervix DU21DZZ
Chest DW22DZZ
Chest Wall DB27DZZ
Colon DD25DZZ
Diaphragm DB28DZZ
Duodenum DD22DZZ
Ear D920DZZ
Esophagus DD20DZZ
Eye D820DZZ
Gallbladder DF21DZZ

Gland

Adrenal DG22DZZ
Parathyroid DG24DZZ
Pituitary DG20DZZ
Thyroid DG25DZZ

Glands, Salivary D926DZZ
Head and Neck DW21DZZ
Ileum DD24DZZ
Jejunum DD23DZZ
Kidney DT20DZZ
Larynx D92BDZZ
Liver DF20DZZ
Lung DB22DZZ

Lymphatics

Abdomen D726DZZ
Axillary D724DZZ
Inguinal D728DZZ
Neck D723DZZ
Pelvis D727DZZ
Thorax D725DZZ

Mediastinum DB26DZZ
Mouth D924DZZ
Nasopharynx D92DDZZ
Neck and Head DW21DZZ
Nerve, Peripheral D027DZZ
Nose D921DZZ
Ovary DU20DZZ

Stereotactic Radiosurgery (continued)

Other Photon (continued)

Palate

Hard D928DZZ
Soft D929DZZ

Pancreas DF23DZZ
Parathyroid Gland DG24DZZ
Pelvic Region DW26DZZ
Pharynx D92CDZZ
Pineal Body DG21DZZ
Pituitary Gland DG20DZZ
Pleura DB25DZZ
Prostate DV20DZZ
Rectum DD27DZZ
Sinuses D927DZZ
Spinal Cord D026DZZ
Spleen D722DZZ
Stomach DD21DZZ
Testis DV21DZZ
Thymus D721DZZ
Thyroid Gland DG25DZZ
Tongue D925DZZ
Trachea DB20DZZ
Ureter DT21DZZ
Urethra DT23DZZ
Uterus DU22DZZ

Ovary DU20

Palate

Hard D928
Soft D929

Pancreas DF23
Parathyroid Gland DG24

Particulate

Abdomen DW23HZZ
Adrenal Gland DG22HZZ
Bile Ducts DF22HZZ
Bladder DT22HZZ
Bone Marrow D720HZZ
Brain D020HZZ
Brain Stem D021HZZ

Breast

Left DM20HZZ
Right DM21HZZ

Bronchus DB21HZZ
Cervix DU21HZZ
Chest DW22HZZ
Chest Wall DB27HZZ
Colon DD25HZZ
Diaphragm DB28HZZ
Duodenum DD22HZZ
Ear D920HZZ
Esophagus DD20HZZ
Eye D820HZZ
Gallbladder DF21HZZ

Gland

Adrenal DG22HZZ
Parathyroid DG24HZZ
Pituitary DG20HZZ
Thyroid DG25HZZ

Glands, Salivary D926HZZ
Head and Neck DW21HZZ
Ileum DD24HZZ
Jejunum DD23HZZ
Kidney DT20HZZ
Larynx D92BHZZ
Liver DF20HZZ
Lung DB22HZZ

Lymphatics

Abdomen D726HZZ
Axillary D724HZZ
Inguinal D728HZZ
Neck D723HZZ
Pelvis D727HZZ
Thorax D725HZZ

Mediastinum DB26HZZ
Mouth D924HZZ
Nasopharynx D92DHZZ
Neck and Head DW21HZZ
Nerve, Peripheral D027HZZ
Nose D921HZZ
Ovary DU20HZZ

Stereotactic Radiosurgery (continued)

Particulate (continued)

Palate

Hard D928HZZ
Soft D929HZZ

Pancreas DF23HZZ
Parathyroid Gland DG24HZZ
Pelvic Region DW26HZZ
Pharynx D92CHZZ
Pineal Body DG21HZZ
Pituitary Gland DG20HZZ
Pleura DB25HZZ
Prostate DV20HZZ
Rectum DD27HZZ
Sinuses D927HZZ
Spinal Cord D026HZZ
Spleen D722HZZ
Stomach DD21HZZ
Testis DV21HZZ
Thymus D721HZZ
Thyroid Gland DG25HZZ
Tongue D925HZZ
Trachea DB20HZZ
Ureter DT21HZZ
Urethra DT23HZZ
Uterus DU22HZZ

Pelvic Region DW26
Pharynx D92C
Pineal Body DG21
Pituitary Gland DG20
Pleura DB25
Prostate DV20
Rectum DD27
Sinuses D927
Spinal Cord D026
Spleen D722
Stomach DD21
Testis DV21
Thymus D721
Thyroid Gland DG25
Tongue D925
Trachea SB20
Ureter DT21
Urethra DT23
Uterus DU22

Sternoclavicular ligament

use Bursa and Ligament, Shoulder, Left

use Bursa and Ligament, Shoulder, Right

Sternocleidomastoid artery

use Artery, Thyroid, Left
use Artery, Thyroid, Right

Sternocleidomastoid muscle

use Muscle, Neck, Left
use Muscle, Neck, Right

Sternocostal ligament

use Sternum Bursa and Ligament

Sternotomy

see Division, Sternum 0P80
see Drainage, Sternum 0P90

Stimulation, cardiac

Cardioversion 5A2204Z

Electrophysiologic testing

see Measurement, Cardiac 4A02

Stimulator Generator

Insertion of device in

Abdomen 0JH8
Back 0JH7
Chest 0JH6

Multiple Array

Abdomen 0JH8
Back 0JH7
Chest 0JH6

Multiple Array Rechargeable

Abdomen 0JH8
Back 0JH7
Chest 0JH6

Removal of device from, Subcutaneous Tissue and Fascia, Trunk 0JPT

Stimulator Generator (continued)

Revision of device in, Subcutaneous Tissue and Fascia, Trunk 0JWT

Single Array

Abdomen 0JH8
Back 0JH7
Chest 0JH6

Single Array Rechargeable

Abdomen 0JH8
Back 0JH7
Chest 0JH6

Stimulator Lead

Insertion of device in

Anal Sphincter 0DHR

Artery

Left 03HL
Right 03HK

Bladder 0THB

Muscle

Lower 0KHY
Upper 0KHX

Stomach 0DH6
Ureter 0TH9

Removal of device from

Anal Sphincter 0DPR
Artery, Upper 03PY
Bladder 0TPB

Muscle

Lower 0KPY
Upper 0KPX

Stomach 0DP6
Ureter 0TP9

Revision of device in

Anal Sphincter 0DWR
Artery, Upper 03WY
Bladder 0TWB

Muscle

Lower 0KWY
Upper 0KWX

Stomach 0DW6
Ureter 0TW9

Stoma

Excision

Abdominal Wall 0WBFXZ2
Neck 0WB6XZ2

Repair

Abdominal Wall 0WQFXZ2
Neck 0WQ6XZ2

Stomatoplasty

see Repair, Mouth and Throat 0CQ
see Replacement, Mouth and Throat 0CR
see Supplement, Mouth and Throat 0CU

Stomatorrhaphy

see Repair, Mouth and Throat 0CQ

Stratos LV

use Cardiac Resynchronization Pacemaker Pulse Generator in 0JH

Stress test

4A02XM4
4A12XM4

Stripping

see Extraction

Study

Electrophysiologic stimulation, cardiac

see Measurement, Cardiac 4A02

Ocular motility 4A07X7Z

Pulmonary airway flow measurement

see Measurement, Respiratory 4A09

Visual acuity 4A07X0Z

Styloglossus muscle

use Muscle, Tongue, Palate, Pharynx

Stylomandibular ligament

use Bursa and Ligament, Head and Neck

Stylopharyngeus muscle
use Muscle, Tongue, Palate, Pharynx
Subacromial bursa
use Bursa and Ligament, Shoulder, Left
use Bursa and Ligament, Shoulder, Right
Subaortic (common iliac) lymph node
use Lymphatic, Pelvis
Subarachnoid space, spinal
use Spinal Canal
Subclavicular (apical) lymph node
use Lymphatic, Axillary, Left
use Lymphatic, Axillary, Right
Subclavius muscle
use Muscle, Thorax, Left
use Muscle, Thorax, Right
Subclavius nerve
use Nerve, Brachial Plexus
Subcostal artery
use Upper Artery
Subcostal muscle
use Muscle, Thorax, Left
use Muscle, Thorax, Right
Subcostal nerve
use Nerve, Thoracic
Subcutaneous injection reservoir, port
use Vascular Access Device, Totally
Implantable in Subcutaneous
Tissue and Fascia
Subcutaneous Defibrillator Lead
Insertion of device in,
Subcutaneous Tissue and
Fascia, Chest 0JH6
Removal of device from,
Subcutaneous Tissue and
Fascia, Trunk 0JPT
Revision of device in,
Subcutaneous Tissue and
Fascia, Trunk 0JWT
Subcutaneous injection reservoir, pump
use Infusion Device, Pump in
Subcutaneous Tissue and Fascia
Subdermal progesterone implant
use Contraceptive Device in
Subcutaneous Tissue and Fascia
Subdural space, spinal
use Spinal Canal
Submandibular ganglion
use Nerve, Facial
use Nerve, Head and Neck
Sympathetic
Submandibular gland
use Gland, Submaxillary, Left
use Gland, Submaxillary, Right
Submandibular lymph node
use Lymphatic, Head
Submandibular space
use Subcutaneous Tissue and
Fascia, Face
Submaxillary ganglion
use Nerve, Head and Neck
Sympathetic
Submaxillary lymph node
use Lymphatic, Head
Submental artery
use Artery, Face
Submental lymph node
use Lymphatic, Head
Submucous (Meissner's) plexus
use Nerve, Abdominal Sympathetic
Suboccipital nerve
use Nerve, Cervical
Suboccipital venous plexus
use Vein, Vertebral, Left
use Vein, Vertebral, Right
Subparotid lymph node
use Lymphatic, Head
Subscapular (posterior) lymph node
use Lymphatic, Axillary, Left
use Lymphatic, Axillary, Right

Subscapular aponeurosis
use Subcutaneous Tissue and Fascia,
Upper Arm, Left
use Subcutaneous Tissue and Fascia,
Upper Arm, Right
Subscapular artery
use Artery, Axillary, Left
use Artery, Axillary, Right
Subscapularis muscle
use Muscle, Shoulder, Left
use Muscle, Shoulder, Right
Substance Abuse Treatment
Counseling
Family, for substance abuse,
Other Family Counseling
HZ63ZZZ
Group
12-Step HZ43ZZZ
Behavioral HZ41ZZZ
Cognitive HZ40ZZZ
Cognitive-Behavioral
HZ42ZZZ
Confrontational HZ48ZZZ
Continuing Care HZ49ZZZ
Infectious Disease
Post-Test HZ4CZZZ
Pre-Test HZ4CZZZ
Interpersonal HZ44ZZZ
Motivational Enhancement
HZ47ZZZ
Psychoeducation HZ46ZZZ
Spiritual HZ4BZZZ
Vocational HZ45ZZZ
Individual
12-Step HZ33ZZZ
Behavioral HZ31ZZZ
Cognitive HZ30ZZZ
Cognitive-Behavioral
HZ32ZZZ
Confrontational HZ38ZZZ
Continuing Care HZ39ZZZ
Infectious Disease
Post-Test HZ3CZZZ
Pre-Test HZ3CZZZ
Interpersonal HZ34ZZZ
Motivational Enhancement
HZ37ZZZ
Psychoeducation HZ36ZZZ
Spiritual HZ3BZZZ
Vocational HZ35ZZZ
Detoxification Services, for
substance abuse HZ2ZZZZ
Medication Management
Antabuse HZ83ZZZ
Bupropion HZ87ZZZ
Clonidine HZ86ZZZ
Levo-alpha-acetyl-methadol
(LAAM) HZ82ZZZ
Methadone Maintenance
HZ81ZZZ
Naloxone HZ85ZZZ
Naltrexone HZ84ZZZ
Nicotine Replacement HZ80ZZZ
Other Replacement Medication
HZ89ZZZ
Psychiatric Medication HZ88ZZZ
Pharmacotherapy
Antabuse HZ93ZZZ
Bupropion HZ97ZZZ
Clonidine HZ96ZZZ
Levo-alpha-acetyl-methadol
(LAAM) HZ92ZZZ
Methadone Maintenance
HZ91ZZZ
Naloxone HZ95ZZZ
Naltrexone HZ94ZZZ
Nicotine Replacement
HZ90ZZZ
Psychiatric Medication HZ98ZZZ
Replacement Medication, Other
HZ99ZZZ

Substance Abuse
Treatment (continued)
Psychotherapy
12-Step HZ53ZZZ
Behavioral HZ51ZZZ
Cognitive HZ50ZZZ
Cognitive-Behavioral HZ52ZZZ
Confrontational HZ58ZZZ
Interactive HZ55ZZZ
Interpersonal HZ54ZZZ
Motivational Enhancement
HZ57ZZZ
Psychoanalysis HZ5BZZZ
Psychodynamic HZ5CZZZ
Psychoeducation HZ56ZZZ
Psychophysiological HZ5DZZZ
Supportive HZ59ZZZ
Substantia nigra
use Basal Ganglia
Subtalar (talocalcaneal) joint
use Joint, Tarsal, Left
use Joint, Tarsal, Right
Subtalar ligament
use Bursa and Ligament, Foot, Left
use Bursa and Ligament, Foot, Right
Subthalamic nucleus
use Basal Ganglia
Suction curettage (D&C), nonobstetric
see Extraction, Endometrium 0UDB
Suction curettage, obstetric post-delivery
see Extraction, Products of
Conception, Retained 10D1
Superficial circumflex iliac vein
use Vein, Saphenous, Left
use Vein, Saphenous, Right
Superficial epigastric artery
use Artery, Femoral, Left
use Artery, Femoral, Right
Superficial epigastric vein
use Vein, Saphenous, Left
use Vein, Saphenous, Right
Superficial Inferior Epigastric Artery
Flap
Replacement
Bilateral 0HRV078
Left 0HRU078
Right 0HRT078
Transfer
Left 0KXG
Right 0KXF
Superficial palmar arch
use Artery, Hand, Left
use Artery, Hand, Right
Superficial palmar venous arch
use Vein, Hand, Left
use Vein, Hand, Right
Superficial temporal artery
use Artery, Temporal, Left
use Artery, Temporal, Right
Superficial transverse perineal muscle
use Muscle, Perineum
Superior cardiac nerve
use Nerve, Thoracic Sympathetic
Superior cerebellar vein
use Vein, Intracranial
Superior cerebral vein
use Vein, Intracranial
Superior clunic (cluneal) nerve
use Nerve, Lumbar
Superior epigastric artery
use Artery, Internal Mammary,
Left
use Artery, Internal Mammary,
Right
Superior genicular artery
use Artery, Popliteal, Left
use Artery, Popliteal, Right
Superior gluteal artery
use Artery, Internal Iliac, Left
use Artery, Internal Iliac, Right

Superior gluteal nerve
use Nerve, Lumbar Plexus
Superior hypogastric plexus
use Nerve, Abdominal Sympathetic
Superior labial artery
use Artery, Face
Superior laryngeal artery
use Artery, Thyroid, Left
use Artery, Thyroid, Right
Superior laryngeal nerve
use Nerve, Vagus
Superior longitudinal muscle
use Muscle, Tongue, Palate,
Pharynx
Superior mesenteric ganglion
use Nerve, Abdominal Sympathetic
Superior mesenteric lymph node
use Lymphatic, Mesenteric
Superior mesenteric plexus
use Nerve, Abdominal Sympathetic
Superior oblique muscle
use Muscle, Extraocular, Left
use Muscle, Extraocular, Right
Superior olivary nucleus
use Pons
Superior rectal artery
use Artery, Inferior Mesenteric
Superior rectal vein
use Vein, Inferior Mesenteric
Superior rectus muscle
use Muscle, Extraocular, Left
use Muscle, Extraocular, Right
Superior tarsal plate
use Eyelid, Upper, Left
use Eyelid, Upper, Right
Superior thoracic artery
use Artery, Axillary, Left
use Artery, Axillary, Right
Superior thyroid artery
use External Carotid Artery, Left
use External Carotid Artery, Right
use Thyroid, Left
use Thyroid, Right
Superior turbinate
use Turbinate, Nasal
Superior ulnar collateral artery
use Artery, Brachial, Left
use Artery, Brachial, Right
Supersaturated Oxygen therapy
5A0512C
5A0522C
Supplement
Abdominal Wall 0WUF
Acetabulum
Left 0QU5
Right 0QU4
Ampulla of Vater 0FUC
Anal Sphincter 0DUR
Ankle Region
Left 0YUL
Right 0YUK
Anus 0DUQ
Aorta
Abdominal 04U0
Thoracic
Ascending/Arch 02UX
Descending 02UW
Arm
Lower
Left 0XUF
Right 0XUD
Upper
Left 0XU9
Right 0XU8
Artery
Anterior Tibial
Left 04UQ
Right 04UP
Axillary
Left 03U6
Right 03U5

Septum (continued)
    Ventricular 02UM
Shoulder Region
    Left 0XU3
    Right 0XU2
Sinus
    Accessory 09UP
    Ethmoid
        Left 09UV
        Right 09UU
    Frontal
        Left 09UT
        Right 09US
    Mastoid
        Left 09UC
        Right 09UB
    Maxillary
        Left 09UR
        Right 09UQ
    Sphenoid
        Left 09UX
        Right 09UW
Skull 0NU0
Spinal Meninges 00UT
Sternum 0PU0
Stomach 0DU6
    Pylorus 0DU7
Subcutaneous Tissue and Fascia
    Abdomen 0JU8
    Back 0JU7
    Buttock 0JU9
    Chest 0JU6
    Face 0JU1
    Foot
        Left 0JUR
        Right 0JUQ
    Hand
        Left 0JUK
        Right 0JUJ
    Lower Arm
        Left 0JUH
        Right 0JUG
    Lower Leg
        Left 0JUP
        Right 0JUN
    Neck
        Left 0JU5
        Right 0JU4
    Pelvic Region 0JUC
    Perineum 0JUB
    Scalp 0JU0
    Upper Arm
        Left 0JUF
        Right 0JUD
    Upper Leg
        Left 0JUM
        Right 0JUL
Tarsal
    Left 0QUM
    Right 0QUL
Tendon
    Abdomen
        Left 0LUG
        Right 0LUF
    Ankle
        Left 0LUT
        Right 0LUS
    Foot
        Left 0LUW
        Right 0LUV
    Hand
        Left 0LU8
        Right 0LU7
    Head and Neck 0LU0
    Hip
        Left 0LUK
        Right 0LUJ
    Knee
        Left 0LUR

Tendon (continued)
    Knee (continued)
        Right 0LUQ
    Lower Arm and
        Wrist
        Left 0LU6
        Right 0LU5
    Lower Leg
        Left 0LUP
        Right 0LUN
    Perineum 0LUH
    Shoulder
        Left 0LU2
        Right 0LU1
    Thorax
        Left 0LUD
        Right 0LUC
    Trunk
        Left 0LUB
        Right 0LU9
    Upper Arm
        Left 0LU4
        Right 0LU3
    Upper Leg
        Left 0LUM
        Right 0LUL
Testis
    Bilateral 0VUC0
    Left 0VUB0
    Right 0VU90
Thumb
    Left 0XUM
    Right 0XUL
Tibia
    Left 0QUH
    Right 0QUG
Toe
    1st
        Left 0YUQ
        Right 0YUP
    2nd
        Left 0YUS
        Right 0YUR
    3rd
        Left 0YUU
        Right 0YUT
    4th
        Left 0YUW
        Right 0YUV
    5th
        Left 0YUY
        Right 0YUX
Tongue 0CU7
Trachea 0BU1
Tunica Vaginalis
    Left 0VU7
    Right 0VU6
Turbinate, Nasal 09UL
Tympanic Membrane
    Left 09U8
    Right 09U7
Ulna
    Left 0PUL
    Right 0PUK
Ureter
    Left 0TU7
    Right 0TU6
Urethra 0TUD
Uterine Supporting Structure 0UU4
Uvula 0CUN
Vagina 0UUG
Valve
    Aortic 02UF
    Mitral 02UG
    Pulmonary 02UH
    Tricuspid 02UJ
Vas Deferens
    Bilateral 0VUQ
    Left 0VUP

Vas Deferens (continued)
    Right 0VUN
Vein
    Axillary
        Left 05U8
        Right 05U7
    Azygos 05U0
    Basilic
        Left 05UC
        Right 05UB
    Brachial
        Left 05UA
        Right 05U9
    Cephalic
        Left 05UF
        Right 05UD
    Colic 06U7
    Common Iliac
        Left 06UD
        Right 06UC
    Esophageal 06U3
    External Iliac
        Left 06UG
        Right 06UF
    External Jugular
        Left 05UQ
        Right 05UP
    Face
        Left 05UV
        Right 05UT
    Femoral
        Left 06UN
        Right 06UM
    Foot
        Left 06UV
        Right 06UT
    Gastric 06U2
    Hand
        Left 05UH
        Right 05UG
    Hemiazygos 05U1
    Hepatic 06U4
    Hypogastric
        Left 06UJ
        Right 06UH
    Inferior Mesenteric 06U6
    Innominate
        Left 05U4
        Right 05U3
    Internal Jugular
        Left 05UN
        Right 05UM
    Intracranial 05UL
    Lower 06UY
    Portal 06U8
    Pulmonary
        Left 02UT
        Right 02US
    Renal
        Left 06UB
        Right 06U9
    Saphenous
        Left 06UQ
        Right 06UP
    Splenic 06U1
    Subclavian
        Left 05U6
        Right 05U5
    Superior Mesenteric 06U5
    Upper 05UY
    Vertebral
        Left 05US
        Right 05UR
Vena Cava
    Inferior 06U0
    Superior 02UV
Ventricle
    Left 02UL
    Right 02UK

Vertebra
    Cervical 0PU3
    Lumbar 0QU0
        Mechanically Expandable
            (Paired) Synthetic
            Substitute XNU0356
    Thoracic 0PU4
        Mechanically Expandable
            (Paired) Synthetic
            Substitute XNU4356
Vesicle
    Bilateral 0VU3
    Left 0VU2
    Right 0VU1
Vocal Cord
    Left 0CUV
    Right 0CUT
Vulva 0UUM
Wrist Region
    Left 0XUH
    Right 0XUG
Supraclavicular (Virchow's) lymph node
    use Lymphatic, Neck, Left
    use Lymphatic, Neck, Right
Supraclavicular nerve
    use Nerve, Cervical Plexus
Suprahyoid lymph node
    use Lymphatic, Head
Suprahyoid muscle
    use Muscle, Neck, Left
    use Muscle, Neck, Right
Suprainguinal lymph node
    use Lymphatic, Pelvis
Supraorbital vein
    use Vein, Face, Left
    use Vein, Face, Right
Suprarenal gland
    use Gland, Adrenal
    use Gland, Adrenal, Bilateral
    use Gland, Adrenal, Left
    use Gland, Adrenal, Right
Suprarenal plexus
    use Nerve, Abdominal Sympathetic
Suprascapular nerve
    use Nerve, Brachial Plexus
Supraspinatus fascia
    use Subcutaneous Tissue and Fascia,
        Upper Arm, Left
    use Subcutaneous Tissue and Fascia,
        Upper Arm, Right
Supraspinatus muscle
    use Muscle, Shoulder, Left
    use Muscle, Shoulder, Right
Supraspinous ligament
    use Bursa and Ligament, Lower Spine
    use Bursa and Ligament, Upper Spine
Suprasternal notch
    use Sternum
Supratrochlear lymph node
    use Lymphatic, Upper Extremity, Left
    use Lymphatic, Upper Extremity,
        Right
Sural artery
    use Artery, Popliteal, Left
    use Artery, Popliteal, Right
Surpass Streamline™ Flow Diverter
    use Intraluminal Device, Flow
        Diverter in 03V
Suspension
    Bladder Neck
        see Reposition, Bladder Neck
        0TSC
    Kidney
        see Reposition, Urinary System
        0TS
    Urethra
        see Reposition, Urinary System
        0TS

Suspension *(continued)*
Urethrovesical
  see Reposition, Bladder Neck
    0TSC
Uterus
  see Reposition, Uterus 0US9
Vagina
  see Reposition, Vagina
    0USG
Sustained Release Drug-eluting
  Intraluminal Device
Dilation
  Anterior Tibial
    Left X27Q385
    Right X27P385
  Femoral
    Left X27J385
    Right X27H385
  Peroneal
    Left X27U385
    Right X27T385
  Popliteal
    Left Distal X27N385
    Left Proximal X27L385
    Right Distal X27M385
    Right Proximal X27K385
  Posterior Tibial
    Left X27S385
    Right X27R385
Four or More
  Anterior Tibial
    Left X27Q3C5
    Right X27P3C5
  Femoral
    Left X27J3C5
    Right X27H3C5
  Peroneal
    Left X27U3C5
    Right X27T3C5
  Popliteal
    Left Distal X27N3C5
    Left Proximal X27L3C5
    Right Distal X27M3C5
    Right Proximal X27K3C5
  Posterior Tibial
    Left X27S3C5
    Right X27R3C5
Three
  Anterior Tibial
    Left X27Q3B5
    Right X27P3B5
  Femoral
    Left X27J3B5
    Right X27H3B5
  Peroneal
    Left X27U3B5
    Right X27T3B5
  Popliteal
    Left Distal X27N3B5
    Left Proximal X27L3B5
    Right Distal X27M3B5
    Right Proximal X27K3B5
  Posterior Tibial
    Left X27S3B5
    Right X27R3B5
Two
  Anterior Tibial
    Left X27Q395
    Right X27P395
  Femoral
    Left X27J395
    Right X27H395
  Peroneal
    Left X27U395
    Right X27T395
  Popliteal
    Left Distal X27N395
    Left Proximal X27L395
    Right Distal X27M395
    Right Proximal X27K395

Sustained Release Drug-
  eluting Intraluminal
  Device *(continued)*
Two *(continued)*
  Posterior Tibial
    Left X27S395
    Right X27R395
Suture
Laceration repair
  see Repair
Ligation
  see Occlusion
Suture Removal
Extremity
  Lower 8E0YXY8
  Upper 8E0XXY8
Head and Neck Region 8E09XY8
Trunk Region 8E0WXY8
Sutureless valve, Perceval
use Zooplastic Tissue, Rapid
  Deployment Technique in New
  Technology
Sweat gland
use Skin
Sympathectomy
see Excision, Peripheral Nervous
  System 01B
SynCardia Total Artificial Heart
use Synthetic Substitute
Synchra CRT-P
use Cardiac Resynchronization
  Pacemaker Pulse Generator
  in 0JH
SynchroMed pump
use Infusion Device, Pump in
  Subcutaneous Tissue and Fascia
Synechiotomy, iris
see Release, Eye 08N
Synovectomy
Lower joint
  see Excision, Lower Joints 0SB
Upper joint
  see Excision, Upper Joints 0RB
Systemic Nuclear Medicine Therapy
Abdomen CW70
Anatomical Regions, Multiple
  CW7YYZZ
Chest CW73
Thyroid CW7G
Whole Body CW7N
Synthetic Human Angiotensin II XW0

T

Tagraxofusp-erzs Antineoplastic XW0
Takedown
Arteriovenous shunt
  see Removal of device from,
    Upper Arteries 03P
Arteriovenous shunt, with creation
  of new shunt
  see Bypass, Upper Arteries 031
Stoma
  see Excision
  see Reposition
Talent® Converter
use Intraluminal Device
Talent® Occluder
use Intraluminal Device
Talent® Stent Graft (abdominal)
  (thoracic)
use Intraluminal Device
Talocalcaneal (subtalar) joint
use Joint, Tarsal, Left
use Joint, Tarsal, Right
Talocalcaneal ligament
use Bursa and Ligament, Foot,
  Left
use Bursa and Ligament, Foot,
  Right

Talocalcaneonavicular joint
use Joint, Tarsal, Left
use Joint, Tarsal, Right
Talocalcaneonavicular ligament
use Bursa and Ligament, Foot, Left
use Bursa and Ligament, Foot, Right
Talocrural joint
use Joint, Ankle, Left
use Joint, Ankle, Right
Talofibular ligament
use Bursa and Ligament, Ankle, Left
use Bursa and Ligament, Ankle,
  Right
Talus bone
use Tarsal, Left
use Tarsal, Right
TandemHeart® System
use Short-term External Heart
  Assist System in Heart and
  Great Vessels
Tarsectomy
see Excision, Lower Bones 0QB
see Resection, Lower Bones 0QT
Tarsometatarsal ligament
use Bursa and Ligament, Foot, Left
use Bursa and Ligament, Foot,
  Right
Tarsorrhaphy
see Repair, Eye 08Q
Tattooing
Cornea 3E0CXMZ
Skin
  see Introduction of substance in
    or on, Skin 3E00
TAXUS® Liberté® Paclitaxel-eluting
  Coronary Stent System
use Intraluminal Device, Drug-
  eluting in Heart and Great
  Vessels
TBNA (transbronchial needle
  aspiration)
Fluid or gas
  see Drainage, Respiratory
    System 0B9
Tissue biopsy
  see Extraction, Respiratory
    System 0BD
TECENTRIQ®
use Atezolizumab Antineoplastic
Telemetry 4A12X4Z
Ambulatory 4A12X45
Temperature gradient study
  4A0ZXKZ
Temporal lobe
use Cerebral Hemisphere
Temporalis muscle
use Muscle, Head
Temporoparietalis muscle
use Muscle, Head
Tendolysis
see Release, Tendons 0LN
Tendonectomy
see Excision, Tendons 0LB
see Resection, Tendons 0LT
Tendonoplasty, tenoplasty
see Repair, Tendons 0LQ
see Replacement, Tendons 0LR
see Supplement, Tendons 0LU
Tendorrhaphy
see Repair, Tendons 0LQ
Tendototomy
see Division, Tendons 0L8
see Drainage, Tendons 0L9
Tenectomy, tenonectomy
see Excision, Tendons 0LB
see Resection, Tendons 0LT
Tenolysis
see Release, Tendons 0LN
Tenontorrhaphy
see Repair, Tendons 0LQ

Tenontotomy
see Division, Tendons 0L8
see Drainage, Tendons 0L9
Tenorrhaphy
see Repair, Tendons 0LQ
Tenosynovectomy
see Excision, Tendons 0LB
see Resection, Tendons 0LT
Tenotomy
see Division, Tendons 0L8
see Drainage, Tendons 0L9
Tensor fasciae latae muscle
use Muscle, Hip, Left
use Muscle, Hip, Right
Tensor veli palatini muscle
use Muscle, Tongue, Palate, Pharynx
Tenth cranial nerve
use Nerve, Vagus
Tentorium cerebelli
use Dura Mater
Teres major muscle
use Muscle, Shoulder, Left
use Muscle, Shoulder, Right
Teres minor muscle
use Muscle, Shoulder, Left
use Muscle, Shoulder, Right
Termination of pregnancy
Aspiration curettage 10A07ZZ
Dilation and curettage 10A07ZZ
Hysterotomy 10A00ZZ
Intra-amniotic injection 10A03ZZ
Laminaria 10A07ZW
Vacuum 10A07Z6
Testectomy
see Excision, Male Reproductive
  System 0VB
see Resection, Male Reproductive
  System 0VT
Testicular artery
use Aorta, Abdominal
Testing
Glaucoma 4A07XBZ
Hearing
  see Hearing Assessment,
    Diagnostic Audiology F13
Mental health
  see Psychological Tests
Muscle function, electromyography
  (EMG)
  see Measurement,
    Musculoskeletal 4A0F
Muscle function, manual
  see Motor Function Assessment,
    Rehabilitation F01
Neurophysiologic monitoring, intra-
  operative
  see Monitoring, Physiological
    Systems 4A1
Range of motion
  see Motor Function Assessment,
    Rehabilitation F01
Vestibular function
  see Vestibular Assessment,
    Diagnostic Audiology F15
Thalamectomy
see Excision, Thalamus 00B9
Thalamotomy
see Drainage, Thalamus 0099
Thenar muscle
use Muscle, Hand, Left
use Muscle, Hand, Right
Therapeutic Massage
Musculoskeletal System
  8E0KX1Z
Reproductive System
  Prostate 8E0VX1C
  Rectum 8E0VX1D
Therapeutic occlusion coil(s)
use Intraluminal Device
Thermography 4A0ZXKZ

Thermotherapy, prostate
see Destruction, Prostate 0V50
Third cranial nerve
use Nerve, Oculomotor
Third occipital nerve
use Nerve, Cervical
Third ventricle
use Cerebral Ventricle
Thoracectomy
see Excision, Anatomical Regions,
General 0WB
Thoracentesis
see Drainage, Anatomical Regions,
General 0W9
Thoracic aortic plexus
use Nerve, Thoracic Sympathetic
Thoracic esophagus
use Esophagus, Middle
Thoracic facet joint
use Joint, Thoracic Vertebral
Thoracic ganglion
use Nerve, Thoracic Sympathetic
Thoracoacromial artery
use Artery, Axillary, Left
use Artery, Axillary, Right
Thoracocentesis
see Drainage, Anatomical Regions,
General 0W9
Thoracolumbar facet joint
use Joint, Thoracolumbar Vertebral
Thoracoplasty
see Repair, Anatomical Regions,
General 0WQ
see Supplement, Anatomical
Regions, General 0WU
Thoracostomy tube
use Drainage Device
Thoracostomy, for lung collapse
see Drainage, Respiratory System 0B9
Thoracotomy
see Drainage, Anatomical Regions,
General 0W9
**Thoratec IVAD (Implantable
Ventricular Assist Device)**
use Implantable Heart Assist System
in Heart and Great Vessels
**Thoratec Paracorporeal Ventricular
Assist Device**
use Short-term External Heart Assist
System in Heart and Great
Vessels
Thrombectomy
see Extirpation
Thrombolysis, Ultrasound assisted
see Fragmentation, Artery
Thymectomy
see Excision, Lymphatic and Hemic
Systems 07B
see Resection, Lymphatic and
Hemic Systems 07T
Thymopexy
see Repair, Lymphatic and Hemic
Systems 07Q
see Reposition, Lymphatic and
Hemic Systems 07S
Thymus gland
use Thymus
Thyroarytenoid muscle
use Muscle, Neck, Left
use Muscle, Neck, Right
Thyrocervical trunk
use Artery, Thyroid, Left
use Artery, Thyroid, Right
Thyroid cartilage
use Larynx
Thyroidectomy
see Excision, Endocrine System
0GB
see Resection, Endocrine System
0GT
Thyroidorrhaphy
see Repair, Endocrine System 0GQ

Thyroidoscopy 0GJK4ZZ
Thyroidotomy
see Drainage, Endocrine System 0G9
Tibial insert
use Liner in Lower Joints
Tibialis anterior muscle
use Muscle, Lower Leg, Left
use Muscle, Lower Leg, Right
Tibialis posterior muscle
use Muscle, Lower Leg, Left
use Muscle, Lower Leg, Right
Tibiofemoral joint
use Joint, Knee, Left
use Joint, Knee, Left, Tibial Surface
use Joint, Knee, Right
use Joint, Knee, Right, Tibial Surface
Tibioperoneal trunk
use Popliteal Artery, Left
use Popliteal Artery, Right
Tisagenlecleucel
use Engineered Autologous
Chimeric Antigen Receptor
T-cell Immunotherapy
Tissue bank graft
use Nonautologous Tissue Substitute
Tissue Expander
Insertion of device in
Breast
Bilateral 0HHV
Left 0HHU
Right 0HHT
Nipple
Left 0HHX
Right 0HHW
Subcutaneous Tissue and Fascia
Abdomen 0JH8
Back 0JH7
Buttock 0JH9
Chest 0JH6
Face 0JH1
Foot
Left 0JHR
Right 0JHQ
Hand
Left 0JHK
Right 0JHJ
Lower Arm
Left 0JHH
Right 0JHG
Lower Leg
Left 0JHP
Right 0JHN
Neck
Left 0JH5
Right 0JH4
Pelvic Region 0JHC
Perineum 0JHB
Scalp 0JH0
Upper Arm
Left 0JHF
Right 0JHD
Upper Leg
Left 0JHM
Right 0JHL
Removal of device from
Breast
Left 0HPU
Right 0HPT
Subcutaneous Tissue and Fascia
Head and Neck 0JPS
Lower Extremity 0JPW
Trunk 0JPT
Upper Extremity 0JPV
Revision of device in
Breast
Left 0HWU
Right 0HWT
Subcutaneous Tissue and Fascia
Head and Neck 0JWS
Lower Extremity 0JWW
Trunk 0JWT
Upper Extremity 0JWV

Tissue expander (inflatable)(injectable)
use Tissue Expander in Skin and
Breast
use Tissue Expander in
Subcutaneous Tissue and Fascia
**Tissue Plasminogen Activator (tPA)
(r-tPA)**
use Thrombolytic Other
**Titanium Sternal Fixation System
(TSFS)**
use Internal Fixation Device, Rigid
Plate in 0PS
use Internal Fixation Device, Rigid
Plate in 0PH
Tocilizumab XW0
**Tomographic (Tomo) Nuclear
Medicine Imaging**
Abdomen CW20
Abdomen and Chest CW24
Abdomen and Pelvis CW21
Anatomical Regions, Multiple
CW2YYZZ
Bladder, Kidneys and Ureters CT23
Brain C020
Breast CH2YYZZ
Bilateral CH22
Left CH21
Right CH20
Bronchi and Lungs CB22
Central Nervous System C02YYZZ
Cerebrospinal Fluid C025
Chest CW23
Chest and Abdomen CW24
Chest and Neck CW26
Digestive System CD2YYZZ
Endocrine System CG2YYZZ
Extremity
Lower CW2D
Bilateral CP2F
Left CP2D
Right CP2C
Upper CW2M
Bilateral CP2B
Left CP29
Right CP28
Gallbladder CF24
Gastrointestinal Tract CD27
Gland, Parathyroid CG21
Head and Neck CW2B
Heart C22YYZZ
Right and Left C226
Hepatobiliary System and Pancreas
CF2YYZZ
Kidneys, Ureters and Bladder CT23
Liver CF25
Liver and Spleen CF26
Lungs and Bronchi CB22
Lymphatics and Hematologic
System C72YYZZ
Musculoskeletal System, Other
CP2YYZZ
Myocardium C22G
Neck and Chest CW26
Neck and Head CW2B
Pancreas and Hepatobiliary System
CF2YYZZ
Pelvic Region CW2J
Pelvis CP26
Pelvis and Abdomen CW21
Pelvis and Spine CP27
Respiratory System CB2YYZZ
Skin CH2YYZZ
Skull CP21
Skull and Cervical Spine CP23
Spine
Cervical CP22
Cervical and Skull CP23
Lumbar CP2H
Thoracic CP2G
Thoracolumbar CP2J
Spine and Pelvis CP27
Spleen C722

**Tomographic (Tomo) Nuclear
Medicine Imaging** *(continued)*
Spleen and Liver CF26
Subcutaneous Tissue CH2YYZZ
Thorax CP24
Ureters, Kidneys and Bladder CT23
Urinary System CT2YYZZ
Tomography, computerized
see Computerized Tomography
(CT Scan)
Tongue, base of
use Pharynx
Tonometry 4A07XBZ
Tonsillectomy
see Excision, Mouth and Throat 0CB
see Resection, Mouth and Throat 0CT
Tonsillotomy
see Drainage, Mouth and Throat 0C9
**Total Anomalous Pulmonary Venous
Return (TAPVR) repair**
see Bypass, Atrium, Left 0217
see Bypass, Vena Cava, Superior
021V
Total artificial (replacement) heart
use Synthetic Substitute
Total parenteral nutrition (TPN)
see Introduction of Nutritional
Substance
Trachectomy
see Excision, Trachea 0BB1
see Resection, Trachea 0BT1
Trachelectomy
see Excision, Cervix 0UBC
see Resection, Cervix 0UTC
Trachelopexy
see Repair, Cervix 0UQC
see Reposition, Cervix 0USC
Tracheloplasty
see Repair, Cervix 0UQC
Trachelorrhaphy
see Repair, Cervix 0UQC
Trachelotomy
see Drainage, Cervix 0U9C
Tracheobronchial lymph node
use Lymphatic, Thorax
Tracheoesophageal fistulization
0B110D6
Tracheolysis
see Release, Respiratory System
0BN
Tracheoplasty
see Repair, Respiratory System 0BQ
see Supplement, Respiratory System
0BU
Tracheorrhaphy
see Repair, Respiratory System 0BQ
Tracheoscopy 0BJ18ZZ
Tracheostomy
see Bypass, Respiratory System 0B1
Tracheostomy Device
Bypass, Trachea 0B11
Change device in, Trachea
0B21XFZ
Removal of device from, Trachea
0BP1
Revision of device in, Trachea 0BW1
Tracheostomy tube
use Tracheostomy Device in
Respiratory System
Tracheotomy
see Drainage, Respiratory System 0B9
Traction
Abdominal Wall 2W63X
Arm
Lower
Left 2W6DX
Right 2W6CX
Upper
Left 2W6BX
Right 2W6AX
Back 2W65X
Chest Wall 2W64X

Transfusion (continued)
  Vein (continued)
    Central (continued)
      Blood (continued)
        Frozen 3024
        White Cells 3024
        Whole 3024
        Bone Marrow 3024
        Factor IX 3024
        Fibrinogen 3024
        Globulin 3024
        Hematopoietic Stem/
          Progenitor Cells
          (HSPC), Genetically
          Modified 3024
        Plasma
          Fresh 3024
          Frozen 3024
        Plasma Cryoprecipitate 3024
        Serum Albumin 3024
        Stem Cells
          Cord Blood 3024
          Embryonic 3024
          Hematopoietic 3024
          T-cell Depleted
            Hematopoietic 3024
    Peripheral
      Antihemophilic Factors
        3023
      Blood
        Platelets 3023
        Red Cells 3023
        Frozen 3023
        White Cells 3023
        Whole 3023
      Bone Marrow 3023
      Factor IX 3023
      Fibrinogen 3023
      Globulin 3023
      Hematopoietic Stem/
        Progenitor Cells
        (HSPC), Genetically
        Modified 3023
      Plasma
        Fresh 3023
        Frozen 3023
      Plasma Cryoprecipitate 3023
      Serum Albumin 3023
      Stem Cells
        Cord Blood 3023X
        Embryonic 3023
        Hematopoietic 3023
        T-cell Depleted
          Hematopoietic 3023

Transplant
  see Transplantation
Transplantation
  Bone marrow
    see Transfusion, Circulatory
      302
  Esophagus 0DY50Z
  Face 0WY20Z
  Hand
    Left 0XYK0Z
    Right 0XYJ0Z
  Heart 02YA0Z
  Hematopoietic cell
    see Transfusion, Circulatory
      302
  Intestine
    Large 0DYE0Z
    Small 0DY80Z
  Kidney
    Left 0TY10Z
    Right 0TY00Z
  Liver 0FY00Z
  Lung
    Bilateral 0BYM0Z
    Left 0BYL0Z
    Lower Lobe
      Left 0BYJ0Z
      Right 0BYF0Z

Transplantation (continued)
  Lung (continued)
    Middle Lobe, Right 0BYD0Z
    Right 0BYK0Z
    Upper Lobe
      Left 0BYG0Z
      Right 0BYC0Z
  Lung Lingula 0BYH0Z
  Ovary
    Left 0UY10Z
    Right 0UY00Z
  Pancreas 0FYG0Z
  Penis 0VYS0Z
  Products of Conception 10Y0
  Scrotum 0VY50Z
  Spleen 07YP0Z
  Stem cell
    see Transfusion, Circulatory 302
  Stomach 0DY60Z
  Thymus 07YM0Z
  Uterus 0UY90Z
Transposition
  see Bypass
  see Reposition
  see Transfer
Transversalis fascia
  use Subcutaneous Tissue and Fascia,
    Trunk
Transverse acetabular ligament
  use Bursa and Ligament, Hip, Left
  use Bursa and Ligament, Hip, Right
Transverse (cutaneous) cervical nerve
  use Nerve, Cervical Plexus
Transverse facial artery
  use Artery, Temporal, Left
  use Artery, Temporal, Right
Transverse foramen
  use Cervical Vertebra
Transverse humeral ligament
  use Bursa and Ligament, Shoulder,
    Left
  use Bursa and Ligament, Shoulder,
    Right
Transverse ligament of atlas
  use Bursa and Ligament, Head and
    Neck
Transverse process
  use Cervical Vertebra
  use Thoracic Vertebra
  use Lumbar Vertebra
Transverse Rectus Abdominis
  Myocutaneous Flap
  Replacement
    Bilateral 0HRV076
    Left 0HRU076
    Right 0HRT076
  Transfer
    Left 0KXL
    Right 0KXK
Transverse scapular ligament
  use Bursa and Ligament, Shoulder,
    Left
  use Bursa and Ligament, Shoulder,
    Right
Transverse thoracis muscle
  use Muscle, Thorax, Left
  use Muscle, Thorax, Right
Transversospinalis muscle
  use Muscle, Trunk, Left
  use Muscle, Trunk, Right
Transversus abdominis muscle
  use Muscle, Abdomen, Left
  use Muscle, Abdomen, Right
Trapezium bone
  use Carpal, Left
  use Carpal, Right
Trapezius muscle
  use Muscle, Trunk, Left
  use Muscle, Trunk, Right
Trapezoid bone
  use Carpal, Left
  use Carpal, Right

Triceps brachii muscle
  use Muscle, Upper Arm, Left
  use Muscle, Upper Arm, Right
Tricuspid annulus
  use Valve, Tricuspid
Trifacial nerve
  use Nerve, Trigeminal
Trifecta™ Valve (aortic)
  use Zooplastic Tissue in Heart and
    Great Vessels
Trigone of bladder
  use Bladder
TriGuard 3™ CEPD (cerebral
  embolic protection device)
  X2A6325
Trimming, excisional
  see Excision
Triquetral bone
  use Carpal, Left
  use Carpal, Right
Trochanteric bursa
  use Bursa and Ligament, Hip, Left
  use Bursa and Ligament, Hip, Right
TUMT (Transurethral microwave
  thermotherapy of prostate)
  0V507ZZ
TUNA (transurethral needle ablation
  of prostate) 0V507ZZ
Tunneled central venous catheter
  use Vascular Access Device
    Tunneled in Subcutaneous
    Tissue and Fascia
Tunneled spinal (intrathecal) catheter
  use Infusion Device
Turbinectomy
  see Excision, Ear, Nose, Sinus 09B
  see Resection, Ear, Nose, Sinus 09T
Turbinoplasty
  see Repair, Ear, Nose, Sinus 09Q
  see Replacement, Ear, Nose, Sinus 09R
  see Supplement, Ear, Nose, Sinus 09U
Turbinotomy
  see Division, Ear, Nose, Sinus 098
  see Drainage, Ear, Nose, Sinus 099
TURP (transurethral resection of
  prostate)
  see Excision, Prostate 0VB0
  see Resection, Prostate 0VT0
Twelfth cranial nerve
  use Nerve, Hypoglossal
Two lead pacemaker
  use Pacemaker, Dual Chamber in 0JH
Tympanic cavity
  use Ear, Middle, Left
  use Ear, Middle, Right
Tympanic nerve
  use Nerve, Glossopharyngeal
Tympanic part of temporal bone
  use Bone, Temporal, Left
  use Bone, Temporal, Right
Tympanogram
  see Hearing Assessment, Diagnostic
    Audiology F13
Tympanoplasty
  see Repair, Ear, Nose, Sinus 09Q
  see Replacement, Ear, Nose, Sinus 09R
  see Supplement, Ear, Nose, Sinus
    09U
Tympanosympathectomy
  see Excision, Nerve, Head and Neck
    Sympathetic 01BK
Tympanotomy
  see Drainage, Ear, Nose, Sinus 099
TYRX Antibacterial Envelope
  use Anti-infective Envelope

U

Ulnar collateral carpal ligament
  use Bursa and Ligament, Wrist, Left
  use Bursa and Ligament, Wrist,
    Right

Ulnar collateral ligament
  use Bursa and Ligament, Elbow,
    Left
  use Bursa and Ligament, Elbow,
    Right
Ulnar notch
  use Radius, Left
  use Radius, Right
Ulnar vein
  use Vein, Brachial, Left
  use Vein, Brachial, Right
Ultrafiltration
  Hemodialysis
    see Performance, Urinary
      5A1D
  Therapeutic plasmapheresis
    see Pheresis, Circulatory
      6A55
Ultraflex™ Precision Colonic Stent
  System
  use Intraluminal Device
ULTRAPRO Hernia System
  (UHS)
  use Synthetic Substitute
ULTRAPRO Partially Absorbable
  Lightweight Mesh
  use Synthetic Substitute
ULTRAPRO Plug
  use Synthetic Substitute
Ultrasonic osteogenic stimulator
  use Bone Growth Stimulator in
    Head and Facial Bones
  use Bone Growth Stimulator in
    Lower Bones
  use Bone Growth Stimulator in
    Upper Bones
Ultrasonography
  Abdomen BW40ZZZ
  Abdomen and Pelvis BW41ZZZ
  Abdominal Wall BH49ZZZ
  Aorta
    Abdominal, Intravascular
      B440ZZ3
    Thoracic, Intravascular
      B340ZZ3
  Appendix BD48ZZZ
  Artery
    Brachiocephalic-Subclavian,
      Right, Intravascular
      B341ZZ3
    Celiac and Mesenteric,
      Intravascular B44KZZ3
    Common Carotid
      Bilateral, Intravascular
        B345ZZ3
      Left, Intravascular B344ZZ3
      Right, Intravascular
        B343ZZ3
    Coronary
      Multiple B241YZZ
        Intravascular B241ZZ3
        Transesophageal
          B241ZZ4
      Single B240YZZ
        Intravascular B240ZZ3
        Transesophageal
          B240ZZ4
    Femoral, Intravascular
      B44LZZ3
    Inferior Mesenteric,
      Intravascular B445ZZ3
    Internal Carotid
      Bilateral, Intravascular
        B348ZZ3
      Left, Intravascular
        B347ZZ3
      Right, Intravascular
        B346ZZ3
    Intra-Abdominal, Other,
      Intravascular B44BZZ3
    Intracranial, Intravascular
      B34RZZ3

Ultrasonography (continued)
  Artery (continued)
    Lower Extremity
      Bilateral, Intravascular
        B44HZZ3
      Left, Intravascular
        B44GZZ3
      Right, Intravascular
        B44FZZ3
    Mesenteric and Celiac,
      Intravascular B44KZZ3
    Ophthalmic, Intravascular
      B34VZZ3
    Penile, Intravascular
      B44NZZ3
    Pulmonary
      Left, Intravascular
        B34TZZ3
      Right, Intravascular
        B34SZZ3
    Renal
      Bilateral, Intravascular
        B448ZZ3
      Left, Intravascular
        B447ZZ3
      Right, Intravascular
        B446ZZ3
    Subclavian, Left, Intravascular
      B342ZZ3
    Superior Mesenteric,
      Intravascular B444ZZ3
    Upper Extremity
      Bilateral, Intravascular
        B34KZZ3
      Left, Intravascular
        B34JZZ3
      Right, Intravascular
        B34HZZ3
  Bile Duct BF40ZZZ
  Bile Duct and Gallbladder
    BF43ZZZ
  Bladder BT40ZZZ
    and Kidney BT4JZZZ
  Brain B040ZZZ
  Breast
    Bilateral BH42ZZZ
    Left BH41ZZZ
    Right BH40ZZZ
  Chest Wall BH4BZZZ
  Coccyx BR4FZZZ
  Connective Tissue
    Lower Extremity BL41ZZZ
    Upper Extremity BL40ZZZ
  Duodenum BD49ZZZ
  Elbow
    Left, Densitometry BP4HZZ1
    Right, Densitometry BP4GZZ1
  Esophagus BD41ZZZ
  Extremity
    Lower BH48ZZZ
    Upper BH47ZZZ
  Eye
    Bilateral B847ZZZ
    Left B846ZZZ
    Right B845ZZZ
  Fallopian Tube
    Bilateral BU42
    Left BU41
    Right BU40
  Fetal Umbilical Cord BY47ZZZ
  Fetus
    First Trimester, Multiple
      Gestation BY4BZZZ
    Second Trimester, Multiple
      Gestation BY4DZZZ
    Single
      First Trimester BY49ZZZ
      Second Trimester
        BY4CZZZ
      Third Trimester BY4FZZZ
    Third Trimester, Multiple
      Gestation BY4GZZZ

Ultrasonography (continued)
  Gallbladder BF42ZZZ
  Gallbladder and Bile Duct BF43ZZZ
  Gastrointestinal Tract BD47ZZZ
  Gland
    Adrenal
      Bilateral BG42ZZZ
      Left BG41ZZZ
      Right BG40ZZZ
    Parathyroid BG43ZZZ
    Thyroid BG44ZZZ
  Hand
    Left, Densitometry BP4PZZ1
    Right, Densitometry BP4NZZ1
  Head and Neck BH4CZZZ
  Heart
    Left B245YZZ
      Intravascular B245ZZ3
      Transesophageal B245ZZ4
    Pediatric B24DYZZ
      Intravascular B24DZZ3
      Transesophageal
        B24DZZ4
    Right B244YZZ
      Intravascular B244ZZ3
      Transesophageal B244ZZ4
    Right and Left B246YZZ
      Intravascular B246ZZ3
      Transesophageal B246ZZ4
  Heart with Aorta B24BYZZ
    Intravascular B24BZZ3
    Transesophageal B24BZZ4
  Hepatobiliary System, All
    BF4CZZZ
  Hip
    Bilateral BQ42ZZZ
    Left BQ41ZZZ
    Right BQ40ZZZ
  Kidney
    and Bladder BT4JZZZ
    Bilateral BT43ZZZ
    Left BT42ZZZ
    Right BT41ZZZ
    Transplant BT49ZZZ
  Knee
    Bilateral BQ49ZZZ
    Left BQ48ZZZ
    Right BQ47ZZZ
  Liver BF45ZZZ
  Liver and Spleen BF46ZZZ
  Mediastinum BB4CZZZ
  Neck BW4FZZZ
  Ovary
    Bilateral BU45
    Left BU44
    Right BU43
  Ovary and Uterus BU4C
  Pancreas BF47ZZZ
  Pelvic Region BW4GZZZ
  Pelvis and Abdomen BW41ZZZ
  Penis BV4BZZZ
  Pericardium B24CYZZ
    Intravascular B24CZZ3
    Transesophageal B24CZZ4
  Placenta BY48ZZZ
  Pleura BB4BZZZ
  Prostate and Seminal Vesicle
    BV49ZZZ
  Rectum BD4CZZZ
  Sacrum BR4FZZZ
  Scrotum BV44ZZZ
  Seminal Vesicle and Prostate
    BV49ZZZ
  Shoulder
    Left, Densitometry BP49ZZ1
    Right, Densitometry BP48ZZ1
  Spinal Cord B04BZZZ
  Spine
    Cervical BR40ZZZ
    Lumbar BR49ZZZ
    Thoracic BR47ZZZ
  Spleen and Liver BF46ZZZ

Ultrasonography (continued)
  Stomach BD42ZZZ
  Tendon
    Lower Extremity BL43ZZZ
    Upper Extremity BL42ZZZ
  Ureter
    Bilateral BT48ZZZ
    Left BT47ZZZ
    Right BT46ZZZ
  Urethra BT45ZZZ
  Uterus BU46
  Uterus and Ovary BU4C
  Vein
    Jugular
      Left, Intravascular
        B544ZZ3
      Right, Intravascular
        B543ZZ3
    Lower Extremity
      Bilateral, Intravascular
        B54DZZ3
      Left, Intravascular B54CZZ3
      Right, Intravascular
        B54BZZ3
    Portal, Intravascular B54TZZ3
    Renal
      Bilateral, Intravascular
        B54LZZ3
      Left, Intravascular
        B54KZZ3
      Right, Intravascular
        B54JZZ3
    Spanchnic, Intravascular
      B54TZZ3
    Subclavian
      Left, Intravascular
        B547ZZ3
      Right, Intravascular
        B546ZZ3
    Upper Extremity
      Bilateral, Intravascular
        B54PZZ3
      Left, Intravascular B54NZZ3
      Right, Intravascular
        B54MZZ3
  Vena Cava
    Inferior, Intravascular B549ZZ3
    Superior, Intravascular B548ZZ3
  Wrist
    Left, Densitometry BP4MZZ1
    Right, Densitometry BP4LZZ1
Ultrasound bone healing system
  use Bone Growth Stimulator in
    Head and Facial Bones
  use Bone Growth Stimulator in
    Lower Bones
  use Bone Growth Stimulator in
    Upper Bones
Ultrasound Therapy
  Heart 6A75
  No Qualifier 6A75
  Vessels
    Head and Neck 6A75
    Other 6A75
    Peripheral 6A75
Ultraviolet Light Therapy, Skin 6A80
Umbilical artery
  use Artery, Internal Iliac, Left
  use Artery, Internal Iliac, Right
  use Artery, Lower
Uniplanar external fixator
  use External Fixation Device,
    Monoplanar in 0PH
  use External Fixation Device,
    Monoplanar in 0PS
  use External Fixation Device,
    Monoplanar in 0QH
  use External Fixation Device,
    Monoplanar in 0QS
Upper GI series
  see Fluoroscopy, Gastrointestinal,
    Upper BD15

Ureteral orifice
  use Ureter
  use Ureter, Left
  use Ureter, Right
  use Ureters, Bilateral
Ureterectomy
  see Excision, Urinary System 0TB
  see Resection, Urinary System 0TT
Ureterocolostomy
  see Bypass, Urinary System 0T1
Ureterocystostomy
  see Bypass, Urinary System 0T1
Ureteroenterostomy
  see Bypass, Urinary System 0T1
Ureteroileostomy
  see Bypass, Urinary System 0T1
Ureterolithotomy
  see Extirpation, Urinary System
    0TC
Ureterolysis
  see Release, Urinary System 0TN
Ureteroneocystostomy
  see Bypass, Urinary System 0T1
  see Reposition, Urinary System 0TS
Ureteropelvic junction (UPJ)
  use Kidney Pelvis, Left
  use Kidney Pelvis, Right
Ureteropexy
  see Repair, Urinary System 0TQ
  see Reposition, Urinary System
    0TS
Ureteroplasty
  see Repair, Urinary System 0TQ
  see Replacement, Urinary System
    0TR
  see Supplement, Urinary System
    0TU
Ureteroplication
  see Restriction, Urinary System 0TV
Ureteropyelography
  see Fluoroscopy, Urinary System
    BT1
Ureterorrhaphy
  see Repair, Urinary System 0TQ
Ureteroscopy 0TJ98ZZ
Ureterostomy
  see Bypass, Urinary System 0T1
  see Drainage, Urinary System 0T9
Ureterotomy
  see Drainage, Urinary System 0T9
Ureteroureterostomy
  see Bypass, Urinary System 0T1
Ureterovesical orifice
  use Ureter
  use Ureters, Bilateral
  use Ureter, Left
  use Ureter, Right
Urethral catheterization, indwelling
  0T9B70Z
Urethrectomy
  see Excision, Urethra 0TBD
  see Resection, Urethra 0TTD
Urethrolithotomy
  see Extirpation, Urethra 0TCD
Urethrolysis
  see Release, Urethra 0TND
Urethropexy
  see Repair, Urethra 0TQD
  see Reposition, Urethra 0TSD
Urethroplasty
  see Repair, Urethra 0TQD
  see Replacement, Urethra 0TRD
  see Supplement, Urethra 0TUD
Urethrorrhaphy
  see Repair, Urethra 0TQD
Urethroscopy 0TJD8ZZ
Urethrotomy
  see Drainage, Urethra 0T9D
Uridine Triacetate XW0DX82
Urinary incontinence stimulator lead
  use Stimulator Lead in Urinary
    System

Urography
   see Fluoroscopy, Urinary System
      BT1
Ustekinumab
   use Other New Technology
      Therapeutic Substance
Uterine Artery
   use Artery, Internal Iliac, Left
   use Artery, Internal Iliac, Right
Uterine artery embolization (UAE)
   see Occlusion, Lower Arteries 04L
Uterine cornu
   use Uterus
Uterine tube
   use Fallopian Tube, Left
   use Fallopian Tube, Right
Uterine vein
   use Vein, Hypogastric, Left
   use Vein, Hypogastric, Right
Uvulectomy
   see Excision, Uvula 0CBN
   see Resection, Uvula 0CTN
Uvulorrhaphy
   see Repair, Uvula 0CQN
Uvulotomy
   see Drainage, Uvula 0C9N

V

V-Wave Interatrial Shunt System
   use Synthetic Substitute
Vabomere™
   use Meropenem-vaboractam Anti-
      infective
Vaccination
   see Introduction of Serum, Toxoid,
      and Vaccine
Vacuum extraction, obstetric
      10D07Z6
Vaginal artery
   use Artery, Internal Iliac, Left
   use Artery, Internal Iliac, Right
Vaginal pessary
   use Intraluminal Device, Pessary
      in Female Reproductive
      System
Vaginal vein
   use Vein, Hypogastric, Left
   use Vein, Hypogastric, Right
Vaginectomy
   see Excision, Vagina 0UBG
   see Resection, Vagina
      0UTG
Vaginofixation
   see Repair, Vagina 0UQG
   see Reposition, Vagina 0USG
Vaginoplasty
   see Repair, Vagina 0UQG
   see Supplement, Vagina 0UUG
Vaginorrhaphy
   see Repair, Vagina 0UQG
Vaginoscopy 0UJH8ZZ
Vaginotomy
   see Drainage, Female Reproductive
      System 0U9
Vagotomy
   see Division, Nerve, Vagus 008Q
Valiant Thoracic Stent Graft
   use Intraluminal Device
Valvotomy, valvulotomy
   see Division, Heart and Great
      Vessels 028
   see Release, Heart and Great Vessels
      02N
Valvuloplasty
   see Repair, Heart and Great Vessels
      02Q
   see Replacement, Heart and Great
      Vessels 02R
   see Supplement, Heart and Great
      Vessels 02U

Valvuloplasty, Alfieri Stitch
   see Restriction, Valve, Mitral 02VG
Vascular Access Device
   Totally Implantable
      Insertion of device in
         Abdomen 0JH8
         Chest 0JH6
         Lower Arm
            Left 0JHH
            Right 0JHG
         Lower Leg
            Left 0JHP
            Right 0JHN
         Upper Arm
            Left 0JHF
            Right 0JHD
         Upper Leg
            Left 0JHM
            Right 0JHL
      Removal of device from
         Lower Extremity 0JPW
         Trunk 0JPT
         Upper Extremity 0JPV
      Revision of device in
         Lower Extremity 0JWW
         Trunk 0JWT
         Upper Extremity 0JWV
   Tunneled
      Insertion of device in
         Abdomen 0JH8
         Chest 0JH6
         Lower Arm
            Left 0JHH
            Right 0JHG
         Lower Leg
            Left 0JHP
            Right 0JHN
         Upper Arm
            Left 0JHF
            Right 0JHD
         Upper Leg
            Left 0JHM
            Right 0JHL
      Removal of device from
         Lower Extremity 0JPW
         Trunk 0JPT
         Upper Extremity 0JPV
      Revision of device in
         Lower Extremity 0JWW
         Trunk 0JWT
         Upper Extremity 0JWV
Vasectomy
   see Excision, Male Reproductive
      System 0VB
Vasography
   see Fluoroscopy, Male Reproductive
      System BV1
   see Plain Radiography, Male
      Reproductive System BV0
Vasoligation
   see Occlusion, Male Reproductive
      System 0VL
Vasorrhaphy
   see Repair, Male Reproductive
      System 0VQ
Vasostomy
   see Bypass, Male Reproductive
      System 0V1
Vasotomy
   Drainage
      see Drainage, Male
         Reproductive System 0V9
      see Occlusion, Male
         Reproductive System 0VL
   With ligation
Vasovasostomy
   see Repair, Male Reproductive
      System 0VQ
Vastus intermedius muscle
   use Muscle, Upper Leg, Left
   use Muscle, Upper Leg, Right

Vastus lateralis muscle
   use Muscle, Upper Leg, Left
   use Muscle, Upper Leg, Right
Vastus medialis muscle
   use Muscle, Upper Leg, Left
   use Muscle, Upper Leg, Right
VCG (vectorcardiogram)
   see Measurement, Cardiac 4A02
Vectra® Vascular Access Graft
   use Vascular Access Device,
      Tunneled in Subcutaneous
      Tissue and Fascia
Veklury *use* Remdesivir Anti-infective
Venclexta®
   use Venetoclax Antineoplastic
Venetoclax Antineoplastic XW0DXR5
Venectomy
   see Excision, Lower Veins 06B
   see Excision, Upper Veins 05B
Venography
   see Fluoroscopy, Veins B51
   see Plain Radiography, Veins B50
Venorrhaphy
   see Repair, Lower Veins 06Q
   see Repair, Upper Veins 05Q
Venotripsy
   see Occlusion, Lower Veins 06L
   see Occlusion, Upper Veins 05L
Ventricular fold
   use Larynx
Ventriculoatriostomy
   see Bypass, Central Nervous System
      and Cranial Nerves 001
Ventriculocisternostomy
   see Bypass, Central Nervous System
      and Cranial Nerves 001
Ventriculogram, cardiac
   Combined left and right heart
      see Fluoroscopy, Heart, Right
         and Left B216
   Left ventricle
      see Fluoroscopy, Heart, Left B215
   Right ventricle
      see Fluoroscopy, Heart, Right
         B214
Ventriculopuncture, through
   previously implanted
   catheter 8C01X6J
Ventriculoscopy 00J04ZZ
Ventriculostomy
   External drainage
      see Drainage, Cerebral Ventricle
         0096
   Internal shunt
      see Bypass, Cerebral Ventricle
         0016
Ventriculovenostomy
   see Bypass, Cerebral Ventricle
      0016
Ventrio™ Hernia Patch
   use Synthetic Substitute
VEP (visual evoked potential)
   4A07X0Z
Vermiform appendix
   use Appendix
Vermilion border
   use Lip, Lower
   use Lip, Upper
Versa
   use Pacemaker, Dual Chamber in 0JH
Version, obstetric
   External 10S0XZZ
   Internal 10S07ZZ
Vertebral arch
   use Vertebra, Cervical
   use Vertebra, Lumbar
   use Vertebra, Thoracic
Vertebral body
   use Cervical Vertebra
   use Thoracic Vertebra
   use Lumbar Vertebra

Vertebral canal
   use Spinal Canal
Vertebral foramen
   use Vertebra, Cervical
   use Vertebra, Lumbar
   use Vertebra, Thoracic
Vertebral lamina
   use Vertebra, Cervical
   use Vertebra, Lumbar
   use Vertebra, Thoracic
Vertebral pedicle
   use Vertebra, Cervical
   use Vertebra, Lumbar
   use Vertebra, Thoracic
Vesical vein
   use Vein, Hypogastric, Left
   use Vein, Hypogastric, Right
Vesicotomy
   see Drainage, Urinary System 0T9
Vesiculectomy
   see Excision, Male Reproductive
      System 0VB
   see Resection, Male Reproductive
      System 0VT
Vesiculogram, seminal
   see Plain Radiography, Male
      Reproductive System BV0
Vesiculotomy
   see Drainage, Male Reproductive
      System 0V9
Vestibular (Scarpa's) ganglion
   use Nerve, Acoustic
Vestibular Assessment F15Z
Vestibular nerve
   use Nerve, Acoustic
Vestibular Treatment F0C
Vestibulocochlear nerve
   use Nerve, Acoustic
VH-IVUS (virtual histology
   intravascular ultrasound)
   see Ultrasonography, Heart
      B24
Virchow's (supraclavicular) lymph
   node
   use Lymphatic, Neck, Left
   use Lymphatic, Neck, Right
Virtuoso (II) (DR) (VR)
   use Defibrillator Generator in 0JH
Vistogard®
   use Uridine Triacetate
Vitrectomy
   see Excision, Eye 08B
   see Resection, Eye 08T
Vitreous body
   use Vitreous, Left
   use Vitreous, Right
Viva (XT)(S)
   use Cardiac Resynchronization
      Defibrillator Pulse Generator
      in 0JH
Vocal fold
   use Vocal Cord, Left
   use Vocal Cord, Right
Vocational
   Assessment
   Retraining
      see Activities of Daily Living
         Assessment, Rehabilitation
         F02
      see Activities of Daily Living
         Treatment, Rehabilitation
         F08
Volar (palmar) digital vein
   use Vein, Hand, Left
   use Vein, Hand, Right
Volar (palmar) metacarpal
   vein
   use Vein, Hand, Left
   use Vein, Hand, Right
Vomer bone
   use Septum, Nasal

Vomer of nasal septum
use Bone, Nasal
Voraxaze
Glucarpidase
Vulvectomy
see Excision, Female Reproductive
System 0UB
see Resection, Female Reproductive
System 0UT
VYXEOS™
use Cytarabine and Daunorubicin
Liposome Antineoplastic

W

WALLSTENT® Endoprosthesis
use Intraluminal Device
Washing
see Irrigation
WavelinQ EndoAVF system
Radial Artery, Left 031C
Radial Artery, Right 031B
Ulnar Artery, Left 031A
Ulnar Artery, Right 0319
Wedge resection, pulmonary
see Excision, Respiratory System
0BB
**Whole Blood Nucleic Acid-base
Microbial Detection** XXE5XM5
Window
see Drainage
Wiring, dental 2W31X9Z

X

X-ray
see Plain Radiography
X-STOP® Spacer
use Spinal Stabilization Device,
Interspinous Process in 0RH
use Spinal Stabilization Device,
Interspinous Process in 0SH
Xact Carotid Stent System
use Intraluminal Device
XENLETA™
use Lefamulin Anti-infective
Xenograft
use Zooplastic Tissue in Heart and
Great Vessels
**XIENCE Everolimus Eluting
Coronary Stent System**
use Intraluminal Device, Drug-
eluting in Heart and Great
Vessels
Xiphoid process
use Sternum
XLIF® System
use Interbody Fusion Device in
Lower Joints
XOSPATA®
use Gilteritinib Antineoplastic

Y

Yoga Therapy 8E0ZXY4

Z

Z-plasty, skin for scar contracture
see Release, Skin and Breast
0HN
Zenith AAA Endovascular Graft
use Intraluminal Device
**Zenith® Fenestrated AAA
Endovascular Graft**
use Intraluminal Device, Branched
or Fenestrated, One or Two
Arteries in 04V
use Intraluminal Device, Branched
or Fenestrated, Three or More
Arteries in 04V
Zenith Flex® AAA Endovascular Graft
use Intraluminal Device
**Zenith TX2® TAA Endovascular
Graft**
use Intraluminal Device
**Zenith® Renu™ AAA Ancillary
Graft**
use Intraluminal Device
ZERBAXA®
use Ceftolozane/Tazobactam Anti-
infective
**Zilver® PTX® (paclitaxel) Drug-
Eluting Peripheral Stent**
use Intraluminal Device, Drug-
eluting in Lower Arteries
use Intraluminal Device, Drug-
eluting in Upper Arteries

**Zimmer® NexGen® LPS Mobile
Bearing Knee**
use Synthetic Substitute
**Zimmer® NexGen® LPS-Flex Mobile
Knee**
use Synthetic Substitute
ZINPLAVA™
use Bezlotoxumab Monoclonal
AntibodyZonule of Zinn
Zonule of Zinn
use Lens, Left
use Lens, Right
**Zooplastic Tissue, Rapid
Deployment Technique,
Replacement** X2RF
**Zotarolimus-eluting coronary
stent**
use Intraluminal Device, Drug-
eluting in Heart and Great
Vessels
ZULRESSO™
use Brexanolone
Zygomatic process of frontal bone
use Bone, Frontal
**Zygomatic process of temporal
bone**
use Bone, Temporal, Left
use Bone, Temporal, Right
Zygomaticus muscle
use Muscle, Facial
Zyvox
use Oxazolidinones

Within each section of ICD-10-PCS the characters have different meanings. The seven character meanings for the Medical and Surgical section are illustrated here through the procedure example of *Percutaneous needle core biopsy of the right kidney*.

Section	Body System	Root Operation	Body Part	Approach	Device	Qualifier
Med/Surg	Urinary	Excision	Kidney, Right	Percutaneous	None	Diagnostic
0	T	B	0	3	Z	X

Section (Character 1)

All Medical and Surgical procedure codes have a first character value of 0.

Body System (Character 2)

The alphanumeric character for the body system is placed in the second position. The following are the body systems applicable to the Medical and Surgical section.

Character Value	Character Value Description
0	Central Nervous System and Cranial Nerves
1	Peripheral Nervous System
2	Heart and Great Vessels
3	Upper Arteries
4	Lower Arteries
5	Upper Veins
6	Lower Veins
7	Lymphatic and Hemic Systems
8	Eye
9	Ear, Nose, Sinus
B	Respiratory System
C	Mouth and Throat
D	Gastrointestinal System
F	Hepatobiliary System and Pancreas
G	Endocrine System
H	Skin and Breast
J	Subcutaneous Tissue and Fascia
K	Muscles
L	Tendons
M	Bursae and Ligaments
N	Head and Facial Bones
P	Upper Bones
Q	Lower Bones
R	Upper Joints
S	Lower Joints
T	Urinary System
U	Female Reproductive System
V	Male Reproductive System
W	Anatomical Regions, General
X	Anatomical Regions, Upper Extremities
Y	Anatomical Regions, Lower Extremities

Root Operations (Character 3)

The alphanumeric character value for root operations is placed in the third position. Listed below are the root operations applicable to the Medical and Surgical section with their associated meaning.

Character Value	Root Operation	Root Operation Definition
0	Alteration	Modifying the anatomic structure of a body part without affecting the function of the body part
1	Bypass	Altering the route of passage of the contents of a tubular body part
2	Change	Taking out or off a device from a body part and putting back an identical or similar device in or on the same body part without cutting or puncturing the skin or a mucous membrane
3	Control	Stopping, or attempting to stop, postprocedural or other acute bleeding
4	Creation	Making a new genital structure that does not take over the function of a body part
5	Destruction	Physical eradication of all or a portion of a body part by the direct use of energy, force, or a destructive agent
6	Detachment	Cutting off all or a portion of the upper or lower extremities
7	Dilation	Expanding an orifice or the lumen of a tubular body part
8	Division	Cutting into a body part, without draining fluids and/or gases from the body part, in order to separate or transect a body part
9	Drainage	Taking or letting out fluids and/or gases from a body part
B	Excision	Cutting out or off, without replacement, a portion of a body part
C	Extirpation	Taking or cutting out solid matter from a body part
D	Extraction	Pulling or stripping out or off all or a portion of a body part by the use of force
F	Fragmentation	Breaking solid matter in a body part into pieces
G	Fusion	Joining together portions of an articular body part rendering the articular body part immobile
H	Insertion	Putting in a nonbiological appliance that monitors, assists, performs, or prevents a physiological function but does not physically take the place of a body part
J	Inspection	Visually and/or manually exploring a body part
K	Map	Locating the route of passage of electrical impulses and/or locating functional areas in a body part
L	Occlusion	Completely closing an orifice or the lumen of a tubular body part
M	Reattachment	Putting back in or on all or a portion of a separated body part to its normal location or other suitable location
N	Release	Freeing a body part from an abnormal physical constraint by cutting or by the use of force
P	Removal	Taking out or off a device from a body part
Q	Repair	Restoring, to the extent possible, a body part to its normal anatomic structure and function
R	Replacement	Putting in or on biological or synthetic material that physically takes the place and/or function of all or a portion of a body part
S	Reposition	Moving to its normal location, or other suitable location, all or a portion of a body part
T	Resection	Cutting out or off, without replacement, all of a body part
V	Restriction	Partially closing an orifice or the lumen of a tubular body part
W	Revision	Correcting, to the extent possible, a portion of a malfunctioning device or the position of a displaced device
U	Supplement	Putting in or on biological or synthetic material that physically reinforces and/or augments the function of a portion of a body part
X	Transfer	Moving, without taking out, all or a portion of a body part to another location to take over the function of all or a portion of a body part
Y	Transplantation	Putting in or on all or a portion of a living body part taken from another individual or animal to physically take the place and/or function of all or a portion of a similar body part

Body Part (Character 4)

For each body system the applicable body part character values will be available for procedure code construction. An example of a body part for this section is the Large Intestines.

Approach (Character 5)

The approach is the technique used to reach the procedure site. The following are the approach character values for the Medical and Surgical section with the associated definitions.

Character Value	Approach	Approach Definition
0	Open	Cutting through the skin or mucous membrane and any other body layers necessary to expose the site of the procedure
3	Percutaneous	Entry, by puncture or minor incision, of instrumentation through the skin or mucous membrane and any other body layers necessary to reach the site of the procedure
4	Percutaneous Endoscopic	Entry, by puncture or minor incision, of instrumentation through the skin or mucous membrane and any other body layers necessary to reach and visualize the site of the procedure
7	Via Natural or Artificial Opening	Entry of instrumentation through a natural or artificial external opening to reach the site of the procedure
8	Via Natural or Artificial Opening Endoscopic	Entry of instrumentation through a natural or artificial external opening to reach and visualize the site of the procedure
F	Via Natural or Artificial Opening Percutaneous Endoscopic	Entry of instrumentation through a natural or artificial external opening to reach and visualize the site of the procedure, and entry, by puncture or minor incision, of instrumentation through the skin or mucous membrane and any other body layers necessary to aid in the performance of the procedure
X	External	Procedures performed directly on the skin or mucous membrane and procedures performed indirectly by the application of external force through the skin or mucous membrane

Device (Character 6)

Depending on the procedure performed there may or may not be a device used. There are several types of devices included in the Medical and Surgical section that fall into one of the four following categories.

- Electronic Appliances
- Grafts and Prostheses
- Implants
- Simple or Mechanical Appliances

When a device is not utilized during the procedure, the character value of Z should be reported.

If a coder is unsure of which option to select for the device utilized during the procedure, Appendix E can be used to guide the selection. For example, if the coder is in Table 02R (replacement of heart and great vessels) the coder can locate the device categories in Appendix E (Autologous Tissue Substitute, Zooplastic Tissue, Synthetic Substitute, and Nonautologous Tissue Substitue). For each of these categories brand name devices and other devices are listed. The coder should select the category in which the device utilized during the procedure is listed.

Qualifier (Character 7)

The qualifier represents an additional attribute for the procedure when applicable. In the preceding example of *Percutaneous needle core biopsy of the right kidney*, the qualifier of X was used to report that the biopsy procedure was diagnostic in nature. If there is no qualifier for a procedure, the Z character value should be reported.

Important Definitions for the Medical and Surgical Section

Medical Surgical Root Operation	Qualifier	Definition
Detachment of Upper and Lower Extremities (0X6 and 0Y6) Arms and Legs	1 – High	Amputation at the proximal portion of the shaft of the humerus or femur
	2 – Mid	Amputation at the middle portion of the shaft of the humerus or femur
	3 – Low	Amputation at the distal portion of the shaft of the humerus or femur
Detachment of Upper and Lower Extremities (0X6 and 0Y6) Fingers, Thumbs, and Toes	0 – Complete	Amputation at the metacarpophalangeal/metatarsal-phalangeal joint
	1 – High	Amputation anywhere along the proximal phalanx
	2 – Mid	Amputation through the proximal interphalangeal joint or anywhere along the middle phalanx
	3 – Low	Amputation through the distal interphalangeal joint or anywhere along the distal phalanx
Transplantation	0 – Allogeneic	Being genetically different although belonging to or obtained from the same species*
	1 – Syngeneic	Genetically identical or closely related, so as to allow tissue transplant; immunologically compatible*
	2 – Zooplastic	Surgical transfer of tissue from an animal to a human*

*Taken from The Free Dictionary by Farlex at www.thefreedictionary.com

Medical and Surgical Section Guidelines (section 0)

B2. Body System

General guidelines

B2.1a The procedure codes in Anatomical Regions, General, Anatomical Regions, Upper Extremities and Anatomical Regions, Lower Extremities can be used when the procedure is performed on an anatomical region rather than a specific body part, or on the rare occasion when no information is available to support assignment of a code to a specific body part.

Examples: Chest tube drainage of the pleural cavity is coded to the root operation Drainage found in the body system Anatomical Regions, General. Suture repair of the abdominal wall is coded to the root operation Repair in the body system Anatomical Regions, General. Amputation of the foot is coded to the root operation Detachment in the body system Anatomical Regions, Lower Extremities.

B2.1b Where the general body part values "upper" and "lower" are provided as an option in the Upper Arteries, Lower Arteries, Upper Veins, Lower Veins, Muscles and Tendons body systems, "upper" or "lower" specifies body parts located above or below the diaphragm respectively.

Example: Vein body parts above the diaphragm are found in the Upper Veins body system; vein body parts below the diaphragm are found in the Lower Veins body system.

B3. Root Operation

General guidelines

B3.1a In order to determine the appropriate root operation, the full definition of the root operation as contained in the PCS Tables must be applied.

B3.1b Components of a procedure specified in the root operation definition or explanation as integral to that root operation are not coded separately. Procedural steps necessary to reach the operative site and close the operative site, including anastomosis of a tubular body part, are also not coded separately.

Examples: Resection of a joint as part of a joint replacement procedure is included in the root operation definition of Replacement and is not coded separately. Laparotomy performed to reach the site of an open liver biopsy is not coded separately. In a resection of sigmoid colon with anastomosis of descending colon to rectum, the anastomosis is not coded separately.

Multiple procedures

B3.2 During the same operative episode, multiple procedures are coded if:

    a. The same root operation is performed on different body parts as defined by distinct values of the body part character.

        Examples: Diagnostic excision of liver and pancreas are coded separately. Excision of lesion in the ascending colon and excision of lesion in the transverse colon are coded separately.

    b. The same root operation is repeated at different body sites that are included in the same body part value.

        Examples: Excision of the sartorius muscle and excision of the gracilis muscle are both included in the upper leg muscle body part value, and multiple procedures are coded. Extraction of multiple toenails are coded separately.

    c. Multiple root operations with distinct objectives are performed on the same body part.

        Example: Destruction of sigmoid lesion and bypass of sigmoid colon are coded separately.

    d. The intended root operation is attempted using one approach but is converted to a different approach.

        Example: Laparoscopic cholecystectomy converted to an open cholecystectomy is coded as percutaneous endoscopic Inspection and open Resection.

Discontinued or incomplete procedures

B3.3 If the intended procedure is discontinued or otherwise not complete, code the procedure to the root operation performed. If a procedure is discontinued before any other root operation is performed, code the root operation Inspection of the body part or anatomical region inspected.

Example: A planned aortic valve replacement procedure is discontinued after the initial thoracotomy and before any incision is made in the heart muscle, when the patient becomes hemodynamically unstable. This procedure is coded as an open Inspection of the mediastinum.

Biopsy procedures

B3.4a Biopsy procedures are coded using the root operations Excision, Extraction, or Drainage and the qualifier Diagnostic.

Examples: Fine needle aspiration biopsy of lung is coded to the root operation Drainage with the qualifier Diagnostic. Biopsy of bone marrow is coded to the root operation Extraction with the qualifier Diagnostic. Lymph node sampling for biopsy is coded to the root operation Excision with the qualifier Diagnostic.

Biopsy followed by more definitive treatment

B3.4b If a diagnostic Excision, Extraction, or Drainage procedure (biopsy) is followed by a more definitive procedure, such as Destruction, Excision or Resection at the same procedure site, both the biopsy and the more definitive treatment are coded.

Example: Biopsy of breast followed by partial mastectomy at the same procedure site, both the biopsy and the partial mastectomy procedure are coded.

Overlapping body layers

B3.5 If root operations Excision, Extraction, Repair or Inspection are performed on overlapping layers of the musculoskeletal system, the body part specifying the deepest layer is coded.

Example: Excisional debridement that includes skin and subcutaneous tissue and muscle is coded to the muscle body part.

Bypass procedures

B3.6a Bypass procedures are coded by identifying the body part bypassed "from" and the body part bypassed "to." The fourth character body part specifies the body part bypassed from, and the qualifier specifies the body part bypassed to.

Example: Bypass from stomach to jejunum, stomach is the body part and jejunum is the qualifier.

B3.6b Coronary artery bypass procedures are coded differently than other bypass procedures as described in the previous guideline. Rather than identifying the body part bypassed from, the body part identifies the number of coronary artery sites bypassed to, and the qualifier specifies the vessel bypassed from.

Example: Aortocoronary artery bypass of the left anterior descending coronary artery and the obtuse marginal coronary artery is classified in the body part axis of classification as two coronary arteries and the qualifier specifies the aorta as the body part bypassed from.

B3.6c If multiple coronary arteries are bypassed, a separate procedure is coded for each coronary artery that uses a different device and/or qualifier.

Example: Aortocoronary artery bypass and internal mammary coronary artery bypass are coded separately.

Control vs. more definitive root operations

B3.7 The root operation Control is defined as, "Stopping, or attempting to stop, postprocedural or other acute bleeding." If an attempt to stop postprocedural or other acute bleeding is initially unsuccessful, and to stop the bleeding requires performing a more definitive root operation, such as Bypass, Detachment, Excision, Extraction, Reposition, Replacement, or Resection, then the more definitive root operation is coded instead of Control.

Example: Resection of spleen to stop bleeding is coded to Resection instead of Control.

Excision vs. Resection

B3.8 PCS contains specific body parts for anatomical subdivisions of a body part, such as lobes of the lungs or liver and regions of the intestine. Resection of the specific body part is coded whenever all of the body part is cut out or off, rather than coding Excision of a less specific body part.

Example: Left upper lung lobectomy is coded to Resection of Upper Lung Lobe, Left rather than Excision of Lung, Left.

Excision for graft

B3.9 If an autograft is obtained from a different procedure site in order to complete the objective of the procedure, a separate procedure is coded, except when the seventh character qualifier value in the ICD-10-PCS table fully specifies the site from which the autograft was obtained.

Examples: Coronary bypass with excision of saphenous vein graft, excision of saphenous vein is coded separately. Replacement of breast with autologous deep inferior epigastric artery perforator (DIEP) flap, excision of the DIEP flap is not coded separately. The seventh character qualifier value Deep Inferior Epigastric Artery Perforator Flap in the Replacement table fully specifies the site of the autograft harvest.

Fusion procedures of the spine

B3.10a The body part coded for a spinal vertebral joint(s) rendered immobile by a spinal fusion procedure is classified by the level of the spine (e.g. thoracic). There are distinct body part values for a single vertebral joint and for multiple vertebral joints at each spinal level.

Example: Body part values specify Lumbar Vertebral Joint, Lumbar Vertebral Joints, 2 or More and Lumbosacral Vertebral Joint.

B3.10b If multiple vertebral joints are fused, a separate procedure is coded for each vertebral joint that uses a different device and/or qualifier.

Example: Fusion of lumbar vertebral joint, posterior approach, anterior column and fusion of lumbar vertebral joint, posterior approach, posterior column are coded separately.

B3.10c Combinations of devices and materials are often used on a vertebral joint to render the joint immobile. When combinations of devices are used on the same vertebral joint, the device value coded for the procedure is as follows:

- If an interbody fusion device is used to render the joint immobile (containing bone graft or bone graft substitute), the procedure is coded with the device value Interbody Fusion Device

- If bone graft is the only device used to render the joint immobile, the procedure is coded with the device value Nonautologous Tissue Substitute or Autologous Tissue Substitute
  - If a mixture of autologous and nonautologous bone graft (with or without biological or synthetic extenders or binders) is used to render the joint immobile, code the procedure with the device value Autologous Tissue Substitute

Examples: Fusion of a vertebral joint using a cage style interbody fusion device containing morsellized bone graft is coded to the device Interbody Fusion Device. Fusion of a vertebral joint using a bone dowel interbody fusion device made of cadaver bone and packed with a mixture of local morsellized bone and demineralized bone matrix is coded to the device Interbody Fusion Device. Fusion of a vertebral joint using both autologous bone graft and bone bank bone graft is coded to the device Autologous Tissue Substitute.

Inspection procedures

B3.11a Inspection of a body part(s) performed in order to achieve the objective of a procedure is not coded separately.

Example: Fiberoptic bronchoscopy performed for irrigation of bronchus, only the irrigation procedure is coded.

B3.11b If multiple tubular body parts are inspected, the most distal body part inspected is coded. If multiple non-tubular body parts in a region are inspected, the body part that specifies the entire area inspected is coded.

Examples: Cystoureteroscopy with inspection of bladder and ureters is coded to the ureter body part value. Exploratory laparotomy with general inspection of abdominal contents is coded to the peritoneal cavity body part value.

B3.11c When both an Inspection procedure and another procedure are performed on the same body part during the same episode, if the Inspection procedure is performed using a different approach than the other procedure, the Inspection procedure is coded separately.

Example: Endoscopic Inspection of the duodenum is coded separately when open Excision of the duodenum is performed during the same procedural episode.

Occlusion vs. Restriction for vessel embolization procedures

B3.12 If the objective of an embolization procedure is to completely close a vessel, the root operation Occlusion is coded. If the objective of an embolization procedure is to narrow the lumen of a vessel, the root operation Restriction is coded.

Examples: Tumor embolization is coded to the root operation Occlusion, because the objective of the procedure is to cut off the blood supply to the vessel. Embolization of a cerebral aneurysm is coded to the root operation Restriction, because the objective of the procedure is not to close off the vessel entirely, but to narrow the lumen of the vessel at the site of the aneurysm where it is abnormally wide.

Release procedures

B3.13 In the root operation Release, the body part value coded is the body part being freed and not the tissue being manipulated or cut to free the body part.

Example: Lysis of intestinal adhesions is coded to the specific intestine body part value.

Release vs. Division

B3.14 If the sole objective of the procedure is freeing a body part without cutting the body part, the root operation is Release. If the sole objective of the procedure is separating or transecting a body part, the root operation is Division.

Example: Freeing a nerve root from surrounding scar tissue to relieve pain is coded to the root operation Release. Severing a nerve root to relieve pain is coded to the root operation Division.

Reposition for fracture treatment

B3.15 Reduction of a displaced fracture is coded to the root operation Reposition and the application of a cast or splint in conjunction with the Reposition procedure is not coded separately. Treatment of a nondisplaced fracture is coded to the procedure performed.

Examples: Putting a pin in a nondisplaced fracture is coded to the root operation Insertion. Casting of a nondisplaced fracture is coded to the root operation Immobilization in the Placement section.

Transplantation vs. Administration

B3.16 Putting in a mature and functioning living body part taken from another individual or animal is coded to the root operation Transplantation. Putting in autologous or nonautologous cells is coded to the Administration section.

Example: Putting in autologous or nonautologous bone marrow, pancreatic islet cells or stem cells is coded to the Administration section.

Transfer procedures using multiple tissue layers

B3.17 The root operation Transfer contains qualifiers that can be used to specify when a transfer flap is composed of more than one tissue layer, such as a musculocutaneous flap. For procedures involving transfer of multiple tissue layers including skin, subcutaneous tissue, fascia or muscle, the procedure is coded to the body part value that describes the deepest tissue layer in the flap, and the qualifier can be used to describe the other tissue layer(s) in the transfer flap.

Example: A musculocutaneous flap transfer is coded to the appropriate body part value in the body system Muscles, and the qualifier is used to describe the additional tissue layer(s) in the transfer flap.

Excision/Resection followed by replacement

B3.18 If an Excision or Resection of a body part is followed by a Replacement procedure, code both procedures to identify each distinct objective, except when the Excision or Resection is considered integral and preparatory for the Replacement procedure.

Examples: Mastectomy followed by reconstruction, both Resection and Replacement of the breast are coded to fully capture the distinct objectives of the procedures performed. Maxillectomy with obturator reconstruction, both Excision and Replacement of the maxilla are coded to fully capture the distinct objectives of the procedures performed. Excisional debridement of tendon with skin graft, both the Excision of the tendon and the Replacement of the skin with a graft are coded to fully capture the distinct objectives of the procedures performed. Esophagectomy followed by reconstruction with colonic interposition, both the Resection and the Transfer of the large intestine to function as the esophagus are coded to fully capture the distinct objectives of the procedures performed.

Examples: Resection of a joint as part of a joint replacement procedure is considered integral and preparatory for the Replacement of the joint and the Resection is not coded separately. Resection of a valve as part of a valve replacement procedure is considered integral and preparatory for the valve Replacement and the Resection is not coded separately.

B4. Body Part

General guidelines

B4.1a If a procedure is performed on a portion of a body part that does not have a separate body part value, code the body part value corresponding to the whole body part.

Example: A procedure performed on the alveolar process of the mandible is coded to the mandible body part.

B4.1b If the prefix "peri" is combined with a body part to identify the site of the procedure, and the site of the procedure is not further specified, then the procedure is coded to the body part named. This guideline applies only when a more specific body part value is not available.

Examples: A procedure site identified as perirenal is coded to the kidney body part when the site of the procedure is not further specified. A procedure site described in the documentation as peri-urethral tissue, and the documentation also indicates that it is the vulvar tissue and not the urethral tissue that is the site of the procedure, then the procedure is coded to the vulva body part. A procedure site documented as involving the periosteum is coded to the corresponding bone body part.

B4.1c If a procedure is performed on a continuous section of a tubular body part, code the body part value corresponding to the furthest anatomical site from the point of entry.

Example: A procedure performed on a continuous section of artery from the femoral artery to the external iliac artery with the point of entry at the femoral artery is coded to the external iliac body part.

Branches of body parts

B4.2 Where a specific branch of a body part does not have its own body part value in PCS, the body part is typically coded to the closest proximal branch that has a specific body part value. In the cardiovascular body systems, if a general body part is available in the correct root operation table, and coding to a proximal branch would require assigning a code in a different body system, the procedure is coded using the general body part value.

Examples: A procedure performed on the mandibular branch of the trigeminal nerve is coded to the trigeminal nerve body part value. Occlusion of the bronchial artery is coded to the body part value Upper Artery in the body system Upper Arteries, and not to the body part value Thoracic Aorta, Descending in the body system Heart and Great Vessels.

Bilateral body part values

B4.3 Bilateral body part values are available for a limited number of body parts. If the identical procedure is performed on contralateral body parts, and a bilateral body part value exists for that body part, a single procedure is coded using the bilateral body part value. If no bilateral body part value exists, each procedure is coded separately using the appropriate body part value.

Examples: The identical procedure performed on both fallopian tubes is coded once using the body part value Fallopian Tube, Bilateral. The identical procedure performed on both knee joints is coded twice using the body part values Knee Joint, Right and Knee Joint, Left.

Coronary arteries

B4.4 The coronary arteries are classified as a single body part that is further specified by number of arteries treated. One procedure code specifying multiple arteries is used when the same procedure is performed, including the same device and qualifier values.

Examples: Angioplasty of two distinct coronary arteries with placement of two stents is coded as Dilation of Coronary Artery, Two Arteries, with Two Intraluminal Devices. Angioplasty of two distinct coronary arteries, one with stent placed and one without, is coded separately as Dilation of Coronary Artery, One Artery with Intraluminal Device, and Dilation of Coronary Artery, One Artery with no device.

Tendons, ligaments, bursae and fascia near a joint

B4.5 Procedures performed on tendons, ligaments, bursae and fascia supporting a joint are coded to the body part in the respective body system that is the focus of the procedure. Procedures performed on joint structures themselves are coded to the body part in the joint body systems.

Examples: Repair of the anterior cruciate ligament of the knee is coded to the knee bursae and ligament body part in the Bursae and Ligaments body system. Knee arthroscopy with shaving of articular cartilage is coded to the knee joint body part in the Lower Joints body system.

Skin, subcutaneous tissue and fascia overlying a joint

B4.6 If a procedure is performed on the skin, subcutaneous tissue or fascia overlying a joint, the procedure is coded to the following body part:

- Shoulder is coded to Upper Arm
- Elbow is coded to Lower Arm
- Wrist is coded to Lower Arm
- Hip is coded to Upper Leg
- Knee is coded to Lower Leg
- Ankle is coded to Foot

Fingers and toes

B4.7 If a body system does not contain a separate body part value for fingers, procedures performed on the fingers are coded to the body part value for the hand. If a body system does not contain a separate body part value for toes, procedures performed on the toes are coded to the body part value for the foot.

Example: Excision of finger muscle is coded to one of the hand muscle body part values in the Muscles body system.

Upper and lower intestinal tract

B4.8 In the Gastrointestinal body system, the general body part values Upper Intestinal Tract and Lower Intestinal Tract are provided as an option for the root operations Change, Inspection, Removal and Revision. Upper Intestinal Tract includes the portion of the gastrointestinal tract from the esophagus down to and including the duodenum, and Lower Intestinal Tract includes the portion of the gastrointestinal tract from the jejunum down to and including the rectum and anus.

Example: In the root operation Change table, change of a device in the jejunum is coded using the body part Lower Intestinal Tract.

B5. Approach

Open approach with percutaneous endoscopic assistance

B5.2a Procedures performed using the open approach with percutaneous endoscopic assistance are coded to the approach Open.

Example: Laparoscopic-assisted sigmoidectomy is coded to the approach Open.

Percutaneous endoscopic approach with extension of incision

B5.2b Procedures performed using the percutaneous endoscopic approach, with incision or extension of an incision to assist in the removal of all or a portion of a body part or to anastomose a tubular body part to complete the procedure, are coded to the approach value Percutaneous Endoscopic.

Examples: Laparoscopic sigmoid colectomy with extension of stapling port for removal of specimen and direct anastomosis is coded to the approach value Percutaneous Endoscopic. Laparoscopic nephrectomy with midline incision for removing the resected kidney is coded to the approach value Percutaneous Endoscopic. Robotic-assisted laparoscopic prostatectomy with extension of incision for removal of the resected prostate is coded to the approach value Percutaneous Endoscopic.

External approach

B5.3a Procedures performed within an orifice on structures that are visible without the aid of any instrumentation are coded to the approach External.

Example: Resection of tonsils is coded to the approach External.

B5.3b Procedures performed indirectly by the application of external force through the intervening body layers are coded to the approach External.

Example: Closed reduction of fracture is coded to the approach External.

Percutaneous procedure via device

B5.4 Procedures performed percutaneously via a device placed for the procedure are coded to the approach Percutaneous.

Example: Fragmentation of kidney stone performed via percutaneous nephrostomy is coded to the approach Percutaneous.

B6. Device

General guidelines

B6.1a A device is coded only if a device remains after the procedure is completed. If no device remains, the device value No Device is coded. In limited root operations, the classification provides the qualifier values Temporary and Intraoperative, for specific procedures involving clinically significant devices, where the purpose of the device is to be utilized for a brief duration during the procedure or current inpatient stay. If a device that is intended to remain after the procedure is completed requires removal before the end of the operative episode in which it was inserted (for example, the device size is inadequate or a complication occurs), both the insertion and removal of the device should be coded.

B6.1b Materials such as sutures, ligatures, radiological markers and temporary post-operative wound drains are considered integral to the performance of a procedure and are not coded as devices.

B6.1c Procedures performed on a device only and not on a body part are specified in the root operations Change, Irrigation, Removal and Revision, and are coded to the procedure performed.

Example: Irrigation of percutaneous nephrostomy tube is coded to the root operation Irrigation of indwelling device in the Administration section.

Drainage device

B6.2 A separate procedure to put in a drainage device is coded to the root operation Drainage with the device value Drainage Device.

Coding Guidelines Reference

Coding Guidelines References

The tables below link ICD-10-PCS coding guidelines to Medical and Surgical section root operations, specific body system tables, and body systems. The guidelines identified in each table are provided in order to remind users to reference the coding guidelines prior to code reporting. The tables provide coding guideline references at the body system and root operation level. It is imperative to review the ICD-10-PCS coding guidelines to ensure the procedure code being reported is accurate and complete.

Root Operation References

Root Operation	Character Value	Coding Guideline(s)
Bypass	1	B3.6a
Change	2	B6.1c
Control	3	B3.7
Division	8	B3.14
Drainage	9	B3.4a, B3.4b, B6.2
Excision	B	B3.4a, B3.4b, B3.8, B3.9, B3.18
Extraction	D	B3.4a, B3.4b
Inspection	J	B3.11a, B3.11b, B3.11c
Occlusion	L	B3.12
Release	N	B3.13, B3.14
Removal	P	B6.1c
Replacement	R	B3.18
Resection	T	B3.8, B3.18
Restriction	V	B3.12
Revision	W	B6.1c
Transplantation	Y	B3.16

Table References

Table	Body System	Root Operation	Coding Guideline(s)
021	Heart and Great Vessels	Bypass	B3.6b, B3.6c, B4.4
027	Heart and Great Vessels	Dilation	B4.4
02C	Heart and Great Vessels	Extirpation	B4.4

Continued →

Table	Body System	Root Operation	Coding Guideline(s)
02Q	Heart and Great Vessels	Repair	B4.4
0HB	Skin and Breast	Excision	B3.5
0HJ	Skin and Breast	Inspection	B3.5
0HQ	Skin and Breast	Repair	B3.5
0HX	Skin and Breast	Transfer	B3.17
0JB	Subcutaneous Tissue and Fascia	Excision	B3.5
0JJ	Subcutaneous Tissue and Fascia	Inspection	B3.5
0JQ	Subcutaneous Tissue and Fascia	Repair	B3.5
0JX	Subcutaneous Tissue and Fascia	Transfer	B3.17
0KB	Muscles	Excision	B3.5
0KJ	Muscles	Inspection	B3.5
0KQ	Muscles	Repair	B3.5
0KX	Muscles	Transfer	B3.17
0LB	Tendons	Excision	B3.5
0LJ	Tendons	Inspection	B3.5
0LQ	Tendons	Repair	B3.5
0MB	Bursae and Ligaments	Excision	B3.5
0MJ	Bursae and Ligaments	Inspection	B3.5
0MQ	Bursae and Ligaments	Repair	B3.5
0NB	Head and Facial Bones	Excision	B3.5
0NJ	Head and Facial Bones	Inspection	B3.5
0NQ	Head and Facial Bones	Repair	B3.5
0NS	Head and Facial Bones	Reposition	B3.15
0PB	Upper Bones	Excision	B3.5
0PJ	Upper Bones	Inspection	B3.5
0PQ	Upper Bones	Repair	B3.5
0PS	Upper Bones	Reposition	B3.15
0QB	Lower Bones	Excision	B3.5
0QJ	Lower Bones	Inspection	B3.5
0QQ	Lower Bones	Repair	B3.5
0QS	Lower Bones	Reposition	B3.15
0RB	Upper Joints	Excision	B3.5
0RG	Upper Joints	Fusion	B3.10a, B3.10b, B3.10c
0RJ	Upper Joints	Inspection	B3.5
0RQ	Upper Joints	Repair	B3.5
0SB	Lower Joints	Excision	B3.5
0SG	Lower Joints	Fusion	B3.10a, B3.10b, B3.10c
0SJ	Lower Joints	Inspection	B3.5
0SQ	Lower Joints	Repair	B3.5
0UD	Female Reproductive System	Extraction	C2

Body System References

Body System	Character Value	Coding Guideline(s)
Gastrointestinal System	D	B4.8
Subcutaneous Tissue and Fascia	J	B4.5, B4.6
Tendons	L	B4.5
Bursae and Ligaments	M	B4.5
Upper Joints	R	B4.5
Lower Joints	S	B4.5

Medial Views of Cerebrum

Sagittal section of brain in situ

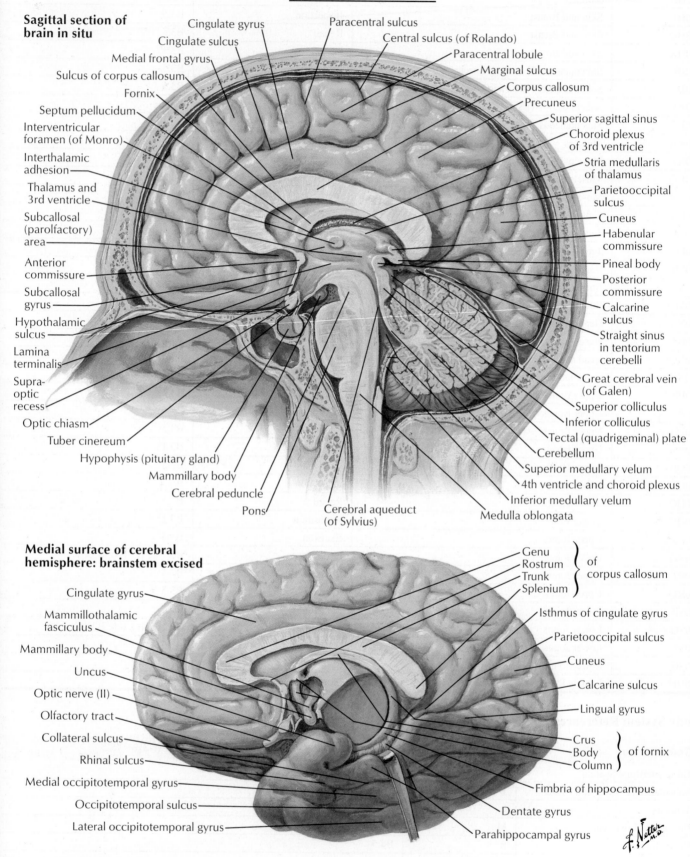

Cingulate gyrus
Cingulate sulcus
Medial frontal gyrus
Sulcus of corpus callosum
Fornix
Septum pellucidum
Interventricular foramen (of Monro)
Interthalamic adhesion
Thalamus and 3rd ventricle
Subcallosal (parolfactory) area
Anterior commissure
Subcallosal gyrus
Hypothalamic sulcus
Lamina terminalis
Supra-optic recess
Optic chiasm
Tuber cinereum
Hypophysis (pituitary gland)
Mammillary body
Cerebral peduncle
Pons
Cerebral aqueduct (of Sylvius)

Paracentral sulcus
Central sulcus (of Rolando)
Paracentral lobule
Marginal sulcus
Corpus callosum
Precuneus
Superior sagittal sinus
Choroid plexus of 3rd ventricle
Stria medullaris of thalamus
Parietooccipital sulcus
Cuneus
Habenular commissure
Pineal body
Posterior commissure
Calcarine sulcus
Straight sinus in tentorium cerebelli
Great cerebral vein (of Galen)
Superior colliculus
Inferior colliculus
Tectal (quadrigeminal) plate
Cerebellum
Superior medullary velum
4th ventricle and choroid plexus
Inferior medullary velum
Medulla oblongata

Medial surface of cerebral hemisphere: brainstem excised

Cingulate gyrus
Mammillothalamic fasciculus
Mammillary body
Uncus
Optic nerve (II)
Olfactory tract
Collateral sulcus
Rhinal sulcus
Medial occipitotemporal gyrus
Occipitotemporal sulcus
Lateral occipitotemporal gyrus

Genu
Rostrum
Trunk
Splenium
} of corpus callosum

Isthmus of cingulate gyrus
Parietooccipital sulcus
Cuneus
Calcarine sulcus
Lingual gyrus
Crus
Body
Column
} of fornix
Fimbria of hippocampus
Dentate gyrus
Parahippocampal gyrus

F. Netter M.D.

Cranial Nerves: Schema

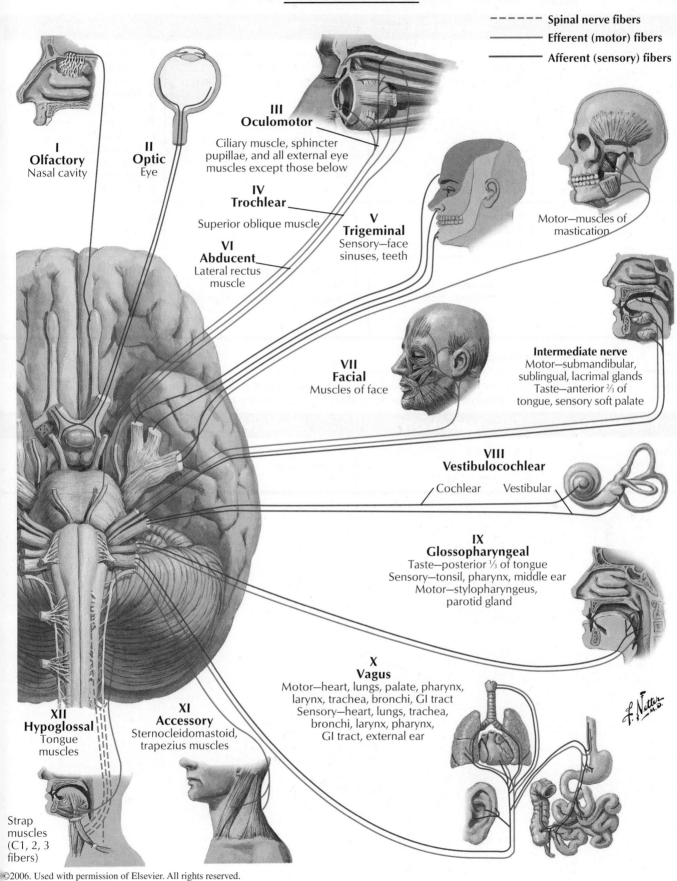

- - - - - Spinal nerve fibers
───── Efferent (motor) fibers
───── Afferent (sensory) fibers

III
Oculomotor
Ciliary muscle, sphincter pupillae, and all external eye muscles except those below

I
Olfactory
Nasal cavity

II
Optic
Eye

IV
Trochlear
Superior oblique muscle

V
Trigeminal
Sensory—face sinuses, teeth

VI
Abducent
Lateral rectus muscle

Motor—muscles of mastication

VII
Facial
Muscles of face

Intermediate nerve
Motor—submandibular, sublingual, lacrimal glands
Taste—anterior ⅔ of tongue, sensory soft palate

VIII
Vestibulocochlear
Cochlear   Vestibular

IX
Glossopharyngeal
Taste—posterior ⅓ of tongue
Sensory—tonsil, pharynx, middle ear
Motor—stylopharyngeus, parotid gland

X
Vagus
Motor—heart, lungs, palate, pharynx, larynx, trachea, bronchi, GI tract
Sensory—heart, lungs, trachea, bronchi, larynx, pharynx, GI tract, external ear

XII
Hypoglossal
Tongue muscles

XI
Accessory
Sternocleidomastoid, trapezius muscles

Strap muscles (C1, 2, 3 fibers)

Medical and Surgical, Central Nervous System and Cranial Nerves

Central Nervous System and Cranial Nerves Tables 001–00X

Section	0	Medical and Surgical
Body System	0	Central Nervous System and Cranial Nerves
Operation	1	**Bypass:** Altering the route of passage of the contents of a tubular body part

Body Part (4th)	Approach (5th)	Device (6th)	Qualifier (7th)
6 Cerebral Ventricle	0 Open 3 Percutaneous 4 Percutaneous Endoscopic	7 Autologous Tissue Substitute J Synthetic Substitute K Nonautologous Tissue Substitute	0 Nasopharynx 1 Mastoid Sinus 2 Atrium 3 Blood Vessel 4 Pleural Cavity 5 Intestine 6 Peritoneal Cavity 7 Urinary Tract 8 Bone Marrow A Subgaleal Space B Cerebral Cisterns
6 Cerebral Ventricle	0 Open 3 Percutaneous 4 Percutaneous Endoscopic	Z No Device	B Cerebral Cisterns
U Spinal Canal	0 Open 3 Percutaneous 4 Percutaneous Endoscopic	7 Autologous Tissue Substitute J Synthetic Substitute K Nonautologous Tissue Substitute	2 Atrium 4 Pleural Cavity 6 Peritoneal Cavity 7 Urinary Tract 9 Fallopian Tube

Section	0	Medical and Surgical
Body System	0	Central Nervous System and Cranial Nerves
Operation	2	**Change:** Taking out or off a device from a body part and putting back an identical or similar device in or on the same body part without cutting or puncturing the skin or a mucous membrane

Body Part (4th)	Approach (5th)	Device (6th)	Qualifier (7th)
0 Brain E Cranial Nerve U Spinal Canal	X External	0 Drainage Device Y Other Device	Z No Qualifier

Section	0	Medical and Surgical
Body System	0	Central Nervous System and Cranial Nerves
Operation	5	Destruction: Physical eradication of all or a portion of a body part by the direct use of energy, force, or a destructive agent

Body Part (4th)	Approach (5th)	Device (6th)	Qualifier (7th)
0 Brain 1 Cerebral Meninges 2 Dura Mater 6 Cerebral Ventricle 7 Cerebral Hemisphere 8 Basal Ganglia 9 Thalamus A Hypothalamus B Pons C Cerebellum D Medulla Oblongata F Olfactory Nerve G Optic Nerve H Oculomotor Nerve J Trochlear Nerve K Trigeminal Nerve L Abducens Nerve M Facial Nerve N Acoustic Nerve P Glossopharyngeal Nerve Q Vagus Nerve R Accessory Nerve S Hypoglossal Nerve T Spinal Meninges W Cervical Spinal Cord X Thoracic Spinal Cord Y Lumbar Spinal Cord	0 Open 3 Percutaneous 4 Percutaneous Endoscopic	Z No Device	Z No Qualifier

Section	0	Medical and Surgical
Body System	0	Central Nervous System and Cranial Nerves
Operation	7	Dilation: Expanding an orifice or the lumen of a tubular body part

Body Part (4th)	Approach (5th)	Device (6th)	Qualifier (7th)
6 Cerebral Ventricle	0 Open 3 Percutaneous 4 Percutaneous Endoscopic	Z No Device	Z No Qualifie

Section	0	Medical and Surgical
Body System	0	Central Nervous System and Cranial Nerves
Operation	8	Division: Cutting into a body part, without draining fluids and/or gases from the body part, in order to separate or transect a body part

Body Part (4th)	Approach (5th)	Device (6th)	Qualifier (7th)
0 Brain 7 Cerebral Hemisphere 8 Basal Ganglia F Olfactory Nerve G Optic Nerve H Oculomotor Nerve J Trochlear Nerve K Trigeminal Nerve L Abducens Nerve M Facial Nerve N Acoustic Nerve P Glossopharyngeal Nerve Q Vagus Nerve R Accessory Nerve S Hypoglossal Nerve W Cervical Spinal Cord X Thoracic Spinal Cord Y Lumbar Spinal Cord	0 Open 3 Percutaneous 4 Percutaneous Endoscopic	Z No Device	Z No Qualifier

Section	0	Medical and Surgical
Body System	0	Central Nervous System and Cranial Nerves
Operation	9	Drainage: Taking or letting out fluids and/or gases from a body part

Body Part (4th)	Approach (5th)	Device (6th)	Qualifier (7th)
0 Brain 1 Cerebral Meninges 2 Dura Mater 3 Epidural Space, Intracranial 4 Subdural Space, Intracranial 5 Subarachnoid Space, Intracranial 6 Cerebral Ventricle 7 Cerebral Hemisphere 8 Basal Ganglia 9 Thalamus A Hypothalamus B Pons C Cerebellum D Medulla Oblongata F Olfactory Nerve G Optic Nerve H Oculomotor Nerve J Trochlear Nerve K Trigeminal Nerve L Abducens Nerve M Facial Nerve N Acoustic Nerve P Glossopharyngeal Nerve Q Vagus Nerve R Accessory Nerve S Hypoglossal Nerve T Spinal Meninges U Spinal Canal W Cervical Spinal Cord X Thoracic Spinal Cord Y Lumbar Spinal Cord	0 Open 3 Percutaneous 4 Percutaneous Endoscopic	0 Drainage Device	Z No Qualifier
0 Brain 1 Cerebral Meninges 2 Dura Mater 3 Epidural Space, Intracranial 4 Subdural Space, Intracranial 5 Subarachnoid Space, Intracranial 6 Cerebral Ventricle 7 Cerebral Hemisphere 8 Basal Ganglia 9 Thalamus A Hypothalamus B Pons C Cerebellum D Medulla Oblongata F Olfactory Nerve G Optic Nerve H Oculomotor Nerve J Trochlear Nerve K Trigeminal Nerve L Abducens Nerve M Facial Nerve N Acoustic Nerve P Glossopharyngeal Nerve Q Vagus Nerve R Accessory Nerve S Hypoglossal Nerve T Spinal Meninges U Spinal Canal W Cervical Spinal Cord X Thoracic Spinal Cord Y Lumbar Spinal Cord	0 Open 3 Percutaneous 4 Percutaneous Endoscopic	Z No Device	X Diagnostic Z No Qualifier

Section	0	Medical and Surgical
Body System	0	Central Nervous System and Cranial Nerves
Operation	B	Excision: Cutting out or off, without replacement, a portion of a body part

Body Part (4th)	Approach (5th)	Device (6th)	Qualifier (7th)
0 Brain	0 Open	Z No Device	X Diagnostic
1 Cerebral Meninges	3 Percutaneous		Z No Qualifier
2 Dura Mater	4 Percutaneous Endoscopic		
6 Cerebral Ventricle			
7 Cerebral Hemisphere			
8 Basal Ganglia			
9 Thalamus			
A Hypothalamus			
B Pons			
C Cerebellum			
D Medulla Oblongata			
F Olfactory Nerve			
G Optic Nerve			
H Oculomotor Nerve			
J Trochlear Nerve			
K Trigeminal Nerve			
L Abducens Nerve			
M Facial Nerve			
N Acoustic Nerve			
P Glossopharyngeal Nerve			
Q Vagus Nerve			
R Accessory Nerve			
S Hypoglossal Nerve			
T Spinal Meninges			
W Cervical Spinal Cord			
X Thoracic Spinal Cord			
Y Lumbar Spinal Cord			

Section	0	Medical and Surgical
Body System	0	Central Nervous System and Cranial Nerves
Operation	C	Extirpation: Taking or cutting out solid matter from a body part

Body Part (4th)	Approach (5th)	Device (6th)	Qualifier (7th)
0 Brain	0 Open	Z No Device	Z No Qualifier
1 Cerebral Meninges	3 Percutaneous		
2 Dura Mater	4 Percutaneous Endoscopic		
3 Epidural Space, Intracranial			
4 Subdural Space, Intracranial			
5 Subarachnoid Space, Intracranial			
6 Cerebral Ventricle			
7 Cerebral Hemisphere			
8 Basal Ganglia			
9 Thalamus			
A Hypothalamus			
B Pons			
C Cerebellum			
D Medulla Oblongata			
F Olfactory Nerve			
G Optic Nerve			
H Oculomotor Nerve			
J Trochlear Nerve			
K Trigeminal Nerve			
L Abducens Nerve			
M Facial Nerve			
N Acoustic Nerve			
P Glossopharyngeal Nerve			
Q Vagus Nerve			
R Accessory Nerve			
S Hypoglossal Nerve			
T Spinal Meninges			
U Spinal Canal			
W Cervical Spinal Cord			
X Thoracic Spinal Cord			
Y Lumbar Spinal Cord			

Section	0	Medical and Surgical
Body System	0	Central Nervous System and Cranial Nerves
Operation	D	Extraction: Pulling or stripping out or off all or a portion of a body part by the use of force

Body Part (4th)	Approach (5th)	Device (6th)	Qualifier (7th)
1 Cerebral Meninges	0 Open	Z No Device	Z No Qualifier
2 Dura Mater	3 Percutaneous		
F Olfactory Nerve	4 Percutaneous Endoscopic		
G Optic Nerve			
H Oculomotor Nerve			
J Trochlear Nerve			
K Trigeminal Nerve			
L Abducens Nerve			
M Facial Nerve			
N Acoustic Nerve			
P Glossopharyngeal Nerve			
Q Vagus Nerve			
R Accessory Nerve			
S Hypoglossal Nerve			
T Spinal Meninges			

Section	0	Medical and Surgical
Body System	0	Central Nervous System and Cranial Nerves
Operation	F	Fragmentation: Breaking solid matter in a body part into pieces

Body Part (4th)	Approach (5th)	Device (6th)	Qualifier (7th)
3 Epidural Space, Intracranial 4 Subdural Space, Intracranial 5 Subarachnoid Space, Intracranial 6 Cerebral Ventricle U Spinal Canal	0 Open 3 Percutaneous 4 Percutaneous Endoscopic X External	Z No Device	Z No Qualifier

Section	0	Medical and Surgical
Body System	0	Central Nervous System and Cranial Nerves
Operation	H	Insertion: Putting in a nonbiological appliance that monitors, assists, performs, or prevents a physiological function but does not physically take the place of a body part

Body Part (4th)	Approach (5th)	Device (6th)	Qualifier (7th)
0 Brain	0 Open	1 Radioactive Element 2 Monitoring Device 3 Infusion Device 4 Radioactive Element, Cesium-131 Collagen Implant M Neurostimulator Lead Y Other Device	Z No Qualifier
0 Brain	3 Percutaneous 4 Percutaneous Endoscopic	1 Radioactive Element 2 Monitoring Device 3 Infusion Device M Neurostimulator Lead Y Other Device	Z No Qualifier
6 Cerebral Ventricle E Cranial Nerve U Spinal Canal V Spinal Cord	0 Open 3 Percutaneous 4 Percutaneous Endoscopic	1 Radioactive Element 2 Monitoring Device 3 Infusion Device M Neurostimulator Lead Y Other Device	Z No Qualifier

Section	0	Medical and Surgical
Body System	0	Central Nervous System and Cranial Nerves
Operation	J	Inspection: Visually and/or manually exploring a body part

Body Part (4th)	Approach (5th)	Device (6th)	Qualifier (7th)
0 Brain E Cranial Nerve U Spinal Canal V Spinal Cord	0 Open 3 Percutaneous 4 Percutaneous Endoscopic	Z No Device	Z No Qualifier

Section	0	Medical and Surgical
Body System	0	Central Nervous System and Cranial Nerves
Operation	K	Map: Locating the route of passage of electrical impulses and/or locating functional areas in a body part

Body Part (4th)	Approach (5th)	Device (6th)	Qualifier (7th)
0 Brain 7 Cerebral Hemisphere 8 Basal Ganglia 9 Thalamus A Hypothalamus B Pons C Cerebellum D Medulla Oblongata	0 Open 3 Percutaneous 4 Percutaneous Endoscopic	Z No Device	Z No Qualifier

Section	0	Medical and Surgical
Body System	0	Central Nervous System and Cranial Nerves
Operation	N	Release: Freeing a body part from an abnormal physical constraint by cutting or by the use of force

Body Part (4th)	Approach (5th)	Device (6th)	Qualifier (7th)
0 Brain 1 Cerebral Meninges 2 Dura Mater 6 Cerebral Ventricle 7 Cerebral Hemisphere 8 Basal Ganglia 9 Thalamus A Hypothalamus B Pons C Cerebellum D Medulla Oblongata F Olfactory Nerve G Optic Nerve H Oculomotor Nerve J Trochlear Nerve K Trigeminal Nerve L Abducens Nerve M Facial Nerve N Acoustic Nerve P Glossopharyngeal Nerve Q Vagus Nerve R Accessory Nerve S Hypoglossal Nerve T Spinal Meninges W Cervical Spinal Cord X Thoracic Spinal Cord Y Lumbar Spinal Cord	0 Open 3 Percutaneous 4 Percutaneous Endoscopic	Z No Device	Z No Qualifier

Section	0	Medical and Surgical
Body System	0	Central Nervous System and Cranial Nerves
Operation	P	Removal: Taking out or off a device from a body part

Body Part (4th)	Approach (5th)	Device (6th)	Qualifier (7th)
0 Brain V Spinal Cord	0 Open 3 Percutaneous 4 Percutaneous Endoscopic	0 Drainage Device 2 Monitoring Device 3 Infusion Device 7 Autologous Tissue Substitute J Synthetic Substitute K Nonautologous Tissue Substitute M Neurostimulator Lead Y Other Device	Z No Qualifier
0 Brain V Spinal Cord	X External	0 Drainage Device 2 Monitoring Device 3 Infusion Device M Neurostimulator Lead	Z No Qualifier
6 Cerebral Ventricle U Spinal Canal	0 Open 3 Percutaneous 4 Percutaneous Endoscopic	0 Drainage Device 2 Monitoring Device 3 Infusion Device J Synthetic Substitute M Neurostimulator Lead Y Other Device	Z No Qualifier
6 Cerebral Ventricle U Spinal Canal	X External	0 Drainage Device 2 Monitoring Device 3 Infusion Device M Neurostimulator Lead	Z No Qualifier

Continued →

Section	0	Medical and Surgical
Body System	0	Central Nervous System and Cranial Nerves
Operation	P	Removal: Taking out or off a device from a body part

Body Part (4th)	Approach (5th)	Device (6th)	Qualifier (7th)
E Cranial Nerve	0 Open 3 Percutaneous 4 Percutaneous Endoscopic	0 Drainage Device 2 Monitoring Device 3 Infusion Device 7 Autologous Tissue Substitute M Neurostimulator Lead Y Other Device	Z No Qualifier
E Cranial Nerve	X External	0 Drainage Device 2 Monitoring Device 3 Infusion Device M Neurostimulator Lead	Z No Qualifier

Section	0	Medical and Surgical
Body System	0	Central Nervous System and Cranial Nerves
Operation	Q	Repair: Restoring, to the extent possible, a body part to its normal anatomic structure and function

Body Part (4th)	Approach (5th)	Device (6th)	Qualifier (7th)
0 Brain 1 Cerebral Meninges 2 Dura Mater 6 Cerebral Ventricle 7 Cerebral Hemisphere 8 Basal Ganglia 9 Thalamus A Hypothalamus B Pons C Cerebellum D Medulla Oblongata F Olfactory Nerve G Optic Nerve H Oculomotor Nerve J Trochlear Nerve K Trigeminal Nerve L Abducens Nerve M Facial Nerve N Acoustic Nerve P Glossopharyngeal Nerve Q Vagus Nerve R Accessory Nerve S Hypoglossal Nerve T Spinal Meninges W Cervical Spinal Cord X Thoracic Spinal Cord Y Lumbar Spinal Cord	0 Open 3 Percutaneous 4 Percutaneous Endoscopic	Z No Device	Z No Qualifier

Section	0	Medical and Surgical
Body System	0	Central Nervous System and Cranial Nerves
Operation	R	Replacement: Putting in or on biological or synthetic material that physically takes the place and/or function of all or a portion of a body part

Body Part (4th)	Approach (5th)	Device (6th)	Qualifier (7th)
1 Cerebral Meninges 2 Dura Mater 6 Cerebral Ventricle F Olfactory Nerve G Optic Nerve H Oculomotor Nerve J Trochlear Nerve K Trigeminal Nerve L Abducens Nerve M Facial Nerve N Acoustic Nerve P Glossopharyngeal Nerve Q Vagus Nerve R Accessory Nerve S Hypoglossal Nerve T Spinal Meninges	0 Open 4 Percutaneous Endoscopic	7 Autologous Tissue Substitute J Synthetic Substitute K Nonautologous Tissue Substitute	Z No Qualifier

Section	0	Medical and Surgical
Body System	0	Central Nervous System and Cranial Nerves
Operation	S	Reposition: Moving to its normal location, or other suitable location, all or a portion of a body part

Body Part (4th)	Approach (5th)	Device (6th)	Qualifier (7th)
F Olfactory Nerve G Optic Nerve H Oculomotor Nerve J Trochlear Nerve K Trigeminal Nerve L Abducens Nerve M Facial Nerve N Acoustic Nerve P Glossopharyngeal Nerve Q Vagus Nerve R Accessory Nerve S Hypoglossal Nerve W Cervical Spinal Cord X Thoracic Spinal Cord Y Lumbar Spinal Cord	0 Open 3 Percutaneous 4 Percutaneous Endoscopic	Z No Device	Z No Qualifier

Section	0	Medical and Surgical
Body System	0	Central Nervous System and Cranial Nerves
Operation	T	Resection: Cutting out or off, without replacement, all of a body part

Body Part (4th)	Approach (5th)	Device (6th)	Qualifier (7th)
7 Cerebral Hemisphere	0 Open 3 Percutaneous 4 Percutaneous Endoscopic	Z No Device	Z No Qualifier

Section	0	Medical and Surgical
Body System	0	Central Nervous System and Cranial Nerves
Operation	U	Supplement: Putting in or on biological or synthetic material that physically reinforces and/or augments the function of a portion of a body part

Body Part (4th)	Approach (5th)	Device (6th)	Qualifier (7th)
1 Cerebral Meninges 2 Dura Mater 6 Cerebral Ventricle F Olfactory Nerve G Optic Nerve H Oculomotor Nerve J Trochlear Nerve K Trigeminal Nerve L Abducens Nerve M Facial Nerve N Acoustic Nerve P Glossopharyngeal Nerve Q Vagus Nerve R Accessory Nerve S Hypoglossal Nerve T Spinal Meninges	0 Open 3 Percutaneous 4 Percutaneous Endoscopic	7 Autologous Tissue Substitute J Synthetic Substitute K Nonautologous Tissue Substitute	Z No Qualifier

Section	0	Medical and Surgical
Body System	0	Central Nervous System and Cranial Nerves
Operation	W	Revision: Correcting, to the extent possible, a portion of a malfunctioning device or the position of a displaced device

Body Part (4th)	Approach (5th)	Device (6th)	Qualifier (7th)
0 Brain V Spinal Cord	0 Open 3 Percutaneous 4 Percutaneous Endoscopic	0 Drainage Device 2 Monitoring Device 3 Infusion Device 7 Autologous Tissue Substitute J Synthetic Substitute K Nonautologous Tissue Substitute M Neurostimulator Lead Y Other Device	Z No Qualifier
0 Brain V Spinal Cord	X External	0 Drainage Device 2 Monitoring Device 3 Infusion Device 7 Autologous Tissue Substitute J Synthetic Substitute K Nonautologous Tissue Substitute M Neurostimulator Lead	Z No Qualifier
6 Cerebral Ventricle U Spinal Canal	0 Open 3 Percutaneous 4 Percutaneous Endoscopic	0 Drainage Device 2 Monitoring Device 3 Infusion Device J Synthetic Substitute M Neurostimulator Lead Y Other Device	Z No Qualifier
6 Cerebral Ventricle U Spinal Canal	X External	0 Drainage Device 2 Monitoring Device 3 Infusion Device J Synthetic Substitute M Neurostimulator Lead	Z No Qualifier

Continued →

Section	0	Medical and Surgical	00W Continued
Body System	0	Central Nervous System and Cranial Nerves	
Operation	W	Revision: Correcting, to the extent possible, a portion of a malfunctioning device or the position of a displaced device	

Body Part (4th)	Approach (5th)	Device (6th)	Qualifier (7th)
E Cranial Nerve	0 Open 3 Percutaneous 4 Percutaneous Endoscopic	0 Drainage Device 2 Monitoring Device 3 Infusion Device 7 Autologous Tissue Substitute M Neurostimulator Lead Y Other Device	Z No Qualifier
E Cranial Nerve	X External	0 Drainage Device 2 Monitoring Device 3 Infusion Device 7 Autologous Tissue Substitute M Neurostimulator Lead	Z No Qualifier

Section	0	Medical and Surgical
Body System	0	Central Nervous System and Cranial Nerves
Operation	X	Transfer: Moving, without taking out, all or a portion of a body part to another location to take over the function of all or a portion of a body part

Body Part (4th)	Approach (5th)	Device (6th)	Qualifier (7th)
F Olfactory Nerve G Optic Nerve H Oculomotor Nerve J Trochlear Nerve K Trigeminal Nerve L Abducens Nerve M Facial Nerve N Acoustic Nerve P Glossopharyngeal Nerve Q Vagus Nerve R Accessory Nerve S Hypoglossal Nerve	0 Open 4 Percutaneous Endoscopic	Z No Device	F Olfactory Nerve G Optic Nerve H Oculomotor Nerve J Trochlear Nerve K Trigeminal Nerve L Abducens Nerve M Facial Nerve N Acoustic Nerve P Glossopharyngeal Nerve Q Vagus Nerve R Accessory Nerve S Hypoglossal Nerve

AHA Coding Clinic

00163J6 Bypass Cerebral Ventricle to Peritoneal Cavity with Synthetic Substitute, Percutaneous Approach—AHA CC: 2Q, 2013, 36-37

00163JA Bypass Cerebral Ventricle to Subgaleal Space with Synthetic Substitute, Percutaneous Approach—AHA CC: 4Q, 2019, 22

001U0J2 Bypass Spinal Canal to Atrium with Synthetic Substitute, Open Approach—AHA CC: 4Q, 2018, 86

00764AA Dilation of Cerebral Ventricle, Percutaneous Endoscopic Approach—AHA CC: 4Q, 2017, 40-41

009430Z Drainage of Intracranial Subdural Space with Drainage Device, Percutaneous Approach—AHA CC: 3Q, 2015, 11-12

009630Z Drainage of Cerebral Ventricle with Drainage Device, Percutaneous Approach—AHA CC: 3Q, 2015, 12-13

009U00Z Drainage of Spinal Canal with Drainage Device, Open Approach—AHA CC: 4Q, 2018, 85

009U3ZX Drainage of Spinal Canal, Percutaneous Approach, Diagnostic—AHA CC: 1Q, 2014, 8

009W00Z Drainage of Cervical Spinal Cord with Drainage Device, Open Approach—AHA CC: 2Q, 2015, 30

00B00ZX Excision of Brain, Open Approach, Diagnostic—AHA CC: 1Q, 2015, 12-13

00B70ZZ Excision of Cerebral Hemisphere, Open Approach—AHA CC: 4Q, 2014, 34-35; 2Q, 2016, 18

00BM0ZZ Excision of Facial Nerve, Open Approach—AHA CC: 2Q, 2016, 12-14

00BR0ZZ Excision of Accessory Nerve, Open Approach—AHA CC: 2Q, 2016, 12-14

00BS0ZZ Excision of Hypoglossal Nerve, Open Approach—AHA CC: 2Q, 2016, 12-14

00BY0ZZ Excision of Lumbar Spinal Cord, Open Approach—AHA CC: 3Q, 2014, 24

00C00ZZ Extirpation of Matter from Brain, Open Approach—AHA CC: 1Q, 2015, 12-13; 4Q, 2016, 27-28

00C04ZZ Extirpation of Matter from Brain, Percutaneous Endoscopic Approach—AHA CC: 2Q, 2019, 36-37

00C40ZZ Extirpation of Matter from Intracranial Subdural Space, Open Approach—AHA CC: 3Q, 2015, 10-11; 2Q, 2016, 29; 3Q, 2019, 4-5

00C74ZZ Extirpation of Matter from Cerebral Hemisphere, Percutaneous Endoscopic Approach—AHA CC: 3Q, 2015, 13

00CU0ZZ Extirpation of Matter from Spinal Canal, Open Approach—AHA CC: 4Q, 2017, 48

00D20ZZ Extraction of Dura Mater, Open Approach—AHA CC: 3Q, 2015, 13-14

00H633Z Insertion of Infusion Device into Cerebral Ventricle, Percutaneous Approach—AHA CC: 2Q, 2020, 15-16

00HU03Z Insertion of Infusion Device into Spinal Canal, Open Approach—AHA CC: 2Q, 2020, 16-17

00HU33Z Insertion of Infusion Device into Spinal Canal, Percutaneous Approach—AHA CC: 3Q, 2014, 19-20

00J00ZZ Inspection of Brain, Open Approach—AHA CC: 2Q, 2019, 36-37

00JU3ZZ Inspection of Spinal Canal, Percutaneous Approach—AHA CC: 1Q, 2017, 50

00N00ZZ Release Brain, Open Approach—AHA CC: 2Q, 2016, 29

00N70ZZ Release Cerebral Hemisphere, Open Approach—AHA CC: 3Q, 2018, 30

00NC0ZZ Release Cerebellum, Open Approach—AHA CC: 3Q, 2017, 10-11

00NM4ZZ Release Facial Nerve, Percutaneous Endoscopic Approach—AHA CC: 4Q, 2018, 10

00NW0ZZ Release Cervical Spinal Cord, Open Approach—AHA CC: 2Q, 2015, 20-22; 2Q, 2017, 23-24

00NW3ZZ Release Cervical Spinal Cord, Percutaneous Approach—AHA CC: 2Q, 2019, 19-20

00NY0ZZ Release Lumbar Spinal Cord, Open Approach—AHA CC: 3Q, 2014, 24; 1Q, 2019, 28-29

00PU03Z Removal of Infusion Device from Spinal Canal, Open Approach—AHA CC: 3Q, 2014, 19-20

00Q20ZZ Repair Dura Mater, Open Approach—AHA CC: 3Q, 2013, 25; 3Q, 2014, 7-8

00SM0ZZ Reposition Facial Nerve, Open Approach—AHA CC: 4Q, 2014, 35

00U20KZ Supplement Dura Mater with Nonautologous Tissue Substitute, Open Approach—AHA CC: 3Q, 2017, 10-11; 1Q, 2018, 9

00UT0KZ Supplement Spinal Meninges with Nonautologous Tissue Substitute, Open Approach—AHA CC: 3Q, 2014, 24

Peripheral Nervous System

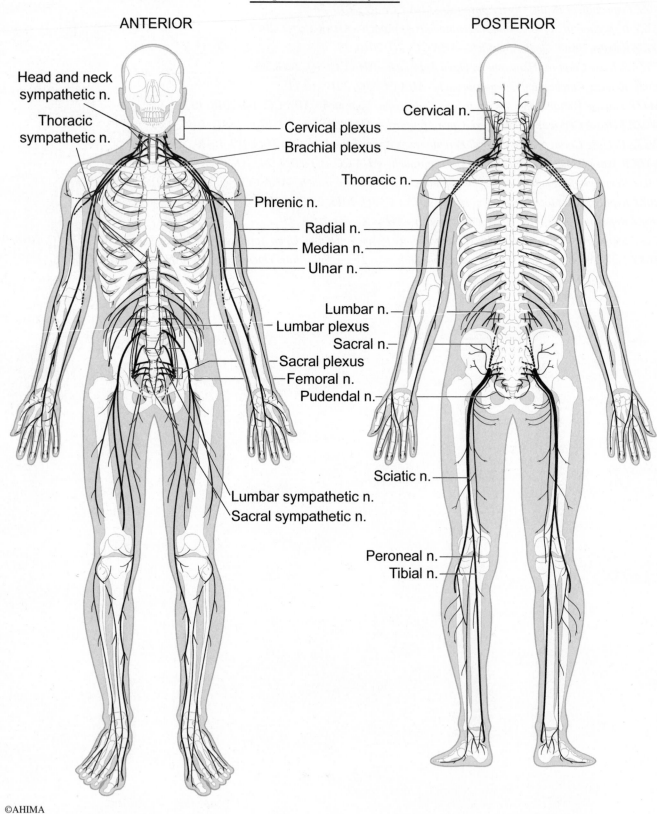

ANTERIOR   POSTERIOR

Head and neck
sympathetic n.

Thoracic
sympathetic n.

Cervical n.

Cervical plexus

Brachial plexus

Thoracic n.

Phrenic n.

Radial n.

Median n.

Ulnar n.

Lumbar n.

Lumbar plexus

Sacral n.

Sacral plexus

Femoral n.

Pudendal n.

Lumbar sympathetic n.

Sacral sympathetic n.

Sciatic n.

Peroneal n.

Tibial n.

©AHIMA

Spinal Column

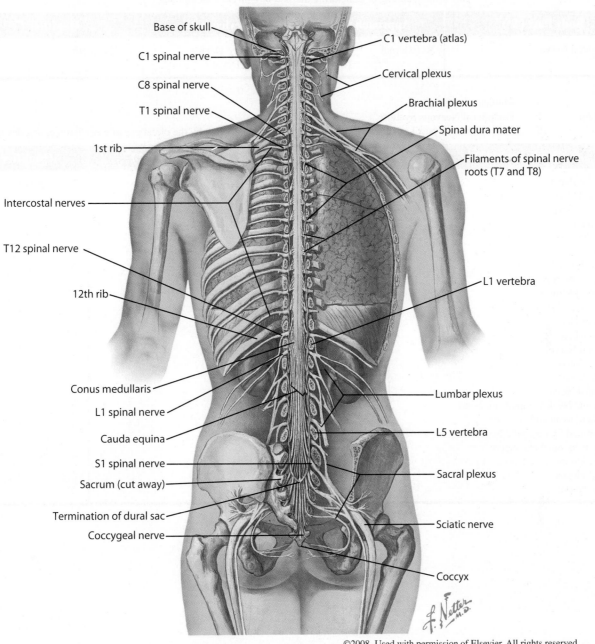

Base of skull

C1 spinal nerve

C8 spinal nerve

T1 spinal nerve

1st rib

Intercostal nerves

T12 spinal nerve

12th rib

Conus medullaris

L1 spinal nerve

Cauda equina

S1 spinal nerve

Sacrum (cut away)

Termination of dural sac

Coccygeal nerve

C1 vertebra (atlas)

Cervical plexus

Brachial plexus

Spinal dura mater

Filaments of spinal nerve roots (T7 and T8)

L1 vertebra

Lumbar plexus

L5 vertebra

Sacral plexus

Sciatic nerve

Coccyx

Peripheral Nervous System Tables 012–01X

Section   **0**   **Medical and Surgical**
Body System   **1**   **Peripheral Nervous System**
Operation   **2**   **Change:** Taking out or off a device from a body part and putting back an identical or similar device in or on the same body part without cutting or puncturing the skin or a mucous membrane

Body Part (4ᵗʰ)	Approach (5ᵗʰ)	Device (6ᵗʰ)	Qualifier (7ᵗʰ)
Y Peripheral Nerve	X External	0 Drainage Device Y Other Device	Z No Qualifier

Section   **0**   **Medical and Surgical**
Body System   **1**   **Peripheral Nervous System**
Operation   **5**   **Destruction:** Physical eradication of all or a portion of a body part by the direct use of energy, force, or a destructive agent

Body Part (4ᵗʰ)	Approach (5ᵗʰ)	Device (6ᵗʰ)	Qualifier (7ᵗʰ)
0 Cervical Plexus 1 Cervical Nerve 2 Phrenic Nerve 3 Brachial Plexus 4 Ulnar Nerve 5 Median Nerve 6 Radial Nerve 8 Thoracic Nerve 9 Lumbar Plexus A Lumbosacral Plexus B Lumbar Nerve C Pudendal Nerve D Femoral Nerve F Sciatic Nerve G Tibial Nerve H Peroneal Nerve K Head and Neck Sympathetic Nerve L Thoracic Sympathetic Nerve M Abdominal Sympathetic Nerve N Lumbar Sympathetic Nerve P Sacral Sympathetic Nerve Q Sacral Plexus R Sacral Nerve	0 Open 3 Percutaneous 4 Percutaneous Endoscopic	Z No Device	Z No Qualifier

Section	0	Medical and Surgical
Body System	1	Peripheral Nervous System
Operation	8	**Division:** Cutting into a body part, without draining fluids and/or gases from the body part, in order to separate or transect a body part

Body Part (4th)	Approach (5th)	Device (6th)	Qualifier (7th)
0 Cervical Plexus 1 Cervical Nerve 2 Phrenic Nerve 3 Brachial Plexus 4 Ulnar Nerve 5 Median Nerve 6 Radial Nerve 8 Thoracic Nerve 9 Lumbar Plexus A Lumbosacral Plexus B Lumbar Nerve C Pudendal Nerve D Femoral Nerve F Sciatic Nerve G Tibial Nerve H Peroneal Nerve K Head and Neck Sympathetic Nerve L Thoracic Sympathetic Nerve M Abdominal Sympathetic Nerve N Lumbar Sympathetic Nerve P Sacral Sympathetic Nerve Q Sacral Plexus R Sacral Nerve	0 Open 3 Percutaneous 4 Percutaneous Endoscopic	Z No Device	Z No Qualifier

Section	0	Medical and Surgical
Body System	1	Peripheral Nervous System
Operation	9	**Drainage:** Taking or letting out fluids and/or gases from a body part

Body Part (4th)	Approach (5th)	Device (6th)	Qualifier (7th)
0 Cervical Plexus 1 Cervical Nerve 2 Phrenic Nerve 3 Brachial Plexus 4 Ulnar Nerve 5 Median Nerve 6 Radial Nerve 8 Thoracic Nerve 9 Lumbar Plexus A Lumbosacral Plexus B Lumbar Nerve C Pudendal Nerve D Femoral Nerve F Sciatic Nerve G Tibial Nerve H Peroneal Nerve K Head and Neck Sympathetic Nerve L Thoracic Sympathetic Nerve M Abdominal Sympathetic Nerve N Lumbar Sympathetic Nerve P Sacral Sympathetic Nerve Q Sacral Plexus R Sacral Nerve	0 Open 3 Percutaneous 4 Percutaneous Endoscopic	0 Drainage Device	Z No Qualifier

Continued →

Section	0	Medical and Surgical
Body System	1	Peripheral Nervous System
Operation	9	**Drainage:** Taking or letting out fluids and/or gases from a body part

Body Part (4th)	Approach (5th)	Device (6th)	Qualifier (7th)
0 Cervical Plexus	0 Open	Z No Device	X Diagnostic
1 Cervical Nerve	3 Percutaneous		Z No Qualifier
2 Phrenic Nerve	4 Percutaneous		
3 Brachial Plexus	Endoscopic		
4 Ulnar Nerve			
5 Median Nerve			
6 Radial Nerve			
8 Thoracic Nerve			
9 Lumbar Plexus			
A Lumbosacral Plexus			
B Lumbar Nerve			
C Pudendal Nerve			
D Femoral Nerve			
F Sciatic Nerve			
G Tibial Nerve			
H Peroneal Nerve			
K Head and Neck Sympathetic Nerve			
L Thoracic Sympathetic Nerve			
M Abdominal Sympathetic Nerve			
N Lumbar Sympathetic Nerve			
P Sacral Sympathetic Nerve			
Q Sacral Plexus			
R Sacral Nerve			

Section	0	Medical and Surgical
Body System	1	Peripheral Nervous System
Operation	B	**Excision:** Cutting out or off, without replacement, a portion of a body part

Body Part (4th)	Approach (5th)	Device (6th)	Qualifier (7th)
0 Cervical Plexus	0 Open	Z No Device	X Diagnostic
1 Cervical Nerve	3 Percutaneous		Z No Qualifier
2 Phrenic Nerve	4 Percutaneous		
3 Brachial Plexus	Endoscopic		
4 Ulnar Nerve			
5 Median Nerve			
6 Radial Nerve			
8 Thoracic Nerve			
9 Lumbar Plexus			
A Lumbosacral Plexus			
B Lumbar Nerve			
C Pudendal Nerve			
D Femoral Nerve			
F Sciatic Nerve			
G Tibial Nerve			
H Peroneal Nerve			
K Head and Neck Sympathetic Nerve			
L Thoracic Sympathetic Nerve			
M Abdominal Sympathetic Nerve			
N Lumbar Sympathetic Nerve			
P Sacral Sympathetic Nerve			
Q Sacral Plexus			
R Sacral Nerve			

Section	0	Medical and Surgical
Body System	1	Peripheral Nervous System
Operation	C	Extirpation: Taking or cutting out solid matter from a body part

Body Part (4th)	Approach (5th)	Device (6th)	Qualifier (7th)
0 Cervical Plexus	0 Open	Z No Device	Z No Qualifier
1 Cervical Nerve	3 Percutaneous		
2 Phrenic Nerve	4 Percutaneous		
3 Brachial Plexus	Endoscopic		
4 Ulnar Nerve			
5 Median Nerve			
6 Radial Nerve			
8 Thoracic Nerve			
9 Lumbar Plexus			
A Lumbosacral Plexus			
B Lumbar Nerve			
C Pudendal Nerve			
D Femoral Nerve			
F Sciatic Nerve			
G Tibial Nerve			
H Peroneal Nerve			
K Head and Neck Sympathetic Nerve			
L Thoracic Sympathetic Nerve			
M Abdominal Sympathetic Nerve			
N Lumbar Sympathetic Nerve			
P Sacral Sympathetic Nerve			
Q Sacral Plexus			
R Sacral Nerve			

Section	0	Medical and Surgical
Body System	1	Peripheral Nervous System
Operation	D	Extraction: Pulling or stripping out or off all or a portion of a body part by the use of force

Body Part (4th)	Approach (5th)	Device (6th)	Qualifier (7th)
0 Cervical Plexus	0 Open	Z No Device	Z No Qualifier
1 Cervical Nerve	3 Percutaneous		
2 Phrenic Nerve	4 Percutaneous		
3 Brachial Plexus	Endoscopic		
4 Ulnar Nerve			
5 Median Nerve			
6 Radial Nerve			
8 Thoracic Nerve			
9 Lumbar Plexus			
A Lumbosacral Plexus			
B Lumbar Nerve			
C Pudendal Nerve			
D Femoral Nerve			
F Sciatic Nerve			
G Tibial Nerve			
H Peroneal Nerve			
K Head and Neck Sympathetic Nerve			
L Thoracic Sympathetic Nerve			
M Abdominal Sympathetic Nerve			
N Lumbar Sympathetic Nerve			
P Sacral Sympathetic Nerve			
Q Sacral Plexus			
R Sacral Nerve			

Section	0	Medical and Surgical
Body System	1	Peripheral Nervous System
Operation	H	**Insertion:** Putting in a nonbiological appliance that monitors, assists, performs, or prevents a physiological function but does not physically take the place of a body part

Body Part (4th)	Approach (5th)	Device (6th)	Qualifier (7th)
Y Peripheral Nerve	0 Open 3 Percutaneous 4 Percutaneous Endoscopic	1 Radioactive Element 2 Monitoring Device M Neurostimulator Lead Y Other Device	Z No Qualifier

Section	0	Medical and Surgical
Body System	1	Peripheral Nervous System
Operation	J	**Inspection:** Visually and/or manually exploring a body part

Body Part (4th)	Approach (5th)	Device (6th)	Qualifier (7th)
Y Peripheral Nerve	0 Open 3 Percutaneous 4 Percutaneous Endoscopic	Z No Device	Z No Qualifier

Section	0	Medical and Surgical
Body System	1	Peripheral Nervous System
Operation	N	**Release:** Freeing a body part from an abnormal physical constraint by cutting or by the use of force

Body Part (4th)	Approach (5th)	Device (6th)	Qualifier (7th)
0 Cervical Plexus 1 Cervical Nerve 2 Phrenic Nerve 3 Brachial Plexus 4 Ulnar Nerve 5 Median Nerve 6 Radial Nerve 8 Thoracic Nerve 9 Lumbar Plexus A Lumbosacral Plexus B Lumbar Nerve C Pudendal Nerve D Femoral Nerve F Sciatic Nerve G Tibial Nerve H Peroneal Nerve K Head and Neck Sympathetic Nerve L Thoracic Sympathetic Nerve M Abdominal Sympathetic Nerve N Lumbar Sympathetic Nerve P Sacral Sympathetic Nerve Q Sacral Plexus R Sacral Nerve	0 Open 3 Percutaneous 4 Percutaneous Endoscopic	Z No Device	Z No Qualifier

Section	0	Medical and Surgical
Body System	1	Peripheral Nervous System
Operation	P	**Removal:** Taking out or off a device from a body part

Body Part (4th)	Approach (5th)	Device (6th)	Qualifier (7th)
Y Peripheral Nerve	0 Open 3 Percutaneous 4 Percutaneous Endoscopic	0 Drainage Device 2 Monitoring Device 7 Autologous Tissue Substitute M Neurostimulator Lead Y Other Device	Z No Qualifier
Y Peripheral Nerve	X External	0 Drainage Device 2 Monitoring Device M Neurostimulator Lead	Z No Qualifier

Section	0	Medical and Surgical
Body System	1	Peripheral Nervous System
Operation	Q	**Repair:** Restoring, to the extent possible, a body part to its normal anatomic structure and function

Body Part (4th)	Approach (5th)	Device (6th)	Qualifier (7th)
0 Cervical Plexus	0 Open	Z No Device	Z No Qualifier
1 Cervical Nerve	3 Percutaneous		
2 Phrenic Nerve	4 Percutaneous		
3 Brachial Plexus	Endoscopic		
4 Ulnar Nerve			
5 Median Nerve			
6 Radial Nerve			
8 Thoracic Nerve			
9 Lumbar Plexus			
A Lumbosacral Plexus			
B Lumbar Nerve			
C Pudendal Nerve			
D Femoral Nerve			
F Sciatic Nerve			
G Tibial Nerve			
H Peroneal Nerve			
K Head and Neck Sympathetic Nerve			
L Thoracic Sympathetic Nerve			
M Abdominal Sympathetic Nerve			
N Lumbar Sympathetic Nerve			
P Sacral Sympathetic Nerve			
Q Sacral Plexus			
R Sacral Nerve			

Section	0	Medical and Surgical
Body System	1	Peripheral Nervous System
Operation	R	**Replacement:** Putting in or on biological or synthetic material that physically takes the place and/or function of all or a portion of a body part

Body Part (4th)	Approach (5th)	Device (6th)	Qualifier (7th)
1 Cervical Nerve	0 Open	7 Autologous Tissue	Z No Qualifier
2 Phrenic Nerve	4 Percutaneous	Substitute	
4 Ulnar Nerve	Endoscopic	J Synthetic Substitute	
5 Median Nerve		K Nonautologous Tissue	
6 Radial Nerve		Substitute	
8 Thoracic Nerve			
B Lumbar Nerve			
C Pudendal Nerve			
D Femoral Nerve			
F Sciatic Nerve			
G Tibial Nerve			
H Peroneal Nerve			
R Sacral Nerve			

Section	0	Medical and Surgical
Body System	1	Peripheral Nervous System
Operation	S	Reposition: Moving to its normal location, or other suitable location, all or a portion of a body part

Body Part (4th)	Approach (5th)	Device (6th)	Qualifier (7th)
0 Cervical Plexus 1 Cervical Nerve 2 Phrenic Nerve 3 Brachial Plexus 4 Ulnar Nerve 5 Median Nerve 6 Radial Nerve 8 Thoracic Nerve 9 Lumbar Plexus A Lumbosacral Plexus B Lumbar Nerve C Pudendal Nerve D Femoral Nerve F Sciatic Nerve G Tibial Nerve H Peroneal Nerve Q Sacral Plexus R Sacral Nerve	0 Open 3 Percutaneous 4 Percutaneous Endoscopic	Z No Device	Z No Qualifier

Section	0	Medical and Surgical
Body System	1	Peripheral Nervous System
Operation	U	Supplement: Putting in or on biological or synthetic material that physically reinforces and/or augments the function of a portion of a body part

Body Part (4th)	Approach (5th)	Device (6th)	Qualifier (7th)
1 Cervical Nerve 2 Phrenic Nerve 4 Ulnar Nerve 5 Median Nerve 6 Radial Nerve 8 Thoracic Nerve B Lumbar Nerve C Pudendal Nerve D Femoral Nerve F Sciatic Nerve G Tibial Nerve H Peroneal Nerve R Sacral Nerve	0 Open 3 Percutaneous 4 Percutaneous Endoscopic	7 Autologous Tissue Substitute J Synthetic Substitute K Nonautologous Tissue Substitute	Z No Qualifier

Section	0	Medical and Surgical
Body System	1	Peripheral Nervous System
Operation	W	Revision: Correcting, to the extent possible, a portion of a malfunctioning device or the position of a displaced device

Body Part (4th)	Approach (5th)	Device (6th)	Qualifier (7th)
Y Peripheral Nerve	0 Open 3 Percutaneous 4 Percutaneous Endoscopic	0 Drainage Device 2 Monitoring Device 7 Autologous Tissue Substitute M Neurostimulator Lead Y Other Device	Z No Qualifier
Y Peripheral Nerve	X External	0 Drainage Device 2 Monitoring Device 7 Autologous Tissue Substitute M Neurostimulator Lead	Z No Qualifier

Section	0	Medical and Surgical
Body System	1	Peripheral Nervous System
Operation	X	Transfer: Moving, without taking out, all or a portion of a body part to another location to take over the function of all or a portion of a body part

Body Part (4ᵗʰ)	Approach (5ᵗʰ)	Device (6ᵗʰ)	Qualifier (7ᵗʰ)
1 Cervical Nerve 2 Phrenic Nerve	0 Open 4 Percutaneous Endoscopic	Z No Device	1 Cervical Nerve 2 Phrenic Nerve
4 Ulnar Nerve 5 Median Nerve 6 Radial Nerve	0 Open 4 Percutaneous Endoscopic	Z No Device	4 Ulnar Nerve 5 Median Nerve 6 Radial Nerve
8 Thoracic Nerve	0 Open 4 Percutaneous Endoscopic	Z No Device	8 Thoracic Nerve
B Lumbar Nerve C Pudendal Nerve	0 Open 4 Percutaneous Endoscopic	Z No Device	B Lumbar Nerve C Perineal Nerve
D Femoral Nerve F Sciatic Nerve G Tibial Nerve H Peroneal Nerve	0 Open 4 Percutaneous Endoscopic	Z No Device	D Femoral Nerve F Sciatic Nerve G Tibial Nerve H Peroneal Nerve

AHA Coding Clinic

01BL0ZZ Excision of Thoracic Sympathetic Nerve, Open Approach—AHA CC: 2Q, 2017, 19-20

01N10ZZ Release Cervical Nerve, Open Approach—AHA CC: 2Q, 2016, 17

01N30ZZ Release Brachial Plexus, Open Approach—AHA CC: 2Q, 2016, 23

01N50ZZ Release Median Nerve, Open Approach—AHA CC: 3Q, 2014, 33-34

01NB0ZZ Release Lumbar Nerve, Open Approach—AHA CC: 2Q, 2015, 34; 2Q, 2016, 16; 2Q, 2018, 22-23; 1Q, 2019, 28-29

01NR0ZZ Release Sacral Nerve, Open Approach—AHA CC: 1Q, 2019, 28-29

01U50KZ Supplement Median Nerve with Nonautologous Tissue Substitute, Open Approach—AHA CC: 4Q, 2017, 62

01U80KZ Supplement Thoracic Nerve with Nonautologous Tissue Substitute, Open Approach—AHA CC: 3Q, 2019, 32-33

Atria, Ventricles and Interventricular Septum

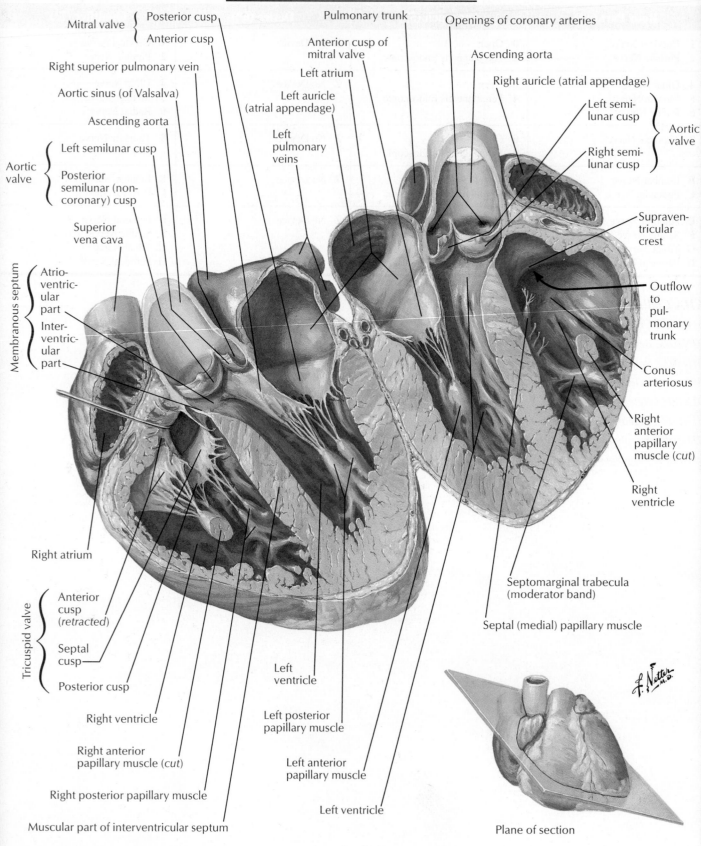

Mitral valve { Posterior cusp / Anterior cusp

Right superior pulmonary vein

Aortic sinus (of Valsalva)

Ascending aorta

Aortic valve { Left semilunar cusp / Posterior semilunar (non-coronary) cusp

Superior vena cava

Membranous septum { Atrio-ventric-ular part / Inter-ventric-ular part

Right atrium

Tricuspid valve { Anterior cusp (retracted) / Septal cusp / Posterior cusp

Right ventricle

Right anterior papillary muscle (cut)

Right posterior papillary muscle

Muscular part of interventricular septum

Pulmonary trunk

Anterior cusp of mitral valve

Left atrium

Left auricle (atrial appendage)

Left pulmonary veins

Openings of coronary arteries

Ascending aorta

Right auricle (atrial appendage)

Aortic valve { Left semilunar cusp / Right semilunar cusp

Supraventricular crest

Outflow to pulmonary trunk

Conus arteriosus

Right anterior papillary muscle (cut)

Right ventricle

Septomarginal trabecula (moderator band)

Septal (medial) papillary muscle

Left ventricle

Left posterior papillary muscle

Left anterior papillary muscle

Left ventricle

Plane of section

Arteries and Veins of the Heart; Arteries and Cardiac Veins

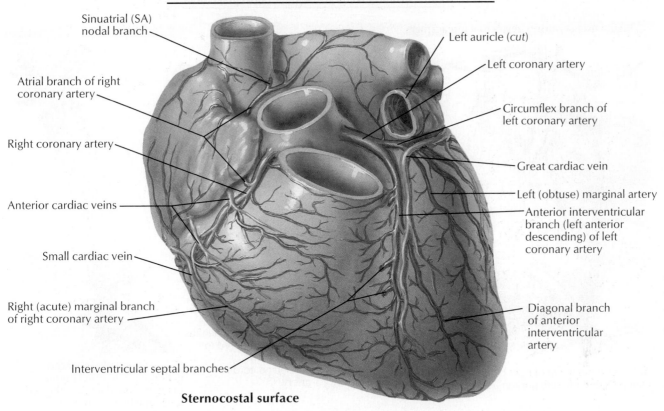

Sinuatrial (SA) nodal branch

Atrial branch of right coronary artery

Right coronary artery

Anterior cardiac veins

Small cardiac vein

Right (acute) marginal branch of right coronary artery

Interventricular septal branches

Left auricle (*cut*)

Left coronary artery

Circumflex branch of left coronary artery

Great cardiac vein

Left (obtuse) marginal artery

Anterior interventricular branch (left anterior descending) of left coronary artery

Diagonal branch of anterior interventricular artery

Sternocostal surface

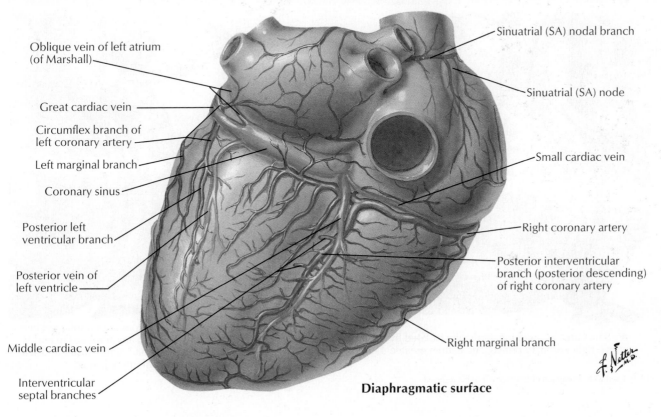

Oblique vein of left atrium (of Marshall)

Great cardiac vein

Circumflex branch of left coronary artery

Left marginal branch

Coronary sinus

Posterior left ventricular branch

Posterior vein of left ventricle

Middle cardiac vein

Interventricular septal branches

Sinuatrial (SA) nodal branch

Sinuatrial (SA) node

Small cardiac vein

Right coronary artery

Posterior interventricular branch (posterior descending) of right coronary artery

Right marginal branch

Diaphragmatic surface

Medical and Surgical, Heart and Great Vessels

125

Right coronary-artery segmental replacement

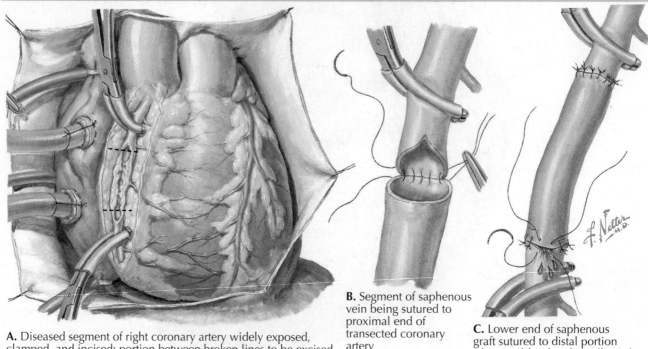

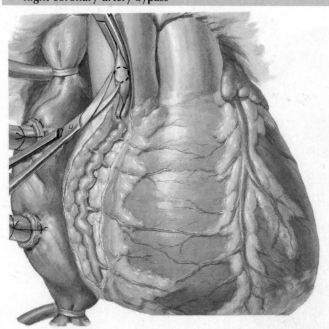

A. Diseased segment of right coronary artery widely exposed, clamped, and incised; portion between broken lines to be excised

B. Segment of saphenous vein being sutured to proximal end of transected coronary artery

C. Lower end of saphenous graft sutured to distal portion of artery; blood and air allowed to escape by loosening distal clamp prior to final closure

Right coronary-artery bypass

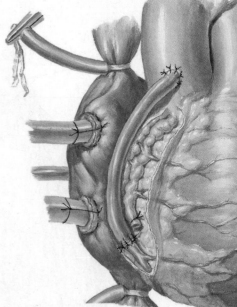

A′. Small area of aorta longitudinally isolated by clamp above right coronary orifice, and ostium created therein

B′. Segment of saphenous vein implanted into new aortic ostium and anastomosed to end of divided right coronary artery distal to diseased area; proximal end of artery ligated

Section   **0**   **Medical and Surgical**
Body System   **2**   **Heart and Great Vessels**
Operation   **1**   **Bypass:** Altering the route of passage of the contents of a tubular body part

Body Part (4ᵗʰ)	Approach (5ᵗʰ)	Device (6ᵗʰ)	Qualifier (7ᵗʰ)
0 Coronary Artery, One Artery 1 Coronary Artery, Two Arteries 2 Coronary Artery, Three Arteries 3 Coronary Artery, Four or More Arteries	0 Open	8 Zooplastic Tissue 9 Autologous Venous Tissue A Autologous Arterial Tissue J Synthetic Substitute K Nonautologous Tissue Substitute	3 Coronary Artery 8 Internal Mammary, Right 9 Internal Mammary, Left C Thoracic Artery F Abdominal Artery W Aorta
0 Coronary Artery, One Artery 1 Coronary Artery, Two Arteries 2 Coronary Artery, Three Arteries 3 Coronary Artery, Four or More Arteries	0 Open	Z No Device	3 Coronary Artery 8 Internal Mammary, Right 9 Internal Mammary, Left C Thoracic Artery F Abdominal Artery
0 Coronary Artery, One Artery 1 Coronary Artery, Two Arteries 2 Coronary Artery, Three Arteries 3 Coronary Artery, Four or More Arteries	3 Percutaneous	4 Intraluminal Device, Drug-eluting D Intraluminal Device	4 Coronary Vein
0 Coronary Artery, One Artery 1 Coronary Artery, Two Arteries 2 Coronary Artery, Three Arteries 3 Coronary Artery, Four or More Arteries	4 Percutaneous Endoscopic	4 Intraluminal Device, Drug-eluting D Intraluminal Device	4 Coronary Vein
0 Coronary Artery, One Artery 1 Coronary Artery, Two Arteries 2 Coronary Artery, Three Arteries 3 Coronary Artery, Four or More Arteries	4 Percutaneous Endoscopic	8 Zooplastic Tissue 9 Autologous Venous Tissue A Autologous Arterial Tissue J Synthetic Substitute K Nonautologous Tissue Substitute	3 Coronary Artery 8 Internal Mammary, Right 9 Internal Mammary, Left C Thoracic Artery F Abdominal Artery W Aorta
0 Coronary Artery, One Artery 1 Coronary Artery, Two Arteries 2 Coronary Artery, Three Arteries 3 Coronary Artery, Four or More Arteries	4 Percutaneous Endoscopic	Z No Device	3 Coronary Artery 8 Internal Mammary, Right 9 Internal Mammary, Left C Thoracic Artery F Abdominal Artery
6 Atrium, Right	0 Open 4 Percutaneous Endoscopic	8 Zooplastic Tissue 9 Autologous Venous Tissue A Autologous Arterial Tissue J Synthetic Substitute K Nonautologous Tissue Substitute	P Pulmonary Trunk Q Pulmonary Artery, Right R Pulmonary Artery, Left
6 Atrium, Right	0 Open 4 Percutaneous Endoscopic	Z No Device	7 Atrium, Left P Pulmonary Trunk Q Pulmonary Artery, Right R Pulmonary Artery, Left
6 Atrium, Right	3 Percutaneous	Z No Device	7 Atrium, Left
7 Atrium, Left	0 Open 4 Percutaneous Endoscopic	8 Zooplastic Tissue 9 Autologous Venous Tissue A Autologous Arterial Tissue J Synthetic Substitute K Nonautologous Tissue Substitute Z No Device	P Pulmonary Trunk Q Pulmonary Artery, Right R Pulmonary Artery, Left S Pulmonary Vein, Right T Pulmonary Vein, Left U Pulmonary Vein, Confluence
7 Atrium	3 Percutaneous	J Synthetic Substitute	6 Atrium, Right
K Ventricle, Right L Ventricle, Left	0 Open 4 Percutaneous Endoscopic	8 Zooplastic Tissue 9 Autologous Venous Tissue A Autologous Arterial Tissue J Synthetic Substitute K Nonautologous Tissue Substitute	P Pulmonary Trunk Q Pulmonary Artery, Right R Pulmonary Artery, Left

Continued →

Section	0	Medical and Surgical
Body System	2	Heart and Great Vessels
Operation	1	**Bypass:** Altering the route of passage of the contents of a tubular body part

Body Part (4th)	Approach (5th)	Device (6th)	Qualifier (7th)
K Ventricle, Right **L** Ventricle, Left	**0** Open **4** Percutaneous Endoscopic	**Z** No Device	**5** Coronary Circulation **8** Internal Mammary, Right **9** Internal Mammary, Left **C** Thoracic Artery **F** Abdominal Artery **P** Pulmonary Trunk **Q** Pulmonary Artery, Right **R** Pulmonary Artery, Left **W** Aorta
P Pulmonary Trunk **Q** Right Pulmonary Artery **R** Left Pulmonary Artery	**0** Open **4** Percutaneous Endoscopic	**8** Zooplastic Tissue **9** Autologous Venous Tissue **A** Autologous Arterial Tissue **J** Synthetic Substitute **K** Nonautologous Tissue Substitute	**A** Innominate Artery **B** Subclavin **D** Carotid
V Superior Vena Cava	**0** Open **4** Percutaneous Endoscopic	**8** Zooplastic Tissue **9** Autologous Venous Tissue **A** Autologous Arterial Tissue **J** Synthetic Substitute **K** Nonautologous Tissue Substitute **Z** No Device	**P** Pulmonary Trunk **Q** Pulmonary Artery, Right **R** Pulmonary Artery, Left **S** Pulmonary Vein, Right **T** Pulmonary Vein, Left **U** Pulmonary Vein, Confluence
W Thoracic Aorta, Descending	**0** Open	**8** Zooplastic Tissue **9** Autologous Venous Tissue **A** Autologous Arterial Tissue **J** Synthetic Substitute **K** Nonautologous Tissue Substitute	**A** Innominate Artery **B** Subclavian **D** Carotid **F** Abdominal Artery **G** Axillary Artery **H** Brachial Artery **P** Pulmonary Trunk **Q** Pulmonary Artery, Right **R** Pulmonary Artery, Left **V** Lower Extremity Artery
W Thoracic Aorta, Descending	**0** Open	**Z** No Device	**A** Innominate Artery **B** Subclavian **D** Carotid **P** Pulmonary Trunk **Q** Pulmonary Artery, Right **R** Pulmonary Artery, Left
W Thoracic Aorta, Descending	**4** Percutaneous Endoscopic	**8** Zooplastic Tissue **9** Autologous Venous Tissue **A** Autologous Arterial Tissue **J** Synthetic Substitute **K** Nonautologous Tissue Substitute **Z** No Device	**A** Innominate Artery **B** Subclavian **D** Carotid **P** Pulmonary Trunk **Q** Pulmonary Artery, Right **R** Pulmonary Artery, Left
X Thoracic Aorta, Ascending/Arch	**0** Open **4** Percutaneous Endoscopic	**8** Zooplastic Tissue **9** Autologous Venous Tissue **A** Autologous Arterial Tissue **J** Synthetic Substitute **K** Nonautologous Tissue Substitute **Z** No Device	**A** Innominate Artery **B** Subclavian **D** Carotid **P** Pulmonary Trunk **Q** Pulmonary Artery, Right **R** Pulmonary Artery, Left

Section	0	Medical and Surgical
Body System	2	Heart and Great Vessels
Operation	4	**Creation:** Putting in or on biological or synthetic material to form a new body part that to the extent possible replicates the anatomic structure or function of an absent body part

Body Part (4th)	Approach (5th)	Device (6th)	Qualifier (7th)
F Aortic Valve	**0** Open	**7** Autologous Tissue Substitute **8** Zooplastic Tissue **J** Synthetic Substitute **K** Nonautologous Tissue Substitute	**J** Truncal Valve
G Mitral Valve **J** Tricuspid Valve	**0** Open	**7** Autologous Tissue Substitute **8** Zooplastic Tissue **J** Synthetic Substitute **K** Nonautologous Tissue Substitute	**2** Common Atrioventricular Valve

Section	0	Medical and Surgical
Body System	2	Heart and Great Vessels
Operation	5	Destruction: Physical eradication of all or a portion of a body part by the direct use of energy, force, or a destructive agent

Body Part (4th)	Approach (5th)	Device (6th)	Qualifier (7th)
4 Coronary Vein 5 Atrial Septum 6 Atrium, Right 8 Conduction Mechanism 9 Chordae Tendineae D Papillary Muscle F Aortic Valve G Mitral Valve H Pulmonary Valve J Tricuspid Valve K Ventricle, Right L Ventricle, Left M Ventricular Septum N Pericardium P Pulmonary Trunk Q Pulmonary Artery, Right R Pulmonary Artery, Left S Pulmonary Vein, Right T Pulmonary Vein, Left V Superior Vena Cava W Thoracic Aorta, Descending X Thoracic Aorta, Ascending/Arch	0 Open 3 Percutaneous 4 Percutaneous Endoscopic	Z No Device	Z No Qualifier
7 Atrium, Left	0 Open 3 Percutaneous 4 Percutaneous Endoscopic	Z No Device	K Left Atrial Appendage Z No Qualifier

Section	0	Medical and Surgical
Body System	2	Heart and Great Vessels
Operation	7	Dilation: Expanding an orifice or the lumen of a tubular body part

Body Part (4th)	Approach (5th)	Device (6th)	Qualifier (7th)
0 Coronary Artery, One Artery 1 Coronary Artery, Two Arteries 2 Coronary Artery, Three Arteries 3 Coronary Artery, Four or More Arteries	0 Open 3 Percutaneous 4 Percutaneous Endoscopic	4 Intraluminal Device, Drug-eluting 5 Intraluminal Device, Drug-eluting, Two 6 Intraluminal Device, Drug-eluting, Three 7 Intraluminal Device, Drug-eluting, Four or More D Intraluminal Device E Intraluminal Devices, Two F Intraluminal Devices, Three G Intraluminal Devices, Four or More T Intraluminal Device, Radioactive Z No Device	6 Bifurcation Z No Qualifier
F Aortic Valve G Mitral Valve H Pulmonary Valve J Tricuspid Valve K Ventricle, Right L Ventricle, Left P Pulmonary Trunk Q Pulmonary Artery, Right S Pulmonary Vein, Right T Pulmonary Vein, Left V Superior Vena Cava W Thoracic Aorta, Descending X Thoracic Aorta, Ascending/Arch	0 Open 3 Percutaneous 4 Percutaneous Endoscopic	4 Intraluminal Device, Drug-eluting D Intraluminal Device Z No Device	Z No Qualifier
R Pulmonary Artery, Left	0 Open 3 Percutaneous 4 Percutaneous Endoscopic	4 Intraluminal Device, Drug-eluting D Intraluminal Device Z No Device	T Ductus Arteriosus Z No Qualifier

Section   **0**   **Medical and Surgical**
Body System   **2**   **Heart and Great Vessels**
Operation   **8**   **Division:** Cutting into a body part, without draining fluids and/or gases from the body part, in order to separate or transect a body part

Body Part (4ᵗʰ)	Approach (5ᵗʰ)	Device (6ᵗʰ)	Qualifier (7ᵗʰ)
8 Conduction Mechanism 9 Chordae Tendineae D Papillary Muscle	0 Open 3 Percutaneous 4 Percutaneous Endoscopic	Z No Device	Z No Qualifier

Section   **0**   **Medical and Surgical**
Body System   **2**   **Heart and Great Vessels**
Operation   **B**   **Excision:** Cutting out or off, without replacement, a portion of a body part

Body Part (4ᵗʰ)	Approach (5ᵗʰ)	Device (6ᵗʰ)	Qualifier (7ᵗʰ)
4 Coronary Vein 5 Atrial Septum 6 Atrium, Right 8 Conduction Mechanism 9 Chordae Tendineae D Papillary Muscle F Aortic Valve G Mitral Valve H Pulmonary Valve J Tricuspid Valve K Ventricle, Right L Ventricle, Left M Ventricular Septum N Pericardium P Pulmonary Trunk Q Pulmonary Artery, Right R Pulmonary Artery, Left S Pulmonary Vein, Right T Pulmonary Vein, Left V Superior Vena Cava W Thoracic Aorta, Descending X Thoracic Aorta, Ascending/Arch	0 Open 3 Percutaneous 4 Percutaneous Endoscopic	Z No Device	X Diagnostic Z No Qualifier
7 Atrium, Left	0 Open 3 Percutaneous 4 Percutaneous Endoscopic	Z No Device	K Left Atrial Appendage X Diagnostic Z No Qualifier

Section   **0**   **Medical and Surgical**
Body System   **2**   **Heart and Great Vessels**
Operation   **C**   **Extirpation:** Taking or cutting out solid matter from a body part

Body Part (4ᵗʰ)	Approach (5ᵗʰ)	Device (6ᵗʰ)	Qualifier (7ᵗʰ)
0 Coronary Artery, One Artery 1 Coronary Artery, Two Arteries 2 Coronary Artery, Three Arteries 3 Coronary Artery, Four or More Arteries	0 Open 3 Percutaneous 4 Percutaneous Endoscopic	Z No Device	6 Bifurcation Z No Qualifier

Continued →

Section	0	Medical and Surgical
Body System	2	Heart and Great Vessels
Operation	C	**Extirpation:** Taking or cutting out solid matter from a body part

Body Part (4th)	Approach (5th)	Device (6th)	Qualifier (7th)
4 Coronary Vein 5 Atrial Septum 6 Atrium, Right 7 Atrium, Left 8 Conduction Mechanism 9 Chordae Tendineae D Papillary Muscle F Aortic Valve G Mitral Valve H Pulmonary Valve J Tricuspid Valve K Ventricle, Right L Ventricle, Left M Ventricular Septum N Pericardium P Pulmonary Trunk Q Pulmonary Artery, Right R Pulmonary Artery, Left S Pulmonary Vein, Right T Pulmonary Vein, Left V Superior Vena Cava W Thoracic Aorta, Descending X Thoracic Aorta, Ascending/Arch	0 Open 3 Percutaneous 4 Percutaneous Endoscopic	Z No Device	Z No Qualifier

Section	0	Medical and Surgical
Body System	2	Heart and Great Vessels
Operation	F	**Fragmentation:** Breaking solid matter in a body part into pieces

Body Part (4th)	Approach (5th)	Device (6th)	Qualifier (7th)
N Pericardium	0 Open 3 Percutaneous 4 Percutaneous Endoscopic X External	Z No Device	Z No Qualifier
P Pulmonary Trunk Q Pulmonary Artery, Right R Pulmonary Artery, Left S Pulmonary Vein, Right T Pulmonary Vein, Left	3 Percutaneous	Z No Device	0 Ultrasonic Z No Qualifier

Section	0	Medical and Surgical
Body System	2	Heart and Great Vessels
Operation	H	**Insertion:** Putting in a nonbiological appliance that monitors, assists, performs, or prevents a physiological function but does not physically take the place of a body part

Body Part (4th)	Approach (5th)	Device (6th)	Qualifier (7th)
0 Coronary Artery, One Artery 1 Coronary Artery, Two Arteries 2 Coronary Artery, Three Arteries 3 Coronary Artery, Four or More Arteries	0 Open 3 Percutaneous 4 Percutaneous Endoscopic	D Intraluminal Device Y Other Device	Z No Qualifier
4 Coronary Vein 6 Atrium, Right 7 Atrium, Left K Ventricle, Right L Ventricle, Left	0 Open 3 Percutaneous 4 Percutaneous Endoscopic	0 Monitoring Device, Pressure Sensor 2 Monitoring Device 3 Infusion Device D Intraluminal Device J Cardiac Lead, Pacemaker K Cardiac Lead, Defibrillator M Cardiac Lead N Intracardiac Pacemaker Y Other Device	Z No Qualifier

Continued →

Section	0	Medical and Surgical	
Body System	2	Heart and Great Vessels	
Operation	H	Insertion: Putting in a nonbiological appliance that monitors, assists, performs, or prevents a physiological function but does not physically take the place of a body part	

Body Part (4th)	Approach (5th)	Device (6th)	Qualifier (7th)
A Heart	0 Open 3 Percutaneous 4 Percutaneous Endoscopic	Q Implantable Heart Assist System Y Other Device	Z No Qualifier
A Heart	0 Open 3 Percutaneous 4 Percutaneous Endoscopic	R Short-term External Heart Assist System	J Intraoperative S Biventricular Z No Qualifier
N Pericardium	0 Open 3 Percutaneous 4 Percutaneous Endoscopic	0 Monitoring Device, Pressure Sensor 2 Monitoring Device J Cardiac Lead, Pacemaker K Cardiac Lead, Defibrillator M Cardiac Lead Y Other Device	Z No Qualifier
P Pulmonary Trunk Q Pulmonary Artery, Right R Pulmonary Artery, Left S Pulmonary Vein, Right T Pulmonary Vein, Left V Superior Vena Cava W Thoracic Aorta, Descending	0 Open 3 Percutaneous 4 Percutaneous Endoscopic	0 Monitoring Device, Pressure Sensor 2 Monitoring Device 3 Infusion Device D Intraluminal Device Y Other Device	Z No Qualifier
X Thoracic Aorta, Ascending/Arch	0 Open 3 Percutaneous 4 Percutaneous Endoscopic	0 Monitoring Device, Pressure Sensor 2 Monitoring Device 3 Infusion Device D Intraluminal Device	Z No Qualifier

Section	0	Medical and Surgical
Body System	2	Heart and Great Vessels
Operation	J	Inspection: Visually and/or manually exploring a body part

Body Part (4th)	Approach (5th)	Device (6th)	Qualifier (7th)
A Heart Y Great Vessel	0 Open 3 Percutaneous 4 Percutaneous Endoscopic	Z No Device	Z No Qualifier

Section	0	Medical and Surgical
Body System	2	Heart and Great Vessels
Operation	K	Map: Locating the route of passage of electrical impulses and/or locating functional areas in a body part

Body Part (4th)	Approach (5th)	Device (6th)	Qualifier (7th)
8 Conduction Mechanism	0 Open 3 Percutaneous 4 Percutaneous Endoscopic	Z No Device	Z No Qualifier

Section	0	Medical and Surgical
Body System	2	Heart and Great Vessels
Operation	L	Occlusion: Completely closing an orifice or the lumen of a tubular body part

Body Part (4th)	Approach (5th)	Device (6th)	Qualifier (7th)
7 Atrium, Left	0 Open 3 Percutaneous 4 Percutaneous Endoscopic	C Extraluminal Device D Intraluminal Device Z No Device	K Left Atrial Appendage
H Pulmonary Valve P Pulmonary Trunk Q Pulmonary Artery, Right S Pulmonary Vein, Right T Pulmonary Vein, Left V Superior Vena Cava	0 Open 3 Percutaneous 4 Percutaneous Endoscopic	C Extraluminal Device D Intraluminal Device Z No Device	Z No Qualifier

Continued →

Section	0	Medical and Surgical
Body System	2	Heart and Great Vessels
Operation	L	Occlusion: Completely closing an orifice or the lumen of a tubular body part

Body Part (4th)	Approach (5th)	Device (6th)	Qualifier (7th)
R Pulmonary Artery, Left	0 Open 3 Percutaneous 4 Percutaneous Endoscopic	C Extraluminal Device D Intraluminal Device Z No Device	T Ductus Arteriosus Z No Qualifier
W Thoracic Aorta, Descending	3 Percutaneous	D Intraluminal Device	J Temporary

Section	0	Medical and Surgical
Body System	2	Heart and Great Vessels
Operation	N	Release: Freeing a body part from an abnormal physical constraint by cutting or by the use of force

Body Part (4th)	Approach (5th)	Device (6th)	Qualifier (7th)
0 Coronary Artery, One Artery 1 Coronary Artery, Two Arteries 2 Coronary Artery, Three Arteries 3 Coronary Artery, Four or More Arteries 4 Coronary Vein 5 Atrial Septum 6 Atrium, Right 7 Atrium, Left 8 Conduction Mechanism 9 Chordae Tendineae D Papillary Muscle F Aortic Valve G Mitral Valve H Pulmonary Valve J Tricuspid Valve K Ventricle, Right L Ventricle, Left M Ventricular Septum N Pericardium P Pulmonary Trunk Q Pulmonary Artery, Right R Pulmonary Artery, Left S Pulmonary Vein, Right T Pulmonary Vein, Left V Superior Vena Cava W Thoracic Aorta, Descending X Thoracic Aorta, Ascending/Arch	0 Open 3 Percutaneous 4 Percutaneous Endoscopic	Z No Device	Z No Qualifier

Section	0	Medical and Surgical
Body System	2	Heart and Great Vessels
Operation	P	Removal: Taking out or off a device from a body part

Body Part (4th)	Approach (5th)	Device (6th)	Qualifier (7th)
A Heart	0 Open 3 Percutaneous 4 Percutaneous Endoscopic	2 Monitoring Device 3 Infusion Device 7 Autologous Tissue Substitute 8 Zooplastic Tissue C Extraluminal Device D Intraluminal Device J Synthetic Substitute K Nonautologous Tissue Substitute M Cardiac Lead N Intracardiac Pacemaker Q Implantable Heart Assist System Y Other Device	Z No Qualifier

Continued →

Section	0	Medical and Surgical
Body System	2	Heart and Great Vessels
Operation	P	Removal: Taking out or off a device from a body part

Body Part (4th)	Approach (5th)	Device (6th)	Qualifier (7th)
A Heart	0 Open 3 Percutaneous 4 Percutaneous Endoscopic	R Short-term External Heart Assist System	S Biventricular Z No Qualifier
A Heart	X External	2 Monitoring Device 3 Infusion Device D Intraluminal Device M Cardiac Lead	Z No Qualifier
Y Great Vessel	0 Open 3 Percutaneous 4 Percutaneous Endoscopic	2 Monitoring Device 3 Infusion Device 7 Autologous Tissue Substitute 8 Zooplastic Tissue C Extraluminal Device D Intraluminal Device J Synthetic Substitute K Nonautologous Tissue Substitute Y Other Device	Z No Qualifier
Y Great Vessel	X External	2 Monitoring Device 3 Infusion Device D Intraluminal Device	Z No Qualifier

Section	0	Medical and Surgical
Body System	2	Heart and Great Vessels
Operation	Q	Repair: Restoring, to the extent possible, a body part to its normal anatomic structure and function

Body Part (4th)	Approach (5th)	Device (6th)	Qualifier (7th)
0 Coronary Artery, One Artery 1 Coronary Artery, Two Arteries 2 Coronary Artery, Three Arteries 3 Coronary Artery, Four or More Arteries 4 Coronary Vein 5 Atrial Septum 6 Atrium, Right 7 Atrium, Left 8 Conduction Mechanism 9 Chordae Tendineae A Heart B Heart, Right C Heart, Left D Papillary Muscle H Pulmonary Valve K Ventricle, Right L Ventricle, Left M Ventricular Septum N Pericardium P Pulmonary Trunk Q Pulmonary Artery, Right R Pulmonary Artery, Left S Pulmonary Vein, Right T Pulmonary Vein, Left V Superior Vena Cava W Thoracic Aorta, Descending X Thoracic Aorta, Ascending/Arch	0 Open 3 Percutaneous 4 Percutaneous Endoscopic	Z No Device	Z No Qualifier
F Aortic Valve	0 Open 3 Percutaneous 4 Percutaneous Endoscopic	Z No Device	J Truncal Valve Z No Qualifier

Continued →

Section	0	Medical and Surgical
Body System	2	Heart and Great Vessels
Operation	Q	Removal: Taking out or off a device from a body part

Body Part (4th)	Approach (5th)	Device (6th)	Qualifier (7th)
G Mitral Valve	0 Open 3 Percutaneous 4 Percutaneous Endoscopic	Z No Device	E Atrioventricular Valve, Left Z No Qualifier
J Tricuspid Valve	0 Open 3 Percutaneous 4 Percutaneous Endoscopic	Z No Device	G Atrioventricular Valve, Right Z No Qualifier

Section	0	Medical and Surgical
Body System	2	Heart and Great Vessels
Operation	R	Replacement: Putting in or on biological or synthetic material that physically takes the place and/or function of all or a portion of a body part

Body Part (4th)	Approach (5th)	Device (6th)	Qualifier (7th)
5 Atrial Septum 6 Atrium, Right 7 Atrium, Left 9 Chordae Tendineae D Papillary Muscle K Ventricle, Right L Ventricle, Left M Ventricular Septum N Pericardium P Pulmonary Trunk Q Pulmonary Artery, Right R Pulmonary Artery, Left S Pulmonary Vein, Right T Pulmonary Vein, Left V Superior Vena Cava W Thoracic Aorta, Descending X Thoracic Aorta, Ascending/Arch	0 Open 4 Percutaneous Endoscopic	7 Autologous Tissue Substitute 8 Zooplastic Tissue J Synthetic Substitute K Nonautologous Tissue Substitute	Z No Qualifier
F Aortic Valve G Mitral Valve H Pulmonary Valve J Tricuspid Valve	0 Open 4 Percutaneous Endoscopic	7 Autologous Tissue Substitute 8 Zooplastic Tissue J Synthetic Substitute K Nonautologous Tissue Substitute	Z No Qualifier
F Aortic Valve G Mitral Valve H Pulmonary Valve J Tricuspid Valve	3 Percutaneous	7 Autologous Tissue Substitute 8 Zooplastic Tissue J Synthetic Substitute K Nonautologous Tissue Substitute	H Transapical Z No Qualifier

Section	0	Medical and Surgical
Body System	2	Heart and Great Vessels
Operation	S	Reposition: Moving to its normal location, or other suitable location, all or a portion of a body part

Body Part (4th)	Approach (5th)	Device (6th)	Qualifier (7th)
0 Coronary Artery, One Artery 1 Coronary Artery, Two Arteries P Pulmonary Trunk Q Pulmonary Artery, Right R Pulmonary Artery, Left S Pulmonary Vein, Right T Pulmonary Vein, Left V Superior Vena Cava W Thoracic Aorta, Descending X Thoracic Aorta, Ascending/Arch	0 Open	Z No Device	Z No Qualifier

Section	0	Medical and Surgical
Body System	2	Heart and Great Vessels
Operation	T	Resection: Cutting out or off, without replacement, all of a body part

Body Part (4th)	Approach (5th)	Device (6th)	Qualifier (7th)
5 Atrial Septum 8 Conduction Mechanism 9 Chordae Tendineae D Papillary Muscle H Pulmonary Valve M Ventricular Septum N Pericardium	0 Open 3 Percutaneous 4 Percutaneous Endoscopic	Z No Device	Z No Qualifier

Section	0	Medical and Surgical
Body System	2	Heart and Great Vessels
Operation	U	Supplement: Putting in or on biological or synthetic material that physically reinforces and/or augments the function of a portion of a body part

Body Part (4th)	Approach (5th)	Device (6th)	Qualifier (7th)
0 Coronary Artery, One Artery 1 Coronary Artery, Two Arteries 2 Coronary Artery, Three Arteries 3 Coronary Artery, Four or More Arteries 5 Atrial Septum 6 Atrium, Right 7 Atrium, Left 9 Chordae Tendineae A Heart D Papillary Muscle H Pulmonary Valve K Ventricle, Right L Ventricle, Left M Ventricular Septum N Pericardium P Pulmonary Trunk Q Pulmonary Artery, Right R Pulmonary Artery, Left S Pulmonary Vein, Right T Pulmonary Vein, Left V Superior Vena Cava W Thoracic Aorta, Descending X Thoracic Aorta, Ascending/Arch	0 Open 3 Percutaneous 4 Percutaneous Endoscopic	7 Autologous Tissue Substitute 8 Zooplastic Tissue J Synthetic Substitute K Nonautologous Tissue Substitute	Z No Qualifier
F Aortic Valve	0 Open 3 Percutaneous 4 Percutaneous Endoscopic	7 Autologous Tissue Substitute 8 Zooplastic Tissue J Synthetic Substitute K Nonautologous Tissue Substitute	J Truncal Valve Z No Qualifier
G Mitral Valve	0 Open 4 Percutaneous Endoscopic	7 Autologous Tissue Substitute 8 Zooplastic Tissue J Synthetic Substitute K Nonautologous Tissue Substitute	E Atrioventricular Valve, Left Z No Qualifier
G Mitral Valve	3 Percutaneous	7 Autologous Tissue Substitute 8 Zooplastic Tissue K Nonautologous Tissue Substitute	E Atrioventricular Valve, Left Z No Qualifier
G Mitral Valve	3 Percutaneous	J Synthetic Substitute	E Atrioventricular Valve, Left H Transapical Z No Qualifier
J Tricuspid Valve	0 Open 3 Percutaneous 4 Percutaneous Endoscopic	7 Autologous Tissue Substitute 8 Zooplastic Tissue J Synthetic Substitute K Nonautologous Tissue Substitute	G Atrioventricular Valve, Right Z No Qualifier

Section	0	Medical and Surgical
Body System	2	Heart and Great Vessels
Operation	V	Restriction: Partially closing an orifice or the lumen of a tubular body part

Body Part (4th)	Approach (5th)	Device (6th)	Qualifier (7th)
A Heart	0 Open 3 Percutaneous 4 Percutaneous Endoscopic	C Extraluminal Device Z No Device	Z No Qualifier
G Mitral Valve	0 Open 3 Percutaneous 4 Percutaneous Endoscopic	Z No Device	Z No Qualifier
P Pulmonary Trunk Q Pulmonary Artery, Right S Pulmonary Vein, Right T Pulmonary Vein, Left V Superior Vena Cava	0 Open 3 Percutaneous 4 Percutaneous Endoscopic	C Extraluminal Device D Intraluminal Device Z No Device	Z No Qualifier
R Pulmonary Artery, Left	0 Open 3 Percutaneous 4 Percutaneous Endoscopic	C Extraluminal Device D Intraluminal Device Z No Device	T Ductus Arteriosus Z No Qualifier
W Thoracic Aorta, Descending X Thoracic Aorta, Ascending/ Arch	0 Open 3 Percutaneous 4 Percutaneous Endoscopic	C Extraluminal Device D Intraluminal Device E Intraluminal Device, Branched or Fenestrated, One or Two Arteries F Intraluminal Device, Branched or Fenestrated, Three or More Arteries Z No Device	Z No Qualifier

Section	0	Medical and Surgical
Body System	2	Heart and Great Vessels
Operation	W	Revision: Correcting, to the extent possible, a portion of a malfunctioning device or the position of a displaced device

Body Part (4th)	Approach (5th)	Device (6th)	Qualifier (7th)
5 Atrial Septum M Ventricular Septum	0 Open 4 Percutaneous Endoscopic	J Synthetic Substitute	Z No Qualifier
A Heart	0 Open 3 Percutaneous 4 Percutaneous Endoscopic	2 Monitoring Device 3 Infusion Device 7 Autologous Tissue Substitute 8 Zooplastic Tissue C Extraluminal Device D Intraluminal Device J Synthetic Substitute K Nonautologous Tissue Substitute M Cardiac Lead N Intracardiac Pacemaker Q Implantable Heart Assist System Y Other Device	Z No Qualifier

Continued →

Section	0	Medical and Surgical
Body System	2	Heart and Great Vessels
Operation	W	Revision: Correcting, to the extent possible, a portion of a malfunctioning device or the position of a displaced device

Body Part (4th)	Approach (5th)	Device (6th)	Qualifier (7th)
A Heart	0 Open 3 Percutaneous 4 Percutaneous Endoscopic	R Short-term External Heart Assist System	S Biventricular Z No Qualifier
A Heart	X External	2 Monitoring Device 3 Infusion Device 7 Autologous Tissue Substitute 8 Zooplastic Tissue C Extraluminal Device D Intraluminal Device J Synthetic Substitute K Nonautologous Tissue Substitute M Cardiac Lead N Intracardiac Pacemaker Q Implantable Heart Assist System	Z No Qualifier
A Heart	X External	R Short-term External Heart Assist System	S Biventricular Z No Qualifier
F Aortic Valve G Mitral Valve H Pulmonary Valve J Tricuspid Valve	0 Open 3 Percutaneous 4 Percutaneous Endoscopic	7 Autologous Tissue Substitute 8 Zooplastic Tissue J Synthetic Substitute K Nonautologous Tissue Substitute	Z No Qualifier
Y Great Vessel	0 Open 3 Percutaneous 4 Percutaneous Endoscopic	2 Monitoring Device 3 Infusion Device 7 Autologous Tissue Substitute 8 Zooplastic Tissue C Extraluminal Device D Intraluminal Device J Synthetic Substitute K Nonautologous Tissue Substitute Y Other Device	Z No Qualifier
Y Great Vessel	X External	2 Monitoring Device 3 Infusion Device 7 Autologous Tissue Substitute 8 Zooplastic Tissue C Extraluminal Device D Intraluminal Device J Synthetic Substitute K Nonautologous Tissue Substitute	Z No Qualifier

Section	0	Medical and Surgical
Body System	2	Heart and Great Vessels
Operation	Y	Transplantation: Putting in or on all or a portion of a living body part taken from another individual or animal to physically take the place and/or function of all or a portion of a similar body part

Body Part (4th)	Approach (5th)	Device (6th)	Qualifier (7th)
A Heart	0 Open	Z No Device	0 Allogeneic 1 Syngeneic 2 Zooplastic

AHA Coding Clinic

0210098 Bypass Coronary Artery, One Artery from Right Internal Mammary with Autologous Venous Tissue, Open Approach—AHA CC: 3Q, 2018, 8-9

021009W Bypass Coronary Artery, One Artery from Aorta with Autologous Venous Tissue, Open Approach—AHA CC: 1Q, 2014, 10-11

02100AW Bypass Coronary Artery, One Artery from Aorta with Autologous Arterial Tissue, Open Approach—AHA CC: 4Q, 2016, 83-84

02100Z9 Bypass Coronary Artery, One Artery from Left Internal Mammary, Open Approach—AHA CC: 3Q, 2014, 8, 20-21; 1Q, 2016, 27-28; 4Q, 2016, 83-84

021109W Bypass Coronary Artery, Two Arteries from Aorta with Autologous VenousTissue, Open Approach—AHA CC: 3Q, 2014, 20-21; 4Q, 2016, 83-84

021209W Bypass Coronary Artery, Three Arteries from Aorta with Autologous Venous Tissue, Open Approach—AHA CC: 1Q, 2016, 27-28

02160JQ Bypass Right Atrium to Right Pulmonary Artery with Synthetic Substitute, Open Approach—AHA CC: 3Q, 2014, 29

02163Z7 Bypass Right Atrium to Left Atrium, Percutaneous Approach—AHA CC: 4Q, 2017, 56

02170ZU Bypass Left Atrium to Pulmonary Vein Confluence, Open Approach—AHA CC: 4Q, 2016, 108-109

021K0JP Bypass Right Ventricle to Pulmonary Trunk with Synthetic Substitute, Open Approach—AHA CC: 1Q, 2017, 19-20; 1Q, 2020, 24-25

021K0JQ Bypass Right Ventricle to Right Pulmonary Artery with Synthetic Substitute, Open Approach—AHA CC: 3Q, 2014, 30

021K0KP Bypass Right Ventricle to Pulmonary Trunk with Nonautologous Tissue Substitute, Open Approach—AHA CC: 3Q, 2015, 16-17; 4Q, 2015. 22-23, 25

021V08S Bypass Superior Vena Cava to Right Pulmonary Vein with Zooplastic Tissue, Open Approach—AHA CC: 4Q, 2016, 145

021V09S Bypass Superior Vena Cava to Right Pulmonary Vein with Autologous Venous Tissue, Open Approach—AHA CC: 4Q, 2016, 144

021W0JQ Bypass Thoracic Aorta, Descending to Right Pulmonary Artery with Synthetic Substitute, Open Approach—AHA CC: 3Q, 2014, 3

021W0JV Bypass Thoracic Aorta, Descending to Lower Extremity Artery with Synthetic Substitute, Open Approach—AHA CC: 4Q, 2018, 46

021X0JA Bypass Thoracic Aorta, Ascending/Arch to Innominate Artery with Synthetic Substitute, Open Approach—AHA CC: 3Q, 2019, 30-31; 4Q, 2019, 23; 1Q, 2020, 37

021X0JD Bypass Thoracic Aorta, Ascending/Arch to Carotid with Synthetic Substitute, Open Approach—AHA CC: 3Q, 2019, 30-31

02570ZK Destruction of Left Atrial Appendage, Open Approach—AHA CC: 3Q, 2014, 20-21

02580ZZ Destruction of Conduction Mechanism, Open Approach—AHA CC: 3Q, 2016, 44

02583ZZ Destruction of Conduction Mechanism, Percutaneous Approach—AHA CC: 3Q, 2014, 19; 4Q, 2014, 47-48; 3Q, 2016, 43-44; 1Q, 2020, 32-33

02584ZZ Destruction of Conduction Mechanism, Percutaneous Endoscopic Approach—AHA CC: 1Q, 2020, 32-33

025M3ZZ Destruction of Ventricular Septum, Percutaneous Approach—AHA CC: 3Q, 2018, 27

025N0ZZ Destruction of Pericardium, Open Approach—AHA CC: 2Q, 2016, 17-18

0270346 Dilation of Coronary Artery, One Artery, Bifurcation, with Drug-eluting Intraluminal Device, Percutaneous Approach—AHA CC: 2Q, 2015, 4-5; 4Q, 2016, 88

027034Z Dilation of Coronary Artery, One Artery with Drug-eluting Intraluminal Device, Percutaneous Approach—AHA CC: 2Q, 2014, 4; 2Q, 2015, 3-4; 4Q, 2015, 13-14; 4Q, 2019, 39-40

027037Z Dilation of Coronary Artery, One Artery with Four or More Drug-eluting Intraluminal Devices, Percutaneous Approach—AHA CC: 4Q, 2016, 85-86

02703DZ Dilation of Coronary Artery, One Artery with Intraluminal Device, Percutaneous Approach—AHA CC: 2Q, 2015, 4

02703EZ Dilation of Coronary Artery, One Artery with Two Intraluminal Devices, Percutaneous Approach—AHA CC: 4Q, 2016, 84-85

02703ZZ Dilation of Coronary Artery, One Artery, Percutaneous Approach—AHA CC: 3Q, 2015, 10; 4Q, 2016, 88, 3Q, 2018, 7-8

027134Z Dilation of Coronary Artery, Two Arteries with Drug-eluting Intraluminal Device, Percutaneous Approach—AHA CC: 2Q, 2015, 5

0271356 Dilation of Coronary Artery, Two Arteries, Bifurcation, with Two Drug-eluting Intraluminal Devices, Percutaneous Approach—AHA CC: 4Q, 2016, 87

027136Z Dilation of Coronary Artery, Two Arteries with Three Drug-eluting Intraluminal Devices, Percutaneous Approach—AHA CC: 4Q, 2016, 84-85

027234Z Dilation of Coronary Artery, Three Arteries with Drug-eluting Intraluminal Device, Percutaneous Approach—AHA CC: 2Q, 2015, 3

027H0ZZ Dilation of Pulmonary Valve, Open Approach—AHA CC: 1Q, 2016, 16-17

027L0ZZ Dilation of Left Ventricle, Open Approach—AHA CC: 4Q, 2017, 33

027Q0DZ Dilation of Right Pulmonary Artery with Intraluminal Device, Open Approach—AHA CC: 3Q, 2015, 16-17

027V3ZZ Dilation of Superior Vena Cava, Percutaneous Approach—AHA CC: 3Q, 2018, 10

02BG0ZZ Excision of Mitral Valve, Open Approach—AHA CC: 2Q, 2015, 23-24

02BK3ZX Excision of Right Ventricle, Percutaneous Approach, Diagnostic—AHA CC: 3Q, 2019, 32

02BN0ZZ Excision of Pericardium, Open Approach—AHA CC: 2Q, 2019, 20-21

02CG0ZZ Extirpation of Matter from Mitral Valve, Open Approach—AHA CC: 2Q, 2016, 24-25

02H13DZ Insertion of Intraluminal Device into Coronary Artery, Two Arteries, Percutaneous Approach—AHA CC: 4Q, 2019, 24

02H633Z Insertion of Infusion Device into Right Atrium, Percutaneous Approach—AHA CC: 2Q, 2016, 15-16; 2Q, 2017, 24-26

02H63KZ Insertion of Cardiac Lead into Right Atrium, Percutaneous Approach—AHA CC: 2Q, 2018, 19

02H73DZ Insertion of Intraluminal Device into Left Atrium, Percutaneous Approach—AHA CC: 4Q, 2017, 104-105

02HA0QZ Insertion of Implantable Heart Assist System into Heart, Open Approach—AHA CC: 1Q, 2019, 24

02HA3RJ Insertion of Short-term External Heart Assist System into Heart, Intraoperative, Percutaneous Approach—AHA CC: 4Q, 2017, 43-44

02HA3RS Insertion of Biventricular Short-term External Heart Assist System into Heart, Percutaneous Approach—AHA CC: 4Q, 2016, 138-139

02HA3RZ Insertion of Short-term External Heart Assist System into Heart, Percutaneous Approach—AHA CC: 1Q, 2017, 11-12; 4Q, 2017, 44-45

02HK3DZ Insertion of Intraluminal Device into Right Ventricle, Percutaneous Approach—AHA CC: 2Q, 2015, 31-32

02HL0DZ Insertion of Intraluminal Device into Left Ventricle, Open Approach—AHA CC: 3Q, 2019, 19-20

02HL3JZ Insertion of Pacemaker Lead into Left Ventricle, Percutaneous Approach—AHA CC: 3Q, 2019, 23

02HP32Z Insertion of Monitoring Device into Pulmonary Trunk, Percutaneous Approach—AHA CC: 3Q, 2015, 35

02HV33Z Insertion of Infusion Device into Superior Vena Cava, Percutaneous Approach—AHA CC: 3Q, 2013, 18; 2Q, 2015, 33-34; 4Q, 2015, 14-15, 28-32; 4Q, 2017, 63-64

02JA3ZZ Inspection of Heart, Percutaneous Approach—AHA CC: 3Q, 2015, 9

02L70CK Occlusion of Left Atrial Appendage with Extraluminal Device, Open Approach—AHA CC: 3Q, 2014, 20-21

02L73DK Occlusion of Left Atrial Appendage with Intraluminal Device, Percutaneous Approach—AHA CC: 4Q, 2018, 94

02LQ3DZ Occlusion of Right Pulmonary Artery with Intraluminal Device, Percutaneous Approach—AHA CC: 4Q, 2017, 34

02LR0ZT Occlusion of Ductus Arteriosus, Open Approach—AHA CC: 4Q, 2015, 23-24

02LS3DZ Occlusion of Right Pulmonary Vein with Intraluminal Device, Percutaneous Approach—AHA CC: 2Q, 2016, 26; 4Q, 2017, 34

02N00ZZ Release Coronary Artery, One Artery, Open Approach—AHA CC: 2Q, 2019, 13-14

02NK0ZZ Release Right Ventricle, Open Approach—AHA CC: 3Q, 2014, 16-17

02NN0ZZ Release Pericardium, Open Approach—AHA CC: 2Q, 2019, 20-21

02PA0QZ Removal of Implantable Heart Assist System from Heart, Open Approach—AHA CC: 1Q, 2019, 24

02PA0RZ Removal of Short-term External Heart Assist System from Heart, Open Approach—AHA CC: 1Q, 2017, 13-14

02PA3DZ Removal of Intraluminal Device from Heart, Percutaneous Approach—AHA CC: 4Q, 2017, 104-105

02PA3MZ Removal of Cardiac Lead from Heart, Percutaneous Approach—AHA CC: 3Q, 2015, 33

02PA3NZ Removal of Intracardiac Pacemaker from Heart, Percutaneous Approach—AHA CC: 4Q, 2016, 96-97

02PA3RZ Removal of Short-term External Heart Assist System from Heart, Percutaneous Approach—AHA CC: 4Q, 2016, 139; 1Q, 2017, 11-12; 4Q, 2017, 44-45; 4Q, 2018, 54

02PY33Z Removal of Infusion Device from Great Vessel, Percutaneous Approach—AHA CC: 4Q, 2015, 31-32; 2Q, 2016, 15-16; 2Q, 2017, 24-26

02PY3JZ Removal of Synthetic Substitute from Great Vessel, Percutaneous Approach—AHA CC: 4Q, 2018, 85

02PYX3Z Removal of Infusion Device from Great Vessel, External Approach—AHA CC: 3Q, 2016, 19

02Q50ZZ Repair Atrial Septum, Open Approach—AHA CC: 4Q, 2015, 23-24

02QS0ZZ Repair Right Pulmonary Vein, Open Approach—AHA CC: 1Q, 2017, 18-19

02QT0ZZ Repair Left Pulmonary Vein, Open Approach—AHA CC: 1Q, 2017, 18-19

02QW0ZZ Repair Thoracic Aorta, Descending, Open Approach—AHA CC: 3Q, 2015, 16

02RF38Z Replacement of Aortic Valve with Zooplastic Tissue, Percutaneous Approach—AHA CC: 1Q, 2019, 31-32

02RF3JZ Replacement of Aortic Valve with Synthetic Substitute, Percutaneous Approach—AHA CC: 4Q, 2019, 24

02RG08Z Replacement of Mitral Valve with Zooplastic Tissue, Open Approach—AHA CC: 3Q, 2019, 23-24

02RJ3JZ Replacement of Tricuspid Valve with Synthetic Substitute, Percutaneous Approach—AHA CC: 4Q, 2017, 56

02RJ48Z Replacement of Tricuspid Valve with Zooplastic Tissue, Percutaneous Endoscopic Approach—AHA CC: 3Q, 2016, 32

02RK0JZ Replacement of Right Ventricle with Synthetic Substitute, Open Approach—AHA CC: 1Q, 2017, 13-14

02RL0JZ Replacement of Left Ventricle with Synthetic Substitute, Open Approach—AHA CC: 1Q, 2017, 13-14

02RW0KZ Replacement of Thoracic Aorta, Descending with Nonautologous Tissue Substitute, Open Approach—AHA CC: 1Q, 2014, 10-11

02RX0JZ Replacement of Thoracic Aorta, Ascending/Arch with Synthetic Substitute, Open Approach—AHA CC: 3Q, 2019, 24; 1Q, 2020, 25-26

02S10ZZ Reposition Coronary Artery, Two Arteries, Open Approach—AHA CC: 4Q, 2016, 103-104

02SP0ZZ Reposition Pulmonary Trunk, Open Approach—AHA CC: 4Q, 2015, 23-24; 4Q, 2016, 103-104

02SW0ZZ Reposition Thoracic Aorta, Descending, Open Approach—AHA CC: 4Q, 2015, 23-24

02SX0ZZ Reposition Thoracic Aorta, Ascending/Arch, Open Approach—AHA CC: 4Q, 2016, 103-104

02U03JZ Supplement Coronary Artery, One Artery with Synthetic Substitute, Percutaneous Approach—AHA CC: 4Q, 2019, 25-26

02U607Z Supplement Right Atrium with Autologous Tissue Substitute, Open Approach—AHA CC: 3Q, 2017, 7-8

02U707Z Supplement Left Atrium with Autologous Tissue Substitute, Open Approach— AHA CC: 3Q, 2017, 7-8

02UF08Z Supplement Aortic Valve with Zooplastic Tissue, Open Approach—AHA CC: 4Q, 2015, 25

02UG08Z Supplement Mitral Valve with Zooplastic Tissue, Open Approach—AHA CC: 4Q, 2017, 36

02UG0JZ Supplement Mitral Valve with Synthetic Substitute, Open Approach—AHA CC: 2Q, 2015, 23-24

02UM08Z Supplement Ventricular Septum with Zooplastic Tissue, Open Approach—AHA CC: 4Q, 2015, 25

02UM0JZ Supplement Ventricular Septum with Synthetic Substitute, Open Approach—AHA CC: 3Q, 2014, 16-17; 4Q, 2015, 22-23

02UP07Z Supplement Pulmonary Trunk with Autologous Tissue Substitute, Open Approach—AHA CC: 2Q, 2016, 23-24

02UP08Z Supplement Pulmonary Trunk with Zooplastic Tissue, Open Approach—AHA CC: 1Q, 2020, 24-25

02UQ0KZ Supplement Right Pulmonary Artery with Nonautologous Tissue Substitute, Open Approach—AHA CC: 3Q, 2015, 16-17

02UR07Z Supplement Left Pulmonary Artery with Autologous Tissue Substitute, Open Approach—AHA CC: 2Q, 2016, 23-24

02UR0KZ Supplement Left Pulmonary Artery with Nonautologous Tissue Substitute, Open Approach—AHA CC: 3Q, 2015, 16-17

02UW07Z Supplement Thoracic Aorta, Descending with Autologous Tissue Substitute, Open Approach—AHA CC: 4Q, 2015, 23-24

02UW0JZ Supplement Thoracic Aorta, Descending with Synthetic Substitute, Open Approach—AHA CC: 2Q, 2016, 26-27

02UX0KZ Supplement Thoracic Aorta, Ascending/Arch with Nonautologous Tissue Substitute, Open Approach—AHA CC: 1Q, 2017, 19-20

02VG0ZZ Restriction of Mitral Valve, Open Approach—AHA CC: 4Q, 2017, 36

02VW0DZ Restriction of Thoracic Aorta, Descending with Intraluminal Device, Open Approach—AHA CC: 1Q, 2020, 25-26

02VW3DZ Restriction of Thoracic Aorta, Descending with Intraluminal Device, Percutaneous Approach—AHA CC: 4Q, 2016, 92-93

02WA3JZ Revision of Synthetic Substitute in Heart, Percutaneous Approach—AHA CC: 3Q, 2014, 31-32

02WA3MZ Revision of Cardiac Lead in Heart, Percutaneous Approach—AHA CC: 3Q, 2015, 32

02WA3NZ Revision of Intracardiac Pacemaker in Heart, Percutaneous Approach—AHA CC: 4Q, 2016, 96

02WAXRZ Revision of Short-term External Heart Assist System in Heart, External Approach—AHA CC: 1Q, 2018, 17

02WY33Z Revision of Infusion Device in Great Vessel, Percutaneous Approach—AHA CC: 3Q, 2018, 9-10

02YA0Z0 Transplantation of Heart, Allogeneic, Open Approach—AHA CC: 3Q, 2013, 18-19

Arteries

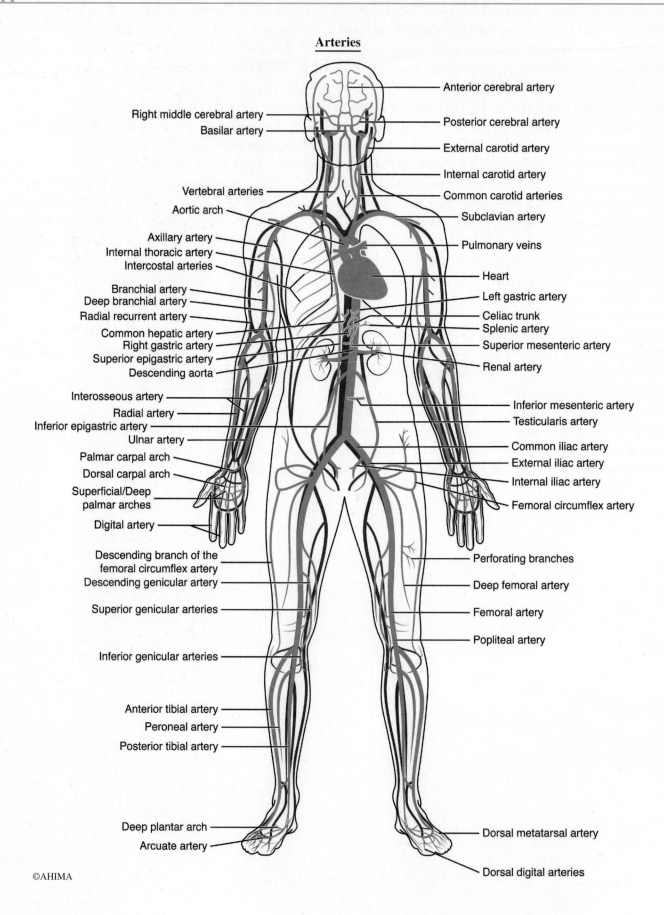

Anterior cerebral artery

Right middle cerebral artery

Posterior cerebral artery

Basilar artery

External carotid artery

Internal carotid artery

Vertebral arteries

Common carotid arteries

Aortic arch

Subclavian artery

Axillary artery

Pulmonary veins

Internal thoracic artery

Intercostal arteries

Heart

Branchial artery

Left gastric artery

Deep branchial artery

Celiac trunk

Radial recurrent artery

Splenic artery

Common hepatic artery

Superior mesenteric artery

Right gastric artery

Superior epigastric artery

Renal artery

Descending aorta

Interosseous artery

Inferior mesenteric artery

Radial artery

Testicularis artery

Inferior epigastric artery

Ulnar artery

Common iliac artery

Palmar carpal arch

External iliac artery

Dorsal carpal arch

Internal iliac artery

Superficial/Deep palmar arches

Femoral circumflex artery

Digital artery

Descending branch of the femoral circumflex artery

Perforating branches

Descending genicular artery

Deep femoral artery

Superior genicular arteries

Femoral artery

Popliteal artery

Inferior genicular arteries

Anterior tibial artery

Peroneal artery

Posterior tibial artery

Deep plantar arch

Dorsal metatarsal artery

Arcuate artery

Dorsal digital arteries

©AHIMA

Arterial Anastomosis Around Elbow

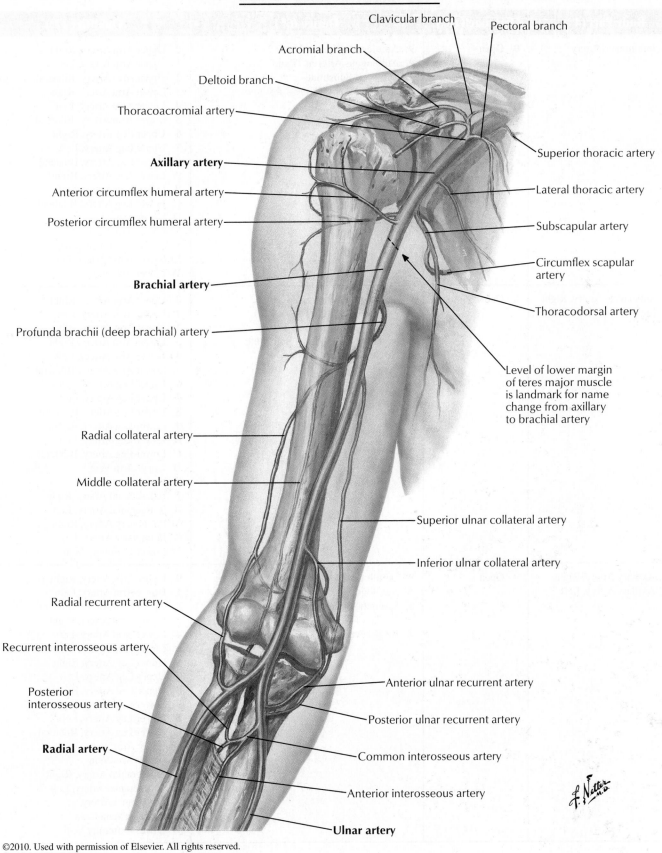

Clavicular branch

Pectoral branch

Acromial branch

Deltoid branch

Thoracoacromial artery

Axillary artery

Anterior circumflex humeral artery

Posterior circumflex humeral artery

Brachial artery

Profunda brachii (deep brachial) artery

Radial collateral artery

Middle collateral artery

Radial recurrent artery

Recurrent interosseous artery

Posterior interosseous artery

Radial artery

Superior thoracic artery

Lateral thoracic artery

Subscapular artery

Circumflex scapular artery

Thoracodorsal artery

Level of lower margin of teres major muscle is landmark for name change from axillary to brachial artery

Superior ulnar collateral artery

Inferior ulnar collateral artery

Anterior ulnar recurrent artery

Posterior ulnar recurrent artery

Common interosseous artery

Anterior interosseous artery

Ulnar artery

Section   0   **Medical and Surgical**
Body System   3   **Upper Arteries**
Operation   1   **Bypass:** Altering the route of passage of the contents of a tubular body part

Body Part (4th)	Approach (5th)	Device (6th)	Qualifier (7th)
2 Innominate Artery	0 Open	9 Autologous Venous Tissue A Autologous Arterial Tissue J Synthetic Substitute K Nonautologous Tissue Substitute Z No Device	0 Upper Arm Artery, Right 1 Upper Arm Artery, Left 2 Upper Arm Artery, Bilateral 3 Lower Arm Artery, Right 4 Lower Arm Artery, Left 5 Lower Arm Artery, Bilateral 6 Upper Leg Artery, Right 7 Upper Leg Artery, Left 8 Upper Leg Artery, Bilateral 9 Lower Leg Artery, Right B Lower Leg Artery, Left C Lower Leg Artery, Bilateral D Upper Arm Vein F Lower Arm Vein J Extracranial Artery, Right K Extracranial Artery, Left W Lower Extremity Vein
3 Subclavian Artery, Right 4 Subclavian Artery, Left	0 Open	9 Autologous Venous Tissue A Autologous Arterial Tissue J Synthetic Substitute K Nonautologous Tissue Substitute Z No Device	0 Upper Arm Artery, Right 1 Upper Arm Artery, Left 2 Upper Arm Artery, Bilateral 3 Lower Arm Artery, Right 4 Lower Arm Artery, Left 5 Lower Arm Artery, Bilateral 6 Upper Leg Artery, Right 7 Upper Leg Artery, Left 8 Upper Leg Artery, Bilateral 9 Lower Leg Artery, Right B Lower Leg Artery, Left C Lower Leg Artery, Bilateral D Upper Arm Vein F Lower Arm Vein J Extracranial Artery, Right K Extracranial Artery, Left M Pulmonary Artery, Right N Pulmonary Artery, Left W Lower Extremity Vein
5 Axillary Artery, Right 6 Axillary Artery, Left	0 Open	9 Autologous Venous Tissue A Autologous Arterial Tissue J Synthetic Substitute K Nonautologous Tissue Substitute Z No Device	0 Upper Arm Artery, Right 1 Upper Arm Artery, Left 2 Upper Arm Artery, Bilateral 3 Lower Arm Artery, Right 4 Lower Arm Artery, Left 5 Lower Arm Artery, Bilateral 6 Upper Leg Artery, Right 7 Upper Leg Artery, Left 8 Upper Leg Artery, Bilateral 9 Lower Leg Artery, Right B Lower Leg Artery, Left C Lower Leg Artery, Bilateral D Upper Arm Vein F Lower Arm Vein J Extracranial Artery, Right K Extracranial Artery, Left T Abdominal Artery V Superior Vena Cava W Lower Extremity Vein

Continued ➡

Body Part (4th)	Approach (5th)	Device (6th)	Qualifier (7th)
7 Brachial Artery, Right	0 Open	9 Autologous Venous Tissue A Autologous Arterial Tissue J Synthetic Substitute K Nonautologous Tissue Substitute Z No Device	0 Upper Arm Artery, Right 3 Lower Arm Artery, Right D Upper Arm Vein F Lower Arm Vein V Superior Vena Cava W Lower Extremity Vein
8 Brachial Artery, Left	0 Open	9 Autologous Venous Tissue A Autologous Arterial Tissue J Synthetic Substitute K Nonautologous Tissue Substitute Z No Device	1 Upper Arm Artery, Left 4 Lower Arm Artery, Left D Upper Arm Vein F Lower Arm Vein V Superior Vena Cava W Lower Extremity Vein
9 Ulnar Artery, Right B Radial Artery, Right	0 Open	9 Autologous Venous Tissue A Autologous Arterial Tissue J Synthetic Substitute K Nonautologous Tissue Substitute Z No Device	3 Lower Arm Artery, Right F Lower Arm Vein
9 Ulnar Artery, Right B Radial Artery, Right	3 Percutaneous	Z No Device	F Lower Arm Vein
A Ulnar Artery, Left C Radial Artery, Left	0 Open	9 Autologous Venous Tissue A Autologous Arterial Tissue J Synthetic Substitute K Nonautologous Tissue Substitute Z No Device	4 Lower Arm Artery, Left F Lower Arm Vein
A Ulnar Artery, Left C Radial Artery, Left	3 Percutaneous	Z No Device	F Lower Arm Vein
G Intracranial Artery S Temporal Artery, Right T Temporal Artery, Left	0 Open	9 Autologous Venous Tissue A Autologous Arterial Tissue J Synthetic Substitute K Nonautologous Tissue Substitute Z No Device	G Intracranial Artery
H Common Carotid Artery, Right J Common Carotid Artery, Left	0 Open	9 Autologous Venous Tissue A Autologous Arterial Tissue J Synthetic Substitute K Nonautologous Tissue Substitute Z No Device	G Intracranial Artery J Extracranial Artery, Right K Extracranial Artery, Left Y Upper Artery
K Internal Carotid Artery, Right L Internal Carotid Artery, Left M External Carotid Artery, Right N External Carotid Artery, Left	0 Open	9 Autologous Venous Tissue A Autologous Arterial Tissue J Synthetic Substitute K Nonautologous Tissue Substitute Z No Device	J Extracranial Artery, Right K Extracranial Artery, Left

Section	0	**Medical and Surgical**
Body System	3	**Upper Arteries**
Operation	5	**Destruction:** Physical eradication of all or a portion of a body part by the direct use of energy, force, or a destructive agent

Body Part (4th)	Approach (5th)	Device (6th)	Qualifier (7th)
0 Internal Mammary Artery, Right 1 Internal Mammary Artery, Left 2 Innominate Artery 3 Subclavian Artery, Right 4 Subclavian Artery, Left 5 Axillary Artery, Right 6 Axillary Artery, Left 7 Brachial Artery, Right 8 Brachial Artery, Left 9 Ulnar Artery, Right A Ulnar Artery, Left B Radial Artery, Right C Radial Artery, Left D Hand Artery, Right F Hand Artery, Left G Intracranial Artery H Common Carotid Artery, Right J Common Carotid Artery, Left K Internal Carotid Artery, Right L Internal Carotid Artery, Left M External Carotid Artery, Right N External Carotid Artery, Left P Vertebral Artery, Right Q Vertebral Artery, Left R Face Artery S Temporal Artery, Right T Temporal Artery, Left U Thyroid Artery, Right V Thyroid Artery, Left Y Upper Artery	0 Open 3 Percutaneous 4 Percutaneous Endoscopic	Z No Device	Z No Qualifier

Section	0	Medical and Surgical
Body System	3	Upper Arteries
Operation	7	Dilation: Expanding an orifice or the lumen of a tubular body part

Body Part (4th)	Approach (5th)	Device (6th)	Qualifier (7th)
0 Internal Mammary Artery, Right 1 Internal Mammary Artery, Left 2 Innominate Artery 3 Subclavian Artery, Right 4 Subclavian Artery, Left 5 Axillary Artery, Right 6 Axillary Artery, Left 7 Brachial Artery, Right 8 Brachial Artery, Left 9 Ulnar Artery, Right A Ulnar Artery, Left B Radial Artery, Right C Radial Artery, Left	0 Open 3 Percutaneous 4 Percutaneous Endoscopic	4 Intraluminal Device, Drug-eluting 5 Intraluminal Device, Drug-eluting, Two 6 Intraluminal Device, Drug-eluting, Three 7 Intraluminal Device, Drug-eluting, Four or More E Intraluminal Devices, Two F Intraluminal Devices, Three G Intraluminal Devices, Four or More	Z No Qualifier
0 Internal Mammary Artery, Right 1 Internal Mammary Artery, Left 2 Innominate Artery 3 Subclavian Artery, Right 4 Subclavian Artery, Left 5 Axillary Artery, Right 6 Axillary Artery, Left 7 Brachial Artery, Right 8 Brachial Artery, Left 9 Ulnar Artery, Right A Ulnar Artery, Left B Radial Artery, Right C Radial Artery, Left	0 Open 3 Percutaneous 4 Percutaneous Endoscopic	D Intraluminal Device Z No Device	1 Drug-Coated Balloon Z No Qualifier
D Hand Artery, Right F Hand Artery, Left G Intracranial Artery H Common Carotid Artery, Right J Common Carotid Artery, Left K Internal Carotid Artery, Right L Internal Carotid Artery, Left M External Carotid Artery, Right N External Carotid Artery, Left P Vertebral Artery, Right Q Vertebral Artery, Left R Face Artery S Temporal Artery, Right T Temporal Artery, Left U Thyroid Artery, Right V Thyroid Artery, Left Y Upper Artery	0 Open 3 Percutaneous 4 Percutaneous Endoscopic	4 Intraluminal Device, Drug-eluting 5 Intraluminal Device, Drug-eluting, Two 6 Intraluminal Device, Drug-eluting, Three 7 Intraluminal Device, Drug-eluting, Four or More D Intraluminal Device E Intraluminal Device, Two F Intraluminal Device, Three G Intraluminal Device, Four or More Z No Device	Z No Qualifier

Section	0	Medical and Surgical
Body System	3	Upper Arteries
Operation	9	**Drainage:** Taking or letting out fluids and/or gases from a body part

Body Part (4ᵗʰ)	Approach (5ᵗʰ)	Device (6ᵗʰ)	Qualifier (7ᵗʰ)
0 Internal Mammary Artery, Right 1 Internal Mammary Artery, Left 2 Innominate Artery 3 Subclavian Artery, Right 4 Subclavian Artery, Left 5 Axillary Artery, Right 6 Axillary Artery, Left 7 Brachial Artery, Right 8 Brachial Artery, Left 9 Ulnar Artery, Right A Ulnar Artery, Left B Radial Artery, Right C Radial Artery, Left D Hand Artery, Right F Hand Artery, Left G Intracranial Artery H Common Carotid Artery, Right J Common Carotid Artery, Left K Internal Carotid Artery, Right L Internal Carotid Artery, Left M External Carotid Artery, Right N External Carotid Artery, Left P Vertebral Artery, Right Q Vertebral Artery, Left R Face Artery S Temporal Artery, Right T Temporal Artery, Left U Thyroid Artery, Right V Thyroid Artery, Left Y Upper Artery	0 Open 3 Percutaneous 4 Percutaneous Endoscopic	0 Drainage Device	Z No Qualifier
0 Internal Mammary Artery, Right 1 Internal Mammary Artery, Left 2 Innominate Artery 3 Subclavian Artery, Right 4 Subclavian Artery, Left 5 Axillary Artery, Right 6 Axillary Artery, Left 7 Brachial Artery, Right 8 Brachial Artery, Left 9 Ulnar Artery, Right A Ulnar Artery, Left B Radial Artery, Right C Radial Artery, Left D Hand Artery, Right F Hand Artery, Left G Intracranial Artery H Common Carotid Artery, Right J Common Carotid Artery, Left K Internal Carotid Artery, Right L Internal Carotid Artery, Left M External Carotid Artery, Right N External Carotid Artery, Left P Vertebral Artery, Right Q Vertebral Artery, Left R Face Artery S Temporal Artery, Right T Temporal Artery, Left U Thyroid Artery, Right V Thyroid Artery, Left Y Upper Artery	0 Open 3 Percutaneous 4 Percutaneous Endoscopic	Z No Device	X Diagnostic Z No Qualifier

Section	0	Medical and Surgical
Body System	3	Upper Arteries
Operation	B	**Excision:** Cutting out or off, without replacement, a portion of a body part

Body Part (4th)	Approach (5th)	Device (6th)	Qualifier (7th)
0 Internal Mammary Artery, Right	0 Open	Z No Device	X Diagnostic
1 Internal Mammary Artery, Left	3 Percutaneous		Z No Qualifier
2 Innominate Artery	4 Percutaneous Endoscopic		
3 Subclavian Artery, Right			
4 Subclavian Artery, Left			
5 Axillary Artery, Right			
6 Axillary Artery, Left			
7 Brachial Artery, Right			
8 Brachial Artery, Left			
9 Ulnar Artery, Right			
A Ulnar Artery, Left			
B Radial Artery, Right			
C Radial Artery, Left			
D Hand Artery, Right			
F Hand Artery, Left			
G Intracranial Artery			
H Common Carotid Artery, Right			
J Common Carotid Artery, Left			
K Internal Carotid Artery, Right			
L Internal Carotid Artery, Left			
M External Carotid Artery, Right			
N External Carotid Artery, Left			
P Vertebral Artery, Right			
Q Vertebral Artery, Left			
R Face Artery			
S Temporal Artery, Right			
T Temporal Artery, Left			
U Thyroid Artery, Right			
V Thyroid Artery, Left			
Y Upper Artery			

Section	0	Medical and Surgical
Body System	3	Upper Arteries
Operation	C	**Extirpation:** Taking or cutting out solid matter from a body part

Body Part (4th)	Approach (5th)	Device (6th)	Qualifier (7th)
0 Internal Mammary Artery, Right	0 Open	Z No Device	Z No Qualifier
1 Internal Mammary Artery, Left	3 Percutaneous		
2 Innominate Artery	4 Percutaneous Endoscopic		
3 Subclavian Artery, Right			
4 Subclavian Artery, Left			
5 Axillary Artery, Right			
6 Axillary Artery, Left			
7 Brachial Artery, Right			
8 Brachial Artery, Left			
9 Ulnar Artery, Right			
A Ulnar Artery, Left			
B Radial Artery, Right			
C Radial Artery, Left			
D Hand Artery, Right			
F Hand Artery, Left			
R Face Artery			
S Temporal Artery, Right			
T Temporal Artery, Left			
U Thyroid Artery, Right			
V Thyroid Artery, Left			
Y Upper Artery			

Continued →

Section	0	Medical and Surgical
Body System	3	Upper Arteries
Operation	C	**Extirpation:** Taking or cutting out solid matter from a body part

Body Part (4th)	Approach (5th)	Device (6th)	Qualifier (7th)
G Intracranial Artery H Common Carotid Artery, Right J Common Carotid Artery, Left K Internal Carotid Artery, Right L Internal Carotid Artery, Left M External Carotid Artery, Right N External Carotid Artery, Left P Vertebral Artery, Right Q Vertebral Artery, Left	0 Open 4 Percutaneous Endoscopic	Z No Device	Z No Qualifier
G Intracranial Artery H Common Carotid Artery, Right J Common Carotid Artery, Left K Internal Carotid Artery, Right L Internal Carotid Artery, Left M External Carotid Artery, Right N External Carotid Artery, Left P Vertebral Artery, Right Q Vertebral Artery, Left	3 Percutaneous	Z No Device	7 Stent Retriever Z No Qualifier

Section	0	Medical and Surgical
Body System	3	Upper Arteries
Operation	F	**Fragmentation:** Breaking solid matter in a body part into pieces

Body Part (4th)	Approach (5th)	Device (6th)	Qualifier (7th)
2 Innominate Artery 3 Subclavian Artery, Right 4 Subclavian Artery, Left 5 Axillary Artery, Right 6 Axillary Artery, Left 7 Brachial Artery, Right 8 Brachial Artery, Left 9 Ulnar Artery, Right A Ulnar Artery, Left B Radial Artery, Right C Radial Artery, Left Y Upper Artery	3 Percutaneous	Z No Device	0 Ultrasonic Z No Qualifier

Section	0	Medical and Surgical
Body System	3	Upper Arteries
Operation	H	**Insertion:** Putting in a nonbiological appliance that monitors, assists, performs, or prevents a physiological function but does not physically take the place of a body part

Body Part (4th)	Approach (5th)	Device (6th)	Qualifier (7th)
0 Internal Mammary Artery, Right 1 Internal Mammary Artery, Left 2 Innominate Artery 3 Subclavian Artery, Right 4 Subclavian Artery, Left 5 Axillary Artery, Right 6 Axillary Artery, Left 7 Brachial Artery, Right 8 Brachial Artery, Left 9 Ulnar Artery, Right A Ulnar Artery, Left B Radial Artery, Right C Radial Artery, Left D Hand Artery, Right F Hand Artery, Left G Intracranial Artery H Common Carotid Artery, Right J Common Carotid Artery, Left M External Carotid Artery, Right N External Carotid Artery, Left P Vertebral Artery, Right Q Vertebral Artery, Left R Face Artery S Temporal Artery, Right T Temporal Artery, Left U Thyroid Artery, Right V Thyroid Artery, Left	0 Open 3 Percutaneous 4 Percutaneous Endoscopic	3 Infusion Device D Intraluminal Device	Z No Qualifier
K Internal Carotid Artery, Right L Internal Carotid Artery, Left	0 Open 3 Percutaneous 4 Percutaneous Endoscopic	3 Infusion Device D Intraluminal Device M Stimulator Lead	Z No Qualifier
Y Upper Artery	0 Open 3 Percutaneous 4 Percutaneous Endoscopic	2 Monitoring Device 3 Infusion Device D Intraluminal Device Y Other Device	Z No Qualifier

Section	0	Medical and Surgical
Body System	3	Upper Arteries
Operation	J	**Inspection:** Visually and/or manually exploring a body part

Body Part (4th)	Approach (5th)	Device (6th)	Qualifier (7th)
Y Upper Artery	0 Open 3 Percutaneous 4 Percutaneous Endoscopic X External	Z No Device	Z No Qualifier

Section	0	Medical and Surgical
Body System	3	Upper Arteries
Operation	L	Occlusion: Completely closing an orifice or the lumen of a tubular body part

Body Part (4th)	Approach (5th)	Device (6th)	Qualifier (7th)
0 Internal Mammary Artery, Right 1 Internal Mammary Artery, Left 2 Innominate Artery 3 Subclavian Artery, Right 4 Subclavian Artery, Left 5 Axillary Artery, Right 6 Axillary Artery, Left 7 Brachial Artery, Right 8 Brachial Artery, Left 9 Ulnar Artery, Right A Ulnar Artery, Left B Radial Artery, Right C Radial Artery, Left D Hand Artery, Right F Hand Artery, Left R Face Artery S Temporal Artery, Right T Temporal Artery, Left U Thyroid Artery, Right V Thyroid Artery, Left Y Upper Artery	0 Open 3 Percutaneous 4 Percutaneous Endoscopic	C Extraluminal Device D Intraluminal Device Z No Device	Z No Qualifier
G Intracranial Artery H Common Carotid Artery, Right J Common Carotid Artery, Left K Internal Carotid Artery, Right L Internal Carotid Artery, Left M External Carotid Artery, Right N External Carotid Artery, Left P Vertebral Artery, Right Q Vertebral Artery, Left	0 Open 3 Percutaneous 4 Percutaneous Endoscopic	B Intraluminal Device, Bioactive C Extraluminal Device D Intraluminal Device Z No Device	Z No Qualifier

Section	0	Medical and Surgical
Body System	3	Upper Arteries
Operation	N	Release: Freeing a body part from an abnormal physical constraint by cutting or by the use of force

Body Part (4th)	Approach (5th)	Device (6th)	Qualifier (7th)
0 Internal Mammary Artery, Right 1 Internal Mammary Artery, Left 2 Innominate Artery 3 Subclavian Artery, Right 4 Subclavian Artery, Left 5 Axillary Artery, Right 6 Axillary Artery, Left 7 Brachial Artery, Right 8 Brachial Artery, Left 9 Ulnar Artery, Right A Ulnar Artery, Left B Radial Artery, Right C Radial Artery, Left D Hand Artery, Right F Hand Artery, Left G Intracranial Artery H Common Carotid Artery, Right J Common Carotid Artery, Left K Internal Carotid Artery, Right L Internal Carotid Artery, Left M External Carotid Artery, Right N External Carotid Artery, Left P Vertebral Artery, Right Q Vertebral Artery, Left R Face Artery S Temporal Artery, Right T Temporal Artery, Left U Thyroid Artery, Right V Thyroid Artery, Left Y Upper Artery	0 Open 3 Percutaneous 4 Percutaneous Endoscopic	Z No Device	Z No Qualifier

Section	0	Medical and Surgical
Body System	3	Upper Arteries
Operation	P	**Removal:** Taking out or off a device from a body part

Body Part (4th)	Approach (5th)	Device (6th)	Qualifier (7th)
Y Upper Artery	**0** Open **3** Percutaneous **4** Percutaneous Endoscopic	**0** Drainage Device **2** Monitoring Device **3** Infusion Device **7** Autologous Tissue Substitute **C** Extraluminal Device **D** Intraluminal Device **J** Synthetic Substitute **K** Nonautologous Tissue Substitute **M** Stimulator Lead **Y** Other Device	**Z** No Qualifier
Y Upper Artery	**X** External	**0** Drainage Device **2** Monitoring Device **3** Infusion Device **D** Intraluminal Device **M** Stimulator Lead	**Z** No Qualifier

Section	0	Medical and Surgical
Body System	3	Upper Arteries
Operation	Q	**Repair:** Restoring, to the extent possible, a body part to its normal anatomic structure and function

Body Part (4th)	Approach (5th)	Device (6th)	Qualifier (7th)
0 Internal Mammary Artery, Right **1** Internal Mammary Artery, Left **2** Innominate Artery **3** Subclavian Artery, Right **4** Subclavian Artery, Left **5** Axillary Artery, Right **6** Axillary Artery, Left **7** Brachial Artery, Right **8** Brachial Artery, Left **9** Ulnar Artery, Right **A** Ulnar Artery, Left **B** Radial Artery, Right **C** Radial Artery, Left **D** Hand Artery, Right **F** Hand Artery, Left **G** Intracranial Artery **H** Common Carotid Artery, Right **J** Common Carotid Artery, Left **K** Internal Carotid Artery, Right **L** Internal Carotid Artery, Left **M** External Carotid Artery, Right **N** External Carotid Artery, Left **P** Vertebral Artery, Right **Q** Vertebral Artery, Left **R** Face Artery **S** Temporal Artery, Right **T** Temporal Artery, Left **U** Thyroid Artery, Right **V** Thyroid Artery, Left **Y** Upper Artery	**0** Open **3** Percutaneous **4** Percutaneous Endoscopic	**Z** No Device	**Z** No Qualifier

Section	0	Medical and Surgical
Body System	3	Upper Arteries
Operation	R	**Replacement:** Putting in or on biological or synthetic material that physically takes the place and/or function of all or a portion of a body part

Body Part (4th)	Approach (5th)	Device (6th)	Qualifier (7th)
0 Internal Mammary Artery, Right 1 Internal Mammary Artery, Left 2 Innominate Artery 3 Subclavian Artery, Right 4 Subclavian Artery, Left 5 Axillary Artery, Right 6 Axillary Artery, Left 7 Brachial Artery, Right 8 Brachial Artery, Left 9 Ulnar Artery, Right A Ulnar Artery, Left B Radial Artery, Right C Radial Artery, Left D Hand Artery, Right F Hand Artery, Left G Intracranial Artery H Common Carotid Artery, Right J Common Carotid Artery, Left K Internal Carotid Artery, Right L Internal Carotid Artery, Left M External Carotid Artery, Right N External Carotid Artery, Left P Vertebral Artery, Right Q Vertebral Artery, Left R Face Artery S Temporal Artery, Right T Temporal Artery, Left U Thyroid Artery, Right V Thyroid Artery, Left Y Upper Artery	0 Open 4 Percutaneous Endoscopic	7 Autologous Tissue Substitute J Synthetic Substitute K Nonautologous Tissue Substitute	Z No Qualifier

Section	0	Medical and Surgical
Body System	3	Upper Arteries
Operation	S	**Reposition:** Moving to its normal location, or other suitable location, all or a portion of a body part

Body Part (4th)	Approach (5th)	Device (6th)	Qualifier (7th)
0 Internal Mammary Artery, Right 1 Internal Mammary Artery, Left 2 Innominate Artery 3 Subclavian Artery, Right 4 Subclavian Artery, Left 5 Axillary Artery, Right 6 Axillary Artery, Left 7 Brachial Artery, Right 8 Brachial Artery, Left 9 Ulnar Artery, Right A Ulnar Artery, Left B Radial Artery, Right C Radial Artery, Left D Hand Artery, Right F Hand Artery, Left G Intracranial Artery H Common Carotid Artery, Right J Common Carotid Artery, Left K Internal Carotid Artery, Right L Internal Carotid Artery, Left M External Carotid Artery, Right N External Carotid Artery, Left P Vertebral Artery, Right Q Vertebral Artery, Left R Face Artery S Temporal Artery, Right T Temporal Artery, Left U Thyroid Artery, Right V Thyroid Artery, Left Y Upper Artery	0 Open 3 Percutaneous 4 Percutaneous Endoscopic	Z No Device	Z No Qualifier

Section	0	Medical and Surgical
Body System	3	Upper Arteries
Operation	U	Supplement: Putting in or on biological or synthetic material that physically reinforces and/or augments the function of a portion of a body part

Body Part (4th)	Approach (5th)	Device (6th)	Qualifier (7th)
0 Internal Mammary Artery, Right	0 Open	7 Autologous Tissue Substitute	Z No Qualifier
1 Internal Mammary Artery, Left	3 Percutaneous	J Synthetic Substitute	
2 Innominate Artery	4 Percutaneous Endoscopic	K Nonautologous Tissue Substitute	
3 Subclavian Artery, Right			
4 Subclavian Artery, Left			
5 Axillary Artery, Right			
6 Axillary Artery, Left			
7 Brachial Artery, Right			
8 Brachial Artery, Left			
9 Ulnar Artery, Right			
A Ulnar Artery, Left			
B Radial Artery, Right			
C Radial Artery, Left			
D Hand Artery, Right			
F Hand Artery, Left			
G Intracranial Artery			
H Common Carotid Artery, Right			
J Common Carotid Artery, Left			
K Internal Carotid Artery, Right			
L Internal Carotid Artery, Left			
M External Carotid Artery, Right			
N External Carotid Artery, Left			
P Vertebral Artery, Right			
Q Vertebral Artery, Left			
R Face Artery			
S Temporal Artery, Right			
T Temporal Artery, Left			
U Thyroid Artery, Right			
V Thyroid Artery, Left			
Y Upper Artery			

Section	0	Medical and Surgical
Body System	3	Upper Arteries
Operation	V	Restriction: Partially closing an orifice or the lumen of a tubular body part

Body Part (4th)	Approach (5th)	Device (6th)	Qualifier (7th)
0 Internal Mammary Artery, Right 1 Internal Mammary Artery, Left 2 Innominate Artery 3 Subclavian Artery, Right 4 Subclavian Artery, Left 5 Axillary Artery, Right 6 Axillary Artery, Left 7 Brachial Artery, Right 8 Brachial Artery, Left 9 Ulnar Artery, Right A Ulnar Artery, Left B Radial Artery, Right C Radial Artery, Left D Hand Artery, Right F Hand Artery, Left R Face Artery S Temporal Artery, Right T Temporal Artery, Left U Thyroid Artery, Right V Thyroid Artery, Left Y Upper Artery	0 Open 3 Percutaneous 4 Percutaneous Endoscopic	C Extraluminal Device D Intraluminal Device Z No Device	Z No Qualifier
G Intracranial Artery H Common Carotid Artery, Right J Common Carotid Artery, Left K Internal Carotid Artery, Right L Internal Carotid Artery, Left M External Carotid Artery, Right N External Carotid Artery, Left P Vertebral Artery, Right Q Vertebral Artery, Left	0 Open 3 Percutaneous 4 Percutaneous Endoscopic	B Intraluminal Device, Bioactive C Extraluminal Device D Intraluminal Device H Intraluminal Device, Flow Diverter Z No Device	Z No Qualifier

Section	0	Medical and Surgical
Body System	3	Upper Arteries
Operation	W	Revision: Correcting, to the extent possible, a portion of a malfunctioning device or the position of a displaced device

Body Part (4th)	Approach (5th)	Device (6th)	Qualifier (7th)
Y Upper Artery	0 Open 3 Percutaneous 4 Percutaneous Endoscopic	0 Drainage Device 2 Monitoring Device 3 Infusion Device 7 Autologous Tissue Substitute C Extraluminal Device D Intraluminal Device J Synthetic Substitute K Nonautologous Tissue Substitute M Stimulator Lead Y Other Device	Z No Qualifier
Y Upper Artery	X External	0 Drainage Device 2 Monitoring Device 3 Infusion Device 7 Autologous Tissue Substitute C Extraluminal Device D Intraluminal Device J Synthetic Substitute K Nonautologous Tissue Substitute M Neurostimulator Lead	Z No Qualifier

AHA Coding Clinic

03170ZD Bypass Right Brachial Artery to Upper Arm Vein, Open Approach—AHA CC: 4Q, 2013, 125-126

03180JD Bypass Left Brachial Artery to Upper Arm Vein with Synthetic Substitute, Open Approach—AHA CC: 3Q, 2016, 37-38

031C0ZF Bypass Left Radial Artery to Lower Arm Vein, Open Approach—AHA CC: 1Q, 2013, 27-28

031J0JJ Bypass Left Common Carotid Artery to Right Extracranial Artery with Synthetic Substitute, Open Approach—AHA CC: 4Q, 2017, 65

031J0ZK Bypass Left Common Carotid Artery to Left Extracranial Artery, Open Approach—AHA CC: 2Q, 2017, 22

037K3DZ Dilation of Right Internal Carotid Artery with Intraluminal Device, Percutaneous Approach—AHA CC: 3Q, 2019, 29-30

03BN0ZZ Excision of Left External Carotid Artery, Open Approach—AHA CC: 2Q, 2016, 12-14

03CK0ZZ Extirpation of Matter from Right Internal Carotid Artery, Open Approach—AHA CC: 2Q, 2016, 11-12

03CN0ZZ Extirpation of Matter from Left External Carotid Artery, Open Approach—AHA CC: 4Q, 2017, 65

03H40DZ Insertion of Intraluminal Device into Left Subclavian Artery, Open Approach—AHA CC: 1Q, 2020, 25-27

03HY32Z Insertion of Monitoring Device into Upper Artery, Percutaneous Approach—AHA CC: 2Q, 2016, 32-33

03JY0ZZ Inspection of Upper Artery, Open Approach—AHA CC: 1Q, 2015, 29

03LG0CZ Occlusion of Intracranial Artery with Extraluminal Device, Open Approach—AHA CC: 2Q, 2016, 30

03LG3DZ Occlusion of Intracranial Artery with Intraluminal Device, Percutaneous Approach—AHA CC: 4Q, 2014, 37

03QH0ZZ Repair Right Common Carotid Artery, Open Approach—AHA CC: 1Q, 2017, 31-32

03SS0ZZ Reposition Right Temporal Artery, Open Approach—AHA CC: 3Q, 2015, 27-28

03UK0JZ Supplement Right Internal Carotid Artery with Synthetic Substitute, Open Approach—AHA CC: 2Q, 2016, 11-12

03VG0CZ Restriction of Intracranial Artery with Extraluminal Device, Open Approach—AHA CC: 1Q, 2019, 22

03VG3DZ Restriction of Intracranial Artery with Intraluminal Device, Percutaneous Approach—AHA CC: 1Q, 2016, 19-20

03VM3DZ Restriction of Right External Carotid Artery with Intraluminal Device, Percutaneous Approach—AHA CC: 4Q, 2016, 26

03WY0JZ Revision of Synthetic Substitute in Upper Artery, Open Approach—AHA CC: 3Q, 2016, 39-40

03WY3DZ Revision of Intraluminal Device in Upper Artery, Percutaneous Approach—AHA CC: 1Q, 2015, 32-33

Arteries

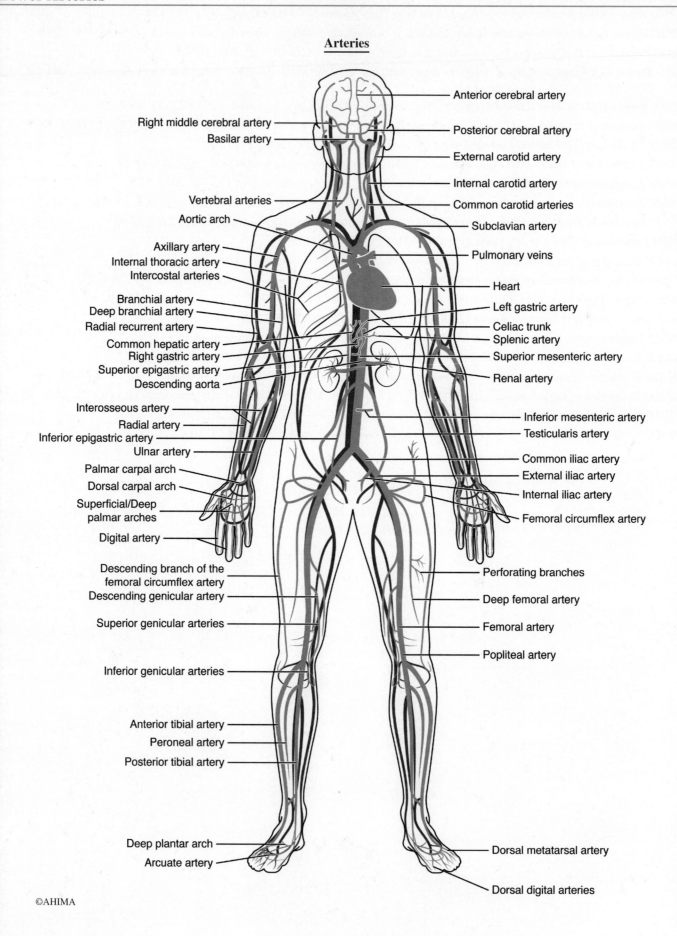

Anterior cerebral artery

Right middle cerebral artery

Posterior cerebral artery

Basilar artery

External carotid artery

Internal carotid artery

Vertebral arteries

Common carotid arteries

Aortic arch

Subclavian artery

Axillary artery

Pulmonary veins

Internal thoracic artery

Intercostal arteries

Heart

Branchial artery

Left gastric artery

Deep branchial artery

Celiac trunk

Radial recurrent artery

Splenic artery

Common hepatic artery

Superior mesenteric artery

Right gastric artery

Superior epigastric artery

Renal artery

Descending aorta

Interosseous artery

Inferior mesenteric artery

Radial artery

Testicularis artery

Inferior epigastric artery

Ulnar artery

Common iliac artery

Palmar carpal arch

External iliac artery

Dorsal carpal arch

Internal iliac artery

Superficial/Deep
palmar arches

Femoral circumflex artery

Digital artery

Descending branch of the
femoral circumflex artery

Perforating branches

Descending genicular artery

Deep femoral artery

Superior genicular arteries

Femoral artery

Popliteal artery

Inferior genicular arteries

Anterior tibial artery

Peroneal artery

Posterior tibial artery

Deep plantar arch

Dorsal metatarsal artery

Arcuate artery

Dorsal digital arteries

©AHIMA

Section	0	Medical and Surgical
Body System	4	Lower Arteries
Operation	1	Bypass: Altering the route of passage of the contents of a tubular body part

Body Part (4th)	Approach (5th)	Device (6th)	Qualifier (7th)
0 Abdominal Aorta C Common Iliac Artery, Right D Common Iliac Artery, Left	0 Open 4 Percutaneous Endoscopic	9 Autologous Venous Tissue A Autologous Arterial Tissue J Synthetic Substitute K Nonautologous Tissue Substitute Z No Device	0 Abdominal Aorta 1 Celiac Artery 2 Mesenteric Artery 3 Renal Artery, Right 4 Renal Artery, Left 5 Renal Artery, Bilateral 6 Common Iliac Artery, Right 7 Common Iliac Artery, Left 8 Common Iliac Arteries, Bilateral 9 Internal Iliac Artery, Right B Internal Iliac Artery, Left C Internal Iliac Arteries, Bilateral D External Iliac Artery, Right F External Iliac Artery, Left G External Iliac Arteries, Bilateral H Femoral Artery, Right J Femoral Artery, Left K Femoral Arteries, Bilateral Q Lower Extremity Artery R Lower Artery
3 Hepatic Artery 4 Splenic Artery	0 Open 4 Percutaneous Endoscopic	9 Autologous Venous Tissue A Autologous Arterial Tissue J Synthetic Substitute K Nonautologous Tissue Substitute Z No Device	3 Renal Artery, Right 4 Renal Artery, Left 5 Renal Artery, Bilateral
E Internal Iliac Artery, Right F Internal Iliac Artery, Left H External Iliac Artery, Right J External Iliac Artery, Left	0 Open 4 Percutaneous Endoscopic	9 Autologous Venous Tissue A Autologous Arterial Tissue J Synthetic Substitute K Nonautologous Tissue Substitute Z No Device	9 Internal Iliac Artery, Right B Internal Iliac Artery, Left C Internal Iliac Arteries, Bilateral D External Iliac Artery, Right F External Iliac Artery, Left G External Iliac Arteries, Bilateral H Femoral Artery, Right J Femoral Artery, Left K Femoral Arteries, Bilateral P Foot Artery Q Lower Extremity Artery
K Femoral Artery, Right L Femoral Artery, Left	0 Open 4 Percutaneous Endoscopic	9 Autologous Venous Tissue A Autologous Arterial Tissue J Synthetic Substitute K Nonautologous Tissue Substitute Z No Device	H Femoral Artery, Right J Femoral Artery, Left K Femoral Arteries, Bilateral L Popliteal Artery M Peroneal Artery N Posterior Tibial Artery P Foot Artery Q Lower Extremity Artery S Lower Extremity Vein
K Femoral Artery, Right L Femoral Artery, Left	3 Percutaneous	J Synthetic Substitute	Q Lower Extremity Artery S Lower Extremity Vein
M Popliteal Artery, Right N Popliteal Artery, Left	0 Open 4 Percutaneous Endoscopic	9 Autologous Venous Tissue A Autologous Arterial Tissue J Synthetic Substitute K Nonautologous Tissue Substitute Z No Device	L Popliteal Artery M Peroneal Artery P Foot Artery Q Lower Extremity Artery S Lower Extremity Vein

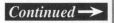
Continued →

Section	0	Medical and Surgical
Body System	4	Lower Arteries
Operation	1	**Bypass:** Altering the route of passage of the contents of a tubular body part

Body Part (4th)	Approach (5th)	Device (6th)	Qualifier (7th)
M Popliteal Artery, Right **N** Popliteal Artery, Left	**3** Percutaneous	**J** Synthetic Substitute	**Q** Lower Extremity Artery **S** Lower Extremity Vein
P Anterior Tibial Artery, Right **Q** Anterior Tibial Artery, Left **R** Posterior Tibial Artery, Right **S** Posterior Tibial Artery, Left	**0** Open **3** Percutaneou **4** Percutaneous Endoscopic	**J** Synthetic Substitute	**Q** Lower Extremity Artery **S** Lower Extremity Vein
T Peroneal Artery, Right **U** Peroneal Artery, Left **V** Foot Artery, Right **W** Foot Artery, Left	**0** Open **4** Percutaneous Endoscopic	**9** Autologous Venous Tissue **A** Autologous Arterial Tissue **J** Synthetic Substitute **K** Nonautologous Tissue Substitute **Z** No Device	**P** Foot Artery **Q** Lower Extremity Artery **S** Lower Extremity Vein
T Peroneal Artery, Right **U** Peroneal Artery, Left **V** Foot Artery, Right **W** Foot Artery, Left	**3** Percutaneous	**J** Synthetic Substitute	**Q** Lower Extremity Artery **S** Lower Extremity Vein

Section	0	Medical and Surgical
Body System	4	Lower Arteries
Operation	5	**Destruction:** Physical eradication of all or a portion of a body part by the direct use of energy, force, or a destructive agent

Body Part (4th)	Approach (5th)	Device (6th)	Qualifier (7th)
0 Abdominal Aorta **1** Celiac Artery **2** Gastric Artery **3** Hepatic Artery **4** Splenic Artery **5** Superior Mesenteric Artery **6** Colic Artery, Right **7** Colic Artery, Left **8** Colic Artery, Middle **9** Renal Artery, Right **A** Renal Artery, Left **B** Inferior Mesenteric Artery **C** Common Iliac Artery, Right **D** Common Iliac Artery, Left **E** Internal Iliac Artery, Right **F** Internal Iliac Artery, Left **H** External Iliac Artery, Right **J** External Iliac Artery, Left **K** Femoral Artery, Right **L** Femoral Artery, Left **M** Popliteal Artery, Right **N** Popliteal Artery, Left **P** Anterior Tibial Artery, Right **Q** Anterior Tibial Artery, Left **R** Posterior Tibial Artery, Right **S** Posterior Tibial Artery, Left **T** Peroneal Artery, Right **U** Peroneal Artery, Left **V** Foot Artery, Right **W** Foot Artery, Left **Y** Lower Artery	**0** Open **3** Percutaneous **4** Percutaneous Endoscopic	**Z** No Device	**Z** No Qualifier

Section	0	Medical and Surgical
Body System	4	Lower Arteries
Operation	7	**Dilation:** Expanding an orifice or the lumen of a tubular body part

Body Part (4th)	Approach (5th)	Device (6th)	Qualifier (7th)
0 Abdominal Aorta 1 Celiac Artery 2 Gastric Artery 3 Hepatic Artery 4 Splenic Artery 5 Superior Mesenteric Artery 6 Colic Artery, Right 7 Colic Artery, Left 8 Colic Artery, Middle 9 Renal Artery, Right A Renal Artery, Left B Inferior Mesenteric Artery C Common Iliac Artery, Right D Common Iliac Artery, Left E Internal Iliac Artery, Right F Internal Iliac Artery, Left H External Iliac Artery, Right J External Iliac Artery, Left K Femoral Artery, Right L Femoral Artery, Left M Popliteal Artery, Right N Popliteal Artery, Left P Anterior Tibial Artery, Right Q Anterior Tibial Artery, Left R Posterior Tibial Artery, Right S Posterior Tibial Artery, Left T Peroneal Artery, Right U Peroneal Artery, Left V Foot Artery, Right W Foot Artery, Left Y Lower Artery	0 Open 3 Percutaneous 4 Percutaneous Endoscopic	4 Intraluminal Device, Drug-eluting D Intraluminal Device Z No Device	1 Drug-Coated Balloon Z No Qualifier
0 Abdominal Aorta 1 Celiac Artery 2 Gastric Artery 3 Hepatic Artery 4 Splenic Artery 5 Superior Mesenteric Artery 6 Colic Artery, Right 7 Colic Artery, Left 8 Colic Artery, Middle 9 Renal Artery, Right A Renal Artery, Left B Inferior Mesenteric Artery C Common Iliac Artery, Right D Common Iliac Artery, Left E Internal Iliac Artery, Right F Internal Iliac Artery, Left H External Iliac Artery, Right J External Iliac Artery, Left K Femoral Artery, Right L Femoral Artery, Left M Popliteal Artery, Right N Popliteal Artery, Left P Anterior Tibial Artery, Right Q Anterior Tibial Artery, Left R Posterior Tibial Artery, Right S Posterior Tibial Artery, Left T Peroneal Artery, Right U Peroneal Artery, Left V Foot Artery, Right W Foot Artery, Left Y Lower Artery	0 Open 3 Percutaneous 4 Percutaneous Endoscopic	5 Intraluminal Device, Drug-eluting, Two 6 Intraluminal Device, Drug-eluting, Three 7 Intraluminal Device, Drug-eluting, Four or More E Intraluminal Devices, Two F Intraluminal Devices, Three G Intraluminal Devices, Four or More	Z No Qualifier

Section	0	Medical and Surgical
Body System	4	Lower Arteries
Operation	9	Drainage: Taking or letting out fluids and/or gases from a body part

Body Part (4th)	Approach (5th)	Device (6th)	Qualifier (7th)
0 Abdominal Aorta 1 Celiac Artery 2 Gastric Artery 3 Hepatic Artery 4 Splenic Artery 5 Superior Mesenteric Artery 6 Colic Artery, Right 7 Colic Artery, Left 8 Colic Artery, Middle 9 Renal Artery, Right A Renal Artery, Left B Inferior Mesenteric Artery C Common Iliac Artery, Right D Common Iliac Artery, Left E Internal Iliac Artery, Right F Internal Iliac Artery, Left H External Iliac Artery, Right J External Iliac Artery, Left K Femoral Artery, Right L Femoral Artery, Left M Popliteal Artery, Right N Popliteal Artery, Left P Anterior Tibial Artery, Right Q Anterior Tibial Artery, Left R Posterior Tibial Artery, Right S Posterior Tibial Artery, Left T Peroneal Artery, Right U Peroneal Artery, Left V Foot Artery, Right W Foot Artery, Left Y Lower Artery	0 Open 3 Percutaneous 4 Percutaneous Endoscopic	0 Drainage Device	Z No Qualifier
0 Abdominal Aorta 1 Celiac Artery 2 Gastric Artery 3 Hepatic Artery 4 Splenic Artery 5 Superior Mesenteric Artery 6 Colic Artery, Right 7 Colic Artery, Left 8 Colic Artery, Middle 9 Renal Artery, Right A Renal Artery, Left B Inferior Mesenteric Artery C Common Iliac Artery, Right D Common Iliac Artery, Left E Internal Iliac Artery, Right F Internal Iliac Artery, Left H External Iliac Artery, Right J External Iliac Artery, Left K Femoral Artery, Right L Femoral Artery, Left M Popliteal Artery, Right N Popliteal Artery, Left P Anterior Tibial Artery, Right Q Anterior Tibial Artery, Left R Posterior Tibial Artery, Right S Posterior Tibial Artery, Left T Peroneal Artery, Right U Peroneal Artery, Left V Foot Artery, Right W Foot Artery, Left Y Lower Artery	0 Open 3 Percutaneous 4 Percutaneous Endoscopic	Z No Device	X Diagnostic Z No Qualifier

Section	0	Medical and Surgical
Body System	4	Lower Arteries
Operation	B	**Excision:** Cutting out or off, without replacement, a portion of a body part

Body Part (4th)	Approach (5th)	Device (6th)	Qualifier (7th)
0 Abdominal Aorta 1 Celiac Artery 2 Gastric Artery 3 Hepatic Artery 4 Splenic Artery 5 Superior Mesenteric Artery 6 Colic Artery, Right 7 Colic Artery, Left 8 Colic Artery, Middle 9 Renal Artery, Right A Renal Artery, Left B Inferior Mesenteric Artery C Common Iliac Artery, Right D Common Iliac Artery, Left E Internal Iliac Artery, Right F Internal Iliac Artery, Left H External Iliac Artery, Right J External Iliac Artery, Left K Femoral Artery, Right L Femoral Artery, Left M Popliteal Artery, Right N Popliteal Artery, Left P Anterior Tibial Artery, Right Q Anterior Tibial Artery, Left R Posterior Tibial Artery, Right S Posterior Tibial Artery, Left T Peroneal Artery, Right U Peroneal Artery, Left V Foot Artery, Right W Foot Artery, Left Y Lower Artery	0 Open 3 Percutaneous 4 Percutaneous Endoscopic	Z No Device	X Diagnostic Z No Qualifier

Section	0	Medical and Surgical
Body System	4	Lower Arteries
Operation	C	**Extirpation:** Taking or cutting out solid matter from a body part

Body Part (4th)	Approach (5th)	Device (6th)	Qualifier (7th)
0 Abdominal Aorta 1 Celiac Artery 2 Gastric Artery 3 Hepatic Artery 4 Splenic Artery 5 Superior Mesenteric Artery 6 Colic Artery, Right 7 Colic Artery, Left 8 Colic Artery, Middle 9 Renal Artery, Right A Renal Artery, Left B Inferior Mesenteric Artery C Common Iliac Artery, Right D Common Iliac Artery, Left E Internal Iliac Artery, Right F Internal Iliac Artery, Left H External Iliac Artery, Right J External Iliac Artery, Left K Femoral Artery, Right L Femoral Artery, Left M Popliteal Artery, Right N Popliteal Artery, Left P Anterior Tibial Artery, Right Q Anterior Tibial Artery, Left R Posterior Tibial Artery, Right S Posterior Tibial Artery, Left T Peroneal Artery, Right U Peroneal Artery, Left V Foot Artery, Right W Foot Artery, Left Y Lower Artery	0 Open 3 Percutaneous 4 Percutaneous Endoscopic	Z No Device	Z No Qualifier

Section	0	Medical and Surgical
Body System	4	Lower Arteries
Operation	F	**Fragmentation:** Breaking solid matter in a body part into pieces

Body Part (4th)	Approach (5th)	Device (6th)	Qualifier (7th)
C Common Iliac Artery, Right D Common Iliac Artery, Left E Internal Iliac Artery, Right F Internal Iliac Artery, Left H External Iliac Artery, Right J External Iliac Artery, Left K Femoral Artery, Right L Femoral Artery, Left M Popliteal Artery, Right N Popliteal Artery, Left P Anterior Tibial Artery, Right Q Anterior Tibial Artery, Left R Posterior Tibial Artery, Right S Posterior Tibial Artery, Left T Peroneal Artery, Right U Peroneal Artery, Left Y Lower Artery	3 Percutaneous	Z No Device	0 Ultrasonic Z No Qualifier

Section	0	Medical and Surgical
Body System	4	Lower Arteries
Operation	H	Insertion: Putting in a nonbiological appliance that monitors, assists, performs, or prevents a physiological function but does not physically take the place of a body part

Body Part (4th)	Approach (5th)	Device (6th)	Qualifier (7th)
0 Abdominal Aorta	**0** Open **3** Percutaneous **4** Percutaneous Endoscopic	**2** Monitoring Device **3** Infusion Device **D** Intraluminal Device	**Z** No Qualifier
1 Celiac Artery **2** Gastric Artery **3** Hepatic Artery **4** Splenic Artery **5** Superior Mesenteric Artery **6** Colic Artery, Right **7** Colic Artery, Left **8** Colic Artery, Middle **9** Renal Artery, Right **A** Renal Artery, Left **B** Inferior Mesenteric Artery **C** Common Iliac Artery, Right **D** Common Iliac Artery, Left **E** Internal Iliac Artery, Right **F** Internal Iliac Artery, Left **H** External Iliac Artery, Right **J** External Iliac Artery, Left **K** Femoral Artery, Right **L** Femoral Artery, Left **M** Popliteal Artery, Right **N** Popliteal Artery, Left **P** Anterior Tibial Artery, Right **Q** Anterior Tibial Artery, Left **R** Posterior Tibial Artery, Right **S** Posterior Tibial Artery, Left **T** Peroneal Artery, Right **U** Peroneal Artery, Left **V** Foot Artery, Right **W** Foot Artery, Left	**0** Open **3** Percutaneous **4** Percutaneous Endoscopic	**3** Infusion Device **D** Intraluminal Device	**Z** No Qualifier
Y Lower Artery	**0** Open **3** Percutaneous **4** Percutaneous Endoscopic	**2** Monitoring Device **3** Infusion Device **D** Intraluminal Device **Y** Other Device	**Z** No Qualifier

Section	0	Medical and Surgical
Body System	4	Lower Arteries
Operation	J	Inspection: Visually and/or manually exploring a body part

Body Part (4th)	Approach (5th)	Device (6th)	Qualifier (7th)
Y Lower Artery	**0** Open **3** Percutaneous **4** Percutaneous Endoscopic **X** External	**Z** No Device	**Z** No Qualifier

Section	0	Medical and Surgical
Body System	4	Lower Arteries
Operation	L	Occlusion: Completely closing an orifice or the lumen of a tubular body part

Body Part (4th)	Approach (5th)	Device (6th)	Qualifier (7th)
0 Abdominal Aorta	0 Open 4 Percutaneous Endoscopic	C Extraluminal Device D Intraluminal Device Z No Device	Z No Qualifier
0 Abdominal Aorta	3 Percutaneous	C Extraluminal Device Z No Device	Z No Qualifier
0 Abdominal Aorta	3 Percutaneous	D Intraluminal Device	J Temporary Z No Qualifier
1 Celiac Artery 2 Gastric Artery 3 Hepatic Artery 4 Splenic Artery 5 Superior Mesenteric Artery 6 Colic Artery, Right 7 Colic Artery, Left 8 Colic Artery, Middle 9 Renal Artery, Right A Renal Artery, Left B Inferior Mesenteric Artery C Common Iliac Artery, Right D Common Iliac Artery, Left H External Iliac Artery, Right J External Iliac Artery, Left K Femoral Artery, Right L Femoral Artery, Left M Popliteal Artery, Right N Popliteal Artery, Left P Anterior Tibial Artery, Right Q Anterior Tibial Artery, Left R Posterior Tibial Artery, Right S Posterior Tibial Artery, Left T Peroneal Artery, Right U Peroneal Artery, Left V Foot Artery, Right W Foot Artery, Left Y Lower Artery	0 Open 3 Percutaneous 4 Percutaneous Endoscopic	C Extraluminal Device D Intraluminal Device Z No Device	Z No Qualifier
E Internal Iliac Artery, Right	0 Open 3 Percutaneous 4 Percutaneous Endoscopic	C Extraluminal Device D Intraluminal Device Z No Device	T Uterine Artery, Right Z No Qualifier
F Internal Iliac Artery, Left	0 Open 3 Percutaneous 4 Percutaneous Endoscopic	C Extraluminal Device D Intraluminal Device Z No Device	U Uterine Artery, Left Z No Qualifier

Section   0   **Medical and Surgical**
Body System   4   **Lower Arteries**
Operation   N   **Release:** Freeing a body part from an abnormal physical constraint by cutting or by the use of force

Body Part (4ᵗʰ)	Approach (5ᵗʰ)	Device (6ᵗʰ)	Qualifier (7ᵗʰ)
0 Abdominal Aorta 1 Celiac Artery 2 Gastric Artery 3 Hepatic Artery 4 Splenic Artery 5 Superior Mesenteric Artery 6 Colic Artery, Right 7 Colic Artery, Left 8 Colic Artery, Middle 9 Renal Artery, Right A Renal Artery, Left B Inferior Mesenteric Artery C Common Iliac Artery, Right D Common Iliac Artery, Left E Internal Iliac Artery, Right F Internal Iliac Artery, Left H External Iliac Artery, Right J External Iliac Artery, Left K Femoral Artery, Right L Femoral Artery, Left M Popliteal Artery, Right N Popliteal Artery, Left P Anterior Tibial Artery, Right Q Anterior Tibial Artery, Left R Posterior Tibial Artery, Right S Posterior Tibial Artery, Left T Peroneal Artery, Right U Peroneal Artery, Left V Foot Artery, Right W Foot Artery, Left Y Lower Artery	0 Open 3 Percutaneous 4 Percutaneous Endoscopic	Z No Device	Z No Qualifier

Section   0   **Medical and Surgical**
Body System   4   **Lower Arteries**
Operation   P   **Removal:** Taking out or off a device from a body part

Body Part (4ᵗʰ)	Approach (5ᵗʰ)	Device (6ᵗʰ)	Qualifier (7ᵗʰ)
Y Lower Artery	0 Open 3 Percutaneous 4 Percutaneous Endoscopic	0 Drainage Device 2 Monitoring Device 3 Infusion Device 7 Autologous Tissue Substitute C Extraluminal Device D Intraluminal Device J Synthetic Substitute K Nonautologous Tissue Substitute Y Other Device	Z No Qualifier
Y Lower Artery	X External	0 Drainage Device 1 Radioactive Element 2 Monitoring Device 3 Infusion Device D Intraluminal Device	Z No Qualifier

Section	0	Medical and Surgical
Body System	4	Lower Arteries
Operation	Q	**Repair:** Restoring, to the extent possible, a body part to its normal anatomic structure and function

Body Part (4ᵗʰ)	Approach (5ᵗʰ)	Device (6ᵗʰ)	Qualifier (7ᵗʰ)
0 Abdominal Aorta	0 Open	**Z** No Device	**Z** No Qualifier
1 Celiac Artery	3 Percutaneous		
2 Gastric Artery	4 Percutaneous		
3 Hepatic Artery	Endoscopic		
4 Splenic Artery			
5 Superior Mesenteric Artery			
6 Colic Artery, Right			
7 Colic Artery, Left			
8 Colic Artery, Middle			
9 Renal Artery, Right			
A Renal Artery, Left			
B Inferior Mesenteric Artery			
C Common Iliac Artery, Right			
D Common Iliac Artery, Left			
E Internal Iliac Artery, Right			
F Internal Iliac Artery, Left			
H External Iliac Artery, Right			
J External Iliac Artery, Left			
K Femoral Artery, Right			
L Femoral Artery, Left			
M Popliteal Artery, Right			
N Popliteal Artery, Left			
P Anterior Tibial Artery, Right			
Q Anterior Tibial Artery, Left			
R Posterior Tibial Artery, Right			
S Posterior Tibial Artery, Left			
T Peroneal Artery, Right			
U Peroneal Artery, Left			
V Foot Artery, Right			
W Foot Artery, Left			
Y Lower Artery			

Section	0	Medical and Surgical
Body System	4	Lower Arteries
Operation	R	**Replacement:** Putting in or on biological or synthetic material that physically takes the place and/or function of all or a portion of a body part

Body Part (4th)	Approach (5th)	Device (6th)	Qualifier (7th)
0 Abdominal Aorta	0 Open	7 Autologous Tissue Substitute	Z No Qualifier
1 Celiac Artery	4 Percutaneous Endoscopic	J Synthetic Substitute	
2 Gastric Artery		K Nonautologous Tissue Substitute	
3 Hepatic Artery			
4 Splenic Artery			
5 Superior Mesenteric Artery			
6 Colic Artery, Right			
7 Colic Artery, Left			
8 Colic Artery, Middle			
9 Renal Artery, Right			
A Renal Artery, Left			
B Inferior Mesenteric Artery			
C Common Iliac Artery, Right			
D Common Iliac Artery, Left			
E Internal Iliac Artery, Right			
F Internal Iliac Artery, Left			
H External Iliac Artery, Right			
J External Iliac Artery, Left			
K Femoral Artery, Right			
L Femoral Artery, Left			
M Popliteal Artery, Right			
N Popliteal Artery, Left			
P Anterior Tibial Artery, Right			
Q Anterior Tibial Artery, Left			
R Posterior Tibial Artery, Right			
S Posterior Tibial Artery, Left			
T Peroneal Artery, Right			
U Peroneal Artery, Left			
V Foot Artery, Right			
W Foot Artery, Left			
Y Lower Artery			

Section	0	Medical and Surgical
Body System	4	Lower Arteries
Operation	S	Reposition: Moving to its normal location, or other suitable location, all or a portion of a body part

Body Part (4th)	Approach (5th)	Device (6th)	Qualifier (7th)
0 Abdominal Aorta	0 Open	Z No Device	Z No Qualifier
1 Celiac Artery	3 Percutaneous		
2 Gastric Artery	4 Percutaneous Endoscopic		
3 Hepatic Artery			
4 Splenic Artery			
5 Superior Mesenteric Artery			
6 Colic Artery, Right			
7 Colic Artery, Left			
8 Colic Artery, Middle			
9 Renal Artery, Right			
A Renal Artery, Left			
B Inferior Mesenteric Artery			
C Common Iliac Artery, Right			
D Common Iliac Artery, Left			
E Internal Iliac Artery, Right			
F Internal Iliac Artery, Left			
H External Iliac Artery, Right			
J External Iliac Artery, Left			
K Femoral Artery, Right			
L Femoral Artery, Left			
M Popliteal Artery, Right			
N Popliteal Artery, Left			
P Anterior Tibial Artery, Right			
Q Anterior Tibial Artery, Left			
R Posterior Tibial Artery, Right			
S Posterior Tibial Artery, Left			
T Peroneal Artery, Right			
U Peroneal Artery, Left			
V Foot Artery, Right			
W Foot Artery, Left			
Y Lower Artery			

Section	0	Medical and Surgical
Body System	4	Lower Arteries
Operation	U	Supplement: Putting in or on biological or synthetic material that physically reinforces and/or augments the function of a portion of a body part

Body Part (4th)	Approach (5th)	Device (6th)	Qualifier (7th)
0 Abdominal Aorta 1 Celiac Artery 2 Gastric Artery 3 Hepatic Artery 4 Splenic Artery 5 Superior Mesenteric Artery 6 Colic Artery, Right 7 Colic Artery, Left 8 Colic Artery, Middle 9 Renal Artery, Right A Renal Artery, Left B Inferior Mesenteric Artery C Common Iliac Artery, Right D Common Iliac Artery, Left E Internal Iliac Artery, Right F Internal Iliac Artery, Left H External Iliac Artery, Right J External Iliac Artery, Left K Femoral Artery, Right L Femoral Artery, Left M Popliteal Artery, Right N Popliteal Artery, Left P Anterior Tibial Artery, Right Q Anterior Tibial Artery, Left R Posterior Tibial Artery, Right S Posterior Tibial Artery, Left T Peroneal Artery, Right U Peroneal Artery, Left V Foot Artery, Right W Foot Artery, Left Y Lower Artery	0 Open 3 Percutaneous 4 Percutaneous Endoscopic	7 Autologous Tissue Substitute J Synthetic Substitute K Nonautologous Tissue Substitute	Z No Qualifier

Section	0	Medical and Surgical
Body System	4	Lower Arteries
Operation	V	Restriction: Partially closing an orifice or the lumen of a tubular body part

Body Part (4th)	Approach (5th)	Device (6th)	Qualifier (7th)
0 Abdominal Aorta	0 Open 3 Percutaneous 4 Percutaneous Endoscopic	C Extraluminal Device E Intraluminal Device, Branched or Fenestrated, One or Two Arteries F Intraluminal Device, Branched or Fenestrated, Three or More Arteries Z No Device	Z No Qualifier
0 Abdominal Aorta	0 Open 3 Percutaneous 4 Percutaneous Endoscopic	D Intraluminal Device	J Temporary Z No Qualifier

Continued →

Section	0	Medical and Surgical
Body System	4	Lower Arteries
Operation	V	**Restriction:** Partially closing an orifice or the lumen of a tubular body part

Body Part (4th)	Approach (5th)	Device (6th)	Qualifier (7th)
1 Celiac Artery 2 Gastric Artery 3 Hepatic Artery 4 Splenic Artery 5 Superior Mesenteric Artery 6 Colic Artery, Right 7 Colic Artery, Left 8 Colic Artery, Middle 9 Renal Artery, Right A Renal Artery, Left B Inferior Mesenteric Artery E Internal Iliac Artery, Right F Internal Iliac Artery, Left H External Iliac Artery, Right J External Iliac Artery, Left K Femoral Artery, Right L Femoral Artery, Left M Popliteal Artery, Right N Popliteal Artery, Left P Anterior Tibial Artery, Right Q Anterior Tibial Artery, Left R Posterior Tibial Artery, Right S Posterior Tibial Artery, Left T Peroneal Artery, Right U Peroneal Artery, Left V Foot Artery, Right W Foot Artery, Left Y Lower Artery	0 Open 3 Percutaneous 4 Percutaneous Endoscopic	C Extraluminal Device D Intraluminal Device Z No Device	Z No Qualifier
C Common Iliac Artery, Right D Common Iliac Artery, Left	0 Open 3 Percutaneous 4 Percutaneous Endoscopic	C Extraluminal Device D Intraluminal Device E Intraluminal Device, Branched or Fenestrated, One or Two Arteries Z No Device	Z No Qualifier

Section	0	Medical and Surgical
Body System	4	Lower Arteries
Operation	W	**Revision:** Correcting, to the extent possible, a portion of a malfunctioning device or the position of a displaced device

Body Part (4th)	Approach (5th)	Device (6th)	Qualifier (7th)
Y Lower Artery	0 Open 3 Percutaneous 4 Percutaneous Endoscopic	0 Drainage Device 2 Monitoring Device 3 Infusion Device 7 Autologous Tissue Substitute C Extraluminal Device D Intraluminal Device J Synthetic Substitute K Nonautologous Tissue Substitute Y Other Device	Z No Qualifier
Y Lower Artery	X External	0 Drainage Device 2 Monitoring Device 3 Infusion Device 7 Autologous Tissue Substitute C Extraluminal Device D Intraluminal Device J Synthetic Substitute K Nonautologus Tissue Substitute	Z No Qualifier

04100Z3 Bypass Abdominal Aorta to Right Renal Artery, Open Approach—AHA CC: 3Q, 2015, 28

04130Z3 Bypass Hepatic Artery to Right Renal Artery, Open Approach—AHA CC: 4Q, 2017, 47

04140Z4 Bypass Splenic Artery to Left Renal Artery, Open Approach—AHA CC: 3Q, 2015, 28; 4Q, 2017, 47

041C0J2 Bypass Right Common Iliac Artery to Mesenteric Artery with Synthetic Substitute, Open Approach—AHA CC: 3Q, 2017, 16

041C0J5 Bypass Right Common Iliac Artery to Bilateral Renal Artery with Synthetic Substitute, Open Approach—AHA CC: 3Q, 2017, 16

041K09N Bypass Right Femoral Artery to Posterior Tibial Artery with Autologous Venous Tissue, Open Approach—AHA CC: 3Q, 2017, 5-6

041K0JL Bypass Right Femoral Artery to Popliteal Artery with Synthetic Substitute, Open Approach—AHA CC: 3Q, 2018, 25

041K0JN Bypass Right Femoral Artery to Posterior Tibial Artery with Synthetic Substitute, Open Approach—AHA CC: 2Q, 2016, 18-19; 3Q, 2017, 5-6

041M09P Bypass Right Popliteal Artery to Foot Artery with Autologous Venous Tissue, Open Approach—AHA CC: 1Q, 2017, 32-33

047K3D1 Dilation of Right Femoral Artery with Intraluminal Device, using Drug-Coated Balloon, Percutaneous Approach—AHA CC: 4Q, 2015, 7,15

047K3Z6 Dilation of Right Femoral Artery, Bifurcation, Percutaneous Approach—AHA CC: 4Q, 2016, 88-89

047L3Z1 Dilation of Left Femoral Artery using Drug-Coated Balloon, Percutaneous Approach—AHA CC: 4Q, 2015, 15

04CJ0ZZ Extirpation of Matter from Left External Iliac Artery, Open Approach—AHA CC: 1Q, 2016, 31

04CK3Z6 Extirpation of Matter from Right Femoral Artery, Bifurcation, Percutaneous Approach—AHA CC: 4Q, 2016, 88-89

04CL3ZZ Extirpation of Matter from Left Femoral Artery, Percutaneous Approach—AHA CC: 1Q, 2015, 36

04H13DZ Insertion of Intraluminal Device into Celiac Artery, Percutaneous Approach—AHA CC: 1Q, 2019, 23

04H53DZ Insertion of Intraluminal Device into Superior Mesenteric Artery, Percutaneous Approach—AHA CC: 1Q, 2019, 23

04H93DZ Insertion of Intraluminal Device into Right Renal Artery, Percutaneous Approach—AHA CC: 1Q, 2019, 23

04HA3DZ Insertion of Intraluminal Device into Left Renal Artery, Percutaneous Approach—AHA CC: 1Q, 2019, 23

04HY32Z Insertion of Monitoring Device into Lower Artery, Percutaneous Approach—AHA CC: 1Q, 2017, 30

04HY33Z Insertion of Infusion Device into Lower Artery, Percutaneous Approach—AHA CC: 3Q, 2019, 20-21

04L33DZ Occlusion of Hepatic Artery with Intraluminal Device, Percutaneous Approach—AHA CC: 3Q, 2014, 26-27

04L73DZ Occlusion of Left Colic Artery with Intraluminal Device, Percutaneous Approach—AHA CC: 1Q, 2014, 24

04LB3DZ Occlusion of Inferior Mesenteric Artery with Intraluminal Device, Percutaneous Approach—AHA CC: 1Q, 2014, 24

04LE3DT Occlusion of Right Uterine Artery with Intraluminal Device, Percutaneous Approach—AHA CC: 2Q, 2015, 27

04LH0CZ Occlusion of Right External Iliac Artery with Extraluminal Device, Open Approach—AHA CC: 2Q, 2018, 18-19

04LJ0CZ Occlusion of Left External Iliac Artery with Extraluminal Device, Open Approach—AHA CC: 2Q, 2018, 18-19

04N10ZZ Release Celiac Artery, Open Approach—AHA CC: 2Q, 2015, 28

04PY33Z Removal of Infusion Device from Lower Artery, Percutaneous Approach—AHA CC: 3Q, 2019, 20-21

04QK0ZZ Repair Right Femoral Artery, Open Approach—AHA CC: 1Q, 2014, 21-22

04R10JZ Replacement of Celiac Artery with Synthetic Substitute, Open Approach—AHA CC: 2Q, 2015, 28

04UJ0KZ Supplement Left External Iliac Artery with Nonautologous Tissue Substitute, Open Approach—AHA CC: 1Q, 2016, 31

04UK0KZ Supplement Right Femoral Artery with Nonautologous Tissue Substitute, Open Approach—AHA CC: 4Q, 2014, 37-38

04UK3JZ Supplement Right Femoral Artery with Synthetic Substitute, Percutaneous Approach—AHA CC: 1Q, 2014, 22-23

04UR07Z Supplement Right Posterior Tibial Artery with Autologous Tissue Substitute, Open Approach—AHA CC: 2Q, 2016, 18-19

04V00DZ Restriction of Abdominal Aorta with Intraluminal Device, Open Approach—AHA CC: 1Q, 2019, 22

04V03DZ Restriction of Abdominal Aorta with Intraluminal Device, Percutaneous Approach—AHA CC: 1Q, 2014, 9; 3Q, 2016, 39

04V03E6 Restriction of Abdominal Aorta, Bifurcation, with Branched or Fenestrated Intraluminal Device, One or Two Arteries, Percutaneous Approach—AHA CC: 4Q, 2016, 91-92

04V03F6 Restriction of Abdominal Aorta, Bifurcation, with Branched or Fenestrated Intraluminal Device, Three or More Arteries, Percutaneous Approach—AHA CC: 4Q, 2016, 92-94

04VC3EZ Restriction of Right Common Iliac Artery with Branched or Fenestrated Intraluminal Device, One or Two Arteries, Percutaneous Approach—AHA CC: 4Q, 2016, 93-94

04VD3EZ Restriction of Left Common Iliac Artery with Branched or Fenestrated Intraluminal Device, One or Two Arteries, Percutaneous Approach—AHA CC: 4Q, 2016, 93-94

04WY07Z Revision of Autologous Tissue Substitute in Lower Artery, Open Approach—AHA CC: 1Q, 2015, 36-37

04WY0JZ Revision of Synthetic Substitute in Lower Artery, Open Approach—AHA CC: 2Q, 2019, 14-15

04WY37Z Revision of Autologous Tissue Substitute in Lower Artery, Percutaneous Approach—AHA CC: 1Q, 2014, 22

04WY3DZ Revision of Intraluminal Device in Lower Artery, Percutaneous Approach—AHA CC: 1Q, 2014, 9-10

Veins

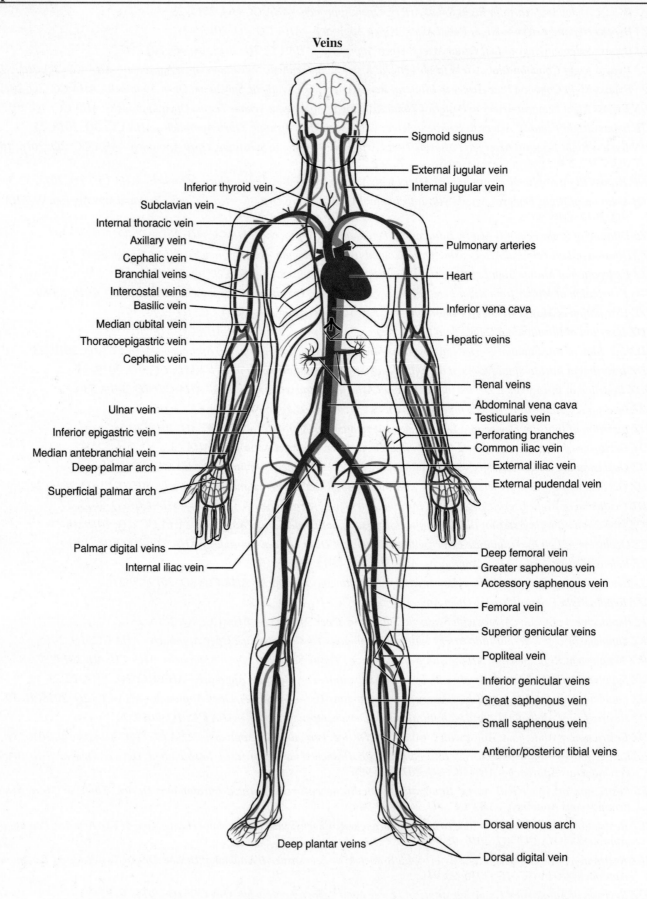

Sigmoid signus

External jugular vein

Internal jugular vein

Inferior thyroid vein

Subclavian vein

Internal thoracic vein

Axillary vein

Cephalic vein

Branchial veins

Intercostal veins

Basilic vein

Median cubital vein

Thoracoepigastric vein

Cephalic vein

Pulmonary arteries

Heart

Inferior vena cava

Hepatic veins

Renal veins

Abdominal vena cava

Testicularis vein

Perforating branches

Common iliac vein

External iliac vein

External pudendal vein

Ulnar vein

Inferior epigastric vein

Median antebranchial vein

Deep palmar arch

Superficial palmar arch

Palmar digital veins

Internal iliac vein

Deep femoral vein

Greater saphenous vein

Accessory saphenous vein

Femoral vein

Superior genicular veins

Popliteal vein

Inferior genicular veins

Great saphenous vein

Small saphenous vein

Anterior/posterior tibial veins

Dorsal venous arch

Deep plantar veins

Dorsal digital vein

Upper Veins Tables 051–05W

051–055

Section	0	Medical and Surgical
Body System	5	Upper Veins
Operation	1	**Bypass:** Altering the route of passage of the contents of a tubular body part

Body Part (4th)	Approach (5th)	Device (6th)	Qualifier (7th)
0 Azygos Vein	0 Open	7 Autologous Tissue Substitute	Y Upper Vein
1 Hemiazygos Vein	4 Percutaneous Endoscopic	9 Autologous Venous Tissue	
3 Innominate Vein, Right		A Autologous Arterial Tissue	
4 Innominate Vein, Left		J Synthetic Substitute	
5 Subclavian Vein, Right		K Nonautologous Tissue Substitute	
6 Subclavian Vein, Left		Z No Device	
7 Axillary Vein, Right			
8 Axillary Vein, Left			
9 Brachial Vein, Right			
A Brachial Vein, Left			
B Basilic Vein, Right			
C Basilic Vein, Left			
D Cephalic Vein, Right			
F Cephalic Vein, Left			
G Hand Vein, Right			
H Hand Vein, Left			
L Intracranial Vein			
M Internal Jugular Vein, Right			
N Internal Jugular Vein, Left			
P External Jugular Vein, Right			
Q External Jugular Vein, Left			
R Vertebral Vein, Right			
S Vertebral Vein, Left			
T Face Vein, Right			
V Face Vein, Left			

Section	0	Medical and Surgical
Body System	5	Upper Veins
Operation	5	**Destruction:** Physical eradication of all or a portion of a body part by the direct use of energy, force, or a destructive agent

Body Part (4th)	Approach (5th)	Device (6th)	Qualifier (7th)
0 Azygos Vein	0 Open	Z No Device	Z No Qualifier
1 Hemiazygos Vein	3 Percutaneous		
3 Innominate Vein, Right	4 Percutaneous Endoscopic		
4 Innominate Vein, Left			
5 Subclavian Vein, Right			
6 Subclavian Vein, Left			
7 Axillary Vein, Right			
8 Axillary Vein, Left			
9 Brachial Vein, Right			
A Brachial Vein, Left			
B Basilic Vein, Right			
C Basilic Vein, Left			
D Cephalic Vein, Right			
F Cephalic Vein, Left			
G Hand Vein, Right			
H Hand Vein, Left			
L Intracranial Vein			
M Internal Jugular Vein, Right			
N Internal Jugular Vein, Left			
P External Jugular Vein, Right			
Q External Jugular Vein, Left			
R Vertebral Vein, Right			
S Vertebral Vein, Left			
T Face Vein, Right			
V Face Vein, Left			
Y Upper Vein			

Section	0	Medical and Surgical
Body System	5	Upper Veins
Operation	7	**Dilation:** Expanding an orifice or the lumen of a tubular body part

Body Part (4th)	Approach (5th)	Device (6th)	Qualifier (7th)
0 Azygos Vein 1 Hemiazygos Vein G Hand Vein, Right H Hand Vein, Left L Intracranial Vein M Internal Jugular Vein, Right N Internal Jugular Vein, Left P External Jugular Vein, Right Q External Jugular Vein, Left R Vertebral Vein, Right S Vertebral Vein, Left T Face Vein, Right V Face Vein, Left Y Upper Vein	0 Open 3 Percutaneous 4 Percutaneous Endoscopic	D Intraluminal Device Z No Device	Z No Qualifier
3 Innominate Vein, Right 4 Innominate Vein, Left 5 Subclavian Vein, Right 6 Subclavian Vein, Left 7 Axillary Vein, Right 8 Axillary Vein, Left 9 Brachial Vein, Right A Brachial Vein, Left B Basilic Vein, Right C Basilic Vein, Left D Cephalic Vein, Right F Cephalic Vein, Left	0 Open 3 Percutaneous 4 Percutaneous Endoscopic	D Intraluminal Device Z No Device	1 Drug-Coated Balloon Z No Qualifier

Section	0	Medical and Surgical
Body System	5	Upper Veins
Operation	9	**Drainage:** Taking or letting out fluids and/or gases from a body part

Body Part (4th)	Approach (5th)	Device (6th)	Qualifier (7th)
0 Azygos Vein 1 Hemiazygos Vein 3 Innominate Vein, Right 4 Innominate Vein, Left 5 Subclavian Vein, Right 6 Subclavian Vein, Left 7 Axillary Vein, Right 8 Axillary Vein, Left 9 Brachial Vein, Right A Brachial Vein, Left B Basilic Vein, Right C Basilic Vein, Left D Cephalic Vein, Right F Cephalic Vein, Left G Hand Vein, Right H Hand Vein, Left L Intracranial Vein M Internal Jugular Vein, Right N Internal Jugular Vein, Left P External Jugular Vein, Right Q External Jugular Vein, Left R Vertebral Vein, Right S Vertebral Vein, Left T Face Vein, Right V Face Vein, Left Y Upper Vein	0 Open 3 Percutaneous 4 Percutaneous Endoscopic	0 Drainage Device	Z No Qualifier

Continued →

Section	0	Medical and Surgical
Body System	5	Upper Veins
Operation	9	Drainage: Taking or letting out fluids and/or gases from a body part

Body Part (4th)	Approach (5th)	Device (6th)	Qualifier (7th)
0 Azygos Vein 1 Hemiazygos Vein 3 Innominate Vein, Right 4 Innominate Vein, Left 5 Subclavian Vein, Right 6 Subclavian Vein, Left 7 Axillary Vein, Right 8 Axillary Vein, Left 9 Brachial Vein, Right A Brachial Vein, Left B Basilic Vein, Right C Basilic Vein, Left D Cephalic Vein, Right F Cephalic Vein, Left G Hand Vein, Right H Hand Vein, Left L Intracranial Vein M Internal Jugular Vein, Right N Internal Jugular Vein, Left P External Jugular Vein, Right Q External Jugular Vein, Left R Vertebral Vein, Right S Vertebral Vein, Left T Face Vein, Right V Face Vein, Left Y Upper Vein	0 Open 3 Percutaneous 4 Percutaneous Endoscopic	Z No Device	X Diagnostic Z No Qualifier

Section	0	Medical and Surgical
Body System	5	Upper Veins
Operation	B	Excision: Cutting out or off, without replacement, a portion of a body part

Body Part (4th)	Approach (5th)	Device (6th)	Qualifier (7th)
0 Azygos Vein 1 Hemiazygos Vein 3 Innominate Vein, Right 4 Innominate Vein, Left 5 Subclavian Vein, Right 6 Subclavian Vein, Left 7 Axillary Vein, Right 8 Axillary Vein, Left 9 Brachial Vein, Right A Brachial Vein, Left B Basilic Vein, Right C Basilic Vein, Left D Cephalic Vein, Right F Cephalic Vein, Left G Hand Vein, Right H Hand Vein, Left L Intracranial Vein M Internal Jugular Vein, Right N Internal Jugular Vein, Left P External Jugular Vein, Right Q External Jugular Vein, Left R Vertebral Vein, Right S Vertebral Vein, Left T Face Vein, Right V Face Vein, Left Y Upper Vein	0 Open 3 Percutaneous 4 Percutaneous Endoscopic	Z No Device	X Diagnostic Z No Qualifier

Section	0	Medical and Surgical
Body System	5	Upper Veins
Operation	C	**Extirpation:** Taking or cutting out solid matter from a body part

Body Part (4th)	Approach (5th)	Device (6th)	Qualifier (7th)
0 Azygos Vein	0 Open	Z No Device	Z No Qualifier
1 Hemiazygos Vein	3 Percutaneous		
3 Innominate Vein, Right	4 Percutaneous Endoscopic		
4 Innominate Vein, Left			
5 Subclavian Vein, Right			
6 Subclavian Vein, Left			
7 Axillary Vein, Right			
8 Axillary Vein, Left			
9 Brachial Vein, Right			
A Brachial Vein, Left			
B Basilic Vein, Right			
C Basilic Vein, Left			
D Cephalic Vein, Right			
F Cephalic Vein, Left			
G Hand Vein, Right			
H Hand Vein, Left			
L Intracranial Vein			
M Internal Jugular Vein, Right			
N Internal Jugular Vein, Left			
P External Jugular Vein, Right			
Q External Jugular Vein, Left			
R Vertebral Vein, Right			
S Vertebral Vein, Left			
T Face Vein, Right			
V Face Vein, Left			
Y Upper Vein			

Section	0	Medical and Surgical
Body System	5	Upper Veins
Operation	D	**Extraction:** Pulling or stripping out or off all or a portion of a body part by the use of force

Body Part (4th)	Approach (5th)	Device (6th)	Qualifier (7th)
9 Brachial Vein, Right	0 Open	Z No Device	Z No Qualifier
A Brachial Vein, Left	3 Percutaneous		
B Basilic Vein, Right			
C Basilic Vein, Left			
D Cephalic Vein, Right			
F Cephalic Vein, Left			
G Hand Vein, Right			
H Hand Vein, Left			
Y Upper Vein			

Section	0	Medical and Surgical
Body System	5	Upper Veins
Operation	F	**Fragmentation:** Breaking solid matter in a body part into pieces

Body Part (4th)	Approach (5th)	Device (6th)	Qualifier (7th)
3 Innominate Vein, Right	3 Percutaneous	Z No Device	0 Ultrasonic
4 Innominate Vein, Left			Z No Qualifier
5 Subclavian Vein, Right			
6 Subclavian Vein, Left			
7 Axillary Vein, Right			
8 Axillary Vein, Left			
9 Brachial Vein, Right			
A Brachial Vein, Left			
B Basilic Vein, Right			
C Basilic Vein, Left			
D Cephalic Vein, Right			
F Cephalic Vein, Left			
Y Upper Vein			

Section	0	Medical and Surgical
Body System	5	Upper Veins
Operation	H	**Insertion:** Putting in a nonbiological appliance that monitors, assists, performs, or prevents a physiological function but does not physically take the place of a body part

Body Part (4ᵗʰ)	Approach (5ᵗʰ)	Device (6ᵗʰ)	Qualifier (7ᵗʰ)
0 Azygos Vein	**0** Open **3** Percutaneous **4** Percutaneous Endoscopic	**2** Monitoring Device **3** Infusion Device **D** Intraluminal Device **M** Neurostimulator Lead	**Z** No Qualifier
1 Hemiazygos Vein **5** Subclavian Vein, Right **6** Subclavian Vein, Left **7** Axillary Vein, Right **8** Axillary Vein, Left **9** Brachial Vein, Right **A** Brachial Vein, Left **B** Basilic Vein, Right **C** Basilic Vein, Left **D** Cephalic Vein, Right **F** Cephalic Vein, Left **G** Hand Vein, Right **H** Hand Vein, Left **L** Intracranial Vein **M** Internal Jugular Vein, Right **N** Internal Jugular Vein, Left **P** External Jugular Vein, Right **Q** External Jugular Vein, Left **R** Vertebral Vein, Right **S** Vertebral Vein, Left **T** Face Vein, Right **V** Face Vein, Left	**0** Open **3** Percutaneous **4** Percutaneous Endoscopic	**3** Infusion Device **D** Intraluminal Device	**Z** No Qualifier
3 Innominate Vein, Right **4** Innominate Vein, Left	**0** Open **3** Percutaneous **4** Percutaneous Endoscopic	**3** Infusion Device **D** Intraluminal Device **M** Neurostimulator Lead	**Z** No Qualifier
Y Upper Vein	**0** Open **3** Percutaneous **4** Percutaneous Endoscopic	**2** Monitoring Device **3** Infusion Device **D** Intraluminal Device **Y** Other Device	**Z** No Qualifier

Section	0	Medical and Surgical
Body System	5	Upper Veins
Operation	J	**Inspection:** Visually and/or manually exploring a body part

Body Part (4ᵗʰ)	Approach (5ᵗʰ)	Device (6ᵗʰ)	Qualifier (7ᵗʰ)
Y Upper Vein	**0** Open **3** Percutaneous **4** Percutaneous Endoscopic **X** External	**Z** No Device	**Z** No Qualifier

Section	0	Medical and Surgical
Body System	5	Upper Veins
Operation	L	Occlusion: Completely closing an orifice or the lumen of a tubular body part

Body Part (4th)	Approach (5th)	Device (6th)	Qualifier (7th)
0 Azygos Vein	0 Open	C Extraluminal Device	Z No Qualifier
1 Hemiazygos Vein	3 Percutaneous	D Intraluminal Device	
3 Innominate Vein, Right	4 Percutaneous Endoscopic	Z No Device	
4 Innominate Vein, Left			
5 Subclavian Vein, Right			
6 Subclavian Vein, Left			
7 Axillary Vein, Right			
8 Axillary Vein, Left			
9 Brachial Vein, Right			
A Brachial Vein, Left			
B Basilic Vein, Right			
C Basilic Vein, Left			
D Cephalic Vein, Right			
F Cephalic Vein, Left			
G Hand Vein, Right			
H Hand Vein, Left			
L Intracranial Vein			
M Internal Jugular Vein, Right			
N Internal Jugular Vein, Left			
P External Jugular Vein, Right			
Q External Jugular Vein, Left			
R Vertebral Vein, Right			
S Vertebral Vein, Left			
T Face Vein, Right			
V Face Vein, Left			
Y Upper Vein			

Section	0	Medical and Surgical
Body System	5	Upper Veins
Operation	N	Release: Freeing a body part from an abnormal physical constraint by cutting or by the use of force

Body Part (4th)	Approach (5th)	Device (6th)	Qualifier (7th)
0 Azygos Vein	0 Open	Z No Device	Z No Qualifier
1 Hemiazygos Vein	3 Percutaneous		
3 Innominate Vein, Right	4 Percutaneous Endoscopic		
4 Innominate Vein, Left			
5 Subclavian Vein, Right			
6 Subclavian Vein, Left			
7 Axillary Vein, Right			
8 Axillary Vein, Left			
9 Brachial Vein, Right			
A Brachial Vein, Left			
B Basilic Vein, Right			
C Basilic Vein, Left			
D Cephalic Vein, Right			
F Cephalic Vein, Left			
G Hand Vein, Right			
H Hand Vein, Left			
L Intracranial Vein			
M Internal Jugular Vein, Right			
N Internal Jugular Vein, Left			
P External Jugular Vein, Right			
Q External Jugular Vein, Left			
R Vertebral Vein, Right			
S Vertebral Vein, Left			
T Face Vein, Right			
V Face Vein, Left			
Y Upper Vein			

Section   0   **Medical and Surgical**
Body System   5   **Upper Veins**
Operation   P   **Removal:** Taking out or off a device from a body part

Body Part (4ᵗʰ)	Approach (5ᵗʰ)	Device (6ᵗʰ)	Qualifier (7ᵗʰ)
0 Azygos Vein	**0** Open **3** Percutaneous **4** Percutaneous Endoscopic **X** External	**2** Monitoring Device **M** Neurostimulator Lead	**Z** No Qualifier
3 Innominate Vein, Right **4** Innominate Vein, Left	**0** Open **3** Percutaneous **4** Percutaneous Endoscopic **X** External	**M** Neurostimulator Lead	**Z** No Qualifier
Y Upper Vein	**0** Open **3** Percutaneous **4** Percutaneous Endoscopic	**0** Drainage Device **2** Monitoring Device **3** Infusion Device **7** Autologous Tissue Substitute **C** Extraluminal Device **D** Intraluminal Device **J** Synthetic Substitute **K** Nonautologous Tissue Substitute **Y** Other Device	**Z** No Qualifier
Y Upper Vein	**X** External	**0** Drainage Device **2** Monitoring Device **3** Infusion Device **D** Intraluminal Device	**Z** No Qualifier

Section   0   **Medical and Surgical**
Body System   5   **Upper Veins**
Operation   Q   **Repair:** Restoring, to the extent possible, a body part to its normal anatomic structure and function

Body Part (4ᵗʰ)	Approach (5ᵗʰ)	Device (6ᵗʰ)	Qualifier (7ᵗʰ)
0 Azygos Vein **1** Hemiazygos Vein **3** Innominate Vein, Right **4** Innominate Vein, Left **5** Subclavian Vein, Right **6** Subclavian Vein, Left **7** Axillary Vein, Right **8** Axillary Vein, Left **9** Brachial Vein, Right **A** Brachial Vein, Left **B** Basilic Vein, Right **C** Basilic Vein, Left **D** Cephalic Vein, Right **F** Cephalic Vein, Left **G** Hand Vein, Right **H** Hand Vein, Left **L** Intracranial Vein **M** Internal Jugular Vein, Right **N** Internal Jugular Vein, Left **P** External Jugular Vein, Right **Q** External Jugular Vein, Left **R** Vertebral Vein, Right **S** Vertebral Vein, Left **T** Face Vein, Right **V** Face Vein, Left **Y** Upper Vein	**0** Open **3** Percutaneous **4** Percutaneous Endoscopic	**Z** No Device	**Z** No Qualifier

Section	0	Medical and Surgical
Body System	5	Upper Veins
Operation	R	**Replacement:** Putting in or on biological or synthetic material that physically takes the place and/or function of all or a portion of a body part

Body Part (4th)	Approach (5th)	Device (6th)	Qualifier (7th)
0 Azygos Vein 1 Hemiazygos Vein 3 Innominate Vein, Right 4 Innominate Vein, Left 5 Subclavian Vein, Right 6 Subclavian Vein, Left 7 Axillary Vein, Right 8 Axillary Vein, Left 9 Brachial Vein, Right A Brachial Vein, Left B Basilic Vein, Right C Basilic Vein, Left D Cephalic Vein, Right F Cephalic Vein, Left G Hand Vein, Right H Hand Vein, Left L Intracranial Vein M Internal Jugular Vein, Right N Internal Jugular Vein, Left P External Jugular Vein, Right Q External Jugular Vein, Left R Vertebral Vein, Right S Vertebral Vein, Left T Face Vein, Right V Face Vein, Left Y Upper Vein	0 Open 4 Percutaneous Endoscopic	7 Autologous Tissue Substitute J Synthetic Substitute K Nonautologous Tissue Substitute	Z No Qualifier

Section	0	Medical and Surgical
Body System	5	Upper Veins
Operation	S	**Reposition:** Moving to its normal location, or other suitable location, all or a portion of a body part

Body Part (4th)	Approach (5th)	Device (6th)	Qualifier (7th)
0 Azygos Vein 1 Hemiazygos Vein 3 Innominate Vein, Right 4 Innominate Vein, Left 5 Subclavian Vein, Right 6 Subclavian Vein, Left 7 Axillary Vein, Right 8 Axillary Vein, Left 9 Brachial Vein, Right A Brachial Vein, Left B Basilic Vein, Right C Basilic Vein, Left D Cephalic Vein, Right F Cephalic Vein, Left G Hand Vein, Right H Hand Vein, Left L Intracranial Vein M Internal Jugular Vein, Right N Internal Jugular Vein, Left P External Jugular Vein, Right Q External Jugular Vein, Left R Vertebral Vein, Right S Vertebral Vein, Left T Face Vein, Right V Face Vein, Left Y Upper Vein	0 Open 3 Percutaneous 4 Percutaneous Endoscopic	Z No Device	Z No Qualifier

Section	0	Medical and Surgical
Body System	5	Upper Veins
Operation	U	Supplement: Putting in or on biological or synthetic material that physically reinforces and/or augments the function of a portion of a body part

Body Part (4th)	Approach (5th)	Device (6th)	Qualifier (7th)
0 Azygos Vein	0 Open	7 Autologous Tissue Substitute	Z No Qualifier
1 Hemiazygos Vein	3 Percutaneous	J Synthetic Substitute	
3 Innominate Vein, Right	4 Percutaneous Endoscopic	K Nonautologous Tissue Substitute	
4 Innominate Vein, Left			
5 Subclavian Vein, Right			
6 Subclavian Vein, Left			
7 Axillary Vein, Right			
8 Axillary Vein, Left			
9 Brachial Vein, Right			
A Brachial Vein, Left			
B Basilic Vein, Right			
C Basilic Vein, Left			
D Cephalic Vein, Right			
F Cephalic Vein, Left			
G Hand Vein, Right			
H Hand Vein, Left			
L Intracranial Vein			
M Internal Jugular Vein, Right			
N Internal Jugular Vein, Left			
P External Jugular Vein, Right			
Q External Jugular Vein, Left			
R Vertebral Vein, Right			
S Vertebral Vein, Left			
T Face Vein, Right			
V Face Vein, Left			
Y Upper Vein			

Section	0	Medical and Surgical
Body System	5	Upper Veins
Operation	V	Restriction: Partially closing an orifice or the lumen of a tubular body part

Body Part (4th)	Approach (5th)	Device (6th)	Qualifier (7th)
0 Azygos Vein	0 Open	C Extraluminal Device	Z No Qualifier
1 Hemiazygos Vein	3 Percutaneous	D Intraluminal Device	
3 Innominate Vein, Right	4 Percutaneous Endoscopic	Z No Device	
4 Innominate Vein, Left			
5 Subclavian Vein, Right			
6 Subclavian Vein, Left			
7 Axillary Vein, Right			
8 Axillary Vein, Left			
9 Brachial Vein, Right			
A Brachial Vein, Left			
B Basilic Vein, Right			
C Basilic Vein, Left			
D Cephalic Vein, Right			
F Cephalic Vein, Left			
G Hand Vein, Right			
H Hand Vein, Left			
L Intracranial Vein			
M Internal Jugular Vein, Right			
N Internal Jugular Vein, Left			
P External Jugular Vein, Right			
Q External Jugular Vein, Left			
R Vertebral Vein, Right			
S Vertebral Vein, Left			
T Face Vein, Right			
V Face Vein, Left			
Y Upper Vein			

Section	0	Medical and Surgical
Body System	5	Upper Veins
Operation	W	Revision: Correcting, to the extent possible, a portion of a malfunctioning device or the position of a displaced device

Body Part (4th)	Approach (5th)	Device (6th)	Qualifier (7th)
0 Azygos Vein	**0** Open **3** Percutaneous **4** Percutaneous Endoscopic **X** External	**2** Monitoring Device **M** Neurostimulator Lead	**Z** No Qualifier
3 Innominate Vein, Right **4** Innominate Vein, Left	**0** Open **3** Percutaneous **4** Percutaneous Endoscopic **X** External	**M** Neurostimulator Lead	**Z** No Qualifier
Y Upper Vein	**0** Open **3** Percutaneous **4** Percutaneous Endoscopic	**0** Drainage Device **2** Monitoring Device **3** Infusion Device **7** Autologous Tissue Substitute **C** Extraluminal Device **D** Intraluminal Device **J** Synthetic Substitute **K** Nonautologous Tissue Substitute **Y** Other Device	**Z** No Qualifier
Y Upper Vein	**X** External	**0** Drainage Device **2** Monitoring Device **3** Infusion Device **7** Autologous Tissue Substitute **C** Extraluminal Device **D** Intraluminal Device **J** Synthetic Substitute **K** Nonautologus Tissue Substitute	**Z** No Qualifier

AHA Coding Clinic

051Q49Y Bypass Left External Jugular Vein to Upper Vein with Autologous Venous Tissue, Percutaneous Endoscopic Approach—AHA CC: 1Q, 2020, 28-29

059430Z Drainage of Left Innominate Vein with Drainage Device, Percutaneous Approach—AHA CC: 3Q, 2018, 7

05BL0ZZ Excision of Intracranial Vein, Open Approach—AHA CC: 1Q, 2020, 24

05BN0ZZ Excision of Left Internal Jugular Vein, Open Approach—AHA CC: 2Q, 2016, 12-14

05BQ0ZZ Excision of Left External Jugular Vein, Open Approach—AHA CC: 2Q, 2016, 12-14

05H032Z Insertion of Monitoring Device into Azygos Vein, Percutaneous Approach—AHA CC: 4Q, 2016, 98-99

05H43MZ Insertion of Neurostimulator Lead into Left Innominate Vein, Percutaneous Approach—AHA CC: 4Q, 2016, 98-99

05Q40ZZ Repair Left Innominate Vein, Open Approach—AHA CC: 3Q, 2017, 15-16

05SD0ZZ Reposition Right Cephalic Vein, Open Approach—AHA CC: 4Q, 2013, 125-126

Veins

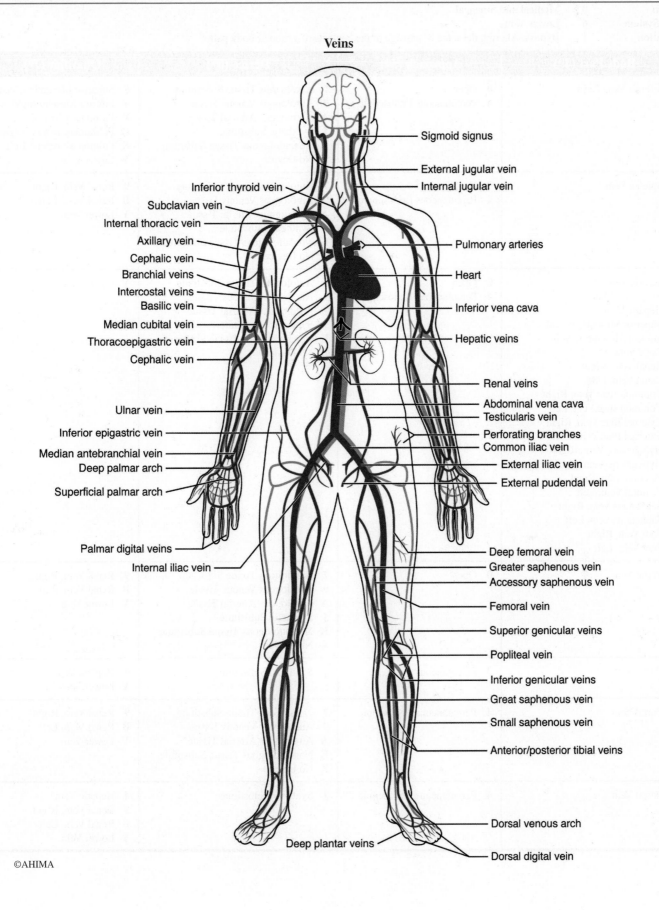

Sigmoid signus

External jugular vein

Internal jugular vein

Inferior thyroid vein

Subclavian vein

Internal thoracic vein

Axillary vein

Cephalic vein

Branchial veins

Intercostal veins

Basilic vein

Median cubital vein

Thoracoepigastric vein

Cephalic vein

Pulmonary arteries

Heart

Inferior vena cava

Hepatic veins

Renal veins

Abdominal vena cava

Testicularis vein

Perforating branches

Common iliac vein

External iliac vein

External pudendal vein

Ulnar vein

Inferior epigastric vein

Median antebranchial vein

Deep palmar arch

Superficial palmar arch

Palmar digital veins

Internal iliac vein

Deep femoral vein

Greater saphenous vein

Accessory saphenous vein

Femoral vein

Superior genicular veins

Popliteal vein

Inferior genicular veins

Great saphenous vein

Small saphenous vein

Anterior/posterior tibial veins

Dorsal venous arch

Deep plantar veins

Dorsal digital vein

©AHIMA

Medical and Surgical, Lower Veins

Lower Veins Tables 061–06W

Section	0	**Medical and Surgical**
Body System	6	**Lower Veins**
Operation	1	**Bypass:** Altering the route of passage of the contents of a tubular body part

Body Part (4ᵗʰ)	Approach (5ᵗʰ)	Device (6ᵗʰ)	Qualifier (7ᵗʰ)
0 Inferior Vena Cava	0 Open 4 Percutaneous Endoscopic	7 Autologous Tissue Substitute 9 Autologous Venous Tissue A Autologous Arterial Tissue J Synthetic Substitute K Nonautologous Tissue Substitute Z No Device	5 Superior Mesenteric Vein 6 Inferior Mesenteric Vein P Pulmonary Trunk Q Pulmonary Artery, Right R Pulmonary Artery, Left Y Lower Vein
1 Splenic Vein	0 Open 4 Percutaneous Endoscopic	7 Autologous Tissue Substitute 9 Autologous Venous Tissue A Autologous Arterial Tissue J Synthetic Substitute K Nonautologous Tissue Substitute Z No Device	9 Renal Vein, Right B Renal Vein, Left Y Lower Vein
2 Gastric Vein 3 Esophageal Vein 4 Hepatic Vein 5 Superior Mesenteric Vein 6 Inferior Mesenteric Vein 7 Colic Vein 9 Renal Vein, Right B Renal Vein, Left C Common Iliac Vein, Right D Common Iliac Vein, Left F External Iliac Vein, Right G External Iliac Vein, Left H Hypogastric Vein, Right J Hypogastric Vein, Left M Femoral Vein, Right N Femoral Vein, Left P Saphenous Vein, Right Q Saphenous Vein, Left T Foot Vein, Right V Foot Vein, Left	0 Open 4 Percutaneous Endoscopic	7 Autologous Tissue Substitute 9 Autologous Venous Tissue A Autologous Arterial Tissue J Synthetic Substitute K Nonautologous Tissue Substitute Z No Device	Y Lower Vein
8 Portal Vein	0 Open	7 Autologous Tissue Substitute 9 Autologous Venous Tissue A Autologous Arterial Tissue J Synthetic Substitute K Nonautologous Tissue Substitute Z No Device	9 Renal Vein, Right B Renal Vein, Left Y Lower Vein
8 Portal Vein	3 Percutaneous	J Synthetic Substitute	4 Hepatic Vein Y Lower Vein
8 Portal Vein	4 Percutaneous Endoscopic	7 Autologous Tissue Substitute 9 Autologous Venous Tissue A Autologous Arterial Tissue K Nonautologous Tissue Substitute Z No Device	9 Renal Vein, Right B Renal Vein, Left Y Lower Vein
8 Portal Vein	4 Percutaneous Endoscopic	J Synthetic Substitute	4 Hepatic Vein 9 Renal Vein, Right B Renal Vein, Left Y Lower Vein

Section	0	Medical and Surgical
Body System	6	Lower Veins
Operation	5	Destruction: Physical eradication of all or a portion of a body part by the direct use of energy, force, or a destructive agent

Body Part (4th)	Approach (5th)	Device (6th)	Qualifier (7th)
0 Inferior Vena Cava 1 Splenic Vein 2 Gastric Vein 3 Esophageal Vein 4 Hepatic Vein 5 Superior Mesenteric Vein 6 Inferior Mesenteric Vein 7 Colic Vein 8 Portal Vein 9 Renal Vein, Right B Renal Vein, Left C Common Iliac Vein, Right D Common Iliac Vein, Left F External Iliac Vein, Right G External Iliac Vein, Left H Hypogastric Vein, Right J Hypogastric Vein, Left M Femoral Vein, Right N Femoral Vein, Left P Saphenous Vein, Right Q Saphenous Vein, Left T Foot Vein, Right V Foot Vein, Left	0 Open 3 Percutaneous 4 Percutaneous Endoscopic	Z No Device	Z No Qualifier
Y Lower Vein	0 Open 3 Percutaneous 4 Percutaneous Endoscopic	Z No Device	C Hemorrhoidal Plexus Z No Qualifier

Section	0	Medical and Surgical
Body System	6	Lower Veins
Operation	7	Dilation: Expanding an orifice or the lumen of a tubular body part

Body Part (4th)	Approach (5th)	Device (6th)	Qualifier (7th)
0 Inferior Vena Cava 1 Splenic Vein 2 Gastric Vein 3 Esophageal Vein 4 Hepatic Vein 5 Superior Mesenteric Vein 6 Inferior Mesenteric Vein 7 Colic Vein 8 Portal Vein 9 Renal Vein, Right B Renal Vein, Left C Common Iliac Vein, Right D Common Iliac Vein, Left F External Iliac Vein, Right G External Iliac Vein, Left H Hypogastric Vein, Right J Hypogastric Vein, Left M Femoral Vein, Right N Femoral Vein, Left P Saphenous Vein, Right Q Saphenous Vein, Left T Foot Vein, Right V Foot Vein, Left Y Lower Vein	0 Open 3 Percutaneous 4 Percutaneous Endoscopic	D Intraluminal Device Z No Device	Z No Qualifier

Section	0	Medical and Surgical
Body System	6	Lower Veins
Operation	9	**Drainage:** Taking or letting out fluids and/or gases from a body part

Body Part (4th)	Approach (5th)	Device (6th)	Qualifier (7th)
0 Inferior Vena Cava	0 Open	0 Drainage Device	Z No Qualifier
1 Splenic Vein	3 Percutaneous		
2 Gastric Vein	4 Percutaneous Endoscopic		
3 Esophageal Vein			
4 Hepatic Vein			
5 Superior Mesenteric Vein			
6 Inferior Mesenteric Vein			
7 Colic Vein			
8 Portal Vein			
9 Renal Vein, Right			
B Renal Vein, Left			
C Common Iliac Vein, Right			
D Common Iliac Vein, Left			
F External Iliac Vein, Right			
G External Iliac Vein, Left			
H Hypogastric Vein, Right			
J Hypogastric Vein, Left			
M Femoral Vein, Right			
N Femoral Vein, Left			
P Saphenous Vein, Right			
Q Saphenous Vein, Left			
T Foot Vein, Right			
V Foot Vein, Left			
Y Lower Vein			
0 Inferior Vena Cava	0 Open	Z No Device	X Diagnostic
1 Splenic Vein	3 Percutaneous		Z No Qualifier
2 Gastric Vein	4 Percutaneous Endoscopic		
3 Esophageal Vein			
4 Hepatic Vein			
5 Superior Mesenteric Vein			
6 Inferior Mesenteric Vein			
7 Colic Vein			
8 Portal Vein			
9 Renal Vein, Right			
B Renal Vein, Left			
C Common Iliac Vein, Right			
D Common Iliac Vein, Left			
F External Iliac Vein, Right			
G External Iliac Vein, Left			
H Hypogastric Vein, Right			
J Hypogastric Vein, Left			
M Femoral Vein, Right			
N Femoral Vein, Left			
P Saphenous Vein, Right			
Q Saphenous Vein, Left			
T Foot Vein, Right			
V Foot Vein, Left			
Y Lower Vein			

Section   **0**   **Medical and Surgical**
Body System   **6**   **Lower Veins**
Operation   **B**   **Excision:** Cutting out or off, without replacement, a portion of a body part

Body Part (4ᵗʰ)	Approach (5ᵗʰ)	Device (6ᵗʰ)	Qualifier (7ᵗʰ)
0 Inferior Vena Cava	0 Open	Z No Device	X Diagnostic
1 Splenic Vein	3 Percutaneous		Z No Qualifier
2 Gastric Vein	4 Percutaneous Endoscopic		
3 Esophageal Vein			
4 Hepatic Vein			
5 Superior Mesenteric Vein			
6 Inferior Mesenteric Vein			
7 Colic Vein			
8 Portal Vein			
9 Renal Vein, Right			
B Renal Vein, Left			
C Common Iliac Vein, Right			
D Common Iliac Vein, Left			
F External Iliac Vein, Right			
G External Iliac Vein, Left			
H Hypogastric Vein, Right			
J Hypogastric Vein, Left			
M Femoral Vein, Right			
N Femoral Vein, Left			
P Saphenous Vein, Right			
Q Saphenous Vein, Left			
T Foot Vein, Right			
V Foot Vein, Left			
Y Lower Vein	0 Open	Z No Device	C Hemorrhoidal Plexus
	3 Percutaneous		X Diagnostic
	4 Percutaneous Endoscopic		Z No Qualifier

Section   **0**   **Medical and Surgical**
Body System   **6**   **Lower Veins**
Operation   **C**   **Extirpation:** Taking or cutting out solid matter from a body part

Body Part (4ᵗʰ)	Approach (5ᵗʰ)	Device (6ᵗʰ)	Qualifier (7ᵗʰ)
0 Inferior Vena Cava	0 Open	Z No Device	Z No Qualifier
1 Splenic Vein	3 Percutaneous		
2 Gastric Vein	4 Percutaneous Endoscopic		
3 Esophageal Vein			
4 Hepatic Vein			
5 Superior Mesenteric Vein			
6 Inferior Mesenteric Vein			
7 Colic Vein			
8 Portal Vein			
9 Renal Vein, Right			
B Renal Vein, Left			
C Common Iliac Vein, Right			
D Common Iliac Vein, Left			
F External Iliac Vein, Right			
G External Iliac Vein, Left			
H Hypogastric Vein, Right			
J Hypogastric Vein, Left			
M Femoral Vein, Right			
N Femoral Vein, Left			
P Saphenous Vein, Right			
Q Saphenous Vein, Left			
T Foot Vein, Right			
V Foot Vein, Left			
Y Lower Vein			

Section	0	Medical and Surgical
Body System	6	Lower Veins
Operation	D	**Extraction:** Pulling or stripping out or off all or a portion of a body part by the use of force

Body Part (4ᵗʰ)	Approach (5ᵗʰ)	Device (6ᵗʰ)	Qualifier (7ᵗʰ)
M Femoral Vein, Right N Femoral Vein, Left P Saphenous Vein, Right Q Saphenous Vein, Left T Foot Vein, Right V Foot Vein, Left Y Lower Vein	0 Open 3 Percutaneous 4 Percutaneous Endoscopic	Z No Device	Z No Qualifier

Section	0	Medical and Surgical
Body System	6	Lower Veins
Operation	F	**Fragmentation:** Breaking solid matter in a body part into pieces

Body Part (4ᵗʰ)	Approach (5ᵗʰ)	Device (6ᵗʰ)	Qualifier (7ᵗʰ)
C Common Iliac Vein, Right D Common Iliac Vein, Left F External Iliac Vein, Right G External Iliac Vein, Left H Hypogastric Vein, Right J Hypogastric Vein, Left M Femoral Vein, Right N Femoral Vein, Left P Saphenous Vein, Right Q Saphenous Vein, Left Y Lower Vein	3 Percutaneous	Z No Device	0 Ultrasonic Z No Qualifier

Section	0	Medical and Surgical
Body System	6	Lower Veins
Operation	H	**Insertion:** Putting in a nonbiological appliance that monitors, assists, performs, or prevents a physiological function but does not physically take the place of a body part

Body Part (4ᵗʰ)	Approach (5ᵗʰ)	Device (6ᵗʰ)	Qualifier (7ᵗʰ)
0 Inferior Vena Cava	0 Open 3 Percutaneous	3 Infusion Device	T Via Umbilical Vein Z No Qualifier
0 Inferior Vena Cava	0 Open 3 Percutaneous	D Intraluminal Device	Z No Qualifier
0 Inferior Vena Cava	4 Percutaneous Endoscopic	3 Infusion Device D Intraluminal Device	Z No Qualifier

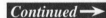

Continued →

Section 0 Medical and Surgical
Body System 6 Lower Veins
Operation H Insertion: Putting in a nonbiological appliance that monitors, assists, performs, or prevents a physiological function but does not physically take the place of a body part

Body Part (4th)	Approach (5th)	Device (6th)	Qualifier (7th)
1 Splenic Vein 2 Gastric Vein 3 Esophageal Vein 4 Hepatic Vein 5 Superior Mesenteric Vein 6 Inferior Mesenteric Vein 7 Colic Vein 8 Portal Vein 9 Renal Vein, Right B Renal Vein, Left C Common Iliac Vein, Right D Common Iliac Vein, Left F External Iliac Vein, Right G External Iliac Vein, Left H Hypogastric Vein, Right J Hypogastric Vein, Left M Femoral Vein, Right N Femoral Vein, Left P Saphenous Vein, Right Q Saphenous Vein, Left T Foot Vein, Right V Foot Vein, Left	0 Open 3 Percutaneous 4 Percutaneous Endoscopic	3 Infusion Device D Intraluminal Device	Z No Qualifier
Y Lower Vein	0 Open 3 Percutaneous 4 Percutaneous Endoscopic	2 Monitoring Device 3 Infusion Device D Intraluminal Device Y Other Device	Z No Qualifier

Section 0 Medical and Surgical
Body System 6 Lower Veins
Operation J Inspection: Visually and/or manually exploring a body part

Body Part (4th)	Approach (5th)	Device (6th)	Qualifier (7th)
Y Lower Vein	0 Open 3 Percutaneous 4 Percutaneous Endoscopic X External	Z No Device	Z No Qualifier

Section	0	Medical and Surgical
Body System	6	Lower Veins
Operation	L	Occlusion: Completely closing an orifice or the lumen of a tubular body part

Body Part (4th)	Approach (5th)	Device (6th)	Qualifier (7th)
0 Inferior Vena Cava 1 Splenic Vein 4 Hepatic Vein 5 Superior Mesenteric Vein 6 Inferior Mesenteric Vein 7 Colic Vein 8 Portal Vein 9 Renal Vein, Right B Renal Vein, Left C Common Iliac Vein, Right D Common Iliac Vein, Left F External Iliac Vein, Right G External Iliac Vein, Left H Hypogastric Vein, Right J Hypogastric Vein, Left M Femoral Vein, Right N Femoral Vein, Left P Saphenous Vein, Right Q Saphenous Vein, Left T Foot Vein, Right V Foot Vein, Left	0 Open 3 Percutaneous 4 Percutaneous Endoscopic	C Extraluminal Device D Intraluminal Device Z No Device	Z No Qualifier
2 Gastric Vein 3 Esophageal Vein	0 Open 3 Percutaneous 4 Percutaneous Endoscopic 7 Via Natural or Artificial Opening 8 Via Natural or Artificial Opening Endoscopic	C Extraluminal Device D Intraluminal Device Z No Device	Z No Qualifier
Y Lower Vein	0 Open 3 Percutaneous 4 Percutaneous Endoscopic	C Extraluminal Device D Intraluminal Device Z No Device	C Hemorrhoidal Plexus Z No Qualifier

Section	0	Medical and Surgical
Body System	6	Lower Veins
Operation	N	Release: Freeing a body part from an abnormal physical constraint by cutting or by the use of force

Body Part (4th)	Approach (5th)	Device (6th)	Qualifier (7th)
0 Inferior Vena Cava 1 Splenic Vein 2 Gastric Vein 3 Esophageal Vein 4 Hepatic Vein 5 Superior Mesenteric Vein 6 Inferior Mesenteric Vein 7 Colic Vein 8 Portal Vein 9 Renal Vein, Right B Renal Vein, Left C Common Iliac Vein, Right D Common Iliac Vein, Left F External Iliac Vein, Right G External Iliac Vein, Left H Hypogastric Vein, Right J Hypogastric Vein, Left M Femoral Vein, Right N Femoral Vein, Left P Saphenous Vein, Right Q Saphenous Vein, Left T Foot Vein, Right V Foot Vein, Left Y Lower Vein	0 Open 3 Percutaneous 4 Percutaneous Endoscopic	Z No Device	Z No Qualifier

Section	0	Medical and Surgical
Body System	6	Lower Veins
Operation	P	**Removal:** Taking out or off a device from a body part

Body Part (4th)	Approach (5th)	Device (6th)	Qualifier (7th)
Y Lower Vein	**0** Open **3** Percutaneous **4** Percutaneous Endoscopic	**0** Drainage Device **2** Monitoring Device **3** Infusion Device **7** Autologous Tissue Substitute **C** Extraluminal Device **D** Intraluminal Device **J** Synthetic Substitute **K** Nonautologous Tissue Substitute **Y** Other Device	**Z** No Qualifier
Y Lower Vein	**X** External	**0** Drainage Device **2** Monitoring Device **3** Infusion Device **D** Intraluminal Device	**Z** No Qualifier

Section	0	Medical and Surgical
Body System	6	Lower Veins
Operation	Q	**Repair:** Restoring, to the extent possible, a body part to its normal anatomic structure and function

Body Part (4th)	Approach (5th)	Device (6th)	Qualifier (7th)
0 Inferior Vena Cava **1** Splenic Vein **2** Gastric Vein **3** Esophageal Vein **4** Hepatic Vein **5** Superior Mesenteric Vein **6** Inferior Mesenteric Vein **7** Colic Vein **8** Portal Vein **9** Renal Vein, Right **B** Renal Vein, Left **C** Common Iliac Vein, Right **D** Common Iliac Vein, Left **F** External Iliac Vein, Right **G** External Iliac Vein, Left **H** Hypogastric Vein, Right **J** Hypogastric Vein, Left **M** Femoral Vein, Right **N** Femoral Vein, Left **P** Saphenous Vein, Right **Q** Saphenous Vein, Left **T** Foot Vein, Right **V** Foot Vein, Left **Y** Lower Vein	**0** Open **3** Percutaneous **4** Percutaneous Endoscopic	**Z** No Device	**Z** No Qualifier

Section	0	Medical and Surgical
Body System	6	Lower Veins
Operation	R	**Replacement:** Putting in or on biological or synthetic material that physically takes the place and/or function of all or a portion of a body part

Body Part (4th)	Approach (5th)	Device (6th)	Qualifier (7th)
0 Inferior Vena Cava	0 Open	7 Autologous Tissue Substitute	Z No Qualifier
1 Splenic Vein	4 Percutaneous Endoscopic	J Synthetic Substitute	
2 Gastric Vein		K Nonautologous Tissue Substitute	
3 Esophageal Vein			
4 Hepatic Vein			
5 Superior Mesenteric Vein			
6 Inferior Mesenteric Vein			
7 Colic Vein			
8 Portal Vein			
9 Renal Vein, Right			
B Renal Vein, Left			
C Common Iliac Vein, Right			
D Common Iliac Vein, Left			
F External Iliac Vein, Right			
G External Iliac Vein, Left			
H Hypogastric Vein, Right			
J Hypogastric Vein, Left			
M Femoral Vein, Right			
N Femoral Vein, Left			
P Saphenous Vein, Right			
Q Saphenous Vein, Left			
T Foot Vein, Right			
V Foot Vein, Left			
Y Lower Vein			

Section	0	Medical and Surgical
Body System	6	Lower Veins
Operation	S	**Reposition:** Moving to its normal location, or other suitable location, all or a portion of a body part

Body Part (4th)	Approach (5th)	Device (6th)	Qualifier (7th)
0 Inferior Vena Cava	0 Open	Z No Device	Z No Qualifier
1 Splenic Vein	3 Percutaneous		
2 Gastric Vein	4 Percutaneous Endoscopic		
3 Esophageal Vein			
4 Hepatic Vein			
5 Superior Mesenteric Vein			
6 Inferior Mesenteric Vein			
7 Colic Vein			
8 Portal Vein			
9 Renal Vein, Right			
B Renal Vein, Left			
C Common Iliac Vein, Right			
D Common Iliac Vein, Left			
F External Iliac Vein, Right			
G External Iliac Vein, Left			
H Hypogastric Vein, Right			
J Hypogastric Vein, Left			
M Femoral Vein, Right			
N Femoral Vein, Left			
P Saphenous Vein, Right			
Q Saphenous Vein, Left			
T Foot Vein, Right			
V Foot Vein, Left			
Y Lower Vein			

Section	0	Medical and Surgical
Body System	6	Lower Veins
Operation	U	**Supplement:** Putting in or on biological or synthetic material that physically reinforces and/or augments the function of a portion of a body part

Body Part (4th)	Approach (5th)	Device (6th)	Qualifier (7th)
0 Inferior Vena Cava 1 Splenic Vein 2 Gastric Vein 3 Esophageal Vein 4 Hepatic Vein 5 Superior Mesenteric Vein 6 Inferior Mesenteric Vein 7 Colic Vein 8 Portal Vein 9 Renal Vein, Right B Renal Vein, Left C Common Iliac Vein, Right D Common Iliac Vein, Left F External Iliac Vein, Right G External Iliac Vein, Left H Hypogastric Vein, Right J Hypogastric Vein, Left M Femoral Vein, Right N Femoral Vein, Left P Saphenous Vein, Right Q Saphenous Vein, Left T Foot Vein, Right V Foot Vein, Left Y Lower Vein	0 Open 3 Percutaneous 4 Percutaneous Endoscopic	7 Autologous Tissue Substitute J Synthetic Substitute K Nonautologous Tissue Substitute	Z No Qualifier

Section	0	Medical and Surgical
Body System	6	Lower Veins
Operation	V	**Restriction:** Partially closing an orifice or the lumen of a tubular body part

Body Part (4th)	Approach (5th)	Device (6th)	Qualifier (7th)
0 Inferior Vena Cava 1 Splenic Vein 2 Gastric Vein 3 Esophageal Vein 4 Hepatic Vein 5 Superior Mesenteric Vein 6 Inferior Mesenteric Vein 7 Colic Vein 8 Portal Vein 9 Renal Vein, Right B Renal Vein, Left C Common Iliac Vein, Right D Common Iliac Vein, Left F External Iliac Vein, Right G External Iliac Vein, Left H Hypogastric Vein, Right J Hypogastric Vein, Left M Femoral Vein, Right N Femoral Vein, Left P Saphenous Vein, Right Q Saphenous Vein, Left T Foot Vein, Right V Foot Vein, Left Y Lower Vein	0 Open 3 Percutaneous 4 Percutaneous Endoscopic	C Extraluminal Device D Intraluminal Device Z No Device	Z No Qualifier

Section	0	Medical and Surgical
Body System	6	Lower Veins
Operation	W	**Revision:** Correcting, to the extent possible, a portion of a malfunctioning device or the position of a displaced device

Body Part (4th)	Approach (5th)	Device (6th)	Qualifier (7th)
Y Lower Vein	**0** Open **3** Percutaneous **4** Percutaneous Endoscopic **X** External	**0** Drainage Device **2** Monitoring Device **3** Infusion Device **7** Autologous Tissue Substitute **C** Extraluminal Device **D** Intraluminal Device **J** Synthetic Substitute **K** Nonautologous Tissue Substitute **Y** Other Device	**Z** No Qualifier
Y Lower Vein	**X** External	**0** Drainage Device **2** Monitoring Device **3** Infusion Device **7** Autologous Tissue Substitute **C** Extraluminal Device **D** Intraluminal Device **J** Synthetic Substitute **K** Nonautologus Tissue Substitute	**Z** No Qualifier

AHA Coding Clinic

06100JP Bypass Inferior Vena Cava to Pulmonary Trunk with Synthetic Substitute, Open Approach—AHA CC: 4Q, 2017, 37-38

06BP0ZZ Excision of Right Saphenous Vein, Open Approach—AHA CC: 1Q, 2014, 10-11; 2Q, 2016, 18-19; 1Q, 2017, 31-32; 3Q. 2017, 5-6

06BP4ZZ Excision of Right Saphenous Vein, Percutaneous Endoscopic Approach—AHA CC: 3Q, 2014, 20-21

06BQ0ZZ Excision of Left Saphenous Vein, Open Approach—AHA CC: 1Q, 2017, 32-33; 1Q, 2020, 28-29

06BQ4ZZ Excision of Left Saphenous Vein, Percutaneous Endoscopic Approach—AHA CC: 3Q, 2014, 20-21; 1Q, 2016, 27-28

06H033T Insertion of Infusion Device, Via Umbilical Vein, into Inferior Vena Cava, Percutaneous Approach—AHA CC: 1Q, 2017, 31

06H033Z Insertion of Infusion Device into Inferior Vena Cava, Percutaneous Approach—AHA CC: 3Q, 2013, 18-19

06HY33Z Insertion of Infusion Device into Lower Vein, Percutaneous Approach—AHA CC: 1Q, 2017, 31

06L34CZ Occlusion of Esophageal Vein with Extraluminal Device, Percutaneous Endoscopic Approach—AHA CC: 4Q, 2013, 112-113

06L38CZ Occlusion of Esophageal Vein with Extraluminal Device, Via Natural or Artificial Opening Endoscopic—AHA CC: 4Q, 2017, 57-58

06LF0CZ Occlusion of Right External Iliac Vein with Extraluminal Device, Open Approach—AHA CC: 2Q, 2018, 18-19

06LG0CZ Occlusion of Left External Iliac Vein with Extraluminal Device, Open Approach—AHA CC: 2Q, 2018, 18-19

06V03DZ Restriction of Inferior Vena Cava with Intraluminal Device, Percutaneous Approach—AHA CC: 3Q, 2018, 11

06WY3DZ Revision of Intraluminal Device in Lower Vein, Percutaneous Approach—AHA CC: 3Q, 2014, 25-26

06WY3JZ Revision of Synthetic Substitute in Lower Vein, Percutaneous Approach—AHA CC: 1Q, 2018, 10; 2Q, 2019, 39

Lymph Vessels and Nodes of Head and Neck; Lymphatic Drainage of Mouth and Pharynx

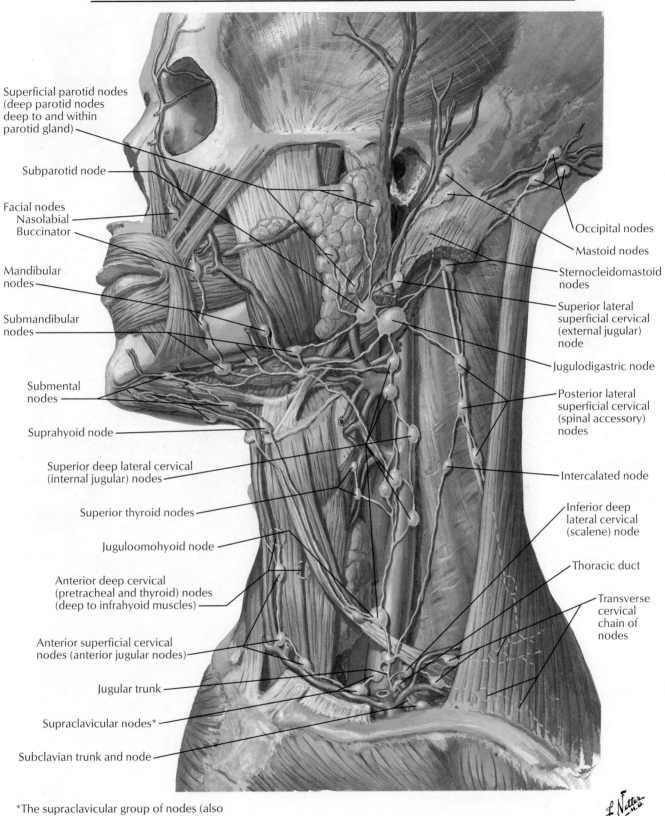

Superficial parotid nodes (deep parotid nodes deep to and within parotid gland)

Subparotid node

Facial nodes
Nasolabial
Buccinator

Mandibular nodes

Submandibular nodes

Submental nodes

Suprahyoid node

Superior deep lateral cervical (internal jugular) nodes

Superior thyroid nodes

Juguloomohyoid node

Anterior deep cervical (pretracheal and thyroid) nodes (deep to infrahyoid muscles)

Anterior superficial cervical nodes (anterior jugular nodes)

Jugular trunk

Supraclavicular nodes*

Subclavian trunk and node

Occipital nodes

Mastoid nodes

Sternocleidomastoid nodes

Superior lateral superficial cervical (external jugular) node

Jugulodigastric node

Posterior lateral superficial cervical (spinal accessory) nodes

Intercalated node

Inferior deep lateral cervical (scalene) node

Thoracic duct

Transverse cervical chain of nodes

*The supraclavicular group of nodes (also known as the lower deep cervical group), especially on the left, are also sometimes referred to as the signal or sentinel lymph nodes of Virchow or Troisier, especially when sufficiently enlarged and palpable. These nodes (or a single node) are so termed because they may be the first recognized presumptive evidence of malignant disease in the viscera.

Lymph Vessels and Nodes of Mammary Gland Lymphatic Drainage

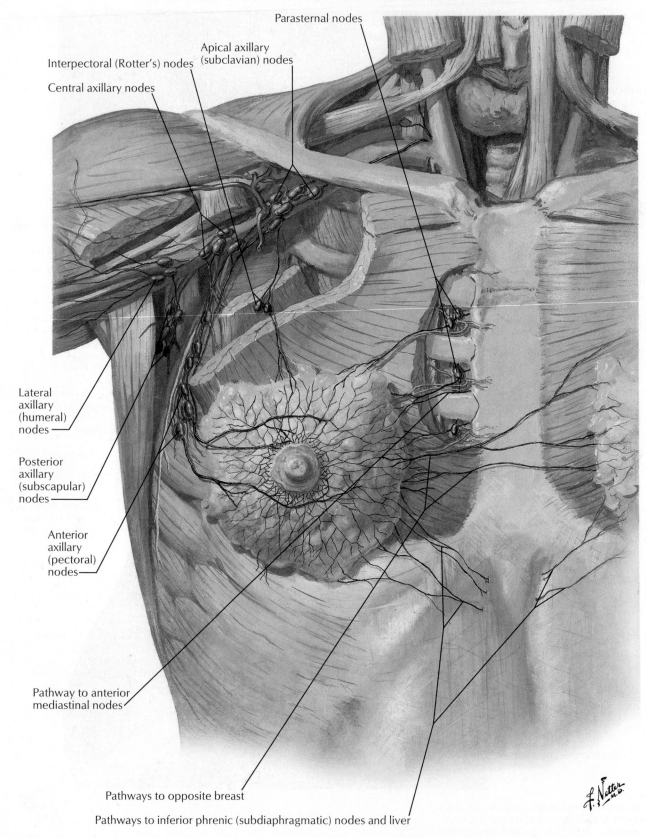

Parasternal nodes

Apical axillary (subclavian) nodes

Interpectoral (Rotter's) nodes

Central axillary nodes

Lateral axillary (humeral) nodes

Posterior axillary (subscapular) nodes

Anterior axillary (pectoral) nodes

Pathway to anterior mediastinal nodes

Pathways to opposite breast

Pathways to inferior phrenic (subdiaphragmatic) nodes and liver

Lymphatic and Hemic Systems Tables 072–07Y

Section	0	Medical and Surgical
Body System	7	Lymphatic and Hemic Systems
Operation	2	**Change:** Taking out or off a device from a body part and putting back an identical or similar device in or on the same body part without cutting or puncturing the skin or a mucous membrane

Body Part (4th)	Approach (5th)	Device (6th)	Qualifier (7th)
K Thoracic Duct L Cisterna Chyli M Thymus N Lymphatic P Spleen T Bone Marrow	X External	0 Drainage Device Y Other Device	Z No Qualifier

Section	0	Medical and Surgical
Body System	7	Lymphatic and Hemic Systems
Operation	5	**Destruction:** Physical eradication of all or a portion of a body part by the direct use of energy, force, or a destructive agent

Body Part (4th)	Approach (5th)	Device (6th)	Qualifier (7th)
0 Lymphatic, Head 1 Lymphatic, Right Neck 2 Lymphatic, Left Neck 3 Lymphatic, Right Upper Extremity 4 Lymphatic, Left Upper Extremity 5 Lymphatic, Right Axillary 6 Lymphatic, Left Axillary 7 Lymphatic, Thorax 8 Lymphatic, Internal Mammary, Right 9 Lymphatic, Internal Mammary, Left B Lymphatic, Mesenteric C Lymphatic, Pelvis D Lymphatic, Aortic F Lymphatic, Right Lower Extremity G Lymphatic, Left Lower Extremity H Lymphatic, Right Inguinal J Lymphatic, Left Inguinal K Thoracic Duct L Cisterna Chyli M Thymus P Spleen	0 Open 3 Percutaneous 4 Percutaneous Endoscopic	Z No Device	Z No Qualifier

Section	0	Medical and Surgical
Body System	7	Lymphatic and Hemic Systems
Operation	9	Drainage: Taking or letting out fluids and/or gases from a body part

Body Part (4th)	Approach (5th)	Device (6th)	Qualifier (7th)
0 Lymphatic, Head 1 Lymphatic, Right Neck 2 Lymphatic, Left Neck 3 Lymphatic, Right Upper Extremity 4 Lymphatic, Left Upper Extremity 5 Lymphatic, Right Axillary 6 Lymphatic, Left Axillary 7 Lymphatic, Thorax 8 Lymphatic, Internal Mammary, Right 9 Lymphatic, Internal Mammary, Left B Lymphatic, Mesenteric C Lymphatic, Pelvis D Lymphatic, Aortic F Lymphatic, Right Lower Extremity G Lymphatic, Left Lower Extremity H Lymphatic, Right Inguinal J Lymphatic, Left Inguinal K Thoracic Duct L Cisterna Chyli	0 Open 3 Percutaneous 4 Percutaneous Endoscopic 8 Via Natural or Artificial Opening Endoscopic	0 Drainage Device	Z No Qualifier
0 Lymphatic, Head 1 Lymphatic, Right Neck 2 Lymphatic, Left Neck 3 Lymphatic, Right Upper Extremity 4 Lymphatic, Left Upper Extremity 5 Lymphatic, Right Axillary 6 Lymphatic, Left Axillary 7 Lymphatic, Thorax 8 Lymphatic, Internal Mammary, Right 9 Lymphatic, Internal Mammary, Left B Lymphatic, Mesenteric C Lymphatic, Pelvis D Lymphatic, Aortic F Lymphatic, Right Lower Extremity G Lymphatic, Left Lower Extremity H Lymphatic, Right Inguinal J Lymphatic, Left Inguinal K Thoracic Duct L Cisterna Chyli	0 Open 3 Percutaneous 4 Percutaneous Endoscopic 8 Via Natural or Artificial Opening Endoscopic	Z No Device	X Diagnostic Z No Qualifier
M Thymus P Spleen T Bone Marrow	0 Open 3 Percutaneous 4 Percutaneous Endoscopic	0 Drainage Device	Z No Qualifier
M Thymus P Spleen T Bone Marrow	0 Open 3 Percutaneous 4 Percutaneous Endoscopic	Z No Device	X No Diagnostic Z No Qualifier

Section	0	Medical and Surgical
Body System	7	Lymphatic and Hemic Systems
Operation	B	**Excision:** Cutting out or off, without replacement, a portion of a body part

Body Part (4th)	Approach (5th)	Device (6th)	Qualifier (7th)
0 Lymphatic, Head	0 Open	Z No Device	X Diagnostic
1 Lymphatic, Right Neck	3 Percutaneous		Z No Qualifier
2 Lymphatic, Left Neck	4 Percutaneous Endoscopic		
3 Lymphatic, Right Upper Extremity			
4 Lymphatic, Left Upper Extremity			
5 Lymphatic, Right Axillary			
6 Lymphatic, Left Axillary			
7 Lymphatic, Thorax			
8 Lymphatic, Internal Mammary, Right			
9 Lymphatic, Internal Mammary, Left			
B Lymphatic, Mesenteric			
C Lymphatic, Pelvis			
D Lymphatic, Aortic			
F Lymphatic, Right Lower Extremity			
G Lymphatic, Left Lower Extremity			
H Lymphatic, Right Inguinal			
J Lymphatic, Left Inguinal			
K Thoracic Duct			
L Cisterna Chyli			
M Thymus			
P Spleen			

Section	0	Medical and Surgical
Body System	7	Lymphatic and Hemic Systems
Operation	C	**Extirpation:** Taking or cutting out solid matter from a body part

Body Part (4th)	Approach (5th)	Device (6th)	Qualifier (7th)
0 Lymphatic, Head	0 Open	Z No Device	Z No Qualifier
1 Lymphatic, Right Neck	3 Percutaneous		
2 Lymphatic, Left Neck	4 Percutaneous Endoscopic		
3 Lymphatic, Right Upper Extremity			
4 Lymphatic, Left Upper Extremity			
5 Lymphatic, Right Axillary			
6 Lymphatic, Left Axillary			
7 Lymphatic, Thorax			
8 Lymphatic, Internal Mammary, Right			
9 Lymphatic, Internal Mammary, Left			
B Lymphatic, Mesenteric			
C Lymphatic, Pelvis			
D Lymphatic, Aortic			
F Lymphatic, Right Lower Extremity			
G Lymphatic, Left Lower Extremity			
H Lymphatic, Right Inguinal			
J Lymphatic, Left Inguinal			
K Thoracic Duct			
L Cisterna Chyli			
M Thymus			
P Spleen			

Section	0	Medical and Surgical
Body System	7	Lymphatic and Hemic Systems
Operation	D	**Extraction:** Pulling or stripping out or off all or a portion of a body part by the use of force

Body Part (4ᵗʰ)	Approach (5ᵗʰ)	Device (6ᵗʰ)	Qualifier (7ᵗʰ)
0 Lymphatic, Head 1 Lymphatic, Right Neck 2 Lymphatic, Left Neck 3 Lymphatic, Right Upper Extremity 4 Lymphatic, Left Upper Extremity 5 Lymphatic, Right Axillary 6 Lymphatic, Left Axillary 7 Lymphatic, Thorax 8 Lymphatic, Internal Mammary, Right 9 Lymphatic, Internal Mammary, Left B Lymphatic, Mesenteric C Lymphatic, Pelvis D Lymphatic, Aortic F Lymphatic, Right Lower Extremity G Lymphatic, Left Lower Extremity H Lymphatic, Right Inguinal J Lymphatic, Left Inguinal K Thoracic Duct L Cisterna Chyli	3 Percutaneous 4 Percutaneous Endoscopic 8 Via Natural or Artificial Opening Endoscopic	Z No Device	X Diagnostic
M Thymus P Spleen	3 Percutaneous 4 Percutaneous Endoscopic	Z No Device	X No Diagnostic
Q Bone Marrow, Sternum R Bone Marrow, Iliac S Bone Marrow, Vertebral	0 Open 3 Percutaneous	Z No Device	X Diagnostic Z No Qualifier

Section	0	Medical and Surgical
Body System	7	Lymphatic and Hemic Systems
Operation	H	**Insertion:** Putting in a nonbiological appliance that monitors, assists, performs, or prevents a physiological function but does not physically take the place of a body part

Body Part (4ᵗʰ)	Approach (5ᵗʰ)	Device (6ᵗʰ)	Qualifier (7ᵗʰ)
K Thoracic Duct L Cisterna Chyli M Thymus N Lymphatic P Spleen T Bone Marrow	0 Open 3 Percutaneous 4 Percutaneous Endoscopic	1 Radioactive Element 3 Infusion Device Y Other Device	Z No Qualifier

Section	0	Medical and Surgical
Body System	7	Lymphatic and Hemic Systems
Operation	J	**Inspection:** Visually and/or manually exploring a body part

Body Part (4ᵗʰ)	Approach (5ᵗʰ)	Device (6ᵗʰ)	Qualifier (7ᵗʰ)
K Thoracic Duct L Cisterna Chyli M Thymus T Bone Marrow	0 Open 3 Percutaneous 4 Percutaneous Endoscopic	Z No Device	Z No Qualifier
N Lymphatic	0 Open 3 Percutaneous 4 Percutaneous Endoscopic 8 Via Natural or Artificial Opening Endoscopic X External	Z No Device	Z No Qualifier
P Spleen	0 Open 3 Percutaneous 4 Percutaneous Endoscopic X External	Z No Device	Z No Qualifier

Section	0	Medical and Surgical
Body System	7	Lymphatic and Hemic Systems
Operation	L	**Occlusion:** Completely closing an orifice or the lumen of a tubular body part

Body Part (4th)	Approach (5th)	Device (6th)	Qualifier (7th)
0 Lymphatic, Head	**0** Open	**C** Extraluminal Device	**Z** No Qualifier
1 Lymphatic, Right Neck	**3** Percutaneous	**D** Intraluminal Device	
2 Lymphatic, Left Neck	**4** Percutaneous Endoscopic	**Z** No Device	
3 Lymphatic, Right Upper Extremity			
4 Lymphatic, Left Upper Extremity			
5 Lymphatic, Right Axillary			
6 Lymphatic, Left Axillary			
7 Lymphatic, Thorax			
8 Lymphatic, Internal Mammary, Right			
9 Lymphatic, Internal Mammary, Left			
B Lymphatic, Mesenteric			
C Lymphatic, Pelvis			
D Lymphatic, Aortic			
F Lymphatic, Right Lower Extremity			
G Lymphatic, Left Lower Extremity			
H Lymphatic, Right Inguinal			
J Lymphatic, Left Inguinal			
K Thoracic Duct			
L Cisterna Chyli			

Section	0	Medical and Surgical
Body System	7	Lymphatic and Hemic Systems
Operation	N	**Release:** Freeing a body part from an abnormal physical constraint by cutting or by the use of force

Body Part (4th)	Approach (5th)	Device (6th)	Qualifier (7th)
0 Lymphatic, Head	**0** Open	**Z** No Device	**Z** No Qualifier
1 Lymphatic, Right Neck	**3** Percutaneous		
2 Lymphatic, Left Neck	**4** Percutaneous Endoscopic		
3 Lymphatic, Right Upper Extremity			
4 Lymphatic, Left Upper Extremity			
5 Lymphatic, Right Axillary			
6 Lymphatic, Left Axillary			
7 Lymphatic, Thorax			
8 Lymphatic, Internal Mammary, Right			
9 Lymphatic, Internal Mammary, Left			
B Lymphatic, Mesenteric			
C Lymphatic, Pelvis			
D Lymphatic, Aortic			
F Lymphatic, Right Lower Extremity			
G Lymphatic, Left Lower Extremity			
H Lymphatic, Right Inguinal			
J Lymphatic, Left Inguinal			
K Thoracic Duct			
L Cisterna Chyli			
M Thymus			
P Spleen			

Section	0	Medical and Surgical
Body System	7	Lymphatic and Hemic Systems
Operation	P	Removal: Taking out or off a device from a body part

Body Part (4th)	Approach (5th)	Device (6th)	Qualifier (7th)
K Thoracic Duct L Cisterna Chyli N Lymphatic	0 Open 3 Percutaneous 4 Percutaneous Endoscopic	0 Drainage Device 3 Infusion Device 7 Autologous Tissue Substitute C Extraluminal Device D Intraluminal Device J Synthetic Substitute K Nonautologous Tissue Substitute Y Other Device	Z No Qualifier
K Thoracic Duct L Cisterna Chyli N Lymphatic	X External	0 Drainage Device 3 Infusion Device D Intraluminal Device	Z No Qualifier
M Thymus P Spleen	0 Open 3 Percutaneous 4 Percutaneous Endoscopic	0 Drainage Device 3 Infusion Device Y Other Device	Z No Qualifier
M Thymus P Spleen	X External	0 Drainage Device 3 Infusion Device	Z No Qualifier
T Bone Marrow	0 Open 3 Percutaneous 4 Percutaneous Endoscopic X External	0 Drainage Device	Z No Qualifier

Section	0	Medical and Surgical
Body System	7	Lymphatic and Hemic Systems
Operation	Q	Repair: Restoring, to the extent possible, a body part to its normal anatomic structure and function

Body Part (4th)	Approach (5th)	Device (6th)	Qualifier (7th)
0 Lymphatic, Head 1 Lymphatic, Right Neck 2 Lymphatic, Left Neck 3 Lymphatic, Right Upper Extremity 4 Lymphatic, Left Upper Extremity 5 Lymphatic, Right Axillary 6 Lymphatic, Left Axillary 7 Lymphatic, Thorax 8 Lymphatic, Internal Mammary, Right 9 Lymphatic, Internal Mammary, Left B Lymphatic, Mesenteric C Lymphatic, Pelvis D Lymphatic, Aortic F Lymphatic, Right Lower Extremity G Lymphatic, Left Lower Extremity H Lymphatic, Right Inguinal J Lymphatic, Left Inguinal K Thoracic Duct L Cisterna Chyli	0 Open 3 Percutaneous 4 Percutaneous Endoscopic 8 Via Natural or Artificial Opening Endoscopic	Z No Device	Z No Qualifier
M Thymus P Spleen	0 Open 3 Percutaneous 4 Percutaneous Endoscopic	Z No Device	Z No Qualifier

Section	0	Medical and Surgical
Body System	7	Lymphatic and Hemic Systems
Operation	S	**Reposition:** Moving to its normal location, or other suitable location, all or a portion of a body part

Body Part (4th)	Approach (5th)	Device (6th)	Qualifier (7th)
M Thymus P Spleen	0 Open	Z No Device	Z No Qualifier

Section	0	Medical and Surgical
Body System	7	Lymphatic and Hemic Systems
Operation	T	**Resection:** Cutting out or off, without replacement, all of a body part

Body Part (4th)	Approach (5th)	Device (6th)	Qualifier (7th)
0 Lymphatic, Head 1 Lymphatic, Right Neck 2 Lymphatic, Left Neck 3 Lymphatic, Right Upper Extremity 4 Lymphatic, Left Upper Extremity 5 Lymphatic, Right Axillary 6 Lymphatic, Left Axillary 7 Lymphatic, Thorax 8 Lymphatic, Internal Mammary, Right 9 Lymphatic, Internal Mammary, Left B Lymphatic, Mesenteric C Lymphatic, Pelvis D Lymphatic, Aortic F Lymphatic, Right Lower Extremity G Lymphatic, Left Lower Extremity H Lymphatic, Right Inguinal J Lymphatic, Left Inguinal K Thoracic Duct L Cisterna Chyli M Thymus P Spleen	0 Open 4 Percutaneous Endoscopic	Z No Device	Z No Qualifier

Section	0	Medical and Surgical
Body System	7	Lymphatic and Hemic Systems
Operation	U	**Supplement:** Putting in or on biological or synthetic material that physically reinforces and/or augments the function of a portion of a body part

Body Part (4th)	Approach (5th)	Device (6th)	Qualifier (7th)
0 Lymphatic, Head 1 Lymphatic, Right Neck 2 Lymphatic, Left Neck 3 Lymphatic, Right Upper Extremity 4 Lymphatic, Left Upper Extremity 5 Lymphatic, Right Axillary 6 Lymphatic, Left Axillary 7 Lymphatic, Thorax 8 Lymphatic, Internal Mammary, Right 9 Lymphatic, Internal Mammary, Left B Lymphatic, Mesenteric C Lymphatic, Pelvis D Lymphatic, Aortic F Lymphatic, Right Lower Extremity G Lymphatic, Left Lower Extremity H Lymphatic, Right Inguinal J Lymphatic, Left Inguinal K Thoracic Duct L Cisterna Chyli	0 Open 4 Percutaneous Endoscopic	7 Autologous Tissue Substitute J Synthetic Substitute K Nonautologous Tissue Substitute	Z No Qualifier

Section	0	Medical and Surgical
Body System	7	Lymphatic and Hemic Systems
Operation	V	Restriction: Partially closing an orifice or the lumen of a tubular body part

Body Part (4th)	Approach (5th)	Device (6th)	Qualifier (7th)
0 Lymphatic, Head 1 Lymphatic, Right Neck 2 Lymphatic, Left Neck 3 Lymphatic, Right Upper Extremity 4 Lymphatic, Left Upper Extremity 5 Lymphatic, Right Axillary 6 Lymphatic, Left Axillary 7 Lymphatic, Thorax 8 Lymphatic, Internal Mammary, Right 9 Lymphatic, Internal Mammary, Left B Lymphatic, Mesenteric C Lymphatic, Pelvis D Lymphatic, Aortic F Lymphatic, Right Lower Extremity G Lymphatic, Left Lower Extremity H Lymphatic, Right Inguinal J Lymphatic, Left Inguinal K Thoracic Duct L Cisterna Chyli	0 Open 3 Percutaneous 4 Percutaneous Endoscopic	C Extraluminal Device D Intraluminal Device Z No Device	Z No Qualifier

Section	0	Medical and Surgical
Body System	7	Lymphatic and Hemic Systems
Operation	W	Revision: Correcting, to the extent possible, a portion of a malfunctioning device or the position of a displaced device

Body Part (4th)	Approach (5th)	Device (6th)	Qualifier (7th)
K Thoracic Duct L Cisterna Chyli N Lymphatic	0 Open 3 Percutaneous 4 Percutaneous Endoscopic	0 Drainage Device 3 Infusion Device 7 Autologous Tissue Substitute C Extraluminal Device D Intraluminal Device J Synthetic Substitute K Nonautologous Tissue Substitute Y Other Device	Z No Qualifier
K Thoracic Duct L Cisterna Chyli N Lymphatic	X External	0 Drainage Device 3 Infusion Device 7 Autologous Tissue Substitute C Extraluminal Device D Intraluminal Device J Synthetic Substitute K Nonautologous Tissue Substitute	Z No Qualifier
M Thymus P Spleen	0 Open 3 Percutaneous 4 Percutaneous Endoscopic	0 Drainage Device 3 Infusion Device Y Other Device	Z No Qualifier
M Thymus P Spleen	X External	0 Drainage Device 3 Infusion Device	Z No Qualifier
T Bone Marrow	0 Open 3 Percutaneous 4 Percutaneous Endoscopic X External	0 Drainage Device	Z No Qualifier

Section	0	Medical and Surgical
Body System	7	Lymphatic and Hemic Systems
Operation	Y	**Transplantation:** Putting in or on all or a portion of a living body part taken from another individual or animal to physically take the place and/or function of all or a portion of a similar body part

Body Part (4ᵗʰ)	Approach (5ᵗʰ)	Device (6ᵗʰ)	Qualifier (7ᵗʰ)
M Thymus **P** Spleen	**0** Open	**Z** No Device	**0** Allogeneic **1** Syngeneic **2** Zooplastic

AHA Coding Clinic

07B74ZX Excision of Thorax Lymphatic, Percutaneous Endoscopic Approach, Diagnostic—AHA CC: 1Q, 2014, 20-21, 26; 3Q, 2014, 10-11

07BB0ZZ Excision of Mesenteric Lymphatic, Open Approach—AHA CC: 1Q, 2019, 6-7

07BD0ZZ Excision of Aortic Lymphatic, Open Approach—AHA CC: 1Q, 2019, 6-7

07Q60ZZ Repair Left Axillary Lymphatic, Open Approach—AHA CC: 1Q, 2017, 34

07T10ZZ Resection of Right Neck Lymphatic, Open Approach—AHA CC: 3Q, 2014, 9-10

07T20ZZ Resection of Left Neck Lymphatic, Open Approach—AHA CC: 3Q, 2014, 9-10; 2Q, 2016, 12-14

07T50ZZ Resection of Right Axillary Lymphatic, Open Approach—AHA CC: 1Q, 2016, 30

07TM0ZZ Resection of Thymus, Open Approach—AHA CC: 3Q, 2014, 16-17

07TP0ZZ Resection of Spleen, Open Approach—AHA CC: 4Q, 2015, 13

07YM0Z0 Transplantation of Thymus, Allogeneic, Open Approach—AHA CC: 3Q, 2019, 29

Anatomy of the Eyeball

Horizontal section

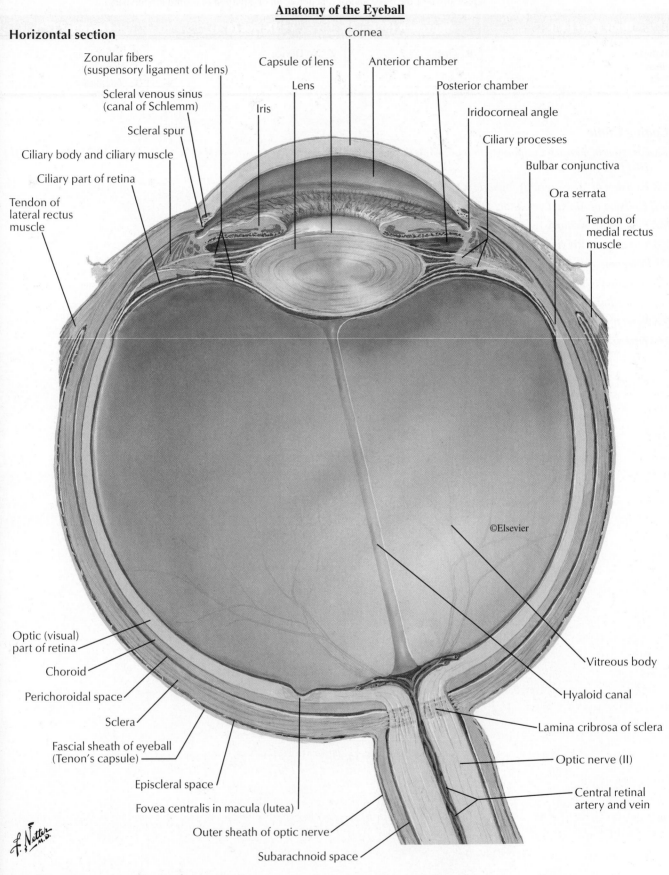

Zonular fibers (suspensory ligament of lens)

Scleral venous sinus (canal of Schlemm)

Scleral spur

Ciliary body and ciliary muscle

Ciliary part of retina

Tendon of lateral rectus muscle

Capsule of lens

Lens

Iris

Cornea

Anterior chamber

Posterior chamber

Iridocorneal angle

Ciliary processes

Bulbar conjunctiva

Ora serrata

Tendon of medial rectus muscle

©Elsevier

Optic (visual) part of retina

Choroid

Perichoroidal space

Sclera

Fascial sheath of eyeball (Tenon's capsule)

Episcleral space

Fovea centralis in macula (lutea)

Outer sheath of optic nerve

Subarachnoid space

Vitreous body

Hyaloid canal

Lamina cribrosa of sclera

Optic nerve (II)

Central retinal artery and vein

Eyelid

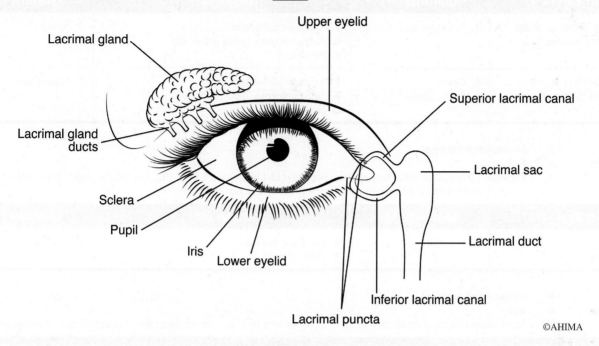

Upper eyelid

Lacrimal gland

Superior lacrimal canal

Lacrimal gland ducts

Lacrimal sac

Sclera

Pupil

Iris

Lower eyelid

Lacrimal duct

Inferior lacrimal canal

Lacrimal puncta

©AHIMA

Eye Muscles

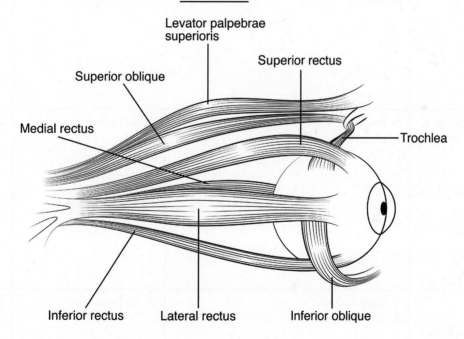

Levator palpebrae superioris

Superior rectus

Superior oblique

Medial rectus

Trochlea

Inferior rectus

Lateral rectus

Inferior oblique

Eye Tables 080–08X

Section	0	Medical and Surgical
Body System	8	Eye
Operation	0	**Alteration:** Modifying the anatomic structure of a body part without affecting the function of the body part

Body Part (4th)	Approach (5th)	Device (6th)	Qualifier (7th)
N Upper Eyelid, Right P Upper Eyelid, Left Q Lower Eyelid, Right R Lower Eyelid, Left	0 Open 3 Percutaneous X External	7 Autologous Tissue Substitute J Synthetic Substitute K Nonautologous Tissue Substitute Z No Device	Z No Qualifier

Section	0	Medical and Surgical
Body System	8	Eye
Operation	1	**Bypass:** Altering the route of passage of the contents of a tubular body part

Body Part (4ᵗʰ)	Approach (5ᵗʰ)	Device (6ᵗʰ)	Qualifier (7ᵗʰ)
2 Anterior Chamber, Right 3 Anterior Chamber, Left	3 Percutaneous	J Synthetic Substitute K Nonautologous Tissue Substitute Z No Device	4 Sclera
X Lacrimal Duct, Right Y Lacrimal Duct, Left	0 Open 3 Percutaneous	J Synthetic Substitute K Nonautologous Tissue Substitute Z No Device	3 Nasal Cavity

Section	0	Medical and Surgical
Body System	8	Eye
Operation	2	**Change:** Taking out or off a device from a body part and putting back an identical or similar device in or on the same body part without cutting or puncturing the skin or a mucous membrane

Body Part (4ᵗʰ)	Approach (5ᵗʰ)	Device (6ᵗʰ)	Qualifier (7ᵗʰ)
0 Eye, Right 1 Eye, Left	X External	0 Drainage Device Y Other Device	Z No Qualifier

Section	0	Medical and Surgical
Body System	8	Eye
Operation	5	**Destruction:** Physical eradication of all or a portion of a body part by the direct use of energy, force, or a destructive agent

Body Part (4ᵗʰ)	Approach (5ᵗʰ)	Device (6ᵗʰ)	Qualifier (7ᵗʰ)
0 Eye, Right 1 Eye, Left 6 Sclera, Right 7 Sclera, Left 8 Cornea, Right 9 Cornea, Left S Conjunctiva, Right T Conjunctiva, Left	X External	Z No Device	Z No Qualifier
2 Anterior Chamber, Right 3 Anterior Chamber, Left 4 Vitreous, Right 5 Vitreous, Left C Iris, Right D Iris, Left E Retina, Right F Retina, Left G Retinal Vessel, Right H Retinal Vessel, Left J Lens, Right K Lens, Left	3 Percutaneous	Z No Device	Z No Qualifier
A Choroid, Right B Choroid, Left L Extraocular Muscle, Right M Extraocular Muscle, Left V Lacrimal Gland, Right W Lacrimal Gland, Left	0 Open 3 Percutaneous	Z No Device	Z No Qualifier
N Upper Eyelid, Right P Upper Eyelid, Left Q Lower Eyelid, Right R Lower Eyelid, Left	0 Open 3 Percutaneous X External	Z No Device	Z No Qualifier
X Lacrimal Duct, Right Y Lacrimal Duct, Left	0 Open 3 Percutaneous 7 Via Natural or Artificial Opening 8 Via Natural or Artificial Opening Endoscopic	Z No Device	Z No Qualifier

Section 0 **Medical and Surgical**
Body System 8 **Eye**
Operation 7 **Dilation:** Expanding an orifice or the lumen of a tubular body part

Body Part (4th)	Approach (5th)	Device (6th)	Qualifier (7th)
X Lacrimal Duct, Right **Y** Lacrimal Duct, Left	**0** Open **3** Percutaneous **7** Via Natural or Artificial Opening **8** Via Natural or Artificial Opening Endoscopic	**D** Intraluminal Device **Z** No Device	**Z** No Qualifier

Section 0 **Medical and Surgical**
Body System 8 **Eye**
Operation 9 **Drainage:** Taking or letting out fluids and/or gases from a body part

Body Part (4th)	Approach (5th)	Device (6th)	Qualifier (7th)
0 Eye, Right **1** Eye, Left **6** Sclera, Right **7** Sclera, Left **8** Cornea, Right **9** Cornea, Left **S** Conjunctiva, Right **T** Conjunctiva, Left	**X** External	**0** Drainage Device	**Z** No Qualifier
0 Eye, Right **1** Eye, Left **6** Sclera, Right **7** Sclera, Left **8** Cornea, Right **9** Cornea, Left **S** Conjunctiva, Right **T** Conjunctiva, Left	**X** External	**Z** No Device	**X** Diagnostic **Z** No Qualifier
2 Anterior Chamber, Right **3** Anterior Chamber, Left **4** Vitreous, Right **5** Vitreous, Left **C** Iris, Right **D** Iris, Left **E** Retina, Right **F** Retina, Left **G** Retinal Vessel, Right **H** Retinal Vessel, Left **J** Lens, Right **K** Lens, Left	**3** Percutaneous	**0** Drainage Device	**Z** No Qualifier
2 Anterior Chamber, Right **3** Anterior Chamber, Left **4** Vitreous, Right **5** Vitreous, Left **C** Iris, Right **D** Iris, Left **E** Retina, Right **F** Retina, Left **G** Retinal Vessel, Right **H** Retinal Vessel, Left **J** Lens, Right **K** Lens, Left	**3** Percutaneous	**Z** No Device	**X** Diagnostic **Z** No Qualifier
A Choroid, Right **B** Choroid, Left **L** Extraocular Muscle, Right **M** Extraocular Muscle, Left **V** Lacrimal Gland, Right **W** Lacrimal Gland, Left	**0** Open **3** Percutaneous	**0** Drainage Device	**Z** No Qualifier

Continued →

Section 0 **Medical and Surgical**
Body System 8 **Eye**
Operation 9 **Drainage:** Taking or letting out fluids and/or gases from a body part

Body Part (4ᵗʰ)	Approach (5ᵗʰ)	Device (6ᵗʰ)	Qualifier (7ᵗʰ)
A Choroid, Right B Choroid, Left L Extraocular Muscle, Right M Extraocular Muscle, Left V Lacrimal Gland, Right W Lacrimal Gland, Left	0 Open 3 Percutaneous	Z No Device	X Diagnostic Z No Qualifier
N Upper Eyelid, Right P Upper Eyelid, Left Q Lower Eyelid, Right R Lower Eyelid, Left	0 Open 3 Percutaneous X External	0 Drainage Device	Z No Qualifier
N Upper Eyelid, Right P Upper Eyelid, Left Q Lower Eyelid, Right R Lower Eyelid, Left	0 Open 3 Percutaneous X External	Z No Device	X Diagnostic Z No Qualifier
X Lacrimal Duct, Right Y Lacrimal Duct, Left	0 Open 3 Percutaneous 7 Via Natural or Artificial Opening 8 Via Natural or Artificial Opening Endoscopic	0 Drainage Device	Z No Qualifier
X Lacrimal Duct, Right Y Lacrimal Duct, Left	0 Open 3 Percutaneous 7 Via Natural or Artificial Opening 8 Via Natural or Artificial Opening Endoscopic	Z No Device	X Diagnostic Z No Qualifier

Section 0 **Medical and Surgical**
Body System 8 **Eye**
Operation B **Excision:** Cutting out or off, without replacement, a portion of a body part

Body Part (4ᵗʰ)	Approach (5ᵗʰ)	Device (6ᵗʰ)	Qualifier (7ᵗʰ)
0 Eye, Right 1 Eye, Left N Upper Eyelid, Right P Upper Eyelid, Left Q Lower Eyelid, Right R Lower Eyelid, Left	0 Open 3 Percutaneous X External	Z No Device	X Diagnostic Z No Qualifier
4 Vitreous, Right 5 Vitreous, Left C Iris, Right D Iris, Left E Retina, Right F Retina, Left J Lens, Right K Lens, Left	3 Percutaneous	Z No Device	X Diagnostic Z No Qualifier
6 Sclera, Right 7 Sclera, Left 8 Cornea, Right 9 Cornea, Left S Conjunctiva, Right T Conjunctiva, Left	X External	Z No Device	X Diagnostic Z No Qualifier

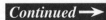
Continued →

Medical and Surgical, Eye Tables

Section 0 Medical and Surgical

Body System 8 Eye

Operation B **Excision:** Cutting out or off, without replacement, a portion of a body part

Body Part (4th)	Approach (5th)	Device (6th)	Qualifier (7th)
A Choroid, Right B Choroid, Left L Extraocular Muscle, Right M Extraocular Muscle, Left V Lacrimal Gland, Right W Lacrimal Gland, Left	0 Open 3 Percutaneous	Z No Device	X Diagnostic Z No Qualifier
X Lacrimal Duct, Right Y Lacrimal Duct, Left	0 Open 3 Percutaneous 7 Via Natural or Artificial Opening 8 Via Natural or Artificial Opening Endoscopic	Z No Device	X Diagnostic Z No Qualifier

Section 0 Medical and Surgical

Body System 8 Eye

Operation C **Extirpation:** Taking or cutting out solid matter from a body part

Body Part (4th)	Approach (5th)	Device (6th)	Qualifier (7th)
0 Eye, Right 1 Eye, Left 6 Sclera, Right 7 Sclera, Left 8 Cornea, Right 9 Cornea, Left S Conjunctiva, Right T Conjunctiva, Left	X External	Z No Device	Z No Qualifier
2 Anterior Chamber, Right 3 Anterior Chamber, Left 4 Vitreous, Right 5 Vitreous, Left C Iris, Right D Iris, Left E Retina, Right F Retina, Left G Retinal Vessel, Right H Retinal Vessel, Left J Lens, Right K Lens, Left	3 Percutaneous X External	Z No Device	Z No Qualifier
A Choroid, Right B Choroid, Left L Extraocular Muscle, Right M Extraocular Muscle, Left N Upper Eyelid, Right P Upper Eyelid, Left Q Lower Eyelid, Right R Lower Eyelid, Left V Lacrimal Gland, Right W Lacrimal Gland, Left	0 Open 3 Percutaneous X External	Z No Device	Z No Qualifier
X Lacrimal Duct, Right Y Lacrimal Duct, Left	0 Open 3 Percutaneous 7 Via Natural or Artificial Opening 8 Via Natural or Artificial Opening Endoscopic	Z No Device	Z No Qualifier

Section	0	Medical and Surgical
Body System	8	Eye
Operation	D	**Extraction:** Pulling or stripping out or off all or a portion of a body part by the use of force

Body Part (4th)	Approach (5th)	Device (6th)	Qualifier (7th)
8 Cornea, Right 9 Cornea, Left	X External	Z No Device	X Diagnostic Z No Qualifier
J Lens, Right K Lens, Left	3 Percutaneous	Z No Device	Z No Qualifier

Section	0	Medical and Surgical
Body System	8	Eye
Operation	F	**Fragmentation:** Breaking solid matter in a body part into pieces

Body Part (4th)	Approach (5th)	Device (6th)	Qualifier (7th)
4 Vitreous, Right 5 Vitreous, Left	3 Percutaneous X External	Z No Device	Z No Qualifier

Section	0	Medical and Surgical
Body System	8	Eye
Operation	H	**Insertion:** Putting in a nonbiological appliance that monitors, assists, performs, or prevents a physiological function but does not physically take the place of a body part

Body Part (4th)	Approach (5th)	Device (6th)	Qualifier (7th)
0 Eye, Right 1 Eye, Left	0 Open	5 Epiretinal Visual Prosthesis Y Other Device	Z No Qualifier
0 Eye, Right 1 Eye, Left	3 Percutaneous	1 Radioactive Element 3 Infusion Device Y Other Device	Z No Qualifier
0 Eye, Right 1 Eye, Left	7 Via Natural or Artificial Opening 8 Via Natural or Artificial Opening Endoscopic	Y Other Device	Z No Qualifier
0 Eye, Right 1 Eye, Left	X External	1 Radioactive Element 3 Infusion Device	Z No Qualifier

Section	0	Medical and Surgical
Body System	8	Eye
Operation	J	**Inspection:** Visually and/or manually exploring a body part

Body Part (4th)	Approach (5th)	Device (6th)	Qualifier (7th)
0 Eye, Right 1 Eye, Left J Lens, Right K Lens, Left	X External	Z No Device	Z No Qualifier
L Extraocular Muscle, Right M Extraocular Muscle, Left	0 Open X External	Z No Device	Z No Qualifier

Section	0	Medical and Surgical
Body System	8	Eye
Operation	L	**Occlusion:** Completely closing an orifice or the lumen of a tubular body part

Body Part (4th)	Approach (5th)	Device (6th)	Qualifier (7th)
X Lacrimal Duct, Right Y Lacrimal Duct, Left	0 Open 3 Percutaneous	C Extraluminal Device D Intraluminal Device Z No Device	Z No Qualifier
X Lacrimal Duct, Right Y Lacrimal Duct, Left	7 Via Natural or Artificial Opening 8 Via Natural or Artificial Opening Endoscopic	D Intraluminal Device Z No Device	Z No Qualifier

Section 0 **Medical and Surgical**
Body System 8 **Eye**
Operation M **Reattachment:** Putting back in or on all or a portion of a separated body part to its normal location or other suitable location

Body Part (4th)	Approach (5th)	Device (6th)	Qualifier (7th)
N Upper Eyelid, Right P Upper Eyelid, Left Q Lower Eyelid, Right R Lower Eyelid, Left	X External	Z No Device	Z No Qualifier

Section 0 **Medical and Surgical**
Body System 8 **Eye**
Operation N **Release:** Freeing a body part from an abnormal physical constraint by cutting or by the use of force

Body Part (4th)	Approach (5th)	Device (6th)	Qualifier (7th)
0 Eye, Right 1 Eye, Left 6 Sclera, Right 7 Sclera, Left 8 Cornea, Right 9 Cornea, Left S Conjunctiva, Right T Conjunctiva, Left	X External	Z No Device	Z No Qualifier
2 Anterior Chamber, Right 3 Anterior Chamber, Left 4 Vitreous, Right 5 Vitreous, Left C Iris, Right D Iris, Left E Retina, Right F Retina, Left G Retinal Vessel, Right H Retinal Vessel, Left J Lens, Right K Lens, Left	3 Percutaneous	Z No Device	Z No Qualifier
A Choroid, Right B Choroid, Left L Extraocular Muscle, Right M Extraocular Muscle, Left V Lacrimal Gland, Right W Lacrimal Gland, Left	0 Open 3 Percutaneous	Z No Device	Z No Qualifier
N Upper Eyelid, Right P Upper Eyelid, Left Q Lower Eyelid, Right R Lower Eyelid, Left	0 Open 3 Percutaneous X External	Z No Device	Z No Qualifier
X Lacrimal Duct, Right Y Lacrimal Duct, Left	0 Open 3 Percutaneous 7 Via Natural or Artificial Opening 8 Via Natural or Artificial Opening Endoscopic	Z No Device	Z No Qualifier

Section	0	Medical and Surgical
Body System	8	Eye
Operation	P	**Removal:** Taking out or off a device from a body part

Body Part (4th)	Approach (5th)	Device (6th)	Qualifier (7th)
0 Eye, Right 1 Eye, Left	0 Open 3 Percutaneous 7 Via Natural or Artificial Opening 8 Via Natural or Artificial Opening Endoscopic	0 Drainage Device 1 Radioactive Element 3 Infusion Device 7 Autologous Tissue Substitute C Extraluminal Device D Intraluminal Device J Synthetic Substitute K Nonautologous Tissue Substitute Y Other Device	Z No Qualifier
0 Eye, Right 1 Eye, Left	X External	0 Drainage Device 1 Radioactive Element 3 Infusion Device 7 Autologous Tissue Substitute C Extraluminal Device D Intraluminal Device J Synthetic Substitute K Nonautologous Tissue Substitute	Z No Qualifier
J Lens, Right K Lens, Left	3 Percutaneous	J Synthetic Substitute Y Other Device	Z No Qualifier
L Extraocular Muscle, Right M Extraocular Muscle, Left	0 Open 3 Percutaneous	0 Drainage Device 7 Autologous Tissue Substitute J Synthetic Substitute K Nonautologous Tissue Substitute Y Other Device	Z No Qualifier

Section	0	Medical and Surgical
Body System	8	Eye
Operation	Q	**Repair:** Restoring, to the extent possible, a body part to its normal anatomic structure and function

Body Part (4th)	Approach (5th)	Device (6th)	Qualifier (7th)
0 Eye, Right 1 Eye, Left 6 Sclera, Right 7 Sclera, Left 8 Cornea, Right 9 Cornea, Left S Conjunctiva, Right T Conjunctiva, Left	X External	Z No Device	Z No Qualifier
2 Anterior Chamber, Right 3 Anterior Chamber, Left 4 Vitreous, Right 5 Vitreous, Left C Iris, Right D Iris, Left E Retina, Right F Retina, Left G Retinal Vessel, Right H Retinal Vessel, Left J Lens, Right K Lens, Left	3 Percutaneous	Z No Device	Z No Qualifier

Continued →

Section | 0 | Medical and Surgical
Body System | 8 | Eye
Operation | Q | **Repair:** Restoring, to the extent possible, a body part to its normal anatomic structure and function

Body Part (4th)	Approach (5th)	Device (6th)	Qualifier (7th)
A Choroid, Right B Choroid, Left L Extraocular Muscle, Right M Extraocular Muscle, Left V Lacrimal Gland, Right W Lacrimal Gland, Left	0 Open 3 Percutaneous	Z No Device	Z No Qualifier
N Upper Eyelid, Right P Upper Eyelid, Left Q Lower Eyelid, Right R Lower Eyelid, Left	0 Open 3 Percutaneous X External	Z No Device	Z No Qualifier
X Lacrimal Duct, Right Y Lacrimal Duct, Left	0 Open 3 Percutaneous 7 Via Natural or Artificial Opening 8 Via Natural or Artificial Opening Endoscopic	Z No Device	Z No Qualifier

Section | 0 | Medical and Surgical
Body System | 8 | Eye
Operation | R | **Replacement:** Putting in or on biological or synthetic material that physically takes the place and/or function of all or a portion of a body part

Body Part (4th)	Approach (5th)	Device (6th)	Qualifier (7th)
0 Eye, Right 1 Eye, Left A Choroid, Right B Choroid, Left	0 Open 3 Percutaneous	7 Autologous Tissue Substitute J Synthetic Substitute K Nonautologous Tissue Substitute	Z No Qualifier
4 Vitreous, Right 5 Vitreous, Left C Iris, Right D Iris, Left G Retinal Vessel, Right H Retinal Vessel, Left	3 Percutaneous	7 Autologous Tissue Substitute J Synthetic Substitute K Nonautologous Tissue Substitute	Z No Qualifier
6 Sclera, Right 7 Sclera, Left S Conjunctiva, Right T Conjunctiva, Left	X External	7 Autologous Tissue Substitute J Synthetic Substitute K Nonautologous Tissue Substitute	Z No Qualifier
8 Cornea, Right 9 Cornea, Left	3 Percutaneous X External	7 Autologous Tissue Substitute J Synthetic Substitute K Nonautologous Tissue Substitute	Z No Qualifier
J Lens, Right K Lens, Left	3 Percutaneous	0 Synthetic Substitute, Intraocular Telescope 7 Autologous Tissue Substitute J Synthetic Substitute K Nonautologous Tissue Substitute	Z No Qualifier
N Upper Eyelid, Right P Upper Eyelid, Left Q Lower Eyelid, Right R Lower Eyelid, Left	0 Open 3 Percutaneous X External	7 Autologous Tissue Substitute J Synthetic Substitute K Nonautologous Tissue Substitute	Z No Qualifier
X Lacrimal Duct, Right Y Lacrimal Duct, Left	0 Open 3 Percutaneous 7 Via Natural or Artificial Opening 8 Via Natural or Artificial Opening Endoscopic	7 Autologous Tissue Substitute J Synthetic Substitute K Nonautologous Tissue Substitute	Z No Qualifier

Section	0	Medical and Surgical
Body System	8	Eye
Operation	S	Reposition: Moving to its normal location, or other suitable location, all or a portion of a body part

Body Part (4th)	Approach (5th)	Device (6th)	Qualifier (7th)
C Iris, Right D Iris, Left G Retinal Vessel, Right H Retinal Vessel, Left J Lens, Right K Lens, Left	3 Percutaneous	Z No Device	Z No Qualifier
L Extraocular Muscle, Right M Extraocular Muscle, Left V Lacrimal Gland, Right W Lacrimal Gland, Left	0 Open 3 Percutaneous	Z No Device	Z No Qualifier
N Upper Eyelid, Right P Upper Eyelid, Left Q Lower Eyelid, Right R Lower Eyelid, Left	0 Open 3 Percutaneous X External	Z No Device	Z No Qualifier
X Lacrimal Duct, Right Y Lacrimal Duct, Left	0 Open 3 Percutaneous 7 Via Natural or Artificial Opening 8 Via Natural or Artificial Opening Endoscopic	Z No Device	Z No Qualifier

Section	0	Medical and Surgical
Body System	8	Eye
Operation	T	Resection: Cutting out or off, without replacement, all of a body part

Body Part (4th)	Approach (5th)	Device (6th)	Qualifier (7th)
0 Eye, Right 1 Eye, Left 8 Cornea, Right 9 Cornea, Left	X External	Z No Device	Z No Qualifier
4 Vitreous, Right 5 Vitreous, Left C Iris, Right D Iris, Left J Lens, Right K Lens, Left	3 Percutaneous	Z No Device	Z No Qualifier
L Extraocular Muscle, Right M Extraocular Muscle, Left V Lacrimal Gland, Right W Lacrimal Gland, Left	0 Open 3 Percutaneous	Z No Device	Z No Qualifier
N Upper Eyelid, Right P Upper Eyelid, Left Q Lower Eyelid, Right R Lower Eyelid, Left	0 Open X External	Z No Device	Z No Qualifier
X Lacrimal Duct, Right Y Lacrimal Duct, Left	0 Open 3 Percutaneous 7 Via Natural or Artificial Opening 8 Via Natural or Artificial Opening Endoscopic	Z No Device	Z No Qualifier

Section   0   **Medical and Surgical**
Body System   8   **Eye**
Operation   U   **Supplement:** Putting in or on biological or synthetic material that physically reinforces and/or augments the function of a portion of a body part

Body Part (4th)	Approach (5th)	Device (6th)	Qualifier (7th)
0 Eye, Right 1 Eye, Left C Iris, Right D Iris, Left E Retina, Right F Retina, Left G Retinal Vessel, Right H Retinal Vessel, Left L Extraocular Muscle, Right M Extraocular Muscle, Left	0 Open 3 Percutaneous	7 Autologous Tissue Substitute J Synthetic Substitute K Nonautologous Tissue Substitute	Z No Qualifier
8 Cornea, Right 9 Cornea, Left N Upper Eyelid, Right P Upper Eyelid, Left Q Lower Eyelid, Right R Lower Eyelid, Left	0 Open 3 Percutaneous X External	7 Autologous Tissue Substitute J Synthetic Substitute K Nonautologous Tissue Substitute	Z No Qualifier
X Lacrimal Duct, Right Y Lacrimal Duct, Left	0 Open 3 Percutaneous 7 Via Natural or Artificial Opening 8 Via Natural or Artificial Opening Endoscopic	7 Autologous Tissue Substitute J Synthetic Substitute K Nonautologous Tissue Substitute	Z No Qualifier

Section   0   **Medical and Surgical**
Body System   8   **Eye**
Operation   V   **Restriction:** Partially closing an orifice or the lumen of a tubular body part

Body Part (4th)	Approach (5th)	Device (6th)	Qualifier (7th)
X Lacrimal Duct, Right Y Lacrimal Duct, Left	0 Open 3 Percutaneous	C Extraluminal Device D Intraluminal Device Z No Device	Z No Qualifier
X Lacrimal Duct, Right Y Lacrimal Duct, Left	7 Via Natural or Artificial Opening 8 Via Natural or Artificial Opening Endoscopic	D Intraluminal Device Z No Device	Z No Qualifier

Section   0   **Medical and Surgical**
Body System   8   **Eye**
Operation   W   **Revision:** Correcting, to the extent possible, a portion of a malfunctioning device or the position of a displaced device

Body Part (4th)	Approach (5th)	Device (6th)	Qualifier (7th)
0 Eye, Right 1 Eye, Left	0 Open 3 Percutaneous 7 Via Natural or Artificial Opening 8 Via Natural or Artificial Opening Endoscopic	0 Drainage Device 3 Infusion Device 7 Autologous Tissue Substitute C Extraluminal Device D Intraluminal Device J Synthetic Substitute K Nonautologous Tissue Substitute Y Other Device	Z No Qualifier
0 Eye, Right 1 Eye, Left	X External	0 Drainage Device 3 Infusion Device 7 Autologous Tissue Substitute C Extraluminal Device D Intraluminal Device J Synthetic Substitute K Nonautologous Tissue Substitute	Z No Qualifier

Continued →

Section	0	Medical and Surgical
Body System	8	Eye
Operation	W	**Revision:** Correcting, to the extent possible, a portion of a malfunctioning device or the position of a displaced device

Body Part (4th)	Approach (5th)	Device (6th)	Qualifier (7th)
J Lens, Right **K** Lens, Left	**3** Percutaneous	**J** Synthetic Substitute **Y** Other Device	**Z** No Qualifier
J Lens, Right **K** Lens, Left	**X** External	**J** Synthetic Substitute	**Z** No Qualifier
L Extraocular Muscle, Right **M** Extraocular Muscle, Left	**0** Open **3** Percutaneous	**0** Drainage Device **7** Autologous Tissue Substitute **J** Synthetic Substitute **K** Nonautologous Tissue Substitute **Y** Other Device	**Z** No Qualifier

Section	0	Medical and Surgical
Body System	8	Eye
Operation	X	**Transfer:** Moving, without taking out, all or a portion of a body part to another location to take over the function of all or a portion of a body part

Body Part (4th)	Approach (5th)	Device (6th)	Qualifier (7th)
L Extraocular Muscle, Right **M** Extraocular Muscle, Left	**0** Open **3** Percutaneous	**Z** No Device	**Z** No Qualifier

AHA Coding Clinic

08133J4 Bypass Left Anterior Chamber to Sclera with Synthetic Substitute, Percutaneous Approach—AHA CC: 1Q, 2019, 27-28

08923ZZ Drainage of Right Anterior Chamber, Percutaneous Approach—AHA CC: 2Q, 2016, 21-22

08B43ZZ Excision of Right Vitreous, Percutaneous Approach—AHA CC: 4Q, 2014, 36-37

08B53ZZ Excision of Left Vitreous, Percutaneous Approach—AHA CC: 4Q, 2014, 35-36

08J0XZZ Inspection of Right Eye, External Approach—AHA CC: 1Q, 2015, 35-36

08NC3ZZ Release Right Iris, Percutaneous Approach—AHA CC: 2Q, 2015, 24-25

08Q7XZZ Repair Left Sclera, External Approach—AHA CC: 3Q, 2018, 13

08Q9XZZ Repair Left Cornea, External Approach—AHA CC: 3Q, 2018, 13

08R8XKZ Replacement of Right Cornea with Nonautologous Tissue Substitute, External Approach—AHA CC: 2Q, 2015, 24-26

08T1XZZ Resection of Left Eye, External Approach—AHA CC: 2Q, 2015, 12-13

08TM0ZZ Resection of Left Extraocular Muscle, Open Approach—AHA CC: 2Q, 2015, 12-13

08TR0ZZ Resection of Left Lower Eyelid, Open Approach—AHA CC: 2Q, 2015, 12-13

08U9XKZ Supplement Left Cornea with Nonautologous Tissue Substitute, External Approach—AHA CC: 3Q, 2014, 31

Nose and Sinuses

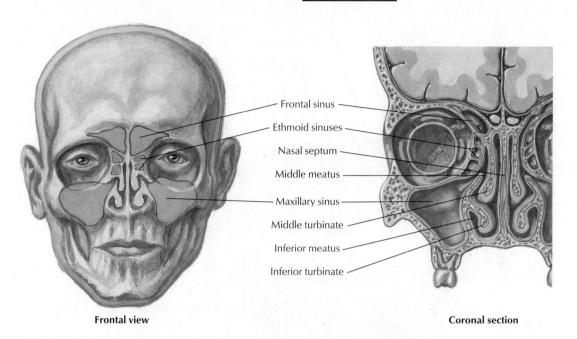

Frontal sinus
Ethmoid sinuses
Nasal septum
Middle meatus
Maxillary sinus
Middle turbinate
Inferior meatus
Inferior turbinate

Frontal view

Coronal section

Anatomy of nasal cavity and sinuses

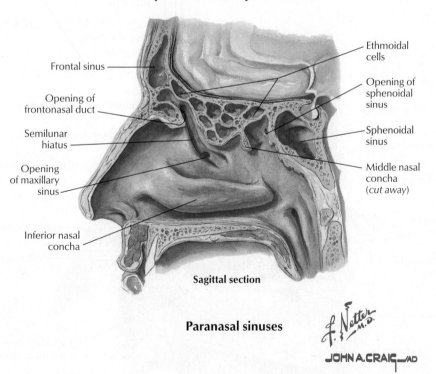

Frontal sinus

Opening of
frontonasal duct

Semilunar
hiatus

Opening
of maxillary
sinus

Inferior nasal
concha

Ethmoidal
cells

Opening of
sphenoidal
sinus

Sphenoidal
sinus

Middle nasal
concha
(*cut away*)

Sagittal section

Paranasal sinuses

Lateral Wall of Nasal Cavity

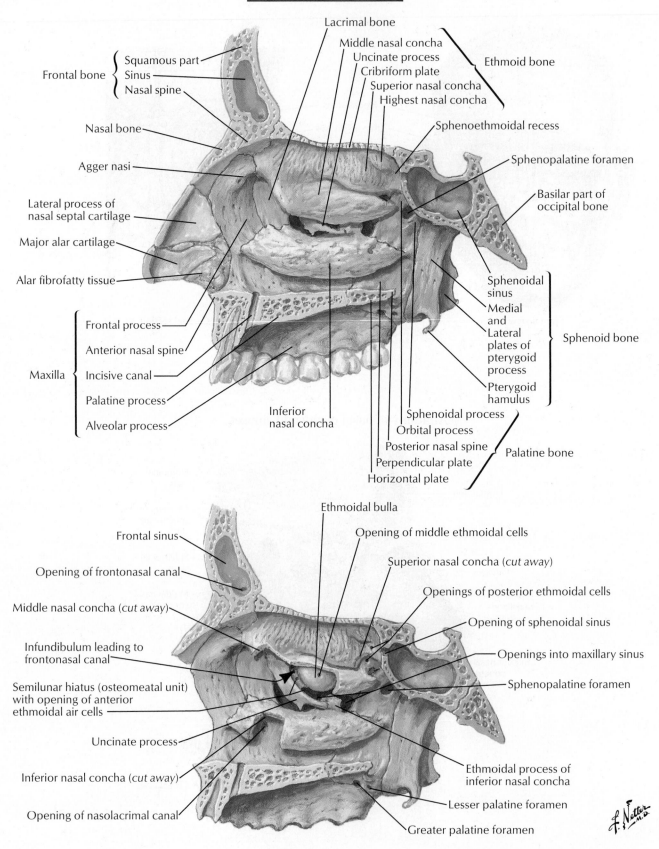

Lacrimal bone

Middle nasal concha

Uncinate process

Cribriform plate

Superior nasal concha

Highest nasal concha

Ethmoid bone

Frontal bone { Squamous part, Sinus, Nasal spine }

Sphenoethmoidal recess

Nasal bone

Agger nasi

Sphenopalatine foramen

Basilar part of occipital bone

Lateral process of nasal septal cartilage

Major alar cartilage

Alar fibrofatty tissue

Sphenoidal sinus

Medial and Lateral plates of pterygoid process

Sphenoid bone

Maxilla { Frontal process, Anterior nasal spine, Incisive canal, Palatine process, Alveolar process }

Pterygoid hamulus

Inferior nasal concha

Sphenoidal process

Orbital process

Posterior nasal spine

Perpendicular plate

Horizontal plate

Palatine bone

Ethmoidal bulla

Opening of middle ethmoidal cells

Frontal sinus

Superior nasal concha (cut away)

Opening of frontonasal canal

Openings of posterior ethmoidal cells

Middle nasal concha (cut away)

Opening of sphenoidal sinus

Infundibulum leading to frontonasal canal

Openings into maxillary sinus

Semilunar hiatus (osteomeatal unit) with opening of anterior ethmoidal air cells

Sphenopalatine foramen

Uncinate process

Inferior nasal concha (cut away)

Ethmoidal process of inferior nasal concha

Lesser palatine foramen

Opening of nasolacrimal canal

Greater palatine foramen

Pathway of Sound Reception

Frontal section

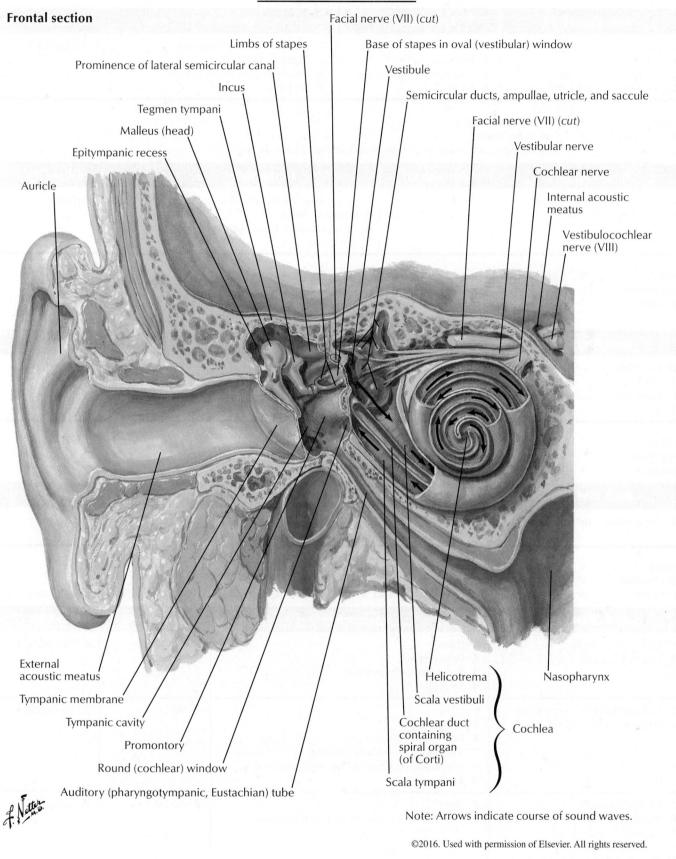

Facial nerve (VII) (*cut*)

Limbs of stapes

Base of stapes in oval (vestibular) window

Prominence of lateral semicircular canal

Vestibule

Incus

Semicircular ducts, ampullae, utricle, and saccule

Tegmen tympani

Facial nerve (VII) (*cut*)

Malleus (head)

Vestibular nerve

Epitympanic recess

Cochlear nerve

Auricle

Internal acoustic meatus

Vestibulocochlear nerve (VIII)

External acoustic meatus

Helicotrema

Nasopharynx

Tympanic membrane

Scala vestibuli

Tympanic cavity

Cochlear duct containing spiral organ (of Corti)

Cochlea

Promontory

Scala tympani

Round (cochlear) window

Auditory (pharyngotympanic, Eustachian) tube

Note: Arrows indicate course of sound waves.

Ear, Nose, Sinus Tables 090–09W

Section	0	Medical and Surgical
Body System	9	Ear, Nose, Sinus
Operation	0	Alteration: Modifying the anatomic structure of a body part without affecting the function of the body part

Body Part (4th)	Approach (5th)	Device (6th)	Qualifier (7th)
0 External Ear, Right 1 External Ear, Left 2 External Ear, Bilateral K Nasal Mucosa and Soft Tissue	0 Open 3 Percutaneous 4 Percutaneous Endoscopic X External	7 Autologous Tissue Substitute J Synthetic Substitute K Nonautologous Tissue Substitute Z No Device	Z No Qualifier

Section	0	Medical and Surgical
Body System	9	Ear, Nose, Sinus
Operation	1	Bypass: Altering the route of passage of the contents of a tubular body part

Body Part (4th)	Approach (5th)	Device (6th)	Qualifier (7th)
D Inner Ear, Right E Inner Ear, Left	0 Open	7 Autologous Tissue Substitute J Synthetic Substitute K Nonautologous Tissue Substitute Z No Device	0 Endolymphatic

Section	0	Medical and Surgical
Body System	9	Ear, Nose, Sinus
Operation	2	Change: Taking out or off a device from a body part and putting back an identical or similar device in or on the same body part without cutting or puncturing the skin or a mucous membrane

Body Part (4th)	Approach (5th)	Device (6th)	Qualifier (7th)
H Ear, Right J Ear, Left K Nasal Mucosa and Soft Tissue Y Sinus	X External	0 Drainage Device Y Other Device	Z No Qualifier

Section	0	Medical and Surgical
Body System	9	Ear, Nose, Sinus
Operation	3	Control: Stopping, or attempting to stop, postprocedural or other acute bleeding

Body Part (4th)	Approach (5th)	Device (6th)	Qualifier (7th)
K Nasal Mucosa and Soft Tissue	7 Via Natural or Artificial Opening 8 Via Natural or Artificial Opening Endoscopic	Z No Device	Z No Qualifier

Section	0	Medical and Surgical
Body System	9	Ear, Nose, Sinus
Operation	5	Destruction: Physical eradication of all or a portion of a body part by the direct use of energy, force, or a destructive agent

Body Part (4th)	Approach (5th)	Device (6th)	Qualifier (7th)
0 External Ear, Right 1 External Ear, Left	0 Open 3 Percutaneous 4 Percutaneous Endoscopic X External	Z No Device	Z No Qualifier
3 External Auditory Canal, Right 4 External Auditory Canal, Left	0 Open 3 Percutaneous 4 Percutaneous Endoscopic 7 Via Natural or Artificial Opening 8 Via Natural or Artificial Opening Endoscopic X External	Z No Device	Z No Qualifier
5 Middle Ear, Right 6 Middle Ear, Left 9 Auditory Ossicle, Right A Auditory Ossicle, Left D Inner Ear, Right E Inner Ear, Left	0 Open 8 Via Natural or Artificial Opening Endoscopic	Z No Device	Z No Qualifier

Continued →

Section	0	Medical and Surgical
Body System	9	Ear, Nose, Sinus
Operation	5	**Destruction:** Physical eradication of all or a portion of a body part by the direct use of energy, force, or a destructive agent

Body Part (4ᵗʰ)	Approach (5ᵗʰ)	Device (6ᵗʰ)	Qualifier (7ᵗʰ)
7 Tympanic Membrane, Right 8 Tympanic Membrane, Left F Eustachian Tube, Right G Eustachian Tube, Left L Nasal Turbinate N Nasopharynx	0 Open 3 Percutaneous 4 Percutaneous Endoscopic 7 Via Natural or Artificial Opening 8 Via Natural or Artificial Opening Endoscopic	Z No Device	Z No Qualifier
B Mastoid Sinus, Right C Mastoid Sinus, Left M Nasal Septum P Accessory Sinus Q Maxillary Sinus, Right R Maxillary Sinus, Left S Frontal Sinus, Right T Frontal Sinus, Left U Ethmoid Sinus, Right V Ethmoid Sinus, Left W Sphenoid Sinus, Right X Sphenoid Sinus, Left	0 Open 3 Percutaneous 4 Percutaneous Endoscopic 8 Via Natural or Artificial Opening Endoscopic	Z No Device	Z No Qualifier
K Nasal Mucosa and Soft Tissue	0 Open 3 Percutaneous 4 Percutaneous Endoscopic 8 Via Natural or Artificial Opening Endoscopic X External	Z No Device	Z No Qualifier

Section	0	Medical and Surgical
Body System	9	Ear, Nose, Sinus
Operation	7	**Dilation:** Expanding an orifice or the lumen of a tubular body part

Body Part (4ᵗʰ)	Approach (5ᵗʰ)	Device (6ᵗʰ)	Qualifier (7ᵗʰ)
F Eustachian Tube, Right G Eustachian Tube, Left	0 Open 7 Via Natural or Artificial Opening 8 Via Natural or Artificial Opening Endoscopic	D Intraluminal Device Z No Device	Z No Qualifier
F Eustachian Tube, Right G Eustachian Tube, Left	3 Percutaneous 4 Percutaneous Endoscopic	Z No Device	Z No Qualifier

Section	0	Medical and Surgical
Body System	9	Ear, Nose, Sinus
Operation	8	**Division:** Cutting into a body part, without draining fluids and/or gases from the body part, in order to separate or transect a body part

Body Part (4ᵗʰ)	Approach (5ᵗʰ)	Device (6ᵗʰ)	Qualifier (7ᵗʰ)
L Nasal Turbinate	0 Open 3 Percutaneous 4 Percutaneous Endoscopic 7 Via Natural or Artificial Opening 8 Via Natural or Artificial Opening Endoscopic	Z No Device	Z No Qualifier

Section	0	Medical and Surgical
Body System	9	Ear, Nose, Sinus
Operation	9	**Drainage:** Taking or letting out fluids and/or gases from a body part

Body Part (4ᵗʰ)	Approach (5ᵗʰ)	Device (6ᵗʰ)	Qualifier (7ᵗʰ)
0 External Ear, Right 1 External Ear, Left	0 Open 3 Percutaneous 4 Percutaneous Endoscopic X External	0 Drainage Device	Z No Qualifier
0 External Ear, Right 1 External Ear, Left	0 Open 3 Percutaneous 4 Percutaneous Endoscopic X External	Z No Device	X Diagnostic Z No Qualifier
3 External Auditory Canal, Right 4 External Auditory Canal, Left K Nasal Mucosa and Soft Tissue	0 Open 3 Percutaneous 4 Percutaneous Endoscopic 7 Via Natural or Artificial Opening 8 Via Natural or Artificial Opening Endoscopic X External	0 Drainage Device	Z No Qualifier
3 External Auditory Canal, Right 4 External Auditory Canal, Left K Nasal Mucosa and Soft Tissue	0 Open 3 Percutaneous 4 Percutaneous Endoscopic 7 Via Natural or Artificial Opening 8 Via Natural or Artificial Opening Endoscopic X External	Z No Device	X Diagnostic Z No Qualifier
5 Middle Ear, Right 6 Middle Ear, Left 9 Auditory Ossicle, Right A Auditory Ossicle, Left D Inner Ear, Right E Inner Ear, Left	0 Open 7 Via Natural or Artificial Opening 8 Via Natural or Artificial Opening Endoscopic	0 Drainage Device	Z No Qualifier
5 Middle Ear, Right 6 Middle Ear, Left 9 Auditory Ossicle, Right A Auditory Ossicle, Left D Inner Ear, Right E Inner Ear, Left	0 Open 7 Via Natural or Artificial Opening 8 Via Natural or Artificial Opening Endoscopic	Z No Device	X Diagnostic Z No Qualifier
7 Tympanic Membrane, Right 8 Tympanic Membrane, Left B Mastoid Sinus, Right C Mastoid Sinus, Left F Eustachian Tube, Right G Eustachian Tube, Left L Nasal Turbinate M Nasal Septum N Nasopharynx P Accessory Sinus Q Maxillary Sinus, Right R Maxillary Sinus, Left S Frontal Sinus, Right T Frontal Sinus, Left U Ethmoid Sinus, Right V Ethmoid Sinus, Left W Sphenoid Sinus, Right X Sphenoid Sinus, Left	0 Open 3 Percutaneous 4 Percutaneous Endoscopic 7 Via Natural or Artificial Opening 8 Via Natural or Artificial Opening Endoscopic	0 Drainage Device	Z No Qualifier

Continued →

Section	0	Medical and Surgical
Body System	9	Ear, Nose, Sinus
Operation	9	Drainage: Taking or letting out fluids and/or gases from a body part

Body Part (4th)	Approach (5th)	Device (6th)	Qualifier (7th)
7 Tympanic Membrane, Right 8 Tympanic Membrane, Left B Mastoid Sinus, Right C Mastoid Sinus, Left F Eustachian Tube, Right G Eustachian Tube, Left L Nasal Turbinate M Nasal Septum N Nasopharynx P Accessory Sinus Q Maxillary Sinus, Right R Maxillary Sinus, Left S Frontal Sinus, Right T Frontal Sinus, Left U Ethmoid Sinus, Right V Ethmoid Sinus, Left W Sphenoid Sinus, Right X Sphenoid Sinus, Left	0 Open 3 Percutaneous 4 Percutaneous Endoscopic 7 Via Natural or Artificial Opening 8 Via Natural or Artificial Opening Endoscopic	Z No Device	X Diagnostic Z No Qualifier

Section	0	Medical and Surgical
Body System	9	Ear, Nose, Sinus
Operation	B	Excision: Cutting out or off, without replacement, a portion of a body part

Body Part (4th)	Approach (5th)	Device (6th)	Qualifier (7th)
0 External Ear, Right 1 External Ear, Left	0 Open 3 Percutaneous 4 Percutaneous Endoscopic X External	Z No Device	X Diagnostic Z No Qualifier
3 External Auditory Canal, Right 4 External Auditory Canal, Left	0 Open 3 Percutaneous 4 Percutaneous Endoscopic 7 Via Natural or Artificial Opening 8 Via Natural or Artificial Opening Endoscopic X External	Z No Device	X Diagnostic Z No Qualifier
5 Middle Ear, Right 6 Middle Ear, Left 9 Auditory Ossicle, Right A Auditory Ossicle, Left D Inner Ear, Right E Inner Ear, Left	0 Open 8 Via Natural or Artificial Opening Endoscopic	Z No Device	X Diagnostic Z No Qualifier
7 Tympanic Membrane, Right 8 Tympanic Membrane, Left F Eustachian Tube, Right G Eustachian Tube, Left L Nasal Turbinate N Nasopharynx	0 Open 3 Percutaneous 4 Percutaneous Endoscopic 7 Via Natural or Artificial Opening 8 Via Natural or Artificial Opening Endoscopic	Z No Device	X Diagnostic Z No Qualifier
B Mastoid Sinus, Right C Mastoid Sinus, Left M Nasal Septum P Accessory Sinus Q Maxillary Sinus, Right R Maxillary Sinus, Left S Frontal Sinus, Right T Frontal Sinus, Left U Ethmoid Sinus, Right V Ethmoid Sinus, Left W Sphenoid Sinus, Right X Sphenoid Sinus, Left	0 Open 3 Percutaneous 4 Percutaneous Endoscopic 8 Via Natural or Artificial Opening Endoscopic	Z No Device	X Diagnostic Z No Qualifier

Continued →

Section	0	Medical and Surgical
Body System	9	Ear, Nose, Sinus
Operation	B	Excision: Cutting out or off, without replacement, a portion of a body part

Body Part (4th)	Approach (5th)	Device (6th)	Qualifier (7th)
K Nasal Mucosa and Soft Tissue	0 Open 3 Percutaneous 4 Percutaneous Endoscopic 8 Via Natural or Artificial Opening Endoscopic X External	Z No Device	X Diagnostic Z No Qualifier

Section	0	Medical and Surgical
Body System	9	Ear, Nose, Sinus
Operation	C	Extirpation: Taking or cutting out solid matter from a body part

Body Part (4th)	Approach (5th)	Device (6th)	Qualifier (7th)
0 External Ear, Right 1 External Ear, Left	0 Open 3 Percutaneous 4 Percutaneous Endoscopic X External	Z No Device	Z No Qualifier
3 External Auditory Canal, Right 4 External Auditory Canal, Left	0 Open 3 Percutaneous 4 Percutaneous Endoscopic 7 Via Natural or Artificial Opening 8 Via Natural or Artificial Opening Endoscopic X External	Z No Device	Z No Qualifier
5 Middle Ear, Right 6 Middle Ear, Left 9 Auditory Ossicle, Right A Auditory Ossicle, Left D Inner Ear, Right E Inner Ear, Left	0 Open 8 Via Natural or Artificial Opening Endoscopic	Z No Device	Z No Qualifier
7 Tympanic Membrane, Right 8 Tympanic Membrane, Left F Eustachian Tube, Right G Eustachian Tube, Left L Nasal Turbinate N Nasopharynx	0 Open 3 Percutaneous 4 Percutaneous Endoscopic 7 Via Natural or Artificial Opening 8 Via Natural or Artificial Opening Endoscopic	Z No Device	Z No Qualifier
B Mastoid Sinus, Right C Mastoid Sinus, Left M Nasal Septum P Accessory Sinus Q Maxillary Sinus, Right R Maxillary Sinus, Left S Frontal Sinus, Right T Frontal Sinus, Left U Ethmoid Sinus, Right V Ethmoid Sinus, Left W Sphenoid Sinus, Right X Sphenoid Sinus, Left	0 Open 3 Percutaneous 4 Percutaneous Endoscopic 8 Via Natural or Artificial Opening Endoscopic	Z No Device	Z No Qualifier
K Nasal Mucosa and Soft Tissue	0 Open 3 Percutaneous 4 Percutaneous Endoscopic 8 Via Natural or Artificial Opening Endoscopic X External	Z No Device	Z No Qualifier

Section	0	Medical and Surgical
Body System	9	Ear, Nose, Sinus
Operation	D	**Extraction:** Pulling or stripping out or off all or a portion of a body part by the use of force

Body Part (4th)	Approach (5th)	Device (6th)	Qualifier (7th)
7 Tympanic Membrane, Right 8 Tympanic Membrane, Left L Nasal Turbinate	0 Open 3 Percutaneous 4 Percutaneous Endoscopic 7 Via Natural or Artificial Opening 8 Via Natural or Artificial Opening Endoscopic	Z No Device	Z No Qualifier
9 Auditory Ossicle, Right A Auditory Ossicle, Left	0 Open	Z No Device	Z No Qualifier
B Mastoid Sinus, Right C Mastoid Sinus, Left M Nasal Septum P Accessory Sinus Q Maxillary Sinus, Right R Maxillary Sinus, Left S Frontal Sinus, Right T Frontal Sinus, Left U Ethmoid Sinus, Right V Ethmoid Sinus, Left W Sphenoid Sinus, Right X Sphenoid Sinus, Left	0 Open 3 Percutaneous 4 Percutaneous Endoscopic	Z No Device	Z No Qualifier

Section	0	Medical and Surgical
Body System	9	Ear, Nose, Sinus
Operation	H	**Insertion:** Putting in a nonbiological appliance that monitors, assists, performs, or prevents a physiological function but does not physically take the place of a body part

Body Part (4th)	Approach (5th)	Device (6th)	Qualifier (7th)
D Inner Ear, Right E Inner Ear, Left	0 Open 3 Percutaneous 4 Percutaneous Endoscopic	1 Radioactive Element 4 Hearing Device, Bone Conduction 5 Hearing Device, Single Channel Cochlear Prosthesis 6 Hearing Device, Multiple Channel Cochlear Prosthesis S Hearing Device	Z No Qualifier
H Ear, Right J Ear, Left K Nasal Mucosa and Soft Tissue Y Sinus	0 Open 3 Percutaneous 4 Percutaneous Endoscopic 7 Via Natural or Artificial Opening 8 Via Natural or Artificial Opening Endoscopic	1 Radioactive Element Y Other Device	Z No Qualifier
N Nasopharynx	7 Via Natural or Artificial Opening 8 Via Natural or Artificial Opening Endoscopic	1 Radioactive Element B Intraluminal Device, Airway	Z No Qualifier

Section	0	Medical and Surgical
Body System	9	Ear, Nose, Sinus
Operation	J	**Inspection:** Visually and/or manually exploring a body part

Body Part (4th)	Approach (5th)	Device (6th)	Qualifier (7th)
7 Tympanic Membrane, Right 8 Tympanic Membrane, Left H Ear, Right J Ear, Left	0 Open 3 Percutaneous 4 Percutaneous Endoscopic 7 Via Natural or Artificial Opening 8 Via Natural or Artificial Opening Endoscopic X External	Z No Device	Z No Qualifier
D Inner Ear, Right E Inner Ear, Left K Nose Y Sinus	0 Open 3 Percutaneous 4 Percutaneous Endoscopic 8 Via Natural or Artificial Opening Endoscopic X External	Z No Device	Z No Qualifier

Section   0   Medical and Surgical
Body System   9   Ear, Nose, Sinus
Operation   M   **Reattachment:** Putting back in or on all or a portion of a separated body part to its normal location or other suitable location

Body Part (4th)	Approach (5th)	Device (6th)	Qualifier (7th)
0 External Ear, Right 1 External Ear, Left K Nasal Mucosa and Soft Tissue	X External	Z No Device	Z No Qualifier

Section   0   Medical and Surgical
Body System   9   Ear, Nose, Sinus
Operation   N   **Release:** Freeing a body part from an abnormal physical constraint by cutting or by the use of force

Body Part (4th)	Approach (5th)	Device (6th)	Qualifier (7th)
0 External Ear, Right 1 External Ear, Left	0 Open 3 Percutaneous 4 Percutaneous Endoscopic X External	Z No Device	Z No Qualifier
3 External Auditory Canal, Right 4 External Auditory Canal, Left	0 Open 3 Percutaneous 4 Percutaneous Endoscopic 7 Via Natural or Artificial Opening 8 Via Natural or Artificial Opening Endoscopic X External	Z No Device	Z No Qualifier
5 Middle Ear, Right 6 Middle Ear, Left 9 Auditory Ossicle, Right A Auditory Ossicle, Left D Inner Ear, Right E Inner Ear, Left	0 Open 8 Via Natural or Artificial Opening Endoscopic	Z No Device	Z No Qualifier
7 Tympanic Membrane, Right 8 Tympanic Membrane, Left F Eustachian Tube, Right G Eustachian Tube, Left L Nasal Turbinate N Nasopharynx	0 Open 3 Percutaneous 4 Percutaneous Endoscopic 7 Via Natural or Artificial Opening 8 Via Natural or Artificial Opening Endoscopic	Z No Device	Z No Qualifier
B Mastoid Sinus, Right C Mastoid Sinus, Left M Nasal Septum P Accessory Sinus Q Maxillary Sinus, Right R Maxillary Sinus, Left S Frontal Sinus, Right T Frontal Sinus, Left U Ethmoid Sinus, Right V Ethmoid Sinus, Left W Sphenoid Sinus, Right X Sphenoid Sinus, Left	0 Open 3 Percutaneous 4 Percutaneous Endoscopic 8 Via Natural or Artificial Opening Endoscopic	Z No Device	Z No Qualifier
K Nasal Mucosa and Soft Tissue	0 Open 3 Percutaneous 4 Percutaneous Endoscopic 8 Via Natural or Artificial Opening Endoscopic X External	Z No Device	Z No Qualifier

Section   0   **Medical and Surgical**
Body System   9   **Ear, Nose, Sinus**
Operation   P   **Removal:** Taking out or off a device from a body part

Body Part (4ᵗʰ)	Approach (5ᵗʰ)	Device (6ᵗʰ)	Qualifier (7ᵗʰ)
7 Tympanic Membrane, Right 8 Tympanic Membrane, Left	0 Open 7 Via Natural or Artificial Opening 8 Via Natural or Artificial Opening Endoscopic X External	0 Drainage Device	Z No Qualifier
D Inner Ear, Right E Inner Ear, Left	0 Open 7 Via Natural or Artificial Opening 8 Via Natural or Artificial Opening Endoscopic	S Hearing Device	Z No Qualifier
H Ear, Right J Ear, Left K Nasal Mucosa and Soft Tissue	0 Open 3 Percutaneous 4 Percutaneous Endoscopic 7 Via Natural or Artificial Opening 8 Via Natural or Artificial Opening Endoscopic	0 Drainage Device 7 Autologous Tissue Substitute D Intraluminal Device J Synthetic Substitute K Nonautologous Tissue Substitute Y Other Device	Z No Qualifier
H Ear, Right J Ear, Left K Nasal Mucosa and Soft Tissue	X External	0 Drainage Device 7 Autologous Tissue Substitute D Intraluminal Device J Synthetic Substitute K Nonautologous Tissue Substitute	Z No Qualifier
Y Sinus	0 Open 3 Percutaneous 4 Percutaneous Endoscopic	0 Drainage Device Y Other Device	Z No Qualifier
Y Sinus	7 Via Natural or Artificial Opening 8 Via Natural or Artificial Opening Endoscopic	Y Other Device	Z No Qualifier
Y Sinus	X External	0 Drainage Device	Z No Qualifier

Section   0   **Medical and Surgical**
Body System   9   **Ear, Nose, Sinus**
Operation   Q   **Repair:** Restoring, to the extent possible, a body part to its normal anatomic structure and function

Body Part (4ᵗʰ)	Approach (5ᵗʰ)	Device (6ᵗʰ)	Qualifier (7ᵗʰ)
0 External Ear, Right 1 External Ear, Left 2 External Ear, Bilateral	0 Open 3 Percutaneous 4 Percutaneous Endoscopic X External	Z No Device	Z No Qualifier
3 External Auditory Canal, Right 4 External Auditory Canal, Left F Eustachian Tube, Right G Eustachian Tube, Left	0 Open 3 Percutaneous 4 Percutaneous Endoscopic 7 Via Natural or Artificial Opening 8 Via Natural or Artificial Opening Endoscopic X External	Z No Device	Z No Qualifier
5 Middle Ear, Right 6 Middle Ear, Left 9 Auditory Ossicle, Right A Auditory Ossicle, Left D Inner Ear, Right E Inner Ear, Left	0 Open 8 Via Natural or Artificial Opening Endoscopic	Z No Device	Z No Qualifier
7 Tympanic Membrane, Right 8 Tympanic Membrane, Left L Nasal Turbinate N Nasopharynx	0 Open 3 Percutaneous 4 Percutaneous Endoscopic 7 Via Natural or Artificial Opening 8 Via Natural or Artificial Opening Endoscopic	Z No Device	Z No Qualifier

Continued →

Section	0	Medical and Surgical
Body System	9	Ear, Nose, Sinus
Operation	Q	Repair: Restoring, to the extent possible, a body part to its normal anatomic structure and function

Body Part (4th)	Approach (5th)	Device (6th)	Qualifier (7th)
B Mastoid Sinus, Right C Mastoid Sinus, Left M Nasal Septum P Accessory Sinus Q Maxillary Sinus, Right R Maxillary Sinus, Left S Frontal Sinus, Right T Frontal Sinus, Left U Ethmoid Sinus, Right V Ethmoid Sinus, Left W Sphenoid Sinus, Right X Sphenoid Sinus, Left	0 Open 3 Percutaneous 4 Percutaneous Endoscopic 8 Via Natural or Artificial Opening Endoscopic	Z No Device	Z No Qualifier
K Nasal Mucosa and Soft Tissue	0 Open 3 Percutaneous 4 Percutaneous Endoscopic 8 Via Natural or Artificial Opening Endoscopic X External	Z No Device	Z No Qualifier

Section	0	Medical and Surgical
Body System	9	Ear, Nose, Sinus
Operation	R	Replacement: Putting in or on biological or synthetic material that physically takes the place and/or function of all or a portion of a body part

Body Part (4th)	Approach (5th)	Device (6th)	Qualifier (7th)
0 External Ear, Right 1 External Ear, Left 2 External Ear, Bilateral K Nasal Mucosa and Soft Tissue	0 Open X External	7 Autologous Tissue Substitute J Synthetic Substitute K Nonautologous Tissue Substitute	Z No Qualifier
5 Middle Ear, Right 6 Middle Ear, Left 9 Auditory Ossicle, Right A Auditory Ossicle, Left D Inner Ear, Right E Inner Ear, Left	0 Open	7 Autologous Tissue Substitute J Synthetic Substitute K Nonautologous Tissue Substitute	Z No Qualifier
7 Tympanic Membrane, Right 8 Tympanic Membrane, Left N Nasopharynx	0 Open 7 Via Natural or Artificial Opening 8 Via Natural or Artificial Opening Endoscopic	7 Autologous Tissue Substitute J Synthetic Substitute K Nonautologous Tissue Substitute	Z No Qualifier
L Nasal Turbinate	0 Open 3 Percutaneous 4 Percutaneous Endoscopic 7 Via Natural or Artificial Opening 8 Via Natural or Artificial Opening Endoscopic	7 Autologous Tissue Substitute J Synthetic Substitute K Nonautologous Tissue Substitute	Z No Qualifier
M Nasal Septum	0 Open 3 Percutaneous 4 Percutaneous Endoscopic	7 Autologous Tissue Substitute J Synthetic Substitute K Nonautologous Tissue Substitute	Z No Qualifier

Section	0	Medical and Surgical
Body System	9	Ear, Nose, Sinus
Operation	S	Reposition: Moving to its normal location, or other suitable location, all or a portion of a body part

Body Part (4th)	Approach (5th)	Device (6th)	Qualifier (7th)
0 External Ear, Right 1 External Ear, Left 2 External Ear, Bilateral K Nasal Mucosa and Soft Tissue	0 Open 4 Percutaneous Endoscopic X External	Z No Device	Z No Qualifier
7 Tympanic Membrane, Right 8 Tympanic Membrane, Left F Eustachian Tube, Right G Eustachian Tube, Left L Nasal Turbinate	0 Open 4 Percutaneous Endoscopic 7 Via Natural or Artificial Opening 8 Via Natural or Artificial Opening Endoscopic	Z No Device	Z No Qualifier
9 Auditory Ossicle, Right A Auditory Ossicle, Left M Nasal Septum	0 Open 4 Percutaneous Endoscopic	Z No Device	Z No Qualifier

Section	0	Medical and Surgical
Body System	9	Ear, Nose, Sinus
Operation	T	Resection: Cutting out or off, without replacement, all of a body part

Body Part (4th)	Approach (5th)	Device (6th)	Qualifier (7th)
0 External Ear, Right 1 External Ear, Left	0 Open 4 Percutaneous Endoscopic X External	Z No Device	Z No Qualifier
5 Middle Ear, Right 6 Middle Ear, Left 9 Auditory Ossicle, Right A Auditory Ossicle, Left D Inner Ear, Right E Inner Ear, Left	0 Open 8 Via Natural or Artificial Opening Endoscopic	Z No Device	Z No Qualifier
7 Tympanic Membrane, Right 8 Tympanic Membrane, Left F Eustachian Tube, Right G Eustachian Tube, Left L Nasal Turbinate N Nasopharynx	0 Open 4 Percutaneous Endoscopic 7 Via Natural or Artificial Opening 8 Via Natural or Artificial Opening Endoscopic	Z No Device	Z No Qualifier
B Mastoid Sinus, Right C Mastoid Sinus, Left M Nasal Septum P Accessory Sinus Q Maxillary Sinus, Right R Maxillary Sinus, Left S Frontal Sinus, Right T Frontal Sinus, Left U Ethmoid Sinus, Right V Ethmoid Sinus, Left W Sphenoid Sinus, Right X Sphenoid Sinus, Left	0 Open 4 Percutaneous Endoscopic 8 Via Natural or Artificial Opening Endoscopic	Z No Device	Z No Qualifier
K Nasal Mucosa and Soft Tissue	0 Open 4 Percutaneous Endoscopic 8 Via Natural or Artificial Opening Endoscopic X External	Z No Device	Z No Qualifier

Section 0 **Medical and Surgical**
Body System 9 **Ear, Nose, Sinus**
Operation U **Supplement:** Putting in or on biological or synthetic material that physically reinforces and/or augments the function of a portion of a body part

Body Part (4ᵗʰ)	Approach (5ᵗʰ)	Device (6ᵗʰ)	Qualifier (7ᵗʰ)
0 External Ear, Right 1 External Ear, Left 2 External Ear, Bilateral	0 Open X External	7 Autologous Tissue Substitute J Synthetic Substitute K Nonautologous Tissue Substitute	Z No Qualifier
5 Middle Ear, Right 6 Middle Ear, Left 9 Auditory Ossicle, Right A Auditory Ossicle, Left D Inner Ear, Right E Inner Ear, Left	0 Open 8 Via Natural or Artificial Opening Endoscopic	7 Autologous Tissue Substitute J Synthetic Substitute K Nonautologous Tissue Substitute	Z No Qualifier
7 Tympanic Membrane, Right 8 Tympanic Membrane, Left N Nasopharynx	0 Open 7 Via Natural or Artificial Opening 8 Via Natural or Artificial Opening Endoscopic	7 Autologous Tissue Substitute J Synthetic Substitute K Nonautologous Tissue Substitute	Z No Qualifier
B Mastoid Sinus, Right C Mastoid Sinus, Left L Nasal Turbinate P Accessory Sinus Q Maxillary Sinus, Right R Maxillary Sinus, Left S Frontal Sinus, Right T Frontal Sinus, Left U Ethmoid Sinus, Right V Ethmoid Sinus, Left W Sphenoid Sinus, Right X Sphenoid Sinus, Left	0 Open 3 Percutaneous 4 Percutaneous Endoscopic 7 Via Natural or Artificial Opening 8 Via Natural or Artificial Opening Endoscopic	7 Autologous Tissue Substitute J Synthetic Substitute K Nonautologous Tissue Substitute	Z No Qualifier
K Nasal Mucosa and Soft Tissue	0 Open 8 Via Natural or Artificial Opening Endoscopic X External	7 Autologous Tissue Substitute J Synthetic Substitute K Nonautologous Tissue Substitute	Z No Qualifier
M Nasal Septum	0 Open 3 Percutaneous 4 Percutaneous Endoscopic 8 Via Natural or Artificial Opening Endoscopic	7 Autologous Tissue Substitute J Synthetic Substitute K Nonautologous Tissue Substitute	Z No Qualifier

Section 0 **Medical and Surgical**
Body System 9 **Ear, Nose, Sinus**
Operation W **Revision:** Correcting, to the extent possible, a portion of a malfunctioning device or the position of a displaced device

Body Part (4ᵗʰ)	Approach (5ᵗʰ)	Device (6ᵗʰ)	Qualifier (7ᵗʰ)
7 Tympanic Membrane, Right 8 Tympanic Membrane, Left 9 Auditory Ossicle, Right A Auditory Ossicle, Left	0 Open 7 Via Natural or Artificial Opening 8 Via Natural or Artificial Opening Endoscopic	7 Autologous Tissue Substitute J Synthetic Substitute K Nonautologous Tissue Substitute	Z No Qualifier
D Inner Ear, Right E Inner Ear, Left	0 Open 7 Via Natural or Artificial Opening 8 Via Natural or Artificial Opening Endoscopic	S Hearing Device	Z No Qualifier
H Ear, Right J Ear, Left K Nasal Mucosa and Soft Tissue	0 Open 3 Percutaneous 4 Percutaneous Endoscopic 7 Via Natural or Artificial Opening 8 Via Natural or Artificial Opening Endoscopic	0 Drainage Device 7 Autologous Tissue Substitute D Intraluminal Device J Synthetic Substitute K Nonautologous Tissue Substitute Y Other Device	Z No Qualifier

Continued →

Section	0	**Medical and Surgical**
Body System	9	**Ear, Nose, Sinus**
Operation	W	**Revision:** Correcting, to the extent possible, a portion of a malfunctioning device or the position of a displaced device

Body Part (4th)	Approach (5th)	Device (6th)	Qualifier (7th)
H Ear, Right **J** Ear, Left **K** Nasal Mucosa and Soft Tissue	**X** External	**0** Drainage Device **7** Autologous Tissue Substitute **D** Intraluminal Device **J** Synthetic Substitute **K** Nonautologous Tissue Substitute	**Z** No Qualifier
Y Sinus	**0** Open **3** Percutaneous **4** Percutaneous Endoscopic	**0** Drainage Device **Y** Other Device	**Z** No Qualifier
Y Sinus	**7** Via Natural or Artificial Opening **8** Via Natural or Artificial Opening Endoscopic	**Y** Other Device	**Z** No Qualifier
Y Sinus	**X** External	**0** Drainage Device	**Z** No Qualifier

AHA Coding Clinic

093K8ZZ Control Bleeding in Nasal Mucosa and Soft Tissue, Via Natural or Artificial Opening Endoscopic—AHA CC: 4Q, 2018, 38

09QKXZZ Repair Nasal Mucosa and Soft Tissue, External Approach—AHA CC: 4Q, 2014, 20-21

09QT4ZZ Repair Left Frontal Sinus, Percutaneous Endoscopic Approach—AHA CC: 4Q, 2013, 114

09QW0ZZ Repair Right Sphenoid Sinus, Open Approach—AHA CC: 3Q, 2014, 22-23

09QX0ZZ Repair Left Sphenoid Sinus, Open Approach—AHA CC: 3Q, 2014, 22-23

Topography of Lungs: Anterior View

Thyroid cartilage

Cricoid cartilage

Thyroid gland

Trachea

Cervical (cupula, or dome, of) parietal pleura

Jugular (suprasternal) notch

Sternoclavicular joint

Apex of lung

Clavicle

Arch of aorta

1st rib and costal cartilage

Cardiac notch of left lung

Right border of heart

Left border of heart

Horizontal fissure of right lung (often incomplete)

Right nipple

Left nipple

Costomediastinal recess of pleural cavity

Oblique fissure of right lung

Oblique fissure of left lung

Costodiaphragmatic recess of pleural cavity

Costodiaphragmatic recess of pleural cavity

Spleen

Inferior border of right lung

Inferior border of left lung

Pleural reflection

Left dome of diaphragm

Gallbladder

Pleural reflection

Stomach

Right dome of diaphragm

Liver

Xiphoid process

Bare area of pericardium

Medical and Surgical, Respiratory System

Structure of the Trachea and Major Bronchi

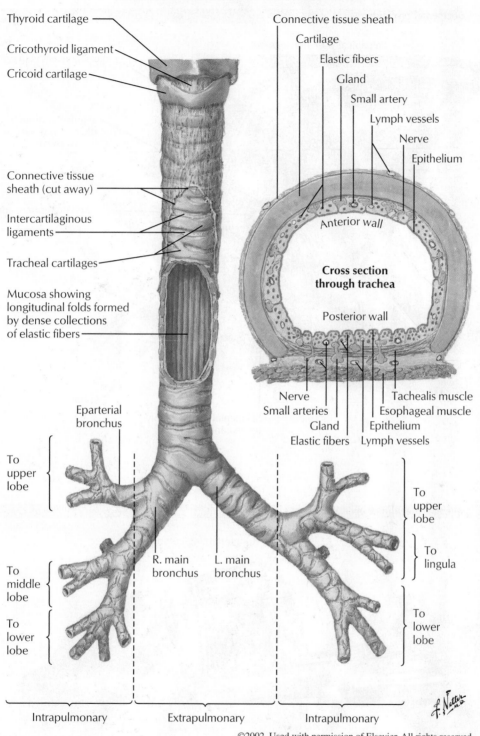

Thyroid cartilage

Cricothyroid ligament

Cricoid cartilage

Connective tissue sheath (cut away)

Intercartilaginous ligaments

Tracheal cartilages

Mucosa showing longitudinal folds formed by dense collections of elastic fibers

Connective tissue sheath

Cartilage

Elastic fibers

Gland

Small artery

Lymph vessels

Nerve

Epithelium

Anterior wall

Cross section through trachea

Posterior wall

Nerve

Small arteries

Gland

Elastic fibers

Tachealis muscle

Esophageal muscle

Epithelium

Lymph vessels

Eparterial bronchus

To upper lobe

To middle lobe

To lower lobe

R. main bronchus

L. main bronchus

To upper lobe

To lingula

To lower lobe

Intrapulmonary

Extrapulmonary

Intrapulmonary

Medical and Surgical, Respiratory System

Sublobar Resection and Surgical Lung Biopsy

Left apical-posterior segment

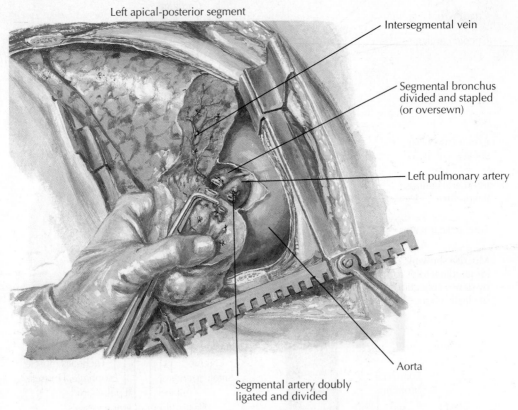

Intersegmental vein

Segmental bronchus divided and stapled (or oversewn)

Left pulmonary artery

Aorta

Segmental artery doubly ligated and divided

Wedge resection or open lung biopsy

Using stapling-cutting device

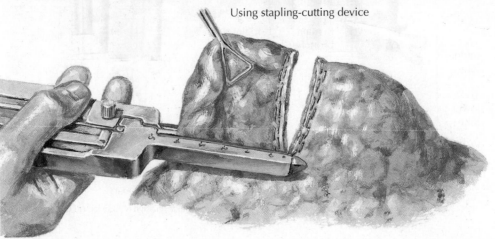

Respiratory System Tables 0B1–0BY

Section	0	Medical and Surgical
Body System	B	Respiratory System
Operation	1	**Bypass:** Altering the route of passage of the contents of a tubular body part

Body Part (4th)	Approach (5th)	Device (6th)	Qualifier (7th)
1 Trachea	0 Open	D Intraluminal Device	6 Esophagus
1 Trachea	0 Open	F Tracheostomy Device Z No Device	4 Cutaneous
1 Trachea	3 Percutaneous 4 Percutaneous Endoscopic	F Tracheostomy Device Z No Device	4 Cutaneous

Section	0	Medical and Surgical
Body System	B	Respiratory System
Operation	2	**Change:** Taking out or off a device from a body part and putting back an identical or similar device in or on the same body part without cutting or puncturing the skin or a mucous membrane

Body Part (4th)	Approach (5th)	Device (6th)	Qualifier (7th)
0 Tracheobronchial Tree K Lung, Right L Lung, Left Q Pleura T Diaphragm	X External	0 Drainage Device Y Other Device	Z No Qualifier
1 Trachea	X External	0 Drainage Device E Intraluminal Device, Endotracheal Airway F Tracheostomy Device Y Other Device	Z No Qualifier

Section	0	Medical and Surgical
Body System	B	Respiratory System
Operation	5	**Destruction:** Physical eradication of all or a portion of a body part by the direct use of energy, force, or a destructive agent

Body Part (4th)	Approach (5th)	Device (6th)	Qualifier (7th)
1 Trachea 2 Carina 3 Main Bronchus, Right 4 Upper Lobe Bronchus, Right 5 Middle Lobe Bronchus, Right 6 Lower Lobe Bronchus, Right 7 Main Bronchus, Left 8 Upper Lobe Bronchus, Left 9 Lingula Bronchus B Lower Lobe Bronchus, Left C Upper Lung Lobe, Right D Middle Lung Lobe, Right F Lower Lung Lobe, Right G Upper Lung Lobe, Left H Lung Lingula J Lower Lung Lobe, Left K Lung, Right L Lung, Left M Lungs, Bilateral	0 Open 3 Percutaneous 4 Percutaneous Endoscopic 7 Via Natural or Artificial Opening 8 Via Natural or Artificial Opening Endoscopic	Z No Device	Z No Qualifier
N Pleura, Right P Pleura, Left T Diaphragm	0 Open 3 Percutaneous 4 Percutaneous Endoscopic	Z No Device	Z No Qualifier

Section	0	Medical and Surgical
Body System	B	Respiratory System
Operation	7	**Dilation:** Expanding an orifice or the lumen of a tubular body part

Body Part (4th)	Approach (5th)	Device (6th)	Qualifier (7th)
1 Trachea 2 Carina 3 Main Bronchus, Right 4 Upper Lobe Bronchus, Right 5 Middle Lobe Bronchus, Right 6 Lower Lobe Bronchus, Right 7 Main Bronchus, Left 8 Upper Lobe Bronchus, Left 9 Lingula Bronchus B Lower Lobe Bronchus, Left	0 Open 3 Percutaneous 4 Percutaneous Endoscopic 7 Via Natural or Artificial Opening 8 Via Natural or Artificial Opening Endoscopic	D Intraluminal Device Z No Device	Z No Qualifier

Section	0	Medical and Surgical
Body System	B	Respiratory System
Operation	9	**Drainage:** Taking or letting out fluids and/or gases from a body part

Body Part (4th)	Approach (5th)	Device (6th)	Qualifier (7th)
1 Trachea 2 Carina 3 Main Bronchus, Right 4 Upper Lobe Bronchus, Right 5 Middle Lobe Bronchus, Right 6 Lower Lobe Bronchus, Right 7 Main Bronchus, Left 8 Upper Lobe Bronchus, Left 9 Lingula Bronchus B Lower Lobe Bronchus, Left C Upper Lung Lobe, Right D Middle Lung Lobe, Right F Lower Lung Lobe, Right G Upper Lung Lobe, Left H Lung Lingula J Lower Lung Lobe, Left K Lung, Right L Lung, Left M Lungs, Bilateral	0 Open 3 Percutaneous 4 Percutaneous Endoscopic 7 Via Natural or Artificial Opening 8 Via Natural or Artificial Opening Endoscopic	0 Drainage Device	Z No Qualifier
1 Trachea 2 Carina 3 Main Bronchus, Right 4 Upper Lobe Bronchus, Right 5 Middle Lobe Bronchus, Right 6 Lower Lobe Bronchus, Right 7 Main Bronchus, Left 8 Upper Lobe Bronchus, Left 9 Lingula Bronchus B Lower Lobe Bronchus, Left C Upper Lung Lobe, Right D Middle Lung Lobe, Right F Lower Lung Lobe, Right G Upper Lung Lobe, Left H Lung Lingula J Lower Lung Lobe, Left K Lung, Right L Lung, Left M Lungs, Bilateral	0 Open 3 Percutaneous 4 Percutaneous Endoscopic 7 Via Natural or Artificial Opening 8 Via Natural or Artificial Opening Endoscopic	Z No Device	X Diagnostic Z No Qualifier
N Pleura, Right P Pleura, Left	0 Open 3 Percutaneous 4 Percutaneous Endoscopic 8 Via Natural or Artificial Opening Endoscopic	0 Drainage Device	Z No Qualifier

Continued →

Section **0** **Medical and Surgical**
Body System **B** **Respiratory System**
Operation **9** **Drainage:** Taking or letting out fluids and/or gases from a body part

Body Part (4th)	Approach (5th)	Device (6th)	Qualifier (7th)
N Pleura, Right P Pleura, Left	0 Open 3 Percutaneous 4 Percutaneous Endoscopic 8 Via Natural or Artificial Opening Endoscopic	Z No Device	X Diagnostic Z No Qualifier
T Diaphragm	0 Open 3 Percutaneous 4 Percutaneous Endoscopic	0 Drainage Device	Z No Qualifier
T Diaphragm	0 Open 3 Percutaneous 4 Percutaneous Endoscopic	Z No Device	X Diagnostic Z No Qualifier

Section **0** **Medical and Surgical**
Body System **B** **Respiratory System**
Operation **B** **Excision:** Cutting out or off, without replacement, a portion of a body part

Body Part (4th)	Approach (5th)	Device (6th)	Qualifier (7th)
1 Trachea 2 Carina 3 Main Bronchus, Right 4 Upper Lobe Bronchus, Right 5 Middle Lobe Bronchus, Right 6 Lower Lobe Bronchus, Right 7 Main Bronchus, Left 8 Upper Lobe Bronchus, Left 9 Lingula Bronchus B Lower Lobe Bronchus, Left C Upper Lung Lobe, Right D Middle Lung Lobe, Right F Lower Lung Lobe, Right G Upper Lung Lobe, Left H Lung Lingula J Lower Lung Lobe, Left K Lung, Right L Lung, Left M Lungs, Bilateral	0 Open 3 Percutaneous 4 Percutaneous Endoscopic 7 Via Natural or Artificial Opening 8 Via Natural or Artificial Opening Endoscopic	Z No Device	X Diagnostic Z No Qualifier
N Pleura, Right P Pleura, Left	0 Open 3 Percutaneous 4 Percutaneous Endoscopic 8 Via Natural or Artificial Opening Endoscopic	Z No Device	X Diagnostic Z No Qualifier
T Diaphragm	0 Open 3 Percutaneous 4 Percutaneous Endoscopic	Z No Device	X Diagnostic Z No Qualifier

Section	0	Medical and Surgical
Body System	B	Respiratory System
Operation	C	**Extirpation:** Taking or cutting out solid matter from a body part

Body Part (4ᵗʰ)	Approach (5ᵗʰ)	Device (6ᵗʰ)	Qualifier (7ᵗʰ)
1 Trachea 2 Carina 3 Main Bronchus, Right 4 Upper Lobe Bronchus, Right 5 Middle Lobe Bronchus, Right 6 Lower Lobe Bronchus, Right 7 Main Bronchus, Left 8 Upper Lobe Bronchus, Left 9 Lingula Bronchus B Lower Lobe Bronchus, Left C Upper Lung Lobe, Right D Middle Lung Lobe, Right F Lower Lung Lobe, Right G Upper Lung Lobe, Left H Lung Lingula J Lower Lung Lobe, Left K Lung, Right L Lung, Left M Lungs, Bilateral	0 Open 3 Percutaneous 4 Percutaneous Endoscopic 7 Via Natural or Artificial Opening 8 Via Natural or Artificial Opening Endoscopic	Z No Device	Z No Qualifier
N Pleura, Right P Pleura, Left T Diaphragm	0 Open 3 Percutaneous 4 Percutaneous Endoscopic	Z No Device	Z No Qualifier

Section	0	Medical and Surgical
Body System	B	Respiratory System
Operation	D	**Extraction:** Pulling or stripping out or off all or a portion of a body part by the use of force

Body Part (4ᵗʰ)	Approach (5ᵗʰ)	Device (6ᵗʰ)	Qualifier (7ᵗʰ)
1 Trachea 2 Carina 3 Main Bronchus, Right 4 Upper Lobe Bronchus, Right 5 Middle Lobe Bronchus, Right 6 Lower Lobe Bronchus, Right 7 Main Bronchus, Left 8 Upper Lobe Bronchus, Left 9 Lingula Bronchus B Lower Lobe Bronchus, Left C Upper Lung Lobe, Right D Middle Lung Lobe, Right F Lower Lung Lobe, Right G Upper Lung Lobe, Left H Lung Lingula J Lower Lung Lobe, Left K Lung, Right L Lung, Left M Lung, Bilateral	4 Percutaneous Endoscopic 8 Via Natural or Artificial Opening Endoscopic	Z No Device	X Diagnostic
N Pleura, Right P Pleura, Left	0 Open 3 Percutaneous 4 Percutaneous Endoscopic	Z No Device	X Diagnostic Z No Qualifier

242

Section 0 **Medical and Surgical**
Body System B **Respiratory System**
Operation F **Fragmentation:** Breaking solid matter in a body part into pieces

Body Part (4th)	Approach (5th)	Device (6th)	Qualifier (7th)
1 Trachea 2 Carina 3 Main Bronchus, Right 4 Upper Lobe Bronchus, Right 5 Middle Lobe Bronchus, Right 6 Lower Lobe Bronchus, Right 7 Main Bronchus, Left 8 Upper Lobe Bronchus, Left 9 Lingula Bronchus B Lower Lobe Bronchus, Left	0 Open 3 Percutaneous 4 Percutaneous Endoscopic 7 Via Natural or Artificial Opening 8 Via Natural or Artificial Opening Endoscopic X External	Z No Device	Z No Qualifier

Section 0 **Medical and Surgical**
Body System B **Respiratory System**
Operation H **Insertion:** Putting in a nonbiological appliance that monitors, assists, performs, or prevents a physiological function but does not physically take the place of a body part

Body Part (4th)	Approach (5th)	Device (6th)	Qualifier (7th)
0 Tracheobronchial Tree	0 Open 3 Percutaneous 4 Percutaneous Endoscopic 7 Via Natural or Artificial Opening 8 Via Natural or Artificial Opening Endoscopic	1 Radioactive Element 2 Monitoring Device 3 Infusion Device D Intraluminal Device Y Other Device	Z No Qualifier
1 Trachea	0 Open	2 Monitoring Device D Intraluminal Device Y Other Device	Z No Qualifier
1 Trachea	3 Percutaneous	D Intraluminal Device E Intraluminal Device, Endotracheal Airway Y Other Device	Z No Qualifier
1 Trachea	4 Percutaneous Endoscopic	D Intraluminal Device Y Other Device	Z No Qualifier
1 Trachea	7 Via Natural or Artificial Opening 8 Via Natural or Artificial Opening Endoscopic	2 Monitoring Device D Intraluminal Device E Intraluminal Device, Endotracheal Airway Y Other Device	Z No Qualifier
3 Main Bronchus, Right 4 Upper Lobe Bronchus, Right 5 Middle Lobe Bronchus, Right 6 Lower Lobe Bronchus, Right 7 Main Bronchus, Left 8 Upper Lobe Bronchus, Left 9 Lingula Bronchus B Lower Lobe Bronchus, Left	0 Open 3 Percutaneous 4 Percutaneous Endoscopic 7 Via Natural or Artificial Opening 8 Via Natural or Artificial Opening Endoscopic	G Intraluminal Device, Endobronchial Valve	Z No Qualifier
K Lung, Right L Lung, Left	0 Open 3 Percutaneous 4 Percutaneous Endoscopic 7 Via Natural or Artificial Opening 8 Via Natural or Artificial Opening Endoscopic	1 Radioactive Element 2 Monitoring Device 3 Infusion Device Y Other Device	Z No Qualifier
Q Pleura	0 Open 3 Percutaneous 4 Percutaneous Endoscopic 7 Via Natural or Artificial Opening 8 Via Natural or Artificial Opening Endoscopic	Y Other Device	Z No Qualifier

Continued →

Section 0 **Medical and Surgical**
Body System B **Respiratory System**
Operation H **Insertion:** Putting in a nonbiological appliance that monitors, assists, performs, or prevents a physiological function but does not physically take the place of a body part

Body Part (4th)	Approach (5th)	Device (6th)	Qualifier (7th)
T Diaphragm	0 Open 3 Percutaneous 4 Percutaneous Endoscopic	2 Monitoring Device M Diaphragmatic Pacemaker Lead Y Other Device	Z No Qualifier
T Diaphragm	7 Via Natural or Artificial Opening 8 Via Natural or Artificial Opening Endoscopic	Y Other Device	Z No Qualifier

Section 0 **Medical and Surgical**
Body System B **Respiratory System**
Operation J **Inspection:** Visually and/or manually exploring a body part

Body Part (4th)	Approach (5th)	Device (6th)	Qualifier (7th)
0 Tracheobronchial Tree 1 Trachea K Lung, Right L Lung, Left Q Pleura T Diaphragm	0 Open 3 Percutaneous 4 Percutaneous Endoscopic 7 Via Natural or Artificial Opening 8 Via Natural or Artificial Opening Endoscopic X External	Z No Device	Z No Qualifier

Section 0 **Medical and Surgical**
Body System B **Respiratory System**
Operation L **Occlusion:** Completely closing an orifice or the lumen of a tubular body part

Body Part (4th)	Approach (5th)	Device (6th)	Qualifier (7th)
1 Trachea 2 Carina 3 Main Bronchus, Right 4 Upper Lobe Bronchus, Right 5 Middle Lobe Bronchus, Right 6 Lower Lobe Bronchus, Right 7 Main Bronchus, Left 8 Upper Lobe Bronchus, Left 9 Lingula Bronchus B Lower Lobe Bronchus, Left	0 Open 3 Percutaneous 4 Percutaneous Endoscopic	C Extraluminal Device D Intraluminal Device Z No Device	Z No Qualifier
1 Trachea 2 Carina 3 Main Bronchus, Right 4 Upper Lobe Bronchus, Right 5 Middle Lobe Bronchus, Right 6 Lower Lobe Bronchus, Right 7 Main Bronchus, Left 8 Upper Lobe Bronchus, Left 9 Lingula Bronchus B Lower Lobe Bronchus, Left	7 Via Natural or Artificial Opening 8 Via Natural or Artificial Opening Endoscopic	D Intraluminal Device Z No Device	Z No Qualifier

Section	0	Medical and Surgical
Body System	B	Respiratory System
Operation	M	**Reattachment:** Putting back in or on all or a portion of a separated body part to its normal location or other suitable location

Body Part (4ᵗʰ)	Approach (5ᵗʰ)	Device (6ᵗʰ)	Qualifier (7ᵗʰ)
1 Trachea 2 Carina 3 Main Bronchus, Right 4 Upper Lobe Bronchus, Right 5 Middle Lobe Bronchus, Right 6 Lower Lobe Bronchus, Right 7 Main Bronchus, Left 8 Upper Lobe Bronchus, Left 9 Lingula Bronchus B Lower Lobe Bronchus, Left C Upper Lung Lobe, Right D Middle Lung Lobe, Right F Lower Lung Lobe, Right G Upper Lung Lobe, Left H Lung Lingula J Lower Lung Lobe, Left K Lung, Right L Lung, Left T Diaphragm	0 Open	Z No Device	Z No Qualifier

Section	0	Medical and Surgical
Body System	B	Respiratory System
Operation	N	**Release:** Freeing a body part from an abnormal physical constraint by cutting or by the use of force

Body Part (4ᵗʰ)	Approach (5ᵗʰ)	Device (6ᵗʰ)	Qualifier (7ᵗʰ)
1 Trachea 2 Carina 3 Main Bronchus, Right 4 Upper Lobe Bronchus, Right 5 Middle Lobe Bronchus, Right 6 Lower Lobe Bronchus, Right 7 Main Bronchus, Left 8 Upper Lobe Bronchus, Left 9 Lingula Bronchus B Lower Lobe Bronchus, Left C Upper Lung Lobe, Right D Middle Lung Lobe, Right F Lower Lung Lobe, Right G Upper Lung Lobe, Left H Lung Lingula J Lower Lung Lobe, Left K Lung, Right L Lung, Left M Lungs, Bilateral	0 Open 3 Percutaneous 4 Percutaneous Endoscopic 7 Via Natural or Artificial Opening 8 Via Natural or Artificial Opening Endoscopic	Z No Device	Z No Qualifier
N Pleura, Right P Pleura, Left T Diaphragm	0 Open 3 Percutaneous 4 Percutaneous Endoscopic	Z No Device	Z No Qualifier

Section	0	Medical and Surgical
Body System	B	Respiratory System
Operation	P	Removal: Taking out or off a device from a body part

Body Part (4th)	Approach (5th)	Device (6th)	Qualifier (7th)
0 Tracheobronchial Tree	0 Open 3 Percutaneous 4 Percutaneous Endoscopic 7 Via Natural or Artificial Opening 8 Via Natural or Artificial Opening Endoscopic	0 Drainage Device 1 Radioactive Element 2 Monitoring Device 3 Infusion Device 7 Autologous Tissue Substitute C Extraluminal Device D Intraluminal Device J Synthetic Substitute K Nonautologous Tissue Substitute Y Other Device	Z No Qualifier
0 Tracheobronchial Tree	X External	0 Drainage Device 1 Radioactive Element 2 Monitoring Device 3 Infusion Device D Intraluminal Device	Z No Qualifier
1 Trachea	0 Open 3 Percutaneous 4 Percutaneous Endoscopic 7 Via Natural or Artificial Opening 8 Via Natural or Artificial Opening Endoscopic	0 Drainage Device 2 Monitoring Device 7 Autologous Tissue Substitute C Extraluminal Device D Intraluminal Device F Tracheostomy Device J Synthetic Substitute K Nonautologous Tissue Substitute	Z No Qualifier
1 Trachea	X External	0 Drainage Device 2 Monitoring Device D Intraluminal Device F Tracheostomy Device	Z No Qualifier
K Lung, Right L Lung, Left	0 Open 3 Percutaneous 4 Percutaneous Endoscopic 7 Via Natural or Artificial Opening 8 Via Natural or Artificial Opening Endoscopic	0 Drainage Device 1 Radioactive Element 2 Monitoring Device 3 Infusion Device Y Other Device	Z No Qualifier
K Lung, Right L Lung, Left	X External	0 Drainage Device 1 Radioactive Element 2 Monitoring Device 3 Infusion Device	Z No Qualifier
Q Pleura	0 Open 3 Percutaneous 4 Percutaneous Endoscopic 7 Via Natural or Artificial Opening 8 Via Natural or Artificial Opening Endoscopic	0 Drainage Device 1 Radioactive Element 2 Monitoring Device Y Other Device	Z No Qualifier
Q Pleura	X External	0 Drainage Device 1 Radioactive Element 2 Monitoring Device	Z No Qualifier
T Diaphragm	0 Open 3 Percutaneous 4 Percutaneous Endoscopic 7 Via Natural or Artificial Opening 8 Via Natural or Artificial Opening Endoscopic	0 Drainage Device 2 Monitoring Device 7 Autologous Tissue Substitute J Synthetic Substitute K Nonautologous Tissue Substitute M Diaphragmatic Pacemaker Lead Y Other Device	Z No Qualifier
T Diaphragm	X External	0 Drainage Device 2 Monitoring Device M Diaphragmatic Pacemaker Lead	Z No Qualifier

Section	0	Medical and Surgical
Body System	B	Respiratory System
Operation	Q	**Repair:** Restoring, to the extent possible, a body part to its normal anatomic structure and function

Body Part (4ᵗʰ)	Approach (5ᵗʰ)	Device (6ᵗʰ)	Qualifier (7ᵗʰ)
1 Trachea 2 Carina 3 Main Bronchus, Right 4 Upper Lobe Bronchus, Right 5 Middle Lobe Bronchus, Right 6 Lower Lobe Bronchus, Right 7 Main Bronchus, Left 8 Upper Lobe Bronchus, Left 9 Lingula Bronchus B Lower Lobe Bronchus, Left C Upper Lung Lobe, Right D Middle Lung Lobe, Right F Lower Lung Lobe, Right G Upper Lung Lobe, Left H Lung Lingula J Lower Lung Lobe, Left K Lung, Right L Lung, Left M Lungs, Bilateral	0 Open 3 Percutaneous 4 Percutaneous Endoscopic 7 Via Natural or Artificial Opening 8 Via Natural or Artificial Opening Endoscopic	Z No Device	Z No Qualifier
N Pleura, Right P Pleura, Left T Diaphragm	0 Open 3 Percutaneous 4 Percutaneous Endoscopic	Z No Device	Z No Qualifier

Section	0	Medical and Surgical
Body System	B	Respiratory
Operation	R	**Replacement:** Putting in or on biological or synthetic material that physically takes the place and/or function of all or a portion of a body part

Body Part (4ᵗʰ)	Approach (5ᵗʰ)	Device (6ᵗʰ)	Qualifier (7ᵗʰ)
1 Trachea 2 Carina 3 Main Bronchus, Right 4 Upper Lobe Bronchus, Right 5 Middle Lobe Bronchus, Right 6 Lower Lobe Bronchus, Right 7 Main Bronchus, Left 8 Upper Lobe Bronchus, Left 9 Lingula Bronchus B Lower Lobe Bronchus, Left T Diaphragm	0 Open 4 Percutaneous Endoscopic	7 Autologous Tissue Substitute J Synthetic Substitute K Nonautologous Tissue Substitute	Z No Qualifier

Section   **0**   **Medical and Surgical**
Body System   **B**   **Respiratory System**
Operation   **S**   **Reposition:** Moving to its normal location, or other suitable location, all or a portion of a body part

Body Part (4th)	Approach (5th)	Device (6th)	Qualifier (7th)
1 Trachea	0 Open	Z No Device	Z No Qualifier
2 Carina			
3 Main Bronchus, Right			
4 Upper Lobe Bronchus, Right			
5 Middle Lobe Bronchus, Right			
6 Lower Lobe Bronchus, Right			
7 Main Bronchus, Left			
8 Upper Lobe Bronchus, Left			
9 Lingula Bronchus			
B Lower Lobe Bronchus, Left			
C Upper Lung Lobe, Right			
D Middle Lung Lobe, Right			
F Lower Lung Lobe, Right			
G Upper Lung Lobe, Left			
H Lung Lingula			
J Lower Lung Lobe, Left			
K Lung, Right			
L Lung, Left			
T Diaphragm			

Section   **0**   **Medical and Surgical**
Body System   **B**   **Respiratory System**
Operation   **T**   **Resection:** Cutting out or off, without replacement, all of a body part

Body Part (4th)	Approach (5th)	Device (6th)	Qualifier (7th)
1 Trachea	0 Open	Z No Device	Z No Qualifier
2 Carina	4 Percutaneous Endoscopic		
3 Main Bronchus, Right			
4 Upper Lobe Bronchus, Right			
5 Middle Lobe Bronchus, Right			
6 Lower Lobe Bronchus, Right			
7 Main Bronchus, Left			
8 Upper Lobe Bronchus, Left			
9 Lingula Bronchus			
B Lower Lobe Bronchus, Left			
C Upper Lung Lobe, Right			
D Middle Lung Lobe, Right			
F Lower Lung Lobe, Right			
G Upper Lung Lobe, Left			
H Lung Lingula			
J Lower Lung Lobe, Left			
K Lung, Right			
L Lung, Left			
M Lungs, Bilateral			
T Diaphragm			

Section 0 **Medical and Surgical**
Body System B **Respiratory System**
Operation U **Supplement:** Putting in or on biological or synthetic material that physically reinforces and/or augments the function of a portion of a body part

Body Part (4th)	Approach (5th)	Device (6th)	Qualifier (7th)
1 Trachea 2 Carina 3 Main Bronchus, Right 4 Upper Lobe Bronchus, Right 5 Middle Lobe Bronchus, Right 6 Lower Lobe Bronchus, Right 7 Main Bronchus, Left 8 Upper Lobe Bronchus, Left 9 Lingula Bronchus B Lower Lobe Bronchus, Left	0 Open 4 Percutaneous Endoscopic 8 Via Natural or Artificial Opening Endoscopic	7 Autologous Tissue Substitute J Synthetic Substitute K Nonautologous Tissue Substitute	Z No Qualifier
T Diaphragm	0 Open 4 Percutaneous Endoscopic	7 Autologous Tissue Substitute J Synthetic Substitute K Nonautologous Tissue Substitute	Z No Qualifier

Section 0 **Medical and Surgical**
Body System B **Respiratory System**
Operation V **Restriction:** Partially closing an orifice or the lumen of a tubular body part

Body Part (4th)	Approach (5th)	Device (6th)	Qualifier (7th)
1 Trachea 2 Carina 3 Main Bronchus, Right 4 Upper Lobe Bronchus, Right 5 Middle Lobe Bronchus, Right 6 Lower Lobe Bronchus, Right 7 Main Bronchus, Left 8 Upper Lobe Bronchus, Left 9 Lingula Bronchus B Lower Lobe Bronchus, Left	0 Open 3 Percutaneous 4 Percutaneous Endoscopic	C Extraluminal Device D Intraluminal Device Z No Device	Z No Qualifier
1 Trachea 2 Carina 3 Main Bronchus, Right 4 Upper Lobe Bronchus, Right 5 Middle Lobe Bronchus, Right 6 Lower Lobe Bronchus, Right 7 Main Bronchus, Left 8 Upper Lobe Bronchus, Left 9 Lingula Bronchus B Lower Lobe Bronchus, Left	7 Via Natural or Artificial Opening 8 Via Natural or Artificial Opening Endoscopic	D Intraluminal Device Z No Device	Z No Qualifier

Section 0 **Medical and Surgical**
Body System B **Respiratory System**
Operation W **Revision:** Correcting, to the extent possible, a portion of a malfunctioning device or the position of a displaced device

Body Part (4th)	Approach (5th)	Device (6th)	Qualifier (7th)
0 Tracheobronchial Tree	0 Open 3 Percutaneous 4 Percutaneous Endoscopic 7 Via Natural or Artificial Opening 8 Via Natural or Artificial Opening Endoscopic	0 Drainage Device 2 Monitoring Device 3 Infusion Device 7 Autologous Tissue Substitute C Extraluminal Device D Intraluminal Device J Synthetic Substitute K Nonautologous Tissue Substitute Y Other Device	Z No Qualifier

Continued →

Section	0	**Medical and Surgical**
Body System	B	**Respiratory System**
Operation	W	**Revision:** Correcting, to the extent possible, a portion of a malfunctioning device or the position of a displaced device

Body Part (4th)	Approach (5th)	Device (6th)	Qualifier (7th)
0 Tracheobronchial Tree	X External	0 Drainage Device 2 Monitoring Device 3 Infusion Device 7 Autologous Tissue Substitute C Extraluminal Device D Intraluminal Device J Synthetic Substitute K Nonautologous Tissue Substitute	Z No Qualifier
1 Trachea	0 Open 3 Percutaneous 4 Percutaneous Endoscopic 7 Via Natural or Artificial Opening 8 Via Natural or Artificial Opening Endoscopic X External	0 Drainage Device 2 Monitoring Device 7 Autologous Tissue Substitute C Extraluminal Device D Intraluminal Device F Tracheostomy Device J Synthetic Substitute K Nonautologous Tissue Substitute	Z No Qualifier
K Lung, Right L Lung, Left	0 Open 3 Percutaneous 4 Percutaneous Endoscopic 7 Via Natural or Artificial Opening 8 Via Natural or Artificial Opening Endoscopic	0 Drainage Device 2 Monitoring Device 3 Infusion Device Y Other Device	Z No Qualifier
K Lung, Right L Lung, Left	X External	0 Drainage Device 2 Monitoring Device 3 Infusion Device	Z No Qualifier
Q Pleura	0 Open 3 Percutaneous 4 Percutaneous Endoscopic 7 Via Natural or Artificial Opening 8 Via Natural or Artificial Opening Endoscopic	0 Drainage Device 2 Monitoring Device Y Other Device	Z No Qualifier
Q Pleura	X External	0 Drainage Device 2 Monitoring Device	Z No Qualifier
T Diaphragm	0 Open 3 Percutaneous 4 Percutaneous Endoscopic 7 Via Natural or Artificial Opening 8 Via Natural or Artificial Opening Endoscopic	0 Drainage Device 2 Monitoring Device 7 Autologous Tissue Substitute J Synthetic Substitute K Nonautologous Tissue Substitute M Diaphragmatic Pacemaker Lead Y Other Device	Z No Qualifier
T Diaphragm	X External	0 Drainage Device 2 Monitoring Device 7 Autologous Tissue Substitute J Synthetic Substitute K Nonautologous Tissue Substitute M Diaphragmatic Pacemaker Lead	Z No Qualifier

Section   0   **Medical and Surgical**
Body System   B   **Respiratory System**
Operation   Y   **Transplantation:** Putting in or on all or a portion of a living body part taken from another individual or animal to physically take the place and/or function of all or a portion of a similar body part

Body Part (4ᵗʰ)	Approach (5ᵗʰ)	Device (6ᵗʰ)	Qualifier (7ᵗʰ)
C Upper Lung Lobe, Right **D** Middle Lung Lobe, Right **F** Lower Lung Lobe, Right **G** Upper Lung Lobe, Left **H** Lung Lingula **J** Lower Lung Lobe, Left **K** Lung, Right **L** Lung, Left **M** Lungs, Bilateral	**0** Open	**Z** No Device	**0** Allogeneic **1** Syngeneic **2** Zooplastic

AHA Coding Clinic

0B5P0ZZ Destruction of Left Pleura, Open Approach—AHA CC: 2Q, 2016, 17-18

0B948ZX Drainage of Right Upper Lobe Bronchus, Via Natural or Artificial Opening Endoscopic, Diagnostic—AHA CC: 1Q, 2016, 26-27

0B988ZX Drainage of Left Upper Lobe Bronchus, Via Natural or Artificial Opening Endoscopic, Diagnostic—AHA CC: 1Q, 2016, 27

0B9J8ZX Drainage of Left Lower Lung Lobe, Via Natural or Artificial Opening Endoscopic, Diagnostic—AHA CC: 1Q, 2016, 26-27; 1Q, 2017, 51

0B9M8ZZ Drainage of Bilateral Lungs, Via Natural or Artificial Opening Endoscopic—AHA CC: 3Q, 2017, 15

0BB10ZZ Excision of Trachea, Open Approach—AHA CC: 1Q, 2015, 15-16

0BB48ZX Excision of Right Upper Lobe Bronchus, Via Natural or Artificial Opening Endoscopic, Diagnostic—AHA CC: 1Q, 2016, 26-27

0BB88ZX Excision of Left Upper Lobe Bronchus, Via Natural or Artificial Opening Endoscopic, Diagnostic—AHA CC: 1Q, 2016, 27

0BBC8ZX Excision of Right Upper Lung Lobe, Via Natural or Artificial Opening Endoscopic, Diagnostic—AHA CC: 1Q, 2016, 26-27

0BBK8ZX Excision of Right Lung, Via Natural or Artificial Opening Endoscopic, Diagnostic—AHA CC: 1Q, 2014, 20-21

0BC58ZZ Extirpation of Matter from Right Middle Lobe Bronchus, Via Natural or Artificial Opening Endoscopic—AHA CC: 3Q, 2017, 14-15

0BH17EZ Insertion of Endotracheal Airway into Trachea, Via Natural or Artificial Opening—AHA CC: 4Q, 2014, 3-15

0BH18EZ Insertion of Endotracheal Airway into Trachea, Via Natural or Artificial Opening Endoscopic—AHA CC: 4Q, 2014, 3-15

0BHB8GZ Insertion of Endobronchial Valve into Left Lower Lobe Bronchus, Via Natural or Artificial Opening Endoscopic—AHA CC: 3Q, 2019, 33-34

0BJL8ZZ Inspection of Left Lung, Via Natural or Artificial Opening Endoscopic—AHA CC: 1Q, 2014, 20

0BJQ4ZZ Inspection of Pleura, Percutaneous Endoscopic Approach—AHA CC: 2Q, 2015, 31

0BN10ZZ Release Trachea, Open Approach—AHA CC: 3Q, 2015, 15-16

0BNL0ZZ Release Left Lung, Open Approach—AHA CC: 3Q, 2018, 28

0BNN0ZZ Release Right Pleura, Open Approach—AHA CC: 2Q, 2019, 20-21

0BU307Z Supplement Right Main Bronchus with Autologous Tissue Substitute, Open Approach—AHA CC: 1Q, 2015, 28-29

Oral Cavity

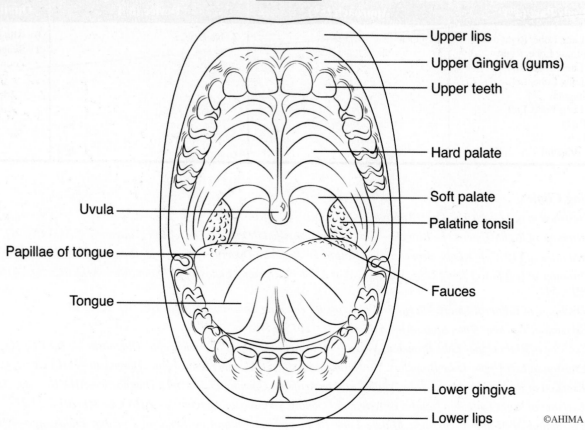

Upper lips

Upper Gingiva (gums)

Upper teeth

Hard palate

Soft palate

Uvula

Palatine tonsil

Papillae of tongue

Fauces

Tongue

Lower gingiva

Lower lips

©AHIMA

Glands of the Oral Cavity

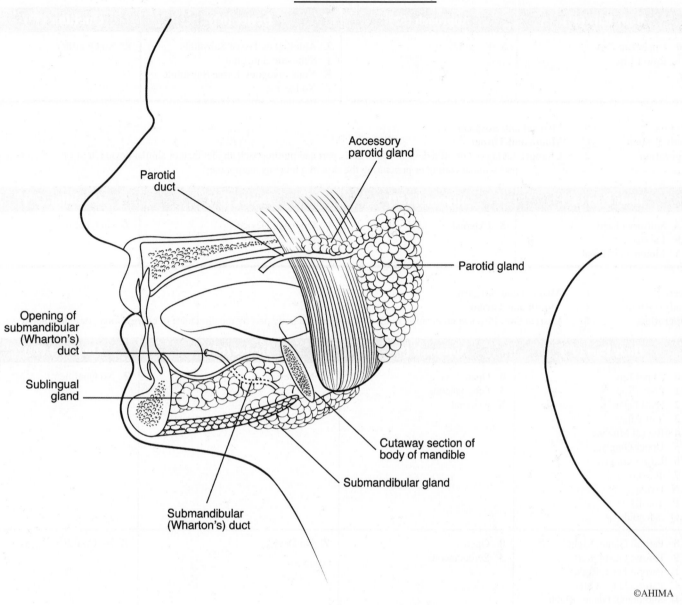

Accessory parotid gland

Parotid duct

Parotid gland

Opening of submandibular (Wharton's) duct

Sublingual gland

Cutaway section of body of mandible

Submandibular gland

Submandibular (Wharton's) duct

©AHIMA

Throat

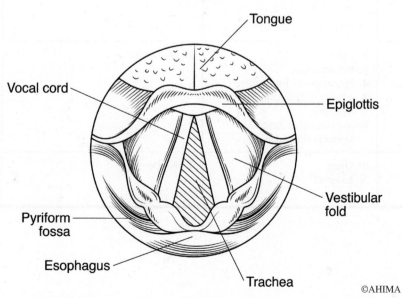

Tongue

Vocal cord

Epiglottis

Pyriform fossa

Vestibular fold

Esophagus

Trachea

©AHIMA

Mouth and Throat Tables 0C0–0CX

Section	0	Medical and Surgical
Body System	C	Mouth and Throat
Operation	0	**Alteration:** Modifying the anatomic structure of a body part without affecting the function of the body part

Body Part (4th)	Approach (5th)	Device (6th)	Qualifier (7th)
0 Upper Lip 1 Lower Lip	X External	7 Autologous Tissue Substitute J Synthetic Substitute K Nonautologous Tissue Substitute Z No Device	Z No Qualifier

Section	0	Medical and Surgical
Body System	C	Mouth and Throat
Operation	2	**Change:** Taking out or off a device from a body part and putting back an identical or similar device in or on the same body part without cutting or puncturing the skin or a mucous membrane

Body Part (4th)	Approach (5th)	Device (6th)	Qualifier (7th)
A Salivary Gland S Larynx Y Mouth and Throat	X External	0 Drainage Device Y Other Device	Z No Qualifier

Section	0	Medical and Surgical
Body System	C	Mouth and Throat
Operation	5	**Destruction:** Physical eradication of all or a portion of a body part by the direct use of energy, force, or a destructive agent

Body Part (4th)	Approach (5th)	Device (6th)	Qualifier (7th)
0 Upper Lip 1 Lower Lip 2 Hard Palate 3 Soft Palate 4 Buccal Mucosa 5 Upper Gingiva 6 Lower Gingiva 7 Tongue N Uvula P Tonsils Q Adenoids	0 Open 3 Percutaneous X External	Z No Device	Z No Qualifier
8 Parotid Gland, Right 9 Parotid Gland, Left B Parotid Duct, Right C Parotid Duct, Left D Sublingual Gland, Right F Sublingual Gland, Left G Submaxillary Gland, Right H Submaxillary Gland, Left J Minor Salivary Gland	0 Open 3 Percutaneous	Z No Device	Z No Qualifier
M Pharynx R Epiglottis S Larynx T Vocal Cord, Right V Vocal Cord, Left	0 Open 3 Percutaneous 4 Percutaneous Endoscopic 7 Via Natural or Artificial Opening 8 Via Natural or Artificial Opening Endoscopic	Z No Device	Z No Qualifier
W Upper Tooth X Lower Tooth	0 Open X External	Z No Device	0 Single 1 Multiple 2 All

Section 0 **Medical and Surgical**
Body System C **Mouth and Throat**
Operation 7 **Dilation:** Expanding an orifice or the lumen of a tubular body part

Body Part (4ᵗʰ)	Approach (5ᵗʰ)	Device (6ᵗʰ)	Qualifier (7ᵗʰ)
B Parotid Duct, Right C Parotid Duct, Left	0 Open 3 Percutaneous 7 Via Natural or Artificial Opening	D Intraluminal Device Z No Device	Z No Qualifier
M Pharynx	7 Via Natural or Artificial Opening 8 Via Natural or Artificial Opening Endoscopic	D Intraluminal Device Z No Device	Z No Qualifier
S Larynx	0 Open 3 Percutaneous 4 Percutaneous Endoscopic 7 Via Natural or Artificial Opening 8 Via Natural or Artificial Opening Endoscopic	D Intraluminal Device Z No Device	Z No Qualifier

Section 0 **Medical and Surgical**
Body System C **Mouth and Throat**
Operation 9 **Drainage:** Taking or letting out fluids and/or gases from a body part

Body Part (4ᵗʰ)	Approach (5ᵗʰ)	Device (6ᵗʰ)	Qualifier (7ᵗʰ)
0 Upper Lip 1 Lower Lip 2 Hard Palate 3 Soft Palate 4 Buccal Mucosa 5 Upper Gingiva 6 Lower Gingiva 7 Tongue N Uvula P Tonsils Q Adenoids	0 Open 3 Percutaneous X External	0 Drainage Device	Z No Qualifier
0 Upper Lip 1 Lower Lip 2 Hard Palate 3 Soft Palate 4 Buccal Mucosa 5 Upper Gingiva 6 Lower Gingiva 7 Tongue N Uvula P Tonsils Q Adenoids	0 Open 3 Percutaneous X External	Z No Device	X Diagnostic Z No Qualifier
8 Parotid Gland, Right 9 Parotid Gland, Left B Parotid Duct, Right C Parotid Duct, Left D Sublingual Gland, Right F Sublingual Gland, Left G Submaxillary Gland, Right H Submaxillary Gland, Left J Minor Salivary Gland	0 Open 3 Percutaneous	0 Drainage Device	Z No Qualifier
8 Parotid Gland, Right 9 Parotid Gland, Left B Parotid Duct, Right C Parotid Duct, Left D Sublingual Gland, Right F Sublingual Gland, Left G Submaxillary Gland, Right H Submaxillary Gland, Left J Minor Salivary Gland	0 Open 3 Percutaneous	Z No Device	X Diagnostic Z No Qualifier

Continued →

Section	0	Medical and Surgical
Body System	C	Mouth and Throat
Operation	9	**Drainage:** Taking or letting out fluids and/or gases from a body part

Body Part (4th)	Approach (5th)	Device (6th)	Qualifier (7th)
M Pharynx R Epiglottis S Larynx T Vocal Cord, Right V Vocal Cord, Left	0 Open 3 Percutaneous 4 Percutaneous Endoscopic 7 Via Natural or Artificial Opening 8 Via Natural or Artificial Opening Endoscopic	0 Drainage Device	Z No Qualifier
M Pharynx R Epiglottis S Larynx T Vocal Cord, Right V Vocal Cord, Left	0 Open 3 Percutaneous 4 Percutaneous Endoscopic 7 Via Natural or Artificial Opening 8 Via Natural or Artificial Opening Endoscopic	Z No Device	X Diagnostic Z No Qualifier
W Upper Tooth X Lower Tooth	0 Open X External	0 Drainage Device Z No Device	0 Single 1 Multiple 2 All

Section	0	Medical and Surgical
Body System	C	Mouth and Throat
Operation	B	**Excision:** Cutting out or off, without replacement, a portion of a body part

Body Part (4th)	Approach (5th)	Device (6th)	Qualifier (7th)
0 Upper Lip 1 Lower Lip 2 Hard Palate 3 Soft Palate 4 Buccal Mucosa 5 Upper Gingiva 6 Lower Gingiva 7 Tongue N Uvula P Tonsils Q Adenoids	0 Open 3 Percutaneous X External	Z No Device	X Diagnostic Z No Qualifier
8 Parotid Gland, Right 9 Parotid Gland, Left B Parotid Duct, Right C Parotid Duct, Left D Sublingual Gland, Right F Sublingual Gland, Left G Submaxillary Gland, Right H Submaxillary Gland, Left J Minor Salivary Gland	0 Open 3 Percutaneous	Z No Device	X Diagnostic Z No Qualifier
M Pharynx R Epiglottis S Larynx T Vocal Cord, Right V Vocal Cord, Left	0 Open 3 Percutaneous 4 Percutaneous Endoscopic 7 Via Natural or Artificial Opening 8 Via Natural or Artificial Opening Endoscopic	Z No Device	X Diagnostic Z No Qualifier
W Upper Tooth X Lower Tooth	0 Open X External	Z No Device	0 Single 1 Multiple 2 All

	Section	0	Medical and Surgical
Body System	C	Mouth and Throat
Operation	C	Extirpation: Taking or cutting out solid matter from a body part

Body Part (4th)	Approach (5th)	Device (6th)	Qualifier (7th)
0 Upper Lip 1 Lower Lip 2 Hard Palate 3 Soft Palate 4 Buccal Mucosa 5 Upper Gingiva 6 Lower Gingiva 7 Tongue N Uvula P Tonsils Q Adenoids	0 Open 3 Percutaneous X External	Z No Device	Z No Qualifier
8 Parotid Gland, Right 9 Parotid Gland, Left B Parotid Duct, Right C Parotid Duct, Left D Sublingual Gland, Right F Sublingual Gland, Left G Submaxillary Gland, Right H Submaxillary Gland, Left J Minor Salivary Gland	0 Open 3 Percutaneous	Z No Device	Z No Qualifier
M Pharynx R Epiglottis S Larynx T Vocal Cord, Right V Vocal Cord, Left	0 Open 3 Percutaneous 4 Percutaneous Endoscopic 7 Via Natural or Artificial Opening 8 Via Natural or Artificial Opening Endoscopic	Z No Device	Z No Qualifier
W Upper Tooth X Lower Tooth	0 Open X External	Z No Device	0 Single 1 Multiple 2 All

	Section	0	Medical and Surgical
Body System	C	Mouth and Throat
Operation	D	Extraction: Pulling or stripping out or off all or a portion of a body part by the use of force

Body Part (4th)	Approach (5th)	Device (6th)	Qualifier (7th)
T Vocal Cord, Right V Vocal Cord, Left	0 Open 3 Percutaneous 4 Percutaneous Endoscopic 7 Via Natural or Artificial Opening 8 Via Natural or Artificial Opening Endoscopic	Z No Device	Z No Qualifier
W Upper Tooth X Lower Tooth	X External	Z No Device	0 Single 1 Multiple 2 All

	Section	0	Medical and Surgical
Body System	C	Mouth and Throat
Operation	F	Fragmentation: Breaking solid matter in a body part into pieces

Body Part (4th)	Approach (5th)	Device (6th)	Qualifier (7th)
B Parotid Duct, Right C Parotid Duct, Left	0 Open 3 Percutaneous 7 Via Natural or Artificial Opening X External	Z No Device	Z No Qualifier

Section	0	Medical and Surgical
Body System	C	Mouth and Throat
Operation	H	**Insertion:** Putting in a nonbiological appliance that monitors, assists, performs, or prevents a physiological function but does not physically take the place of a body part

Body Part (4th)	Approach (5th)	Device (6th)	Qualifier (7th)
7 Tongue	**0** Open **3** Percutaneous **X** External	**1** Radioactive Element	**Z** No Qualifier
A Salivary Gland **S** Larynx	**0** Open **3** Percutaneous **7** Via Natural or Artificial Opening **8** Via Natural or Artificial Opening Endoscopic	**1** Radioactive Element **Y** Other Device	**Z** No Qualifier
Y Mouth and Throat	**0** Open **3** Percutaneous	**1** Radioactive Element **Y** Other Device	**Z** No Qualifier
Y Mouth and Throat	**7** Via Natural or Artificial Opening **8** Via Natural or Artificial Opening Endoscopic	**1** Radioactive Element **B** Intraluminal Device, Airway **Y** Other Device	**Z** No Qualifier

Section	0	Medical and Surgical
Body System	C	Mouth and Throat
Operation	J	**Inspection:** Visually and/or manually exploring a body part

Body Part (4th)	Approach (5th)	Device (6th)	Qualifier (7th)
A SalivaryGland	**0** Open **3** Percutaneous **X** External	**Z** No Device	**Z** No Qualifier
S Larynx **Y** Mouth and Throat	**0** Open **3** Percutaneous **4** Percutaneous Endoscopic **7** Via Natural or Artificial Opening **8** Via Natural or Artificial Opening Endoscopic **X** External	**Z** No Device	**Z** No Qualifier

Section	0	Medical and Surgical
Body System	C	Mouth and Throat
Operation	L	**Occlusion:** Completely closing an orifice or the lumen of a tubular body part

Body Part (4th)	Approach (5th)	Device (6th)	Qualifier (7th)
B Parotid Duct, Right **C** Parotid Duct, Left	**0** Open **3** Percutaneous **4** Percutaneous Endoscopic	**C** Extraluminal Device **D** Intraluminal Device **Z** No Device	**Z** No Qualifier
B Parotid Duct, Right **C** Parotid Duct, Left	**7** Via Natural or Artificial Opening **8** Via Natural or Artificial Opening Endoscopic	**D** Intraluminal Device **Z** No Device	**Z** No Qualifier

Section	0	Medical and Surgical
Body System	C	Mouth and Throat
Operation	M	**Reattachment:** Putting back in or on all or a portion of a separated body part to its normal location or other suitable location

Body Part (4th)	Approach (5th)	Device (6th)	Qualifier (7th)
0 Upper Lip **1** Lower Lip **3** Soft Palate **7** Tongue **N** Uvula	**0** Open	**Z** No Device	**Z** No Qualifier
W Upper Tooth **X** Lower Tooth	**0** Open **X** External	**Z** No Device	**0** Single **1** Multiple **2** All

Section	0	Medical and Surgical
Body System	C	Mouth and Throat
Operation	N	**Release:** Freeing a body part from an abnormal physical constraint by cutting or by the use of force

Body Part (4th)	Approach (5th)	Device (6th)	Qualifier (7th)
0 Upper Lip 1 Lower Lip 2 Hard Palate 3 Soft Palate 4 Buccal Mucosa 5 Upper Gingiva 6 Lower Gingiva 7 Tongue N Uvula P Tonsils Q Adenoids	0 Open 3 Percutaneous X External	Z No Device	Z No Qualifier
8 Parotid Gland, Right 9 Parotid Gland, Left B Parotid Duct, Right C Parotid Duct, Left D Sublingual Gland, Right F Sublingual Gland, Left G Submaxillary Gland, Right H Submaxillary Gland, Left J Minor Salivary Gland	0 Open 3 Percutaneous	Z No Device	Z No Qualifier
M Pharynx R Epiglottis S Larynx T Vocal Cord, Right V Vocal Cord, Left	0 Open 3 Percutaneous 4 Percutaneous Endoscopic 7 Via Natural or Artificial Opening 8 Via Natural or Artificial Opening Endoscopic	Z No Device	Z No Qualifier
W Upper Tooth X Lower Tooth	0 Open X External	Z No Device	0 Single 1 Multiple 2 All

Section	0	Medical and Surgical
Body System	C	Mouth and Throat
Operation	P	**Removal:** Taking out or off a device from a body part

Body Part (4th)	Approach (5th)	Device (6th)	Qualifier (7th)
A Salivary Gland	0 Open 3 Percutaneous	0 Drainage Device C Extraluminal Device Y Other Device	Z No Qualifier
A Salivary Gland	7 Via Natural or Artificial Opening 8 Via Natural or Artificial Opening Endoscopic	Y Other Device	Z No Qualifier
S Larynx	0 Open 3 Percutaneous 7 Via Natural or Artificial Opening 8 Via Natural or Artificial Opening Endoscopic	0 Drainage Device 7 Autologous Tissue Substitute D Intraluminal Device J Synthetic Substitute K Nonautologous Tissue Substitute Y Other Device	Z No Qualifier
S Larynx	X External	0 Drainage Device 7 Autologous Tissue Substitute D Intraluminal Device J Synthetic Substitute K Nonautologous Tissue Substitute	Z No Qualifier

Continued →

Section   0   **Medical and Surgical**
Body System   C   **Mouth and Throat**
Operation   P   **Removal:** Taking out or off a device from a body part

Body Part (4th)	Approach (5th)	Device (6th)	Qualifier (7th)
Y Mouth and Throat	0 Open 3 Percutaneous 7 Via Natural or Artificial Opening 8 Via Natural or Artificial Opening Endoscopic	0 Drainage Device 1 Radioactive Element 7 Autologous Tissue Substitute D Intraluminal Device J Synthetic Substitute K Nonautologous Tissue Substitute Y Other Device	Z No Qualifier
Y Mouth and Throat	X External	0 Drainage Device 1 Radioactive Element 7 Autologous Tissue Substitute D Intraluminal Device J Synthetic Substitute K Nonautologous Tissue Substitute	Z No Qualifier

Section   0   **Medical and Surgical**
Body System   C   **Mouth and Throat**
Operation   Q   **Repair:** Restoring, to the extent possible, a body part to its normal anatomic structure and function

Body Part (4th)	Approach (5th)	Device (6th)	Qualifier (7th)
0 Upper Lip 1 Lower Lip 2 Hard Palate 3 Soft Palate 4 Buccal Mucosa 5 Upper Gingiva 6 Lower Gingiva 7 Tongue N Uvula P Tonsils Q Adenoids	0 Open 3 Percutaneous X External	Z No Device	Z No Qualifier
8 Parotid Gland, Right 9 Parotid Gland, Left B Parotid Duct, Right C Parotid Duct, Left D Sublingual Gland, Right F Sublingual Gland, Left G Submaxillary Gland, Right H Submaxillary Gland, Left J Minor Salivary Gland	0 Open 3 Percutaneous	Z No Device	Z No Qualifier
M Pharynx R Epiglottis S Larynx T Vocal Cord, Right V Vocal Cord, Left	0 Open 3 Percutaneous 4 Percutaneous Endoscopic 7 Via Natural or Artificial Opening 8 Via Natural or Artificial Opening Endoscopic	Z No Device	Z No Qualifier
W Upper Tooth X Lower Tooth	0 Open X External	Z No Device	0 Single 1 Multiple 2 All

Section **0** **Medical and Surgical**
Body System **C** **Mouth and Throat**
Operation **V** **Restriction:** Partially closing an orifice or the lumen of a tubular body part

Body Part (4th)	Approach (5th)	Device (6th)	Qualifier (7th)
B Parotid Duct, Right **C** Parotid Duct, Left	**0** Open **3** Percutaneous	**C** Extraluminal Device **D** Intraluminal Device **Z** No Device	**Z** No Qualifier
B Parotid Duct, Right **C** Parotid Duct, Left	**7** Via Natural or Artificial Opening **8** Via Natural or Artificial Opening Endoscopic	**D** Intraluminal Device **Z** No Device	**Z** No Qualifier

Section **0** **Medical and Surgical**
Body System **C** **Mouth and Throat**
Operation **W** **Revision:** Correcting, to the extent possible, a portion of a malfunctioning device or the position of a displaced device

Body Part (4th)	Approach (5th)	Device (6th)	Qualifier (7th)
A Salivary Gland	**0** Open **3** Percutaneous	**0** Drainage Device **C** Extraluminal Device **Y** Other Device	**Z** No Qualifier
A Salivary Gland	**7** Via Natural or Artificial Opening **8** Via Natural or Artificial Opening Endoscopic	**Y** Other Device	**Z** No Qualifier
A Salivary Gland	**X** External	**0** Drainage Device **C** Extraluminal Device	**Z** No Qualifier
S Larynx	**0** Open **3** Percutaneous **7** Via Natural or Artificial Opening **8** Via Natural or Artificial Opening Endoscopic	**0** Drainage Device **7** Autologous Tissue Substitute **D** Intraluminal Device **J** Synthetic Substitute **K** Nonautologous Tissue Substitute **Y** Other Device	**Z** No Qualifier
S Larynx	**X** External	**0** Drainage Device **7** Autologous Tissue Substitute **D** Intraluminal Device **J** Synthetic Substitute **K** Nonautologous Tissue Substitute	**Z** No Qualifier
Y Mouth and Throat	**0** Open **3** Percutaneous **7** Via Natural or Artificial Opening **8** Via Natural or Artificial Opening Endoscopic	**0** Drainage Device **1** Radioactive Element **7** Autologous Tissue Substitute **D** Intraluminal Device **J** Synthetic Substitute **K** Nonautologous Tissue Substitute **Y** Other Device	**Z** No Qualifier
Y Mouth and Throat	**X** External	**0** Drainage Device **1** Radioactive Element **7** Autologous Tissue Substitute **D** Intraluminal Device **J** Synthetic Substitute **K** Nonautologous Tissue Substitute	**Z** No Qualifier

Section	0	Medical and Surgical
Body System	C	Mouth and Throat
Operation	X	**Transfer:** Moving, without taking out, all or a portion of a body part to another location to take over the function of all or a portion of a body part

Body Part (4th)	Approach (5th)	Device (6th)	Qualifier (7th)
0 Upper Lip	0 Open	Z No Device	Z No Qualifier
1 Lower Lip	X External		
3 Soft Palate			
4 Buccal Mucosa			
5 Upper Gingiva			
6 Lower Gingiva			
7 Tongue			

AHA Coding Clinic

0CB80ZZ Excision of Right Parotid Gland, Open Approach—AHA CC: 3Q, 2014, 21-22

0CBM8ZX Excision of Pharynx, Via Natural or Artificial Opening Endoscopic, Diagnostic—AHA CC: 2Q, 2016, 20

0CBM8ZZ Excision of Pharynx, Via Natural or Artificial Opening Endoscopic—AHA CC: 3Q, 2016, 28-29

0CCH3ZZ Extirpation of Matter from Left Submaxillary Gland, Percutaneous Approach—AHA CC: 2Q, 2016, 20

0CQ50ZZ Repair Upper Gingiva, Open Approach—AHA CC: 1Q, 2017, 20-21

0CR3XJZ Replacement of Soft Palate with Synthetic Substitute, External Approach—AHA CC: 3Q, 2014, 25

0CR4XKZ Replacement of Buccal Mucosa with Nonautologous Tissue Substitute, External Approach—AHA CC: 2Q, 2014, 5-6

0CSR8ZZ Reposition Epiglottis, Via Natural or Artificial Opening Endoscopic—AHA CC: 3Q, 2016, 28-29

0CT90ZZ Resection of Left Parotid Gland, Open Approach—AHA CC: 2Q, 2016, 12-14

0CTW0Z1 Resection of Upper Tooth, Multiple, Open Approach—AHA CC: 3Q, 2014, 23-24

0CTX0Z1 Resection of Lower Tooth, Multiple, Open Approach—AHA CC: 3Q, 2014, 23-24

Gastrointestinal System: Organization

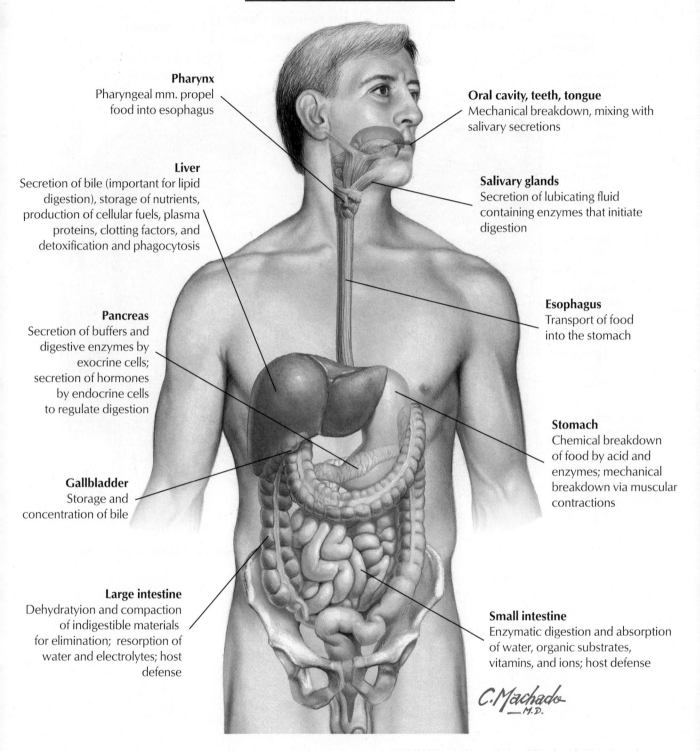

Pharynx
Pharyngeal mm. propel food into esophagus

Oral cavity, teeth, tongue
Mechanical breakdown, mixing with salivary secretions

Liver
Secretion of bile (important for lipid digestion), storage of nutrients, production of cellular fuels, plasma proteins, clotting factors, and detoxification and phagocytosis

Salivary glands
Secretion of lubicating fluid containing enzymes that initiate digestion

Esophagus
Transport of food into the stomach

Pancreas
Secretion of buffers and digestive enzymes by exocrine cells; secretion of hormones by endocrine cells to regulate digestion

Stomach
Chemical breakdown of food by acid and enzymes; mechanical breakdown via muscular contractions

Gallbladder
Storage and concentration of bile

Large intestine
Dehydratyion and compaction of indigestible materials for elimination; resorption of water and electrolytes; host defense

Small intestine
Enzymatic digestion and absorption of water, organic substrates, vitamins, and ions; host defense

C. Machado
_M.D._

Stomach, Liver, Gallbladder

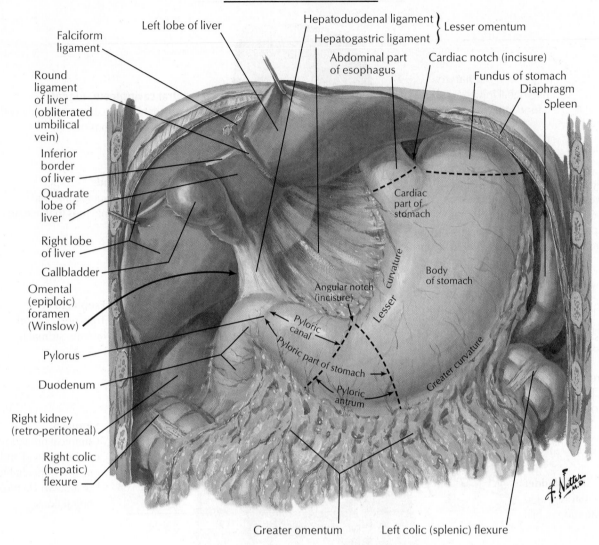

Falciform ligament

Left lobe of liver

Hepatoduodenal ligament } Lesser omentum
Hepatogastric ligament }

Round ligament of liver (obliterated umbilical vein)

Abdominal part of esophagus

Cardiac notch (incisure)

Fundus of stomach
Diaphragm
Spleen

Inferior border of liver

Quadrate lobe of liver

Cardiac part of stomach

Right lobe of liver

Body of stomach

Gallbladder

Angular notch (incisure)

Lesser curvature

Omental (epiploic) foramen (Winslow)

Pyloric canal

Pylorus

Pyloric part of stomach

Greater curvature

Duodenum

Pyloric antrum

Right kidney (retro-peritoneal)

Right colic (hepatic) flexure

Greater omentum

Left colic (splenic) flexure

Large Intestine Structure of Colon

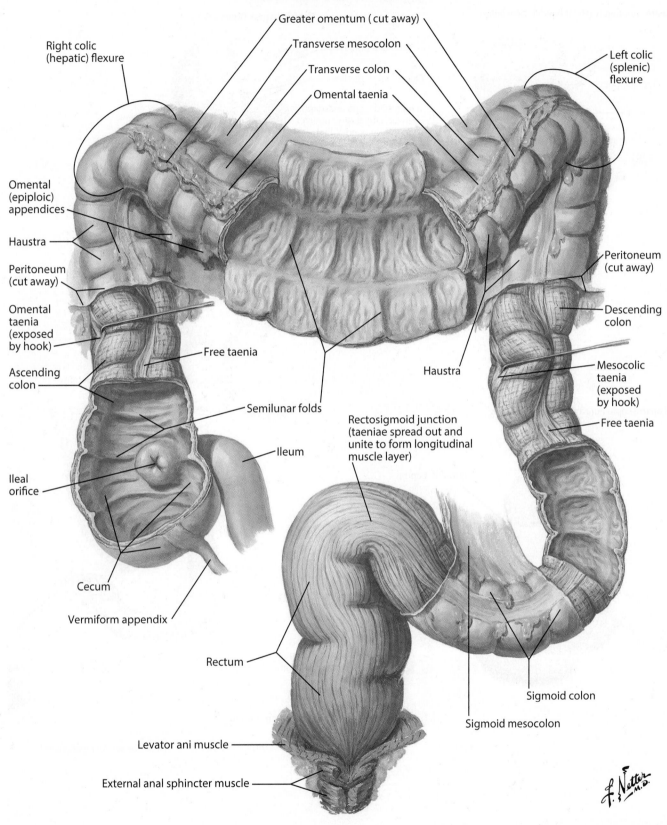

Greater omentum (cut away)

Transverse mesocolon

Transverse colon

Omental taenia

Right colic (hepatic) flexure

Left colic (splenic) flexure

Omental (epiploic) appendices

Haustra

Peritoneum (cut away)

Peritoneum (cut away)

Descending colon

Omental taenia (exposed by hook)

Free taenia

Haustra

Mesocolic taenia (exposed by hook)

Ascending colon

Semilunar folds

Free taenia

Rectosigmoid junction (taeniae spread out and unite to form longitudinal muscle layer)

Ileum

Ileal orifice

Cecum

Vermiform appendix

Rectum

Sigmoid colon

Sigmoid mesocolon

Levator ani muscle

External anal sphincter muscle

F. Netter M.D.

©2014. Used with permission of Elsevier. All rights reserved.

Treatment of Morbid Obesity

Gastric stapling (vertical banded gastroplasty)

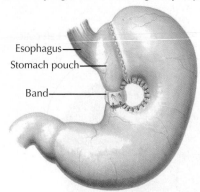

Esophagus

Stomach pouch

Band

Gastric bypass (Roux-en-Y)

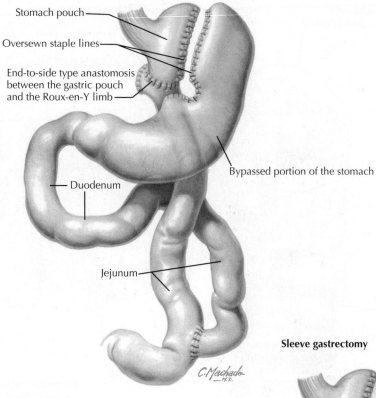

Stomach pouch

Oversewn staple lines

End-to-side type anastomosis
between the gastric pouch
and the Roux-en-Y limb

Bypassed portion of the stomach

Duodenum

Jejunum

C. Machado
M.D.

Sleeve gastrectomy

Laparoscopic adjustable gastric banding

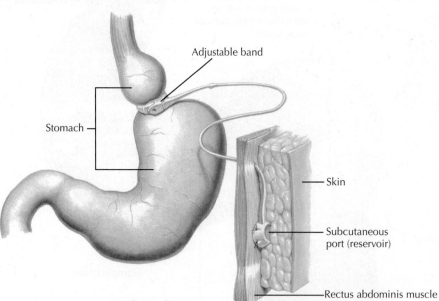

Adjustable band

Stomach

Skin

Subcutaneous
port (reservoir)

Rectus abdominis muscle

K. marzejn

Section   **0**   **Medical and Surgical**
Body System   **D**   **Gastrointestinal System**
Operation   **1**   **Bypass:** Altering the route of passage of the contents of a tubular body part

Body Part (4th)	Approach (5th)	Device (6th)	Qualifier (7th)
1 Esophagus, Upper 2 Esophagus, Middle 3 Esophagus, Lower 5 Esophagus	0 Open 4 Percutaneous Endoscopic 8 Via Natural or Artificial Opening Endoscopic	7 Autologous Tissue Substitute J Synthetic Substitute K Nonautologous Tissue Substitute Z No Device	4 Cutaneous 6 Stomach 9 Duodenum A Jejunum B Ileum
1 Esophagus, Upper 2 Esophagus, Middle 3 Esophagus, Lower 5 Esophagus	3 Percutaneous	J Synthetic Substitute	4 Cutaneous
6 Stomach 9 Duodenum	0 Open 4 Percutaneous Endoscopic 8 Via Natural or Artificial Opening Endoscopic	7 Autologous Tissue Substitute J Synthetic Substitute K Nonautologous Tissue Substitute Z No Device	4 Cutaneous 9 Duodenum A Jejunum B Ileum L Transverse Colon
6 Stomach 9 Duodenum	3 Percutaneous	J Synthetic Substitute	4 Cutaneous
8 Small Intestine	0 Open 4 Percutaneous Endoscopic 8 Via Natural or Artificial Opening Endoscopic	7 Autologous Tissue Substitute J Synthetic Substitute K Nonautologous Tissue Z No Device	4 Cutaneous 8 Small Intestine H Cecum K Ascending Colon L Transverse Colon M Descending Colon N Sigmoid Colon P Rectum Q Anus
A Jejunum	0 Open 4 Percutaneous Endoscopic 8 Via Natural or Artificial Opening Endoscopic	7 Autologous Tissue Substitute J Synthetic Substitute K Nonautologous Tissue Substitute Z No Device	4 Cutaneous A Jejunum B Ileum H Cecum K Ascending Colon L Transverse Colon M Descending Colon N Sigmoid Colon P Rectum Q Anus
A Jejunum	3 Percutaneous	J Synthetic Substitute	4 Cutaneous
B Ileum	0 Open 4 Percutaneous Endoscopic 8 Via Natural or Artificial Opening Endoscopic	7 Autologous Tissue Substitute J Synthetic Substitute K Nonautologous Tissue Substitute Z No Device	4 Cutaneous B Ileum H Cecum K Ascending Colon L Transverse Colon M Descending Colon N Sigmoid Colon P Rectum Q Anus
B Ileum	3 Percutaneous	J Synthetic Substitute	4 Cutaneous
E Large Intestine	0 Open 4 Percutaneous Endoscopic 8 Via Natural or Artificial Opening Endoscopic	7 Autologous Tissue Substitute J Synthetic Substitute K Nonautologous Tissue Z No Device	4 Cutaneous E Large Intestine P Rectum

Section	0	**Medical and Surgical**
Body System	D	**Gastrointestinal System**
Operation	1	**Bypass:** Altering the route of passage of the contents of a tubular body part

Body Part (4th)	Approach (5th)	Device (6th)	Qualifier (7th)
H Cecum	0 Open 4 Percutaneous Endoscopic 8 Via Natural or Artificial Opening Endoscopic	7 Autologous Tissue Substitute J Synthetic Substitute K Nonautologous Tissue Substitute Z No Device	4 Cutaneous H Cecum K Ascending Colon L Transverse Colon M Descending Colon N Sigmoid Colon P Rectum
H Cecum	3 Percutaneous	J Synthetic Substitute	4 Cutaneous
K Ascending Colon	0 Open 4 Percutaneous Endoscopic 8 Via Natural or Artificial Opening Endoscopic	7 Autologous Tissue Substitute J Synthetic Substitute K Nonautologous Tissue Substitute Z No Device	4 Cutaneous K Ascending Colon L Transverse Colon M Descending Colon N Sigmoid Colon P Rectum
K Ascending Colon	3 Percutaneous	J Synthetic Substitute	4 Cutaneous
L Transverse Colon	0 Open 4 Percutaneous Endoscopic 8 Via Natural or Artificial Opening Endoscopic	7 Autologous Tissue Substitute J Synthetic Substitute K Nonautologous Tissue Substitute Z No Device	4 Cutaneous L Transverse Colon M Descending Colon N Sigmoid Colon P Rectum
L Transverse Colon	3 Percutaneous	J Synthetic Substitute	4 Cutaneous
M Descending Colon	0 Open 4 Percutaneous Endoscopic 8 Via Natural or Artificial Opening Endoscopic	7 Autologous Tissue Substitute J Synthetic Substitute K Nonautologous Tissue Substitute Z No Device	4 Cutaneous M Descending Colon N Sigmoid Colon P Rectum
M Descending Colon	3 Percutaneous	J Synthetic Substitute	4 Cutaneous
N Sigmoid Colon	0 Open 4 Percutaneous Endoscopic 8 Via Natural or Artificial Opening Endoscopic	7 Autologous Tissue Substitute J Synthetic Substitute K Nonautologous Tissue Substitute Z No Device	4 Cutaneous N Sigmoid Colon P Rectum
N Sigmoid Colon	3 Percutaneous	J Synthetic Substitute	4 Cutaneous

Section	0	**Medical and Surgical**
Body System	D	**Gastrointestinal System**
Operation	2	**Change:** Taking out or off a device from a body part and putting back an identical or similar device in or on the same body part without cutting or puncturing the skin or a mucous membrane

Body Part (4th)	Approach (5th)	Device (6th)	Qualifier (7th)
0 Upper Intestinal Tract D Lower Intestinal Tract	X External	0 Drainage Device U Feeding Device Y Other Device	Z No Qualifier
U Omentum V Mesentery W Peritoneum	X External	0 Drainage Device Y Other Device	Z No Qualifier

Section	0	Medical and Surgical
Body System	D	Gastrointestinal System
Operation	5	Destruction: Physical eradication of all or a portion of a body part by the direct use of energy, force, or a destructive agent

Body Part (4th)	Approach (5th)	Device (6th)	Qualifier (7th)
1 Esophagus, Upper 2 Esophagus, Middle 3 Esophagus, Lower 4 Esophagogastric Junction 5 Esophagus 6 Stomach 7 Stomach, Pylorus 8 Small Intestine 9 Duodenum A Jejunum B Ileum C Ileocecal Valve E Large Intestine F Large Intestine, Right G Large Intestine, Left H Cecum J Appendix K Ascending Colon L Transverse Colon M Descending Colon N Sigmoid Colon P Rectum	0 Open 3 Percutaneous 4 Percutaneous Endoscopic 7 Via Natural or Artificial Opening 8 Via Natural or Artificial Opening Endoscopic	Z No Device	Z No Qualifier
Q Anus	0 Open 3 Percutaneous 4 Percutaneous Endoscopic 7 Via Natural or Artificial Opening 8 Via Natural or Artificial Opening Endoscopic X External	Z No Device	Z No Qualifier
R Anal Sphincter U Omentum V Mesentery W Peritoneum	0 Open 3 Percutaneous 4 Percutaneous Endoscopic	Z No Device	Z No Qualifier

Section	0	Medical and Surgical
Body System	D	Gastrointestinal System
Operation	7	Dilation: Expanding an orifice or the lumen of a tubular body part

Body Part (4th)	Approach (5th)	Device (6th)	Qualifier (7th)
1 Esophagus, Upper 2 Esophagus, Middle 3 Esophagus, Lower 4 Esophagogastric Junction 5 Esophagus 6 Stomach 7 Stomach, Pylorus 8 Small Intestine 9 Duodenum A Jejunum B Ileum C Ileocecal Valve E Large Intestine F Large Intestine, Right G Large Intestine, Left H Cecum K Ascending Colon L Transverse Colon M Descending Colon N Sigmoid Colon P Rectum Q Anus	0 Open 3 Percutaneous 4 Percutaneous Endoscopic 7 Via Natural or Artificial Opening 8 Via Natural or Artificial Opening Endoscopic	D Intraluminal Device Z No Device	Z No Qualifier

Section   **0**   **Medical and Surgical**
Body System   **D**   **Gastrointestinal System**
Operation   **8**   **Division:** Cutting into a body part, without draining fluids and/or gases from the body part, in order to separate or transect a body part

Body Part (4th)	Approach (5th)	Device (6th)	Qualifier (7th)
4 Esophagogastric Junction 7 Stomach, Pylorus	0 Open 3 Percutaneous 4 Percutaneous Endoscopic 7 Via Natural or Artificial Opening 8 Via Natural or Artificial Opening Endoscopic	Z No Device	Z No Qualifier
R Anal Sphincter	0 Open 3 Percutaneous	Z No Device	Z No Qualifier

Section   **0**   **Medical and Surgical**
Body System   **D**   **Gastrointestinal System**
Operation   **9**   **Drainage:** Taking or letting out fluids and/or gases from a body part

Body Part (4th)	Approach (5th)	Device (6th)	Qualifier (7th)
1 Esophagus, Upper 2 Esophagus, Middle 3 Esophagus, Lower 4 Esophagogastric Junction 5 Esophagus 6 Stomach 7 Stomach, Pylorus 8 Small Intestine 9 Duodenum A Jejunum B Ileum C Ileocecal Valve E Large Intestine F Large Intestine, Right G Large Intestine, Left H Cecum J Appendix K Ascending Colon L Transverse Colon M Descending Colon N Sigmoid Colon P Rectum	0 Open 3 Percutaneous 4 Percutaneous Endoscopic 7 Via Natural or Artificial Opening 8 Via Natural or Artificial Opening Endoscopic	0 Drainage Device	Z No Qualifier
1 Esophagus, Upper 2 Esophagus, Middle 3 Esophagus, Lower 4 Esophagogastric Junction 5 Esophagus 6 Stomach 7 Stomach, Pylorus 8 Small Intestine 9 Duodenum A Jejunum B Ileum C Ileocecal Valve E Large Intestine F Large Intestine, Right G Large Intestine, Left H Cecum J Appendix K Ascending Colon L Transverse Colon M Descending Colon N Sigmoid Colon P Rectum	0 Open 3 Percutaneous 4 Percutaneous Endoscopic 7 Via Natural or Artificial Opening 8 Via Natural or Artificial Opening Endoscopic	Z No Device	X Diagnostic Z No Qualifier

Continued →

Section 0 **Medical and Surgical**
Body System D **Gastrointestinal System**
Operation 9 **Drainage:** Taking or letting out fluids and/or gases from a body part

Body Part (4th)	Approach (5th)	Device (6th)	Qualifier (7th)
Q Anus	0 Open 3 Percutaneous 4 Percutaneous Endoscopic 7 Via Natural or Artificial Opening 8 Via Natural or Artificial Opening Endoscopic X External	0 Drainage Device	Z No Qualifier
Q Anus	0 Open 3 Percutaneous 4 Percutaneous Endoscopic 7 Via Natural or Artificial Opening 8 Via Natural or Artificial Opening Endoscopic X External	Z No Device	X Diagnostic Z No Qualifier
R Anal Sphincter U Omentum V Mesentery W Peritoneum	0 Open 3 Percutaneous 4 Percutaneous Endoscopic	0 Drainage Device	Z No Qualifier
R Anal Sphincter U Omentum V Mesentery W Peritoneum	0 Open 3 Percutaneous 4 Percutaneous Endoscopic	Z No Device	X Diagnostic Z No Qualifier

Section 0 **Medical and Surgical**
Body System D **Gastrointestinal System**
Operation B **Excision:** Cutting out or off, without replacement, a portion of a body part

Body Part (4th)	Approach (5th)	Device (6th)	Qualifier (7th)
1 Esophagus, Upper 2 Esophagus, Middle 3 Esophagus, Lower 4 Esophagogastric Junction 5 Esophagus 7 Stomach, Pylorus 8 Small Intestine 9 Duodenum A Jejunum B Ileum C Ileocecal Valve E Large Intestine F Large Intestine, Right H Cecum J Appendix K Ascending Colon P Rectum	0 Open 3 Percutaneous 4 Percutaneous Endoscopic 7 Via Natural or Artificial Opening 8 Via Natural or Artificial Opening Endoscopic	Z No Device	X Diagnostic Z No Qualifier
6 Stomach	0 Open 3 Percutaneous 4 Percutaneous Endoscopic 7 Via Natural or Artificial Opening 8 Via Natural or Artificial Opening Endoscopic	Z No Device	3 Vertical X Diagnostic Z No Qualifier
G Large Intestine, Left L Transverse Colon M Descending Colon N Sigmoid Colon	0 Open 3 Percutaneous 4 Percutaneous Endoscopic 7 Via Natural or Artificial Opening 8 Via Natural or Artificial Opening Endoscopic	Z No Device	X Diagnostic Z No Qualifier

Continued →

Section	0	Medical and Surgical
Body System	D	Gastrointestinal System
Operation	B	Excision: Cutting out or off, without replacement, a portion of a body part

Body Part (4ᵗʰ)	Approach (5ᵗʰ)	Device (6ᵗʰ)	Qualifier (7ᵗʰ)
G Large Intestine, Left L Transverse Colon M Descending Colon N Sigmoid Colon	F Via Natural or Artificial Opening With Percutaneous Endoscopic Assistance	Z No Device	Z No Qualifier
Q Anus	0 Open 3 Percutaneous 4 Percutaneous Endoscopic 7 Via Natural or Artificial Opening 8 Via Natural or Artificial Opening Endoscopic X External	Z No Device	X Diagnostic Z No Qualifier
R Anal Sphincter U Omentum V Mesentery W Peritoneum	0 Open 3 Percutaneous 4 Percutaneous Endoscopic	Z No Device	X Diagnostic Z No Qualifier

Section	0	Medical and Surgical
Body System	D	Gastrointestinal System
Operation	C	Extirpation: Taking or cutting out solid matter from a body part

Body Part (4ᵗʰ)	Approach (5ᵗʰ)	Device (6ᵗʰ)	Qualifier (7ᵗʰ)
1 Esophagus, Upper 2 Esophagus, Middle 3 Esophagus, Lower 4 Esophagogastric Junction 5 Esophagus 6 Stomach 7 Stomach, Pylorus 8 Small Intestine 9 Duodenum A Jejunum B Ileum C Ileocecal Valve E Large Intestine F Large Intestine, Right G Large Intestine, Left H Cecum J Appendix K Ascending Colon L Transverse Colon M Descending Colon N Sigmoid Colon P Rectum	0 Open 3 Percutaneous 4 Percutaneous Endoscopic 7 Via Natural or Artificial Opening 8 Via Natural or Artificial Opening Endoscopic	Z No Device	Z No Qualifier
Q Anus	0 Open 3 Percutaneous 4 Percutaneous Endoscopic 7 Via Natural or Artificial Opening 8 Via Natural or Artificial Opening Endoscopic X External	Z No Device	Z No Qualifier
R Anal Sphincter U Omentum V Mesentery W Peritoneum	0 Open 3 Percutaneous 4 Percutaneous Endoscopic	Z No Device	Z No Qualifier

Section	0	Medical and Surgical
Body System	D	Gastrointestinal System
Operation	D	**Extraction:** Pulling or stripping out or off all or a portion of a body part by the use of force

Body Part (4th)	Approach (5th)	Device (6th)	Qualifier (7th)
1 Esophagus, Upper 2 Esophagus, Middle 3 Esophagus, Lower 4 Esophagogastric Junction 5 Esophagus 6 Stomach 7 Stomach, Pylorus 8 Small Intestine 9 Duodenum A Jejunum B Ileum C Ileocecal Valve E Large Intestine F Large Intestine, Right G Large Intestine, Left H Cecum J Appendix K Ascending Colon L Transverse Colon M Descending Colon N Sigmoid Colon P Rectum	3 Percutaneous 4 Percutaneous Endoscopic 8 Via Natural or Artificial Opening Endoscopic	Z No Device	X Diagnostic
Q Anus	3 Percutaneous 4 Percutaneous Endoscopic 8 Via Natural or Artificial Opening Endoscopic X External	Z No Device	X Diagnostic

Section	0	Medical and Surgical
Body System	D	Gastrointestinal System
Operation	F	**Fragmentation:** Breaking solid matter in a body part into pieces

Body Part (4th)	Approach (5th)	Device (6th)	Qualifier (7th)
5 Esophagus 6 Stomach 8 Small Intestine 9 Duodenum A Jejunum B Ileum E Large Intestine F Large Intestine, Right G Large Intestine, Left H Cecum J Appendix K Ascending Colon L Transverse Colon M Descending Colon N Sigmoid Colon P Rectum Q Anus	0 Open 3 Percutaneous 4 Percutaneous Endoscopic 7 Via Natural or Artificial Opening 8 Via Natural or Artificial Opening Endoscopic X External	Z No Device	Z No Qualifier

Section	0	Medical and Surgical
Body System	D	Gastrointestinal System
Operation	H	Insertion: Putting in a nonbiological appliance that monitors, assists, performs, or prevents a physiological function but does not physically take the place of a body part

Body Part (4th)	Approach (5th)	Device (6th)	Qualifier (7th)
0 Upper Intestinal Tract **D** Lower Intestinal Tract	**0** Open **3** Percutaneous **4** Percutaneous Endoscopic **7** Via Natural or Artificial Opening **8** Via Natural or Artificial Opening Endoscopic	**Y** Other Device	**Z** No Qualifier
5 Esophagus	**0** Open **3** Percutaneous **4** Percutaneous Endoscopic	**1** Radioactive Element **2** Monitoring Device **3** Infusion Device **D** Intraluminal Device **U** Feeding Device **Y** Other Device	**Z** No Qualifier
5 Esophagus	**7** Via Natural or Artificial Opening **8** Via Natural or Artificial Opening Endoscopic	**1** Radioactive Element **2** Monitoring Device **3** Infusion Device **B** Intraluminal Device, Airway **D** Intraluminal Device **U** Feeding Device **Y** Other Device	**Z** No Qualifier
6 Stomach	**0** Open **3** Percutaneous **4** Percutaneous Endoscopic	**1** Radioactive Element **2** Monitoring Device **3** Infusion Device **D** Intraluminal Device **M** Stimulator Lead **U** Feeding Device **Y** Other Device	**Z** No Qualifier
6 Stomach	**7** Via Natural or Artificial Opening **8** Via Natural or Artificial Opening Endoscopic	**1** Radioactive Element **2** Monitoring Device **3** Infusion Device **D** Intraluminal Device **U** Feeding Device **Y** Other Device	**Z** No Qualifier
8 Small Intestine **9** Duodenum **A** Jejunum **B** Ileum	**0** Open **3** Percutaneous **4** Percutaneous Endoscopic **7** Via Natural or Artificial Opening **8** Via Natural or Artificial Opening Endoscopic	**1** Radioactive Element **2** Monitoring Device **3** Infusion Device **D** Intraluminal Device **U** Feeding Device	**Z** No Qualifier
E Large Intestine **P** Rectum	**0** Open **3** Percutaneous **4** Percutaneous Endoscopic **7** Via Natural or Artificial Opening **8** Via Natural or Artificial Opening Endoscopic	**1** Radioactive Element **D** Intraluminal Device	**Z** No Qualifier
Q Anus	**0** Open **3** Percutaneous **4** Percutaneous Endoscopic	**D** Intraluminal Device **L** Artificial Sphincter	**Z** No Qualifier
Q Anus	**7** Via Natural or Artificial Opening **8** Via Natural or Artificial Opening Endoscopic	**D** Intraluminal Device	**Z** No Qualifier
R Anal Sphincter	**0** Open **3** Percutaneous **4** Percutaneous Endoscopic	**M** Stimulator Lead	**Z** No Qualifier

Section	0	Medical and Surgical
Body System	D	Gastrointestinal System
Operation	J	Inspection: Visually and/or manually exploring a body part

Body Part (4th)	Approach (5th)	Device (6th)	Qualifier (7th)
0 Upper Intestinal Tract 6 Stomach D Lower Intestinal Tract	0 Open 3 Percutaneous 4 Percutaneous Endoscopic 7 Via Natural or Artificial Opening 8 Via Natural or Artificial Opening Endoscopic X External	Z No Device	Z No Qualifier
U Omentum V Mesentery W Peritoneum	0 Open 3 Percutaneous 4 Percutaneous Endoscopic X External	Z No Device	Z No Qualifier

Section	0	Medical and Surgical
Body System	D	Gastrointestinal System
Operation	L	Occlusion: Completely closing an orifice or the lumen of a tubular body part

Body Part (4th)	Approach (5th)	Device (6th)	Qualifier (7th)
1 Esophagus, Upper 2 Esophagus, Middle 3 Esophagus, Lower 4 Esophagogastric Junction 5 Esophagus 6 Stomach 7 Stomach, Pylorus 8 Small Intestine 9 Duodenum A Jejunum B Ileum C Ileocecal Valve E Large Intestine F Large Intestine, Right G Large Intestine, Left H Cecum K Ascending Colon L Transverse Colon M Descending Colon N Sigmoid Colon P Rectum	0 Open 3 Percutaneous 4 Percutaneous Endoscopic	C Extraluminal Device D Intraluminal Device Z No Device	Z No Qualifier
1 Esophagus, Upper 2 Esophagus, Middle 3 Esophagus, Lower 4 Esophagogastric Junction 5 Esophagus 6 Stomach 7 Stomach, Pylorus 8 Small Intestine 9 Duodenum A Jejunum B Ileum C Ileocecal Valve E Large Intestine F Large Intestine, Right G Large Intestine, Left H Cecum K Ascending Colon L Transverse Colon M Descending Colon N Sigmoid Colon P Rectum	7 Via Natural or Artificial Opening 8 Via Natural or Artificial Opening Endoscopic	D Intraluminal Device Z No Device	Z No Qualifier

Continued →

Section	0	Medical and Surgical
Body System	D	Gastrointestinal System
Operation	L	Occlusion: Completely closing an orifice or the lumen of a tubular body part

Body Part (4th)	Approach (5th)	Device (6th)	Qualifier (7th)
Q Anus	0 Open 3 Percutaneous 4 Percutaneous Endoscopic X External	C Extraluminal Device D Intraluminal Device Z No Device	Z No Qualifier
Q Anus	7 Via Natural or Artificial Opening 8 Via Natural or Artificial Opening Endoscopic	D Intraluminal Device Z No Device	Z No Qualifier

Section	0	Medical and Surgical
Body System	D	Gastrointestinal System
Operation	M	Reattachment: Putting back in or on all or a portion of a separated body part to its normal location or other suitable location

Body Part (4th)	Approach (5th)	Device (6th)	Qualifier (7th)
5 Esophagus 6 Stomach 8 Small Intestine 9 Duodenum A Jejunum B Ileum E Large Intestine F Large Intestine, Right G Large Intestine, Left H Cecum K Ascending Colon L Transverse Colon M Descending Colon N Sigmoid Colon P Rectum	0 Open 4 Percutaneous Endoscopic	Z No Device	Z No Qualifier

Section	0	Medical and Surgical
Body System	D	Gastrointestinal System
Operation	N	Release: Freeing a body part from an abnormal physical constraint by cutting or by the use of force

Body Part (4th)	Approach (5th)	Device (6th)	Qualifier (7th)
1 Esophagus, Upper 2 Esophagus, Middle 3 Esophagus, Lower 4 Esophagogastric Junction 5 Esophagus 6 Stomach 7 Stomach, Pylorus 8 Small Intestine 9 Duodenum A Jejunum B Ileum C Ileocecal Valve E Large Intestine F Large Intestine, Right G Large Intestine, Left H Cecum J Appendix K Ascending Colon L Transverse Colon M Descending Colon N Sigmoid Colon P Rectum	0 Open 3 Percutaneous 4 Percutaneous Endoscopic 7 Via Natural or Artificial Opening 8 Via Natural or Artificial Opening Endoscopic	Z No Device	Z No Qualifier

Continued →

Section 0 Medical and Surgical
Body System D Gastrointestinal System
Operation N Release: Freeing a body part from an abnormal physical constraint by cutting or by the use of force

Body Part (4th)	Approach (5th)	Device (6th)	Qualifier (7th)
Q Anus	0 Open 3 Percutaneous 4 Percutaneous Endoscopic 7 Via Natural or Artificial Opening 8 Via Natural or Artificial Opening Endoscopic X External	Z No Device	Z No Qualifier
R Anal Sphincter U Omentum V Mesentery W Peritoneum	0 Open 3 Percutaneous 4 Percutaneous Endoscopic	Z No Device	Z No Qualifier

Section 0 Medical and Surgical
Body System D Gastrointestinal System
Operation P Removal: Taking out or off a device from a body part

Body Part (4th)	Approach (5th)	Device (6th)	Qualifier (7th)
0 Upper Intestinal Tract D Lower Intestinal Tract	0 Open 3 Percutaneous 4 Percutaneous Endoscopic 7 Via Natural or Artificial Opening 8 Via Natural or Artificial Opening Endoscopic	0 Drainage Device 2 Monitoring Device 3 Infusion Device 7 Autologous Tissue Substitute C Extraluminal Device D Intraluminal Device J Synthetic Substitute K Nonautologous Tissue Substitute U Feeding Device Y Other Device	Z No Qualifier
0 Upper Intestinal Tract D Lower Intestinal Tract	X External	0 Drainage Device 2 Monitoring Device 3 Infusion Device D Intraluminal Device U Feeding Device	Z No Qualifier
5 Esophagus	0 Open 3 Percutaneous 4 Percutaneous Endoscopic	1 Radioactive Element 2 Monitoring Device 3 Infusion Device U Feeding Device Y Other Device	Z No Qualifier
5 Esophagus	7 Via Natural or Artificial Opening 8 Via Natural or Artificial Opening Endoscopic	1 Radioactive Element D Intraluminal Device Y Other Device	Z No Qualifier
5 Esophagus	X External	1 Radioactive Element 2 Monitoring Device 3 Infusion Device D Intraluminal Device U Feeding Device	Z No Qualifier

Continued →

Section 0 **Medical and Surgical**
Body System D **Gastrointestinal System**
Operation P **Removal:** Taking out or off a device from a body part

Body Part (4th)	Approach (5th)	Device (6th)	Qualifier (7th)
6 Stomach	0 Open 3 Percutaneous 4 Percutaneous Endoscopic	0 Drainage Device 2 Monitoring Device 3 Infusion Device 7 Autologous Tissue Substitute C Extraluminal Device D Intraluminal Device J Synthetic Substitute K Nonautologous Tissue Substitute M Stimulator Lead U Feeding Device Y Other Device	Z No Qualifier
6 Stomach	7 Via Natural or Artificial Opening 8 Via Natural or Artificial Opening Endoscopic	0 Drainage Device 2 Monitoring Device 3 Infusion Device 7 Autologous Tissue Substitute C Extraluminal Device D Intraluminal Device J Synthetic Substitute K Nonautologous Tissue Substitute U Feeding Device Y Other Device	Z No Qualifier
6 Stomach	X External	0 Drainage Device 2 Monitoring Device 3 Infusion Device D Intraluminal Device U Feeding Device	Z No Qualifier
P Rectum	0 Open 3 Percutaneous 4 Percutaneous Endoscopic 7 Via Natural or Artificial Opening 8 Via Natural or Artificial Opening Endoscopic X External	1 Radioactive Element	Z No Qualifier
Q Anus	0 Open 3 Percutaneous 4 Percutaneous Endoscopic 7 Via Natural or Artificial Opening 8 Via Natural or Artificial Opening Endoscopic	L Artificial Sphincter	Z No Qualifier
R Anal Sphincter	0 Open 3 Percutaneous 4 Percutaneous Endoscopic	M Stimulator Lead	Z No Qualifier
U Omentum V Mesentery W Peritoneum	0 Open 3 Percutaneous 4 Percutaneous Endoscopic	0 Drainage Device 1 Radioactive Element 7 Autologous Tissue Substitute J Synthetic Substitute K Nonautologous Tissue Substitute	Z No Qualifier

Section	0	Medical and Surgical
Body System	D	Gastrointestinal System
Operation	Q	**Repair:** Restoring, to the extent possible, a body part to its normal anatomic structure and function

Body Part (4th)	Approach (5th)	Device (6th)	Qualifier (7th)
1 Esophagus, Upper 2 Esophagus, Middle 3 Esophagus, Lower 4 Esophagogastric Junction 5 Esophagus 6 Stomach 7 Stomach, Pylorus 8 Small Intestine 9 Duodenum A Jejunum B Ileum C Ileocecal Valve E Large Intestine F Large Intestine, Right G Large Intestine, Left H Cecum J Appendix K Ascending Colon L Transverse Colon M Descending Colon N Sigmoid Colon P Rectum	0 Open 3 Percutaneous 4 Percutaneous Endoscopic 7 Via Natural or Artificial Opening 8 Via Natural or Artificial Opening Endoscopic	Z No Device	Z No Qualifier
Q Anus	0 Open 3 Percutaneous 4 Percutaneous Endoscopic 7 Via Natural or Artificial Opening 8 Via Natural or Artificial Opening Endoscopic X External	Z No Device	Z No Qualifier
R Anal Sphincter U Omentum V Mesentery W Peritoneum	0 Open 3 Percutaneous 4 Percutaneous Endoscopic	Z No Device	Z No Qualifier

Section	0	Medical and Surgical
Body System	D	Gastrointestinal System
Operation	R	**Replacement:** Putting in or on biological or synthetic material that physically takes the place and/or function of all or a portion of a body part

Body Part (4th)	Approach (5th)	Device (6th)	Qualifier (7th)
5 Esophagus	0 Open 4 Percutaneous Endoscopic 7 Via Natural or Artificial Opening 8 Via Natural or Artificial Opening Endoscopic	7 Autologous Tissue Substitute J Synthetic Substitute K Nonautologous Tissue Substitute	Z No Qualifier
R Anal Sphincter U Omentum V Mesentery W Peritoneum	0 Open 4 Percutaneous Endoscopic	7 Autologous Tissue Substitute J Synthetic Substitute K Nonautologous Tissue Substitute	Z No Qualifier

Section	0	Medical and Surgical
Body System	D	Gastrointestinal System
Operation	S	Reposition: Moving to its normal location, or other suitable location, all or a portion of a body part

Body Part (4th)	Approach (5th)	Device (6th)	Qualifier (7th)
5 Esophagus 6 Stomach 9 Duodenum A Jejunum B Ileum H Cecum K Ascending Colon L Transverse Colon M Descending Colon N Sigmoid Colon P Rectum Q Anus	0 Open 4 Percutaneous Endoscopic 7 Via Natural or Artificial Opening 8 Via Natural or Artificial Opening Endoscopic X External	Z No Device	Z No Qualifier
8 Small Intestine E Large Intestine	0 Open 4 Percutaneous Endoscopic 7 Via Natural or Artificial Opening 8 Via Natural or Artificial Opening Endoscopic	Z No Device	Z No Qualifier

Section	0	Medical and Surgical
Body System	D	Gastrointestinal System
Operation	T	Resection: Cutting out or off, without replacement, all of a body part

Body Part (4th)	Approach (5th)	Device (6th)	Qualifier (7th)
1 Esophagus, Upper 2 Esophagus, Middle 3 Esophagus, Lower 4 Esophagogastric Junction 5 Esophagus 6 Stomach 7 Stomach, Pylorus 8 Small Intestine 9 Duodenum A Jejunum B Ileum C Ileocecal Valve E Large Intestine F Large Intestine, Right H Cecum J Appendix K Ascending Colon P Rectum Q Anus	0 Open 4 Percutaneous Endoscopic 7 Via Natural or Artificial Opening 8 Via Natural or Artificial Opening Endoscopic	Z No Device	Z No Qualifier
G Large Intestine, Left L Transverse Colon M Descending Colon N Sigmoid Colon	0 Open 4 Percutaneous Endoscopic 7 Via Natural or Artificial Opening 8 Via Natural or Artificial Opening Endoscopic F Via Natural or Artificial Opening With Percutaneous Endoscopic Assistance	Z No Device	Z No Qualifier
R Anal Sphincter U Omentum	0 Open 4 Percutaneous Endoscopic	Z No Device	Z No Qualifier

Section	0	Medical and Surgical
Body System	D	Gastrointestinal System
Operation	U	Supplement: Putting in or on biological or synthetic material that physically reinforces and/or augments the function of a portion of a body part

Body Part (4th)	Approach (5th)	Device (6th)	Qualifier (7th)
1 Esophagus, Upper 2 Esophagus, Middle 3 Esophagus, Lower 4 Esophagogastric Junction 5 Esophagus 6 Stomach 7 Stomach, Pylorus 8 Small Intestine 9 Duodenum A Jejunum B Ileum C Ileocecal Valve E Large Intestine F Large Intestine, Right G Large Intestine, Left H Cecum K Ascending Colon L Transverse Colon M Descending Colon N Sigmoid Colon P Rectum	0 Open 4 Percutaneous Endoscopic 7 Via Natural or Artificial Opening 8 Via Natural or Artificial Opening Endoscopic	7 Autologous Tissue Substitute J Synthetic Substitute K Nonautologous Tissue Substitute	Z No Qualifier
Q Anus	0 Open 4 Percutaneous Endoscopic 7 Via Natural or Artificial Opening 8 Via Natural or Artificial Opening Endoscopic X External	7 Autologous Tissue Substitute J Synthetic Substitute K Nonautologous Tissue Substitute	Z No Qualifier
R Anal Sphincter U Omentum V Mesentery W Peritoneum	0 Open 4 Percutaneous Endoscopic	7 Autologous Tissue Substitute J Synthetic Substitute K Nonautologous Tissue Substitute	Z No Qualifier

Section	0	Medical and Surgical
Body System	D	Gastrointestinal System
Operation	V	Restriction: Partially closing an orifice or the lumen of a tubular body part

Body Part (4th)	Approach (5th)	Device (6th)	Qualifier (7th)
1 Esophagus, Upper 2 Esophagus, Middle 3 Esophagus, Lower 4 Esophagogastric Junction 5 Esophagus 6 Stomach 7 Stomach, Pylorus 8 Small Intestine 9 Duodenum A Jejunum B Ileum C Ileocecal Valve E Large Intestine F Large Intestine, Right G Large Intestine, Left H Cecum K Ascending Colon L Transverse Colon M Descending Colon N Sigmoid Colon P Rectum	0 Open 3 Percutaneous 4 Percutaneous Endoscopic	C Extraluminal Device D Intraluminal Device Z No Device	Z No Qualifier

Continued →

Section	0	Medical and Surgical
Body System	D	Gastrointestinal System
Operation	V	Restriction: Partially closing an orifice or the lumen of a tubular body part

Body Part (4th)	Approach (5th)	Device (6th)	Qualifier (7th)

1 Esophagus, Upper
2 Esophagus, Middle
3 Esophagus, Lower
4 Esophagogastric Junction
5 Esophagus
6 Stomach
7 Stomach, Pylorus
8 Small Intestine
9 Duodenum
A Jejunum
B Ileum
C Ileocecal Valve
E Large Intestine
F Large Intestine, Right
G Large Intestine, Left
H Cecum
K Ascending Colon
L Transverse Colon
M Descending Colon
N Sigmoid Colon
P Rectum
	7 Via Natural or Artificial
	  Opening
	8 Via Natural or Artificial
	  Opening Endoscopic
		D Intraluminal Device
		Z No Device
			Z No Qualifier

Q Anus	0 Open 3 Percutaneous 4 Percutaneous Endoscopic X External	C Extraluminal Device D Intraluminal Device Z No Device	Z No Qualifier

Q Anus	7 Via Natural or Artificial
	  Opening
	8 Via Natural or Artificial
	  Opening Endoscopic
		D Intraluminal Device
		Z No Device
			Z No Qualifier

Section	0	Medical and Surgical
Body System	D	Gastrointestinal System
Operation	W	Revision: Correcting, to the extent possible, a portion of a malfunctioning device or the position of a displaced device

Body Part (4th)	Approach (5th)	Device (6th)	Qualifier (7th)

0 Upper Intestinal
  Tract
D Lower Intestinal
  Tract
	0 Open
	3 Percutaneous
	4 Percutaneous Endoscopic
	7 Via Natural or Artificial Opening
	8 Via Natural or Artificial Opening Endoscopic
		0 Drainage Device
		2 Monitoring Device
		3 Infusion Device
		7 Autologous Tissue Substitute
		C Extraluminal Device
		D Intraluminal Device
		J Synthetic Substitute
		K Nonautologous Tissue Substitute
		U Feeding Device
		Y Other Device
			Z No Qualifier

0 Upper Intestinal
  Tract
D Lower Intestinal
  Tract
	X External	0 Drainage Device
		2 Monitoring Device
		3 Infusion Device
		7 Autologous Tissue Substitute
		C Extraluminal Device
		D Intraluminal Device
		J Synthetic Substitute
		K Nonautologous Tissue Substitute
		U Feeding Device
			Z No Qualifier

Continued →

Body Part (4th)	Approach (5th)	Device (6th)	Qualifier (7th)
5 Esophagus	0 Open 3 Percutaneous 4 Percutaneous Endoscopic	Y Other Device	Z No Qualifier
5 Esophagus	7 Via Natural or Artificial Opening 8 Via Natural or Artificial Opening Endoscopic	D Intraluminal Device Y Other Device	Z No Qualifier
5 Esophagus	X External	D Intraluminal Device	Z No Qualifier
6 Stomach	0 Open 3 Percutaneous 4 Percutaneous Endoscopic	0 Drainage Device 2 Monitoring Device 3 Infusion Device 7 Autologous Tissue Substitute C Extraluminal Device D Intraluminal Device J Synthetic Substitute K Nonautologous Tissue Substitute M Stimulator Lead U Feeding Device Y Other Device	Z No Qualifier
6 Stomach	7 Via Natural or Artificial Opening 8 Via Natural or Artificial Opening Endoscopic	0 Drainage Device 2 Monitoring Device 3 Infusion Device 7 Autologous Tissue Substitute C Extraluminal Device D Intraluminal Device J Synthetic Substitute K Nonautologous Tissue Substitute U Feeding Device Y Other Device	Z No Qualifier
6 Stomach	X External	0 Drainage Device 2 Monitoring Device 3 Infusion Device 7 Autologous Tissue Substitute C Extraluminal Device D Intraluminal Device J Synthetic Substitute K Nonautologous Tissue Substitute U Feeding Device	Z No Qualifier
8 Small Intestine E Large Intestine	0 Open 4 Percutaneous Endoscopic 7 Via Natural or Artificial Opening 8 Via Natural or Artificial Opening Endoscopic	7 Autologous Tissue Substitute J Synthetic Substitute K Nonautologous Tissue Substitute	Z No Qualifier
Q Anus	0 Open 3 Percutaneous 4 Percutaneous Endoscopic 7 Via Natural or Artificial Opening 8 Via Natural or Artificial Opening Endoscopic	L Artificial Sphincter	Z No Qualifier
R Anal Sphincter	0 Open 3 Percutaneous 4 Percutaneous Endoscopic	M Stimulator Lead	Z No Qualifier
U Omentum V Mesentery W Peritoneum	0 Open 3 Percutaneous 4 Percutaneous Endoscopic	0 Drainage Device 7 Autologous Tissue Substitute J Synthetic Substitute K Nonautologous Tissue Substitute	Z No Qualifier

Section	0	Medical and Surgical
Body System	D	Gastrointestinal System
Operation	X	Transfer: Moving, without taking out, all or a portion of a body part to another location to take over the function of all or a portion of a body part

Body Part (4ᵗʰ)	Approach (5ᵗʰ)	Device (6ᵗʰ)	Qualifier (7ᵗʰ)
6 Stomach 8 Small Intestine	0 Open 4 Percutaneous Endoscopic	Z No Device	5 Esophagus
E Large Intestine	0 Open 4 Percutaneous Endoscopic	Z No Device	5 Esophagus 7 Vagina

Section	0	Medical and Surgical
Body System	D	Gastrointestinal System
Operation	Y	Transplantation: Putting in or on all or a portion of a living body part taken from another individual or animal to physically take the place and/or function of all or a portion of a similar body part

Body Part (4ᵗʰ)	Approach (5ᵗʰ)	Device (6ᵗʰ)	Qualifier (7ᵗʰ)
5 Esophagus 6 Stomach 8 Small Intestine E Large Intestine	0 Open	Z No Device	0 Allogeneic 1 Syngeneic 2 Zooplastic

AHA Coding Clinic

0D160ZA Bypass Stomach to Jejunum, Open Approach—AHA CC: 2Q, 2017, 17-18

0D194ZB Bypass Duodenum to Ileum, Percutaneous Endoscopic Approach—AHA CC: 2Q, 2016, 31

0D1N0Z4 Bypass Sigmoid Colon to Cutaneous, Open Approach—AHA CC: 4Q, 2014, 41-42

0D2DXUZ Change Feeding Device in Lower Intestinal Tract, External Approach—AHA CC: 1Q, 2019, 26-27

0D5W0ZZ Destruction of Peritoneum, Open Approach—AHA CC: 1Q, 2017, 34-35

0D768ZZ Dilation of Stomach, Via Natural or Artificial Opening Endoscopic—AHA CC: 4Q, 2014, 40

0D7A8ZZ Dilation of Jejunum, Via Natural or Artificial Opening Endoscopic—AHA CC: 4Q, 2014, 40

0D844ZZ Division of Esophagogastric Junction, Percutaneous Endoscopic Approach—AHA CC: 3Q, 2017, 22-23

0D874ZZ Division of Stomach, Pylorus, Percutaneous Endoscopic Approach—AHA CC: 3Q, 2017, 23-24; 2Q, 2019, 15-16

0D9670Z Drainage of Stomach with Drainage Device, Via Natural or Artificial Opening—AHA CC: 2Q, 2015, 29

0DB28ZX Excision of Middle Esophagus, Via Natural or Artificial Opening Endoscopic, Diagnostic—AHA CC: 1Q, 2016, 24-25

0DB60ZZ Excision of Stomach, Open Approach—AHA CC: 2Q, 2017, 17-18; 1Q, 2019, 4-7

0DB64Z3 Excision of Stomach, Percutaneous Endoscopic Approach, Vertical—AHA CC: 2Q, 2016, 31

0DB90ZZ Excision of Duodenum, Open Approach—AHA CC: 3Q, 2014, 32-33; 1Q, 2019, 4-7

0DBA0ZZ Excision of Jejunum, Open Approach—AHA CC: 1Q, 2019 4-5

0DBA4ZZ Excision of Jejunum, Percutaneous Endoscopic Approach—AHA CC: 2Q, 2019, 15-16

0DBB0ZZ Excision of Ileum, Open Approach—AHA CC: 3Q, 2014, 28-29; 3Q, 2016, 5-6

0DBK8ZZ Excision of Ascending Colon, Via Natural or Artificial Opening Endoscopic—AHA CC: 1Q, 2017, 16

0DBN0ZZ Excision of Sigmoid Colon, Open Approach—AHA CC: 4Q, 2014, 40-41; 1Q, 2019, 27

0DBP0ZZ Excision of Rectum, Open Approach—AHA CC: 1Q, 2019, 27

0DBP7ZZ Excision of Rectum, Via Natural or Artificial Opening—AHA CC: 1Q, 2016, 22

0DD68ZX Extraction of Stomach, Via Natural or Artificial Opening Endoscopic, Diagnostic—AHA CC: 4Q, 2017, 42

0DH63UZ Insertion of Feeding Device into Stomach, Percutaneous Approach—AHA CC: 4Q, 2013, 117

0DH67UZ Insertion of Feeding Device into Stomach, Via Natural or Artificial Opening—AHA CC: 3Q, 2016, 26-27

0DH68YZ Insertion of Monitoring Device into Stomach, Via Natural or Artificial Opening Endoscopic—AHA CC: 2Q, 2019, 18

0DJ07ZZ Inspection of Upper Intestinal Tract, Via Natural or Artificial Opening—AHA CC: 2Q, 2016, 20-21

0DJ08ZZ Inspection of Upper Intestinal Tract, Via Natural or Artificial Opening Endoscopic—AHA CC: 3Q, 2015, 24-25

0DJD0ZZ Inspection of Lower Intestinal Tract, Open Approach—AHA CC: 1Q, 2019, 25-26

0DJD8ZZ Inspection of Lower Intestinal Tract, Via Natural or Artificial Opening Endoscopic—AHA CC: 2Q, 2017, 15-16

0DN50ZZ Release Esophagus, Open Approach—AHA CC: 3Q, 2015, 15-16

0DN80ZZ Release Small Intestine, Open Approach—AHA CC: 4Q, 2017, 49-50

0DNW0ZZ Release Peritoneum, Open Approach—AHA CC: 1Q, 2017, 35

0DP68YZ Removal of Other Device from Stomach, Via Natural or Artificial Opening Endoscopic—AHA CC: 2Q, 2019, 18-19

0DQ64ZZ Repair Stomach, Percutaneous Endoscopic Approach—AHA CC: 2Q, 2019, 15-16

0DQ98ZZ Repair Duodenum, Via Natural or Artificial Opening Endoscopic—AHA CC: 4Q, 2014, 20

0DQP0ZZ Repair Rectum, Open Approach—AHA CC: 1Q, 2016, 7-8

0DQR0ZZ Repair Anal Sphincter, Open Approach—AHA CC: 1Q, 2016, 7-8

0DQV4ZZ Repair Mesentery, Percutaneous Endoscopic Approach— AHA CC: 1Q, 2018, 11-12

0DS80ZZ Reposition Small Intestine, Open Approach—AHA CC: 4Q, 2017, 49-50

0DSB7ZZ Reposition Ileum, Via Natural or Artificial Opening—AHA CC: 3Q, 2017, 9-10

0DSE0ZZ Reposition Large Intestine, Open Approach—AHA CC: 4Q, 2017, 49-50

0DSK7ZZ Reposition Ascending Colon, Via Natural or Artificial Opening—AHA CC: 3Q, 2017, 9-10

0DSM4ZZ Reposition Descending Colon, Percutaneous Endoscopic Approach—AHA CC: 3Q, 2016, 5-6

0DSP0ZZ Reposition Rectum, Open Approach—AHA CC: 3Q, 2017, 17-18; 1Q, 2019, 30-31

0DT30ZZ Resection of Lower Esophagus, Open Approach—AHA CC: 1Q, 2019, 14-15

0DT90ZZ Resection of Duodenum, Open Approach—AHA CC: 1Q, 2019, 4-7

0DTF0ZZ Resection of Right Large Intestine, Open Approach—AHA CC: 3Q, 2014, 6-7; 4Q, 2014, 42-43

0DTH0ZZ Resection of Cecum, Open Approach—AHA CC: 3Q, 2014, 6

0DTJ0ZZ Resection of Appendix, Open Approach—AHA CC: 4Q, 2017, 49-50

0DTP0ZZ Resection of Rectum, Open Approach—AHA CC: 4Q, 2014, 40-41

0DTQ0ZZ Resection of Anus, Open Approach—AHA CC: 4Q, 2014, 40-41

0DUP0JZ Supplement Rectum with Synthetic Substitute, Open Approach—AHA CC: 1Q, 2019, 30-31

0DV40ZZ Restriction of Esophagogastric Junction, Open Approach—AHA CC: 2Q, 2016, 22-23

0DV44ZZ Restriction of Esophagogastric Junction, Percutaneous Endoscopic Approach—AHA CC: 3Q, 2014, 28; 3Q, 2017, 22-23

0DW63CZ Revision of Extraluminal Device in Stomach, Percutaneous Approach—AHA CC: 1Q, 2018, 20

0DX60Z5 Transfer Stomach to Esophagus, Open Approach—AHA CC: 2Q, 2016, 22-23; 2Q, 2017, 18

0DXE0Z5 Transfer Large Intestine to Esophagus, Open Approach—AHA CC: 1Q, 2019, 14-15

0DXE0Z7 Transfer Large Intestine to Vagina, Open Approach—AHA CC: 4Q, 2019, 30

Surfaces and Bed of Liver

Surfaces and Bed of Liver

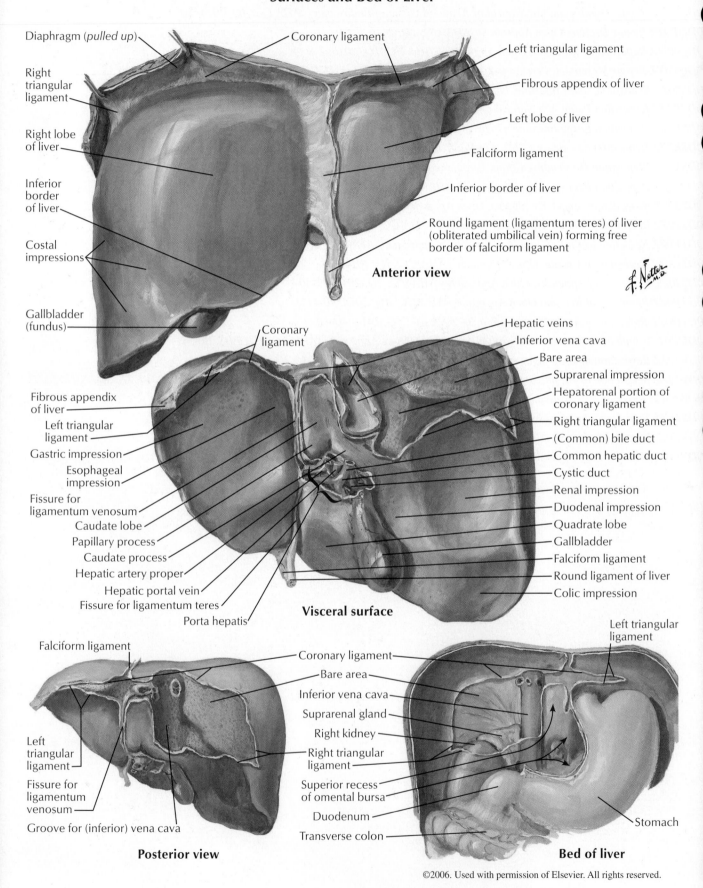

Diaphragm (*pulled up*)

Coronary ligament

Left triangular ligament

Right triangular ligament

Fibrous appendix of liver

Right lobe of liver

Left lobe of liver

Inferior border of liver

Falciform ligament

Inferior border of liver

Costal impressions

Round ligament (ligamentum teres) of liver (obliterated umbilical vein) forming free border of falciform ligament

Gallbladder (fundus)

Anterior view

Coronary ligament

Hepatic veins

Inferior vena cava

Bare area

Suprarenal impression

Fibrous appendix of liver

Hepatorenal portion of coronary ligament

Left triangular ligament

Right triangular ligament

Gastric impression

(Common) bile duct

Esophageal impression

Common hepatic duct

Fissure for ligamentum venosum

Cystic duct

Caudate lobe

Renal impression

Papillary process

Duodenal impression

Caudate process

Quadrate lobe

Hepatic artery proper

Gallbladder

Hepatic portal vein

Falciform ligament

Fissure for ligamentum teres

Round ligament of liver

Porta hepatis

Colic impression

Visceral surface

Falciform ligament

Coronary ligament

Left triangular ligament

Bare area

Inferior vena cava

Suprarenal gland

Right kidney

Left triangular ligament

Right triangular ligament

Fissure for ligamentum venosum

Superior recess of omental bursa

Groove for (inferior) vena cava

Duodenum

Transverse colon

Stomach

Posterior view

Bed of liver

Medical and Surgical, Hepatobiliary System and Pancreas

Pancreas: Anatomy and Histology

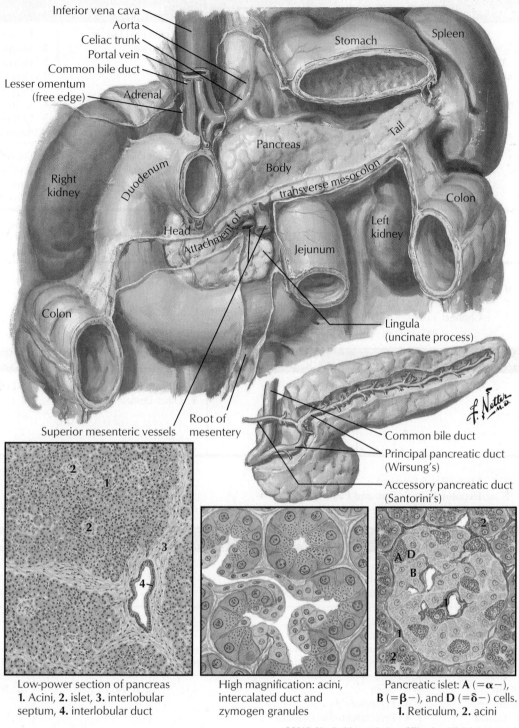

Inferior vena cava
Aorta
Celiac trunk
Portal vein
Common bile duct
Lesser omentum (free edge)
Adrenal
Stomach
Spleen
Pancreas
Body
Tail
trahsverse mesocolon
Right kidney
Duodenum
Colon
Head
Attachment of
Jejunum
Left kidney
Colon
Lingula (uncinate process)
Superior mesenteric vessels
Root of mesentery
Common bile duct
Principal pancreatic duct (Wirsung's)
Accessory pancreatic duct (Santorini's)

Low-power section of pancreas
1. Acini, **2.** islet, **3.** interlobular septum, **4.** interlobular duct

High magnification: acini, intercalated duct and zymogen granules

Pancreatic islet: **A** (=α−), **B** (=β−), and **D** (=δ−) cells.
1. Reticulum, **2.** acini

Hepatobiliary System and Pancreas Tables 0F1–0FY

Section	0	Medical and Surgical
Body System	F	Hepatobiliary System and Pancreas
Operation	1	**Bypass:** Altering the route of passage of the contents of a tubular body part

Body Part (4th)	Approach (5th)	Device (6th)	Qualifier (7th)
4 Gallbladder 5 Hepatic Duct, Right 6 Hepatic Duct, Left 7 Hepatic Duct, Common 8 Cystic Duct 9 Common Bile Duct	0 Open 4 Percutaneous Endoscopic	D Intraluminal Device Z No Device	3 Duodenum 4 Stomach 5 Hepatic Duct, Right 6 Hepatic Duct, Left 7 Hepatic Duct, Caudate 8 Cystic Duct 9 Common Bile Duct B Small Intestine
D Pancreatic Duct	0 Open 4 Percutaneous Endoscopic	D Intraluminal Device Z No Device	3 Duodenum 4 Stomach B Small Intestine C Large Intestine
F Pancreatic Duct, Accessory G Pancreas	0 Open 4 Percutaneous Endoscopic	D Intraluminal Device Z No Device	3 Duodenum B Small Intestine C Large Intestine

Section	0	Medical and Surgical
Body System	F	Hepatobiliary System and Pancreas
Operation	2	**Change:** Taking out or off a device from a body part and putting back an identical or similar device in or on the same body part without cutting or puncturing the skin or a mucous membrane

Body Part (4th)	Approach (5th)	Device (6th)	Qualifier (7th)
0 Liver 4 Gallbladder B Hepatobiliary Duct D Pancreatic Duct G Pancreas	X External	0 Drainage Device Y Other Device	Z No Qualifier

Section	0	Medical and Surgical
Body System	F	Hepatobiliary System and Pancreas
Operation	5	**Destruction:** Physical eradication of all or a portion of a body part by the direct use of energy, force, or a destructive agent

Body Part (4th)	Approach (5th)	Device (6th)	Qualifier (7th)
0 Liver 1 Liver, Right Lobe 2 Liver, Left Lobe	0 Open 3 Percutaneous 4 Percutaneous Endoscopic	Z No Device	F Irreversible Electroporation Z No Qualifier
4 Gallbladder	0 Open 3 Percutaneous 4 Percutaneous Endoscopic 8 Via Natural or Artificial Opening Endoscopic	Z No Device	Z No Qualifier
5 Hepatic Duct, Right 6 Hepatic Duct, Left 7 Hepatic Duct, Common 8 Cystic Duct 9 Common Bile Duct C Ampulla of Vater D Pancreatic Duct F Pancreatic Duct, Accessory	0 Open 3 Percutaneous 4 Percutaneous Endoscopic 7 Via Natural or Artificial Opening 8 Via Natural or Artificial Opening Endoscopic	Z No Device	Z No Qualifier
G Pancreas	0 Open 3 Percutaneous 4 Percutaneous Endoscopic	Z No Device	F Irreversible Electroporation Z No Qualifier
G Pancreas	8 Via Natural or Artificial Opening Endoscopic	Z No Device	Z No Qualifier

Section	0	Medical and Surgical
Body System	F	Hepatobiliary System and Pancreas
Operation	7	**Dilation:** Expanding an orifice or the lumen of a tubular body part

Body Part (4th)	Approach (5th)	Device (6th)	Qualifier (7th)
5 Hepatic Duct, Right 6 Hepatic Duct, Left 7 Hepatic Duct, Common 8 Cystic Duct 9 Common Bile Duct C Ampulla of Vater D Pancreatic Duct F Pancreatic Duct, Accessory	0 Open 3 Percutaneous 4 Percutaneous Endoscopic 7 Via Natural or Artificial Opening 8 Via Natural or Artificial Opening Endoscopic	D Intraluminal Device Z No Device	Z No Qualifier

Section	0	Medical and Surgical
Body System	F	Hepatobiliary System and Pancreas
Operation	8	**Division:** Cutting into a body part, without draining fluids and/or gases from the body part, in order to separate or transect a body part

Body Part (4th)	Approach (5th)	Device (6th)	Qualifier (7th)
G Pancreas	0 Open 3 Percutaneous 4 Percutaneous Endoscopic	Z No Device	Z No Qualifier

Section	0	Medical and Surgical
Body System	F	Hepatobiliary System and Pancreas
Operation	9	**Drainage:** Taking or letting out fluids and/or gases from a body part

Body Part (4th)	Approach (5th)	Device (6th)	Qualifier (7th)
0 Liver 1 Liver, Right Lobe 2 Liver, Left Lobe	0 Open 3 Percutaneous 4 Percutaneous Endoscopic	0 Drainage Device	Z No Qualifier
0 Liver 1 Liver, Right Lobe 2 Liver, Left Lobe	0 Open 3 Percutaneous 4 Percutaneous Endoscopic	Z No Device	X Diagnostic Z No Qualifier
4 Gallbladder G Pancreas	0 Open 3 Percutaneous 4 Percutaneous Endoscopic 8 Via Natural or Artificial Opening Endoscopic	0 Drainage Device	Z No Qualifier
4 Gallbladder G Pancreas	0 Open 3 Percutaneous 4 Percutaneous Endoscopic 8 Via Natural or Artificial Opening Endoscopic	Z No Device	X Diagnostic Z No Qualifier
5 Hepatic Duct, Right 6 Hepatic Duct, Left 7 Hepatic Duct, Common 8 Cystic Duct 9 Common Bile Duct C Ampulla of Vater D Pancreatic Duct F Pancreatic Duct, Accessory	0 Open 3 Percutaneous 4 Percutaneous Endoscopic 7 Via Natural or Artificial Opening 8 Via Natural or Artificial Opening Endoscopic	0 Drainage Device	Z No Qualifier
5 Hepatic Duct, Right 6 Hepatic Duct, Left 7 Hepatic Duct, Common 8 Cystic Duct 9 Common Bile Duct C Ampulla of Vater D Pancreatic Duct F Pancreatic Duct, Accessory	0 Open 3 Percutaneous 4 Percutaneous Endoscopic 7 Via Natural or Artificial Opening 8 Via Natural or Artificial Opening Endoscopic	Z No Device	X Diagnostic Z No Qualifier

Section   0   **Medical and Surgical**
Body System   F   **Hepatobiliary System and Pancreas**
Operation   B   **Excision:** Cutting out or off, without replacement, a portion of a body part

Body Part (4th)	Approach (5th)	Device (6th)	Qualifier (7th)
0 Liver 1 Liver, Right Lobe 2 Liver, Left Lobe	0 Open 3 Percutaneous 4 Percutaneous Endoscopic	Z No Device	X Diagnostic Z No Qualifier
4 Gallbladder G Pancreas	0 Open 3 Percutaneous 4 Percutaneous Endoscopic 8 Via Natural or Artificial Opening Endoscopic	Z No Device	X Diagnostic Z No Qualifier
5 Hepatic Duct, Right 6 Hepatic Duct, Left 7 Hepatic Duct, Common 8 Cystic Duct 9 Common Bile Duct C Ampulla of Vater D Pancreatic Duct F Pancreatic Duct, Accessory	0 Open 3 Percutaneous 4 Percutaneous Endoscopic 7 Via Natural or Artificial Opening 8 Via Natural or Artificial Opening Endoscopic	Z No Device	X Diagnostic Z No Qualifier

Section   0   **Medical and Surgical**
Body System   F   **Hepatobiliary System and Pancreas**
Operation   C   **Extirpation:** Taking or cutting out solid matter from a body part

Body Part (4th)	Approach (5th)	Device (6th)	Qualifier (7th)
0 Liver 1 Liver, Right Lobe 2 Liver, Left Lobe	0 Open 3 Percutaneous 4 Percutaneous Endoscopic	Z No Device	Z No Qualifier
4 Gallbladder G Pancreas	0 Open 3 Percutaneous 4 Percutaneous Endoscopic 8 Via Natural or Artificial Opening Endoscopic	Z No Device	Z No Qualifier
5 Hepatic Duct, Right 6 Hepatic Duct, Left 7 Hepatic Duct, Common 8 Cystic Duct 9 Common Bile Duct C Ampulla of Vater D Pancreatic Duct F Pancreatic Duct, Accessory	0 Open 3 Percutaneous 4 Percutaneous Endoscopic 7 Via Natural or Artificial Opening 8 Via Natural or Artificial Opening Endoscopic	Z No Device	Z No Qualifier

Section   0   **Medical and Surgical**
Body System   F   **Hepatobiliary System and Pancreas**
Operation   D   **Extraction:** Pulling or stripping out or off all or a portion of a body part by the use of force

Body Part (4th)	Approach (5th)	Device (6th)	Qualifier (7th)
0 Liver 1 Liver, Right Lobe 2 Liver, Left Lobe	3 Percutaneous 4 Percutaneous Endoscopic	Z No Device	X Diagnostic
4 Gallbladder 5 Hepatic Duct, Right 6 Hepatic Duct, Left 7 Hepatic Duct, Common 8 Cystic Duct 9 Common Bile Duct C Ampulla of Vater D Pancreatic Duct F Pancreatic Duct, Accessory G Pancreas	3 Percutaneous 4 Percutaneous Endoscopic 8 Via Natural or Artificial Opening Endoscopic	Z No Device	X Diagnostic

Section	0	Medical and Surgical
Body System	F	Hepatobiliary System and Pancreas
Operation	F	Fragmentation: Breaking solid matter in a body part into pieces

Body Part (4th)	Approach (5th)	Device (6th)	Qualifier (7th)
4 Gallbladder 5 Hepatic Duct, Right 6 Hepatic Duct, Left 7 Hepatic Duct, Common 8 Cystic Duct 9 Common Bile Duct C Ampulla of Vater D Pancreatic Duct F Pancreatic Duct, Accessory	0 Open 3 Percutaneous 4 Percutaneous Endoscopic 7 Via Natural or Artificial Opening 8 Via Natural or Artificial Opening Endoscopic X External	Z No Device	Z No Qualifier

Section	0	Medical and Surgical
Body System	F	Hepatobiliary System and Pancreas
Operation	H	Insertion: Putting in a nonbiological appliance that monitors, assists, performs, or prevents a physiological function but does not physically take the place of a body part

Body Part (4th)	Approach (5th)	Device (6th)	Qualifier (7th)
0 Liver 4 Gallbladder G Pancreas	0 Open 3 Percutaneous 4 Percutaneous Endoscopic	1 Radioactive Element 2 Monitoring Device 3 Infusion Device Y Other Device	Z No Qualifier
1 Liver, Right Lobe 2 Liver, Left Lobe	0 Open 3 Percutaneous 4 Percutaneous Endoscopic	2 Monitoring Device 3 Infusion Device	Z No Qualifier
B Hepatobiliary Duct D Pancreatic Duct	0 Open 3 Percutaneous 4 Percutaneous Endoscopic 7 Via Natural or Artificial Opening 8 Via Natural or Artificial Opening Endoscopic	1 Radioactive Element 2 Monitoring Device 3 Infusion Device D Intraluminal Device Y Other Device	Z No Qualifier

Section	0	Medical and Surgical
Body System	F	Hepatobiliary System and Pancreas
Operation	J	Inspection: Visually and/or manually exploring a body part

Body Part (4th)	Approach (5th)	Device (6th)	Qualifier (7th)
0 Liver	0 Open 3 Percutaneous 4 Percutaneous Endoscopic X External	Z No Device	Z No Qualifier
4 Gallbladder G Pancreas	0 Open 3 Percutaneous 4 Percutaneous Endoscopic 8 Via Natural or Artificial Opening Endoscopic X External	Z No Device	Z No Qualifier
B Hepatobiliary Duct D Pancreatic Duct	0 Open 3 Percutaneous 4 Percutaneous Endoscopic 7 Via Natural or Artificial Opening 8 Via Natural or Artificial Opening Endoscopic	Z No Device	Z No Qualifier

Section	0	Medical and Surgical
Body System	F	Hepatobiliary System and Pancreas
Operation	L	**Occlusion:** Completely closing an orifice or the lumen of a tubular body part

Body Part (4th)	Approach (5th)	Device (6th)	Qualifier (7th)
5 Hepatic Duct, Right 6 Hepatic Duct, Left 7 Hepatic Duct, Common 8 Cystic Duct 9 Common Bile Duct C Ampulla of Vater D Pancreatic Duct F Pancreatic Duct, Accessory	0 Open 3 Percutaneous 4 Percutaneous Endoscopic	C Extraluminal Device D Intraluminal Device Z No Device	Z No Qualifier
5 Hepatic Duct, Right 6 Hepatic Duct, Left 7 Hepatic Duct, Common 8 Cystic Duct 9 Common Bile Duct C Ampulla of Vater D Pancreatic Duct F Pancreatic Duct, Accessory	7 Via Natural or Artificial Opening 8 Via Natural or Artificial Opening Endoscopic	D Intraluminal Device Z No Device	Z No Qualifier

Section	0	Medical and Surgical
Body System	F	Hepatobiliary System and Pancreas
Operation	M	**Reattachment:** Putting back in or on all or a portion of a separated body part to its normal location or other suitable location

Body Part (4th)	Approach (5th)	Device (6th)	Qualifier (7th)
0 Liver 1 Liver, Right Lobe 2 Liver, Left Lobe 4 Gallbladder 5 Hepatic Duct, Right 6 Hepatic Duct, Left 7 Hepatic Duct, Common 8 Cystic Duct 9 Common Bile Duct C Ampulla of Vater D Pancreatic Duct F Pancreatic Duct, Accessory G Pancreas	0 Open 4 Percutaneous Endoscopic	Z No Device	Z No Qualifier

Section	0	Medical and Surgical
Body System	F	Hepatobiliary System and Pancreas
Operation	N	**Release:** Freeing a body part from an abnormal physical constraint by cutting or by the use of force

Body Part (4th)	Approach (5th)	Device (6th)	Qualifier (7th)
0 Liver 1 Liver, Right Lobe 2 Liver, Left Lobe	0 Open 3 Percutaneous 4 Percutaneous Endoscopic	Z No Device	Z No Qualifier
4 Gallbladder G Pancreas	0 Open 3 Percutaneous 4 Percutaneous Endoscopic 8 Via Natural or Artificial Opening Endoscopic	Z No Device	Z No Qualifier
5 Hepatic Duct, Right 6 Hepatic Duct, Left 7 Hepatic Duct, Common 8 Cystic Duct 9 Common Bile Duct C Ampulla of Vater D Pancreatic Duct F Pancreatic Duct, Accessory	0 Open 3 Percutaneous 4 Percutaneous Endoscopic 7 Via Natural or Artificial Opening 8 Via Natural or Artificial Opening Endoscopic	Z No Device	Z No Qualifier

Section	0	Medical and Surgical
Body System	F	Hepatobiliary System and Pancreas
Operation	P	Removal: Taking out or off a device from a body part

Body Part (4th)	Approach (5th)	Device (6th)	Qualifier (7th)
0 Liver	0 Open 3 Percutaneous 4 Percutaneous Endoscopic	0 Drainage Device 2 Monitoring Device 3 Infusion Device Y Other Device	Z No Qualifier
0 Liver	X External	0 Drainage Device 2 Monitoring Device 3 Infusion Device	Z No Qualifier
4 Gallbladder G Pancreas	0 Open 3 Percutaneous 4 Percutaneous Endoscopic X External	0 Drainage Device 2 Monitoring Device 3 Infusion Device D Intraluminal Device Y Other Device	Z No Qualifier
4 Gallbladder G Pancreas	X External	0 Drainage Device 2 Monitoring Device 3 Infusion Device D Intraluminal Device	Z No Qualifier
B Hepatobiliary Duct D Pancreatic Duct	0 Open 3 Percutaneous 4 Percutaneous Endoscopic 7 Via Natural or Artificial Opening 8 Via Natural or Artificial Opening Endoscopic	0 Drainage Device 1 Radioactive Element 2 Monitoring Device 3 Infusion Device 7 Autologous Tissue Substitute C Extraluminal Device D Intraluminal Device J Synthetic Substitute K Nonautologous Tissue Substitute Y Other Device	Z No Qualifier
B Hepatobiliary Duct D Pancreatic Duct	X External	0 Drainage Device 1 Radioactive Element 2 Monitoring Device 3 Infusion Device D Intraluminal Device	Z No Qualifier

Section	0	Medical and Surgical
Body System	F	Hepatobiliary System and Pancreas
Operation	Q	Repair: Restoring, to the extent possible, a body part to its normal anatomic structure and function

Body Part (4th)	Approach (5th)	Device (6th)	Qualifier (7th)
0 Liver 1 Liver, Right Lobe 2 Liver, Left Lobe	0 Open 3 Percutaneous 4 Percutaneous Endoscopic	Z No Device	Z No Qualifier
4 Gallbladder G Pancreas	0 Open 3 Percutaneous 4 Percutaneous Endoscopic 8 Via Natural or Artificial Opening Endoscopic	Z No Device	Z No Qualifier
5 Hepatic Duct, Right 6 Hepatic Duct, Left 7 Hepatic Duct, Common 8 Cystic Duct 9 Common Bile Duct C Ampulla of Vater D Pancreatic Duct F Pancreatic Duct, Accessory	0 Open 3 Percutaneous 4 Percutaneous Endoscopic 7 Via Natural or Artificial Opening 8 Via Natural or Artificial Opening Endoscopic	Z No Device	Z No Qualifier

Section	0	Medical and Surgical
Body System	F	Hepatobiliary System and Pancreas
Operation	R	**Replacement:** Putting in or on biological or synthetic material that physically takes the place and/or function of all or a portion of a body part

Body Part (4th)	Approach (5th)	Device (6th)	Qualifier (7th)
5 Hepatic Duct, Right 6 Hepatic Duct, Left 7 Hepatic Duct, Common 8 Cystic Duct 9 Common Bile Duct C Ampulla of Vater D Pancreatic Duct F Pancreatic Duct, Accessory	0 Open 4 Percutaneous Endoscopic 8 Via Natural or Artificial Opening Endoscopic	7 Autologous Tissue Substitute J Synthetic Substitute K Nonautologous Tissue Substitute	Z No Qualifier

Section	0	Medical and Surgical
Body System	F	Hepatobiliary System and Pancreas
Operation	S	**Reposition:** Moving to its normal location, or other suitable location, all or a portion of a body part

Body Part (4th)	Approach (5th)	Device (6th)	Qualifier (7th)
0 Liver 4 Gallbladder 5 Hepatic Duct, Right 6 Hepatic Duct, Left 7 Hepatic Duct, Common 8 Cystic Duct 9 Common Bile Duct C Ampulla of Vater D Pancreatic Duct F Pancreatic Duct, Accessory G Pancreas	0 Open 4 Percutaneous Endoscopic	Z No Device	Z No Qualifier

Section	0	Medical and Surgical
Body System	F	Hepatobiliary System and Pancreas
Operation	T	**Resection:** Cutting out or off, without replacement, all of a body part

Body Part (4th)	Approach (5th)	Device (6th)	Qualifier (7th)
0 Liver 1 Liver, Right Lobe 2 Liver, Left Lobe 4 Gallbladder G Pancreas	0 Open 4 Percutaneous Endoscopic	Z No Device	Z No Qualifier
5 Hepatic Duct, Right 6 Hepatic Duct, Left 7 Hepatic Duct, Common 8 Cystic Duct 9 Common Bile Duct C Ampulla of Vater D Pancreatic Duct F Pancreatic Duct, Accessory	0 Open 4 Percutaneous Endoscopic 7 Via Natural or Artificial Opening 8 Via Natural or Artificial Opening Endoscopic	Z No Device	Z No Qualifier

Section	0	Medical and Surgical
Body System	F	Hepatobiliary System and Pancreas
Operation	U	Supplement: Putting in or on biological or synthetic material that physically reinforces and/or augments the function of a portion of a body part

Body Part (4th)	Approach (5th)	Device (6th)	Qualifier (7th)
5 Hepatic Duct, Right 6 Hepatic Duct, Left 7 Hepatic Duct, Common 8 Cystic Duct 9 Common Bile Duct C Ampulla of Vater D Pancreatic Duct F Pancreatic Duct, Accessory	0 Open 3 Percutaneous 4 Percutaneous Endoscopic 8 Via Natural or Artificial Opening Endoscopic	7 Autologous Tissue Substitute J Synthetic Substitute K Nonautologous Tissue Substitute	Z No Qualifier

Section	0	Medical and Surgical
Body System	F	Hepatobiliary System and Pancreas
Operation	V	Restriction: Partially closing an orifice or the lumen of a tubular body part

Body Part (4th)	Approach (5th)	Device (6th)	Qualifier (7th)
5 Hepatic Duct, Right 6 Hepatic Duct, Left 7 Hepatic Duct, Common 8 Cystic Duct 9 Common Bile Duct C Ampulla of Vater D Pancreatic Duct F Pancreatic Duct, Accessory	0 Open 3 Percutaneous 4 Percutaneous Endoscopic	C Extraluminal Device D Intraluminal Device Z No Device	Z No Qualifier
5 Hepatic Duct, Right 6 Hepatic Duct, Left 7 Hepatic Duct, Common 8 Cystic Duct 9 Common Bile Duct C Ampulla of Vater D Pancreatic Duct F Pancreatic Duct, Accessory	7 Via Natural or Artificial Opening 8 Via Natural or Artificial Opening Endoscopic	D Intraluminal Device Z No Device	Z No Qualifier

Section	0	Medical and Surgical
Body System	F	Hepatobiliary System and Pancreas
Operation	W	Revision: Correcting, to the extent possible, a portion of a malfunctioning device or the position of a displaced device

Body Part (4th)	Approach (5th)	Device (6th)	Qualifier (7th)
0 Liver	0 Open 3 Percutaneous 4 Percutaneous Endoscopic	0 Drainage Device 2 Monitoring Device 3 Infusion Device Y Other Device	Z No Qualifier
0 Liver	X External	0 Drainage Device 2 Monitoring Device 3 Infusion Device	Z No Qualifier
4 Gallbladder G Pancreas	0 Open 3 Percutaneous 4 Percutaneous Endoscopic	0 Drainage Device 2 Monitoring Device 3 Infusion Device D Intraluminal Device Y Other Device	Z No Qualifier
4 Gallbladder G Pancreas	X External	0 Drainage Device 2 Monitoring Device 3 Infusion Device D Intraluminal Device	Z No Qualifier

Continued →

Section	0	Medical and Surgical
Body System	F	Hepatobiliary System and Pancreas
Operation	W	Revision: Correcting, to the extent possible, a portion of a malfunctioning device or the position of a displaced device

Body Part (4th)	Approach (5th)	Device (6th)	Qualifier (7th)
B Hepatobiliary Duct D Pancreatic Duct	0 Open 3 Percutaneous 4 Percutaneous Endoscopic 7 Via Natural or Artificial Opening 8 Via Natural or Artificial Opening Endoscopic	0 Drainage Device 2 Monitoring Device 3 Infusion Device 7 Autologous Tissue Substitute C Extraluminal Device D Intraluminal Device J Synthetic Substitute K Nonautologous Tissue Substitute Y Other Device	Z No Qualifier
B Hepatobiliary Duct D Pancreatic Duct	X External	0 Drainage Device 2 Monitoring Device 3 Infusion Device 7 Autologous Tissue Substitute C Extraluminal Device D Intraluminal Device J Synthetic Substitute K Nonautologous Tissue Substitute	Z No Qualifier

Section	0	Medical and Surgical
Body System	F	Hepatobiliary System and Pancreas
Operation	Y	Transplantation: Putting in or on all or a portion of a living body part taken from another individual or animal to physically take the place and/or function of all or a portion of a similar body part

Body Part (4th)	Approach (5th)	Device (6th)	Qualifier (7th)
0 Liver G Pancreas	0 Open	Z No Device	0 Allogeneic 1 Syngeneic 2 Zooplastic

AHA Coding Clinic

0F5G4ZF Destruction of Pancreas using Irreversible Electroporation, Percutaneous Endoscopic Approach—AHA CC: 4Q, 2018, 39-40

0F798DZ Dilation of Common Bile Duct with Intraluminal Device, Via Natural or Artificial Opening Endoscopic—AHA CC: 3Q, 2014, 15-16; 1Q, 2016, 25

0F7D8DZ Dilation of Pancreatic Duct with Intraluminal Device, Via Natural or Artificial Opening Endoscopic—AHA CC: 1Q, 2016, 25; 3Q, 2016, 27-28

0F9630Z Drainage of Left Hepatic Duct with Drainage Device, Percutaneous Approach—AHA CC: 1Q, 2015, 32

0F9G40Z Drainage of Pancreas with Drainage Device, Percutaneous Endoscopic Approach AHA CC: 3Q, 2014, 15-16

0FB00ZX Excision of Liver, Open Approach, Diagnostic—AHA CC: 3Q, 2016, 41

0FB90ZZ Excision of Common Bile Duct, Open Approach—AHA CC: 1Q, 2019, 4-7

0FB98ZX Excision of Common Bile Duct, Via Natural or Artificial Opening Endoscopic, Diagnostic—AHA CC: 1Q, 2016, 23-25

0FBD8ZX Excision of Pancreatic Duct, Via Natural or Artificial Opening Endoscopic, Diagnostic—AHA CC: 1Q, 2016, 25

0FBG0ZZ Excision of Pancreas, Open Approach—AHA CC: 3Q, 2014, 32-33; 1Q, 2019, 4-8

0FQ00ZZ Repair Liver, Open Approach—AHA CC: 4Q, 2013, 109-111

0FQ90ZZ Repair Common Bile Duct, Open Approach—AHA CC: 3Q, 2016, 27

0FT00ZZ Resection of Liver, Open Approach—AHA CC: 4Q, 2012, 99-101

0FT40ZZ Resection of Gallbladder, Open Approach—AHA CC: 1Q, 2019, 4-5

0FY00Z0 Transplantation of Liver, Allogeneic, Open Approach—AHA CC: 4Q, 2012, 99-101; 3Q, 2014, 13-14

Endocrine System

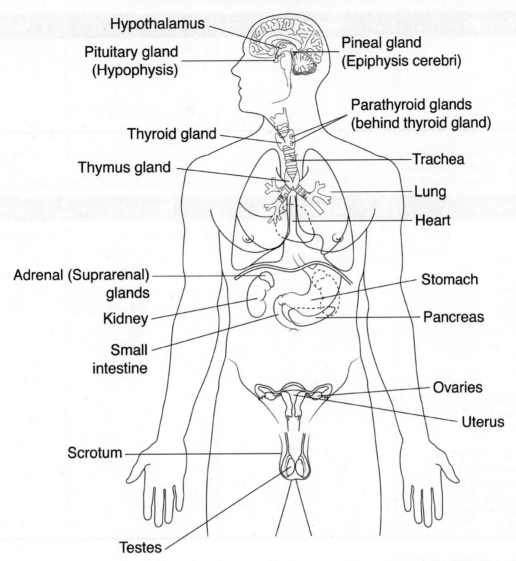

Hypothalamus

Pituitary gland
(Hypophysis)

Pineal gland
(Epiphysis cerebri)

Parathyroid glands
(behind thyroid gland)

Thyroid gland

Thymus gland

Trachea

Lung

Heart

Adrenal (Suprarenal)
glands

Kidney

Small
intestine

Stomach

Pancreas

Ovaries

Uterus

Scrotum

Testes

©AHIMA

Endocrine System Tables 0G2–0GW

Section	0	Medical and Surgical
Body System	G	Endocrine System
Operation	2	**Change:** Taking out or off a device from a body part and putting back an identical or similar device in or on the same body part without cutting or puncturing the skin or a mucous membrane

Body Part (4th)	Approach (5th)	Device (6th)	Qualifier (7th)
0 Pituitary Gland 1 Pineal Body 5 Adrenal Gland K Thyroid Gland R Parathyroid Gland S Endocrine Gland	X External	0 Drainage Device Y Other Device	Z No Qualifier

Section	0	Medical and Surgical
Body System	G	Endocrine System
Operation	5	**Destruction:** Physical eradication of all or a portion of a body part by the direct use of energy, force, or a destructive agent

Body Part (4th)	Approach (5th)	Device (6th)	Qualifier (7th)
0 Pituitary Gland 1 Pineal Body 2 Adrenal Gland, Left 3 Adrenal Gland, Right 4 Adrenal Glands, Bilateral 6 Carotid Body, Left 7 Carotid Body, Right 8 Carotid Bodies, Bilateral 9 Para-aortic Body B Coccygeal Glomus C Glomus Jugulare D Aortic Body F Paraganglion Extremity G Thyroid Gland Lobe, Left H Thyroid Gland Lobe, Right K Thyroid Gland L Superior Parathyroid Gland, Right M Superior Parathyroid Gland, Left N Inferior Parathyroid Gland, Right P Inferior Parathyroid Gland, Left Q Parathyroid Glands, Multiple R Parathyroid Gland	0 Open 3 Percutaneous 4 Percutaneous Endoscopic	Z No Device	Z No Qualifier

Section	0	Medical and Surgical
Body System	G	Endocrine System
Operation	8	**Division:** Cutting into a body part, without draining fluids and/or gases from the body part, in order to separate or transect a body part

Body Part (4th)	Approach (5th)	Device (6th)	Qualifier (7th)
0 Pituitary Gland J Thyroid Gland Isthmus	0 Open 3 Percutaneous 4 Percutaneous Endoscopic	Z No Device	Z No Qualifier

Section	0	Medical and Surgical
Body System	G	Endocrine System
Operation	9	Drainage: Taking or letting out fluids and/or gases from a body part

Body Part (4th)	Approach (5th)	Device (6th)	Qualifier (7th)
0 Pituitary Gland 1 Pineal Body 2 Adrenal Gland, Left 3 Adrenal Gland, Right 4 Adrenal Glands, Bilateral 6 Carotid Body, Left 7 Carotid Body, Right 8 Carotid Bodies, Bilateral 9 Para-aortic Body B Coccygeal Glomus C Glomus Jugulare D Aortic Body F Paraganglion Extremity G Thyroid Gland Lobe, Left H Thyroid Gland Lobe, Right K Thyroid Gland L Superior Parathyroid Gland, Right M Superior Parathyroid Gland, Left N Inferior Parathyroid Gland, Right P Inferior Parathyroid Gland, Left Q Parathyroid Glands, Multiple R Parathyroid Gland	0 Open 3 Percutaneous 4 Percutaneous Endoscopic	0 Drainage Device	Z No Qualifier
0 Pituitary Gland 1 Pineal Body 2 Adrenal Gland, Left 3 Adrenal Gland, Right 4 Adrenal Glands, Bilateral 6 Carotid Body, Left 7 Carotid Body, Right 8 Carotid Bodies, Bilateral 9 Para-aortic Body B Coccygeal Glomus C Glomus Jugulare D Aortic Body F Paraganglion Extremity G Thyroid Gland Lobe, Left H Thyroid Gland Lobe, Right K Thyroid Gland L Superior Parathyroid Gland, Right M Superior Parathyroid Gland, Left N Inferior Parathyroid Gland, Right P Inferior Parathyroid Gland, Left Q Parathyroid Glands, Multiple R Parathyroid Gland	0 Open 3 Percutaneous 4 Percutaneous Endoscopic	Z No Device	X Diagnostic Z No Qualifier

Section	0	Medical and Surgical
Body System	G	Endocrine System
Operation	B	**Excision:** Cutting out or off, without replacement, a portion of a body part

Body Part (4th)	Approach (5th)	Device (6th)	Qualifier (7th)
0 Pituitary Gland 1 Pineal Body 2 Adrenal Gland, Left 3 Adrenal Gland, Right 4 Adrenal Glands, Bilateral 6 Carotid Body, Left 7 Carotid Body, Right 8 Carotid Bodies, Bilateral 9 Para-aortic Body B Coccygeal Glomus C Glomus Jugulare D Aortic Body F Paraganglion Extremity G Thyroid Gland Lobe, Left H Thyroid Gland Lobe, Right J Thyroid Gland Isthmus L Superior Parathyroid Gland, Right M Superior Parathyroid Gland, Left N Inferior Parathyroid Gland, Right P Inferior Parathyroid Gland, Left Q Parathyroid Glands, Multiple R Parathyroid Gland	0 Open 3 Percutaneous 4 Percutaneous Endoscopic	Z No Device	X Diagnostic Z No Qualifier

Section	0	Medical and Surgical
Body System	G	Endocrine System
Operation	C	**Extirpation:** Taking or cutting out solid matter from a body part

Body Part (4th)	Approach (5th)	Device (6th)	Qualifier (7th)
0 Pituitary Gland 1 Pineal Body 2 Adrenal Gland, Left 3 Adrenal Gland, Right 4 Adrenal Glands, Bilateral 6 Carotid Body, Left 7 Carotid Body, Right 8 Carotid Bodies, Bilateral 9 Para-aortic Body B Coccygeal Glomus C Glomus Jugulare D Aortic Body F Paraganglion Extremity G Thyroid Gland Lobe, Left H Thyroid Gland Lobe, Right K Thyroid Gland L Superior Parathyroid Gland, Right M Superior Parathyroid Gland, Left N Inferior Parathyroid Gland, Right P Inferior Parathyroid Gland, Left Q Parathyroid Glands, Multiple R Parathyroid Gland	0 Open 3 Percutaneous 4 Percutaneous Endoscopic	Z No Device	Z No Qualifier

Section	0	Medical and Surgical
Body System	G	Endocrine System
Operation	H	**Insertion:** Putting in a nonbiological appliance that monitors, assists, performs, or prevents a physiological function but does not physically take the place of a body part

Body Part (4th)	Approach (5th)	Device (6th)	Qualifier (7th)
S Endocrine Gland	0 Open 3 Percutaneous 4 Percutaneous Endoscopic	1 Radioactive Element 2 Monitoring Device 3 Infusion Device Y Other Device	Z No Qualifier

Section   **0**   **Medical and Surgical**
Body System   **G**   **Endocrine System**
Operation   **J**   **Inspection:** Visually and/or manually exploring a body part

Body Part (4th)	Approach (5th)	Device (6th)	Qualifier (7th)
0 Pituitary Gland 1 Pineal Body 5 Adrenal Gland K Thyroid Gland R Parathyroid Gland S Endocrine Gland	0 Open 3 Percutaneous 4 Percutaneous Endoscopic	Z No Device	Z No Qualifier

Section   **0**   **Medical and Surgical**
Body System   **G**   **Endocrine System**
Operation   **M**   **Reattachment:** Putting back in or on all or a portion of a separated body part to its normal location or other suitable location

Body Part (4th)	Approach (5th)	Device (6th)	Qualifier (7th)
2 Adrenal Gland, Left 3 Adrenal Gland, Right G Thyroid Gland Lobe, Left H Thyroid Gland Lobe, Right L Superior Parathyroid Gland, Right M Superior Parathyroid Gland, Left N Inferior Parathyroid Gland, Right P Inferior Parathyroid Gland, Left Q Parathyroid Glands, Multiple R Parathyroid Gland	0 Open 4 Percutaneous Endoscopic	Z No Device	Z No Qualifier

Section   **0**   **Medical and Surgical**
Body System   **G**   **Endocrine System**
Operation   **N**   **Release:** Freeing a body part from an abnormal physical constraint by cutting or by the use of force

Body Part (4th)	Approach (5th)	Device (6th)	Qualifier (7th)
0 Pituitary Gland 1 Pineal Body 2 Adrenal Gland, Left 3 Adrenal Gland, Right 4 Adrenal Glands, Bilateral 6 Carotid Body, Left 7 Carotid Body, Right 8 Carotid Bodies, Bilateral 9 Para-aortic Body B Coccygeal Glomus C Glomus Jugulare D Aortic Body F Paraganglion Extremity G Thyroid Gland Lobe, Left H Thyroid Gland Lobe, Right K Thyroid Gland L Superior Parathyroid Gland, Right M Superior Parathyroid Gland, Left N Inferior Parathyroid Gland, Right P Inferior Parathyroid Gland, Left Q Parathyroid Glands, Multiple R Parathyroid Gland	0 Open 3 Percutaneous 4 Percutaneous Endoscopic	Z No Device	Z No Qualifier

Section	0	Medical and Surgical
Body System	G	Endocrine System
Operation	P	Removal: Taking out or off a device from a body part

Body Part (4th)	Approach (5th)	Device (6th)	Qualifier (7th)
0 Pituitary Gland 1 Pineal Body 5 Adrenal Gland K Thyroid Gland R Parathyroid Gland	0 Open 3 Percutaneous 4 Percutaneous Endoscopic X External	0 Drainage Device	Z No Qualifier
S Endocrine Gland	0 Open 3 Percutaneous 4 Percutaneous Endoscopic	0 Drainage Device 2 Monitoring Device 3 Infusion Device Y Other Device	Z No Qualifier
S Endocrine Gland	X External	0 Drainage Device 2 Monitoring Device 3 Infusion Device	Z No Qualifier

Section	0	Medical and Surgical
Body System	G	Endocrine System
Operation	Q	Repair: Restoring, to the extent possible, a body part to its normal anatomic structure and function

Body Part (4th)	Approach (5th)	Device (6th)	Qualifier (7th)
0 Pituitary Gland 1 Pineal Body 2 Adrenal Gland, Left 3 Adrenal Gland, Right 4 Adrenal Glands, Bilateral 6 Carotid Body, Left 7 Carotid Body, Right 8 Carotid Bodies, Bilateral 9 Para-aortic Body B Coccygeal Glomus C Glomus Jugulare D Aortic Body F Paraganglion Extremity G Thyroid Gland Lobe, Left H Thyroid Gland Lobe, Right J Thyroid Gland Isthmus K Thyroid Gland L Superior Parathyroid Gland, Right M Superior Parathyroid Gland, Left N Inferior Parathyroid Gland, Right P Inferior Parathyroid Gland, Left Q Parathyroid Glands, Multiple R Parathyroid Gland	0 Open 3 Percutaneous 4 Percutaneous Endoscopic	Z No Device	Z No Qualifier

Section	0	Medical and Surgical
Body System	G	Endocrine System
Operation	S	Reposition: Moving to its normal location, or other suitable location, all or a portion of a body part

Body Part (4th)	Approach (5th)	Device (6th)	Qualifier (7th)
2 Adrenal Gland, Left 3 Adrenal Gland, Right G Thyroid Gland Lobe, Left H Thyroid Gland Lobe, Right L Superior Parathyroid Gland, Right M Superior Parathyroid Gland, Left N Inferior Parathyroid Gland, Right P Inferior Parathyroid Gland, Left Q Parathyroid Glands, Multiple R Parathyroid Gland	0 Open 4 Percutaneous Endoscopic	Z No Device	Z No Qualifier

Section	0	Medical and Surgical
Body System	G	Endocrine System
Operation	T	**Resection:** Cutting out or off, without replacement, all of a body part

Body Part (4th)	Approach (5th)	Device (6th)	Qualifier (7th)
0 Pituitary Gland **1** Pineal Body **2** Adrenal Gland, Left **3** Adrenal Gland, Right **4** Adrenal Glands, Bilateral **6** Carotid Body, Left **7** Carotid Body, Right **8** Carotid Bodies, Bilateral **9** Para-aortic Body **B** Coccygeal Glomus **C** Glomus Jugulare **D** Aortic Body **F** Paraganglion Extremity **G** Thyroid Gland Lobe, Left **H** Thyroid Gland Lobe, Right **J** Thyroid Gland Isthmus **K** Thyroid Gland **L** Superior Parathyroid Gland, Right **M** Superior Parathyroid Gland, Left **N** Inferior Parathyroid Gland, Right **P** Inferior Parathyroid Gland, Left **Q** Parathyroid Glands, Multiple **R** Parathyroid Gland	**0** Open **4** Percutaneous Endoscopic	**Z** No Device	**Z** No Qualifier

Section	0	Medical and Surgical
Body System	G	Endocrine System
Operation	W	**Revision:** Correcting, to the extent possible, a portion of a malfunctioning device or the position of a displaced device

Body Part (4th)	Approach (5th)	Device (6th)	Qualifier (7th)
0 Pituitary Gland **1** Pineal Body **5** Adrenal Gland **K** Thyroid Gland **R** Parathyroid Gland	**0** Open **3** Percutaneous **4** Percutaneous Endoscopic **X** External	**0** Drainage Device	**Z** No Qualifier
S Endocrine Gland	**0** Open **3** Percutaneous **4** Percutaneous Endoscopic	**0** Drainage Device **2** Monitoring Device **3** Infusion Device **Y** Other Device	**Z** No Qualifier
S Endocrine Gland	**X** External	**0** Drainage Device **2** Monitoring Device **3** Infusion Device	**Z** No Qualifier

AHA Coding Clinic

0GB00ZZ Excision of Pituitary Gland, Open Approach—AHA CC: 3Q, 2014, 22-23

0GBG0ZZ Excision of Left Thyroid Gland Lobe, Open Approach—AHA CC: 2Q, 2017, 20

0GBH0ZZ Excision of Right Thyroid Gland Lobe, Open Approach—AHA CC: 2Q, 2017, 20

Cross-Section of the Skin Showing Layers and Types of Infections

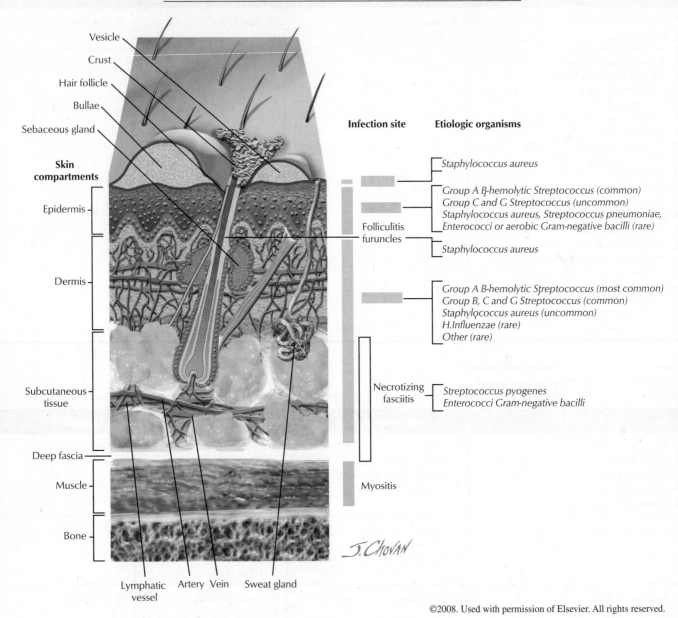

Infection site	Etiologic organisms
	Staphylococcus aureus
Folliculitis furuncles	*Group A β-hemolytic Streptococcus (common)* *Group C and G Streptococcus (uncommon)* *Staphylococcus aureus, Streptococcus pneumoniae,* *Enterococci or aerobic Gram-negative bacilli (rare)*
	Staphylococcus aureus
	Group A B-hemolytic Streptococcus (most common) *Group B, C and G Streptococcus (common)* *Staphylococcus aureus (uncommon)* *H.Influenzae (rare)* *Other (rare)*
Necrotizing fasciitis	*Streptococcus pyogenes* *Enterococci Gram-negative bacilli*
Myositis	

Skin compartments:

- Epidermis
- Dermis
- Subcutaneous tissue
- Deep fascia
- Muscle
- Bone

Labels: Vesicle, Crust, Hair follicle, Bullae, Sebaceous gland, Lymphatic vessel, Artery, Vein, Sweat gland

J. CHOVAN

Breast

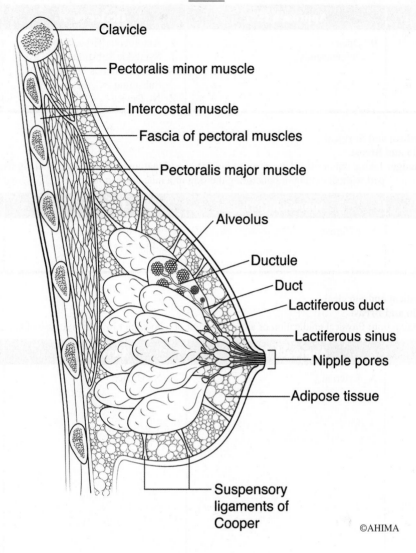

- Clavicle
- Pectoralis minor muscle
- Intercostal muscle
- Fascia of pectoral muscles
- Pectoralis major muscle
- Alveolus
- Ductule
- Duct
- Lactiferous duct
- Lactiferous sinus
- Nipple pores
- Adipose tissue
- Suspensory ligaments of Cooper

©AHIMA

Nail Bed

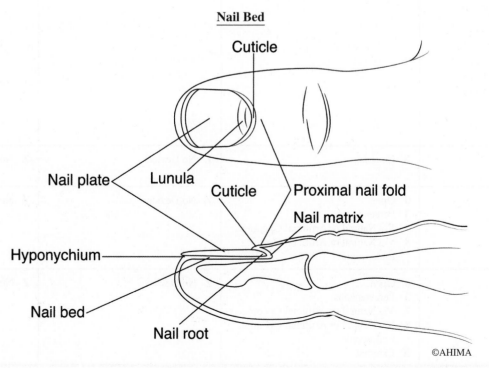

- Cuticle
- Nail plate
- Lunula
- Cuticle
- Proximal nail fold
- Nail matrix
- Hyponychium
- Nail bed
- Nail root

©AHIMA

Section   0   **Medical and Surgical**
Body System   H   **Skin and Breast**
Operation   0   **Alteration:** Modifying the anatomic structure of a body part without affecting the function of the body part

Body Part (4th)	Approach (5th)	Device (6th)	Qualifier (7th)
T Breast, Right U Breast, Left V Breast, Bilateral	0 Open 3 Percutaneous	7 Autologous Tissue Substitute J Synthetic Substitute K Nonautologous Tissue Substitute Z No Device	Z No Qualifier

Section   0   **Medical and Surgical**
Body System   H   **Skin and Breast**
Operation   2   **Change:** Taking out or off a device from a body part and putting back an identical or similar device in or on the same body part without cutting or puncturing the skin or a mucous membrane

Body Part (4th)	Approach (5th)	Device (6th)	Qualifier (7th)
P Skin T Breast, Right U Breast, Left	X External	0 Drainage Device Y Other Device	Z No Qualifier

Section   0   **Medical and Surgical**
Body System   H   **Skin and Breast**
Operation   5   **Destruction:** Physical eradication of all or a portion of a body part by the direct use of energy, force, or a destructive agent

Body Part (4th)	Approach (5th)	Device (6th)	Qualifier (7th)
0 Skin, Scalp 1 Skin, Face 2 Skin, Right Ear 3 Skin, Left Ear 4 Skin, Neck 5 Skin, Chest 6 Skin, Back 7 Skin, Abdomen 8 Skin, Buttock 9 Skin, Perineum A Skin, Inguinal B Skin, Right Upper Arm C Skin, Left Upper Arm D Skin, Right Lower Arm E Skin, Left Lower Arm F Skin, Right Hand G Skin, Left Hand H Skin, Right Upper Leg J Skin, Left Upper Leg K Skin, Right Lower Leg L Skin, Left Lower Leg M Skin, Right Foot N Skin, Left Foot	X External	Z No Device	D Multiple Z No Qualifier
Q Finger Nail R Toe Nail	X External	Z No Device	Z No Qualifier
T Breast, Right U Breast, Left V Breast, Bilateral	0 Open 3 Percutaneous 7 Via Natural or Artificial Opening 8 Via Natural or Artificial Opening Endoscopic	Z No Device	Z No Qualifier
W Nipple, Right X Nipple, Left	0 Open 3 Percutaneous 7 Via Natural or Artificial Opening 8 Via Natural or Artificial Opening Endoscopic X External	Z No Device	Z No Qualifier

Section	0	Medical and Surgical
Body System	H	Skin and Breast
Operation	8	Division: Cutting into a body part, without draining fluids and/or gases from the body part, in order to separate or transect a body part

Body Part (4th)	Approach (5th)	Device (6th)	Qualifier (7th)
0 Skin, Scalp 1 Skin, Face 2 Skin, Right Ear 3 Skin, Left Ear 4 Skin, Neck 5 Skin, Chest 6 Skin, Back 7 Skin, Abdomen 8 Skin, Buttock 9 Skin, Perineum A Skin, Inguinal B Skin, Right Upper Arm C Skin, Left Upper Arm D Skin, Right Lower Arm E Skin, Left Lower Arm F Skin, Right Hand G Skin, Left Hand H Skin, Right Upper Leg J Skin, Left Upper Leg K Skin, Right Lower Leg L Skin, Left Lower Leg M Skin, Right Foot N Skin, Left Foot	X External	Z No Device	Z No Qualifier

Section	0	Medical and Surgical
Body System	H	Skin and Breast
Operation	9	Drainage: Taking or letting out fluids and/or gases from a body part

Body Part (4th)	Approach (5th)	Device (6th)	Qualifier (7th)
0 Skin, Scalp 1 Skin, Face 2 Skin, Right Ear 3 Skin, Left Ear 4 Skin, Neck 5 Skin, Chest 6 Skin, Back 7 Skin, Abdomen 8 Skin, Buttock 9 Skin, Perineum A Skin, Inguinal B Skin, Right Upper Arm C Skin, Left Upper Arm D Skin, Right Lower Arm E Skin, Left Lower Arm F Skin, Right Hand G Skin, Left Hand H Skin, Right Upper Leg J Skin, Left Upper Leg K Skin, Right Lower Leg L Skin, Left Lower Leg M Skin, Right Foot N Skin, Left Foot Q Finger Nail R Toe Nail	X External	0 Drainage Device	Z No Qualifier

Continued →

Section	0	Medical and Surgical
Body System	H	Skin and Breast
Operation	9	Drainage: Taking or letting out fluids and/or gases from a body part

Body Part (4th)	Approach (5th)	Device (6th)	Qualifier (7th)
0 Skin, Scalp **1** Skin, Face **2** Skin, Right Ear **3** Skin, Left Ear **4** Skin, Neck **5** Skin, Chest **6** Skin, Back **7** Skin, Abdomen **8** Skin, Buttock **9** Skin, Perineum **A** Skin, Inguinal **B** Skin, Right Upper Arm **C** Skin, Left Upper Arm **D** Skin, Right Lower Arm **E** Skin, Left Lower Arm **F** Skin, Right Hand **G** Skin, Left Hand **H** Skin, Right Upper Leg **J** Skin, Left Upper Leg **K** Skin, Right Lower Leg **L** Skin, Left Lower Leg **M** Skin, Right Foot **N** Skin, Left Foot **Q** Finger Nail **R** Toe Nail	**X** External	**Z** No Device	**X** Diagnostic **Z** No Qualifier
T Breast, Right **U** Breast, Left **V** Breast, Bilateral	**0** Open **3** Percutaneous **7** Via Natural or Artificial Opening **8** Via Natural or Artificial Opening Endoscopic	**0** Drainage Device	**Z** No Qualifier
T Breast, Right **U** Breast, Left **V** Breast, Bilateral	**0** Open **3** Percutaneous **7** Via Natural or Artificial Opening **8** Via Natural or Artificial Opening Endoscopic	**Z** No Device	**X** Diagnostic **Z** No Qualifier
W Nipple, Right **X** Nipple, Left	**0** Open **3** Percutaneous **7** Via Natural or Artificial Opening **8** Via Natural or Artificial Opening Endoscopic **X** External	**0** Drainage Device	**Z** No Qualifier
W Nipple, Right **X** Nipple, Left	**0** Open **3** Percutaneous **7** Via Natural or Artificial Opening **8** Via Natural or Artificial Opening Endoscopic **X** External	**Z** No Device	**X** Diagnostic **Z** No Qualifier

Section	0	Medical and Surgical
Body System	H	Skin and Breast
Operation	B	**Excision:** Cutting out or off, without replacement, a portion of a body part

Body Part (4th)	Approach (5th)	Device (6th)	Qualifier (7th)
0 Skin, Scalp 1 Skin, Face 2 Skin, Right Ear 3 Skin, Left Ear 4 Skin, Neck 5 Skin, Chest 6 Skin, Back 7 Skin, Abdomen 8 Skin, Buttock 9 Skin, Perineum A Skin, Inguinal B Skin, Right Upper Arm C Skin, Left Upper Arm D Skin, Right Lower Arm E Skin, Left Lower Arm F Skin, Right Hand G Skin, Left Hand H Skin, Right Upper Leg J Skin, Left Upper Leg K Skin, Right Lower Leg L Skin, Left Lower Leg M Skin, Right Foot N Skin, Left Foot Q Finger Nail R Toe Nail	X External	Z No Device	X Diagnostic Z No Qualifier
T Breast, Right U Breast, Left V Breast, Bilateral Y Supernumerary Breast	0 Open 3 Percutaneous 7 Via Natural or Artificial Opening 8 Via Natural or Artificial Opening Endoscopic	Z No Device	X Diagnostic Z No Qualifier
W Nipple, Right X Nipple, Left	0 Open 3 Percutaneous 7 Via Natural or Artificial Opening 8 Via Natural or Artificial Opening Endoscopic X External	Z No Device	X Diagnostic Z No Qualifier

Section	0	Medical and Surgical
Body System	H	Skin and Breast
Operation	C	Extirpation: Taking or cutting out solid matter from a body part

Body Part (4th)	Approach (5th)	Device (6th)	Qualifier (7th)
0 Skin, Scalp 1 Skin, Face 2 Skin, Right Ear 3 Skin, Left Ear 4 Skin, Neck 5 Skin, Chest 6 Skin, Back 7 Skin, Abdomen 8 Skin, Buttock 9 Skin, Perineum A Skin, Inguinal B Skin, Right Upper Arm C Skin, Left Upper Arm D Skin, Right Lower Arm E Skin, Left Lower Arm F Skin, Right Hand G Skin, Left Hand H Skin, Right Upper Leg J Skin, Left Upper Leg K Skin, Right Lower Leg L Skin, Left Lower Leg M Skin, Right Foot N Skin, Left Foot Q Finger Nail R Toe Nail	X External	Z No Device	Z No Qualifier
T Breast, Right U Breast, Left V Breast, Bilateral	0 Open 3 Percutaneous 7 Via Natural or Artificial Opening 8 Via Natural or Artificial Opening Endoscopic	Z No Device	Z No Qualifier
W Nipple, Right X Nipple, Left	0 Open 3 Percutaneous 7 Via Natural or Artificial Opening 8 Via Natural or Artificial Opening Endoscopic X External	Z No Device	Z No Qualifier

Section	0	Medical and Surgical
Body System	H	Skin and Breast
Operation	D	**Extraction:** Pulling or stripping out or off all or a portion of a body part by the use of force

Body Part (4th)	Approach (5th)	Device (6th)	Qualifier (7th)
0 Skin, Scalp 1 Skin, Face 2 Skin, Right Ear 3 Skin, Left Ear 4 Skin, Neck 5 Skin, Chest 6 Skin, Back 7 Skin, Abdomen 8 Skin, Buttock 9 Skin, Perineum A Skin, Inguinal B Skin, Right Upper Arm C Skin, Left Upper Arm D Skin, Right Lower Arm E Skin, Left Lower Arm F Skin, Right Hand G Skin, Left Hand H Skin, Right Upper Leg J Skin, Left Upper Leg K Skin, Right Lower Leg L Skin, Left Lower Leg M Skin, Right Foot N Skin, Left Foot Q Finger Nail R Toe Nail S Hair	X External	Z No Device	Z No Qualifier
T Breast, Right U Breast, Left V Breast, Bilateral Y Supernumerary Breast	0 Open	Z No Device	Z No Qualifier

Section	0	Medical and Surgical
Body System	H	Skin and Breast
Operation	H	**Insertion:** Putting in a nonbiological appliance that monitors, assists, performs, or prevents a physiological function but does not physically take the place of a body part

Body Part (4th)	Approach (5th)	Device (6th)	Qualifier (7th)
P Skin	X External	Y Other Device	Z No Qualifier
T Breast, Right U Breast, Left	0 Open 3 Percutaneous 7 Via Natural or Artificial Opening 8 Via Natural or Artificial Opening Endoscopic	1 Radioactive Element N Tissue Expander Y Other Device	Z No Qualifier
V Breast, Bilateral	0 Open 3 Percutaneous 7 Via Natural or Artificial Opening 8 Via Natural or Artificial Opening Endoscopic	1 Radioactive Element N Tissue Expander	Z No Qualifier
W Nipple, Right X Nipple, Left	0 Open 3 Percutaneous 7 Via Natural or Artificial Opening 8 Via Natural or Artificial Opening Endoscopic	1 Radioactive Element N Tissue Expander	Z No Qualifier
W Nipple, Right X Nipple, Left	X External	1 Radioactive Element	Z No Qualifier

Section	0	Medical and Surgical
Body System	H	Skin and Breast
Operation	J	**Inspection:** Visually and/or manually exploring a body part

Body Part (4th)	Approach (5th)	Device (6th)	Qualifier (7th)
P Skin Q Finger Nail R Toe Nail	X External	Z No Device	Z No Qualifier
T Breast, Right U Breast, Left	0 Open 3 Percutaneous 7 Via Natural or Artificial Opening 8 Via Natural or Artificial Opening Endoscopic	Z No Device	Z No Qualifier

Section	0	Medical and Surgical
Body System	H	Skin and Breast
Operation	M	**Reattachment:** Putting back in or on all or a portion of a separated body part to its normal location or other suitable location

Body Part (4th)	Approach (5th)	Device (6th)	Qualifier (7th)
0 Skin, Scalp 1 Skin, Face 2 Skin, Right Ear 3 Skin, Left Ear 4 Skin, Neck 5 Skin, Chest 6 Skin, Back 7 Skin, Abdomen 8 Skin, Buttock 9 Skin, Perineum A Skin, Inguinal B Skin, Right Upper Arm C Skin, Left Upper Arm D Skin, Right Lower Arm E Skin, Left Lower Arm F Skin, Right Hand G Skin, Left Hand H Skin, Right Upper Leg J Skin, Left Upper Leg K Skin, Right Lower Leg L Skin, Left Lower Leg M Skin, Right Foot N Skin, Left Foot T Breast, Right U Breast, Left V Breast, Bilateral W Nipple, Right X Nipple, Left	X External	Z No Device	Z No Qualifier

Section	0	**Medical and Surgical**
Body System	H	**Skin and Breast**
Operation	N	**Release:** Freeing a body part from an abnormal physical constraint by cutting or by the use of force

Body Part (4th)	Approach (5th)	Device (6th)	Qualifier (7th)
0 Skin, Scalp **1** Skin, Face **2** Skin, Right Ear **3** Skin, Left Ear **4** Skin, Neck **5** Skin, Chest **6** Skin, Back **7** Skin, Abdomen **8** Skin, Buttock **9** Skin, Perineum **A** Skin, Inguinal **B** Skin, Right Upper Arm **C** Skin, Left Upper Arm **D** Skin, Right Lower Arm **E** Skin, Left Lower Arm **F** Skin, Right Hand **G** Skin, Left Hand **H** Skin, Right Upper Leg **J** Skin, Left Upper Leg **K** Skin, Right Lower Leg **L** Skin, Left Lower Leg **M** Skin, Right Foot **N** Skin, Left Foot **Q** Finger Nail **R** Toe Nail	**X** External	**Z** No Device	**Z** No Qualifier
T Breast, Right **U** Breast, Left **V** Breast, Bilateral	**0** Open **3** Percutaneous **7** Via Natural or Artificial Opening **8** Via Natural or Artificial Opening Endoscopic	**Z** No Device	**Z** No Qualifier
W Nipple, Right **X** Nipple, Left	**0** Open **3** Percutaneous **7** Via Natural or Artificial Opening **8** Via Natural or Artificial Opening Endoscopic **X** External	**Z** No Device	**Z** No Qualifier

Section   0   **Medical and Surgical**
Body System   H   **Skin and Breast**
Operation   P   **Removal:** Taking out or off a device from a body part

Body Part (4ᵗʰ)	Approach (5ᵗʰ)	Device (6ᵗʰ)	Qualifier (7ᵗʰ)
P Skin	X External	0 Drainage Device 7 Autologous Tissue Substitute J Synthetic Substitute K Nonautologous Tissue Substitute Y Other Device	Z No Qualifier
Q Finger Nail R Toe Nail	X External	0 Drainage Device 7 Autologous Tissue Substitute J Synthetic Substitute K Nonautologous Tissue Substitute	Z No Qualifier
S Hair	X External	7 Autologous Tissue Substitute J Synthetic Substitute K Nonautologous Tissue Substitute	Z No Qualifier
T Breast, Right U Breast, Left	0 Open 3 Percutaneous 7 Via Natural or Artificial Opening 8 Via Natural or Artificial Opening Endoscopic	0 Drainage Device 1 Radioactive Element 7 Autologous Tissue Substitute J Synthetic Substitute K Nonautologous Tissue Substitute N Tissue Expander Y Other Device	Z No Qualifier

Section   0   **Medical and Surgical**
Body System   H   **Skin and Breast**
Operation   Q   **Repair:** Restoring, to the extent possible, a body part to its normal anatomic structure and function

Body Part (4ᵗʰ)	Approach (5ᵗʰ)	Device (6ᵗʰ)	Qualifier (7ᵗʰ)
0 Skin, Scalp 1 Skin, Face 2 Skin, Right Ear 3 Skin, Left Ear 4 Skin, Neck 5 Skin, Chest 6 Skin, Back 7 Skin, Abdomen 8 Skin, Buttock 9 Skin, Perineum A Skin, Inguinal B Skin, Right Upper Arm C Skin, Left Upper Arm D Skin, Right Lower Arm E Skin, Left Lower Arm F Skin, Right Hand G Skin, Left Hand H Skin, Right Upper Leg J Skin, Left Upper Leg K Skin, Right Lower Leg L Skin, Left Lower Leg M Skin, Right Foot N Skin, Left Foot Q Finger Nail R Toe Nail	X External	Z No Device	Z No Qualifier
T Breast, Right U Breast, Left V Breast, Bilateral Y Supernumerary Breast	0 Open 3 Percutaneous 7 Via Natural or Artificial Opening 8 Via Natural or Artificial Opening Endoscopic	Z No Device	Z No Qualifier

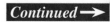

Continued →

Section	0	Medical and Surgical
Body System	H	Skin and Breast
Operation	Q	Repair: Restoring, to the extent possible, a body part to its normal anatomic structure and function

Body Part (4th)	Approach (5th)	Device (6th)	Qualifier (7th)
W Nipple, Right X Nipple, Left	0 Open 3 Percutaneous 7 Via Natural or Artificial Opening 8 Via Natural or Artificial Opening Endoscopic X External	Z No Device	Z No Qualifier

Section	0	Medical and Surgical
Body System	H	Skin and Breast
Operation	R	Replacement: Putting in or on biological or synthetic material that physically takes the place and/or function of all or a portion of a body part

Body Part (4th)	Approach (5th)	Device (6th)	Qualifier (7th)
0 Skin, Scalp 1 Skin, Face 2 Skin, Right Ear 3 Skin, Left Ear 4 Skin, Neck 5 Skin, Chest 6 Skin, Back 7 Skin, Abdomen 8 Skin, Buttock 9 Skin, Perineum A Skin, Inguinal B Skin, Right Upper Arm C Skin, Left Upper Arm D Skin, Right Lower Arm E Skin, Left Lower Arm F Skin, Right Hand G Skin, Left Hand H Skin, Right Upper Leg J Skin, Left Upper Leg K Skin, Right Lower Leg L Skin, Left Lower Leg M Skin, Right Foot N Skin, Left Foot	X External	7 Autologous Tissue Substitute	2 Cell Suspension Technique 3 Full Thickness 4 Partial Thickness
0 Skin, Scalp 1 Skin, Face 2 Skin, Right Ear 3 Skin, Left Ear 4 Skin, Neck 5 Skin, Chest 6 Skin, Back 7 Skin, Abdomen 8 Skin, Buttock 9 Skin, Perineum A Skin, Inguinal B Skin, Right Upper Arm C Skin, Left Upper Arm D Skin, Right Lower Arm E Skin, Left Lower Arm F Skin, Right Hand G Skin, Left Hand H Skin, Right Upper Leg J Skin, Left Upper Leg K Skin, Right Lower Leg L Skin, Left Lower Leg M Skin, Right Foot N Skin, Left Foot	X External	J Synthetic Substitute	3 Full Thickness 4 Partial Thickness Z No Qualifier

Continued →

Section	0	Medical and Surgical			*0HR Continued*

Body System   **H**   **Skin and Breast**

Operation   **R**   **Replacement:** Putting in or on biological or synthetic material that physically takes the place and/or function of all or a portion of a body part

Body Part (4ᵗʰ)	Approach (5ᵗʰ)	Device (6ᵗʰ)	Qualifier (7ᵗʰ)
0 Skin, Scalp **1** Skin, Face **2** Skin, Right Ear **3** Skin, Left Ear **4** Skin, Neck **5** Skin, Chest **6** Skin, Back **7** Skin, Abdomen **8** Skin, Buttock **9** Skin, Perineum **A** Skin, Inguinal **B** Skin, Right Upper Arm **C** Skin, Left Upper Arm **D** Skin, Right Lower Arm **E** Skin, Left Lower Arm **F** Skin, Right Hand **G** Skin, Left Hand **H** Skin, Right Upper Leg **J** Skin, Left Upper Leg **K** Skin, Right Lower Leg **L** Skin, Left Lower Leg **M** Skin, Right Foot **N** Skin, Left Foot	**X** External	**K** Nonautologous Tissue Substitute	**3** Full Thickness **4** Partial Thickness
Q Finger Nail **R** Toe Nail **S** Hair	**X** External	**7** Autologous Tissue Substitute **J** Synthetic Substitute **K** Nonautologous Tissue Substitute	**Z** No Qualifier
T Breast, Right **U** Breast, Left **V** Breast, Bilateral	**0** Open	**7** Autologous Tissue Substitute	**5** Latissimus Dorsi Myocutaneous Flap **6** Transverse Rectus Abdominis Myocutaneous Flap **7** Deep Inferior Epigastric Artery Perforator Flap **8** Superficial Inferior Epigastric Artery Flap **9** Gluteal Artery Perforator Flap **Z** No Qualifier
T Breast, Right **U** Breast, Left **V** Breast, Bilateral	**0** Open	**J** Synthetic Substitute **K** Nonautologous Tissue Substitute	**Z** No Qualifier
T Breast, Right **U** Breast, Left **V** Breast, Bilateral	**3** Percutaneous	**7** Autologous Tissue Substitute **J** Synthetic Substitute **K** Nonautologous Tissue Substitute	**Z** No Qualifier
W Nipple, Right **X** Nipple, Left	**0** Open **3** Percutaneous **X** External	**7** Autologous Tissue Substitute **J** Synthetic Substitute **K** Nonautologous Tissue Substitute	**Z** No Qualifier

Section 0 **Medical and Surgical**
Body System H **Skin and Breast**
Operation S **Reposition:** Moving to its normal location, or other suitable location, all or a portion of a body part

Body Part (4th)	Approach (5th)	Device (6th)	Qualifier (7th)
S Hair W Nipple, Right X Nipple, Left	X External	Z No Device	Z No Qualifier
T Breast, Right U Breast, Left V Breast, Bilateral	0 Open	Z No Device	Z No Qualifier

Section 0 **Medical and Surgical**
Body System H **Skin and Breast**
Operation T **Resection:** Cutting out or off, without replacement, all of a body part

Body Part (4th)	Approach (5th)	Device (6th)	Qualifier (7th)
Q Finger Nail R Toe Nail W Nipple, Right X Nipple, Left	X External	Z No Device	Z No Qualifier
T Breast, Right U Breast, Left V Breast, Bilateral Y Supernumerary Breast	0 Open	Z No Device	Z No Qualifier

Section 0 **Medical and Surgical**
Body System H **Skin and Breast**
Operation U **Supplement:** Putting in or on biological or synthetic material that physically reinforces and/or augments the function of a portion of a body part

Body Part (4th)	Approach (5th)	Device (6th)	Qualifier (7th)
T Breast, Right U Breast, Left V Breast, Bilateral	0 Open 3 Percutaneous 7 Via Natural or Artificial Opening 8 Via Natural or Artificial Opening Endoscopic	7 Autologous Tissue Substitute J Synthetic Substitute K Nonautologous Tissue Substitute	Z No Qualifier
W Nipple, Right X Nipple, Left	0 Open 3 Percutaneous 7 Via Natural or Artificial Opening 8 Via Natural or Artificial Opening Endoscopic X External	7 Autologous Tissue Substitute J Synthetic Substitute K Nonautologous Tissue Substitute	Z No Qualifier

Section	0	Medical and Surgical
Body System	H	Skin and Breast
Operation	W	Revision: Correcting, to the extent possible, a portion of a malfunctioning device or the position of a displaced device

Body Part (4th)	Approach (5th)	Device (6th)	Qualifier (7th)
P Skin	**X** External	**0** Drainage Device **7** Autologous Tissue Substitute **J** Synthetic Substitute **K** Nonautologous Tissue Substitute **Y** Other Device	**Z** No Qualifier
Q Finger Nail **R** Toe Nail	**X** External	**0** Drainage Device **7** Autologous Tissue Substitute **J** Synthetic Substitute **K** Nonautologous Tissue Substitute	**Z** No Qualifier
S Hair	**X** External	**7** Autologous Tissue Substitute **J** Synthetic Substitute **K** Nonautologous Tissue Substitute	**Z** No Qualifier
T Breast, Right **U** Breast, Left	**0** Open **3** Percutaneous **7** Via Natural or Artificial Opening **8** Via Natural or Artificial Opening Endoscopic	**0** Drainage Device **7** Autologous Tissue Substitute **J** Synthetic Substitute **K** Nonautologous Tissue Substitute **N** Tissue Expander **Y** Other Device	**Z** No Qualifier

Section	0	Medical and Surgical
Body System	H	Skin and Breast
Operation	X	Transfer: Moving, without taking out, all or a portion of a body part to another location to take over the function of all or a portion of a body part

Body Part (4th)	Approach (5th)	Device (6th)	Qualifier (7th)
0 Skin, Scalp **1** Skin, Face **2** Skin, Right Ear **3** Skin, Left Ear **4** Skin, Neck **5** Skin, Chest **6** Skin, Back **7** Skin, Abdomen **8** Skin, Buttock **9** Skin, Perineum **A** Skin, Inguinal **B** Skin, Right Upper Arm **C** Skin, Left Upper Arm **D** Skin, Right Lower Arm **E** Skin, Left Lower Arm **F** Skin, Right Hand **G** Skin, Left Hand **H** Skin, Right Upper Leg **J** Skin, Left Upper Leg **K** Skin, Right Lower Leg **L** Skin, Left Lower Leg **M** Skin, Right Foot **N** Skin, Left Foot	**X** External	**Z** No Device	**Z** No Qualifier

AHA Coding Clinic

0HB8XZZ Excision of Buttock Skin, External Approach—AHA CC: 3Q, 2015, 3

0HBHXZZ Excision of Right Upper Leg Skin, External Approach—AHA CC: 1Q, 2020, 31-32

0HBJXZZ Excision of Left Upper Leg Skin, External Approach—AHA CC: 3Q, 2016, 29-30

0HBT0ZZ Excision of Right Breast, Open Approach—AHA CC: 1Q, 2018, 14-15

0HD6XZZ Extraction of Back Skin, External Approach—AHA CC: 3Q, 2015, 5-6

0HDHXZZ Extraction of Right Upper Leg Skin, External Approach—AHA CC: 3Q, 2015, 5

0HHT0NZ Insertion of Tissue Expander into Right Breast, Open Approach—AHA CC: 4Q, 2017, 67

0HHU0YZ *Insertion of Other Device into Left Breast, Open Approach—AHA CC: 4Q, 2013, 107*

0HHV0NZ *Insertion of Tissue Expander into Bilateral Breast, Open Approach—AHA CC: 2Q, 2014, 12*

0HPT07Z *Removal of Autologous Tissue Substitute from Right Breast, Open Approach—AHA CC: 2Q, 2016, 27*

0HPT0NZ *Removal of Tissue Expander from Right Breast, Open Approach—AHA CC: 3Q, 2018, 13-14*

0HPU07Z *Removal of Autologous Tissue Substitute from Left Breast, Open Approach—AHA CC: 2Q, 2016, 27*

0HQ9XZZ *Repair Perineum Skin, External Approach—AHA CC: 1Q, 2016, 7*

0HQEXZZ *Repair Left Lower Arm Skin, External Approach—AHA CC: 4Q, 2014, 31-32*

0HRMXK3 *Replacement of Right Foot Skin with Nonautologous Tissue Substitute, Full Thickness, External Approach—AHA CC: 1Q, 2017, 35-36*

0HRNXK3 *Replacement of Left Foot Skin with Nonautologous Tissue Substitute, Full Thickness, External Approach—AHA CC: 3Q, 2014, 14-15*

0HRU07Z *Replacement of Left Breast with Autologous Tissue Substitute, Open Approach—AHA CC: 1Q, 2020, 27-28*

0HRV077 *Replacement of Bilateral Breast using Deep Inferior Epigastric Artery Perforator Flap, Open Approach—AHA CC: 3Q, 2018, 13-14*

0HTT0ZZ *Resection of Right Breast, Open Approach—AHA CC: 4Q, 2014, 34*

0HTU0ZZ *Resection of Left Breast, Open Approach—AHA CC: 3Q, 2018, 13-14*

Cross-Section of the Skin Showing Layer and Types of Infections

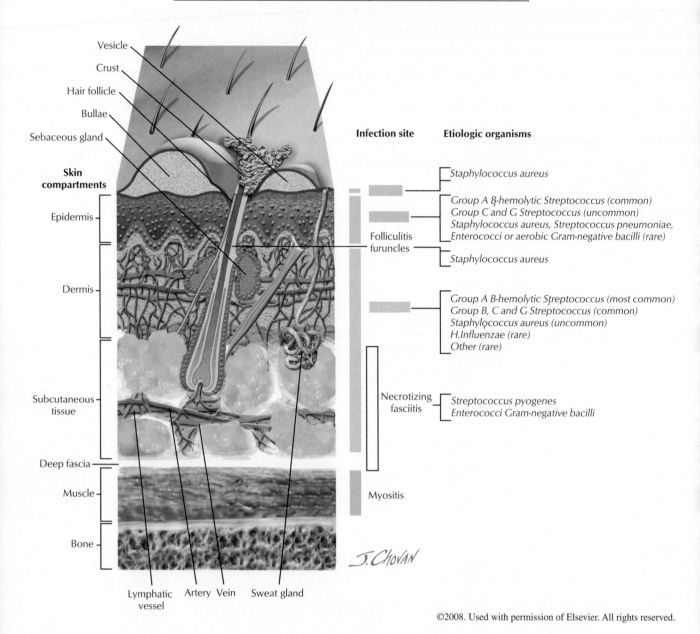

Vesicle

Crust

Hair follicle

Bullae

Sebaceous gland

Skin compartments

Epidermis

Dermis

Subcutaneous tissue

Deep fascia

Muscle

Bone

Lymphatic vessel

Artery Vein

Sweat gland

Infection site

Etiologic organisms

Staphylococcus aureus

Group A β-hemolytic Streptococcus (common)
Group C and G Streptococcus (uncommon)
Staphylococcus aureus, Streptococcus pneumoniae,
Enterococci or aerobic Gram-negative bacilli (rare)

Folliculitis furuncles

Staphylococcus aureus

Group A B-hemolytic Streptococcus (most common)
Group B, C and G Streptococcus (common)
Staphylococcus aureus (uncommon)
H.Influenzae (rare)
Other (rare)

Necrotizing fasciitis

Streptococcus pyogenes
Enterococci Gram-negative bacilli

Myositis

J. CHOVAN

Subcutaneous Tissue and Fascia Tables 0J0–0JX

Section	0	Medical and Surgical
Body System	J	Subcutaneous Tissue and Fascia
Operation	0	Alteration: Modifying the anatomic structure of a body part without affecting the function of the body part

Body Part (4th)	Approach (5th)	Device (6th)	Qualifier (7th)
1 Subcutaneous Tissue and Fascia, Face 4 Subcutaneous Tissue and Fascia, Right Neck 5 Subcutaneous Tissue and Fascia, Left Neck 6 Subcutaneous Tissue and Fascia, Chest 7 Subcutaneous Tissue and Fascia, Back 8 Subcutaneous Tissue and Fascia, Abdomen 9 Subcutaneous Tissue and Fascia, Buttock D Subcutaneous Tissue and Fascia, Right Upper Arm F Subcutaneous Tissue and Fascia, Left Upper Arm G Subcutaneous Tissue and Fascia, Right Lower Arm H Subcutaneous Tissue and Fascia, Left Lower Arm L Subcutaneous Tissue and Fascia, Right Upper Leg M Subcutaneous Tissue and Fascia, Left Upper Leg N Subcutaneous Tissue and Fascia, Right Lower Leg P Subcutaneous Tissue and Fascia, Left Lower Leg	0 Open 3 Percutaneous	Z No Device	Z No Qualifier

Section	0	Medical and Surgical
Body System	J	Subcutaneous Tissue and Fascia
Operation	2	Change: Taking out or off a device from a body part and putting back an identical or similar device in or on the same body part without cutting or puncturing the skin or a mucous membrane

Body Part (4th)	Approach (5th)	Device (6th)	Qualifier (7th)
S Subcutaneous Tissue and Fascia, Head and Neck T Subcutaneous Tissue and Fascia, Trunk V Subcutaneous Tissue and Fascia, Upper Extremity W Subcutaneous Tissue and Fascia, Lower Extremity	X External	0 Drainage Device Y Other Device	Z No Qualifier

Section	0	Medical and Surgical
Body System	J	Subcutaneous Tissue and Fascia
Operation	5	Destruction: Physical eradication of all or a portion of a body part by the direct use of energy, force, or a destructive agent

Body Part (4th)	Approach (5th)	Device (6th)	Qualifier (7th)
0 Subcutaneous Tissue and Fascia, Scalp 1 Subcutaneous Tissue and Fascia, Face 4 Subcutaneous Tissue and Fascia, Right Neck 5 Subcutaneous Tissue and Fascia, Left Neck 6 Subcutaneous Tissue and Fascia, Chest 7 Subcutaneous Tissue and Fascia, Back 8 Subcutaneous Tissue and Fascia, Abdomen 9 Subcutaneous Tissue and Fascia, Buttock B Subcutaneous Tissue and Fascia, Perineum C Subcutaneous Tissue and Fascia, Pelvic Region D Subcutaneous Tissue and Fascia, Right Upper Arm F Subcutaneous Tissue and Fascia, Left Upper Arm G Subcutaneous Tissue and Fascia, Right Lower Arm H Subcutaneous Tissue and Fascia, Left Lower Arm J Subcutaneous Tissue and Fascia, Right Hand K Subcutaneous Tissue and Fascia, Left Hand L Subcutaneous Tissue and Fascia, Right Upper Leg M Subcutaneous Tissue and Fascia, Left Upper Leg N Subcutaneous Tissue and Fascia, Right Lower Leg P Subcutaneous Tissue and Fascia, Left Lower Leg Q Subcutaneous Tissue and Fascia, Right Foot R Subcutaneous Tissue and Fascia, Left Foot	0 Open 3 Percutaneous	Z No Device	Z No Qualifier

Section	0	Medical and Surgical
Body System	J	Subcutaneous Tissue and Fascia
Operation	8	**Division:** Cutting into a body part, without draining fluids and/or gases from the body part, in order to separate or transect a body part

Body Part (4th)	Approach (5th)	Device (6th)	Qualifier (7th)
0 Subcutaneous Tissue and Fascia, Scalp	0 Open	Z No Device	Z No Qualifier
1 Subcutaneous Tissue and Fascia, Face	3 Percutaneous		
4 Subcutaneous Tissue and Fascia, Right Neck			
5 Subcutaneous Tissue and Fascia, Left Neck			
6 Subcutaneous Tissue and Fascia, Chest			
7 Subcutaneous Tissue and Fascia, Back			
8 Subcutaneous Tissue and Fascia, Abdomen			
9 Subcutaneous Tissue and Fascia, Buttock			
B Subcutaneous Tissue and Fascia, Perineum			
C Subcutaneous Tissue and Fascia, Pelvic Region			
D Subcutaneous Tissue and Fascia, Right Upper Arm			
F Subcutaneous Tissue and Fascia, Left Upper Arm			
G Subcutaneous Tissue and Fascia, Right Lower Arm			
H Subcutaneous Tissue and Fascia, Left Lower Arm			
J Subcutaneous Tissue and Fascia, Right Hand			
K Subcutaneous Tissue and Fascia, Left Hand			
L Subcutaneous Tissue and Fascia, Right Upper Leg			
M Subcutaneous Tissue and Fascia, Left Upper Leg			
N Subcutaneous Tissue and Fascia, Right Lower Leg			
P Subcutaneous Tissue and Fascia, Left Lower Leg			
Q Subcutaneous Tissue and Fascia, Right Foot			
R Subcutaneous Tissue and Fascia, Left Foot			
S Subcutaneous Tissue and Fascia, Head and Neck			
T Subcutaneous Tissue and Fascia, Trunk			
V Subcutaneous Tissue and Fascia, Upper Extremity			
W Subcutaneous Tissue and Fascia, Lower Extremity			

Section	0	Medical and Surgical
Body System	J	Subcutaneous Tissue and Fascia
Operation	9	**Drainage:** Taking or letting out fluids and/or gases from a body part

Body Part (4th)	Approach (5th)	Device (6th)	Qualifier (7th)
0 Subcutaneous Tissue and Fascia, Scalp	0 Open	0 Drainage Device	Z No Qualifier
1 Subcutaneous Tissue and Fascia, Face	3 Percutaneous		
4 Subcutaneous Tissue and Fascia, Right Neck			
5 Subcutaneous Tissue and Fascia, Left Neck			
6 Subcutaneous Tissue and Fascia, Chest			
7 Subcutaneous Tissue and Fascia, Back			
8 Subcutaneous Tissue and Fascia, Abdomen			
9 Subcutaneous Tissue and Fascia, Buttock			
B Subcutaneous Tissue and Fascia, Perineum			
C Subcutaneous Tissue and Fascia, Pelvic Region			
D Subcutaneous Tissue and Fascia, Right Upper Arm			
F Subcutaneous Tissue and Fascia, Left Upper Arm			
G Subcutaneous Tissue and Fascia, Right Lower Arm			
H Subcutaneous Tissue and Fascia, Left Lower Arm			
J Subcutaneous Tissue and Fascia, Right Hand			
K Subcutaneous Tissue and Fascia, Left Hand			
L Subcutaneous Tissue and Fascia, Right Upper Leg			
M Subcutaneous Tissue and Fascia, Left Upper Leg			
N Subcutaneous Tissue and Fascia, Right Lower Leg			
P Subcutaneous Tissue and Fascia, Left Lower Leg			
Q Subcutaneous Tissue and Fascia, Right Foot			
R Subcutaneous Tissue and Fascia, Left Foot			

Continued →

Section	0	Medical and Surgical
Body System	J	Subcutaneous Tissue and Fascia
Operation	9	Drainage: Taking or letting out fluids and/or gases from a body part

Body Part (4th)	Approach (5th)	Device (6th)	Qualifier (7th)
0 Subcutaneous Tissue and Fascia, Scalp	0 Open	Z No Device	X Diagnostic
1 Subcutaneous Tissue and Fascia, Face	3 Percutaneous		Z No Qualifier
4 Subcutaneous Tissue and Fascia, Right Neck			
5 Subcutaneous Tissue and Fascia, Left Neck			
6 Subcutaneous Tissue and Fascia, Chest			
7 Subcutaneous Tissue and Fascia, Back			
8 Subcutaneous Tissue and Fascia, Abdomen			
9 Subcutaneous Tissue and Fascia, Buttock			
B Subcutaneous Tissue and Fascia, Perineum			
C Subcutaneous Tissue and Fascia, Pelvic Region			
D Subcutaneous Tissue and Fascia, Right Upper Arm			
F Subcutaneous Tissue and Fascia, Left Upper Arm			
G Subcutaneous Tissue and Fascia, Right Lower Arm			
H Subcutaneous Tissue and Fascia, Left Lower Arm			
J Subcutaneous Tissue and Fascia, Right Hand			
K Subcutaneous Tissue and Fascia, Left Hand			
L Subcutaneous Tissue and Fascia, Right Upper Leg			
M Subcutaneous Tissue and Fascia, Left Upper Leg			
N Subcutaneous Tissue and Fascia, Right Lower Leg			
P Subcutaneous Tissue and Fascia, Left Lower Leg			
Q Subcutaneous Tissue and Fascia, Right Foot			
R Subcutaneous Tissue and Fascia, Left Foot			

Section	0	Medical and Surgical
Body System	J	Subcutaneous Tissue and Fascia
Operation	B	Excision: Cutting out or off, without replacement, a portion of a body part

Body Part (4th)	Approach (5th)	Device (6th)	Qualifier (7th)
0 Subcutaneous Tissue and Fascia, Scalp	0 Open	Z No Device	X Diagnostic
1 Subcutaneous Tissue and Fascia, Face	3 Percutaneous		Z No Qualifier
4 Subcutaneous Tissue and Fascia, Right Neck			
5 Subcutaneous Tissue and Fascia, Left Neck			
6 Subcutaneous Tissue and Fascia, Chest			
7 Subcutaneous Tissue and Fascia, Back			
8 Subcutaneous Tissue and Fascia, Abdomen			
9 Subcutaneous Tissue and Fascia, Buttock			
B Subcutaneous Tissue and Fascia, Perineum			
C Subcutaneous Tissue and Fascia, Pelvic Region			
D Subcutaneous Tissue and Fascia, Right Upper Arm			
F Subcutaneous Tissue and Fascia, Left Upper Arm			
G Subcutaneous Tissue and Fascia, Right Lower Arm			
H Subcutaneous Tissue and Fascia, Left Lower Arm			
J Subcutaneous Tissue and Fascia, Right Hand			
K Subcutaneous Tissue and Fascia, Left Hand			
L Subcutaneous Tissue and Fascia, Right Upper Leg			
M Subcutaneous Tissue and Fascia, Left Upper Leg			
N Subcutaneous Tissue and Fascia, Right Lower Leg			
P Subcutaneous Tissue and Fascia, Left Lower Leg			
Q Subcutaneous Tissue and Fascia, Right Foot			
R Subcutaneous Tissue and Fascia, Left Foot			

Section	0	Medical and Surgical
Body System	J	Subcutaneous Tissue and Fascia
Operation	C	Extirpation: Taking or cutting out solid matter from a body part

Body Part (4th)	Approach (5th)	Device (6th)	Qualifier (7th)
0 Subcutaneous Tissue and Fascia, Scalp 1 Subcutaneous Tissue and Fascia, Face 4 Subcutaneous Tissue and Fascia, Right Neck 5 Subcutaneous Tissue and Fascia, Left Neck 6 Subcutaneous Tissue and Fascia, Chest 7 Subcutaneous Tissue and Fascia, Back 8 Subcutaneous Tissue and Fascia, Abdomen 9 Subcutaneous Tissue and Fascia, Buttock B Subcutaneous Tissue and Fascia, Perineum C Subcutaneous Tissue and Fascia, Pelvic Region D Subcutaneous Tissue and Fascia, Right Upper Arm F Subcutaneous Tissue and Fascia, Left Upper Arm G Subcutaneous Tissue and Fascia, Right Lower Arm H Subcutaneous Tissue and Fascia, Left Lower Arm J Subcutaneous Tissue and Fascia, Right Hand K Subcutaneous Tissue and Fascia, Left Hand L Subcutaneous Tissue and Fascia, Right Upper Leg M Subcutaneous Tissue and Fascia, Left Upper Leg N Subcutaneous Tissue and Fascia, Right Lower Leg P Subcutaneous Tissue and Fascia, Left Lower Leg Q Subcutaneous Tissue and Fascia, Right Foot R Subcutaneous Tissue and Fascia, Left Foot	0 Open 3 Percutaneous	Z No Device	Z No Qualifier

Section	0	Medical and Surgical
Body System	J	Subcutaneous Tissue and Fascia
Operation	D	Extraction: Pulling or stripping out or off all or a portion of a body part by the use of force

Body Part (4th)	Approach (5th)	Device (6th)	Qualifier (7th)
0 Subcutaneous Tissue and Fascia, Scalp 1 Subcutaneous Tissue and Fascia, Face 4 Subcutaneous Tissue and Fascia, Right Neck 5 Subcutaneous Tissue and Fascia, Left Neck 6 Subcutaneous Tissue and Fascia, Chest 7 Subcutaneous Tissue and Fascia, Back 8 Subcutaneous Tissue and Fascia, Abdomen 9 Subcutaneous Tissue and Fascia, Buttock B Subcutaneous Tissue and Fascia, Perineum C Subcutaneous Tissue and Fascia, Pelvic Region D Subcutaneous Tissue and Fascia, Right Upper Arm F Subcutaneous Tissue and Fascia, Left Upper Arm G Subcutaneous Tissue and Fascia, Right Lower Arm H Subcutaneous Tissue and Fascia, Left Lower Arm J Subcutaneous Tissue and Fascia, Right Hand K Subcutaneous Tissue and Fascia, Left Hand L Subcutaneous Tissue and Fascia, Right Upper Leg M Subcutaneous Tissue and Fascia, Left Upper Leg N Subcutaneous Tissue and Fascia, Right Lower Leg P Subcutaneous Tissue and Fascia, Left Lower Leg Q Subcutaneous Tissue and Fascia, Right Foot R Subcutaneous Tissue and Fascia, Left Foot	0 Open 3 Percutaneous	Z No Device	Z No Qualifier

Section	0	Medical and Surgical
Body System	J	Subcutaneous Tissue and Fascia
Operation	H	**Insertion:** Putting in a nonbiological appliance that monitors, assists, performs, or prevents a physiological function but does not physically take the place of a body part

Body Part (4th)	Approach (5th)	Device (6th)	Qualifier (7th)
0 Subcutaneous Tissue and Fascia, Scalp 1 Subcutaneous Tissue and Fascia, Face 4 Subcutaneous Tissue and Fascia, Right Neck 5 Subcutaneous Tissue and Fascia, Left Neck 9 Subcutaneous Tissue and Fascia, Buttock B Subcutaneous Tissue and Fascia, Perineum C Subcutaneous Tissue and Fascia, Pelvic Region J Subcutaneous Tissue and Fascia, Right Hand K Subcutaneous Tissue and Fascia, Left Hand Q Subcutaneous Tissue and Fascia, Right Foot R Subcutaneous Tissue and Fascia, Left Foot	0 Open 3 Percutaneous	N Tissue Expander	Z No Qualifier
6 Subcutaneous Tissue and Fascia, Chest	0 Open 3 Percutaneous	0 Monitoring Device, Hemodynamic 2 Monitoring Device 4 Pacemaker, Single Chamber 5 Pacemaker, Single Chamber Rate Responsive 6 Pacemaker, Dual Chamber 7 Cardiac Resynchronization Pacemaker Pulse Generator 8 Defibrillator Generator 9 Cardiac Resynchronization Defibrillator Pulse Generator A Contractility Modulation Device B Stimulator Generator, Single Array C Stimulator Generator, Single Array Rechargeable D Stimulator Generator, Multiple Array E Stimulator Generator, Multiple Array Rechargeable F Subcutaneous Defibrillator Lead H Contraceptive Device M Stimulator Generator N Tissue Expander P Cardiac Rhythm Related Device V Infusion Device, Pump W Vascular Access Device, Totally Implantable X Vascular Access Device, Tunneled Y Other Device	Z No Qualifier
7 Subcutaneous Tissue and Fascia, Back	0 Open 3 Percutaneous	B Stimulator Generator, Single Array C Stimulator Generator, Single Array Rechargeable D Stimulator Generator, Multiple Array E Stimulator Generator, Multiple Array Rechargeable M Stimulator Generator N Tissue Expander V Infusion Device, Pump Y Other Device	Z No Qualifier

Continued →

Section	0	Medical and Surgical
Body System	J	Subcutaneous Tissue and Fascia
Operation	H	Insertion: Putting in a nonbiological appliance that monitors, assists, performs, or prevents a physiological function but does not physically take the place of a body part

Body Part (4th)	Approach (5th)	Device (6th)	Qualifier (7th)
8 Subcutaneous Tissue and Fascia, Abdomen	0 Open 3 Percutaneous	0 Monitoring Device, Hemodynamic 2 Monitoring Device 4 Pacemaker, Single Chamber 5 Pacemaker, Single Chamber Rate Responsive 6 Pacemaker, Dual Chamber 7 Cardiac Resynchronization Pacemaker Pulse Generator 8 Defibrillator Generator 9 Cardiac Resynchronization Defibrillator Pulse Generator A Contractility Modulation Device B Stimulator Generator, Single Array C Stimulator Generator, Single Array Rechargeable D Stimulator Generator, Multiple Array E Stimulator Generator, Multiple Array Rechargeable H Contraceptive Device M Stimulator Generator N Tissue Expander P Cardiac Rhythm Related Device V Infusion Device, Pump W Vascular Access Device Totally Implantable X Vascular Access Device, Tunneled Y Other Device	Z No Qualifier
D Subcutaneous Tissue and Fascia, Right Upper Arm F Subcutaneous Tissue and Fascia, Left Upper Arm G Subcutaneous Tissue and Fascia, Right Lower Arm H Subcutaneous Tissue and Fascia, Left Lower Arm L Subcutaneous Tissue and Fascia, Right Upper Leg M Subcutaneous Tissue and Fascia, Left Upper Leg N Subcutaneous Tissue and Fascia, Right Lower Leg P Subcutaneous Tissue and Fascia, Left Lower Leg	0 Open 3 Percutaneous	H Contraceptive Device N Tissue Expander V Infusion Device, Pump W Vascular Access Device, Totally Implantable X Vascular Access Device, Tunneled	Z No Qualifier
S Subcutaneous Tissue and Fascia, Head and Neck V Subcutaneous Tissue and Fascia, Upper Extremity W Subcutaneous Tissue and Fascia, Lower Extremity	0 Open 3 Percutaneous	1 Radioactive Element 3 Infusion Device Y Other Device	Z No Qualifier
T Subcutaneous Tissue and Fascia, Trunk	0 Open 3 Percutaneous	1 Radioactive Element 3 Infusion Device V Infusion Device, Pump Y Other Device	Z No Qualifier

Section	0	Medical and Surgical
Body System	J	Subcutaneous Tissue and Fascia
Operation	J	Inspection: Visually and/or manually exploring a body part

Body Part (4th)	Approach (5th)	Device (6th)	Qualifier (7th)
S Subcutaneous Tissue and Fascia, Head and Neck T Subcutaneous Tissue and Fascia, Trunk V Subcutaneous Tissue and Fascia, Upper Extremity W Subcutaneous Tissue and Fascia, Lower Extremity	0 Open 3 Percutaneous X External	Z No Device	Z No Qualifier

Section	0	Medical and Surgical
Body System	J	Subcutaneous Tissue and Fascia
Operation	N	Release: Freeing a body part from an abnormal physical constraint by cutting or by the use of force

Body Part (4th)	Approach (5th)	Device (6th)	Qualifier (7th)
0 Subcutaneous Tissue and Fascia, Scalp 1 Subcutaneous Tissue and Fascia, Face 4 Subcutaneous Tissue and Fascia, Right Neck 5 Subcutaneous Tissue and Fascia, Left Neck 6 Subcutaneous Tissue and Fascia, Chest 7 Subcutaneous Tissue and Fascia, Back 8 Subcutaneous Tissue and Fascia, Abdomen 9 Subcutaneous Tissue and Fascia, Buttock B Subcutaneous Tissue and Fascia, Perineum C Subcutaneous Tissue and Fascia, Pelvic Region D Subcutaneous Tissue and Fascia, Right Upper Arm F Subcutaneous Tissue and Fascia, Left Upper Arm G Subcutaneous Tissue and Fascia, Right Lower Arm H Subcutaneous Tissue and Fascia, Left Lower Arm J Subcutaneous Tissue and Fascia, Right Hand K Subcutaneous Tissue and Fascia, Left Hand L Subcutaneous Tissue and Fascia, Right Upper Leg M Subcutaneous Tissue and Fascia, Left Upper Leg N Subcutaneous Tissue and Fascia, Right Lower Leg P Subcutaneous Tissue and Fascia, Left Lower Leg Q Subcutaneous Tissue and Fascia, Right Foot R Subcutaneous Tissue and Fascia, Left Foot	0 Open 3 Percutaneous X External	Z No Device	Z No Qualifier

Section	0	Medical and Surgical
Body System	J	Subcutaneous Tissue and Fascia
Operation	P	Removal: Taking out or off a device from a body part

Body Part (4th)	Approach (5th)	Device (6th)	Qualifier (7th)
S Subcutaneous Tissue and Fascia, Head and Neck	0 Open 3 Percutaneous	0 Drainage Device 1 Radioactive Element 3 Infusion Device 7 Autologous Tissue Substitute J Synthetic Substitute K Nonautologous Tissue Substitute N Tissue Expander Y Other Device	Z No Qualifier
S Subcutaneous Tissue and Fascia, Head and Neck	X External	0 Drainage Device 1 Radioactive Element 3 Infusion Device	Z No Qualifier
T Subcutaneous Tissue and Fascia, Trunk	0 Open 3 Percutaneous	0 Drainage Device 1 Radioactive Element 2 Monitoring Device 3 Infusion Device 7 Autologous Tissue Substitute F Subcutaneous Defibrillator Lead H Contraceptive Device J Synthetic Substitute K Nonautologous Tissue Substitute M Stimulator Generator N Tissue Expander P Cardiac Rhythm Related Device V Infusion Device, Pump W Vascular Access Device, Totally Implantable X Vascular Access Device, Tunneled Y Other Device	Z No Qualifier

Continued →

Section	0	Medical and Surgical
Body System	J	Subcutaneous Tissue and Fascia
Operation	P	**Removal:** Taking out or off a device from a body part

Body Part (4th)	Approach (5th)	Device (6th)	Qualifier (7th)
T Subcutaneous Tissue and Fascia, Trunk	X External	0 Drainage Device 1 Radioactive Element 2 Monitoring Device 3 Infusion Device H Contraceptive Device V Infusion Device, Pump X Vascular Access Device, Tunneled	Z No Qualifier
V Subcutaneous Tissue and Fascia, Upper Extremity W Subcutaneous Tissue and Fascia, Lower Extremity	0 Open 3 Percutaneous	0 Drainage Device 1 Radioactive Element 3 Infusion Device 7 Autologous Tissue Substitute H Contraceptive Device J Synthetic Substitute K Nonautologous Tissue Substitute N Tissue Expander V Infusion Device, Pump W Vascular Access Device, Totally Implantable X Vascular Access Device, Tunneled Y Other Device	Z No Qualifier
V Subcutaneous Tissue and Fascia, Upper Extremity W Subcutaneous Tissue and Fascia, Lower Extremity	X External	0 Drainage Device 1 Radioactive Element 3 Infusion Device H Contraceptive Device V Infusion Device, Pump X Vascular Access Device, Tunneled	Z No Qualifier

Section	0	Medical and Surgical
Body System	J	Subcutaneous Tissue and Fascia
Operation	Q	**Repair:** Restoring, to the extent possible, a body part to its normal anatomic structure and function

Body Part (4th)	Approach (5th)	Device (6th)	Qualifier (7th)
0 Subcutaneous Tissue and Fascia, Scalp 1 Subcutaneous Tissue and Fascia, Face 4 Subcutaneous Tissue and Fascia, Right Neck 5 Subcutaneous Tissue and Fascia, Left Neck 6 Subcutaneous Tissue and Fascia, Chest 7 Subcutaneous Tissue and Fascia, Back 8 Subcutaneous Tissue and Fascia, Abdomen 9 Subcutaneous Tissue and Fascia, Buttock B Subcutaneous Tissue and Fascia, Perineum C Subcutaneous Tissue and Fascia, Pelvic Region D Subcutaneous Tissue and Fascia, Right Upper Arm F Subcutaneous Tissue and Fascia, Left Upper Arm G Subcutaneous Tissue and Fascia, Right Lower Arm H Subcutaneous Tissue and Fascia, Left Lower Arm J Subcutaneous Tissue and Fascia, Right Hand K Subcutaneous Tissue and Fascia, Left Hand L Subcutaneous Tissue and Fascia, Right Upper Leg M Subcutaneous Tissue and Fascia, Left Upper Leg N Subcutaneous Tissue and Fascia, Right Lower Leg P Subcutaneous Tissue and Fascia, Left Lower Leg Q Subcutaneous Tissue and Fascia, Right Foot R Subcutaneous Tissue and Fascia, Left Foot	0 Open 3 Percutaneous	Z No Device	Z No Qualifier

Section	0	Medical and Surgical
Body System	J	Subcutaneous Tissue and Fascia
Operation	R	**Replacement:** Putting in or on biological or synthetic material that physically takes the place and/or function of all or a portion of a body part

Body Part (4th)	Approach (5th)	Device (6th)	Qualifier (7th)
0 Subcutaneous Tissue and Fascia, Scalp 1 Subcutaneous Tissue and Fascia, Face 4 Subcutaneous Tissue and Fascia, Right Neck 5 Subcutaneous Tissue and Fascia, Left Neck 6 Subcutaneous Tissue and Fascia, Chest 7 Subcutaneous Tissue and Fascia, Back 8 Subcutaneous Tissue and Fascia, Abdomen 9 Subcutaneous Tissue and Fascia, Buttock B Subcutaneous Tissue and Fascia, Perineum C Subcutaneous Tissue and Fascia, Pelvic Region D Subcutaneous Tissue and Fascia, Right Upper Arm F Subcutaneous Tissue and Fascia, Left Upper Arm G Subcutaneous Tissue and Fascia, Right Lower Arm H Subcutaneous Tissue and Fascia, Left Lower Arm J Subcutaneous Tissue and Fascia, Right Hand K Subcutaneous Tissue and Fascia, Left Hand L Subcutaneous Tissue and Fascia, Right Upper Leg M Subcutaneous Tissue and Fascia, Left Upper Leg N Subcutaneous Tissue and Fascia, Right Lower Leg P Subcutaneous Tissue and Fascia, Left Lower Leg Q Subcutaneous Tissue and Fascia, Right Foot R Subcutaneous Tissue and Fascia, Left Foot	0 Open 3 Percutaneous	7 Autologous Tissue Substitute J Synthetic Substitute K Nonautologous Tissue Substitute	Z No Qualifier

Section	0	Medical and Surgical
Body System	J	Subcutaneous Tissue and Fascia
Operation	U	**Supplement:** Putting in or on biological or synthetic material that physically reinforces and/or augments the function of a portion of a body part

Body Part (4th)	Approach (5th)	Device (6th)	Qualifier (7th)
0 Subcutaneous Tissue and Fascia, Scalp 1 Subcutaneous Tissue and Fascia, Face 4 Subcutaneous Tissue and Fascia, Right Neck 5 Subcutaneous Tissue and Fascia, Left Neck 6 Subcutaneous Tissue and Fascia, Chest 7 Subcutaneous Tissue and Fascia, Back 8 Subcutaneous Tissue and Fascia, Abdomen 9 Subcutaneous Tissue and Fascia, Buttock B Subcutaneous Tissue and Fascia, Perineum C Subcutaneous Tissue and Fascia, Pelvic Region D Subcutaneous Tissue and Fascia, Right Upper Arm F Subcutaneous Tissue and Fascia, Left Upper Arm G Subcutaneous Tissue and Fascia, Right Lower Arm H Subcutaneous Tissue and Fascia, Left Lower Arm J Subcutaneous Tissue and Fascia, Right Hand K Subcutaneous Tissue and Fascia, Left Hand L Subcutaneous Tissue and Fascia, Right Upper Leg M Subcutaneous Tissue and Fascia, Left Upper Leg N Subcutaneous Tissue and Fascia, Right Lower Leg P Subcutaneous Tissue and Fascia, Left Lower Leg Q Subcutaneous Tissue and Fascia, Right Foot R Subcutaneous Tissue and Fascia, Left Foot	0 Open 3 Percutaneous	7 Autologous Tissue Substitute J Synthetic Substitute K Nonautologous Tissue Substitute	Z No Qualifier

Section   0   **Medical and Surgical**
Body System   J   **Subcutaneous Tissue and Fascia**
Operation   W   **Revision:** Correcting, to the extent possible, a portion of a malfunctioning device or the position of a displaced device

Body Part (4th)	Approach (5th)	Device (6th)	Qualifier (7th)
S Subcutaneous Tissue and Fascia, Head and Neck	**0** Open **3** Percutaneous	**0** Drainage Device **3** Infusion Device **7** Autologous Tissue Substitute **J** Synthetic Substitute **K** Nonautologous Tissue Substitute **N** Tissue Expander **Y** Other Device	**Z** No Qualifier
S Subcutaneous Tissue and Fascia, Head and Neck	**X** External	**0** Drainage Device **3** Infusion Device **7** Autologous Tissue Substitute **J** Synthetic Substitute **K** Nonautologous Tissue Substitute **N** Tissue Expander	**Z** No Qualifier
T Subcutaneous Tissue and Fascia, Trunk	**0** Open **3** Percutaneous	**0** Drainage Device **2** Monitoring Device **3** Infusion Device **7** Autologous Tissue Substitute **F** Subcutaneous Defibrillator Lead **H** Contraceptive Device **J** Synthetic Substitute **K** Nonautologous Tissue Substitute **M** Stimulator Generator **N** Tissue Expander **P** Cardiac Rhythm Related Device **V** Infusion Device, Pump **W** Vascular Access Device, Totally Implantable **X** Vascular Access Device, Tunneled **Y** Other Device	**Z** No Qualifier
T Subcutaneous Tissue and Fascia, Trunk	**X** External	**0** Drainage Device **2** Monitoring Device **3** Infusion Device **7** Autologous Tissue Substitute **F** Subcutaneous Defibrillator Lead **H** Contraceptive Device **J** Synthetic Substitute **K** Nonautologous Tissue Substitute **M** Stimulator Generator **N** Tissue Expander **P** Cardiac Rhythm Related Device **V** Infusion Device, Pump **W** Vascular Access Device, Totally Implantable **X** Vascular Access Device, Tunneled	**Z** No Qualifier
V Subcutaneous Tissue and Fascia, Upper Extremity **W** Subcutaneous Tissue and Fascia, Lower Extremity	**0** Open **3** Percutaneous	**0** Drainage Device **3** Infusion Device **7** Autologous Tissue Substitute **H** Contraceptive Device **J** Synthetic Substitute **K** Nonautologous Tissue Substitute **N** Tissue Expander **V** Infusion Device, Pump **W** Vascular Access Device, Totally Implantable **X** Vascular Access Device, Tunneled **Y** Other Device	**Z** No Qualifier

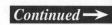
Continued →

Section	0	Medical and Surgical
Body System	J	Subcutaneous Tissue and Fascia
Operation	W	**Revision:** Correcting, to the extent possible, a portion of a malfunctioning device or the position of a displaced device

Body Part (4th)	Approach (5th)	Device (6th)	Qualifier (7th)
V Subcutaneous Tissue and Fascia, Upper Extremity W Subcutaneous Tissue and Fascia, Lower Extremity	X External	0 Drainage Device 3 Infusion Device 7 Autologous Tissue Substitute H Contraceptive Device J Synthetic Substitute K Nonautologous Tissue Substitute N Tissue Expander V Infusion Device, Pump W Vascular Access Device, Totally Implantable X Vascular Access Device, Tunneled	Z No Qualifier

Section	0	Medical and Surgical
Body System	J	Subcutaneous Tissue and Fascia
Operation	X	**Transfer:** Moving, without taking out, all or a portion of a body part to another location to take over the function of all or a portion of a body part

Body Part (4th)	Approach (5th)	Device (6th)	Qualifier (7th)
0 Subcutaneous Tissue and Fascia, Scalp 1 Subcutaneous Tissue and Fascia, Face 4 Subcutaneous Tissue and Fascia, Right Neck 5 Subcutaneous Tissue and Fascia, Left Neck 6 Subcutaneous Tissue and Fascia, Chest 7 Subcutaneous Tissue and Fascia, Back 8 Subcutaneous Tissue and Fascia, Abdomen 9 Subcutaneous Tissue and Fascia, Buttock B Subcutaneous Tissue and Fascia, Perineum C Subcutaneous Tissue and Fascia, Pelvic Region D Subcutaneous Tissue and Fascia, Right Upper Arm F Subcutaneous Tissue and Fascia, Left Upper Arm G Subcutaneous Tissue and Fascia, Right Lower Arm H Subcutaneous Tissue and Fascia, Left Lower Arm J Subcutaneous Tissue and Fascia, Right Hand K Subcutaneous Tissue and Fascia, Left Hand L Subcutaneous Tissue and Fascia, Right Upper Leg M Subcutaneous Tissue and Fascia, Left Upper Leg N Subcutaneous Tissue and Fascia, Right Lower Leg P Subcutaneous Tissue and Fascia, Left Lower Leg Q Subcutaneous Tissue and Fascia, Right Foot R Subcutaneous Tissue and Fascia, Left Foot	0 Open 3 Percutaneous	Z No Device	B Skin and Subcutaneous Tissue C Skin, Subcutaneous Tissue and Fascia Z No Qualifier

AHA Coding Clinic

0J2TXYZ Change Other Device in Trunk Subcutaneous Tissue and Fascia, External Approach—AHA CC: 2Q, 2017, 26; 3Q, 2018, 10

0J910ZZ Drainage of Face Subcutaneous Tissue and Fascia, Open Approach—AHA CC: 3Q, 2018, 16

0J940ZZ Drainage of Right Neck Subcutaneous Tissue and Fascia, Open Approach—AHA CC: 3Q, 2018, 16-17

0J960ZZ Drainage of Chest Subcutaneous Tissue and Fascia, Open Approach—AHA CC: 3Q, 2015, 23-24

0J9C0ZZ Drainage of Pelvic Region Subcutaneous Tissue and Fascia, Open Approach—AHA CC: 3Q, 2015, 23-24

0J9D0ZZ Drainage of Right Upper Arm Subcutaneous Tissue and Fascia, Open Approach—AHA CC: 3Q, 2015, 23-24

0J9F0ZZ Drainage of Left Upper Arm Subcutaneous Tissue and Fascia, Open Approach—AHA CC: 3Q, 2015, 23-24

0J9L0ZZ Drainage of Right Upper Leg Subcutaneous Tissue and Fascia, Open Approach—AHA CC: 3Q, 2015, 23-24

0J9M0ZZ Drainage of Left Upper Leg Subcutaneous Tissue and Fascia, Open Approach—AHA CC: 3Q, 2015, 23-24

0JB70ZZ Excision of Back Subcutaneous Tissue and Fascia, Open Approach—AHA CC: 1Q, 2018, 7-8

0JB80ZZ Excision of Abdomen Subcutaneous Tissue and Fascia, Open Approach—AHA CC: 3Q, 2014, 22-23; 4Q, 2014, 39-40; 1Q, 2020, 31-32

0JB90ZZ Excision of Buttock Subcutaneous Tissue and Fascia, Open Approach—AHA CC: 3Q, 2015, 6-7

0JB93ZZ Excision of Buttock Subcutaneous Tissue and Fascia, Percutaneous Approach—AHA CC: 3Q, 2019, 25

0JBB0ZZ Excision of Perineum Subcutaneous Tissue and Fascia, Open Approach—AHA CC: 1Q, 2015, 29-30

0JBH0ZZ Excision of Left Lower Arm Subcutaneous Tissue and Fascia, Open Approach—AHA CC: 2Q, 2015, 13

0JC80ZZ Extirpation of Matter from Abdomen Subcutaneous Tissue and Fascia, Open Approach—AHA CC: 3Q, 2017, 22

0JD70ZZ Extraction of Back Subcutaneous Tissue and Fascia, Open Approach—AHA CC: 3Q, 2016, 21

0JDC0ZZ Extraction of Pelvic Region Subcutaneous Tissue and Fascia, Open Approach—AHA CC: 1Q, 2015, 23

0JDL0ZZ Extraction of Right Upper Leg Subcutaneous Tissue and Fascia, Open Approach—AHA CC: 1Q, 2016, 40

0JDN0ZZ Extraction of Right Lower Leg Subcutaneous Tissue and Fascia, Open Approach—AHA CC: 3Q, 2016, 20-21

0JDR0ZZ Extraction of Left Foot Subcutaneous Tissue and Fascia, Open Approach—AHA CC: 3Q, 2016, 22

0JH608Z Insertion of Defibrillator Generator into Chest Subcutaneous Tissue and Fascia, Open Approach—AHA CC: 4Q, 2012, 104-106

0JH60MZ Insertion of Stimulator Generator into Chest Subcutaneous Tissue and Fascia, Open Approach—AHA CC: 4Q, 2016, 98-99

0JH60PZ Insertion of Cardiac Rhythm Related Device into Chest Subcutaneous Tissue and Fascia, Open Approach—AHA CC: 4Q, 2012, 104-106

0JH60WZ Insertion of Totally Implantable Vascular Access Device into Chest Subcutaneous Tissue and Fascia, Open Approach—AHA CC: 4Q, 2017, 63-64

0JH60XZ Insertion of Tunneled Vascular Access Device into Chest Subcutaneous Tissue and Fascia, Open Approach—AHA CC: 2Q, 2015, 33-34

0JH63VZ Insertion of Infusion Pump into Chest Subcutaneous Tissue and Fascia, Percutaneous Approach—AHA CC: 4Q, 2015, 14-15

0JH63XZ Insertion of Tunneled Vascular Access Device into Chest Subcutaneous Tissue and Fascia, Percutaneous Approach—AHA CC: 4Q, 2015, 30-32; 2Q, 2016, 15-16; 2Q, 2017, 24-26

0JH80VZ Insertion of Infusion Pump into Abdomen Subcutaneous Tissue and Fascia, Open Approach—AHA CC: 3Q, 2014, 19-20

0JH80WZ Insertion of Totally Implantable Vascular Access Device into Abdomen Subcutaneous Tissue and Fascia, Open Approach— AHA CC: 2Q, 2016, 14

0JHS33Z Insertion of Infusion Device into Head and Neck Subcutaneous Tissue and Fascia, Percutaneous Approach—AHA CC: 2Q, 2020, 15-16

0JHT03Z Insertion of Infusion Device into Trunk Subcutaneous Tissue and Fascia, Open Approach—AHA CC: 2Q, 2020, 16-17

0JHT0YZ Insertion of Other Device into Trunk Subcutaneous Tissue and Fascia, Open Approach—AHA CC: 4Q, 2018, 42-43

0JNL0ZZ Release Right Upper Leg Subcutaneous Tissue and Fascia, Open Approach—AHA CC: 3Q, 2017, 11-12

0JNM0ZZ Release Left Upper Leg Subcutaneous Tissue and Fascia, Open Approach—AHA CC: 3Q, 2017, 11-12

0JNN0ZZ Release Right Lower Leg Subcutaneous Tissue and Fascia, Open Approach—AHA CC: 3Q, 2017, 11-12

0JNP0ZZ Release Left Lower Leg Subcutaneous Tissue and Fascia, Open Approach—AHA CC: 3Q, 2017, 11-12

0JNQ0ZZ Release Right Foot Subcutaneous Tissue and Fascia, Open Approach—AHA CC: 3Q, 2017, 11-12

0JNR0ZZ Release Left Foot Subcutaneous Tissue and Fascia, Open Approach—AHA CC: 3Q, 2017, 11-12

0JPT0NZ Removal of Tissue Expander from Trunk Subcutaneous Tissue and Fascia, Open Approach—AHA CC: 4Q, 2013, 109-111

0JPT0PZ Removal of Cardiac Rhythm Related Device from Trunk Subcutaneous Tissue and Fascia, Open Approach—AHA CC: 4Q, 2012, 104-106

0JPT0VZ Removal of Infusion Pump from Trunk Subcutaneous Tissue and Fascia, Open Approach—AHA CC: 3Q, 2014, 19-20

0JPT0XZ Removal of Tunneled Vascular Access Device from Trunk Subcutaneous Tissue and Fascia, Open Approach—AHA CC: 4Q, 2015, 31-32; 2Q, 2016, 15-16

0JPT3JZ Removal of Synthetic Substitute from Trunk Subcutaneous Tissue and Fascia, Percutaneous Approach—AHA CC: 4Q, 2018, 86

0JPT3YZ Removal of Other Device from Trunk Subcutaneous Tissue and Fascia, Percutaneous Approach—AHA CC: 3Q, 2018, 29

0JQC0ZZ Repair Pelvic Region Subcutaneous Tissue and Fascia, Open Approach—AHA CC: 4Q, 2014, 44-45; 3Q, 2017, 19

0JR107Z Replacement of Face Subcutaneous Tissue and Fascia with Autologous Tissue Substitute, Open Approach—AHA CC: 2Q, 2015, 13

0JU707Z Supplement of Back Subcutaneous Tissue and Fascia with Autologous Tissue Substitute, Open Approach—AHA CC: 1Q, 2018, 7-8

0JUH0KZ Supplement of Left Lower Arm Subcutaneous Tissue and Fascia with Nonautologous Tissue Substitute, Open Approach—AHA CC: 2Q, 2018, 20

0JWS0JZ Revision of Synthetic Substitute in Head and Neck Subcutaneous Tissue and Fascia, Open Approach—AHA CC: 2Q, 2015, 9-10

0JWT0JZ Revision of Synthetic Substitute in Trunk Subcutaneous Tissue and Fascia, Open Approach— AHA CC: 1Q, 2018, 8-9

0JWT0PZ Revision of Cardiac Rhythm Related Device in Trunk Subcutaneous Tissue and Fascia, Open Approach—AHA CC: 4Q, 2012, 104-106

0JWT33Z Revision of Infusion Device in Trunk Subcutaneous Tissue and Fascia, Percutaneous Approach—AHA CC: 4Q, 2015, 33

0JX00ZC Transfer Scalp Subcutaneous Tissue and Fascia with Skin, Subcutaneous Tissue and Fascia, Open Approach—AHA CC: 1Q, 2018, 10

0JX60ZB Transfer Chest Subcutaneous Tissue and Fascia with Skin and Subcutaneous Tissue, Open Approach—AHA CC: 4Q, 2013, 109-111

0JX80ZB Transfer Abdomen Subcutaneous Tissue and Fascia with Skin and Subcutaneous Tissue, Open Approach—AHA CC: 4Q, 2013, 109-111

0JXN0ZC Transfer Right Lower Leg Subcutaneous Tissue and Fascia with Skin, Subcutaneous Tissue and Fascia, Open Approach—AHA CC: 3Q, 2014, 18-19

Muscles

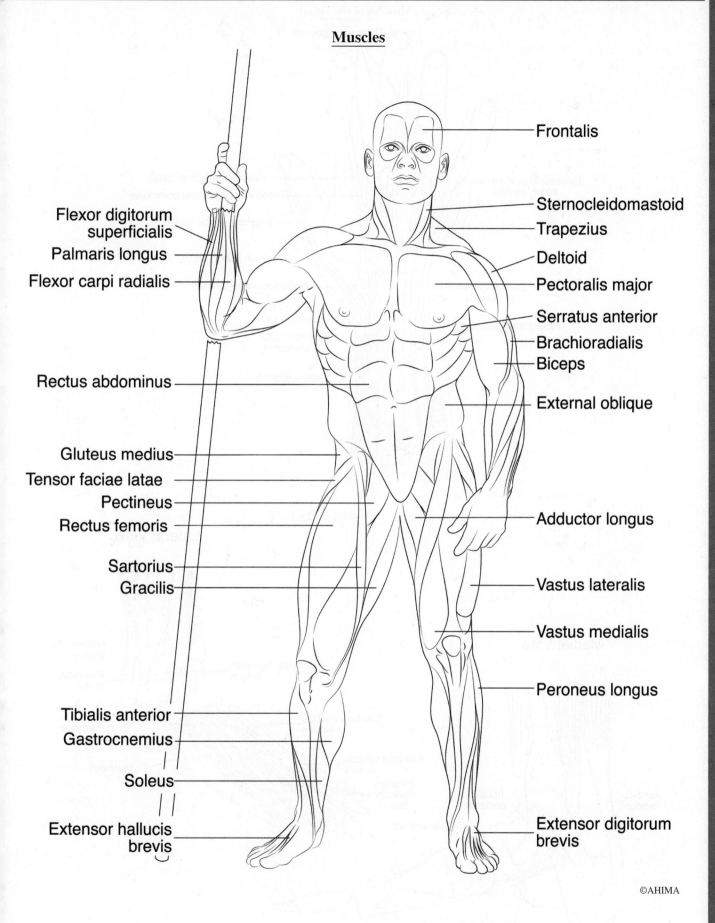

Frontalis

Sternocleidomastoid

Trapezius

Deltoid

Pectoralis major

Serratus anterior

Brachioradialis

Biceps

External oblique

Adductor longus

Vastus lateralis

Vastus medialis

Peroneus longus

Extensor digitorum
brevis

Flexor digitorum
superficialis

Palmaris longus

Flexor carpi radialis

Rectus abdominus

Gluteus medius

Tensor faciae latae

Pectineus

Rectus femoris

Sartorius

Gracilis

Tibialis anterior

Gastrocnemius

Soleus

Extensor hallucis
brevis

©AHIMA

Muscles of the Hand

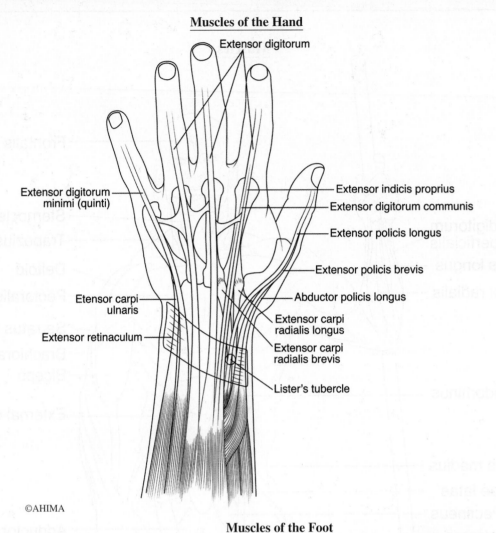

Extensor digitorum

Extensor digitorum minimi (quinti)

Etensor carpi ulnaris

Extensor retinaculum

Extensor indicis proprius

Extensor digitorum communis

Extensor policis longus

Extensor policis brevis

Abductor policis longus

Extensor carpi radialis longus

Extensor carpi radialis brevis

Lister's tubercle

©AHIMA

Muscles of the Foot

Lateral View

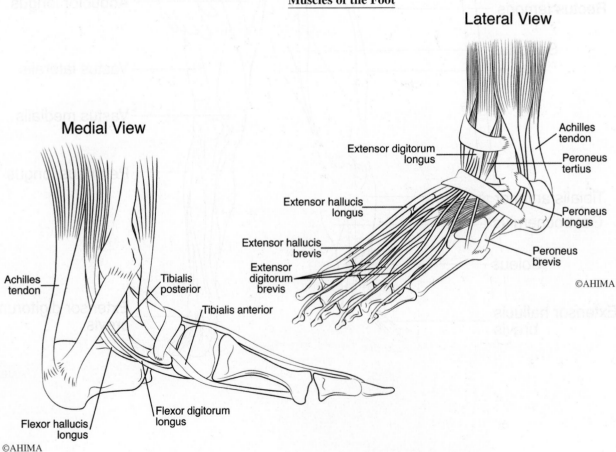

Extensor digitorum longus

Extensor hallucis longus

Extensor hallucis brevis

Extensor digitorum brevis

Achilles tendon

Peroneus tertius

Peroneus longus

Peroneus brevis

©AHIMA

Medial View

Achilles tendon

Tibialis posterior

Tibialis anterior

Flexor hallucis longus

Flexor digitorum longus

©AHIMA

Section   **0**   **Medical and Surgical**
Body System   **K**   **Muscles**
Operation   **2**   **Change:** Taking out or off a device from a body part and putting back an identical or similar device in or on the same body part without cutting or puncturing the skin or a mucous membrane

Body Part (4th)	Approach (5th)	Device (6th)	Qualifier (7th)
X Upper Muscle Y Lower Muscle	X External	0 Drainage Device Y Other Device	Z No Qualifier

Section   **0**   **Medical and Surgical**
Body System   **K**   **Muscles**
Operation   **5**   **Destruction:** Physical eradication of all or a portion of a body part by the direct use of energy, force, or a destructive agent

Body Part (4th)	Approach (5th)	Device (6th)	Qualifier (7th)
0 Head Muscle 1 Facial Muscle 2 Neck Muscle, Right 3 Neck Muscle, Left 4 Tongue, Palate, Pharynx Muscle 5 Shoulder Muscle, Right 6 Shoulder Muscle, Left 7 Upper Arm Muscle, Right 8 Upper Arm Muscle, Left 9 Lower Arm and Wrist Muscle, Right B Lower Arm and Wrist Muscle, Left C Hand Muscle, Right D Hand Muscle, Left F Trunk Muscle, Right G Trunk Muscle, Left H Thorax Muscle, Right J Thorax Muscle, Left K Abdomen Muscle, Right L Abdomen Muscle, Left M Perineum Muscle N Hip Muscle, Right P Hip Muscle, Left Q Upper Leg Muscle, Right R Upper Leg Muscle, Left S Lower Leg Muscle, Right T Lower Leg Muscle, Left V Foot Muscle, Right W Foot Muscle, Left	0 Open 3 Percutaneous 4 Percutaneous Endoscopic	Z No Device	Z No Qualifier

Section	0	**Medical and Surgical**
Body System	K	**Muscles**
Operation	8	**Division:** Cutting into a body part, without draining fluids and/or gases from the body part, in order to separate or transect a body part

Body Part (4ᵗʰ)	Approach (5ᵗʰ)	Device (6ᵗʰ)	Qualifier (7ᵗʰ)
0 Head Muscle 1 Facial Muscle 2 Neck Muscle, Right 3 Neck Muscle, Left 4 Tongue, Palate, Pharynx Muscle 5 Shoulder Muscle, Right 6 Shoulder Muscle, Left 7 Upper Arm Muscle, Right 8 Upper Arm Muscle, Left 9 Lower Arm and Wrist Muscle, Right B Lower Arm and Wrist Muscle, Left C Hand Muscle, Right D Hand Muscle, Left F Trunk Muscle, Right G Trunk Muscle, Left H Thorax Muscle, Right J Thorax Muscle, Left K Abdomen Muscle, Right L Abdomen Muscle, Left M Perineum Muscle N Hip Muscle, Right P Hip Muscle, Left Q Upper Leg Muscle, Right R Upper Leg Muscle, Left S Lower Leg Muscle, Right T Lower Leg Muscle, Left V Foot Muscle, Right W Foot Muscle, Left	0 Open 3 Percutaneous 4 Percutaneous Endoscopic	Z No Device	Z No Qualifier

Section	0	Medical and Surgical
Body System	K	Muscles
Operation	9	**Drainage:** Taking or letting out fluids and/or gases from a body part

Body Part (4th)	Approach (5th)	Device (6th)	Qualifier (7th)
0 Head Muscle 1 Facial Muscle 2 Neck Muscle, Right 3 Neck Muscle, Left 4 Tongue, Palate, Pharynx Muscle 5 Shoulder Muscle, Right 6 Shoulder Muscle, Left 7 Upper Arm Muscle, Right 8 Upper Arm Muscle, Left 9 Lower Arm and Wrist Muscle, Right B Lower Arm and Wrist Muscle, Left C Hand Muscle, Right D Hand Muscle, Left F Trunk Muscle, Right G Trunk Muscle, Left H Thorax Muscle, Right J Thorax Muscle, Left K Abdomen Muscle, Right L Abdomen Muscle, Left M Perineum Muscle N Hip Muscle, Right P Hip Muscle, Left Q Upper Leg Muscle, Right R Upper Leg Muscle, Left S Lower Leg Muscle, Right T Lower Leg Muscle, Left V Foot Muscle, Right W Foot Muscle, Left	0 Open 3 Percutaneous 4 Percutaneous Endoscopic	0 Drainage Device	Z No Qualifier
0 Head Muscle 1 Facial Muscle 2 Neck Muscle, Right 3 Neck Muscle, Left 4 Tongue, Palate, Pharynx Muscle 5 Shoulder Muscle, Right 6 Shoulder Muscle, Left 7 Upper Arm Muscle, Right 8 Upper Arm Muscle, Left 9 Lower Arm and Wrist Muscle, Right B Lower Arm and Wrist Muscle, Left C Hand Muscle, Right D Hand Muscle, Left F Trunk Muscle, Right G Trunk Muscle, Left H Thorax Muscle, Right J Thorax Muscle, Left K Abdomen Muscle, Right L Abdomen Muscle, Left M Perineum Muscle N Hip Muscle, Right P Hip Muscle, Left Q Upper Leg Muscle, Right R Upper Leg Muscle, Left S Lower Leg Muscle, Right T Lower Leg Muscle, Left V Foot Muscle, Right W Foot Muscle, Left	0 Open 3 Percutaneous 4 Percutaneous Endoscopic	Z No Device	X Diagnostic Z No Qualifier

Section   **0**   **Medical and Surgical**
Body System   **K**   **Muscles**
Operation   **B**   **Excision:** Cutting out or off, without replacement, a portion of a body part

Body Part (4th)	Approach (5th)	Device (6th)	Qualifier (7th)
0 Head Muscle	0 Open	Z No Device	X Diagnostic
1 Facial Muscle	3 Percutaneous		Z No Qualifier
2 Neck Muscle, Right	4 Percutaneous Endoscopic		
3 Neck Muscle, Left			
4 Tongue, Palate, Pharynx Muscle			
5 Shoulder Muscle, Right			
6 Shoulder Muscle, Left			
7 Upper Arm Muscle, Right			
8 Upper Arm Muscle, Left			
9 Lower Arm and Wrist Muscle, Right			
B Lower Arm and Wrist Muscle, Left			
C Hand Muscle, Right			
D Hand Muscle, Left			
F Trunk Muscle, Right			
G Trunk Muscle, Left			
H Thorax Muscle, Right			
J Thorax Muscle, Left			
K Abdomen Muscle, Right			
L Abdomen Muscle, Left			
M Perineum Muscle			
N Hip Muscle, Right			
P Hip Muscle, Left			
Q Upper Leg Muscle, Right			
R Upper Leg Muscle, Left			
S Lower Leg Muscle, Right			
T Lower Leg Muscle, Left			
V Foot Muscle, Right			
W Foot Muscle, Left			

Section   **0**   **Medical and Surgical**
Body System   **K**   **Muscles**
Operation   **C**   **Extirpation:** Taking or cutting out solid matter from a body part

Body Part (4th)	Approach (5th)	Device (6th)	Qualifier (7th)
0 Head Muscle	0 Open	Z No Device	Z No Qualifier
1 Facial Muscle	3 Percutaneous		
2 Neck Muscle, Right	4 Percutaneous Endoscopic		
3 Neck Muscle, Left			
4 Tongue, Palate, Pharynx Muscle			
5 Shoulder Muscle, Right			
6 Shoulder Muscle, Left			
7 Upper Arm Muscle, Right			
8 Upper Arm Muscle, Left			
9 Lower Arm and Wrist Muscle, Right			
B Lower Arm and Wrist Muscle, Left			
C Hand Muscle, Right			
D Hand Muscle, Left			
F Trunk Muscle, Right			
G Trunk Muscle, Left			
H Thorax Muscle, Right			
J Thorax Muscle, Left			
K Abdomen Muscle, Right			
L Abdomen Muscle, Left			
M Perineum Muscle			
N Hip Muscle, Right			
P Hip Muscle, Left			
Q Upper Leg Muscle, Right			
R Upper Leg Muscle, Left			
S Lower Leg Muscle, Right			
T Lower Leg Muscle, Left			
V Foot Muscle, Right			
W Foot Muscle, Left			

Section	0	Medical and Surgical
Body System	K	Muscles
Operation	D	**Extraction:** Pulling or stripping out or off all or a portion of a body part by the use of force

Body Part (4th)	Approach (5th)	Device (6th)	Qualifier (7th)
0 Head Muscle	0 Open	Z No Device	Z No Qualifier
1 Facial Muscle			
2 Neck Muscle, Right			
3 Neck Muscle, Left			
4 Tongue, Palate, Pharynx Muscle			
5 Shoulder Muscle, Right			
6 Shoulder Muscle, Left			
7 Upper Arm Muscle, Right			
8 Upper Arm Muscle, Left			
9 Lower Arm and Wrist Muscle, Right			
B Lower Arm and Wrist Muscle, Left			
C Hand Muscle, Right			
D Hand Muscle, Left			
F Trunk Muscle, Right			
G Trunk Muscle, Left			
H Thorax Muscle, Right			
J Thorax Muscle, Left			
K Abdomen Muscle, Right			
L Abdomen Muscle, Left			
M Perineum			
N Hip Muscle, Right			
P Hip Muscle, Left			
Q Upper Leg Muscle, Right			
R Upper Leg Muscle, Left			
S Lower Leg Muscle, Right			
T Lower Leg Muscle, Left			
V Foot Muscle, Right			
W Foot Muscle, Left			

Section	0	Medical and Surgical
Body System	K	Muscles
Operation	H	**Insertion:** Putting in a nonbiological appliance that monitors, assists, performs, or prevents a physiological function but does not physically take the place of a body part

Body Part (4th)	Approach (5th)	Device (6th)	Qualifier (7th)
X Upper Muscle	0 Open	M Stimulator Lead	Z No Qualifier
Y Lower Muscle	3 Percutaneous	Y Other Device	
	4 Percutaneous Endoscopic		

Section	0	Medical and Surgical
Body System	K	Muscles
Operation	J	**Inspection:** Visually and/or manually exploring a body part

Body Part (4th)	Approach (5th)	Device (6th)	Qualifier (7th)
X Upper Muscle	0 Open	Z No Device	Z No Qualifier
Y Lower Muscle	3 Percutaneous		
	4 Percutaneous Endoscopic		
	X External		

Section	0	Medical and Surgical
Body System	K	Muscles
Operation	M	Reattachment: Putting back in or on all or a portion of a separated body part to its normal location or other suitable location

Body Part (4th)	Approach (5th)	Device (6th)	Qualifier (7th)
0 Head Muscle	0 Open	Z No Device	Z No Qualifier
1 Facial Muscle	4 Percutaneous Endoscopic		
2 Neck Muscle, Right			
3 Neck Muscle, Left			
4 Tongue, Palate, Pharynx Muscle			
5 Shoulder Muscle, Right			
6 Shoulder Muscle, Left			
7 Upper Arm Muscle, Right			
8 Upper Arm Muscle, Left			
9 Lower Arm and Wrist Muscle, Right			
B Lower Arm and Wrist Muscle, Left			
C Hand Muscle, Right			
D Hand Muscle, Left			
F Trunk Muscle, Right			
G Trunk Muscle, Left			
H Thorax Muscle, Right			
J Thorax Muscle, Left			
K Abdomen Muscle, Right			
L Abdomen Muscle, Left			
M Perineum Muscle			
N Hip Muscle, Right			
P Hip Muscle, Left			
Q Upper Leg Muscle, Right			
R Upper Leg Muscle, Left			
S Lower Leg Muscle, Right			
T Lower Leg Muscle, Left			
V Foot Muscle, Right			
W Foot Muscle, Left			

Section	0	Medical and Surgical
Body System	K	Muscles
Operation	N	Release: Freeing a body part from an abnormal physical constraint by cutting or by the use of force

Body Part (4th)	Approach (5th)	Device (6th)	Qualifier (7th)
0 Head Muscle	0 Open	Z No Device	Z No Qualifier
1 Facial Muscle	3 Percutaneous		
2 Neck Muscle, Right	4 Percutaneous Endoscopic		
3 Neck Muscle, Left	X External		
4 Tongue, Palate, Pharynx Muscle			
5 Shoulder Muscle, Right			
6 Shoulder Muscle, Left			
7 Upper Arm Muscle, Right			
8 Upper Arm Muscle, Left			
9 Lower Arm and Wrist Muscle, Right			
B Lower Arm and Wrist Muscle, Left			
C Hand Muscle, Right			
D Hand Muscle, Left			
F Trunk Muscle, Right			
G Trunk Muscle, Left			
H Thorax Muscle, Right			
J Thorax Muscle, Left			
K Abdomen Muscle, Right			
L Abdomen Muscle, Left			
M Perineum Muscle			
N Hip Muscle, Right			
P Hip Muscle, Left			
Q Upper Leg Muscle, Right			
R Upper Leg Muscle, Left			
S Lower Leg Muscle, Right			
T Lower Leg Muscle, Left			
V Foot Muscle, Right			
W Foot Muscle, Left			

Section	0	Medical and Surgical
Body System	K	Muscles
Operation	P	**Removal:** Taking out or off a device from a body part

Body Part (4ᵗʰ)	Approach (5ᵗʰ)	Device (6ᵗʰ)	Qualifier (7ᵗʰ)
X Upper Muscle Y Lower Muscle	0 Open 3 Percutaneous 4 Percutaneous Endoscopic	0 Drainage Device 7 Autologous Tissue Substitute J Synthetic Substitute K Nonautologous Tissue Substitute M Stimulator Lead Y Other Device	Z No Qualifier
X Upper Muscle Y Lower Muscle	X External	0 Drainage Device M Stimulator Lead	Z No Qualifier

Section	0	Medical and Surgical
Body System	K	Muscles
Operation	Q	**Repair:** Restoring, to the extent possible, a body part to its normal anatomic structure and function

Body Part (4ᵗʰ)	Approach (5ᵗʰ)	Device (6ᵗʰ)	Qualifier (7ᵗʰ)
0 Head Muscle 1 Facial Muscle 2 Neck Muscle, Right 3 Neck Muscle, Left 4 Tongue, Palate, Pharynx Muscle 5 Shoulder Muscle, Right 6 Shoulder Muscle, Left 7 Upper Arm Muscle, Right 8 Upper Arm Muscle, Left 9 Lower Arm and Wrist Muscle, Right B Lower Arm and Wrist Muscle, Left C Hand Muscle, Right D Hand Muscle, Left F Trunk Muscle, Right G Trunk Muscle, Left H Thorax Muscle, Right J Thorax Muscle, Left K Abdomen Muscle, Right L Abdomen Muscle, Left M Perineum Muscle N Hip Muscle, Right P Hip Muscle, Left Q Upper Leg Muscle, Right R Upper Leg Muscle, Left S Lower Leg Muscle, Right T Lower Leg Muscle, Left V Foot Muscle, Right W Foot Muscle, Left	0 Open 3 Percutaneous 4 Percutaneous Endoscopic	Z No Device	Z No Qualifier

Section	0	Medical and Surgical
Body System	K	Muscles
Operation	R	**Replacement:** Putting in or on biological or synthetic material that physically takes the place and/or function of all or a portion of a body part

Body Part (4th)	Approach (5th)	Device (6th)	Qualifier (7th)
0 Head Muscle 1 Facial Muscle 2 Neck Muscle, Right 3 Neck Muscle, Left 4 Tongue, Palate, Pharynx Muscle 5 Shoulder Muscle, Right 6 Shoulder Muscle, Left 7 Upper Arm Muscle, Right 8 Upper Arm Muscle, Left 9 Lower Arm and Wrist Muscle, Right B Lower Arm and Wrist Muscle, Left C Hand Muscle, Right D Hand Muscle, Left F Trunk Muscle, Right G Trunk Muscle, Left H Thorax Muscle, Right J Thorax Muscle, Left K Abdomen Muscle, Right L Abdomen Muscle, Left M Perineum N Hip Muscle, Right P Hip Muscle, Left Q Upper Leg Muscle, Right R Upper Leg Muscle, Left S Lower Leg Muscle, Right T Lower Leg Muscle, Left V Foot Muscle, Right W Foot Muscle, Left	0 Open 4 Percutaneous Endoscopic	7 Autologous Tissue Substitute J Synthetic Substitute K Nonautologous Tissue Substitute	Z No Qualifier

Section	0	Medical and Surgical
Body System	K	Muscles
Operation	S	**Reposition:** Moving to its normal location, or other suitable location, all or a portion of a body part

Body Part (4th)	Approach (5th)	Device (6th)	Qualifier (7th)
0 Head Muscle 1 Facial Muscle 2 Neck Muscle, Right 3 Neck Muscle, Left 4 Tongue, Palate, Pharynx Muscle 5 Shoulder Muscle, Right 6 Shoulder Muscle, Left 7 Upper Arm Muscle, Right 8 Upper Arm Muscle, Left 9 Lower Arm and Wrist Muscle, Right B Lower Arm and Wrist Muscle, Left C Hand Muscle, Right D Hand Muscle, Left F Trunk Muscle, Right G Trunk Muscle, Left H Thorax Muscle, Right J Thorax Muscle, Left K Abdomen Muscle, Right L Abdomen Muscle, Left M Perineum Muscle N Hip Muscle, Right P Hip Muscle, Left Q Upper Leg Muscle, Right R Upper Leg Muscle, Left S Lower Leg Muscle, Right T Lower Leg Muscle, Left V Foot Muscle, Right W Foot Muscle, Left	0 Open 4 Percutaneous Endoscopic	Z No Device	Z No Qualifier

Section | 0 | Medical and Surgical
Body System | K | Muscles
Operation | T | **Resection:** Cutting out or off, without replacement, all of a body part

Body Part (4ᵗʰ)	Approach (5ᵗʰ)	Device (6ᵗʰ)	Qualifier (7ᵗʰ)
0 Head Muscle	0 Open	Z No Device	Z No Qualifier
1 Facial Muscle	4 Percutaneous Endoscopic		
2 Neck Muscle, Right			
3 Neck Muscle, Left			
4 Tongue, Palate, Pharynx Muscle			
5 Shoulder Muscle, Right			
6 Shoulder Muscle, Left			
7 Upper Arm Muscle, Right			
8 Upper Arm Muscle, Left			
9 Lower Arm and Wrist Muscle, Right			
B Lower Arm and Wrist Muscle, Left			
C Hand Muscle, Right			
D Hand Muscle, Left			
F Trunk Muscle, Right			
G Trunk Muscle, Left			
H Thorax Muscle, Right			
J Thorax Muscle, Left			
K Abdomen Muscle, Right			
L Abdomen Muscle, Left			
M Perineum Muscle			
N Hip Muscle, Right			
P Hip Muscle, Left			
Q Upper Leg Muscle, Right			
R Upper Leg Muscle, Left			
S Lower Leg Muscle, Right			
T Lower Leg Muscle, Left			
V Foot Muscle, Right			
W Foot Muscle, Left			

Section | 0 | Medical and Surgical
Body System | K | Muscles
Operation | U | **Supplement:** Putting in or on biological or synthetic material that physically reinforces and/or augments the function of a portion of a body part

Body Part (4ᵗʰ)	Approach (5ᵗʰ)	Device (6ᵗʰ)	Qualifier (7ᵗʰ)
0 Head Muscle	0 Open	7 Autologous Tissue Substitute	Z No Qualifier
1 Facial Muscle	4 Percutaneous Endoscopic	J Synthetic Substitute	
2 Neck Muscle, Right		K Nonautologous Tissue Substitute	
3 Neck Muscle, Left			
4 Tongue, Palate, Pharynx Muscle			
5 Shoulder Muscle, Right			
6 Shoulder Muscle, Left			
7 Upper Arm Muscle, Right			
8 Upper Arm Muscle, Left			
9 Lower Arm and Wrist Muscle, Right			
B Lower Arm and Wrist Muscle, Left			
C Hand Muscle, Right			
D Hand Muscle, Left			
F Trunk Muscle, Right			
G Trunk Muscle, Left			
H Thorax Muscle, Right			
J Thorax Muscle, Left			
K Abdomen Muscle, Right			
L Abdomen Muscle, Left			
M Perineum Muscle			
N Hip Muscle, Right			
P Hip Muscle, Left			
Q Upper Leg Muscle, Right			
R Upper Leg Muscle, Left			
S Lower Leg Muscle, Right			
T Lower Leg Muscle, Left			
V Foot Muscle, Right			
W Foot Muscle, Left			

Section	0	Medical and Surgical
Body System	K	Muscles
Operation	W	Revision: Correcting, to the extent possible, a portion of a malfunctioning device or the position of a displaced device

Body Part (4th)	Approach (5th)	Device (6th)	Qualifier (7th)
X Upper Muscle Y Lower Muscle	0 Open 3 Percutaneous 4 Percutaneous Endoscopic	0 Drainage Device 7 Autologous Tissue Substitute J Synthetic Substitute K Nonautologous Tissue Substitute M Stimulator Lead Y Other Device	Z No Qualifier
X Upper Muscle Y Lower Muscle	X External	0 Drainage Device 7 Autologous Tissue Substitute J Synthetic Substitute K Nonautologous Tissue Substitute M Stimulator Lead	Z No Qualifier

Section	0	Medical and Surgical
Body System	K	Muscles
Operation	X	Transfer: Moving, without taking out, all or a portion of a body part to another location to take over the function of all or a portion of a body part

Body Part (4th)	Approach (5th)	Device (6th)	Qualifier (7th)
0 Head Muscle 1 Facial Muscle 2 Neck Muscle, Right 3 Neck Muscle, Left 4 Tongue, Palate, Pharynx Muscle 5 Shoulder Muscle, Right 6 Shoulder Muscle, Left 7 Upper Arm Muscle, Right 8 Upper Arm Muscle, Left 9 Lower Arm and Wrist Muscle, Right B Lower Arm and Wrist Muscle, Left C Hand Muscle, Right D Hand Muscle, Left H Thorax Muscle, Right J Thorax Muscle, Left M Perineum Muscle N Hip Muscle, Right P Hip Muscle, Left Q Upper Leg Muscle, Right R Upper Leg Muscle, Left S Lower Leg Muscle, Right T Lower Leg Muscle, Left V Foot Muscle, Right W Foot Muscle, Left	0 Open 4 Percutaneous Endoscopic	Z No Device	0 Skin 1 Subcutaneous Tissue 2 Skin and Subcutaneous Tissue Z No Qualifier
F Trunk Muscle, Right G Trunk Muscle, Left	0 Open 4 Percutaneous Endoscopic	Z No Device	0 Skin 1 Subcutaneous Tissue 2 Skin and Subcutaneous Tissue 5 Latissimus Dorsi Myocutaneous Flap 7 Deep Inferior Epigastric Artery Perforator Flap 8 Superficial Inferior Epigastric Artery Flap 9 Gluteal Artery Perforator Flap Z No Qualifier
K Abdomen Muscle, Right L Abdomen Muscle, Left	0 Open 4 Percutaneous Endoscopic	Z No Device	0 Skin 1 Subcutaneous Tissue 2 Skin and Subcutaneous Tissue 6 Transverse Rectus Abdominis Myocutaneous Flap Z No Qualifier

0K844ZZ Division of Tongue, Palate, Pharynx Muscle, Percutaneous Endoscopic Approach—AHA CC: 2Q, 2020, 25

0KBN0ZZ Excision of Right Hip Muscle, Open Approach—AHA CC: 3Q, 2016, 20

0KBP0ZZ Excision of Left Hip Muscle, Open Approach—AHA CC: 3Q, 2016, 20; 4Q, 2019, 43-44

0KBR0ZZ Excision of Left Upper Leg Muscle, Open Approach—AHA CC: 1Q, 2020, 27-28

0KDS0ZZ Extraction of Right Lower Leg Muscle, Open Approach—AHA CC: 4Q, 2017, 42

0KN84ZZ Release Left Upper Arm Muscle, Percutaneous Endoscopic Approach—AHA CC: 2Q, 2015, 22-23

0KNK0ZZ Release Right Abdomen Muscle, Open Approach—AHA CC: 4Q, 2014, 39-40

0KNL0ZZ Release Left Abdomen Muscle, Open Approach—AHA CC: 4Q, 2014, 39-40

0KNT0ZZ Release Left Lower Leg Muscle, Open Approach—AHA CC: 2Q, 2017, 12-14

0KNV0ZZ Release Right Foot Muscle, Open Approach—AHA CC: 2Q, 2017, 12-14

0KQM0ZZ Repair Perineum Muscle, Open Approach—AHA CC: 4Q, 2013, 120; 1Q, 2016, 7; 2Q, 2016, 34-35

0KT30ZZ Resection of Left Neck Muscle, Open Approach—AHA CC: 2Q, 2016, 12-14

0KTM0ZZ Resection of Perineum Muscle, Open Approach—AHA CC: 4Q, 2014, 40-41; 1Q, 2015, 38

0KX10Z2 Transfer Facial Muscle with Skin and Subcutaneous Tissue, Open Approach—AHA CC: 3Q, 2015, 33

0KX40Z2 Transfer Tongue, Palate, Pharynx Muscle with Skin and Subcutaneous Tissue, Open Approach—AHA CC: 2Q, 2015, 26

0KXF0Z2 Transfer Right Trunk Muscle with Skin and Subcutaneous Tissue, Open Approach—AHA CC: 2Q, 2014, 12

0KXF0Z5 Transfer Right Trunk Muscle, Latissimus Dorsi Myocutaneous Flap, Open Approach—AHA CC: 4Q, 2017, 67

0KXK0Z6 Transfer Right Abdomen Muscle, Transverse Rectus Abdominis Myocutaneous Flap, Open Approach—AHA CC: 4Q, 2014, 41

0KXL0Z6 Transfer Left Abdomen Muscle, Transverse Rectus Abdominis Myocutaneous Flap, Open Approach—AHA CC: 2Q, 2014, 10-11

0KXQ0ZZ Transfer Right Upper Leg Muscle, Open Approach—AHA CC: 3Q, 2016, 30-31

0KXR0ZZ Transfer Left Upper Leg Muscle, Open Approach—AHA CC: 3Q, 2016, 30-31

Shoulder Tendons and Ligaments

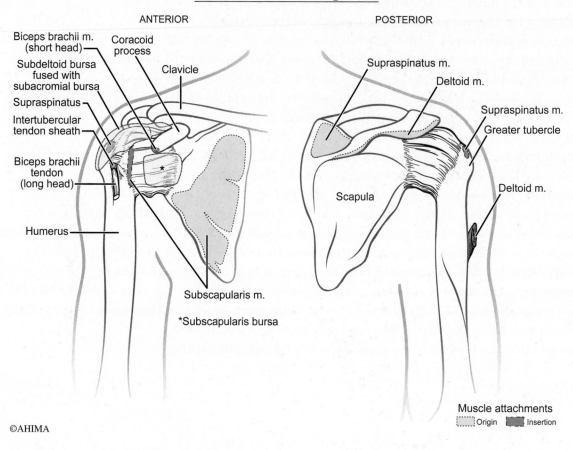

ANTERIOR

Biceps brachii m. (short head)
Coracoid process
Clavicle
Subdeltoid bursa fused with subacromial bursa
Supraspinatus
Intertubercular tendon sheath
Biceps brachii tendon (long head)
Humerus
Subscapularis m.

*Subscapularis bursa

POSTERIOR

Supraspinatus m.
Deltoid m.
Supraspinatus m.
Greater tubercle
Deltoid m.
Scapula

©AHIMA

Muscle attachments
Origin   Insertion

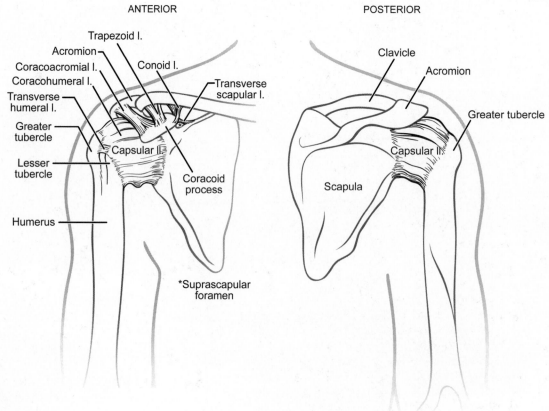

ANTERIOR

Trapezoid l.
Acromion
Coracoacromial l.
Coracohumeral l.
Conoid l.
Transverse humeral l.
Transverse scapular l.
Greater tubercle
Capsular l.
Lesser tubercle
Coracoid process
Humerus

*Suprascapular foramen

POSTERIOR

Clavicle
Acromion
Greater tubercle
Capsular l.
Scapula

©AHIMA

Hip Tendons and Ligaments

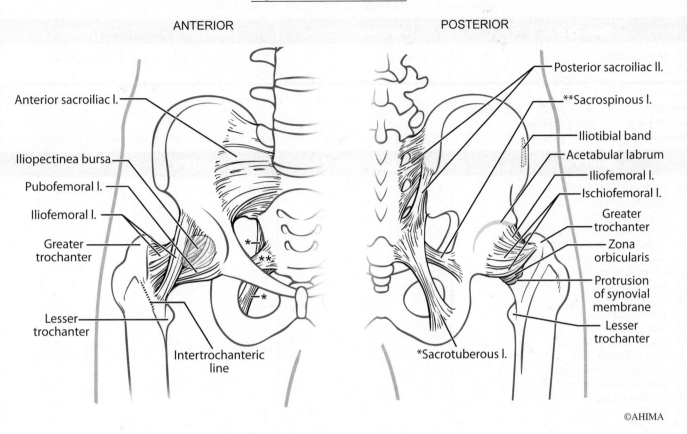

ANTERIOR

POSTERIOR

Anterior sacroiliac l.

Iliopectinea bursa

Pubofemoral l.

Iliofemoral l.

Greater trochanter

Lesser trochanter

Intertrochanteric line

Posterior sacroiliac ll.

**Sacrospinous l.

Iliotibial band

Acetabular labrum

Iliofemoral l.

Ischiofemoral l.

Greater trochanter

Zona orbicularis

Protrusion of synovial membrane

Lesser trochanter

*Sacrotuberous l.

©AHIMA

Knee Tendons and Ligaments

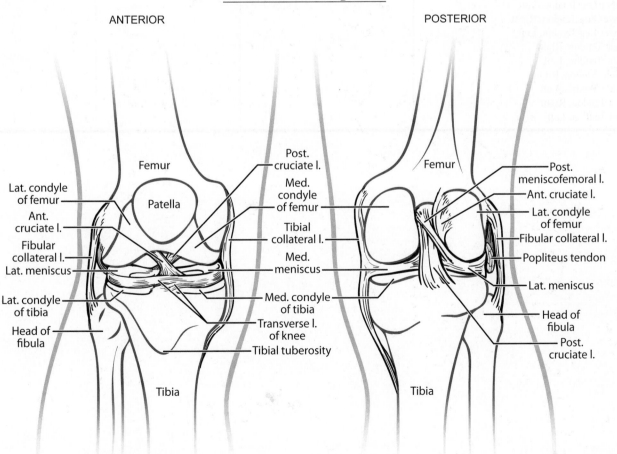

ANTERIOR

POSTERIOR

Femur

Lat. condyle of femur

Ant. cruciate l.

Fibular collateral l.

Lat. meniscus

Lat. condyle of tibia

Head of fibula

Patella

Tibia

Post. cruciate l.

Med. condyle of femur

Tibial collateral l.

Med. meniscus

Med. condyle of tibia

Transverse l. of knee

Tibial tuberosity

Femur

Post. meniscofemoral l.

Ant. cruciate l.

Lat. condyle of femur

Fibular collateral l.

Popliteus tendon

Lat. meniscus

Head of fibula

Post. cruciate l.

Tibia

©AHIMA

Section	0	Medical and Surgical
Body System	L	Tendons
Operation	2	**Change:** Taking out or off a device from a body part and putting back an identical or similar device in or on the same body part without cutting or puncturing the skin or a mucous membrane

Body Part (4th)	Approach (5th)	Device (6th)	Qualifier (7th)
X Upper Tendon Y Lower Tendon	X External	0 Drainage Device Y Other Device	Z No Qualifier

Section	0	Medical and Surgical
Body System	L	Tendons
Operation	5	**Destruction:** Physical eradication of all or a portion of a body part by the direct use of energy, force, or a destructive agent

Body Part (4th)	Approach (5th)	Device (6th)	Qualifier (7th)
0 Head and Neck Tendon 1 Shoulder Tendon, Right 2 Shoulder Tendon, Left 3 Upper Arm Tendon, Right 4 Upper Arm Tendon, Left 5 Lower Arm and Wrist Tendon, Right 6 Lower Arm and Wrist Tendon, Left 7 Hand Tendon, Right 8 Hand Tendon, Left 9 Trunk Tendon, Right B Trunk Tendon, Left C Thorax Tendon, Right D Thorax Tendon, Left F Abdomen Tendon, Right G Abdomen Tendon, Left H Perineum Tendon J Hip Tendon, Right K Hip Tendon, Left L Upper Leg Tendon, Right M Upper Leg Tendon, Left N Lower Leg Tendon, Right P Lower Leg Tendon, Left Q Knee Tendon, Right R Knee Tendon, Left S Ankle Tendon, Right T Ankle Tendon, Left V Foot Tendon, Right W Foot Tendon, Left	0 Open 3 Percutaneous 4 Percutaneous Endoscopic	Z No Device	Z No Qualifier

Section	0	Medical and Surgical
Body System	L	Tendons
Operation	8	Division: Cutting into a body part, without draining fluids and/or gases from the body part, in order to separate or transect a body part

Body Part (4th)	Approach (5th)	Device (6th)	Qualifier (7th)
0 Head and Neck Tendon 1 Shoulder Tendon, Right 2 Shoulder Tendon, Left 3 Upper Arm Tendon, Right 4 Upper Arm Tendon, Left 5 Lower Arm and Wrist Tendon, Right 6 Lower Arm and Wrist Tendon, Left 7 Hand Tendon, Right 8 Hand Tendon, Left 9 Trunk Tendon, Right B Trunk Tendon, Left C Thorax Tendon, Right D Thorax Tendon, Left F Abdomen Tendon, Right G Abdomen Tendon, Left H Perineum Tendon J Hip Tendon, Right K Hip Tendon, Left L Upper Leg Tendon, Right M Upper Leg Tendon, Left N Lower Leg Tendon, Right P Lower Leg Tendon, Left Q Knee Tendon, Right R Knee Tendon, Left S Ankle Tendon, Right T Ankle Tendon, Left V Foot Tendon, Right W Foot Tendon, Left	0 Open 3 Percutaneous 4 Percutaneous Endoscopic	Z No Device	Z No Qualifier

Section	0	Medical and Surgical
Body System	L	Tendons
Operation	9	Drainage: Taking or letting out fluids and/or gases from a body part

Body Part (4th)	Approach (5th)	Device (6th)	Qualifier (7th)
0 Head and Neck Tendon 1 Shoulder Tendon, Right 2 Shoulder Tendon, Left 3 Upper Arm Tendon, Right 4 Upper Arm Tendon, Left 5 Lower Arm and Wrist Tendon, Right 6 Lower Arm and Wrist Tendon, Left 7 Hand Tendon, Right 8 Hand Tendon, Left 9 Trunk Tendon, Right B Trunk Tendon, Left C Thorax Tendon, Right D Thorax Tendon, Left F Abdomen Tendon, Right G Abdomen Tendon, Left H Perineum Tendon J Hip Tendon, Right K Hip Tendon, Left L Upper Leg Tendon, Right M Upper Leg Tendon, Left N Lower Leg Tendon, Right P Lower Leg Tendon, Left Q Knee Tendon, Right R Knee Tendon, Left S Ankle Tendon, Right T Ankle Tendon, Left V Foot Tendon, Right W Foot Tendon, Left	0 Open 3 Percutaneous 4 Percutaneous Endoscopic	0 Drainage Device	Z No Qualifier

Continued →

Section	0	Medical and Surgical
Body System	L	Tendons
Operation	9	**Drainage:** Taking or letting out fluids and/or gases from a body part

Body Part (4th)	Approach (5th)	Device (6th)	Qualifier (7th)
0 Head and Neck Tendon 1 Shoulder Tendon, Right 2 Shoulder Tendon, Left 3 Upper Arm Tendon, Right 4 Upper Arm Tendon, Left 5 Lower Arm and Wrist Tendon, Right 6 Lower Arm and Wrist Tendon, Left 7 Hand Tendon, Right 8 Hand Tendon, Left 9 Trunk Tendon, Right B Trunk Tendon, Left C Thorax Tendon, Right D Thorax Tendon, Left F Abdomen Tendon, Right G Abdomen Tendon, Left H Perineum Tendon J Hip Tendon, Right K Hip Tendon, Left L Upper Leg Tendon, Right M Upper Leg Tendon, Left N Lower Leg Tendon, Right P Lower Leg Tendon, Left Q Knee Tendon, Right R Knee Tendon, Left S Ankle Tendon, Right T Ankle Tendon, Left V Foot Tendon, Right W Foot Tendon, Left	0 Open 3 Percutaneous 4 Percutaneous Endoscopic	Z No Device	X Diagnostic Z No Qualifier

Section	0	Medical and Surgical
Body System	L	Tendons
Operation	B	**Excision:** Cutting out or off, without replacement, a portion of a body part

Body Part (4th)	Approach (5th)	Device (6th)	Qualifier (7th)
0 Head and Neck Tendon 1 Shoulder Tendon, Right 2 Shoulder Tendon, Left 3 Upper Arm Tendon, Right 4 Upper Arm Tendon, Left 5 Lower Arm and Wrist Tendon, Right 6 Lower Arm and Wrist Tendon, Left 7 Hand Tendon, Right 8 Hand Tendon, Left 9 Trunk Tendon, Right B Trunk Tendon, Left C Thorax Tendon, Right D Thorax Tendon, Left F Abdomen Tendon, Right G Abdomen Tendon, Left H Perineum Tendon J Hip Tendon, Right K Hip Tendon, Left L Upper Leg Tendon, Right M Upper Leg Tendon, Left N Lower Leg Tendon, Right P Lower Leg Tendon, Left Q Knee Tendon, Right R Knee Tendon, Left S Ankle Tendon, Right T Ankle Tendon, Left V Foot Tendon, Right W Foot Tendon, Left	0 Open 3 Percutaneous 4 Percutaneous Endoscopic	Z No Device	X Diagnostic Z No Qualifier

Section	0	Medical and Surgical
Body System	L	Tendons
Operation	C	**Extirpation:** Taking or cutting out solid matter from a body part

Body Part (4th)	Approach (5th)	Device (6th)	Qualifier (7th)
0 Head and Neck Tendon	0 Open	Z No Device	Z No Qualifier
1 Shoulder Tendon, Right	3 Percutaneous		
2 Shoulder Tendon, Left	4 Percutaneous Endoscopic		
3 Upper Arm Tendon, Right			
4 Upper Arm Tendon, Left			
5 Lower Arm and Wrist Tendon, Right			
6 Lower Arm and Wrist Tendon, Left			
7 Hand Tendon, Right			
8 Hand Tendon, Left			
9 Trunk Tendon, Right			
B Trunk Tendon, Left			
C Thorax Tendon, Right			
D Thorax Tendon, Left			
F Abdomen Tendon, Right			
G Abdomen Tendon, Left			
H Perineum Tendon			
J Hip Tendon, Right			
K Hip Tendon, Left			
L Upper Leg Tendon, Right			
M Upper Leg Tendon, Left			
N Lower Leg Tendon, Right			
P Lower Leg Tendon, Left			
Q Knee Tendon, Right			
R Knee Tendon, Left			
S Ankle Tendon, Right			
T Ankle Tendon, Left			
V Foot Tendon, Right			
W Foot Tendon, Left			

Section	0	Medical and Surgical
Body System	L	Tendons
Operation	D	**Extraction:** Pulling or stripping out or off all or a portion of a body part by the use of force

Body Part (4th)	Approach (5th)	Device (6th)	Qualifier (7th)
0 Head and Neck Tendon	0 Open	Z No Device	Z No Qualifier
1 Shoulder Tendon, Right			
2 Shoulder Tendon, Left			
3 Upper Arm Tendon, Right			
4 Upper Arm Tendon, Left			
5 Lower Arm and Wrist Tendon, Right			
6 Lower Arm and Wrist Tendon, Left			
7 Hand Tendon, Right			
8 Hand Tendon, Left			
9 Trunk Tendon, Right			
B Trunk Tendon, Left			
C Thorax Tendon, Right			
D Thorax Tendon, Left			
F Abdomen Tendon, Right			
G Abdomen Tendon, Left			
H Perineum Tendon			
J Hip Tendon, Right			
K Hip Tendon, Left			
L Upper Leg Tendon, Right			
M Upper Leg Tendon, Left			
N Lower Leg Tendon, Right			
P Lower Leg Tendon, Left			
Q Knee Tendon, Right			
R Knee Tendon, Left			
S Ankle Tendon, Right			
T Ankle Tendon, Left			
V Foot Tendon, Right			
W Foot Tendon, Left			

Section	0	Medical and Surgical
Body System	L	Tendons
Operation	H	**Inspection:** Putting in a nonbiological appliance that monitors, assists, performs, or prevents a physiological function but does not physically take the place of a body part

Body Part (4th)	Approach (5th)	Device (6th)	Qualifier (7th)
X Upper Tendon Y Lower Tendon	0 Open 3 Percutaneous 4 Percutaneous Endoscopic	Y Other Device	Z No Qualifier

Section	0	Medical and Surgical
Body System	L	Tendons
Operation	J	**Inspection:** Visually and/or manually exploring a body part

Body Part (4th)	Approach (5th)	Device (6th)	Qualifier (7th)
X Upper Tendon Y Lower Tendon	0 Open 3 Percutaneous 4 Percutaneous Endoscopic X External	Z No Device	Z No Qualifier

Section	0	Medical and Surgical
Body System	L	Tendons
Operation	M	**Reattachment:** Putting back in or on all or a portion of a separated body part to its normal location or other suitable location

Body Part (4th)	Approach (5th)	Device (6th)	Qualifier (7th)
0 Head and Neck Tendon 1 Shoulder Tendon, Right 2 Shoulder Tendon, Left 3 Upper Arm Tendon, Right 4 Upper Arm Tendon, Left 5 Lower Arm and Wrist Tendon, Right 6 Lower Arm and Wrist Tendon, Left 7 Hand Tendon, Right 8 Hand Tendon, Left 9 Trunk Tendon, Right B Trunk Tendon, Left C Thorax Tendon, Right D Thorax Tendon, Left F Abdomen Tendon, Right G Abdomen Tendon, Left H Perineum Tendon J Hip Tendon, Right K Hip Tendon, Left L Upper Leg Tendon, Right M Upper Leg Tendon, Left N Lower Leg Tendon, Right P Lower Leg Tendon, Left Q Knee Tendon, Right R Knee Tendon, Left S Ankle Tendon, Right T Ankle Tendon, Left V Foot Tendon, Right W Foot Tendon, Left	0 Open 4 Percutaneous Endoscopic	Z No Device	Z No Qualifier

Section	0	Medical and Surgical
Body System	L	Tendons
Operation	N	**Release:** Freeing a body part from an abnormal physical constraint by cutting or by the use of force

Body Part (4th)	Approach (5th)	Device (6th)	Qualifier (7th)
0 Head and Neck Tendon 1 Shoulder Tendon, Right 2 Shoulder Tendon, Left 3 Upper Arm Tendon, Right 4 Upper Arm Tendon, Left 5 Lower Arm and Wrist Tendon, Right 6 Lower Arm and Wrist Tendon, Left 7 Hand Tendon, Right 8 Hand Tendon, Left 9 Trunk Tendon, Right B Trunk Tendon, Left C Thorax Tendon, Right D Thorax Tendon, Left F Abdomen Tendon, Right G Abdomen Tendon, Left H Perineum Tendon J Hip Tendon, Right K Hip Tendon, Left L Upper Leg Tendon, Right M Upper Leg Tendon, Left N Lower Leg Tendon, Right P Lower Leg Tendon, Left Q Knee Tendon, Right R Knee Tendon, Left S Ankle Tendon, Right T Ankle Tendon, Left V Foot Tendon, Right W Foot Tendon, Left	0 Open 3 Percutaneous 4 Percutaneous Endoscopic X External	Z No Device	Z No Qualifier

Section	0	Medical and Surgical
Body System	L	Tendons
Operation	P	**Removal:** Taking out or off a device from a body part

Body Part (4th)	Approach (5th)	Device (6th)	Qualifier (7th)
X Upper Tendon Y Lower Tendon	0 Open 3 Percutaneous 4 Percutaneous Endoscopic	0 Drainage Device 7 Autologous Tissue Substitute J Synthetic Substitute K Nonautologous Tissue Substitute Y Other Device	Z No Qualifier
X Upper Tendon Y Lower Tendon	X External	0 Drainage Device	Z No Qualifier

Section	0	Medical and Surgical
Body System	L	Tendons
Operation	Q	**Repair:** Restoring, to the extent possible, a body part to its normal anatomic structure and function

Body Part (4th)	Approach (5th)	Device (6th)	Qualifier (7th)
0 Head and Neck Tendon	0 Open	Z No Device	Z No Qualifier
1 Shoulder Tendon, Right	3 Percutaneous		
2 Shoulder Tendon, Left	4 Percutaneous Endoscopic		
3 Upper Arm Tendon, Right			
4 Upper Arm Tendon, Left			
5 Lower Arm and Wrist Tendon, Right			
6 Lower Arm and Wrist Tendon, Left			
7 Hand Tendon, Right			
8 Hand Tendon, Left			
9 Trunk Tendon, Right			
B Trunk Tendon, Left			
C Thorax Tendon, Right			
D Thorax Tendon, Left			
F Abdomen Tendon, Right			
G Abdomen Tendon, Left			
H Perineum Tendon			
J Hip Tendon, Right			
K Hip Tendon, Left			
L Upper Leg Tendon, Right			
M Upper Leg Tendon, Left			
N Lower Leg Tendon, Right			
P Lower Leg Tendon, Left			
Q Knee Tendon, Right			
R Knee Tendon, Left			
S Ankle Tendon, Right			
T Ankle Tendon, Left			
V Foot Tendon, Right			
W Foot Tendon, Left			

Section	0	Medical and Surgical
Body System	L	Tendons
Operation	R	**Replacement:** Putting in or on biological or synthetic material that physically takes the place and/or function of all or a portion of a body part

Body Part (4th)	Approach (5th)	Device (6th)	Qualifier (7th)
0 Head and Neck Tendon	0 Open	7 Autologous Tissue Substitute	Z No Qualifier
1 Shoulder Tendon, Right	4 Percutaneous Endoscopic	J Synthetic Substitute	
2 Shoulder Tendon, Left		K Nonautologous Tissue Substitute	
3 Upper Arm Tendon, Right			
4 Upper Arm Tendon, Left			
5 Lower Arm and Wrist Tendon, Right			
6 Lower Arm and Wrist Tendon, Left			
7 Hand Tendon, Right			
8 Hand Tendon, Left			
9 Trunk Tendon, Right			
B Trunk Tendon, Left			
C Thorax Tendon, Right			
D Thorax Tendon, Left			
F Abdomen Tendon, Right			
G Abdomen Tendon, Left			
H Perineum Tendon			
J Hip Tendon, Right			
K Hip Tendon, Left			
L Upper Leg Tendon, Right			
M Upper Leg Tendon, Left			
N Lower Leg Tendon, Right			
P Lower Leg Tendon, Left			
Q Knee Tendon, Right			
R Knee Tendon, Left			
S Ankle Tendon, Right			
T Ankle Tendon, Left			
V Foot Tendon, Right			
W Foot Tendon, Left			

Section	0	Medical and Surgical
Body System	L	Tendons
Operation	S	**Reposition:** Moving to its normal location, or other suitable location, all or a portion of a body part

Body Part (4th)	Approach (5th)	Device (6th)	Qualifier (7th)
0 Head and Neck Tendon 1 Shoulder Tendon, Right 2 Shoulder Tendon, Left 3 Upper Arm Tendon, Right 4 Upper Arm Tendon, Left 5 Lower Arm and Wrist Tendon, Right 6 Lower Arm and Wrist Tendon, Left 7 Hand Tendon, Right 8 Hand Tendon, Left 9 Trunk Tendon, Right B Trunk Tendon, Left C Thorax Tendon, Right D Thorax Tendon, Left F Abdomen Tendon, Right G Abdomen Tendon, Left H Perineum Tendon J Hip Tendon, Right K Hip Tendon, Left L Upper Leg Tendon, Right M Upper Leg Tendon, Left N Lower Leg Tendon, Right P Lower Leg Tendon, Left Q Knee Tendon, Right R Knee Tendon, Left S Ankle Tendon, Right T Ankle Tendon, Left V Foot Tendon, Right W Foot Tendon, Left	0 Open 4 Percutaneous Endoscopic	Z No Device	Z No Qualifier

Section	0	Medical and Surgical
Body System	L	Tendons
Operation	T	**Resection:** Cutting out or off, without replacement, all of a body part

Body Part (4th)	Approach (5th)	Device (6th)	Qualifier (7th)
0 Head and Neck Tendon 1 Shoulder Tendon, Right 2 Shoulder Tendon, Left 3 Upper Arm Tendon, Right 4 Upper Arm Tendon, Left 5 Lower Arm and Wrist Tendon, Right 6 Lower Arm and Wrist Tendon, Left 7 Hand Tendon, Right 8 Hand Tendon, Left 9 Trunk Tendon, Right B Trunk Tendon, Left C Thorax Tendon, Right D Thorax Tendon, Left F Abdomen Tendon, Right G Abdomen Tendon, Left H Perineum Tendon J Hip Tendon, Right K Hip Tendon, Left L Upper Leg Tendon, Right M Upper Leg Tendon, Left N Lower Leg Tendon, Right P Lower Leg Tendon, Left Q Knee Tendon, Right R Knee Tendon, Left S Ankle Tendon, Right T Ankle Tendon, Left V Foot Tendon, Right W Foot Tendon, Left	0 Open 4 Percutaneous Endoscopic	Z No Device	Z No Qualifier

Section	0	Medical and Surgical
Body System	L	Tendons
Operation	U	**Supplement:** Putting in or on biological or synthetic material that physically reinforces and/or augments the function of a portion of a body part

Body Part (4th)	Approach (5th)	Device (6th)	Qualifier (7th)
0 Head and Neck Tendon	0 Open	7 Autologous Tissue Substitute	Z No Qualifier
1 Shoulder Tendon, Right	4 Percutaneous Endoscopic	J Synthetic Substitute	
2 Shoulder Tendon, Left		K Nonautologous Tissue Substitute	
3 Upper Arm Tendon, Right			
4 Upper Arm Tendon, Left			
5 Lower Arm and Wrist Tendon, Right			
6 Lower Arm and Wrist Tendon, Left			
7 Hand Tendon, Right			
8 Hand Tendon, Left			
9 Trunk Tendon, Right			
B Trunk Tendon, Left			
C Thorax Tendon, Right			
D Thorax Tendon, Left			
F Abdomen Tendon, Right			
G Abdomen Tendon, Left			
H Perineum Tendon			
J Hip Tendon, Right			
K Hip Tendon, Left			
L Upper Leg Tendon, Right			
M Upper Leg Tendon, Left			
N Lower Leg Tendon, Right			
P Lower Leg Tendon, Left			
Q Knee Tendon, Right			
R Knee Tendon, Left			
S Ankle Tendon, Right			
T Ankle Tendon, Left			
V Foot Tendon, Right			
W Foot Tendon, Left			

Section	0	Medical and Surgical
Body System	L	Tendons
Operation	W	**Revision:** Correcting, to the extent possible, a portion of a malfunctioning device or the position of a displaced device

Body Part (4th)	Approach (5th)	Device (6th)	Qualifier (7th)
X Upper Tendon	0 Open	0 Drainage Device	Z No Qualifier
Y Lower Tendon	3 Percutaneous	7 Autologous Tissue Substitute	
	4 Percutaneous Endoscopic	J Synthetic Substitute	
		K Nonautologous Tissue Substitute	
		Y Other Device	
X Upper Tendon	X External	0 Drainage Device	Z No Qualifier
Y Lower Tendon		7 Autologous Tissue Substitute	
		J Synthetic Substitute	
		K Nonautologous Tissue Substitute	

Section	0	Medical and Surgical
Body System	L	Tendons
Operation	X	**Transfer:** Moving, without taking out, all or a portion of a body part to another location to take over the function of all or a portion of a body part

Body Part (4ᵗʰ)	Approach (5ᵗʰ)	Device (6ᵗʰ)	Qualifier (7ᵗʰ)
0 Head and Neck Tendon	0 Open	Z No Device	Z No Qualifier
1 Shoulder Tendon, Right	4 Percutaneous Endoscopic		
2 Shoulder Tendon, Left			
3 Upper Arm Tendon, Right			
4 Upper Arm Tendon, Left			
5 Lower Arm and Wrist Tendon, Right			
6 Lower Arm and Wrist Tendon, Left			
7 Hand Tendon, Right			
8 Hand Tendon, Left			
9 Trunk Tendon, Right			
B Trunk Tendon, Left			
C Thorax Tendon, Right			
D Thorax Tendon, Left			
F Abdomen Tendon, Right			
G Abdomen Tendon, Left			
H Perineum Tendon			
J Hip Tendon, Right			
K Hip Tendon, Left			
L Upper Leg Tendon, Right			
M Upper Leg Tendon, Left			
N Lower Leg Tendon, Right			
P Lower Leg Tendon, Left			
Q Knee Tendon, Right			
R Knee Tendon, Left			
S Ankle Tendon, Right			
T Ankle Tendon, Left			
V Foot Tendon, Right			
W Foot Tendon, Left			

AHA Coding Clinic

0L8J0ZZ Division of Right Hip Tendon, Open Approach—AHA CC: 3Q, 2016, 30-31

0LB60ZZ Excision of Left Lower Arm and Wrist Tendon, Open Approach—AHA CC: 3Q, 2015, 26-27

0LBL0ZZ Excision of Right Upper Leg Tendon, Open Approach—AHA CC: 2Q, 2017, 21-22

0LBP0ZZ Excision of Left Lower Leg Tendon, Open Approach—AHA CC: 3Q, 2014, 18-19

0LBT0ZZ Excision of Left Ankle Tendon, Open Approach—AHA CC: 3Q, 2014, 14-15

0LQ14ZZ Repair Right Shoulder Tendon, Percutaneous Endoscopic Approach—AHA CC: 3Q, 2013, 20-22; 3Q, 2016, 32-33

0LS30ZZ Reposition Right Upper Arm Tendon, Open Approach—AHA CC: 3Q, 2016, 32-33

0LS40ZZ Reposition Left Upper Arm Tendon, Open Approach—AHA CC: 3Q, 2015, 14-15

0LUM0KZ Supplement Left Upper Leg Tendon with Nonautologous Tissue Substitute, Open Approach—AHA CC: 2Q, 2015, 11

0LUQ0KZ Supplement Right Knee Tendon with Nonautologous Tissue Substitute, Open Approach—AHA CC: 2Q, 2015, 11

Bursa of the Knee

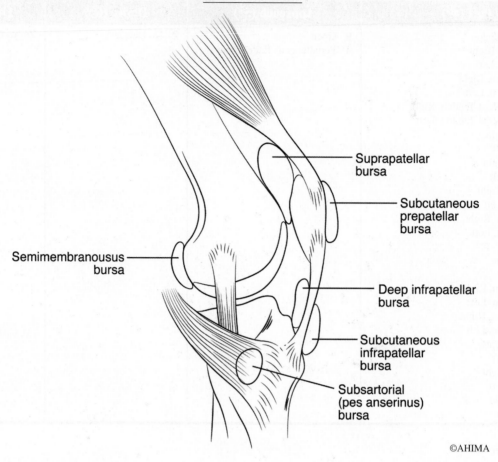

Suprapatellar bursa

Subcutaneous prepatellar bursa

Semimembranousus bursa

Deep infrapatellar bursa

Subcutaneous infrapatellar bursa

Subsartorial (pes anserinus) bursa

©AHIMA

Ligaments of the Knee

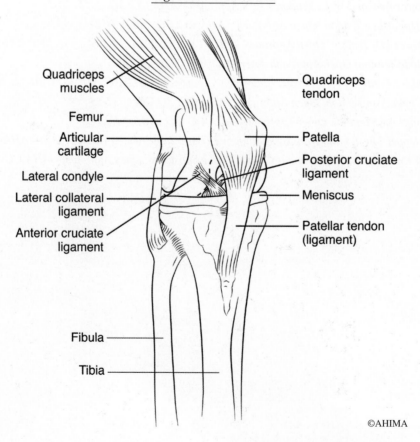

Quadriceps muscles

Femur

Articular cartilage

Lateral condyle

Lateral collateral ligament

Anterior cruciate ligament

Quadriceps tendon

Patella

Posterior cruciate ligament

Meniscus

Patellar tendon (ligament)

Fibula

Tibia

©AHIMA

Shoulder Tendons and Ligaments

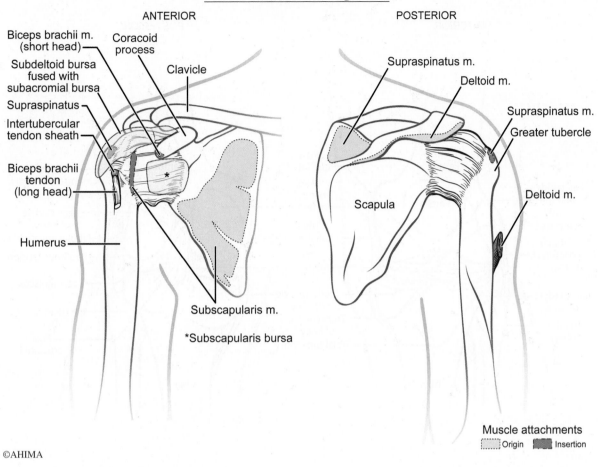

ANTERIOR

Biceps brachii m. (short head)
Coracoid process
Clavicle

Subdeltoid bursa fused with subacromial bursa
Supraspinatus
Intertubercular tendon sheath
Biceps brachii tendon (long head)
Humerus

Subscapularis m.

*Subscapularis bursa

POSTERIOR

Supraspinatus m.
Deltoid m.
Supraspinatus m.
Greater tubercle
Deltoid m.
Scapula

Muscle attachments
Origin   Insertion

©AHIMA

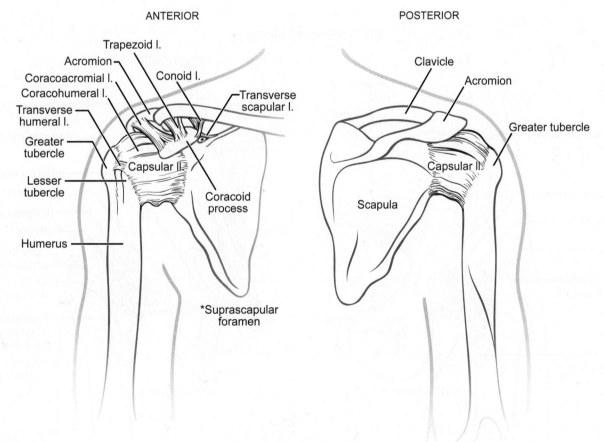

ANTERIOR

Trapezoid l.
Acromion
Conoid l.
Coracoacromial l.
Coracohumeral l.
Transverse scapular l.
Transverse humeral l.
Greater tubercle
Capsular l.
Lesser tubercle
Coracoid process
Humerus

*Suprascapular foramen

POSTERIOR

Clavicle
Acromion
Greater tubercle
Capsular l.
Scapula

©AHIMA

Knee Tendons and Ligaments

ANTERIOR

POSTERIOR

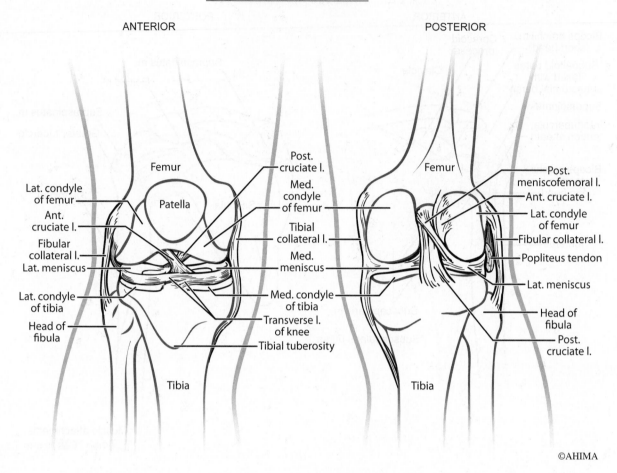

Anterior view labels:
- Femur
- Lat. condyle of femur
- Ant. cruciate l.
- Fibular collateral l.
- Lat. meniscus
- Lat. condyle of tibia
- Head of fibula
- Patella
- Post. cruciate l.
- Med. condyle of femur
- Tibial collateral l.
- Med. meniscus
- Med. condyle of tibia
- Transverse l. of knee
- Tibial tuberosity
- Tibia

Posterior view labels:
- Femur
- Post. meniscofemoral l.
- Ant. cruciate l.
- Lat. condyle of femur
- Fibular collateral l.
- Popliteus tendon
- Lat. meniscus
- Head of fibula
- Post. cruciate l.
- Tibia

©AHIMA

Hip Tendons and Ligaments

ANTERIOR

POSTERIOR

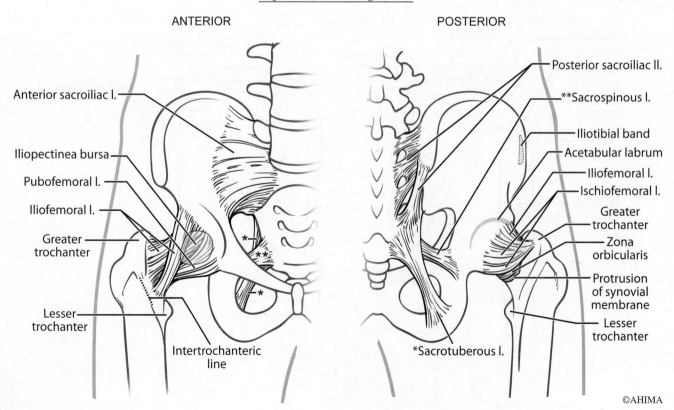

Anterior view labels:
- Anterior sacroiliac l.
- Iliopectinea bursa
- Pubofemoral l.
- Iliofemoral l.
- Greater trochanter
- Lesser trochanter
- Intertrochanteric line
- *
- **
- *

Posterior view labels:
- Posterior sacroiliac ll.
- **Sacrospinous l.
- Iliotibial band
- Acetabular labrum
- Iliofemoral l.
- Ischiofemoral l.
- Greater trochanter
- Zona orbicularis
- Protrusion of synovial membrane
- Lesser trochanter
- *Sacrotuberous l.

©AHIMA

Section	0	**Medical and Surgical**
Body System	M	**Bursae and Ligaments**
Operation	2	**Change:** Taking out or off a device from a body part and putting back an identical or similar device in or on the same body part without cutting or puncturing the skin or a mucous membrane

Body Part (4ᵗʰ)	Approach (5ᵗʰ)	Device (6ᵗʰ)	Qualifier (7ᵗʰ)
X Upper Bursa and Ligament **Y** Lower Bursa and Ligament	**X** External	**0** Drainage Device **Y** Other Device	**Z** No Qualifier

Section	0	**Medical and Surgical**
Body System	M	**Bursae and Ligaments**
Operation	5	**Destruction:** Physical eradication of all or a portion of a body part by the direct use of energy, force, or a destructive agent

Body Part (4ᵗʰ)	Approach (5ᵗʰ)	Device (6ᵗʰ)	Qualifier (7ᵗʰ)
0 Head and Neck Bursa and Ligament **1** Shoulder Bursa and Ligament, Right **2** Shoulder Bursa and Ligament, Left **3** Elbow Bursa and Ligament, Right **4** Elbow Bursa and Ligament, Left **5** Wrist Bursa and Ligament, Right **6** Wrist Bursa and Ligament, Left **7** Hand Bursa and Ligament, Right **8** Hand Bursa and Ligament, Left **9** Upper Extremity Bursa and Ligament, Right **B** Upper Extremity Bursa and Ligament, Left **C** Upper Spine Bursa and Ligament, Right **D** Lower Spine Bursa and Ligament, Left **F** Sternum Bursa and Ligament, Right **G** Rib(s) Bursa and Ligament, Left **H** Abdomen Bursa and Ligament, Right **J** Abdomen Bursa and Ligament, Left **K** Perineum Bursa and Ligament **L** Hip Bursa and Ligament, Right **M** Hip Bursa and Ligament, Left **N** Knee Bursa and Ligament, Right **P** Knee Bursa and Ligament, Left **Q** Ankle Bursa and Ligament, Right **R** Ankle Bursa and Ligament, Left **S** Foot Bursa and Ligament, Right **T** Foot Bursa and Ligament, Left **V** Lower Extremity Bursa and Ligament, Right **W** Lower Extremity Bursa and Ligament, Left	**0** Open **3** Percutaneous **4** Percutaneous Endoscopic	**Z** No Device	**Z** No Qualifier

Section	0	Medical and Surgical
Body System	M	Bursae and Ligaments
Operation	8	**Division:** Cutting into a body part, without draining fluids and/or gases from the body part, in order to separate or transect a body part

Body Part (4th)	Approach (5th)	Device (6th)	Qualifier (7th)
0 Head and Neck Bursa and Ligament 1 Shoulder Bursa and Ligament, Right 2 Shoulder Bursa and Ligament, Left 3 Elbow Bursa and Ligament, Right 4 Elbow Bursa and Ligament, Left 5 Wrist Bursa and Ligament, Right 6 Wrist Bursa and Ligament, Left 7 Hand Bursa and Ligament, Right 8 Hand Bursa and Ligament, Left 9 Upper Extremity Bursa and Ligament, Right B Upper Extremity Bursa and Ligament, Left C Upper Spine Bursa and Ligament, Right D Lower Spine Bursa and Ligament, Left F Sternum Bursa and Ligament, Right G Rib(s) Bursa and Ligament, Left H Abdomen Bursa and Ligament, Right J Abdomen Bursa and Ligament, Left K Perineum Bursa and Ligament L Hip Bursa and Ligament, Right M Hip Bursa and Ligament, Left N Knee Bursa and Ligament, Right P Knee Bursa and Ligament, Left Q Ankle Bursa and Ligament, Right R Ankle Bursa and Ligament, Left S Foot Bursa and Ligament, Right T Foot Bursa and Ligament, Left V Lower Extremity Bursa and Ligament, Right W Lower Extremity Bursa and Ligament, Left	0 Open 3 Percutaneous 4 Percutaneous Endoscopic	Z No Device	Z No Qualifier

Section	0	Medical and Surgical
Body System	M	Bursae and Ligaments
Operation	9	**Drainage:** Taking or letting out fluids and/or gases from a body part

Body Part (4th)	Approach (5th)	Device (6th)	Qualifier (7th)
0 Head and Neck Bursa and Ligament 1 Shoulder Bursa and Ligament, Right 2 Shoulder Bursa and Ligament, Left 3 Elbow Bursa and Ligament, Right 4 Elbow Bursa and Ligament, Left 5 Wrist Bursa and Ligament, Right 6 Wrist Bursa and Ligament, Left 7 Hand Bursa and Ligament, Right 8 Hand Bursa and Ligament, Left 9 Upper Extremity Bursa and Ligament, Right B Upper Extremity Bursa and Ligament, Left C Upper Spine Bursa and Ligament, Right D Lower Spine Bursa and Ligament, Left F Sternum Bursa and Ligament, Right G Rib(s) Bursa and Ligament, Left H Abdomen Bursa and Ligament, Right J Abdomen Bursa and Ligament, Left K Perineum Bursa and Ligament L Hip Bursa and Ligament, Right M Hip Bursa and Ligament, Left N Knee Bursa and Ligament, Right P Knee Bursa and Ligament, Left Q Ankle Bursa and Ligament, Right R Ankle Bursa and Ligament, Left S Foot Bursa and Ligament, Right T Foot Bursa and Ligament, Left V Lower Extremity Bursa and Ligament, Right W Lower Extremity Bursa and Ligament, Left	0 Open 3 Percutaneous 4 Percutaneous Endoscopic	0 Drainage Device	Z No Qualifier

Continued →

Section	0	Medical and Surgical
Body System	M	Bursae and Ligaments
Operation	9	Drainage: Taking or letting out fluids and/or gases from a body part

Body Part (4th)	Approach (5th)	Device (6th)	Qualifier (7th)
0 Head and Neck Bursa and Ligament	0 Open	Z No Device	X Diagnostic
1 Shoulder Bursa and Ligament, Right	3 Percutaneous		Z No Qualifier
2 Shoulder Bursa and Ligament, Left	4 Percutaneous Endoscopic		
3 Elbow Bursa and Ligament, Right			
4 Elbow Bursa and Ligament, Left			
5 Wrist Bursa and Ligament, Right			
6 Wrist Bursa and Ligament, Left			
7 Hand Bursa and Ligament, Right			
8 Hand Bursa and Ligament, Left			
9 Upper Extremity Bursa and Ligament, Right			
B Upper Extremity Bursa and Ligament, Left			
C Upper Spine Bursa and Ligament, Right			
D Lower Spine Bursa and Ligament, Left			
F Sternum Bursa and Ligament, Right			
G Rib(s) Bursa and Ligament, Left			
H Abdomen Bursa and Ligament, Right			
J Abdomen Bursa and Ligament, Left			
K Perineum Bursa and Ligament			
L Hip Bursa and Ligament, Right			
M Hip Bursa and Ligament, Left			
N Knee Bursa and Ligament, Right			
P Knee Bursa and Ligament, Left			
Q Ankle Bursa and Ligament, Right			
R Ankle Bursa and Ligament, Left			
S Foot Bursa and Ligament, Right			
T Foot Bursa and Ligament, Left			
V Lower Extremity Bursa and Ligament, Right			
W Lower Extremity Bursa and Ligament, Left			

Section	0	Medical and Surgical
Body System	M	Bursae and Ligaments
Operation	B	Excision: Cutting out or off, without replacement, a portion of a body part

Body Part (4th)	Approach (5th)	Device (6th)	Qualifier (7th)
0 Head and Neck Bursa and Ligament	0 Open	Z No Device	X Diagnostic
1 Shoulder Bursa and Ligament, Right	3 Percutaneous		Z No Qualifier
2 Shoulder Bursa and Ligament, Left	4 Percutaneous Endoscopic		
3 Elbow Bursa and Ligament, Right			
4 Elbow Bursa and Ligament, Left			
5 Wrist Bursa and Ligament, Right			
6 Wrist Bursa and Ligament, Left			
7 Hand Bursa and Ligament, Right			
8 Hand Bursa and Ligament, Left			
9 Upper Extremity Bursa and Ligament, Right			
B Upper Extremity Bursa and Ligament, Left			
C Upper Spine Bursa and Ligament, Right			
D Lower Spine Bursa and Ligament, Left			
F Sternum Bursa and Ligament, Right			
G Rib(s) Bursa and Ligament, Left			
H Abdomen Bursa and Ligament, Right			
J Abdomen Bursa and Ligament, Left			
K Perineum Bursa and Ligament			
L Hip Bursa and Ligament, Right			
M Hip Bursa and Ligament, Left			
N Knee Bursa and Ligament, Right			
P Knee Bursa and Ligament, Left			
Q Ankle Bursa and Ligament, Right			
R Ankle Bursa and Ligament, Left			
S Foot Bursa and Ligament, Right			
T Foot Bursa and Ligament, Left			
V Lower Extremity Bursa and Ligament, Right			
W Lower Extremity Bursa and Ligament, Left			

Section	0	Medical and Surgical
Body System	M	Bursae and Ligaments
Operation	C	Extirpation: Taking or cutting out solid matter from a body part

Body Part (4th)	Approach (5th)	Device (6th)	Qualifier (7th)
0 Head and Neck Bursa and Ligament	0 Open	Z No Device	Z No Qualifier
1 Shoulder Bursa and Ligament, Right	3 Percutaneous		
2 Shoulder Bursa and Ligament, Left	4 Percutaneous Endoscopic		
3 Elbow Bursa and Ligament, Right			
4 Elbow Bursa and Ligament, Left			
5 Wrist Bursa and Ligament, Right			
6 Wrist Bursa and Ligament, Left			
7 Hand Bursa and Ligament, Right			
8 Hand Bursa and Ligament, Left			
9 Upper Extremity Bursa and Ligament, Right			
B Upper Extremity Bursa and Ligament, Left			
C Upper Spine Bursa and Ligament, Right			
D Trunk Bursa and Ligament, Left			
F Sternum Bursa and Ligament, Right			
G Rib(s) Bursa and Ligament, Left			
H Abdomen Bursa and Ligament, Right			
J Abdomen Bursa and Ligament, Left			
K Perineum Bursa and Ligament			
L Hip Bursa and Ligament, Right			
M Hip Bursa and Ligament, Left			
N Knee Bursa and Ligament, Right			
P Knee Bursa and Ligament, Left			
Q Ankle Bursa and Ligament, Right			
R Ankle Bursa and Ligament, Left			
S Foot Bursa and Ligament, Right			
T Foot Bursa and Ligament, Left			
V Lower Extremity Bursa and Ligament, Right			
W Lower Extremity Bursa and Ligament, Left			

Section	0	Medical and Surgical
Body System	M	Bursae and Ligaments
Operation	D	Extraction: Pulling or stripping out or off all or a portion of a body part by the use of force

Body Part (4th)	Approach (5th)	Device (6th)	Qualifier (7th)
0 Head and Neck Bursa and Ligament	0 Open	Z No Device	Z No Qualifier
1 Shoulder Bursa and Ligament, Right	3 Percutaneous		
2 Shoulder Bursa and Ligament, Left	4 Percutaneous Endoscopic		
3 Elbow Bursa and Ligament, Right			
4 Elbow Bursa and Ligament, Left			
5 Wrist Bursa and Ligament, Right			
6 Wrist Bursa and Ligament, Left			
7 Hand Bursa and Ligament, Right			
8 Hand Bursa and Ligament, Left			
9 Upper Extremity Bursa and Ligament, Right			
B Upper Extremity Bursa and Ligament, Left			
C Upper Spine Bursa and Ligament, Right			
D Lower Spine Bursa and Ligament, Left			
F Sternum Bursa and Ligament, Right			
G Rib(s) Bursa and Ligament, Left			
H Abdomen Bursa and Ligament, Right			
J Abdomen Bursa and Ligament, Left			
K Perineum Bursa and Ligament			
L Hip Bursa and Ligament, Right			
M Hip Bursa and Ligament, Left			
N Knee Bursa and Ligament, Right			
P Knee Bursa and Ligament, Left			
Q Ankle Bursa and Ligament, Right			
R Ankle Bursa and Ligament, Left			
S Foot Bursa and Ligament, Right			
T Foot Bursa and Ligament, Left			
V Lower Extremity Bursa and Ligament, Right			
W Lower Extremity Bursa and Ligament, Left			

Section	0	Medical and Surgical
Body System	M	Bursae and Ligaments
Operation	H	Insertion: Putting in a nonbiological appliance that monitors, assists, performs, or prevents a physiological function but does not physically take the place of a body part

Body Part (4th)	Approach (5th)	Device (6th)	Qualifier (7th)
X Upper Bursa and Ligament Y Lower Bursa and Ligament	0 Open 3 Percutaneous 4 Percutaneous Endoscopic	Y Other Device	Z No Qualifier

Section	0	Medical and Surgical
Body System	M	Bursae and Ligaments
Operation	J	Inspection: Visually and/or manually exploring a body part

Body Part (4th)	Approach (5th)	Device (6th)	Qualifier (7th)
X Upper Bursa and Ligament Y Lower Bursa and Ligament	0 Open 3 Percutaneous 4 Percutaneous Endoscopic X External	Z No Device	Z No Qualifier

Section	0	Medical and Surgical
Body System	M	Bursae and Ligaments
Operation	M	Reattachment: Putting back in or on all or a portion of a separated body part to its normal location or other suitable location

Body Part (4th)	Approach (5th)	Device (6th)	Qualifier (7th)
0 Head and Neck Bursa and Ligament 1 Shoulder Bursa and Ligament, Right 2 Shoulder Bursa and Ligament, Left 3 Elbow Bursa and Ligament, Right 4 Elbow Bursa and Ligament, Left 5 Wrist Bursa and Ligament, Right 6 Wrist Bursa and Ligament, Left 7 Hand Bursa and Ligament, Right 8 Hand Bursa and Ligament, Left 9 Upper Extremity Bursa and Ligament, Right B Upper Extremity Bursa and Ligament, Left C Upper Spine Bursa and Ligament, Right D Lower Spine Bursa and Ligament, Left F Sternum Bursa and Ligament, Right G Rib(s) Bursa and Ligament, Left H Abdomen Bursa and Ligament, Right J Abdomen Bursa and Ligament, Left K Perineum Bursa and Ligament L Hip Bursa and Ligament, Right M Hip Bursa and Ligament, Left N Knee Bursa and Ligament, Right P Knee Bursa and Ligament, Left Q Ankle Bursa and Ligament, Right R Ankle Bursa and Ligament, Left S Foot Bursa and Ligament, Right T Foot Bursa and Ligament, Left V Lower Extremity Bursa and Ligament, Right W Lower Extremity Bursa and Ligament, Left	0 Open 4 Percutaneous Endoscopic	Z No Device	Z No Qualifier

Section 0 **Medical and Surgical**
Body System M **Bursae and Ligaments**
Operation N **Release:** Freeing a body part from an abnormal physical constraint by cutting or by the use of force

Body Part (4th)	Approach (5th)	Device (6th)	Qualifier (7th)
0 Head and Neck Bursa and Ligament	0 Open	Z No Device	Z No Qualifier
1 Shoulder Bursa and Ligament, Right	3 Percutaneous		
2 Shoulder Bursa and Ligament, Left	4 Percutaneous Endoscopic		
3 Elbow Bursa and Ligament, Right	X External		
4 Elbow Bursa and Ligament, Left			
5 Wrist Bursa and Ligament, Right			
6 Wrist Bursa and Ligament, Left			
7 Hand Bursa and Ligament, Right			
8 Hand Bursa and Ligament, Left			
9 Upper Extremity Bursa and Ligament, Right			
B Upper Extremity Bursa and Ligament, Left			
C Upper Spine Bursa and Ligament, Right			
D Lower Spine Bursa and Ligament, Left			
F Sternum Bursa and Ligament, Right			
G Rib(s) Bursa and Ligament, Left			
H Abdomen Bursa and Ligament, Right			
J Abdomen Bursa and Ligament, Left			
K Perineum Bursa and Ligament			
L Hip Bursa and Ligament, Right			
M Hip Bursa and Ligament, Left			
N Knee Bursa and Ligament, Right			
P Knee Bursa and Ligament, Left			
Q Ankle Bursa and Ligament, Right			
R Ankle Bursa and Ligament, Left			
S Foot Bursa and Ligament, Right			
T Foot Bursa and Ligament, Left			
V Lower Extremity Bursa and Ligament, Right			
W Lower Extremity Bursa and Ligament, Left			

Section 0 **Medical and Surgical**
Body System M **Bursae and Ligaments**
Operation P **Removal:** Taking out or off a device from a body part

Body Part (4th)	Approach (5th)	Device (6th)	Qualifier (7th)
X Upper Bursa and Ligament Y Lower Bursa and Ligament	0 Open 3 Percutaneous 4 Percutaneous Endoscopic	0 Drainage Device 7 Autologous Tissue Substitute J Synthetic Substitute K Nonautologous Tissue Substitute Y Other Device	Z No Qualifier
X Upper Bursa and Ligament Y Lower Bursa and Ligament	X External	0 Drainage Device	Z No Qualifier

Section	0	Medical and Surgical
Body System	M	Bursae and Ligaments
Operation	Q	**Repair:** Restoring, to the extent possible, a body part to its normal anatomic structure and function

Body Part (4th)	Approach (5th)	Device (6th)	Qualifier (7th)
0 Head and Neck Bursa and Ligament	0 Open	Z No Device	Z No Qualifier
1 Shoulder Bursa and Ligament, Right	3 Percutaneous		
2 Shoulder Bursa and Ligament, Left	4 Percutaneous Endoscopic		
3 Elbow Bursa and Ligament, Right			
4 Elbow Bursa and Ligament, Left			
5 Wrist Bursa and Ligament, Right			
6 Wrist Bursa and Ligament, Left			
7 Hand Bursa and Ligament, Right			
8 Hand Bursa and Ligament, Left			
9 Upper Extremity Bursa and Ligament, Right			
B Upper Extremity Bursa and Ligament, Left			
C Upper Spine Bursa and Ligament, Right			
D Lower Spine Bursa and Ligament, Left			
F Sternum Bursa and Ligament, Right			
G Rib(s) Bursa and Ligament, Left			
H Abdomen Bursa and Ligament, Right			
J Abdomen Bursa and Ligament, Left			
K Perineum Bursa and Ligament			
L Hip Bursa and Ligament, Right			
M Hip Bursa and Ligament, Left			
N Knee Bursa and Ligament, Right			
P Knee Bursa and Ligament, Left			
Q Ankle Bursa and Ligament, Right			
R Ankle Bursa and Ligament, Left			
S Foot Bursa and Ligament, Right			
T Foot Bursa and Ligament, Left			
V Lower Extremity Bursa and Ligament, Right			
W Lower Extremity Bursa and Ligament, Left			

Section	0	Medical and Surgical
Body System	M	Bursae and Ligaments
Operation	R	**Replacement:** Putting in or on biological or synthetic material that physically takes the place and/or function of all or a portion of a body part

Body Part (4th)	Approach (5th)	Device (6th)	Qualifier (7th)
0 Head and Neck Bursa and Ligament	0 Open	7 Autologous Tissue Substitute	Z No Qualifier
1 Shoulder Bursa and Ligament, Right	4 Percutaneous Endoscopic	J Synthetic Substitute	
2 Shoulder Bursa and Ligament, Left		K Nonautologous Tissue Substitute	
3 Elbow Bursa and Ligament, Right			
4 Elbow Bursa and Ligament, Left			
5 Wrist Bursa and Ligament, Right			
6 Wrist Bursa and Ligament, Left			
7 Hand Bursa and Ligament, Right			
8 Hand Bursa and Ligament, Left			
9 Upper Extremity Bursa and Ligament, Right			
B Upper Extremity Bursa and Ligament, Left			
C Upper Spine Bursa and Ligament			
D Lower Spine Bursa and Ligament			
F Sternum Bursa and Ligament			
G Rib(s) Bursa and Ligament			
H Abdomen Bursa and Ligament, Right			
J Abdomen Bursa and Ligament, Left			
K Perineum Bursa and Ligament			
L Hip Bursa and Ligament, Right			
M Hip Bursa and Ligament, Left			
N Knee Bursa and Ligament, Right			
P Knee Bursa and Ligament, Left			
Q Ankle Bursa and Ligament, Right			
R Ankle Bursa and Ligament, Left			
S Foot Bursa and Ligament, Right			
T Foot Bursa and Ligament, Left			
V Lower Extremity Bursa and Ligament, Right			
W Lower Extremity Bursa and Ligament, Left			

Section	0	Medical and Surgical
Body System	M	Bursae and Ligaments
Operation	S	**Reposition:** Moving to its normal location, or other suitable location, all or a portion of a body part

Body Part (4th)	Approach (5th)	Device (6th)	Qualifier (7th)
0 Head and Neck Bursa and Ligament	0 Open	Z No Device	Z No Qualifier
1 Shoulder Bursa and Ligament, Right	4 Percutaneous Endoscopic		
2 Shoulder Bursa and Ligament, Left			
3 Elbow Bursa and Ligament, Right			
4 Elbow Bursa and Ligament, Left			
5 Wrist Bursa and Ligament, Right			
6 Wrist Bursa and Ligament, Left			
7 Hand Bursa and Ligament, Right			
8 Hand Bursa and Ligament, Left			
9 Upper Extremity Bursa and Ligament, Right			
B Upper Extremity Bursa and Ligament, Left			
C Upper Spine Bursa and Ligament, Right			
D Lower Spine Bursa and Ligament, Left			
F Sternum Bursa and Ligament, Right			
G Rib(s) Bursa and Ligament, Left			
H Abdomen Bursa and Ligament, Right			
J Abdomen Bursa and Ligament, Left			
K Perineum Bursa and Ligament			
L Hip Bursa and Ligament, Right			
M Hip Bursa and Ligament, Left			
N Knee Bursa and Ligament, Right			
P Knee Bursa and Ligament, Left			
Q Ankle Bursa and Ligament, Right			
R Ankle Bursa and Ligament, Left			
S Foot Bursa and Ligament, Right			
T Foot Bursa and Ligament, Left			
V Lower Extremity Bursa and Ligament, Right			
W Lower Extremity Bursa and Ligament, Left			

Section	0	Medical and Surgical
Body System	M	Bursae and Ligaments
Operation	T	**Resection:** Cutting out or off, without replacement, all of a body part

Body Part (4th)	Approach (5th)	Device (6th)	Qualifier (7th)
0 Head and Neck Bursa and Ligament	0 Open	Z No Device	Z No Qualifier
1 Shoulder Bursa and Ligament, Right	4 Percutaneous Endoscopic		
2 Shoulder Bursa and Ligament, Left			
3 Elbow Bursa and Ligament, Right			
4 Elbow Bursa and Ligament, Left			
5 Wrist Bursa and Ligament, Right			
6 Wrist Bursa and Ligament, Left			
7 Hand Bursa and Ligament, Right			
8 Hand Bursa and Ligament, Left			
9 Upper Extremity Bursa and Ligament, Right			
B Upper Extremity Bursa and Ligament, Left			
C Upper Spine Bursa and Ligament, Right			
D Lower Spine Bursa and Ligament, Left			
F Sternum Bursa and Ligament, Right			
G Rib(s) Bursa and Ligament, Left			
H Abdomen Bursa and Ligament, Right			
J Abdomen Bursa and Ligament, Left			
K Perineum Bursa and Ligament			
L Hip Bursa and Ligament, Right			
M Hip Bursa and Ligament, Left			
N Knee Bursa and Ligament, Right			
P Knee Bursa and Ligament, Left			
Q Ankle Bursa and Ligament, Right			
R Ankle Bursa and Ligament, Left			
S Foot Bursa and Ligament, Right			
T Foot Bursa and Ligament, Left			
V Lower Extremity Bursa and Ligament, Right			
W Lower Extremity Bursa and Ligament, Left			

Head and Facial Bones

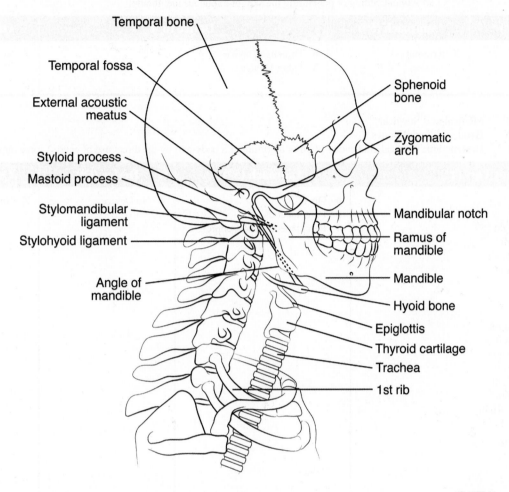

Temporal bone

Temporal fossa

External acoustic
meatus

Styloid process

Mastoid process

Stylomandibular
ligament

Stylohyoid ligament

Angle of
mandible

Sphenoid
bone

Zygomatic
arch

Mandibular notch

Ramus of
mandible

Mandible

Hyoid bone

Epiglottis

Thyroid cartilage

Trachea

1st rib

©AHIMA

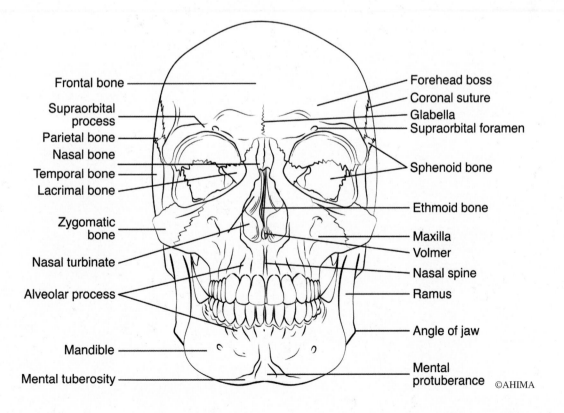

Frontal bone

Supraorbital
process

Parietal bone

Nasal bone

Temporal bone

Lacrimal bone

Zygomatic
bone

Nasal turbinate

Alveolar process

Mandible

Mental tuberosity

Forehead boss

Coronal suture

Glabella

Supraorbital foramen

Sphenoid bone

Ethmoid bone

Maxilla

Volmer

Nasal spine

Ramus

Angle of jaw

Mental
protuberance ©AHIMA

Head and Facial Bones Tables 0N2–0NW

Section	0	Medical and Surgical
Body System	N	Head and Facial Bones
Operation	2	Change: Taking out or off a device from a body part and putting back an identical or similar device in or on the same body part without cutting or puncturing the skin or a mucous membrane

Body Part (4th)	Approach (5th)	Device (6th)	Qualifier (7th)
0 Skull **B** Nasal Bone **W** Facial Bone	**X** External	**0** Drainage Device **Y** Other Device	**Z** No Qualifier

Section	0	Medical and Surgical
Body System	N	Head and Facial Bones
Operation	5	Destruction: Physical eradication of all or a portion of a body part by the direct use of energy, force, or a destructive agent

Body Part (4th)	Approach (5th)	Device (6th)	Qualifier (7th)
0 Skull **1** Frontal Bone **3** Parietal Bone, Right **4** Parietal Bone, Left **5** Temporal Bone, Right **6** Temporal Bone, Left **7** Occipital Bone **B** Nasal Bone **C** Sphenoid Bone **F** Ethmoid Bone, Right **G** Ethmoid Bone, Left **H** Lacrimal Bone, Right **J** Lacrimal Bone, Left **K** Palatine Bone, Right **L** Palatine Bone, Left **M** Zygomatic Bone, Right **N** Zygomatic Bone, Left **P** Orbit, Right **Q** Orbit, Left **R** Maxilla **T** Mandible, Right **V** Mandible, Left **X** Hyoid Bone	**0** Open **3** Percutaneous **4** Percutaneous Endoscopic	**Z** No Device	**Z** No Qualifier

Section   0   **Medical and Surgical**
Body System   N   **Head and Facial Bones**
Operation   8   **Division:** Cutting into a body part, without draining fluids and/or gases from the body part, in order to separate or transect a body part

Body Part (4ᵗʰ)	Approach (5ᵗʰ)	Device (6ᵗʰ)	Qualifier (7ᵗʰ)
0 Skull	0 Open	Z No Device	Z No Qualifier
1 Frontal Bone	3 Percutaneous		
3 Parietal Bone, Right	4 Percutaneous Endoscopic		
4 Parietal Bone, Left			
5 Temporal Bone, Right			
6 Temporal Bone, Left			
7 Occipital Bone			
B Nasal Bone			
C Sphenoid Bone			
F Ethmoid Bone, Right			
G Ethmoid Bone, Left			
H Lacrimal Bone, Right			
J Lacrimal Bone, Left			
K Palatine Bone, Right			
L Palatine Bone, Left			
M Zygomatic Bone, Right			
N Zygomatic Bone, Left			
P Orbit, Right			
Q Orbit, Left			
R Maxilla			
T Mandible, Right			
V Mandible, Left			
X Hyoid Bone			

Section   0   **Medical and Surgical**
Body System   N   **Head and Facial Bones**
Operation   9   **Drainage:** Taking or letting out fluids and/or gases from a body part

Body Part (4ᵗʰ)	Approach (5ᵗʰ)	Device (6ᵗʰ)	Qualifier (7ᵗʰ)
0 Skull	0 Open	0 Drainage Device	Z No Qualifier
1 Frontal Bone	3 Percutaneous		
3 Parietal Bone, Right	4 Percutaneous Endoscopic		
4 Parietal Bone, Left			
5 Temporal Bone, Right			
6 Temporal Bone, Left			
7 Occipital Bone			
B Nasal Bone			
C Sphenoid Bone			
F Ethmoid Bone, Right			
G Ethmoid Bone, Left			
H Lacrimal Bone, Right			
J Lacrimal Bone, Left			
K Palatine Bone, Right			
L Palatine Bone, Left			
M Zygomatic Bone, Right			
N Zygomatic Bone, Left			
P Orbit, Right			
Q Orbit, Left			
R Maxilla			
T Mandible, Right			
V Mandible, Left			
X Hyoid Bone			

Continued ➡

Section	0	Medical and Surgical
Body System	N	Head and Facial Bones
Operation	9	Drainage: Taking or letting out fluids and/or gases from a body part

Body Part (4th)	Approach (5th)	Device (6th)	Qualifier (7th)
0 Skull	0 Open	Z No Device	X Diagnostic
1 Frontal Bone	3 Percutaneous		Z No Qualifier
3 Parietal Bone, Right	4 Percutaneous Endoscopic		
4 Parietal Bone, Left			
5 Temporal Bone, Right			
6 Temporal Bone, Left			
7 Occipital Bone			
B Nasal Bone			
C Sphenoid Bone			
F Ethmoid Bone, Right			
G Ethmoid Bone, Left			
H Lacrimal Bone, Right			
J Lacrimal Bone, Left			
K Palatine Bone, Right			
L Palatine Bone, Left			
M Zygomatic Bone, Right			
N Zygomatic Bone, Left			
P Orbit, Right			
Q Orbit, Left			
R Maxilla			
T Mandible, Right			
V Mandible, Left			
X Hyoid Bone			

Section	0	Medical and Surgical
Body System	N	Head and Facial Bones
Operation	B	Excision: Cutting out or off, without replacement, a portion of a body part

Body Part (4th)	Approach (5th)	Device (6th)	Qualifier (7th)
0 Skull	0 Open	Z No Device	X Diagnostic
1 Frontal Bone	3 Percutaneous		Z No Qualifier
3 Parietal Bone, Right	4 Percutaneous Endoscopic		
4 Parietal Bone, Left			
5 Temporal Bone, Right			
6 Temporal Bone, Left			
7 Occipital Bone			
B Nasal Bone			
C Sphenoid Bone			
F Ethmoid Bone, Right			
G Ethmoid Bone, Left			
H Lacrimal Bone, Right			
J Lacrimal Bone, Left			
K Palatine Bone, Right			
L Palatine Bone, Left			
M Zygomatic Bone, Right			
N Zygomatic Bone, Left			
P Orbit, Right			
Q Orbit, Left			
R Maxilla			
T Mandible, Right			
V Mandible, Left			
X Hyoid Bone			

Section   **0**   **Medical and Surgical**
Body System **N**   **Head and Facial Bones**
Operation   **C**   **Extirpation: Taking or cutting out solid matter from a body part**

Body Part (4th)	Approach (5th)	Device (6th)	Qualifier (7th)
1 Frontal Bone **3** Parietal Bone, Right **4** Parietal Bone, Left **5** Temporal Bone, Right **6** Temporal Bone, Left **7** Occipital Bone **B** Nasal Bone **C** Sphenoid Bone **F** Ethmoid Bone, Right **G** Ethmoid Bone, Left **H** Lacrimal Bone, Right **J** Lacrimal Bone, Left **K** Palatine Bone, Right **L** Palatine Bone, Left **M** Zygomatic Bone, Right **N** Zygomatic Bone, Left **P** Orbit, Right **Q** Orbit, Left **R** Maxilla **T** Mandible, Right **V** Mandible, Left **X** Hyoid Bone	**0** Open **3** Percutaneous **4** Percutaneous Endoscopic	**Z** No Device	**Z** No Qualifier

Section   **0**   **Medical and Surgical**
Body System **N**   **Head and Facial Bones**
Operation   **D**   **Extraction: Pulling or stripping out or off all or a portion of a body part by the use of force**

Body Part (4th)	Approach (5th)	Device (6th)	Qualifier (7th)
0 Skull **1** Frontal Bone **3** Parietal Bone, Right **4** Parietal Bone, Left **5** Temporal Bone, Right **6** Temporal Bone, Left **7** Occipital Bone **B** Nasal Bone **C** Sphenoid Bone **F** Ethmoid Bone, Right **G** Ethmoid Bone, Left **H** Lacrimal Bone, Right **J** Lacrimal Bone, Left **K** Palatine Bone, Right **L** Palatine Bone, Left **M** Zygomatic Bone, Right **N** Zygomatic Bone, Left **P** Orbit, Right **Q** Orbit, Left **R** Maxilla **T** Mandible, Right **V** Mandible, Left **X** Hyoid Bone	**0** Open	**Z** No Device	**Z** No Qualifier

Section	0	Medical and Surgical
Body System	N	Head and Facial Bones
Operation	H	Insertion: Putting in a nonbiological appliance that monitors, assists, performs, or prevents a physiological function but does not physically take the place of a body part

Body Part (4th)	Approach (5th)	Device (6th)	Qualifier (7th)
0 Skull	0 Open	4 Internal Fixation Device 5 External Fixation Device M Bone Growth Stimulator N Neurostimulator Generator	Z No Qualifier
0 Skull	3 Percutaneous 4 Percutaneous Endoscopic	4 Internal Fixation Device 5 External Fixation Device M Bone Growth Stimulator	Z No Qualifier
1 Frontal Bone 3 Parietal Bone, Right 4 Parietal Bone, Left 7 Occipital Bone C Sphenoid Bone F Ethmoid Bone, Right G Ethmoid Bone, Left H Lacrimal Bone, Right J Lacrimal Bone, Left K Palatine Bone, Right L Palatine Bone, Left M Zygomatic Bone, Right N Zygomatic Bone, Left P Orbit, Right Q Orbit, Left X Hyoid Bone	0 Open 3 Percutaneous 4 Percutaneous Endoscopic	4 Internal Fixation Device	Z No Qualifier
5 Temporal Bone, Right 6 Temporal Bone, Left	0 Open 3 Percutaneous 4 Percutaneous Endoscopic	4 Internal Fixation Device S Hearing Device	Z No Qualifier
B Nasal Bone	0 Open 3 Percutaneous 4 Percutaneous Endoscopic	4 Internal Fixation Device M Bone Growth Stimulator	Z No Qualifier
R Maxilla T Mandible, Right V Mandible, Left	0 Open 3 Percutaneous 4 Percutaneous Endoscopic	4 Internal Fixation Device 5 External Fixation Device	Z No Qualifier
W Facial Bone	0 Open 3 Percutaneous 4 Percutaneous Endoscopic	M Bone Growth Stimulator	Z No Qualifier

Section	0	Medical and Surgical
Body System	N	Head and Facial Bones
Operation	J	Inspection: Visually and/or manually exploring a body part

Body Part (4th)	Approach (5th)	Device (6th)	Qualifier (7th)
0 Skull B Nasal Bone W Facial Bone	0 Open 3 Percutaneous 4 Percutaneous Endoscopic X External	Z No Device	Z No Qualifier

Section	0	Medical and Surgical
Body System	N	Head and Facial Bones
Operation	N	Release: Freeing a body part from an abnormal physical constraint by cutting or by the use of force

Body Part (4th)	Approach (5th)	Device (6th)	Qualifier (7th)
1 Frontal Bone 3 Parietal Bone, Right 4 Parietal Bone, Left 5 Temporal Bone, Right 6 Temporal Bone, Left 7 Occipital Bone B Nasal Bone C Sphenoid Bone F Ethmoid Bone, Right G Ethmoid Bone, Left H Lacrimal Bone, Right J Lacrimal Bone, Left K Palatine Bone, Right L Palatine Bone, Left M Zygomatic Bone, Right N Zygomatic Bone, Left P Orbit, Right Q Orbit, Left R Maxilla T Mandible, Right V Mandible, Left X Hyoid Bone	0 Open 3 Percutaneous 4 Percutaneous Endoscopic	Z No Device	Z No Qualifier

Section	0	Medical and Surgical
Body System	N	Head and Facial Bones
Operation	P	Removal: Taking out or off a device from a body part

Body Part (4th)	Approach (5th)	Device (6th)	Qualifier (7th)
0 Skull	0 Open	0 Drainage Device 4 Internal Fixation Device 5 External Fixation Device 7 Autologous Tissue Substitute J Synthetic Substitute K Nonautologous Tissue Substitute M Bone Growth Stimulator N Neurostimulator Generator S Hearing Device	Z No Qualifier
0 Skull	3 Percutaneous 4 Percutaneous Endoscopic	0 Drainage Device 4 Internal Fixation Device 5 External Fixation Device 7 Autologous Tissue Substitute J Synthetic Substitute K Nonautologous Tissue Substitute M Bone Growth Stimulator S Hearing Device	Z No Qualifier
0 Skull	X External	0 Drainage Device 4 Internal Fixation Device 5 External Fixation Device M Bone Growth Stimulator S Hearing Device	Z No Qualifier
B Nasal Bone W Facial Bone	0 Open 3 Percutaneous 4 Percutaneous Endoscopic	0 Drainage Device 4 Internal Fixation Device 7 Autologous Tissue Substitute J Synthetic Substitute K Nonautologous Tissue Substitute M Bone Growth Stimulator	Z No Qualifier
B Nasal Bone W Facial Bone	X External	0 Drainage Device 4 Internal Fixation Device M Bone Growth Stimulator	Z No Qualifier

Section	0	Medical and Surgical
Body System	N	Head and Facial Bones
Operation	Q	**Repair:** Restoring, to the extent possible, a body part to its normal anatomic structure and function

Body Part (4th)	Approach (5th)	Device (6th)	Qualifier (7th)
0 Skull **1** Frontal Bone **3** Parietal Bone, Right **4** Parietal Bone, Left **5** Temporal Bone, Right **6** Temporal Bone, Left **7** Occipital Bone **B** Nasal Bone **C** Sphenoid Bone **F** Ethmoid Bone, Right **G** Ethmoid Bone, Left **H** Lacrimal Bone, Right **J** Lacrimal Bone, Left **K** Palatine Bone, Right **L** Palatine Bone, Left **M** Zygomatic Bone, Right **N** Zygomatic Bone, Left **P** Orbit, Right **Q** Orbit, Left **R** Maxilla **T** Mandible, Right **V** Mandible, Left **X** Hyoid Bone	**0** Open **3** Percutaneous **4** Percutaneous Endoscopic **X** External	**Z** No Device	**Z** No Qualifier

Section	0	Medical and Surgical
Body System	N	Head and Facial Bones
Operation	R	**Replacement:** Putting in or on biological or synthetic material that physically takes the place and/or function of all or a portion of a body part

Body Part (4th)	Approach (5th)	Device (6th)	Qualifier (7th)
0 Skull **1** Frontal Bone **3** Parietal Bone, Right **4** Parietal Bone, Left **5** Temporal Bone, Right **6** Temporal Bone, Left **7** Occipital Bone **B** Nasal Bone **C** Sphenoid Bone **F** Ethmoid Bone, Right **G** Ethmoid Bone, Left **H** Lacrimal Bone, Right **J** Lacrimal Bone, Left **K** Palatine Bone, Right **L** Palatine Bone, Left **M** Zygomatic Bone, Right **N** Zygomatic Bone, Left **P** Orbit, Right **Q** Orbit, Left **R** Maxilla **T** Mandible, Right **V** Mandible, Left **X** Hyoid Bone	**0** Open **3** Percutaneous **4** Percutaneous Endoscopic	**7** Autologous Tissue Substitute **J** Synthetic Substitute **K** Nonautologous Tissue Substitute	**Z** No Qualifier

Section	0	Medical and Surgical
Body System	N	Head and Facial Bones
Operation	S	Reposition: Moving to its normal location, or other suitable location, all or a portion of a body part

Body Part (4th)	Approach (5th)	Device (6th)	Qualifier (7th)
0 Skull R Maxilla T Mandible, Right V Mandible, Left	0 Open 3 Percutaneous 4 Percutaneous Endoscopic	4 Internal Fixation Device 5 External Fixation Device Z No Device	Z No Qualifier
0 Skull R Maxilla T Mandible, Right V Mandible, Left	X External	Z No Device	Z No Qualifier
1 Frontal Bone 3 Parietal Bone, Right 4 Parietal Bone, Left 5 Temporal Bone, Right 6 Temporal Bone, Left 7 Occipital Bone B Nasal Bone C Sphenoid Bone F Ethmoid Bone, Right G Ethmoid Bone, Left H Lacrimal Bone, Right J Lacrimal Bone, Left K Palatine Bone, Right L Palatine Bone, Left M Zygomatic Bone, Right N Zygomatic Bone, Left P Orbit, Right Q Orbit, Left X Hyoid Bone	0 Open 3 Percutaneous 4 Percutaneous Endoscopic	4 Internal Fixation Device Z No Device	Z No Qualifier
1 Frontal Bone 3 Parietal Bone, Right 4 Parietal Bone, Left 5 Temporal Bone, Right 6 Temporal Bone, Left 7 Occipital Bone B Nasal Bone C Sphenoid Bone F Ethmoid Bone, Right G Ethmoid Bone, Left H Lacrimal Bone, Right J Lacrimal Bone, Left K Palatine Bone, Right L Palatine Bone, Left M Zygomatic Bone, Right N Zygomatic Bone, Left P Orbit, Right Q Orbit, Left X Hyoid Bone	X External	Z No Device	Z No Qualifier

Section	0	Medical and Surgical
Body System	N	Head and Facial Bones
Operation	T	**Resection:** Cutting out or off, without replacement, all of a body part

Body Part (4th)	Approach (5th)	Device (6th)	Qualifier (7th)
1 Frontal Bone 3 Parietal Bone, Right 4 Parietal Bone, Left 5 Temporal Bone, Right 6 Temporal Bone, Left 7 Occipital Bone B Nasal Bone C Sphenoid Bone F Ethmoid Bone, Right G Ethmoid Bone, Left H Lacrimal Bone, Right J Lacrimal Bone, Left K Palatine Bone, Right L Palatine Bone, Left M Zygomatic Bone, Right N Zygomatic Bone, Left P Orbit, Right Q Orbit, Left R Maxilla T Mandible, Right V Mandible, Left X Hyoid Bone	0 Open	Z No Device	Z No Qualifier

Section	0	Medical and Surgical
Body System	N	Head and Facial Bones
Operation	U	**Supplement:** Putting in or on biological or synthetic material that physically reinforces and/or augments the function of a portion of a body part

Body Part (4th)	Approach (5th)	Device (6th)	Qualifier (7th)
0 Skull 1 Frontal Bone 3 Parietal Bone, Right 4 Parietal Bone, Left 5 Temporal Bone, Right 6 Temporal Bone, Left 7 Occipital Bone B Nasal Bone C Sphenoid Bone F Ethmoid Bone, Right G Ethmoid Bone, Left H Lacrimal Bone, Right J Lacrimal Bone, Left K Palatine Bone, Right L Palatine Bone, Left M Zygomatic Bone, Right N Zygomatic Bone, Left P Orbit, Right Q Orbit, Left R Maxilla T Mandible, Right V Mandible, Left X Hyoid Bone	0 Open 3 Percutaneous 4 Percutaneous Endoscopic	7 Autologous Tissue Substitute J Synthetic Substitute K Nonautologous Tissue Substitute	Z No Qualifier

Section	0	Medical and Surgical
Body System	N	Head and Facial Bones
Operation	W	**Revision:** Correcting, to the extent possible, a portion of a malfunctioning device or the position of a displaced device

Body Part (4th)	Approach (5th)	Device (6th)	Qualifier (7th)
0 Skull	**0** Open	**0** Drainage Device **4** Internal Fixation Device **5** External Fixation Device **7** Autologous Tissue Substitute **J** Synthetic Substitute **K** Nonautologous Tissue Substitute **M** Bone Growth Stimulator **N** Neurostimulator Generator **S** Hearing Device	**Z** No Qualifier
0 Skull	**3** Percutaneous **4** Percutaneous Endoscopic **X** External	**0** Drainage Device **4** Internal Fixation Device **5** External Fixation Device **7** Autologous Tissue Substitute **J** Synthetic Substitute **K** Nonautologous Tissue Substitute **M** Bone Growth Stimulator **S** Hearing Device	**Z** No Qualifier
B Nasal Bone **W** Facial Bone	**0** Open **3** Percutaneous **4** Percutaneous Endoscopic **X** External	**0** Drainage Device **4** Internal Fixation Device **7** Autologous Tissue Substitute **J** Synthetic Substitute **K** Nonautologous Tissue Substitute **M** Bone Growth Stimulator	**Z** No Qualifier

AHA Coding Clinic

0NBB0ZZ Excision of Nasal Bone, Open Approach—AHA CC: 1Q, 2017, 20-21

0NBQ0ZZ Excision of Left Orbit, Open Approach—AHA CC: 2Q, 2015, 12-13

0NH004Z Insertion of Internal Fixation Device into Skull, Open Approach—AHA CC: 3Q, 2015, 13-14

0NP004Z Removal of Internal Fixation Device from Skull, Open Approach—AHA CC: 3Q, 2015, 13-14

0NR00JZ Replacement of Skull with Synthetic Substitute, Open Approach—AHA CC: 3Q, 2014, 7-8

0NR70JZ Replacement of Occipital Bone with Synthetic Substitute, Open Approach—AHA CC: 3Q, 2017, 17

0NRV07Z Replacement of Left Mandible with Autologous Tissue Substitute, Open Approach—AHA CC: 1Q, 2017, 23-24

0NRV0JZ Replacement of Left Mandible with Synthetic Substitute, Open Approach—AHA CC: 1Q, 2017, 23-24

0NS004Z Reposition Skull with Internal Fixation Device, Open Approach—AHA CC: 3Q, 2017, 22

0NS005Z Reposition Skull with External Fixation Device, Open Approach—AHA CC: 3Q, 2013, 24-25

0NS00ZZ Reposition Skull, Open Approach—AHA CC: 3Q, 2015, 17-18; 2Q, 2016, 30

0NS104Z Reposition Frontal Bone with Internal Fixation Device, Open Approach—AHA CC: 3Q, 2013, 25

0NS504Z Reposition Right Temporal Bone with Internal Fixation Device, Open Approach—AHA CC: 3Q, 2015, 27-28

0NSR04Z Reposition Maxilla with Internal Fixation Device, Open Approach—AHA CC: 3Q, 2014, 23-24

0NSR0ZZ Reposition Maxilla, Open Approach—AHA CC: 1Q, 2017, 20-21

0NU00JZ Supplement Skull with Synthetic Substitute, Open Approach—AHA CC: 3Q, 2013, 24-25

0NUR07Z Supplement Maxilla with Autologous Tissue Substitute, Open Approach—AHA CC: 3Q, 2016, 29-30

Bones - Front and Back Views

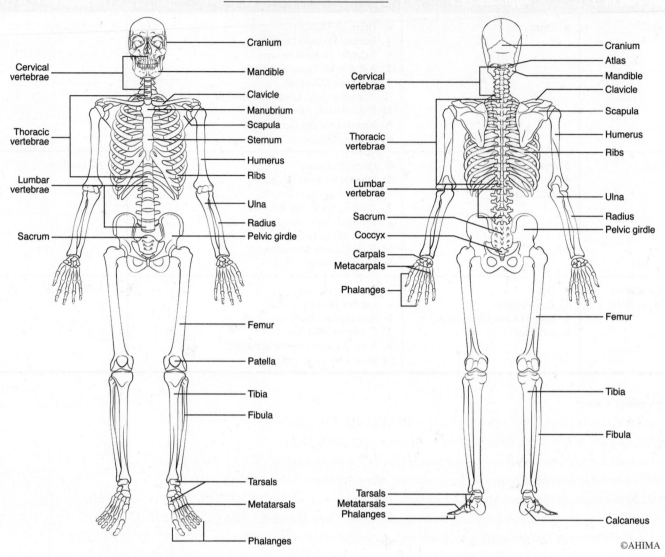

Cranium
Cervical vertebrae
Mandible
Clavicle
Manubrium
Thoracic vertebrae
Scapula
Sternum
Humerus
Ribs
Lumbar vertebrae
Ulna
Radius
Sacrum
Pelvic girdle

Femur

Patella

Tibia

Fibula

Tarsals

Metatarsals

Phalanges

Cranium
Atlas
Cervical vertebrae
Mandible
Clavicle
Scapula
Thoracic vertebrae
Humerus
Ribs
Lumbar vertebrae
Sacrum
Ulna
Coccyx
Radius
Pelvic girdle
Carpals
Metacarpals
Phalanges

Femur

Tibia

Fibula

Tarsals
Metatarsals
Phalanges

Calcaneus

©AHIMA

Vertebral Column

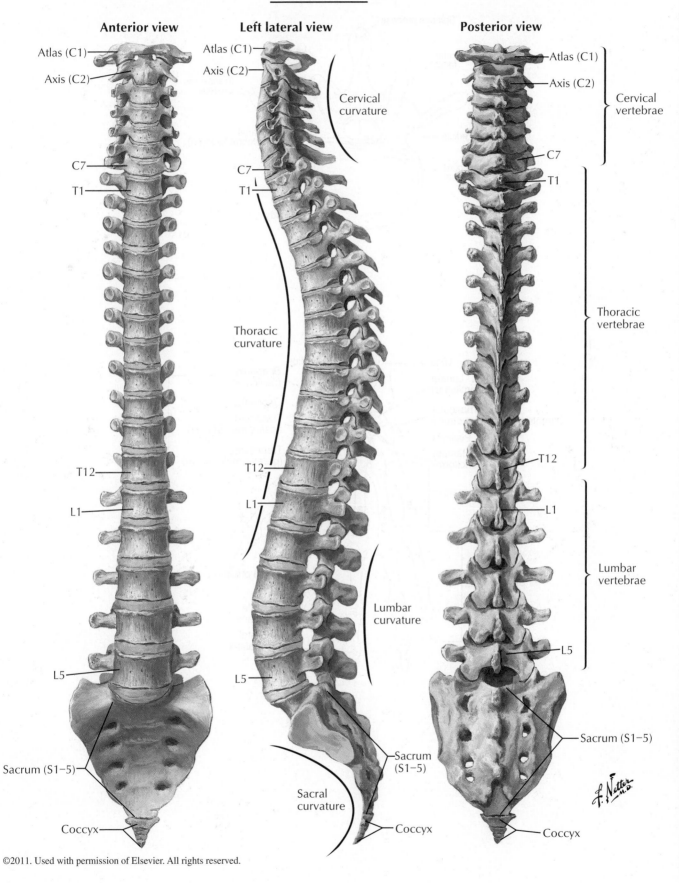

Anterior view

Atlas (C1)
Axis (C2)
C7
T1
T12
L1
L5
Sacrum (S1–5)
Coccyx

Left lateral view

Atlas (C1)
Axis (C2)
Cervical curvature
C7
T1
Thoracic curvature
T12
L1
Lumbar curvature
L5
Sacral curvature
Sacrum (S1–5)
Coccyx

Posterior view

Atlas (C1)
Axis (C2)
Cervical vertebrae
C7
T1
Thoracic vertebrae
T12
L1
Lumbar vertebrae
L5
Sacrum (S1–5)
Coccyx

Medical and Surgical, Upper Bones

Cross-section Spine

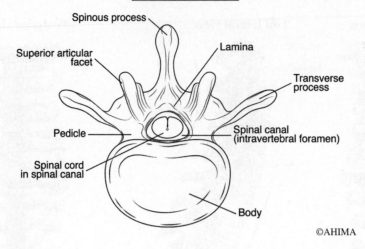

Spinous process

Lamina

Superior articular facet

Transverse process

Pedicle

Spinal canal (intravertebral foramen)

Spinal cord in spinal canal

Body

©AHIMA

Hand Bones

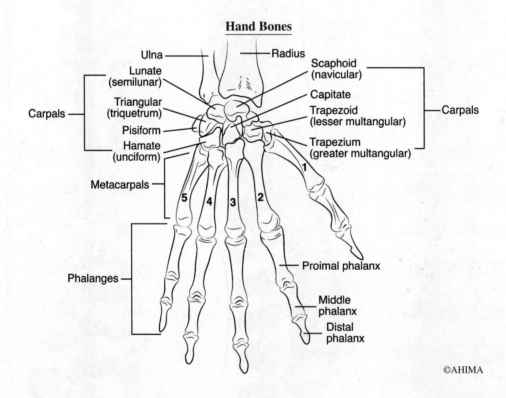

Ulna

Radius

Lunate (semilunar)

Scaphoid (navicular)

Triangular (triquetrum)

Capitate

Carpals

Trapezoid (lesser multangular)

Pisiform

Hamate (unciform)

Trapezium (greater multangular)

Carpals

Metacarpals

1

5 4 3 2

Phalanges

Proimal phalanx

Middle phalanx

Distal phalanx

©AHIMA

Section	0	Medical and Surgical
Body System	P	Upper Bones
Operation	2	**Change:** Taking out or off a device from a body part and putting back an identical or similar device in or on the same body part without cutting or puncturing the skin or a mucous membrane

Body Part (4th)	Approach (5th)	Device (6th)	Qualifier (7th)
Y Upper Bone	**X** External	**0** Drainage Device **Y** Other Device	**Z** No Qualifier

Section	0	Medical and Surgical
Body System	P	Upper Bones
Operation	5	**Destruction:** Physical eradication of all or a portion of a body part by the direct use of energy, force, or a destructive agent

Body Part (4th)	Approach (5th)	Device (6th)	Qualifier (7th)
0 Sternum **1** Ribs, 1 to 2 **2** Ribs, 3 or More **3** Cervical Vertebra **4** Thoracic Vertebra **5** Scapula, Right **6** Scapula, Left **7** Glenoid Cavity, Right **8** Glenoid Cavity, Left **9** Clavicle, Right **B** Clavicle, Left **C** Humeral Head, Right **D** Humeral Head, Left **F** Humeral Shaft, Right **G** Humeral Shaft, Left **H** Radius, Right **J** Radius, Left **K** Ulna, Right **L** Ulna, Left **M** Carpal, Right **N** Carpal, Left **P** Metacarpal, Right **Q** Metacarpal, Left **R** Thumb Phalanx, Right **S** Thumb Phalanx, Left **T** Finger Phalanx, Right **V** Finger Phalanx, Left	**0** Open **3** Percutaneous **4** Percutaneous Endoscopic	**Z** No Device	**Z** No Qualifier

Section   0   **Medical and Surgical**
Body System   P   **Upper Bones**
Operation   8   **Division:** Cutting into a body part, without draining fluids and/or gases from the body part, in order to separate or transect a body part

Body Part (4th)	Approach (5th)	Device (6th)	Qualifier (7th)
0 Sternum	0 Open	Z No Device	Z No Qualifier
1 Ribs, 1 to 2	3 Percutaneous		
2 Ribs, 3 or More	4 Percutaneous Endoscopic		
3 Cervical Vertebra			
4 Thoracic Vertebra			
5 Scapula, Right			
6 Scapula, Left			
7 Glenoid Cavity, Right			
8 Glenoid Cavity, Left			
9 Clavicle, Right			
B Clavicle, Left			
C Humeral Head, Right			
D Humeral Head, Left			
F Humeral Shaft, Right			
G Humeral Shaft, Left			
H Radius, Right			
J Radius, Left			
K Ulna, Right			
L Ulna, Left			
M Carpal, Right			
N Carpal, Left			
P Metacarpal, Right			
Q Metacarpal, Left			
R Thumb Phalanx, Right			
S Thumb Phalanx, Left			
T Finger Phalanx, Right			
V Finger Phalanx, Left			

Section   0   **Medical and Surgical**
Body System   P   **Upper Bones**
Operation   9   **Drainage:** Taking or letting out fluids and/or gases from a body part

Body Part (4th)	Approach (5th)	Device (6th)	Qualifier (7th)
0 Sternum	0 Open	0 Drainage Device	Z No Qualifier
1 Ribs, 1 to 2	3 Percutaneous		
2 Ribs, 3 or More	4 Percutaneous Endoscopic		
3 Cervical Vertebra			
4 Thoracic Vertebra			
5 Scapula, Right			
6 Scapula, Left			
7 Glenoid Cavity, Right			
8 Glenoid Cavity, Left			
9 Clavicle, Right			
B Clavicle, Left			
C Humeral Head, Right			
D Humeral Head, Left			
F Humeral Shaft, Right			
G Humeral Shaft, Left			
H Radius, Right			
J Radius, Left			
K Ulna, Right			
L Ulna, Left			
M Carpal, Right			
N Carpal, Left			
P Metacarpal, Right			
Q Metacarpal, Left			
R Thumb Phalanx, Right			
S Thumb Phalanx, Left			
T Finger Phalanx, Right			
V Finger Phalanx, Left			

Continued →

Section **0** **Medical and Surgical**
Body System **P** **Upper Bones**
Operation **9** **Drainage:** Taking or letting out fluids and/or gases from a body part

Body Part (4th)	Approach (5th)	Device (6th)	Qualifier (7th)
0 Sternum	0 Open	Z No Device	X Diagnostic
1 Ribs, 1 to 2	3 Percutaneous		Z No Qualifier
2 Ribs, 3 or More	4 Percutaneous Endoscopic		
3 Cervical Vertebra			
4 Thoracic Vertebra			
5 Scapula, Right			
6 Scapula, Left			
7 Glenoid Cavity, Right			
8 Glenoid Cavity, Left			
9 Clavicle, Right			
B Clavicle, Left			
C Humeral Head, Right			
D Humeral Head, Left			
F Humeral Shaft, Right			
G Humeral Shaft, Left			
H Radius, Right			
J Radius, Left			
K Ulna, Right			
L Ulna, Left			
M Carpal, Right			
N Carpal, Left			
P Metacarpal, Right			
Q Metacarpal, Left			
R Thumb Phalanx, Right			
S Thumb Phalanx, Left			
T Finger Phalanx, Right			
V Finger Phalanx, Left			

Section **0** **Medical and Surgical**
Body System **P** **Upper Bones**
Operation **B** **Excision:** Cutting out or off, without replacement, a portion of a body part

Body Part (4th)	Approach (5th)	Device (6th)	Qualifier (7th)
0 Sternum	0 Open	Z No Device	X Diagnostic
1 Ribs, 1 to 2	3 Percutaneous		Z No Qualifier
2 Ribs, 3 or More	4 Percutaneous Endoscopic		
3 Cervical Vertebra			
4 Thoracic Vertebra			
5 Scapula, Right			
6 Scapula, Left			
7 Glenoid Cavity, Right			
8 Glenoid Cavity, Left			
9 Clavicle, Right			
B Clavicle, Left			
C Humeral Head, Right			
D Humeral Head, Left			
F Humeral Shaft, Right			
G Humeral Shaft, Left			
H Radius, Right			
J Radius, Left			
K Ulna, Right			
L Ulna, Left			
M Carpal, Right			
N Carpal, Left			
P Metacarpal, Right			
Q Metacarpal, Left			
R Thumb Phalanx, Right			
S Thumb Phalanx, Left			
T Finger Phalanx, Right			
V Finger Phalanx, Left			

Section	0	Medical and Surgical
Body System	P	Upper Bones
Operation	C	Extirpation: Taking or cutting out solid matter from a body part

Body Part (4th)	Approach (5th)	Device (6th)	Qualifier (7th)
0 Sternum	0 Open	Z No Device	Z No Qualifier
1 Ribs, 1 to 2	3 Percutaneous		
2 Ribs, 3 or More	4 Percutaneous Endoscopic		
3 Cervical Vertebra			
4 Thoracic Vertebra			
5 Scapula, Right			
6 Scapula, Left			
7 Glenoid Cavity, Right			
8 Glenoid Cavity, Left			
9 Clavicle, Right			
B Clavicle, Left			
C Humeral Head, Right			
D Humeral Head, Left			
F Humeral Shaft, Right			
G Humeral Shaft, Left			
H Radius, Right			
J Radius, Left			
K Ulna, Right			
L Ulna, Left			
M Carpal, Right			
N Carpal, Left			
P Metacarpal, Right			
Q Metacarpal, Left			
R Thumb Phalanx, Right			
S Thumb Phalanx, Left			
T Finger Phalanx, Right			
V Finger Phalanx, Left			

Section	0	Medical and Surgical
Body System	P	Upper Bones
Operation	D	Extraction: Pulling or stripping out or off all or a portion of a body part by the use of force

Body Part (4th)	Approach (5th)	Device (6th)	Qualifier (7th)
0 Sternum	0 Open	Z No Device	Z No Qualifier
1 Ribs, 1 to 2			
2 Ribs, 3 or More			
3 Cervical Vertebra			
4 Thoracic Vertebra			
5 Scapula, Right			
6 Scapula, Left			
7 Glenoid Cavity, Right			
8 Glenoid Cavity, Left			
9 Clavical, Right			
B Clavical, Left			
C Humeral Head, Right			
D Humeral Head, Left			
F Humeral Shaft, Right			
G Humeral Shaft, Left			
H Radius, Right			
J Radius, Left			
K Ulna, Right			
L Ulna, Left			
M Carpal, Right			
N Carpal, Left			
P Metacarpal, Right			
Q Metacarpal, Left			
R Thumb Phalanx, Right			
S Thumb Phalanx, Left			
T Finger Phalanx, Right			
V Finger Phalanx, Left			

Section   **0**   **Medical and Surgical**
Body System   **P**   **Upper Bones**
Operation   **H**   **Insertion:** Putting in a nonbiological appliance that monitors, assists, performs, or prevents a physiological function but does not physically take the place of a body part

Body Part (4th)	Approach (5th)	Device (6th)	Qualifier (7th)
0 Sternum	0 Open 3 Percutaneous 4 Percutaneous Endoscopic	0 Internal Fixation Device, Rigid Plate 4 Internal Fixation Device	Z No Qualifier
1 Ribs, 1 to 2 2 Ribs, 3 or More 3 Cervical Vertebra 4 Thoracic Vertebra 5 Scapula, Right 6 Scapula, Left 7 Glenoid Cavity, Right 8 Glenoid Cavity, Left 9 Clavicle, Right B Clavicle, Left	0 Open 3 Percutaneous 4 Percutaneous Endoscopic	4 Internal Fixation Device	Z No Qualifier
C Humeral Head, Right D Humeral Head, Left H Radius, Right J Radius, Left K Ulna, Right L Ulna, Left	0 Open 3 Percutaneous 4 Percutaneous Endoscopic	4 Internal Fixation Device 5 External Fixation Device 6 Internal Fixation Device, Intramedullary 8 External Fixation Device, Limb Lengthening B External Fixation Device, Monoplanar C External Fixation Device, Ring D External Fixation Device, Hybrid	Z No Qualifier
F Humeral Shaft, Right G Humeral Shaft, Left	0 Open 3 Percutaneous 4 Percutaneous Endoscopic	4 Internal Fixation Device 5 External Fixation Device 6 Internal Fixation Device, Intramedullary 7 Internal Fixation Device, Intramedullary Limb Lengthening 8 External Fixation Device, Limb Lengthening B External Fixation Device, Monoplanar C External Fixation Device, Ring D External Fixation Device, Hybrid	Z No Qualifier
M Carpal, Right N Carpal, Left P Metacarpal, Right Q Metacarpal, Left R Thumb Phalanx, Right S Thumb Phalanx, Left T Finger Phalanx, Right V Finger Phalanx, Left	0 Open 3 Percutaneous 4 Percutaneous Endoscopic	4 Internal Fixation Device 5 External Fixation Device	Z No Qualifier
Y Upper Bone	0 Open 3 Percutaneous 4 Percutaneous Endoscopic	M Bone Growth Stimulator	Z No Qualifier

Section   **0**   **Medical and Surgical**
Body System   **P**   **Upper Bones**
Operation   **J**   **Inspection:** Visually and/or manually exploring a body part

Body Part (4th)	Approach (5th)	Device (6th)	Qualifier (7th)
Y Upper Bone	0 Open 3 Percutaneous 4 Percutaneous Endoscopic X External	Z No Device	Z No Qualifier

Section	0	Medical and Surgical
Body System	P	Upper Bones
Operation	N	Release: Freeing a body part from an abnormal physical constraint by cutting or by the use of force

Body Part (4th)	Approach (5th)	Device (6th)	Qualifier (7th)
0 Sternum 1 Ribs, 1 to 2 2 Ribs, 3 or More 3 Cervical Vertebra 4 Thoracic Vertebra 5 Scapula, Right 6 Scapula, Left 7 Glenoid Cavity, Right 8 Glenoid Cavity, Left 9 Clavicle, Right B Clavicle, Left C Humeral Head, Right D Humeral Head, Left F Humeral Shaft, Right G Humeral Shaft, Left H Radius, Right J Radius, Left K Ulna, Right L Ulna, Left M Carpal, Right N Carpal, Left P Metacarpal, Right Q Metacarpal, Left R Thumb Phalanx, Right S Thumb Phalanx, Left T Finger Phalanx, Right V Finger Phalanx, Left	0 Open 3 Percutaneous 4 Percutaneous Endoscopic	Z No Device	Z No Qualifier

Section	0	Medical and Surgical
Body System	P	Upper Bones
Operation	P	Removal: Taking out or off a device from a body part

Body Part (4th)	Approach (5th)	Device (6th)	Qualifier (7th)
0 Sternum 1 Ribs, 1 to 2 2 Ribs, 3 or More 3 Cervical Vertebra 4 Thoracic Vertebra 5 Scapula, Right 6 Scapula, Left 7 Glenoid Cavity, Right 8 Glenoid Cavity, Left 9 Clavicle, Right B Clavicle, Left	0 Open 3 Percutaneous 4 Percutaneous Endoscopic	4 Internal Fixation Device 7 Autologous Tissue Substitute J Synthetic Substitute K Nonautologous Tissue Substitute	Z No Qualifier
0 Sternum 1 Ribs, 1 to 2 2 Ribs, 3 or More 3 Cervical Vertebra 4 Thoracic Vertebra 5 Scapula, Right 6 Scapula, Left 7 Glenoid Cavity, Right 8 Glenoid Cavity, Left 9 Clavicle, Right B Clavicle, Left	X External	4 Internal Fixation Device	Z No Qualifier

Continued →

Body Part (4th)	Approach (5th)	Device (6th)	Qualifier (7th)
C Humeral Head, Right D Humeral Head, Left F Humeral Shaft, Right G Humeral Shaft, Left H Radius, Right J Radius, Left K Ulna, Right L Ulna, Left M Carpal, Right N Carpal, Left P Metacarpal, Right Q Metacarpal, Left R Thumb Phalanx, Right S Thumb Phalanx, Left T Finger Phalanx, Right V Finger Phalanx, Left	0 Open 3 Percutaneous 4 Percutaneous Endoscopic	4 Internal Fixation Device 5 External Fixation Device 7 Autologous Tissue Substitute J Synthetic Substitute K Nonautologous Tissue Substitute	Z No Qualifier
C Humeral Head, Right D Humeral Head, Left F Humeral Shaft, Right G Humeral Shaft, Left H Radius, Right J Radius, Left K Ulna, Right L Ulna, Left M Carpal, Right N Carpal, Left P Metacarpal, Right Q Metacarpal, Left R Thumb Phalanx, Right S Thumb Phalanx, Left T Finger Phalanx, Right V Finger Phalanx, Left	X External	4 Internal Fixation Device 5 External Fixation Device	Z No Qualifier
Y Upper Bone	0 Open 3 Percutaneous 4 Percutaneous Endoscopic X External	0 Drainage Device M Bone Growth Stimulator	Z No Qualifier

Section	0	Medical and Surgical
Body System	P	Upper Bones
Operation	Q	**Repair:** Restoring, to the extent possible, a body part to its normal anatomic structure and function

Body Part (4th)	Approach (5th)	Device (6th)	Qualifier (7th)
0 Sternum	0 Open	Z No Device	Z No Qualifier
1 Ribs, 1 to 2	3 Percutaneous		
2 Ribs, 3 or More	4 Percutaneous Endoscopic		
3 Cervical Vertebra	X External		
4 Thoracic Vertebra			
5 Scapula, Right			
6 Scapula, Left			
7 Glenoid Cavity, Right			
8 Glenoid Cavity, Left			
9 Clavicle, Right			
B Clavicle, Left			
C Humeral Head, Right			
D Humeral Head, Left			
F Humeral Shaft, Right			
G Humeral Shaft, Left			
H Radius, Right			
J Radius, Left			
K Ulna, Right			
L Ulna, Left			
M Carpal, Right			
N Carpal, Left			
P Metacarpal, Right			
Q Metacarpal, Left			
R Thumb Phalanx, Right			
S Thumb Phalanx, Left			
T Finger Phalanx, Right			
V Finger Phalanx, Left			

Section	0	Medical and Surgical
Body System	P	Upper Bones
Operation	R	**Replacement:** Putting in or on biological or synthetic material that physically takes the place and/or function of all or a portion of a body part

Body Part (4th)	Approach (5th)	Device (6th)	Qualifier (7th)
0 Sternum	0 Open	7 Autologous Tissue Substitute	Z No Qualifier
1 Ribs, 1 to 2	3 Percutaneous	J Synthetic Substitute	
2 Ribs, 3 or More	4 Percutaneous Endoscopic	K Nonautologous Tissue Substitute	
3 Cervical Vertebra			
4 Thoracic Vertebra			
5 Scapula, Right			
6 Scapula, Left			
7 Glenoid Cavity, Right			
8 Glenoid Cavity, Left			
9 Clavicle, Right			
B Clavicle, Left			
C Humeral Head, Right			
D Humeral Head, Left			
F Humeral Shaft, Right			
G Humeral Shaft, Left			
H Radius, Right			
J Radius, Left			
K Ulna, Right			
L Ulna, Left			
M Carpal, Right			
N Carpal, Left			
P Metacarpal, Right			
Q Metacarpal, Left			
R Thumb Phalanx, Right			
S Thumb Phalanx, Left			
T Finger Phalanx, Right			
V Finger Phalanx, Left			

Section	0	Medical and Surgical
Body System	P	Upper Bones
Operation	S	Reposition: Moving to its normal location, or other suitable location, all or a portion of a body part

Body Part (4th)	Approach (5th)	Device (6th)	Qualifier (7th)
0 Sternum	0 Open 3 Percutaneous 4 Percutaneous Endoscopic	0 Internal Fixation Device, Rigid Plate 4 Internal Fixation Device Z No Device	Z No Qualifier
0 Sternum	X External	Z No Device	Z No Qualifier
1 Ribs, 1 to 2 2 Ribs, 3 or More 3 Cervical Vertebra 4 Thoracic Vertebra 5 Scapula, Right 6 Scapula, Left 7 Glenoid Cavity, Right 8 Glenoid Cavity, Left 9 Clavicle, Right B Clavicle, Left	0 Open 3 Percutaneous 4 Percutaneous Endoscopic	4 Internal Fixation Device Z No Device	Z No Qualifier
1 Ribs, 1 to 2 2 Ribs, 3 or More 3 Cervical Vertebra 4 Thoracic Vertebra 5 Scapula, Right 6 Scapula, Left 7 Glenoid Cavity, Right 8 Glenoid Cavity, Left 9 Clavicle, Right B Clavicle, Left	X External	Z No Device	Z No Qualifier
C Humeral Head, Right D Humeral Head, Left F Humeral Shaft, Right G Humeral Shaft, Left H Radius, Right J Radius, Left K Ulna, Right L Ulna, Left	0 Open 3 Percutaneous 4 Percutaneous Endoscopic	4 Internal Fixation Device 5 External Fixation Device 6 Internal Fixation Device, Intramedullary B External Fixation Device, Monoplanar C External Fixation Device, Ring D External Fixation Device, Hybrid Z No Device	Z No Qualifier
C Humeral Head, Right D Humeral Head, Left F Humeral Shaft, Right G Humeral Shaft, Left H Radius, Right J Radius, Left K Ulna, Right L Ulna, Left	X External	Z No Device	Z No Qualifier
M Carpal, Right N Carpal, Left P Metacarpal, Right Q Metacarpal, Left R Thumb Phalanx, Right S Thumb Phalanx, Left T Finger Phalanx, Right V Finger Phalanx, Left	0 Open 3 Percutaneous 4 Percutaneous Endoscopic	4 Internal Fixation Device 5 External Fixation Device Z No Device	Z No Qualifier
M Carpal, Right N Carpal, Left P Metacarpal, Right Q Metacarpal, Left R Thumb Phalanx, Right S Thumb Phalanx, Left T Finger Phalanx, Right V Finger Phalanx, Left	X External	Z No Device	Z No Qualifier

Section	0	Medical and Surgical
Body System	P	Upper Bones
Operation	T	Resection: Cutting out or off, without replacement, all of a body part

Body Part (4th)	Approach (5th)	Device (6th)	Qualifier (7th)
0 Sternum	0 Open	Z No Device	Z No Qualifier
1 Ribs, 1 to 2			
2 Ribs, 3 or More			
5 Scapula, Right			
6 Scapula, Left			
7 Glenoid Cavity, Right			
8 Glenoid Cavity, Left			
9 Clavicle, Right			
B Clavicle, Left			
C Humeral Head, Right			
D Humeral Head, Left			
F Humeral Shaft, Right			
G Humeral Shaft, Left			
H Radius, Right			
J Radius, Left			
K Ulna, Right			
L Ulna, Left			
M Carpal, Right			
N Carpal, Left			
P Metacarpal, Right			
Q Metacarpal, Left			
R Thumb Phalanx, Right			
S Thumb Phalanx, Left			
T Finger Phalanx, Right			
V Finger Phalanx, Left			

Section	0	Medical and Surgical
Body System	P	Upper Bones
Operation	U	Supplement: Putting in or on biological or synthetic material that physically reinforces and/or augments the function of a portion of a body part

Body Part (4th)	Approach (5th)	Device (6th)	Qualifier (7th)
0 Sternum	0 Open	7 Autologous Tissue Substitute	Z No Qualifier
1 Ribs, 1 to 2	3 Percutaneous	J Synthetic Substitute	
2 Ribs, 3 or More	4 Percutaneous Endoscopic	K Nonautologous Tissue Substitute	
3 Cervical Vertebra			
4 Thoracic Vertebra			
5 Scapula, Right			
6 Scapula, Left			
7 Glenoid Cavity, Right			
8 Glenoid Cavity, Left			
9 Clavicle, Right			
B Clavicle, Left			
C Humeral Head, Right			
D Humeral Head, Left			
F Humeral Shaft, Right			
G Humeral Shaft, Left			
H Radius, Right			
J Radius, Left			
K Ulna, Right			
L Ulna, Left			
M Carpal, Right			
N Carpal, Left			
P Metacarpal, Right			
Q Metacarpal, Left			
R Thumb Phalanx, Right			
S Thumb Phalanx, Left			
T Finger Phalanx, Right			
V Finger Phalanx, Left			

Section	0	Medical and Surgical
Body System	P	Upper Bones
Operation	W	Revision: Correcting, to the extent possible, a portion of a malfunctioning device or the position of a displaced device

Body Part (4th)	Approach (5th)	Device (6th)	Qualifier (7th)
0 Sternum 1 Ribs, 1 to 2 2 Ribs, 3 or More 3 Cervical Vertebra 4 Thoracic Vertebra 5 Scapula, Right 6 Scapula, Left 7 Glenoid Cavity, Right 8 Glenoid Cavity, Left 9 Clavicle, Right B Clavicle, Left	0 Open 3 Percutaneous 4 Percutaneous Endoscopic X External	4 Internal Fixation Device 7 Autologous Tissue Substitute J Synthetic Substitute K Nonautologous Tissue Substitute	Z No Qualifier
C Humeral Head, Right D Humeral Head, Left F Humeral Shaft, Right G Humeral Shaft, Left H Radius, Right J Radius, Left K Ulna, Right L Ulna, Left M Carpal, Right N Carpal, Left P Metacarpal, Right Q Metacarpal, Left R Thumb Phalanx, Right S Thumb Phalanx, Left T Finger Phalanx, Right V Finger Phalanx, Left	0 Open 3 Percutaneous 4 Percutaneous Endoscopic X External	4 Internal Fixation Device 5 External Fixation Device 7 Autologous Tissue Substitute J Synthetic Substitute K Nonautologous Tissue Substitute	Z No Qualifier
Y Upper Bone	0 Open 3 Percutaneous 4 Percutaneous Endoscopic X External	0 Drainage Device M Bone Growth Stimulator	Z No Qualifier

AHA Coding Clinic

0PB10ZZ Excision of 1 to 2 Ribs, Open Approach—AHA CC: 4Q, 2012, 101-102; 4Q, 2013, 109-111

0PB20ZZ Excision of 3 or More Ribs, Open Approach—AHA CC: 4Q, 2013, 109-111

0PB54ZZ Excision of Right Scapula, Percutaneous Endoscopic Approach—AHA CC: 3Q, 2013, 20-22

0PC00ZZ Extirpation of Matter from Sternum, Open Approach—AHA CC: 3Q, 2019, 19

0PH000Z Insertion of Rigid Plate Internal Fixation Device into Sternum, Open Approach—AHA CC: 1Q, 2020, 29-30

0PH304Z Insertion of Internal Fixation Device into Cervical Vertebra, Open Approach—AHA CC: 2Q, 2017, 23-24; 2Q, 2019, 40

0PH404Z Insertion of Internal Fixation Device into Thoracic Vertebra, Open Approach—AHA CC: 4Q, 2014, 28-29

0PH504Z Insertion of Internal Fixation Device into Right Scapula, Open Approach—AHA CC: 4Q, 2018, 12-13

0PP404Z Removal of Internal Fixation Device from Thoracic Vertebra, Open Approach—AHA CC: 4Q, 2014, 28-29

0PRH0JZ Replacement of Right Radius with Synthetic Substitute, Open Approach—AHA CC: 4Q, 2018, 92-93

0PS00ZZ Reposition Sternum, Open Approach—AHA CC: 4Q, 2015, 34

0PS204Z Reposition 3 or More Ribs with Internal Fixation Device, Open Approach—AHA CC: 4Q, 2014, 26; 4Q, 2017, 53

0PS3XZZ Reposition Cervical Vertebra, External Approach—AHA CC: 2Q, 2015, 35

0PS404Z Reposition Thoracic Vertebra with Internal Fixation Device, Open Approach—AHA CC: 1Q, 2020, 33-34

0PS444Z Reposition Thoracic Vertebra with Internal Fixation Device, Percutaneous Endoscopic Approach—AHA CC: 3Q, 2018, 26-27

0PS4XZZ Reposition Thoracic Vertebra, External Approach—AHA CC: 1Q, 2016, 21

0PSJ04Z Reposition Left Radius with Internal Fixation Device, Open Approach—AHA CC: 3Q, 2014, 33-34; 4Q, 2014, 32-33

0PSL04Z Reposition Left Ulna with Internal Fixation Device, Open Approach—AHA CC: 4Q, 2014, 32-33

0PTN0ZZ Resection of Left Carpal, Open Approach—AHA CC: 3Q, 2015, 26-27

0PU00JZ Supplement Sternum with Synthetic Substitute, Open Approach—AHA CC: 4Q, 2013, 109-111

0PU30KZ Supplement Cervical Vertebra with Nonautologous Tissue Substitute, Open Approach—AHA CC: 2Q, 2015, 20-21

0PU507Z Supplement Right Scapula with Autologous Tissue Substitute, Open Approach—AHA CC: 4Q, 2018, 12-13

0PU50KZ Supplement Right Scapula with Nonautologous Tissue Substitute, Open Approach—AHA CC: 4Q, 2018, 12-13

0PW104Z Revision of Internal Fixation Device in 1 to 2 Ribs, Open Approach—AHA CC: 4Q, 2014, 26-27

0PW204Z Revision of Internal Fixation Device in 3 or More Ribs, Open Approach—AHA CC: 4Q, 2014, 26-27

0PW404Z Revision of Internal Fixation Device in Thoracic Vertebra, Open Approach—AHA CC: 4Q, 2014, 27-28

Bones - Front and Back Views

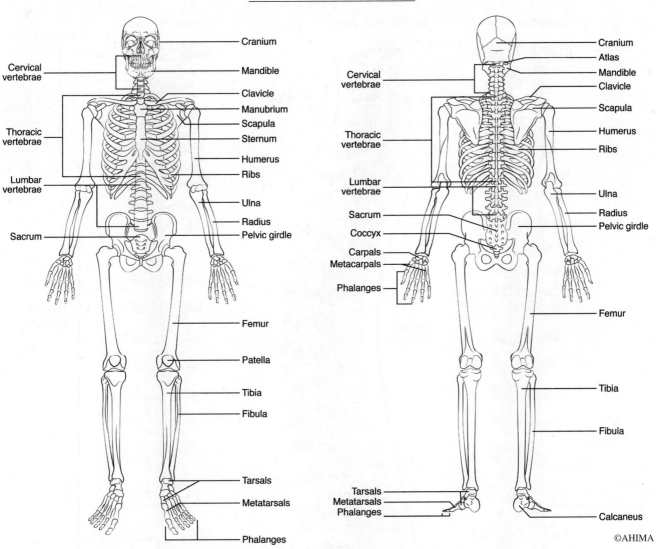

Cranium

Mandible

Cervical vertebrae

Clavicle

Manubrium

Scapula

Sternum

Thoracic vertebrae

Humerus

Ribs

Lumbar vertebrae

Ulna

Radius

Sacrum

Pelvic girdle

Femur

Patella

Tibia

Fibula

Tarsals

Metatarsals

Phalanges

Cranium

Atlas

Mandible

Cervical vertebrae

Clavicle

Scapula

Humerus

Thoracic vertebrae

Ribs

Lumbar vertebrae

Ulna

Sacrum

Radius

Coccyx

Pelvic girdle

Carpals

Metacarpals

Phalanges

Femur

Tibia

Fibula

Tarsals

Metatarsals

Phalanges

Calcaneus

©AHIMA

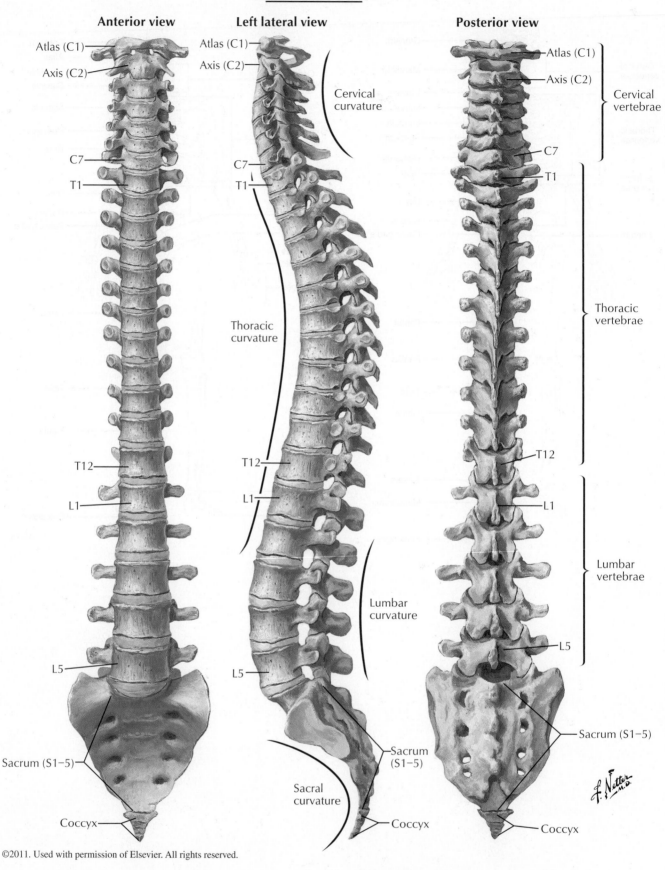

Vertebral Column

Anterior view

Atlas (C1)
Axis (C2)
C7
T1
T12
L1
L5
Sacrum (S1–5)
Coccyx

Left lateral view

Atlas (C1)
Axis (C2)
Cervical curvature
C7
T1
Thoracic curvature
T12
L1
Lumbar curvature
L5
Sacrum (S1–5)
Sacral curvature
Coccyx

Posterior view

Atlas (C1)
Axis (C2)
Cervical vertebrae
C7
T1
Thoracic vertebrae
T12
L1
Lumbar vertebrae
L5
Sacrum (S1–5)
Coccyx

F. Netter M.D.

Lower Bones Tables 0Q2–0QW

Section	0	Medical and Surgical
Body System	Q	Lower Bones
Operation	2	**Change:** Taking out or off a device from a body part and putting back an identical or similar device in or on the same body part without cutting or puncturing the skin or a mucous membrane

Body Part (4th)	Approach (5th)	Device (6th)	Qualifier (7th)
Y Lower Bone	X External	0 Drainage Device Y Other Device	Z No Qualifier

Section	0	Medical and Surgical
Body System	Q	Lower Bones
Operation	5	**Destruction:** Physical eradication of all or a portion of a body part by the direct use of energy, force, or a destructive agent

Body Part (4th)	Approach (5th)	Device (6th)	Qualifier (7th)
0 Lumbar Vertebra 1 Sacrum 2 Pelvic Bone, Right 3 Pelvic Bone, Left 4 Acetabulum, Right 5 Acetabulum, Left 6 Upper Femur, Right 7 Upper Femur, Left 8 Femoral Shaft, Right 9 Femoral Shaft, Left B Lower Femur, Right C Lower Femur, Left D Patella, Right F Patella, Left G Tibia, Right H Tibia, Left J Fibula, Right K Fibula, Left L Tarsal, Right M Tarsal, Left N Metatarsal, Right P Metatarsal, Left Q Toe Phalanx, Right R Toe Phalanx, Left S Coccyx	0 Open 3 Percutaneous 4 Percutaneous Endoscopic	Z No Device	Z No Qualifier

Section	0	Medical and Surgical
Body System	Q	Lower Bones
Operation	8	Division: Cutting into a body part, without draining fluids and/or gases from the body part, in order to separate or transect a body part

Body Part (4th)	Approach (5th)	Device (6th)	Qualifier (7th)
0 Lumbar Vertebra 1 Sacrum 2 Pelvic Bone, Right 3 Pelvic Bone, Left 4 Acetabulum, Right 5 Acetabulum, Left 6 Upper Femur, Right 7 Upper Femur, Left 8 Femoral Shaft, Right 9 Femoral Shaft, Left B Lower Femur, Right C Lower Femur, Left D Patella, Right F Patella, Left G Tibia, Right H Tibia, Left J Fibula, Right K Fibula, Left L Tarsal, Right M Tarsal, Left N Metatarsal, Right P Metatarsal, Left Q Toe Phalanx, Right R Toe Phalanx, Left S Coccyx	0 Open 3 Percutaneous 4 Percutaneous Endoscopic	Z No Device	Z No Qualifier

Section	0	Medical and Surgical
Body System	Q	Lower Bones
Operation	9	Drainage: Taking or letting out fluids and/or gases from a body part

Body Part (4th)	Approach (5th)	Device (6th)	Qualifier (7th)
0 Lumbar Vertebra 1 Sacrum 2 Pelvic Bone, Right 3 Pelvic Bone, Left 4 Acetabulum, Right 5 Acetabulum, Left 6 Upper Femur, Right 7 Upper Femur, Left 8 Femoral Shaft, Right 9 Femoral Shaft, Left B Lower Femur, Right C Lower Femur, Left D Patella, Right F Patella, Left G Tibia, Right H Tibia, Left J Fibula, Right K Fibula, Left L Tarsal, Right M Tarsal, Left N Metatarsal, Right P Metatarsal, Left Q Toe Phalanx, Right R Toe Phalanx, Left S Coccyx	0 Open 3 Percutaneous 4 Percutaneous Endoscopic	0 Drainage Device	Z No Qualifier

Continued →

Section	0	Medical and Surgical
Body System	Q	Lower Bones
Operation	9	**Drainage:** Taking or letting out fluids and/or gases from a body part

Body Part (4th)	Approach (5th)	Device (6th)	Qualifier (7th)
0 Lumbar Vertebra 1 Sacrum 2 Pelvic Bone, Right 3 Pelvic Bone, Left 4 Acetabulum, Right 5 Acetabulum, Left 6 Upper Femur, Right 7 Upper Femur, Left 8 Femoral Shaft, Right 9 Femoral Shaft, Left B Lower Femur, Right C Lower Femur, Left D Patella, Right F Patella, Left G Tibia, Right H Tibia, Left J Fibula, Right K Fibula, Left L Tarsal, Right M Tarsal, Left N Metatarsal, Right P Metatarsal, Left Q Toe Phalanx, Right R Toe Phalanx, Left S Coccyx	0 Open 3 Percutaneous 4 Percutaneous Endoscopic	Z No Device	X Diagnostic Z No Qualifier

Section	0	Medical and Surgical
Body System	Q	Lower Bones
Operation	B	**Excision:** Cutting out or off, without replacement, a portion of a body part

Body Part (4th)	Approach (5th)	Device (6th)	Qualifier (7th)
0 Lumbar Vertebra 1 Sacrum 2 Pelvic Bone, Right 3 Pelvic Bone, Left 4 Acetabulum, Right 5 Acetabulum, Left 6 Upper Femur, Right 7 Upper Femur, Left 8 Femoral Shaft, Right 9 Femoral Shaft, Left B Lower Femur, Right C Lower Femur, Left D Patella, Right F Patella, Left G Tibia, Right H Tibia, Left J Fibula, Right K Fibula, Left L Tarsal, Right M Tarsal, Left N Metatarsal, Right P Metatarsal, Left Q Toe Phalanx, Right R Toe Phalanx, Left S Coccyx	0 Open 3 Percutaneous 4 Percutaneous Endoscopic	Z No Device	X Diagnostic Z No Qualifier

Section	0	Medical and Surgical
Body System	Q	Lower Bones
Operation	C	Extirpation: Taking or cutting out solid matter from a body part

Body Part (4th)	Approach (5th)	Device (6th)	Qualifier (7th)
0 Lumbar Vertebra 1 Sacrum 2 Pelvic Bone, Right 3 Pelvic Bone, Left 4 Acetabulum, Right 5 Acetabulum, Left 6 Upper Femur, Right 7 Upper Femur, Left 8 Femoral Shaft, Right 9 Femoral Shaft, Left B Lower Femur, Right C Lower Femur, Left D Patella, Right F Patella, Left G Tibia, Right H Tibia, Left J Fibula, Right K Fibula, Left L Tarsal, Right M Tarsal, Left N Metatarsal, Right P Metatarsal, Left Q Toe Phalanx, Right R Toe Phalanx, Left S Coccyx	0 Open 3 Percutaneous 4 Percutaneous Endoscopic	Z No Device	Z No Qualifier

Section	0	Medical and Surgical
Body System	Q	Lower Bones
Operation	D	Extraction: Pulling or stripping out or off all or a portion of a body part by the use of force

Body Part (4th)	Approach (5th)	Device (6th)	Qualifier (7th)
0 Lumbar Vertebra 1 Sacrum 2 Pelvic Bone, Right 3 Pelvic Bone, Left 4 Acetabulum, Right 5 Acetabulum, Left 6 Upper Femur, Right 7 Upper Femur, Left 8 Femoral Shaft, Right 9 Femoral Shaft, Left B Lower Femur, Right C Lower Femur, Left D Patella, Right F Patella, Left G Tibia, Right H Tibia, Left J Fibula, Right K Fibula, Left L Tarsal, Right M Tarsal, Left N Metatarsal, Right P Metatarsal, Left Q Toe Phalanx, Right R Toe Phalanx, Left S Coccyx	0 Open	Z No Device	Z No Qualifier

Section	0	Medical and Surgical
Body System	Q	Lower Bones
Operation	H	Insertion: Putting in a nonbiological appliance that monitors, assists, performs, or prevents a physiological function but does not physically take the place of a body part

Body Part (4th)	Approach (5th)	Device (6th)	Qualifier (7th)
0 Lumbar Vertebra 1 Sacrum 2 Pelvic Bone, Right 3 Pelvic Bone, Left 4 Acetabulum, Right 5 Acetabulum, Left D Patella, Right F Patella, Left L Tarsal, Right M Tarsal, Left N Metatarsal, Right P Metatarsal, Left Q Toe Phalanx, Right R Toe Phalanx, Left S Coccyx	0 Open 3 Percutaneous 4 Percutaneous Endoscopic	4 Internal Fixation Device 5 External Fixation Device	Z No Qualifier
6 Upper Femur, Right 7 Upper Femur, Left B Lower Femur, Right C Lower Femur, Left J Fibula, Right K Fibula, Left	0 Open 3 Percutaneous 4 Percutaneous Endoscopic	4 Internal Fixation Device 5 External Fixation Device 6 Internal Fixation Device, Intramedullary 8 External Fixation Device, Limb Lengthening B External Fixation Device, Monoplanar C External Fixation Device, Ring D External Fixation Device, Hybrid	Z No Qualifier
8 Femoral Shaft, Right 9 Femoral Shaft, Left G Tibia, Right H Tibia, Left	0 Open 3 Percutaneous 4 Percutaneous Endoscopic	4 Internal Fixation Device 5 External Fixation Device 6 Internal Fixation Device, Intramedullary 7 Internal Fixation Device, Intramedullary Limb Lengthening 8 External Fixation Device, Limb Lengthening B External Fixation Device, Monoplanar C External Fixation Device, Ring D External Fixation Device, Hybrid	Z No Qualifier
Y Lower Bone	0 Open 3 Percutaneous 4 Percutaneous Endoscopic	M Bone Growth Stimulator	Z No Qualifier

Section	0	Medical and Surgical
Body System	Q	Lower Bones
Operation	J	Inspection: Visually and/or manually exploring a body part

Body Part (4th)	Approach (5th)	Device (6th)	Qualifier (7th)
Y Lower Bone	0 Open 3 Percutaneous 4 Percutaneous Endoscopic X External	Z No Device	Z No Qualifier

Section 0 **Medical and Surgical**
Body System Q **Lower Bones**
Operation N **Release:** Freeing a body part from an abnormal physical constraint by cutting or by the use of force

Body Part (4th)	Approach (5th)	Device (6th)	Qualifier (7th)
0 Lumbar Vertebra	0 Open	Z No Device	Z No Qualifier
1 Sacrum	3 Percutaneous		
2 Pelvic Bone, Right	4 Percutaneous Endoscopic		
3 Pelvic Bone, Left			
4 Acetabulum, Right			
5 Acetabulum, Left			
6 Upper Femur, Right			
7 Upper Femur, Left			
8 Femoral Shaft, Right			
9 Femoral Shaft, Left			
B Lower Femur, Right			
C Lower Femur, Left			
D Patella, Right			
F Patella, Left			
G Tibia, Right			
H Tibia, Left			
J Fibula, Right			
K Fibula, Left			
L Tarsal, Right			
M Tarsal, Left			
N Metatarsal, Right			
P Metatarsal, Left			
Q Toe Phalanx, Right			
R Toe Phalanx, Left			
S Coccyx			

Section 0 **Medical and Surgical**
Body System Q **Lower Bones**
Operation P **Removal:** Taking out or off a device from a body part

Body Part (4th)	Approach (5th)	Device (6th)	Qualifier (7th)
0 Lumbar Vertebra	0 Open	4 Internal Fixation Device	Z No Qualifier
1 Sacrum	3 Percutaneous	5 External Fixation Device	
2 Pelvic Bone, Right	4 Percutaneous Endoscopic	7 Autologous Tissue Substitute	
3 Pelvic Bone, Left		J Synthetic Substitute	
4 Acetabulum, Right		K Nonautologous Tissue Substitute	
5 Acetabulum, Left			
6 Upper Femur, Right			
7 Upper Femur, Left			
8 Femoral Shaft, Right			
9 Femoral Shaft, Left			
B Lower Femur, Right			
C Lower Femur, Left			
D Patella, Right			
F Patella, Left			
G Tibia, Right			
H Tibia, Left			
J Fibula, Right			
K Fibula, Left			
L Tarsal, Right			
M Tarsal, Left			
N Metatarsal, Right			
P Metatarsal, Left			
Q Toe Phalanx, Right			
R Toe Phalanx, Left			
S Coccyx			

Continued →

Section	0	Medical and Surgical
Body System	Q	Lower Bones
Operation	P	Removal: Taking out or off a device from a body part

Body Part (4ᵗʰ)	Approach (5ᵗʰ)	Device (6ᵗʰ)	Qualifier (7ᵗʰ)
0 Lumbar Vertebra 1 Sacrum 2 Pelvic Bone, Right 3 Pelvic Bone, Left 4 Acetabulum, Right 5 Acetabulum, Left 6 Upper Femur, Right 7 Upper Femur, Left 8 Femoral Shaft, Right 9 Femoral Shaft, Left B Lower Femur, Right C Lower Femur, Left D Patella, Right F Patella, Left G Tibia, Right H Tibia, Left J Fibula, Right K Fibula, Left L Tarsal, Right M Tarsal, Left N Metatarsal, Right P Metatarsal, Left Q Toe Phalanx, Right R Toe Phalanx, Left S Coccyx	X External	4 Internal Fixation Device 5 External Fixation Device	Z No Qualifier
Y Lower Bone	0 Open 3 Percutaneous 4 Percutaneous Endoscopic X External	0 Drainage Device M Bone Growth Stimulator	Z No Qualifier

Section	0	Medical and Surgical
Body System	Q	Lower Bones
Operation	Q	Repair: Restoring, to the extent possible, a body part to its normal anatomic structure and function

Body Part (4ᵗʰ)	Approach (5ᵗʰ)	Device (6ᵗʰ)	Qualifier (7ᵗʰ)
0 Lumbar Vertebra 1 Sacrum 2 Pelvic Bone, Right 3 Pelvic Bone, Left 4 Acetabulum, Right 5 Acetabulum, Left 6 Upper Femur, Right 7 Upper Femur, Left 8 Femoral Shaft, Right 9 Femoral Shaft, Left B Lower Femur, Right C Lower Femur, Left D Patella, Right F Patella, Left G Tibia, Right H Tibia, Left J Fibula, Right K Fibula, Left L Tarsal, Right M Tarsal, Left N Metatarsal, Right P Metatarsal, Left Q Toe Phalanx, Right R Toe Phalanx, Left S Coccyx	0 Open 3 Percutaneous 4 Percutaneous Endoscopic X External	Z No Device	Z No Qualifier

Section	**0**	**Medical and Surgical**
Body System	**Q**	**Lower Bones**
Operation	**R**	**Replacement:** Putting in or on biological or synthetic material that physically takes the place and/or function of all or a portion of a body part

Body Part (4ᵗʰ)	Approach (5ᵗʰ)	Device (6ᵗʰ)	Qualifier (7ᵗʰ)
0 Lumbar Vertebra 1 Sacrum 2 Pelvic Bone, Right 3 Pelvic Bone, Left 4 Acetabulum, Right 5 Acetabulum, Left 6 Upper Femur, Right 7 Upper Femur, Left 8 Femoral Shaft, Right 9 Femoral Shaft, Left B Lower Femur, Right C Lower Femur, Left D Patella, Right F Patella, Left G Tibia, Right H Tibia, Left J Fibula, Right K Fibula, Left L Tarsal, Right M Tarsal, Left N Metatarsal, Right P Metatarsal, Left Q Toe Phalanx, Right R Toe Phalanx, Left S Coccyx	0 Open 3 Percutaneous 4 Percutaneous Endoscopic	7 Autologous Tissue Substitute J Synthetic Substitute K Nonautologous Tissue Substitute	Z No Qualifier

Section	**0**	**Medical and Surgical**
Body System	**Q**	**Lower Bones**
Operation	**S**	**Reposition:** Moving to its normal location, or other suitable location, all or a portion of a body part

Body Part (4ᵗʰ)	Approach (5ᵗʰ)	Device (6ᵗʰ)	Qualifier (7ᵗʰ)
0 Lumbar Vertebra 1 Sacrum 4 Acetabulum, Right 5 Acetabulum, Left S Coccyx	0 Open 3 Percutaneous 4 Percutaneous Endoscopic	4 Internal Fixation Device Z No Device	Z No Qualifier
0 Lumbar Vertebra 1 Sacrum 4 Acetabulum, Right 5 Acetabulum, Left S Coccyx	X External	Z No Device	Z No Qualifier
2 Pelvic Bone, Right 3 Pelvic Bone, Left D Patella, Right F Patella, Left L Tarsal, Right M Tarsal, Left Q Toe Phalanx, Right R Toe Phalanx, Left	0 Open 3 Percutaneous 4 Percutaneous Endoscopic	4 Internal Fixation Device 5 External Fixation Device Z No Device	Z No Qualifier
2 Pelvic Bone, Right 3 Pelvic Bone, Left D Patella, Right F Patella, Left L Tarsal, Right M Tarsal, Left Q Toe Phalanx, Right R Toe Phalanx, Left	X External	Z No Device	Z No Qualifier

Continued →

Section 0 **Medical and Surgical**
Body System Q **Lower Bones**
Operation S **Reposition:** Moving to its normal location, or other suitable location, all or a portion of a body part

Body Part (4th)	Approach (5th)	Device (6th)	Qualifier (7th)
6 Upper Femur, Right 7 Upper Femur, Left 8 Femoral Shaft, Right 9 Femoral Shaft, Left B Lower Femur, Right C Lower Femur, Left G Tibia, Right H Tibia, Left J Fibula, Right K Fibula, Left	0 Open 3 Percutaneous 4 Percutaneous Endoscopic	4 Internal Fixation Device 5 External Fixation Device 6 Internal Fixation Device, Intramedullary B External Fixation Device, Monoplanar C External Fixation Device, Ring D External Fixation Device, Hybrid Z No Device	Z No Qualifier
6 Upper Femur, Right 7 Upper Femur, Left 8 Femoral Shaft, Right 9 Femoral Shaft, Left B Lower Femur, Right C Lower Femur, Left G Tibia, Right H Tibia, Left J Fibula, Right K Fibula, Left	X External	Z No Device	Z No Qualifier
N Metatarsal, Right P Metatarsal, Left	0 Open 3 Percutaneous 4 Percutaneous Endoscopic	4 Internal Fixation Device 5 External Fixation Device Z No Device	2 Sesamoid Bone(s) 1st Toe Z No Qualifier
N Metatarsal, Right P Metatarsal, Left	X External	Z No Device	2 Sesamoid Bone(s) 1st Toe Z No Qualifier

Section 0 **Medical and Surgical**
Body System Q **Lower Bones**
Operation T **Resection:** Cutting out or off, without replacement, all of a body part

Body Part (4th)	Approach (5th)	Device (6th)	Qualifier (7th)
2 Pelvic Bone, Right 3 Pelvic Bone, Left 4 Acetabulum, Right 5 Acetabulum, Left 6 Upper Femur, Right 7 Upper Femur, Left 8 Femoral Shaft, Right 9 Femoral Shaft, Left B Lower Femur, Right C Lower Femur, Left D Patella, Right F Patella, Left G Tibia, Right H Tibia, Left J Fibula, Right K Fibula, Left L Tarsal, Right M Tarsal, Left N Metatarsal, Right P Metatarsal, Left Q Toe Phalanx, Right R Toe Phalanx, Left S Coccyx	0 Open	Z No Device	Z No Qualifier

Section 0 **Medical and Surgical**
Body System Q **Lower Bones**
Operation U **Supplement:** Putting in or on biological or synthetic material that physically reinforces and/or augments the function of a portion of a body part

Body Part (4th)	Approach (5th)	Device (6th)	Qualifier (7th)
0 Lumbar Vertebra	0 Open	7 Autologous Tissue Substitute	Z No Qualifier
1 Sacrum	3 Percutaneous	J Synthetic Substitute	
2 Pelvic Bone, Right	4 Percutaneous Endoscopic	K Nonautologous Tissue Substitute	
3 Pelvic Bone, Left			
4 Acetabulum, Right			
5 Acetabulum, Left			
6 Upper Femur, Right			
7 Upper Femur, Left			
8 Femoral Shaft, Right			
9 Femoral Shaft, Left			
B Lower Femur, Right			
C Lower Femur, Left			
D Patella, Right			
F Patella, Left			
G Tibia, Right			
H Tibia, Left			
J Fibula, Right			
K Fibula, Left			
L Tarsal, Right			
M Tarsal, Left			
N Metatarsal, Right			
P Metatarsal, Left			
Q Toe Phalanx, Right			
R Toe Phalanx, Left			
S Coccyx			

Section 0 **Medical and Surgical**
Body System Q **Lower Bones**
Operation W **Revision:** Correcting, to the extent possible, a portion of a malfunctioning device or the position of a displaced device

Body Part (4th)	Approach (5th)	Device (6th)	Qualifier (7th)
0 Lumbar Vertebra	0 Open	4 Internal Fixation Device	Z No Qualifier
1 Sacrum	3 Percutaneous	7 Autologous Tissue Substitute	
4 Acetabulum, Right	4 Percutaneous Endoscopic	J Synthetic Substitute	
5 Acetabulum, Left	X External	K Nonautologous Tissue Substitute	
S Coccyx			
2 Pelvic Bone, Right	0 Open	4 Internal Fixation Device	Z No Qualifier
3 Pelvic Bone, Left	3 Percutaneous	5 External Fixation Device	
6 Upper Femur, Right	4 Percutaneous Endoscopic	7 Autologous Tissue Substitute	
7 Upper Femur, Left	X External	J Synthetic Substitute	
8 Femoral Shaft, Right		K Nonautologous Tissue Substitute	
9 Femoral Shaft, Left			
B Lower Femur, Right			
C Lower Femur, Left			
D Patella, Right			
F Patella, Left			
G Tibia, Right			
H Tibia, Left			
J Fibula, Right			
K Fibula, Left			
L Tarsal, Right			
M Tarsal, Left			
N Metatarsal, Right			
P Metatarsal, Left			
Q Toe Phalanx, Right			
R Toe Phalanx, Left			

Continued →

410

Section 0 **Medical and Surgical**
Body System Q **Lower Bones**
Operation W **Revision:** Correcting, to the extent possible, a portion of a malfunctioning device or the position of a displaced device

0QW Continued

0QW

Body Part (4th)	Approach (5th)	Device (6th)	Qualifier (7th)
Y Lower Bone	**0** Open **3** Percutaneous **4** Percutaneous Endoscopic **X** External	**0** Drainage Device **M** Bone Growth Stimulator	**Z** No Qualifier

AHA Coding Clinic

0Q830ZZ Division of Left Pelvic Bone, Open Approach—AHA CC: 2Q, 2016, 32

0QB10ZZ Excision of Sacrum, Open Approach—AHA CC: 2Q, 2020, 26

0QB20ZZ Excision of Right Pelvic Bone, Open Approach—AHA CC: 2Q, 2014, 6-7: 4Q, 2018, 12-13

0QB30ZZ Excision of Left Pelvic Bone, Open Approach—AHA CC: 2Q, 2019, 19-20

0QB74ZZ Excision of Left Upper Femur, Percutaneous Endoscopic Approach—AHA CC: 4Q, 2014, 25-26

0QBJ0ZZ Excision of Right Fibula, Open Approach—AHA CC: 1Q, 2017, 23-24

0QBK0ZZ Excision of Left Fibula, Open Approach—AHA CC: 2Q, 2013, 39-40

0QBL0ZZ Excision of Right Tarsal, Open Approach—AHA CC: 3Q, 2018, 17-18

0QH204Z Insertion of Internal Fixation Device into Right Pelvic Bone, Open Approach—AHA CC: 1Q, 2017, 21-22

0QH304Z Insertion of Internal Fixation Device into Left Pelvic Bone, Open Approach—AHA CC: 1Q, 2017, 21-22

0QHG04Z Insertion of Internal Fixation Device into Right Tibia, Open Approach—AHA CC: 3Q, 2016, 34-35

0QHJ04Z Insertion of Internal Fixation Device into Right Fibula, Open Approach—AHA CC: 3Q, 2016, 34-35

0QP004Z Removal of Internal Fixation Device from Lumbar Vertebra, Open Approach—AHA CC: 4Q, 2017, 75

0QPG04Z Removal of Internal Fixation Device from Right Tibia, Open Approach—AHA CC: 2Q, 2015, 6-7

0QQ10ZZ Repair Sacrum, Open Approach—AHA CC: 3Q, 2014, 24

0QQ20ZZ Repair Right Pelvic Bone, Open Approach—AHA CC: 1Q, 2018, 15

0QQ30ZZ Repair Left Pelvic Bone, Open Approach—AHA CC: 1Q, 2018, 15

0QS004Z Reposition Lumbar Vertebra with Internal Fixation Device, Open Approach—AHA CC: 1Q, 2020, 33-34

0QS504Z Reposition Left Acetabulum with Internal Fixation Device, Open Approach—AHA CC: 2Q, 2016, 32; 1Q, 2018, 25

0QS904Z Reposition Left Femoral Shaft with Internal Fixation Device, Open Approach—AHA CC: 3Q, 2019, 26

0QSC04Z Reposition Left Lower Femur with Internal Fixation Device, Open Approach—AHA CC: 4Q, 2014, 31

0QSF04Z Reposition Left Patella with Internal Fixation Device, Open Approach—AHA CC: 3Q, 2016, 34-35

0QSH04Z Reposition Left Tibia with Internal Fixation Device, Open Approach—AHA CC: 4Q, 2014, 30-31; 3Q, 2016, 34-35

0QSK0ZZ Reposition Left Fibula, Open Approach—AHA CC: 3Q, 2016, 34-35

0QSL04Z Reposition Right Tarsal with Internal Fixation Device, Open Approach—AHA CC: 1Q, 2018, 13

0QSM04Z Reposition Left Tarsal with Internal Fixation Device, Open Approach—AHA CC: 1Q, 2018, 13

0QT60ZZ Resection of Right Upper Femur, Open Approach—AHA CC: 3Q, 2016, 30-31

0QT70ZZ Resection of Left Upper Femur, Open Approach—AHA CC: 3Q, 2015, 26; 3Q, 2016, 30-31

0QTC0ZZ Resection of Left Lower Femur, Open Approach—AHA CC: 4Q, 2014, 30-31

0QU03JZ Supplement Lumbar Vertebra with Synthetic Substitute, Percutaneous Approach—AHA CC: 2Q, 2014, 12-13; 2Q, 2019, 35

0QU20JZ Supplement Right Pelvic Bone with Synthetic Substitute, Open Approach—AHA CC: 2Q, 2013, 35-36

0QU50JZ Supplement Left Acetabulum with Synthetic Substitute, Open Approach—AHA CC: 3Q, 2015, 18-19

0QU90KZ Supplement Left Femoral Shaft with Nonautologous Tissue Substitute, Open Approach—AHA CC: 3Q, 2019, 26

0QUC0KZ Supplement Left Lower Femur with—Nonautologous Tissue Substitute, Open Approach—AHA CC: 4Q, 2014, 31

0QW034Z Revision of Internal Fixation Device in Lumbar Vertebra, Percutaneous Approach—AHA CC: 4Q, 2017, 75

Intervertebral Joint

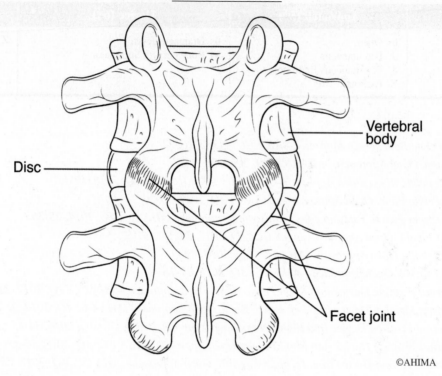

Disc

Vertebral body

Facet joint

©AHIMA

Shoulder

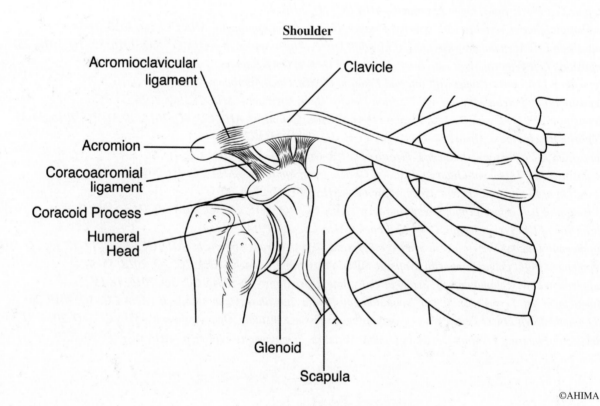

Acromioclavicular ligament

Clavicle

Acromion

Coracoacromial ligament

Coracoid Process

Humeral Head

Glenoid

Scapula

©AHIMA

Anterior Interbody Fusion by Dowel Graft

Cervical Spine Injury: Anterior Interbody Fusion by Dowel Graft (Cloward)

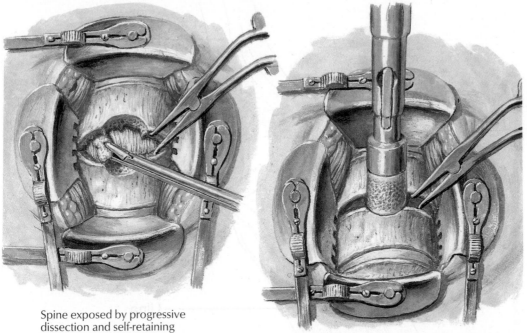

Spine exposed by progressive dissection and self-retaining retractors inserted. Disc, osteophytes and bone fragments removed under direct vision

Dowel bone graft obtained from ilium or bone bank is cut 2 mm wider and 2 mm shorter than drill hole. It is impacted after hole is widened with vertebra spreader

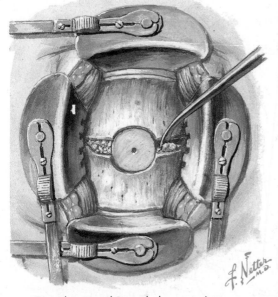

Dowel recessed 2 mm below anterior margin of drill hole. When spreader is removed, graft is locked securely in place. Cortical end plates lateral to dowel are perforated and interspace packed with bone dust removed from drill

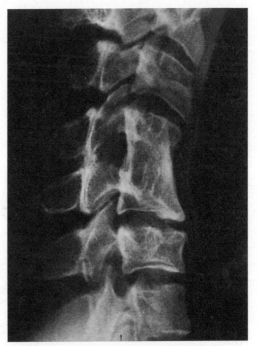

Follow-up x-ray film. Dowel graft fusion of C5-6 with good union

Elbow

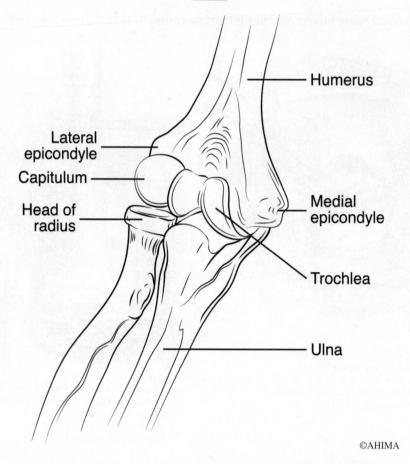

Humerus

Lateral
epicondyle

Capitulum

Head of
radius

Medial
epicondyle

Trochlea

Ulna

©AHIMA

Wrist

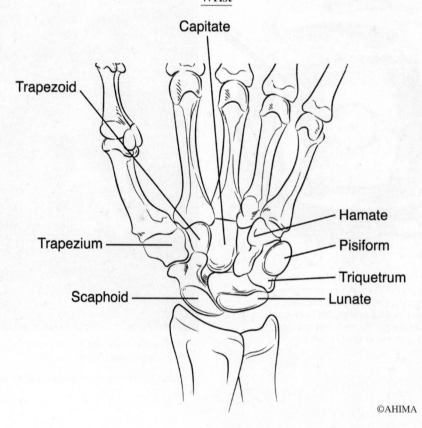

Capitate

Trapezoid

Trapezium

Scaphoid

Hamate

Pisiform

Triquetrum

Lunate

©AHIMA

Section   **0**   **Medical and Surgical**
Body System   **R**   **Upper Joints**
Operation   **2**   **Change:** Taking out or off a device from a body part and putting back an identical or similar device in or on the same body part without cutting or puncturing the skin or a mucous membrane

Body Part (4th)	Approach (5th)	Device (6th)	Qualifier (7th)
Y Upper Joint	**X** External	**0** Drainage Device **Y** Other Device	**Z** No Qualifier

Section   **0**   **Medical and Surgical**
Body System   **R**   **Upper Joints**
Operation   **5**   **Destruction:** Physical eradication of all or a portion of a body part by the direct use of energy, force, or a destructive agent

Body Part (4th)	Approach (5th)	Device (6th)	Qualifier (7th)
0 Occipital-cervical Joint **1** Cervical Vertebral Joint **3** Cervical Vertebral Disc **4** Cervicothoracic Vertebral Joint **5** Cervicothoracic Vertebral Disc **6** Thoracic Vertebral Joint **9** Thoracic Vertebral Disc **A** Thoracolumbar Vertebral Joint **B** Thoracolumbar Vertebral Disc **C** Temporomandibular Joint, Right **D** Temporomandibular Joint, Left **E** Sternoclavicular Joint, Right **F** Sternoclavicular Joint, Left **G** Acromioclavicular Joint, Right **H** Acromioclavicular Joint, Left **J** Shoulder Joint, Right **K** Shoulder Joint, Left **L** Elbow Joint, Right **M** Elbow Joint, Left **N** Wrist Joint, Right **P** Wrist Joint, Left **Q** Carpal Joint, Right **R** Carpal Joint, Left **S** Carpometacarpal Joint, Right **T** Carpometacarpal Joint, Left **U** Metacarpophalangeal Joint, Right **V** Metacarpophalangeal Joint, Left **W** Finger Phalangeal Joint, Right **X** Finger Phalangeal Joint, Left	**0** Open **3** Percutaneous **4** Percutaneous Endoscopic	**Z** No Device	**Z** No Qualifier

Section	0	Medical and Surgical
Body System	R	Upper Joints
Operation	9	**Drainage:** Taking or letting out fluids and/or gases from a body part

Body Part (4th)	Approach (5th)	Device (6th)	Qualifier (7th)
0 Occipital-cervical Joint 1 Cervical Vertebral Joint 3 Cervical Vertebral Disc 4 Cervicothoracic Vertebral Joint 5 Cervicothoracic Vertebral Disc 6 Thoracic Vertebral Joint 9 Thoracic Vertebral Disc A Thoracolumbar Vertebral Joint B Thoracolumbar Vertebral Disc C Temporomandibular Joint, Right D Temporomandibular Joint, Left E Sternoclavicular Joint, Right F Sternoclavicular Joint, Left G Acromioclavicular Joint, Right H Acromioclavicular Joint, Left J Shoulder Joint, Right K Shoulder Joint, Left L Elbow Joint, Right M Elbow Joint, Left N Wrist Joint, Right P Wrist Joint, Left Q Carpal Joint, Right R Carpal Joint, Left S Carpometacarpal Joint, Right T Carpometacarpal Joint, Left U Metacarpophalangeal Joint, Right V Metacarpophalangeal Joint, Left W Finger Phalangeal Joint, Right X Finger Phalangeal Joint, Left	0 Open 3 Percutaneous 4 Percutaneous Endoscopic	0 Drainage Device	Z No Qualifier
0 Occipital-cervical Joint 1 Cervical Vertebral Joint 3 Cervical Vertebral Disc 4 Cervicothoracic Vertebral Joint 5 Cervicothoracic Vertebral Disc 6 Thoracic Vertebral Joint 9 Thoracic Vertebral Disc A Thoracolumbar Vertebral Joint B Thoracolumbar Vertebral Disc C Temporomandibular Joint, Right D Temporomandibular Joint, Left E Sternoclavicular Joint, Right F Sternoclavicular Joint, Left G Acromioclavicular Joint, Right H Acromioclavicular Joint, Left J Shoulder Joint, Right K Shoulder Joint, Left L Elbow Joint, Right M Elbow Joint, Left N Wrist Joint, Right P Wrist Joint, Left Q Carpal Joint, Right R Carpal Joint, Left S Carpometacarpal Joint, Right T Carpometacarpal Joint, Left U Metacarpophalangeal Joint, Right V Metacarpophalangeal Joint, Left W Finger Phalangeal Joint, Right X Finger Phalangeal Joint, Left	0 Open 3 Percutaneous 4 Percutaneous Endoscopic	Z No Device	X Diagnostic Z No Qualifier

Section	0	Medical and Surgical
Body System	R	Upper Joints
Operation	B	Excision: Cutting out or off, without replacement, a portion of a body part

Body Part (4th)	Approach (5th)	Device (6th)	Qualifier (7th)
0 Occipital-cervical Joint	0 Open	Z No Device	X Diagnostic
1 Cervical Vertebral Joint	3 Percutaneous		Z No Qualifier
3 Cervical Vertebral Disc	4 Percutaneous Endoscopic		
4 Cervicothoracic Vertebral Joint			
5 Cervicothoracic Vertebral Disc			
6 Thoracic Vertebral Joint			
9 Thoracic Vertebral Disc			
A Thoracolumbar Vertebral Joint			
B Thoracolumbar Vertebral Disc			
C Temporomandibular Joint, Right			
D Temporomandibular Joint, Left			
E Sternoclavicular Joint, Right			
F Sternoclavicular Joint, Left			
G Acromioclavicular Joint, Right			
H Acromioclavicular Joint, Left			
J Shoulder Joint, Right			
K Shoulder Joint, Left			
L Elbow Joint, Right			
M Elbow Joint, Left			
N Wrist Joint, Right			
P Wrist Joint, Left			
Q Carpal Joint, Right			
R Carpal Joint, Left			
S Carpometacarpal Joint, Right			
T Carpometacarpal Joint, Left			
U Metacarpophalangeal Joint, Right			
V Metacarpophalangeal Joint, Left			
W Finger Phalangeal Joint, Right			
X Finger Phalangeal Joint, Left			

Section	0	Medical and Surgical
Body System	R	Upper Joints
Operation	C	**Extirpation:** Taking or cutting out solid matter from a body part

Body Part (4th)	Approach (5th)	Device (6th)	Qualifier (7th)
0 Occipital-cervical Joint 1 Cervical Vertebral Joint 3 Cervical Vertebral Disc 4 Cervicothoracic Vertebral Joint 5 Cervicothoracic Vertebral Disc 6 Thoracic Vertebral Joint 9 Thoracic Vertebral Disc A Thoracolumbar Vertebral Joint B Thoracolumbar Vertebral Disc C Temporomandibular Joint, Right D Temporomandibular Joint, Left E Sternoclavicular Joint, Right F Sternoclavicular Joint, Left G Acromioclavicular Joint, Right H Acromioclavicular Joint, Left J Shoulder Joint, Right K Shoulder Joint, Left L Elbow Joint, Right M Elbow Joint, Left N Wrist Joint, Right P Wrist Joint, Left Q Carpal Joint, Right R Carpal Joint, Left S Carpometacarpal Joint, Right T Carpometacarpal Joint, Left U Metacarpophalangeal Joint, Right V Metacarpophalangeal Joint, Left W Finger Phalangeal Joint, Right X Finger Phalangeal Joint, Left	0 Open 3 Percutaneous 4 Percutaneous Endoscopic	Z No Device	Z No Qualifier

Section	0	Medical and Surgical
Body System	R	Upper Joints
Operation	G	**Fusion:** Joining together portions of an articular body part rendering the articular body part immobile

Body Part (4th)	Approach (5th)	Device (6th)	Qualifier (7th)
0 Occipital-cervical Joint 1 Cervical Vertebral Joint 2 Cervical Vertebral Joints, 2 or more 4 Cervicothoracic Vertebral Joint 6 Thoracic Vertebral Joint 7 Thoracic Vertebral Joints, 2 to 7 8 Thoracic Vertebral Joints, 8 or more A Thoracolumbar Vertebral Joint	0 Open 3 Percutaneous 4 Percutaneous Endoscopic	7 Autologous Tissue Substitute J Synthetic Substitute K Nonautologous Tissue Substitute	0 Anterior Approach, Anterior Column 1 Posterior Approach, Posterior Column J Posterior Approach, Anterior Column
0 Occipital-cervical Joint 1 Cervical Vertebral Joint 2 Cervical Vertebral Joints, 2 or more 4 Cervicothoracic Vertebral Joint 6 Thoracic Vertebral Joint 7 Thoracic Vertebral Joints, 2 to 7 8 Thoracic Vertebral Joints, 8 or more A Thoracolumbar Vertebral Joint	0 Open 3 Percutaneous 4 Percutaneous Endoscopic	A Interbody Fusion Device	0 Anterior Approach, Anterior Column J Posterior Approach, Anterior Column
C Temporomandibular Joint, Right D Temporomandibular Joint, Left E Sternoclavicular Joint, Right F Sternoclavicular Joint, Left G Acromioclavicular Joint, Right H Acromioclavicular Joint, Left J Shoulder Joint, Right K Shoulder Joint, Left	0 Open 3 Percutaneous 4 Percutaneous Endoscopic	4 Internal Fixation Device 7 Autologous Tissue Substitute J Synthetic Substitute K Nonautologous Tissue Substitute	Z No Qualifier

Continued →

Section	0	Medical and Surgical
Body System	R	Upper Joints
Operation	G	**Fusion:** Joining together portions of an articular body part rendering the articular body part immobile

Body Part (4th)	Approach (5th)	Device (6th)	Qualifier (7th)
L Elbow Joint, Right M Elbow Joint, Left N Wrist Joint, Right P Wrist Joint, Left Q Carpal Joint, Right R Carpal Joint, Left S Carpometacarpal Joint, Right T Carpometacarpal Joint, Left U Metacarpophalangeal Joint, Right V Metacarpophalangeal Joint, Left W Finger Phalangeal Joint, Right X Finger Phalangeal Joint, Left	0 Open 3 Percutaneous 4 Percutaneous Endoscopic	3 Internal Fixation Device, Sustained Compression 4 Internal Fixation Device 5 External Fixation Device 7 Autologous Tissue Substitute J Synthetic Substitute K Nonautologous Tissue Substitute	Z No Qualifier

Section	0	Medical and Surgical
Body System	R	Upper Joints
Operation	H	**Insertion:** Putting in a nonbiological appliance that monitors, assists, performs, or prevents a physiological function but does not physically take the place of a body part

Body Part (4th)	Approach (5th)	Device (6th)	Qualifier (7th)
0 Occipital-cervical Joint 1 Cervical Vertebral Joint 4 Cervicothoracic Vertebral Joint 6 Thoracic Vertebral Joint A Thoracolumbar Vertebral Joint	0 Open 3 Percutaneous 4 Percutaneous Endoscopic	3 Infusion Device 4 Internal Fixation Device 8 Spacer B Spinal Stabilization Device, Interspinous Process C Spinal Stabilization Device, Pedicle-Based D Spinal Stabilization Device, Facet Replacement	Z No Qualifier
3 Cervical Vertebral Disc 5 Cervicothoracic Vertebral Disc 9 Thoracic Vertebral Disc B Thoracolumbar Vertebral Disc	0 Open 3 Percutaneous 4 Percutaneous Endoscopic	3 Infusion Device	Z No Qualifier
C Temporomandibular Joint, Right D Temporomandibular Joint, Left E Sternoclavicular Joint, Right F Sternoclavicular Joint, Left G Acromioclavicular Joint, Right H Acromioclavicular Joint, Left J Shoulder Joint, Right K Shoulder Joint, Left	0 Open 3 Percutaneous 4 Percutaneous Endoscopic	3 Infusion Device 4 Internal Fixation Device 8 Spacer	Z No Qualifier
L Elbow Joint, Right M Elbow Joint, Left N Wrist Joint, Right P Wrist Joint, Left Q Carpal Joint, Right R Carpal Joint, Left S Carpometacarpal Joint, Right T Carpometacarpal Joint, Left U Metacarpophalangeal Joint, Right V Metacarpophalangeal Joint, Left W Finger Phalangeal Joint, Right X Finger Phalangeal Joint, Left	0 Open 3 Percutaneous 4 Percutaneous Endoscopic	3 Infusion Device 4 Internal Fixation Device 5 External Fixation Device 8 Spacer	Z No Qualifier

Section	0	Medical and Surgical
Body System	R	Upper Joints
Operation	J	Inspection: Visually and/or manually exploring a body part

Body Part (4th)	Approach (5th)	Device (6th)	Qualifier (7th)
0 Occipital-cervical Joint	0 Open	Z No Device	Z No Qualifier
1 Cervical Vertebral Joint	3 Percutaneous		
3 Cervical Vertebral Disc	4 Percutaneous Endoscopic		
4 Cervicothoracic Vertebral Joint	X External		
5 Cervicothoracic Vertebral Disc			
6 Thoracic Vertebral Joint			
9 Thoracic Vertebral Disc			
A Thoracolumbar Vertebral Joint			
B Thoracolumbar Vertebral Disc			
C Temporomandibular Joint, Right			
D Temporomandibular Joint, Left			
E Sternoclavicular Joint, Right			
F Sternoclavicular Joint, Left			
G Acromioclavicular Joint, Right			
H Acromioclavicular Joint, Left			
J Shoulder Joint, Right			
K Shoulder Joint, Left			
L Elbow Joint, Right			
M Elbow Joint, Left			
N Wrist Joint, Right			
P Wrist Joint, Left			
Q Carpal Joint, Right			
R Carpal Joint, Left			
S Carpometacarpal Joint, Right			
T Carpometacarpal Joint, Left			
U Metacarpophalangeal Joint, Right			
V Metacarpophalangeal Joint, Left			
W Finger Phalangeal Joint, Right			
X Finger Phalangeal Joint, Left			

Section	0	Medical and Surgical
Body System	R	Upper Joints
Operation	N	Release: Freeing a body part from an abnormal physical constraint by cutting or by the use of force

Body Part (4th)	Approach (5th)	Device (6th)	Qualifier (7th)
0 Occipital-cervical Joint	0 Open	Z No Device	Z No Qualifier
1 Cervical Vertebral Joint	3 Percutaneous		
3 Cervical Vertebral Disc	4 Percutaneous Endoscopic		
4 Cervicothoracic Vertebral Joint	X External		
5 Cervicothoracic Vertebral Disc			
6 Thoracic Vertebral Joint			
9 Thoracic Vertebral Disc			
A Thoracolumbar Vertebral Joint			
B Thoracolumbar Vertebral Disc			
C Temporomandibular Joint, Right			
D Temporomandibular Joint, Left			
E Sternoclavicular Joint, Right			
F Sternoclavicular Joint, Left			
G Acromioclavicular Joint, Right			
H Acromioclavicular Joint, Left			
J Shoulder Joint, Right			
K Shoulder Joint, Left			
L Elbow Joint, Right			
M Elbow Joint, Left			
N Wrist Joint, Right			
P Wrist Joint, Left			
Q Carpal Joint, Right			
R Carpal Joint, Left			
S Carpometacarpal Joint, Right			
T Carpometacarpal Joint, Left			
U Metacarpophalangeal Joint, Right			
V Metacarpophalangeal Joint, Left			
W Finger Phalangeal Joint, Right			
X Finger Phalangeal Joint, Left			

Section	0	Medical and Surgical
Body System	R	Upper Joints
Operation	P	Removal: Taking out or off a device from a body part

Body Part (4th)	Approach (5th)	Device (6th)	Qualifier (7th)
0 Occipital-cervical Joint 1 Cervical Vertebral Joint 4 Cervicothoracic Vertebral Joint 6 Thoracic Vertebral Joint A Thoracolumbar Vertebral Joint	0 Open 3 Percutaneous 4 Percutaneous Endoscopic	0 Drainage Device 3 Infusion Device 4 Internal Fixation Device 7 Autologous Tissue Substitute 8 Spacer A Interbody Fusion Device J Synthetic Substitute K Nonautologous Tissue Substitute	Z No Qualifier
0 Occipital-cervical Joint 1 Cervical Vertebral Joint 4 Cervicothoracic Vertebral Joint 6 Thoracic Vertebral Joint A Thoracolumbar Vertebral Joint	X External	0 Drainage Device 3 Infusion Device 4 Internal Fixation Device	Z No Qualifier
3 Cervical Vertebral Disc 5 Cervicothoracic Vertebral Disc 9 Thoracic Vertebral Disc B Thoracolumbar Vertebral Disc	0 Open 3 Percutaneous 4 Percutaneous Endoscopic	0 Drainage Device 3 Infusion Device 7 Autologous Tissue Substitute J Synthetic Substitute K Nonautologous Tissue Substitute	Z No Qualifier
3 Cervical Vertebral Disc 5 Cervicothoracic Vertebral Disc 9 Thoracic Vertebral Disc B Thoracolumbar Vertebral Disc	X External	0 Drainage Device 3 Infusion Device	Z No Qualifier
C Temporomandibular Joint, Right D Temporomandibular Joint, Left E Sternoclavicular Joint, Right F Sternoclavicular Joint, Left G Acromioclavicular Joint, Right H Acromioclavicular Joint, Left J Shoulder Joint, Right K Shoulder Joint, Left	0 Open 3 Percutaneous 4 Percutaneous Endoscopic	0 Drainage Device 3 Infusion Device 4 Internal Fixation Device 7 Autologous Tissue Substitute 8 Spacer J Synthetic Substitute K Nonautologous Tissue Substitute	Z No Qualifier
C Temporomandibular Joint, Right D Temporomandibular Joint, Left E Sternoclavicular Joint, Right F Sternoclavicular Joint, Left G Acromioclavicular Joint, Right H Acromioclavicular Joint, Left J Shoulder Joint, Right K Shoulder Joint, Left	X External	0 Drainage Device 3 Infusion Device 4 Internal Fixation Device	Z No Qualifier
L Elbow Joint, Right M Elbow Joint, Left N Wrist Joint, Right P Wrist Joint, Left Q Carpal Joint, Right R Carpal Joint, Left S Carpometacarpal Joint, Right T Carpometacarpal Joint, Left U Metacarpophalangeal Joint, Right V Metacarpophalangeal Joint, Left W Finger Phalangeal Joint, Right X Finger Phalangeal Joint, Left	0 Open 3 Percutaneous 4 Percutaneous Endoscopic	0 Drainage Device 3 Infusion Device 4 Internal Fixation Device 5 External Fixation Device 7 Autologous Tissue Substitute 8 Spacer J Synthetic Substitute K Nonautologous Tissue Substitute	Z No Qualifier

Continued →

Section	0	Medical and Surgical
Body System	R	Upper Joints
Operation	P	**Removal:** Taking out or off a device from a body part

Body Part (4th)	Approach (5th)	Device (6th)	Qualifier (7th)
L Elbow Joint, Right M Elbow Joint, Left N Wrist Joint, Right P Wrist Joint, Left Q Carpal Joint, Right R Carpal Joint, Left S Carpometacarpal Joint, Right T Carpometacarpal Joint, Left U Metacarpophalangeal Joint, Right V Metacarpophalangeal Joint, Left W Finger Phalangeal Joint, Right X Finger Phalangeal Joint, Left	X External	0 Drainage Device 3 Infusion Device 4 Internal Fixation Device 5 External Fixation Device	Z No Qualifier

Section	0	Medical and Surgical
Body System	R	Upper Joints
Operation	Q	**Repair:** Restoring, to the extent possible, a body part to its normal anatomic structure and function

Body Part (4th)	Approach (5th)	Device (6th)	Qualifier (7th)
0 Occipital-cervical Joint 1 Cervical Vertebral Joint 3 Cervical Vertebral Disc 4 Cervicothoracic Vertebral Joint 5 Cervicothoracic Vertebral Disc 6 Thoracic Vertebral Joint 9 Thoracic Vertebral Disc A Thoracolumbar Vertebral Joint B Thoracolumbar Vertebral Disc C Temporomandibular Joint, Right D Temporomandibular Joint, Left E Sternoclavicular Joint, Right F Sternoclavicular Joint, Left G Acromioclavicular Joint, Right H Acromioclavicular Joint, Left J Shoulder Joint, Right K Shoulder Joint, Left L Elbow Joint, Right M Elbow Joint, Left N Wrist Joint, Right P Wrist Joint, Left Q Carpal Joint, Right R Carpal Joint, Left S Carpometacarpal Joint, Right T Carpometacarpal Joint, Left U Metacarpophalangeal Joint, Right V Metacarpophalangeal Joint, Left W Finger Phalangeal Joint, Right X Finger Phalangeal Joint, Left	0 Open 3 Percutaneous 4 Percutaneous Endoscopic X External	Z No Device	Z No Qualifier

Section	0	Medical and Surgical
Body System	R	Upper Joints
Operation	R	Replacement: Putting in or on biological or synthetic material that physically takes the place and/or function of all or a portion of a body part

Body Part (4th)	Approach (5th)	Device (6th)	Qualifier (7th)
0 Occipital-cervical Joint 1 Cervical Vertebral Joint 3 Cervical Vertebral Disc 4 Cervicothoracic Vertebral Joint 5 Cervicothoracic Vertebral Disc 6 Thoracic Vertebral Joint 9 Thoracic Vertebral Disc A Thoracolumbar Vertebral Joint B Thoracolumbar Vertebral Disc C Temporomandibular Joint, Right D Temporomandibular Joint, Left E Sternoclavicular Joint, Right F Sternoclavicular Joint, Left G Acromioclavicular Joint, Right H Acromioclavicular Joint, Left L Elbow Joint, Right M Elbow Joint, Left N Wrist Joint, Right P Wrist Joint, Left Q Carpal Joint, Right R Carpal Joint, Left S Carpometacarpal Joint, Right T Carpometacarpal Joint, Left U Metacarpophalangeal Joint, Right V Metacarpophalangeal Joint, Left W Finger Phalangeal Joint, Right X Finger Phalangeal Joint, Left	0 Open	7 Autologous Tissue Substitute J Synthetic Substitute K Nonautologous Tissue Substitute	Z No Qualifier
J Shoulder Joint, Right K Shoulder Joint, Left	0 Open	0 Synthetic Substitute, Reverse Ball and Socket 7 Autologous Tissue Substitute K Nonautologous Tissue Substitute	Z No Qualifier
J Shoulder Joint, Right K Shoulder Joint, Left	0 Open	J Synthetic Substitute	6 Humeral Surface 7 Glenoid Surface Z No Qualifier

Section	0	Medical and Surgical
Body System	R	Upper Joints
Operation	S	Reposition: Moving to its normal location, or other suitable location, all or a portion of a body part

Body Part (4th)	Approach (5th)	Device (6th)	Qualifier (7th)
0 Occipital-cervical Joint 1 Cervical Vertebral Joint 4 Cervicothoracic Vertebral Joint 6 Thoracic Vertebral Joint A Thoracolumbar Vertebral Joint C Temporomandibular Joint, Right D Temporomandibular Joint, Left E Sternoclavicular Joint, Right F Sternoclavicular Joint, Left G Acromioclavicular Joint, Right H Acromioclavicular Joint, Left J Shoulder Joint, Right K Shoulder Joint, Left	0 Open 3 Percutaneous 4 Percutaneous Endoscopic X External	4 Internal Fixation Device Z No Device	Z No Qualifier

Continued →

Section	0	Medical and Surgical
Body System	R	Upper Joints
Operation	S	Reposition: Moving to its normal location, or other suitable location, all or a portion of a body part

Body Part (4th)	Approach (5th)	Device (6th)	Qualifier (7th)
L Elbow Joint, Right M Elbow Joint, Left N Wrist Joint, Right P Wrist Joint, Left Q Carpal Joint, Right R Carpal Joint, Left S Carpometacarpal Joint, Right T Carpometacarpal Joint, Left U Metacarpophalangeal Joint, Right V Metacarpophalangeal Joint, Left W Finger Phalangeal Joint, Right X Finger Phalangeal Joint, Left	0 Open 3 Percutaneous 4 Percutaneous Endoscopic X External	4 Internal Fixation Device 5 External Fixation Device Z No Device	Z No Qualifier

Section	0	Medical and Surgical
Body System	R	Upper Joints
Operation	T	Resection: Cutting out or off, without replacement, all of a body part

Body Part (4th)	Approach (5th)	Device (6th)	Qualifier (7th)
3 Cervical Vertebral Disc 4 Cervicothoracic Vertebral Joint 5 Cervicothoracic Vertebral Disc 9 Thoracic Vertebral Disc B Thoracolumbar Vertebral Disc C Temporomandibular Joint, Right D Temporomandibular Joint, Left E Sternoclavicular Joint, Right F Sternoclavicular Joint, Left G Acromioclavicular Joint, Right H Acromioclavicular Joint, Left J Shoulder Joint, Right K Shoulder Joint, Left L Elbow Joint, Right M Elbow Joint, Left N Wrist Joint, Right P Wrist Joint, Left Q Carpal Joint, Right R Carpal Joint, Left S Carpometacarpal Joint, Right T Carpometacarpal Joint, Left U Metacarpophalangeal Joint, Right V Metacarpophalangeal Joint, Left W Finger Phalangeal Joint, Right X Finger Phalangeal Joint, Left	0 Open	Z No Device	Z No Qualifier

Section	0	Medical and Surgical
Body System	R	Upper Joints
Operation	U	Supplement: Putting in or on biological or synthetic material that physically reinforces and/or augments the function of a portion of a body part

Body Part (4th)	Approach (5th)	Device (6th)	Qualifier (7th)
0 Occipital-cervical Joint 1 Cervical Vertebral Joint 3 Cervical Vertebral Disc 4 Cervicothoracic Vertebral Joint 5 Cervicothoracic Vertebral Disc 6 Thoracic Vertebral Joint 9 Thoracic Vertebral Disc A Thoracolumbar Vertebral Joint B Thoracolumbar Vertebral Disc C Temporomandibular Joint, Right D Temporomandibular Joint, Left E Sternoclavicular Joint, Right F Sternoclavicular Joint, Left G Acromioclavicular Joint, Right H Acromioclavicular Joint, Left J Shoulder Joint, Right K Shoulder Joint, Left L Elbow Joint, Right M Elbow Joint, Left N Wrist Joint, Right P Wrist Joint, Left Q Carpal Joint, Right R Carpal Joint, Left S Carpometacarpal Joint, Right T Carpometacarpal Joint, Left U Metacarpophalangeal Joint, Right V Metacarpophalangeal Joint, Left W Finger Phalangeal Joint, Right X Finger Phalangeal Joint, Left	0 Open 3 Percutaneous 4 Percutaneous Endoscopic	7 Autologous Tissue Substitute J Synthetic Substitute K Nonautologous Tissue Substitute	Z No Qualifier

Section	0	Medical and Surgical
Body System	R	Upper Joints
Operation	W	Revision: Correcting, to the extent possible, a portion of a malfunctioning device or the position of a displaced device

Body Part (4th)	Approach (5th)	Device (6th)	Qualifier (7th)
0 Occipital-cervical Joint 1 Cervical Vertebral Joint 4 Cervicothoracic Vertebral Joint 6 Thoracic Vertebral Joint A Thoracolumbar Vertebral Joint	0 Open 3 Percutaneous 4 Percutaneous Endoscopic X External	0 Drainage Device 3 Infusion Device 4 Internal Fixation Device 7 Autologous Tissue Substitute 8 Spacer A Interbody Fusion Device J Synthetic Substitute K Nonautologous Tissue Substitute	Z No Qualifier
3 Cervical Vertebral Disc 5 Cervicothoracic Vertebral Disc 9 Thoracic Vertebral Disc B Thoracolumbar Vertebral Disc	0 Open 3 Percutaneous 4 Percutaneous Endoscopic X External	0 Drainage Device 3 Infusion Device 7 Autologous Tissue Substitute J Synthetic Substitute K Nonautologous Tissue Substitute	Z No Qualifier
C Temporomandibular Joint, Right D Temporomandibular Joint, Left E Sternoclavicular Joint, Right F Sternoclavicular Joint, Left G Acromioclavicular Joint, Right H Acromioclavicular Joint, Left J Shoulder Joint, Right K Shoulder Joint, Left	0 Open 3 Percutaneous 4 Percutaneous Endoscopic X External	0 Drainage Device 3 Infusion Device 4 Internal Fixation Device 7 Autologous Tissue Substitute 8 Spacer J Synthetic Substitute K Nonautologous Tissue Substitute	Z No Qualifier

Continued →

Section	0	Medical and Surgical					*0RW Continued*
Body System	R	Upper Joints					
Operation	W	Revision: Correcting, to the extent possible, a portion of a malfunctioning device or the position of a displaced device					

Body Part (4th)	Approach (5th)	Device (6th)	Qualifier (7th)
L Elbow Joint, Right **M** Elbow Joint, Left **N** Wrist Joint, Right **P** Wrist Joint, Left **Q** Carpal Joint, Right **R** Carpal Joint, Left **S** Carpometacarpal Joint, Right **T** Carpometacarpal Joint, Left **U** Metacarpophalangeal Joint, Right **V** Metacarpophalangeal Joint, Left **W** Finger Phalangeal Joint, Right **X** Finger Phalangeal Joint, Left	**0** Open **3** Percutaneous **4** Percutaneous Endoscopic **X** External	**0** Drainage Device **3** Infusion Device **4** Internal Fixation Device **5** External Fixation Device **7** Autologous Tissue Substitute **8** Spacer **J** Synthetic Substitute **K** Nonautologous Tissue Substitute	**Z** No Qualifier

AHA Coding Clinic

0RG20A0 Fusion of 2 or more Cervical Vertebral Joints with Interbody Fusion Device, Anterior Approach, Anterior Column, Open Approach—AHA CC: 3Q, 2019, 28

0RG2371 Fusion of 2 or more Cervical Vertebral Joints with Autologous Tissue Substitute, Posterior Approach, Posterior Column, Percutaneous Approach—AHA CC: 2Q, 2019, 19-20

0RG40A0 Fusion of Cervicothoracic Vertebral Joint with Interbody Fusion Device, Anterior Approach, Anterior Column, Open Approach—AHA CC: 1Q, 2013, 29-30; 2Q, 2014, 7-8

0RG7071 Fusion of 2 to 7 Thoracic Vertebral Joints with Autologous Tissue Substitute, Posterior Approach, Posterior Column, Open Approach—AHA CC: 1Q, 2013, 21-23

0RGA071 Fusion of Thoracolumbar Vertebral Joint with Autologous Tissue Substitute, Posterior Approach, Posterior Column, Open Approach—AHA CC: 1Q, 2013, 21-23

0RGW04Z Fusion of Right Finger Phalangeal Joint with Internal Fixation Device, Open Approach—AHA CC: 4Q, 2017, 62

0RHJ04Z Insertion of Internal Fixation Device into Right Shoulder Joint, Open Approach—AHA CC: 3Q, 2016, 32-33

0RNJ4ZZ Release Right Shoulder Joint, Percutaneous Endoscopic Approach—AHA CC: 3Q, 2016, 32-33

0RNK4ZZ Release Left Shoulder Joint, Percutaneous Endoscopic Approach—AHA CC: 2Q, 2015, 22-23

0RQJ4ZZ Repair Right Shoulder Joint, Percutaneous Endoscopic Approach—AHA CC: 1Q, 2016, 30-31

0RRJ00Z Replacement of Right Shoulder Joint with Reverse Ball and Socket Synthetic Substitute, Open Approach—AHA CC: 1Q, 2015, 27

0RRK0J6 Replacement of Left Shoulder Joint with Synthetic Substitute, Humeral Surface, Open Approach—AHA CC: 3Q, 2015, 14-15

0RSH04Z Reposition Left Acromioclavicular Joint with Internal Fixation Device, Open Approach—AHA CC: 3Q, 2019, 26-27

0RSPXZZ Reposition Left Wrist Joint, External Approach—AHA CC: 4Q, 2014, 32-33

0RSR04Z Reposition Left Carpal Joint with Internal Fixation Device, Open Approach—AHA CC: 3Q, 2014, 33-34

0RT50ZZ Resection of Cervicothoracic Vertebral Disc, Open Approach—AHA CC: 2Q, 2014, 7-8

0RUH0KZ Supplement Left Acromioclavicular Joint with Nonautologous Tissue Substitute, Open Approach—AHA CC: 3Q, 2019, 26-27

0RUT07Z Supplement Left Carpometacarpal Joint with Autologous Tissue Substitute, Open Approach—AHA CC: 3Q, 2015, 26-27

Intervertebral Joint

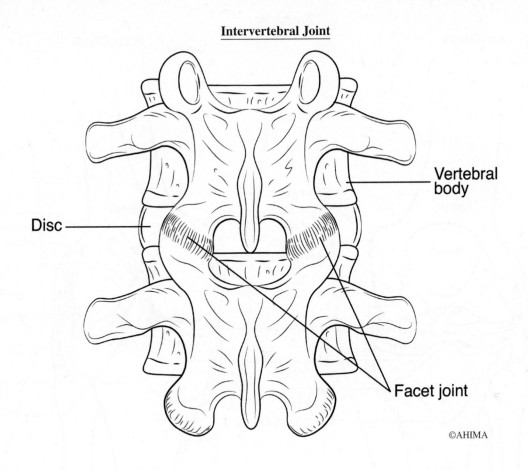

Disc

Vertebral
body

Facet joint

©AHIMA

Hip

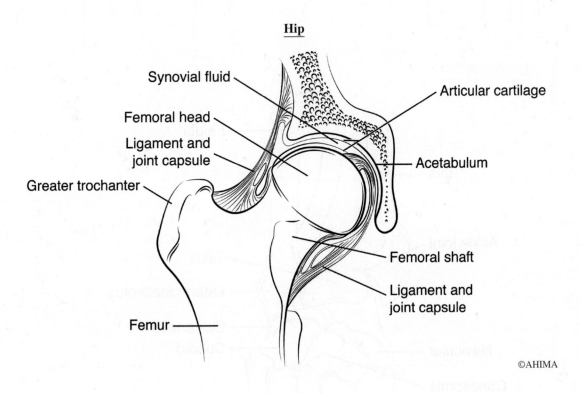

Synovial fluid

Femoral head

Ligament and
joint capsule

Greater trochanter

Femur

Articular cartilage

Acetabulum

Femoral shaft

Ligament and
joint capsule

©AHIMA

Knee Joint

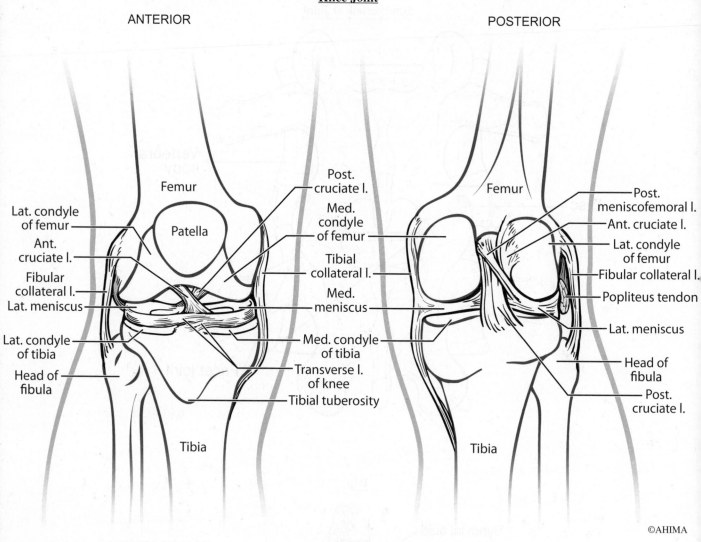

ANTERIOR

POSTERIOR

Femur

Lat. condyle of femur

Ant. cruciate l.

Fibular collateral l.

Lat. meniscus

Lat. condyle of tibia

Head of fibula

Patella

Tibia

Post. cruciate l.

Med. condyle of femur

Tibial collateral l.

Med. meniscus

Med. condyle of tibia

Transverse l. of knee

Tibial tuberosity

Femur

Tibia

Post. meniscofemoral l.

Ant. cruciate l.

Lat. condyle of femur

Fibular collateral l.

Popliteus tendon

Lat. meniscus

Head of fibula

Post. cruciate l.

©AHIMA

Ankle

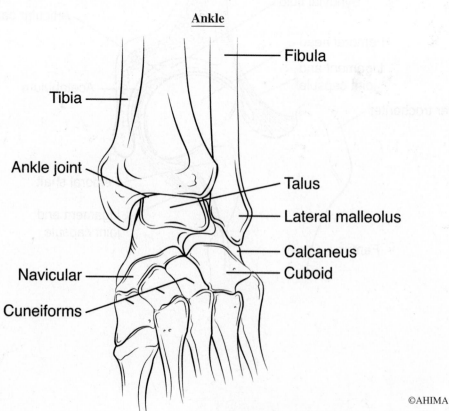

Tibia

Ankle joint

Navicular

Cuneiforms

Fibula

Talus

Lateral malleolus

Calcaneus

Cuboid

©AHIMA

Total Knee Replacement Technique: Steps 1-5

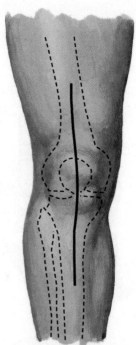

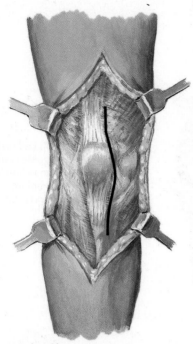

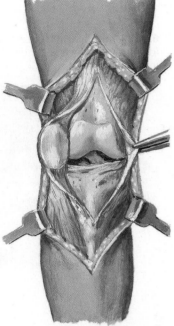

1. Longitudinal 8- to 12-in. skin incision is centered on patella.

2. Capsular incision skirts medial margin of patella and courses distally through periosteum medial to tibial tuberosity.

3. Patella is reflected laterally by raising patellar ligament in continuity with periosteum.

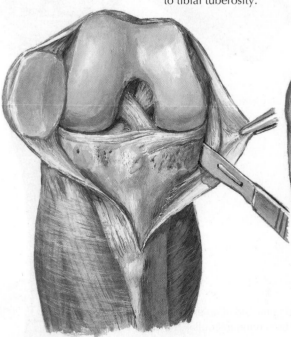

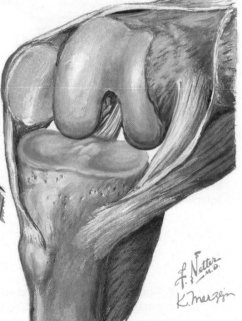

4. If further exposure of the medial knee is needed, a flap can be raised by elevating the deep medial collateral ligament and pes anserinus subperiosteally, aided by external rotation of the tibia.

5. The anterior cruciate ligament and both menisci are excised, and the tibia is subluxated anteriorly.

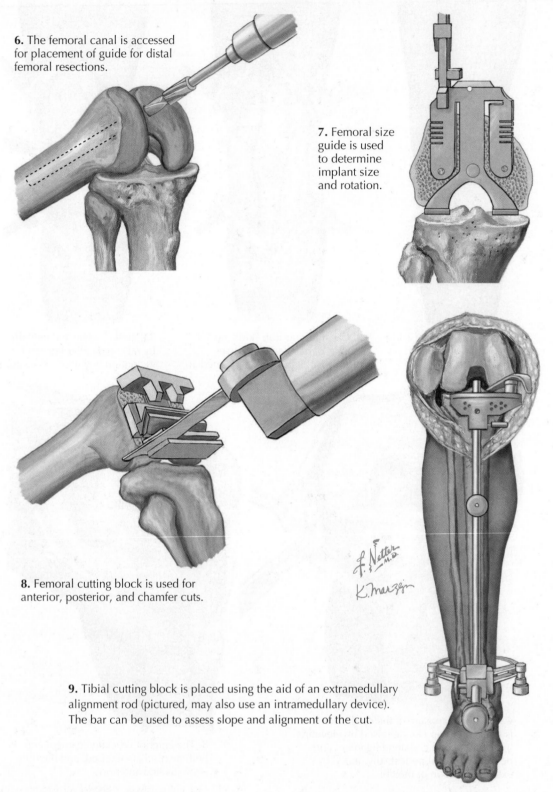

6. The femoral canal is accessed for placement of guide for distal femoral resections.

7. Femoral size guide is used to determine implant size and rotation.

8. Femoral cutting block is used for anterior, posterior, and chamfer cuts.

9. Tibial cutting block is placed using the aid of an extramedullary alignment rod (pictured, may also use an intramedullary device). The bar can be used to assess slope and alignment of the cut.

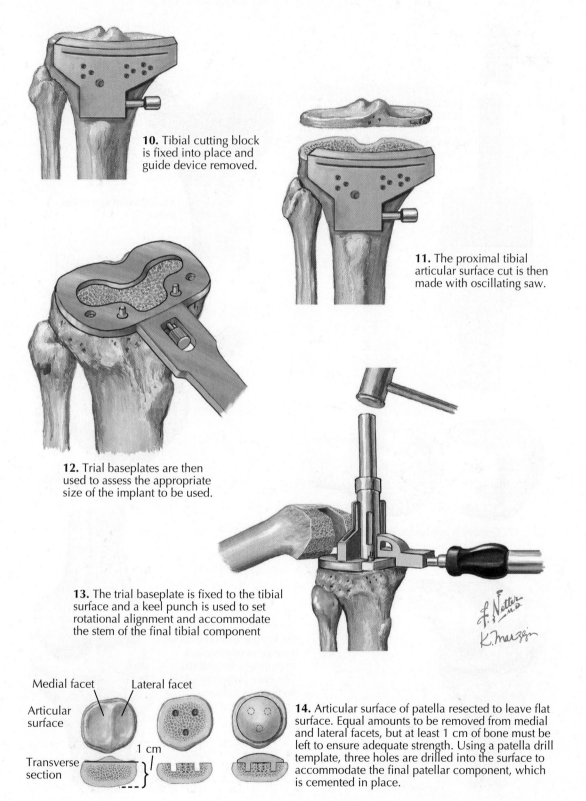

10. Tibial cutting block is fixed into place and guide device removed.

11. The proximal tibial articular surface cut is then made with oscillating saw.

12. Trial baseplates are then used to assess the appropriate size of the implant to be used.

13. The trial baseplate is fixed to the tibial surface and a keel punch is used to set rotational alignment and accommodate the stem of the final tibial component

Medial facet   Lateral facet

Articular surface

Transverse section

1 cm

14. Articular surface of patella resected to leave flat surface. Equal amounts to be removed from medial and lateral facets, but at least 1 cm of bone must be left to ensure adequate strength. Using a patella drill template, three holes are drilled into the surface to accommodate the final patellar component, which is cemented in place.

Medical and Surgical, Lower Joints

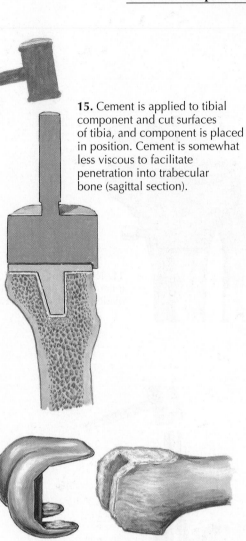

15. Cement is applied to tibial component and cut surfaces of tibia, and component is placed in position. Cement is somewhat less viscous to facilitate penetration into trabecular bone (sagittal section).

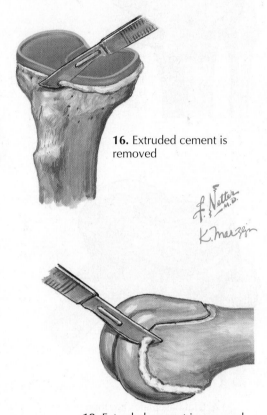

16. Extruded cement is removed

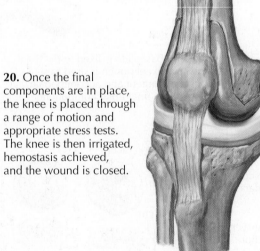

18. Extruded cement is removed

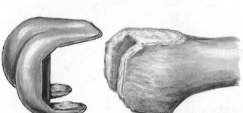

17. Cement is applied to posterior limb of femoral component and spread evenly over beveled ends of femur

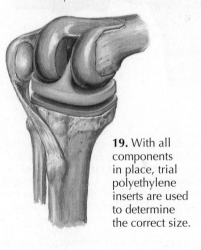

19. With all components in place, trial polyethylene inserts are used to determine the correct size.

20. Once the final components are in place, the knee is placed through a range of motion and appropriate stress tests. The knee is then irrigated, hemostasis achieved, and the wound is closed.

Section	0	Medical and Surgical
Body System	S	Lower Joints
Operation	2	**Change:** Taking out or off a device from a body part and putting back an identical or similar device in or on the same body part without cutting or puncturing the skin or a mucous membrane

Body Part (4th)	Approach (5th)	Device (6th)	Qualifier (7th)
Y Lower Joint	X External	0 Drainage Device Y Other Device	Z No Qualifier

Section	0	Medical and Surgical
Body System	S	Lower Joints
Operation	5	**Destruction:** Physical eradication of all or a portion of a body part by the direct use of energy, force, or a destructive agent

Body Part (4th)	Approach (5th)	Device (6th)	Qualifier (7th)
0 Lumbar Vertebral Joint 2 Lumbar Vertebral Disc 3 Lumbosacral Joint 4 Lumbosacral Disc 5 Sacrococcygeal Joint 6 Coccygeal Joint 7 Sacroiliac Joint, Right 8 Sacroiliac Joint, Left 9 Hip Joint, Right B Hip Joint, Left C Knee Joint, Right D Knee Joint, Left F Ankle Joint, Right G Ankle Joint, Left H Tarsal Joint, Right J Tarsal Joint, Left K Tarsometatarsal Joint, Right L Tarsometatarsal Joint, Left M Metatarsal-Phalangeal Joint, Right N Metatarsal-Phalangeal Joint, Left P Toe Phalangeal Joint, Right Q Toe Phalangeal Joint, Left	0 Open 3 Percutaneous 4 Percutaneous Endoscopic	Z No Device	Z No Qualifier

Section	0	Medical and Surgical
Body System	S	Lower Joints
Operation	9	**Drainage:** Taking or letting out fluids and/or gases from a body part

Body Part (4th)	Approach (5th)	Device (6th)	Qualifier (7th)
0 Lumbar Vertebral Joint 2 Lumbar Vertebral Disc 3 Lumbosacral Joint 4 Lumbosacral Disc 5 Sacrococcygeal Joint 6 Coccygeal Joint 7 Sacroiliac Joint, Right 8 Sacroiliac Joint, Left 9 Hip Joint, Right B Hip Joint, Left C Knee Joint, Right D Knee Joint, Left F Ankle Joint, Right G Ankle Joint, Left H Tarsal Joint, Right J Tarsal Joint, Left K Tarsometatarsal Joint, Right L Tarsometatarsal Joint, Left M Metatarsal-Phalangeal Joint, Right N Metatarsal-Phalangeal Joint, Left P Toe Phalangeal Joint, Right Q Toe Phalangeal Joint, Left	0 Open 3 Percutaneous 4 Percutaneous Endoscopic	0 Drainage Device	Z No Qualifier
0 Lumbar Vertebral Joint 2 Lumbar Vertebral Disc 3 Lumbosacral Joint 4 Lumbosacral Disc 5 Sacrococcygeal Joint 6 Coccygeal Joint 7 Sacroiliac Joint, Right 8 Sacroiliac Joint, Left 9 Hip Joint, Right B Hip Joint, Left C Knee Joint, Right D Knee Joint, Left F Ankle Joint, Right G Ankle Joint, Left H Tarsal Joint, Right J Tarsal Joint, Left K Tarsometatarsal Joint, Right L Tarsometatarsal Joint, Left M Metatarsal-Phalangeal Joint, Right N Metatarsal-Phalangeal Joint, Left P Toe Phalangeal Joint, Right Q Toe Phalangeal Joint, Left	0 Open 3 Percutaneous 4 Percutaneous Endoscopic	Z No Device	X Diagnostic Z No Qualifier

Section	0	Medical and Surgical
Body System	S	Lower Joints
Operation	B	**Excision:** Cutting out or off, without replacement, a portion of a body part

Body Part (4th)	Approach (5th)	Device (6th)	Qualifier (7th)
0 Lumbar Vertebral Joint 2 Lumbar Vertebral Disc 3 Lumbosacral Joint 4 Lumbosacral Disc 5 Sacrococcygeal Joint 6 Coccygeal Joint 7 Sacroiliac Joint, Right 8 Sacroiliac Joint, Left 9 Hip Joint, Right B Hip Joint, Left C Knee Joint, Right D Knee Joint, Left F Ankle Joint, Right G Ankle Joint, Left H Tarsal Joint, Right J Tarsal Joint, Left K Tarsometatarsal Joint, Right L Tarsometatarsal Joint, Left M Metatarsal-Phalangeal Joint, Right N Metatarsal-Phalangeal Joint, Left P Toe Phalangeal Joint, Right Q Toe Phalangeal Joint, Left	0 Open 3 Percutaneous 4 Percutaneous Endoscopic	Z No Device	X Diagnostic Z No Qualifier

Section	0	Medical and Surgical
Body System	S	Lower Joints
Operation	C	**Extirpation:** Taking or cutting out solid matter from a body part

Body Part (4th)	Approach (5th)	Device (6th)	Qualifier (7th)
0 Lumbar Vertebral Joint 2 Lumbar Vertebral Disc 3 Lumbosacral Joint 4 Lumbosacral Disc 5 Sacrococcygeal Joint 6 Coccygeal Joint 7 Sacroiliac Joint, Right 8 Sacroiliac Joint, Left 9 Hip Joint, Right B Hip Joint, Left C Knee Joint, Right D Knee Joint, Left F Ankle Joint, Right G Ankle Joint, Left H Tarsal Joint, Right J Tarsal Joint, Left K Tarsometatarsal Joint, Right L Tarsometatarsal Joint, Left M Metatarsal-Phalangeal Joint, Right N Metatarsal-Phalangeal Joint, Left P Toe Phalangeal Joint, Right Q Toe Phalangeal Joint, Left	0 Open 3 Percutaneous 4 Percutaneous Endoscopic	Z No Device	Z No Qualifier

Section	0	Medical and Surgical
Body System	S	Lower Joints
Operation	G	Fusion: Joining together portions of an articular body part rendering the articular body part immobile

Body Part (4th)	Approach (5th)	Device (6th)	Qualifier (7th)
0 Lumbar Vertebral Joint 1 Lumbar Vertebral Joints, 2 or more 3 Lumbosacral Joint	0 Open 3 Percutaneous 4 Percutaneous Endoscopic	7 Autologous Tissue Substitute J Synthetic Substitute K Nonautologous Tissue Substitute	0 Anterior Approach, Anterior Column 1 Posterior Approach, Posterior Column J Posterior Approach, Anterior Column
0 Lumbar Vertebral Joint 1 Lumbar Vertebral Joints, 2 or more 3 Lumbosacral Joint	0 Open 3 Percutaneous 4 Percutaneous Endoscopic	A Interbody Fusion Device	0 Anterior Approach, Anterior Column J Posterior Approach, Anterior Column
5 Sacrococcygeal Joint 6 Coccygeal Joint 7 Sacroiliac Joint, Right 8 Sacroiliac Joint, Left	0 Open 3 Percutaneous 4 Percutaneous Endoscopic	4 Internal Fixation Device 7 Autologous Tissue Substitute J Synthetic Substitute K Nonautologous Tissue Substitute	Z No Qualifier
9 Hip Joint, Right B Hip Joint, Left C Knee Joint, Right D Knee Joint, Left F Ankle Joint, Right G Ankle Joint, Left H Tarsal Joint, Right J Tarsal Joint, Left K Tarsometatarsal Joint, Right L Tarsometatarsal Joint, Left M Metatarsal-Phalangeal Joint, Right N Metatarsal-Phalangeal Joint, Left P Toe Phalangeal Joint, Right Q Toe Phalangeal Joint, Left	0 Open 3 Percutaneous 4 Percutaneous Endoscopic	3 Internal Fixation Device, Sustained Compression 4 Internal Fixation Device 5 External Fixation Device 7 Autologous Tissue Substitute J Synthetic Substitute K Nonautologous Tissue Substitute	Z No Qualifier

Section	0	Medical and Surgical
Body System	S	Lower Joints
Operation	H	Insertion: Putting in a nonbiological appliance that monitors, assists, performs, or prevents a physiological function but does not physically take the place of a body part

Body Part (4th)	Approach (5th)	Device (6th)	Qualifier (7th)
0 Lumbar Vertebral Joint 3 Lumbosacral Joint	0 Open 3 Percutaneous 4 Percutaneous Endoscopic	3 Infusion Device 4 Internal Fixation Device 8 Spacer B Spinal Stabilization Device, Interspinous Process C Spinal Stabilization Device, Pedicle-Based D Spinal Stabilization Device, Facet Replacement	Z No Qualifier
2 Lumbar Vertebral Disc 4 Lumbosacral Disc	0 Open 3 Percutaneous 4 Percutaneous Endoscopic	3 Infusion Device 8 Spacer	Z No Qualifier
5 Sacrococcygeal Joint 6 Coccygeal Joint 7 Sacroiliac Joint, Right 8 Sacroiliac Joint, Left	0 Open 3 Percutaneous 4 Percutaneous Endoscopic	3 Infusion Device 4 Internal Fixation Device 8 Spacer	Z No Qualifier

Continued →
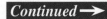

Section 0 **Medical and Surgical**
Body System S **Lower Joints**
Operation H **Insertion:** Putting in a nonbiological appliance that monitors, assists, performs, or prevents a physiological function but does not physically take the place of a body part

Body Part (4th)	Approach (5th)	Device (6th)	Qualifier (7th)
9 Hip Joint, Right	0 Open	3 Infusion Device	Z No Qualifier
B Hip Joint, Left	3 Percutaneous	4 Internal Fixation Device	
C Knee Joint, Right	4 Percutaneous	5 External Fixation Device	
D Knee Joint, Left	Endoscopic	8 Spacer	
F Ankle Joint, Right			
G Ankle Joint, Left			
H Tarsal Joint, Right			
J Tarsal Joint, Left			
K Tarsometatarsal Joint, Right			
L Tarsometatarsal Joint, Left			
M Metatarsal-Phalangeal Joint, Right			
N Metatarsal-Phalangeal Joint, Left			
P Toe Phalangeal Joint, Right			
Q Toe Phalangeal Joint, Left			

Section 0 **Medical and Surgical**
Body System S **Lower Joints**
Operation J **Inspection:** Visually and/or manually exploring a body part

Body Part (4th)	Approach (5th)	Device (6th)	Qualifier (7th)
0 Lumbar Vertebral Joint	0 Open	Z No Device	Z No Qualifier
2 Lumbar Vertebral Disc	3 Percutaneous		
3 Lumbosacral Joint	4 Percutaneous		
4 Lumbosacral Disc	Endoscopic		
5 Sacrococcygeal Joint	X External		
6 Coccygeal Joint			
7 Sacroiliac Joint, Right			
8 Sacroiliac Joint, Left			
9 Hip Joint, Right			
B Hip Joint, Left			
C Knee Joint, Right			
D Knee Joint, Left			
F Ankle Joint, Right			
G Ankle Joint, Left			
H Tarsal Joint, Right			
J Tarsal Joint, Left			
K Tarsometatarsal Joint, Right			
L Tarsometatarsal Joint, Left			
M Metatarsal-Phalangeal Joint, Right			
N Metatarsal-Phalangeal Joint, Left			
P Toe Phalangeal Joint, Right			
Q Toe Phalangeal Joint, Left			

Section	0	Medical and Surgical
Body System	S	Lower Joints
Operation	N	Release: Freeing a body part from an abnormal physical constraint by cutting or by the use of force

Body Part (4th)	Approach (5th)	Device (6th)	Qualifier (7th)
0 Lumbar Vertebral Joint	0 Open	Z No Device	Z No Qualifier
2 Lumbar Vertebral Disc	3 Percutaneous		
3 Lumbosacral Joint	4 Percutaneous Endoscopic		
4 Lumbosacral Disc	X External		
5 Sacrococcygeal Joint			
6 Coccygeal Joint			
7 Sacroiliac Joint, Right			
8 Sacroiliac Joint, Left			
9 Hip Joint, Right			
B Hip Joint, Left			
C Knee Joint, Right			
D Knee Joint, Left			
F Ankle Joint, Right			
G Ankle Joint, Left			
H Tarsal Joint, Right			
J Tarsal Joint, Left			
K Tarsometatarsal Joint, Right			
L Tarsometatarsal Joint, Left			
M Metatarsal-Phalangeal Joint, Right			
N Metatarsal-Phalangeal Joint, Left			
P Toe Phalangeal Joint, Right			
Q Toe Phalangeal Joint, Left			

Section	0	Medical and Surgical
Body System	S	Lower Joints
Operation	P	Removal: Taking out or off a device from a body part

Body Part (4th)	Approach (5th)	Device (6th)	Qualifier (7th)
0 Lumbar Vertebral Joint 3 Lumbosacral Joint	0 Open 3 Percutaneous 4 Percutaneous Endoscopic	0 Drainage Device 3 Infusion Device 4 Internal Fixation Device 7 Autologous Tissue Substitute 8 Spacer A Interbody Fusion Device J Synthetic Substitute K Nonautologous Tissue Substitute	Z No Qualifier
0 Lumbar Vertebral Joint 3 Lumbosacral Joint	X External	0 Drainage Device 3 Infusion Device 4 Internal Fixation Device	Z No Qualifier
2 Lumbar Vertebral Disc 4 Lumbosacral Disc	0 Open 3 Percutaneous 4 Percutaneous Endoscopic	0 Drainage Device 3 Infusion Device 7 Autologous Tissue Substitute J Synthetic Substitute K Nonautologous Tissue Substitute	Z No Qualifier
2 Lumbar Vertebral Disc 4 Lumbosacral Disc	X External	0 Drainage Device 3 Infusion Device	Z No Qualifier
5 Sacrococcygeal Joint 6 Coccygeal Joint 7 Sacroiliac Joint, Right 8 Sacroiliac Joint, Left	0 Open 3 Percutaneous 4 Percutaneous Endoscopic	0 Drainage Device 3 Infusion Device 4 Internal Fixation Device 7 Autologous Tissue Substitute 8 Spacer J Synthetic Substitute K Nonautologous Tissue Substitute	Z No Qualifier

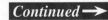
Continued →

Body Part (4th)	Approach (5th)	Device (6th)	Qualifier (7th)
5 Sacrococcygeal Joint 6 Coccygeal Joint 7 Sacroiliac Joint, Right 8 Sacroiliac Joint, Left	X External	0 Drainage Device 3 Infusion Device 4 Internal Fixation Device	Z No Qualifier
9 Hip Joint, Right B Hip Joint, Left	0 Open	0 Drainage Device 3 Infusion Device 4 Internal Fixation Device 5 External Fixation Device 7 Autologous Tissue Substitute 8 Spacer 9 Liner B Resurfacing Device E Articulating Spacer J Synthetic Substitute K Nonautologous Tissue Substitute	Z No Qualifier
9 Hip Joint, Right B Hip Joint, Left	3 Percutaneous 4 Percutaneous Endoscopic	0 Drainage Device 3 Infusion Device 4 Internal Fixation Device 5 External Fixation Device 7 Autologous Tissue Substitute 8 Spacer J Synthetic Substitute K Nonautologous Tissue Substitute	Z No Qualifier
9 Hip Joint, Right B Hip Joint, Left	X External	0 Drainage Device 3 Infusion Device 4 Internal Fixation Device 5 External Fixation Device	Z No Qualifier
A Hip Joint, Acetabular Surface, Right E Hip Joint, Acetabular Surface, Left R Hip Joint, Femoral Surface, Right S Hip Joint, Femoral Surface, Left T Knee Joint, Femoral Surface, Right U Knee Joint, Femoral Surface, Left V Knee Joint, Tibial Surface, Right W Knee Joint, Tibial Surface, Left	0 Open 3 Percutaneous 4 Percutaneous Endoscopic	J Synthetic Substitute	Z No Qualifier
C Knee Joint, Right D Knee Joint, Left	0 Open	0 Drainage Device 3 Infusion Device 4 Internal Fixation Device 5 External Fixation Device 7 Autologous Tissue Substitute 8 Spacer 9 Liner E Articulating Spacer K Nonautologous Tissue Substitute L Synthetic Substitute, Unicondylar Medial M Synthetic Substitute, Unicondylar Lateral N Synthetic Substitute, Unicondylar Patellofemoral	Z No Qualifier
C Knee Joint, Right D Knee Joint, Left	0 Open	J Synthetic Substitute	C Patellar Surface Z No Qualifier

Continued →

Section	0	Medical and Surgical
Body System	S	Lower Joints
Operation	P	Removal: Taking out or off a device from a body part

Body Part (4th)	Approach (5th)	Device (6th)	Qualifier (7th)
C Knee Joint, Right D Knee Joint, Left	3 Percutaneous 4 Percutaneous Endoscopic	0 Drainage Device 3 Infusion Device 4 Internal Fixation Device 5 External Fixation Device 7 Autologous Tissue Substitute 8 Spacer K Nonautologous Tissue Substitute L Synthetic Substitute, Unicondylar Medial M Synthetic Substitute, Unicondylar Lateral N Synthetic Substitute, Unicondylar Patellofemoral	Z No Qualifier
C Knee Joint, Right D Knee Joint, Left	3 Percutaneous 4 Percutaneous Endoscopic	J Synthetic Substitute	C Patellar Surface Z No Qualifier
C Knee Joint, Right D Knee Joint, Left	X External	0 Drainage Device 3 Infusion Device 4 Internal Fixation Device 5 External Fixation Device	Z No Qualifier
F Ankle Joint, Right G Ankle Joint, Left H Tarsal Joint, Right J Tarsal Joint, Left K Tarsometatarsal Joint, Right L Tarsometatarsal Joint, Left M Metatarsal-Phalangeal Joint, Right N Metatarsal-Phalangeal Joint, Left P Toe Phalangeal Joint, Right Q Toe Phalangeal Joint, Left	0 Open 3 Percutaneous 4 Percutaneous Endoscopic	0 Drainage Device 3 Infusion Device 4 Internal Fixation Device 5 External Fixation Device 7 Autologous Tissue Substitute 8 Spacer J Synthetic Substitute K Nonautologous Tissue Substitute	Z No Qualifier
F Ankle Joint, Right G Ankle Joint, Left H Tarsal Joint, Right J Tarsal Joint, Left K Tarsometatarsal Joint, Right L Tarsometatarsal Joint, Left M Metatarsal-Phalangeal Joint, Right N Metatarsal-Phalangeal Joint, Left P Toe Phalangeal Joint, Right Q Toe Phalangeal Joint, Left	X External	0 Drainage Device 3 Infusion Device 4 Internal Fixation Device 5 External Fixation Device	Z No Qualifier

Section	0	Medical and Surgical
Body System	S	Lower Joints
Operation	Q	**Repair:** Restoring, to the extent possible, a body part to its normal anatomic structure and function

Body Part (4th)	Approach (5th)	Device (6th)	Qualifier (7th)
0 Lumbar Vertebral Joint 2 Lumbar Vertebral Disc 3 Lumbosacral Joint 4 Lumbosacral Disc 5 Sacrococcygeal Joint 6 Coccygeal Joint 7 Sacroiliac Joint, Right 8 Sacroiliac Joint, Left 9 Hip Joint, Right B Hip Joint, Left C Knee Joint, Right D Knee Joint, Left F Ankle Joint, Right G Ankle Joint, Left H Tarsal Joint, Right J Tarsal Joint, Left K Tarsometatarsal Joint, Right L Tarsometatarsal Joint, Left M Metatarsal-Phalangeal Joint, Right N Metatarsal-Phalangeal Joint, Left P Toe Phalangeal Joint, Right Q Toe Phalangeal Joint, Left	0 Open 3 Percutaneous 4 Percutaneous Endoscopic X External	Z No Device	Z No Qualifier

Section	0	Medical and Surgical
Body System	S	Lower Joints
Operation	R	**Replacement:** Putting in or on biological or synthetic material that physically takes the place and/or function of all or a portion of a body part

Body Part (4th)	Approach (5th)	Device (6th)	Qualifier (7th)
0 Lumbar Vertebral Joint 2 Lumbar Vertebral Disc 3 Lumbosacral Joint 4 Lumbosacral Disc 5 Sacrococcygeal Joint 6 Coccygeal Joint 7 Sacroiliac Joint, Right 8 Sacroiliac Joint, Left H Tarsal Joint, Right J Tarsal Joint, Left K Tarsometatarsal Joint, Right L Tarsometatarsal Joint, Left M Metatarsal-Phalangeal Joint, Right N Metatarsal-Phalangeal Joint, Left P Toe Phalangeal Joint, Right Q Toe Phalangeal Joint, Left	0 Open	7 Autologous Tissue Substitute J Synthetic Substitute K Nonautologous Tissue Substitute	Z No Qualifier
9 Hip Joint, Right B Hip Joint, Left	0 Open	1 Synthetic Substitute, Metal 2 Synthetic Substitute, Metal on Polyethylene 3 Synthetic Substitute, Ceramic 4 Synthetic Substitute, Ceramic on Polyethylene 6 Synthetic Substitute, Oxidized Zirconium on Polyethylene J Synthetic Substitute	9 Cemented A Uncemented Z No Qualifier
9 Hip Joint, Right B Hip Joint, Left	0 Open	7 Autologous Tissue Substitute E Articulating Spacer K Nonautologous Tissue Substitute	Z No Qualifier
A Hip Joint, Acetabular Surface, Right E Hip Joint, Acetabular Surface, Left	0 Open	0 Synthetic Substitute, Polyethylene 1 Synthetic Substitute, Metal 3 Synthetic Substitute, Ceramic J Synthetic Substitute	9 Cemented A Uncemented Z No Qualifier

Continued →

Section	0	Medical and Surgical
Body System	S	Lower Joints
Operation	R	Replacement: Putting in or on biological or synthetic material that physically takes the place and/or function of all or a portion of a body part

Body Part (4th)	Approach (5th)	Device (6th)	Qualifier (7th)
A Hip Joint, Acetabular Surface, Right E Hip Joint, Acetabular Surface, Left	0 Open	7 Autologous Tissue Substitute K Nonautologous Tissue Substitute	Z No Qualifier
C Knee Joint, Right D Knee Joint, Left	0 Open	6 Synthetic Substitute, Oxidized Zirconium on Polyethylene J Synthetic Substitute L Synthetic Substitute, Unicondylar Medial M Synthetic Substitute, Unicondylar Lateral N Synthetic Substitute, Unicondylar Patellofemoral	9 Cemented A Uncemented Z No Qualifier
C Knee Joint, Right D Knee Joint, Left	0 Open	7 Autologous Tissue Substitute E Articulating Spacer K Nonautologous Tissue Substitute	Z No Qualifier
F Ankle Joint, Right G Ankle Joint, Left T Knee Joint, Femoral Surface, Right U Knee Joint, Femoral Surface, Left V Knee Joint, Tibial Surface, Right W Knee Joint, Tibial Surface, Left	0 Open	7 Autologous Tissue Substitute K Nonautologous Tissue Substitute	Z No Qualifier
F Ankle Joint, Right G Ankle Joint, Left T Knee Joint, Femoral Surface, Right U Knee Joint, Femoral Surface, Left V Knee Joint, Tibial Surface, Right W Knee Joint, Tibial Surface, Left	0 Open	J Synthetic Substitute	9 Cemented A Uncemented Z No Qualifier
R Hip Joint, Femoral Surface, Right S Hip Joint, Femoral Surface, Left	0 Open	1 Synthetic Substitute, Metal 3 Synthetic Substitute, Ceramic J Synthetic Substitute	9 Cemented A Uncemented Z No Qualifier
R Hip Joint, Femoral Surface, Right S Hip Joint, Femoral Surface, Left	0 Open	7 Autologous Tissue Substitute K Nonautologous Tissue Substitute	Z No Qualifier

Section	0	Medical and Surgical
Body System	S	Lower Joints
Operation	S	Reposition: Moving to its normal location, or other suitable location, all or a portion of a body part

Body Part (4th)	Approach (5th)	Device (6th)	Qualifier (7th)
0 Lumbar Vertebral Joint 3 Lumbosacral Joint 5 Sacrococcygeal Joint 6 Coccygeal Joint 7 Sacroiliac Joint, Right 8 Sacroiliac Joint, Left	0 Open 3 Percutaneous 4 Percutaneous Endoscopic X External	4 Internal Fixation Device Z No Device	Z No Qualifier
9 Hip Joint, Right B Hip Joint, Left C Knee Joint, Right D Knee Joint, Left F Ankle Joint, Right G Ankle Joint, Left H Tarsal Joint, Right J Tarsal Joint, Left K Tarsometatarsal Joint, Right L Tarsometatarsal Joint, Left M Metatarsal-Phalangeal Joint, Right N Metatarsal-Phalangeal Joint, Left P Toe Phalangeal Joint, Right Q Toe Phalangeal Joint, Left	0 Open 3 Percutaneous 4 Percutaneous Endoscopic X External	4 Internal Fixation Device 5 External Fixation Device Z No Device	Z No Qualifier

Section   **0**   **Medical and Surgical**
Body System   **S**   **Lower Joints**
Operation   **T**   **Resection:** Cutting out or off, without replacement, all of a body part

Body Part (4ᵗʰ)	Approach (5ᵗʰ)	Device (6ᵗʰ)	Qualifier (7ᵗʰ)
2 Lumbar Vertebral Disc **4** Lumbosacral Disc **5** Sacrococcygeal Joint **6** Coccygeal Joint **7** Sacroiliac Joint, Right **8** Sacroiliac Joint, Left **9** Hip Joint, Right **B** Hip Joint, Left **C** Knee Joint, Right **D** Knee Joint, Left **F** Ankle Joint, Right **G** Ankle Joint, Left **H** Tarsal Joint, Right **J** Tarsal Joint, Left **K** Tarsometatarsal Joint, Right **L** Tarsometatarsal Joint, Left **M** Metatarsal-Phalangeal Joint, Right **N** Metatarsal-Phalangeal Joint, Left **P** Toe Phalangeal Joint, Right **Q** Toe Phalangeal Joint, Left	**0** Open	**Z** No Device	**Z** No Qualifier

Section   **0**   **Medical and Surgical**
Body System   **S**   **Lower Joints**
Operation   **U**   **Supplement:** Putting in or on biological or synthetic material that physically reinforces and/or augments the function of a portion of a body part

Body Part (4ᵗʰ)	Approach (5ᵗʰ)	Device (6ᵗʰ)	Qualifier (7ᵗʰ)
0 Lumbar Vertebral Joint **2** Lumbar Vertebral Disc **3** Lumbosacral Joint **4** Lumbosacral Disc **5** Sacrococcygeal Joint **6** Coccygeal Joint **7** Sacroiliac Joint, Right **8** Sacroiliac Joint, Left **F** Ankle Joint, Right **G** Ankle Joint, Left **H** Tarsal Joint, Right **J** Tarsal Joint, Left **K** Tarsometatarsal Joint, Right **L** Tarsometatarsal Joint, Left **M** Metatarsal-Phalangeal Joint, Right **N** Metatarsal-Phalangeal Joint, Left **P** Toe Phalangeal Joint, Right **Q** Toe Phalangeal Joint, Left	**0** Open **3** Percutaneous **4** Percutaneous Endoscopic	**7** Autologous Tissue Substitute **J** Synthetic Substitute **K** Nonautologous Tissue Substitute	**Z** No Qualifier
9 Hip Joint, Right **B** Hip Joint, Left	**0** Open	**7** Autologous Tissue Substitute **9** Liner **B** Resurfacing Device **J** Synthetic Substitute **K** Nonautologous Tissue Substitute	**Z** No Qualifier
9 Hip Joint, Right **B** Hip Joint, Left	**3** Percutaneous **4** Percutaneous Endoscopic	**7** Autologous Tissue Substitute **J** Synthetic Substitute **K** Nonautologous Tissue Substitute	**Z** No Qualifier
A Hip Joint, Acetabular Surface, Right **E** Hip Joint, Acetabular Surface, Left **R** Hip Joint, Femoral Surface, Right **S** Hip Joint, Femoral Surface, Left	**0** Open	**9** Liner **B** Resurfacing Device	**Z** No Qualifier

Continued →

Section	0	Medical and Surgical
Body System	S	Lower Joints
Operation	U	Supplement: Putting in or on biological or synthetic material that physically reinforces and/or augments the function of a portion of a body part

Body Part (4th)	Approach (5th)	Device (6th)	Qualifier (7th)
C Knee Joint, Right D Knee Joint, Left	0 Open	7 Autologous Tissue Substitute J Synthetic Substitute K Nonautologous Tissue Substitute	Z No Qualifier
C Knee Joint, Right D Knee Joint, Left	0 Open	9 Liner	C Patellar Surface Z No Qualifier
C Knee Joint, Right D Knee Joint, Left	3 Percutaneous 4 Percutaneous Endoscopic	7 Autologous Tissue Substitute J Synthetic Substitute K Nonautologous Tissue Substitute	Z No Qualifier
T Knee Joint, Femoral Surface, Right U Knee Joint, Femoral Surface, Left V Knee Joint, Tibial Surface, Right W Knee Joint, Tibial Surface, Left	0 Open	9 Liner	Z No Qualifier

Section	0	Medical and Surgical
Body System	S	Lower Joints
Operation	W	Revision: Correcting, to the extent possible, a portion of a malfunctioning device or the position of a displaced device

Body Part (4th)	Approach (5th)	Device (6th)	Qualifier (7th)
0 Lumbar Vertebral Joint 3 Lumbosacral Joint	0 Open 3 Percutaneous 4 Percutaneous Endoscopic X External	0 Drainage Device 3 Infusion Device 4 Internal Fixation Device 7 Autologous Tissue Substitute 8 Spacer A Interbody Fusion Device J Synthetic Substitute K Nonautologous Tissue Substitute	Z No Qualifier
2 Lumbar Vertebral Disc 4 Lumbosacral Disc	0 Open 3 Percutaneous 4 Percutaneous Endoscopic X External	0 Drainage Device 3 Infusion Device 7 Autologous Tissue Substitute J Synthetic Substitute K Nonautologous Tissue Substitute	Z No Qualifier
5 Sacrococcygeal Joint 6 Coccygeal Joint 7 Sacroiliac Joint, Right 8 Sacroiliac Joint, Left	0 Open 3 Percutaneous 4 Percutaneous Endoscopic X External	0 Drainage Device 3 Infusion Device 4 Internal Fixation Device 7 Autologous Tissue Substitute 8 Spacer J Synthetic Substitute K Nonautologous Tissue Substitute	Z No Qualifier
9 Hip Joint, Right B Hip Joint, Left	0 Open	0 Drainage Device 3 Infusion Device 4 Internal Fixation Device 5 External Fixation Device 7 Autologous Tissue Substitute 8 Spacer 9 Liner B Resurfacing Device J Synthetic Substitute K Nonautologous Tissue Substitute	Z No Qualifier

Continued →

Body System S Lower Joints
Operation W Revision: Correcting, to the extent possible, a portion of a malfunctioning device or the position of a displaced device

Body Part (4th)	Approach (5th)	Device (6th)	Qualifier (7th)
9 Hip Joint, Right B Hip Joint, Left	3 Percutaneous 4 Percutaneous Endoscopic X External	0 Drainage Device 3 Infusion Device 4 Internal Fixation Device 5 External Fixation Device 7 Autologous Tissue Substitute 8 Spacer J Synthetic Substitute K Nonautologous Tissue Substitute	Z No Qualifier
A Hip Joint, Acetabular Surface, Right E Hip Joint, Acetabular Surface, Left R Hip Joint, Femoral Surface, Right S Hip Joint, Femoral Surface, Left T Knee Joint, Femoral Surface, Right U Knee Joint, Femoral Surface, Left V Knee Joint, Tibial Surface, Right W Knee Joint, Tibial Surface, Left	0 Open 3 Percutaneous 4 Percutaneous Endoscopic X External	J Synthetic Substitute	Z No Qualifier
C Knee Joint, Right D Knee Joint, Left	0 Open	0 Drainage Device 3 Infusion Device 4 Internal Fixation Device 5 External Fixation Device 7 Autologous Tissue Substitute 8 Spacer 9 Liner K Nonautologous Tissue Substitute	Z No Qualifier
C Knee Joint, Right D Knee Joint, Left	0 Open	J Synthetic Substitute	C Patellar Surface Z No Qualifier
C Knee Joint, Right D Knee Joint, Left	3 Percutaneous 4 Percutaneous Endoscopic X External	0 Drainage Device 3 Infusion Device 4 Internal Fixation Device 5 External Fixation Device 7 Autologous Tissue Substitute 8 Spacer K Nonautologous Tissue Substitute	Z No Qualifier
C Knee Joint, Right E Knee Joint, Left	3 Percutaneous 4 Percutaneous Endoscopic X External	J Synthetic Substitute	C Patellar Surface Z No Qualifier
F Ankle Joint, Right G Ankle Joint, Left H Tarsal Joint, Right J Tarsal Joint, Left K Tarsometatarsal Joint, Right L Tarsometatarsal Joint, Left M Metatarsal-Phalangeal Joint, Right N Metatarsal-Phalangeal Joint, Left P Toe Phalangeal Joint, Right Q Toe Phalangeal Joint, Left	0 Open 3 Percutaneous 4 Percutaneous Endoscopic X External	0 Drainage Device 3 Infusion Device 4 Internal Fixation Device 5 External Fixation Device 7 Autologous Tissue Substitute 8 Spacer J Synthetic Substitute K Nonautologous Tissue Substitute	Z No Qualifier

0S9D4ZZ Drainage of Left Knee Joint, Percutaneous Endoscopic Approach— AHA CC: 2Q, 2018, 17

0SB20ZZ Excision of Lumbar Vertebral Disc, Open Approach—AHA CC: 2Q, 2014, 6-7; 2Q, 2016, 16; 4Q, 2017, 76-77

0SB40ZZ Excision of Lumbosacral Disc, Open Approach—AHA CC: 4Q, 2017, 76-77

0SBD4ZZ Excision of Left Knee Joint, Percutaneous Endoscopic Approach—AHA CC: 1Q, 2015, 34

0SG0071 Fusion of Lumbar Vertebral Joint with Autologous Tissue Substitute, Posterior Approach, Posterior Column, Open Approach—
  AHA CC: 1Q, 2013, 21-23; 3Q, 2013, 25-26

0SG00AJ Fusion of Lumbar Vertebral Joint with Interbody Fusion Device, Posterior Approach, Anterior Column, Open Approach—AHA
  CC: 3Q, 2013, 25-26

0SG107J Fusion of 2 or more Lumbar Vertebral Joints with Autologous Tissue Substitute, Posterior Approach, Anterior Column, Open
  Approach—AHA CC: 3Q, 2014, 36

0SGG04Z Fusion of Left Ankle Joint with Internal Fixation Device, Open Approach—AHA CC: 2Q, 2013, 39-40

0SGG07Z Fusion of Left Ankle Joint with Autologous Tissue Substitute, Open Approach—AHA CC: 2Q, 2013, 39-40

0SJG3ZZ Inspection of Left Ankle Joint, Percutaneous Approach—AHA CC: 1Q, 2017, 50

0SNC4ZZ Release Right Knee Joint, Percutaneous Endoscopic Approach—AHA CC: 2Q, 2020, 26-27

0SP909Z Removal of Liner from Right Hip Joint, Open Approach—AHA CC: 2Q, 2015, 19-20; 4Q, 2016, 111-112

0SP90JZ Removal of Synthetic Substitute from Right Hip Joint, Open Approach—AHA CC: 2Q, 2015, 19-20

0SPC0JZ Removal of Synthetic Substitute from Right Knee Joint, Open Approach—AHA CC: 2Q, 2015, 18-19

0SPF0JZ Removal of Synthetic Substitute from Right Ankle Joint, Open Approach—AHA CC: 4Q, 2017, 107-108

0SPG04Z Removal of Internal Fixation Device from Left Ankle Joint, Open Approach—AHA CC: 2Q, 2013, 39-40

0SPR0JZ Removal of Synthetic Substitute from Right Hip Joint, Femoral Surface, Open Approach—AHA CC: 4Q, 2016, 111-112

0SPW0JZ Removal of Synthetic Substitute from Left Knee Joint, Tibial Surface, Open Approach—AHA CC: 2Q, 2018, 16-17

0SQB4ZZ Repair Left Hip Joint, Percutaneous Endoscopic Approach—AHA CC: 4Q, 2014, 25-26

0SRB06Z Replacement of Left Hip Joint with Oxidized Zirconium on Polyethylene Synthetic Substitute, Open Approach—AHA CC: 4Q,
  2017, 39

0SRB0J9 Replacement of Left Hip Joint with Synthetic Substitute, Cemented, Open Approach—AHA CC: 3Q, 2015, 18-19

0SRC0J9 Replacement of Right Knee Joint with Synthetic Substitute, Cemented, Open Approach—AHA CC: 2Q, 2015, 18-19

0SRD0JZ Replacement of Left Knee Joint with Synthetic Substitute, Open Approach—AHA CC: 4Q, 2016, 109-110

0SRD0LZ Replacement of Left Knee Joint with Unicondylar Synthetic Substitute, Open Approach—AHA CC: 4Q, 2016, 110

0SRF0JA Replacement of Right Ankle Joint with Synthetic Substitute, Uncemented, Open Approach—AHA CC: 4Q, 2017, 107-108

0SRR03A Replacement of Right Hip Joint, Femoral Surface with Ceramic Synthetic Substitute, Uncemented, Open Approach—AHA CC:
  2Q, 2015, 19-20

0SRR0J9 Replacement of Right Hip Joint, Femoral Surface with Synthetic Substitute, Cemented, Open Approach—AHA CC: 4Q, 2016,
  111-112

0SRW0JZ Replacement of Left Knee Joint, Tibial Surface with Synthetic Substitute, Open Approach—AHA CC: 2Q, 2018, 16-17

0SSB04Z Reposition Left Hip Joint with Internal Fixation Device, Open Approach—AHA CC: 2Q, 2016, 32

0STD0ZZ Resection of Left Knee Joint, Open Approach—AHA CC: 4Q, 2014, 30-31

0STM0ZZ Resection of Right Metatarsal-Phalangeal Joint, Open Approach—AHA CC: 1Q, 2016, 20-21

0SUA09Z Supplement Right Hip Joint, Acetabular Surface with Liner, Open Approach—AHA CC: 2Q, 2015, 19-20; 4Q, 2016, 111-112

0SWF0JZ Revision of Synthetic Substitute in Right Ankle Joint, Open Approach—AHA CC: 4Q, 2017, 107-108

0SWW0JZ Revision of Synthetic Substitute in Left Knee Joint, Tibial Surface, Open Approach—AHA CC: 4Q, 2016, 112

Urinary System

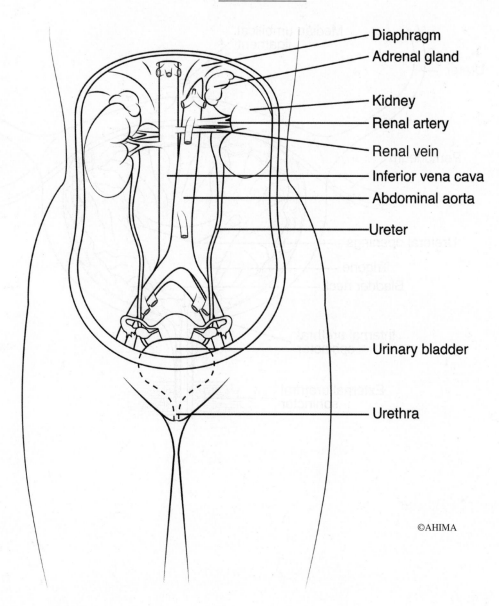

Diaphragm

Adrenal gland

Kidney

Renal artery

Renal vein

Inferior vena cava

Abdominal aorta

Ureter

Urinary bladder

Urethra

©AHIMA

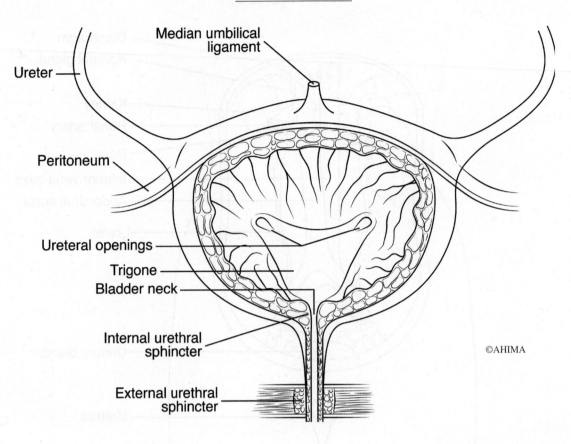

Median umbilical ligament

Ureter

Peritoneum

Ureteral openings

Trigone

Bladder neck

Internal urethral sphincter

External urethral sphincter

©AHIMA

Kidney

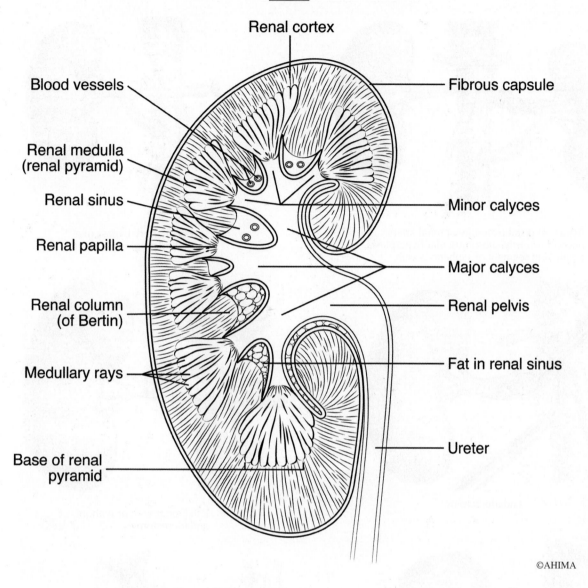

Renal cortex

Blood vessels

Renal medulla
(renal pyramid)

Renal sinus

Renal papilla

Renal column
(of Bertin)

Medullary rays

Base of renal
pyramid

Fibrous capsule

Minor calyces

Major calyces

Renal pelvis

Fat in renal sinus

Ureter

©AHIMA

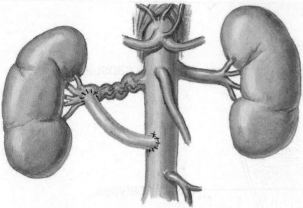

Bypass to distal extremity of renal artery
beyond extensive fibromuscular hyperplasia,
employing segment of saphenous vein

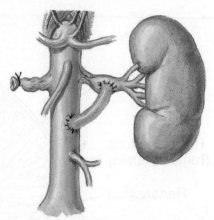

Renal artery bypass plus
contralateral nephrectomy

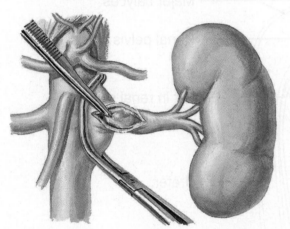

Endarterectomy

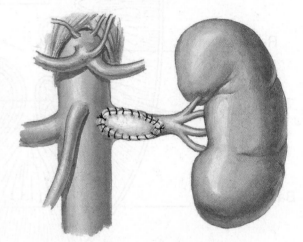

Patch graft with or without
endarterectomy

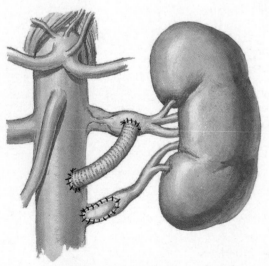

Renal artery bypass plus patch graft
to accessory renal artery

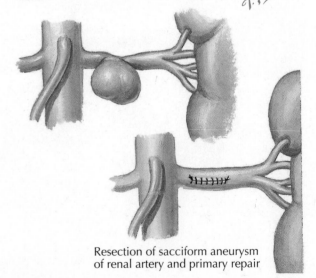

Resection of sacciform aneurysm
of renal artery and primary repair

Section	0	Medical and Surgical
Body System	T	Urinary System
Operation	1	Bypass: Altering the route of passage of the contents of a tubular body part

Body Part (4th)	Approach (5th)	Device (6th)	Qualifier (7th)
3 Kidney Pelvis, Right 4 Kidney Pelvis, Left	0 Open 4 Percutaneous Endoscopic	7 Autologous Tissue Substitute J Synthetic Substitute K Nonautologous Tissue Substitute Z No Device	3 Kidney Pelvis, Right 4 Kidney Pelvis, Left 6 Ureter, Right 7 Ureter, Left 8 Colon 9 Colocutaneous A Ileum B Bladder C Ileocutaneous D Cutaneous
3 Kidney Pelvis, Right 4 Kidney Pelvis, Left	3 Percutaneous	J Synthetic Substitute	D Cutaneous
6 Ureter, Right 7 Ureter, Left 8 Ureters, Bilateral	0 Open 4 Percutaneous Endoscopic	7 Autologous Tissue Substitute J Synthetic Substitute K Nonautologous Tissue Substitute Z No Device	6 Ureter, Right 7 Ureter, Left 8 Colon 9 Colocutaneous A Ileum B Bladder C Ileocutaneous D Cutaneous
6 Ureter, Right 7 Ureter, Left 8 Ureters, Bilateral	3 Percutaneous	J Synthetic Substitute	D Cutaneous
B Bladder	0 Open 4 Percutaneous Endoscopic	7 Autologous Tissue Substitute J Synthetic Substitute K Nonautologous Tissue Substitute Z No Device	9 Colocutaneous C Ileocutaneous D Cutaneous
B Bladder	3 Percutaneous	J Synthetic Substitute	D Cutaneous

Section	0	Medical and Surgical
Body System	T	Urinary System
Operation	2	Change: Taking out or off a device from a body part and putting back an identical or similar device in or on the same body part without cutting or puncturing the skin or a mucous membrane

Body Part (4th)	Approach (5th)	Device (6th)	Qualifier (7th)
5 Kidney 9 Ureter B Bladder D Urethra	X External	0 Drainage Device Y Other Device	Z No Qualifier

Section	0	Medical and Surgical
Body System	T	Urinary System
Operation	5	Destruction: Physical eradication of all or a portion of a body part by the direct use of energy, force, or a destructive agent

Body Part (4th)	Approach (5th)	Device (6th)	Qualifier (7th)
0 Kidney, Right 1 Kidney, Left 3 Kidney Pelvis, Right 4 Kidney Pelvis, Left 6 Ureter, Right 7 Ureter, Left B Bladder C Bladder Neck	0 Open 3 Percutaneous 4 Percutaneous Endoscopic 7 Via Natural or Artificial Opening 8 Via Natural or Artificial Opening Endoscopic	Z No Device	Z No Qualifier

Continued →

Medical and Surgical, Urinary System Tables

Section   **0**   **Medical and Surgical**
Body System   **T**   **Urinary System**
Operation   **5**   **Destruction:** Physical eradication of all or a portion of a body part by the direct use of energy, force, or a destructive agent

Body Part (4th)	Approach (5th)	Device (6th)	Qualifier (7th)
D Urethra	**0** Open **3** Percutaneous **4** Percutaneous Endoscopic **7** Via Natural or Artificial Opening **8** Via Natural or Artificial Opening Endoscopic **X** External	**Z** No Device	**Z** No Qualifier

Section   **0**   **Medical and Surgical**
Body System   **T**   **Urinary System**
Operation   **7**   **Dilation:** Expanding an orifice or the lumen of a tubular body part

Body Part (4th)	Approach (5th)	Device (6th)	Qualifier (7th)
3 Kidney Pelvis, Right **4** Kidney Pelvis, Left **6** Ureter, Right **7** Ureter, Left **8** Ureters, Bilateral **B** Bladder **C** Bladder Neck **D** Urethra	**0** Open **3** Percutaneous **4** Percutaneous Endoscopic **7** Via Natural or Artificial Opening **8** Via Natural or Artificial Opening Endoscopic	**D** Intraluminal Device **Z** No Device	**Z** No Qualifier

Section   **0**   **Medical and Surgical**
Body System   **T**   **Urinary System**
Operation   **8**   **Division:** Cutting into a body part, without draining fluids and/or gases from the body part, in order to separate or transect a body part

Body Part (4th)	Approach (5th)	Device (6th)	Qualifier (7th)
2 Kidneys, Bilateral **C** Bladder Neck	**0** Open **3** Percutaneous **4** Percutaneous Endoscopic	**Z** No Device	**Z** No Qualifier

Section   **0**   **Medical and Surgical**
Body System   **T**   **Urinary System**
Operation   **9**   **Drainage:** Taking or letting out fluids and/or gases from a body part

Body Part (4th)	Approach (5th)	Device (6th)	Qualifier (7th)
0 Kidney, Right **1** Kidney, Left **3** Kidney Pelvis, Right **4** Kidney Pelvis, Left **6** Ureter, Right **7** Ureter, Left **8** Ureters, Bilateral **B** Bladder **C** Bladder Neck	**0** Open **3** Percutaneous **4** Percutaneous Endoscopic **7** Via Natural or Artificial Opening **8** Via Natural or Artificial Opening Endoscopic	**0** Drainage Device	**Z** No Qualifier
0 Kidney, Right **1** Kidney, Left **3** Kidney Pelvis, Right **4** Kidney Pelvis, Left **6** Ureter, Right **7** Ureter, Left **8** Ureters, Bilateral **B** Bladder **C** Bladder Neck	**0** Open **3** Percutaneous **4** Percutaneous Endoscopic **7** Via Natural or Artificial Opening **8** Via Natural or Artificial Opening Endoscopic	**Z** No Device	**X** Diagnostic **Z** No Qualifier

Continued →

Section   **0**   **Medical and Surgical**
Body System   **T**   **Urinary System**
Operation   **9**   **Drainage:** Taking or letting out fluids and/or gases from a body part

Body Part (4th)	Approach (5th)	Device (6th)	Qualifier (7th)
D Urethra	0 Open 3 Percutaneous 4 Percutaneous Endoscopic 7 Via Natural or Artificial Opening 8 Via Natural or Artificial Opening Endoscopic X External	0 Drainage Device	Z No Qualifier
D Urethra	0 Open 3 Percutaneous 4 Percutaneous Endoscopic 7 Via Natural or Artificial Opening 8 Via Natural or Artificial Opening Endoscopic X External	Z No Device	X Diagnostic Z No Qualifier

Section   **0**   **Medical and Surgical**
Body System   **T**   **Urinary System**
Operation   **B**   **Excision:** Cutting out or off, without replacement, a portion of a body part

Body Part (4th)	Approach (5th)	Device (6th)	Qualifier (7th)
0 Kidney, Right 1 Kidney, Left 3 Kidney Pelvis, Right 4 Kidney Pelvis, Left 6 Ureter, Right 7 Ureter, Left B Bladder C Bladder Neck	0 Open 3 Percutaneous 4 Percutaneous Endoscopic 7 Via Natural or Artificial Opening 8 Via Natural or Artificial Opening Endoscopic	Z No Device	X Diagnostic Z No Qualifier
D Urethra	0 Open 3 Percutaneous 4 Percutaneous Endoscopic 7 Via Natural or Artificial Opening 8 Via Natural or Artificial Opening Endoscopic X External	Z No Device	X Diagnostic Z No Qualifier

Section   **0**   **Medical and Surgical**
Body System   **T**   **Urinary System**
Operation   **C**   **Extirpation:** Taking or cutting out solid matter from a body part

Body Part (4th)	Approach (5th)	Device (6th)	Qualifier (7th)
0 Kidney, Right 1 Kidney, Left 3 Kidney Pelvis, Right 4 Kidney Pelvis, Left 6 Ureter, Right 7 Ureter, Left B Bladder C Bladder Neck	0 Open 3 Percutaneous 4 Percutaneous Endoscopic 7 Via Natural or Artificial Opening 8 Via Natural or Artificial Opening Endoscopic	Z No Device	Z No Qualifier
D Urethra	0 Open 3 Percutaneous 4 Percutaneous Endoscopic 7 Via Natural or Artificial Opening 8 Via Natural or Artificial Opening Endoscopic X External	Z No Device	Z No Qualifier

Section	0	Medical and Surgical
Body System	T	Urinary System
Operation	D	Extraction: Pulling or stripping out or off all or a portion of a body part by the use of force

Body Part (4th)	Approach (5th)	Device (6th)	Qualifier (7th)
0 Kidney, Right 1 Kidney, Left	0 Open 3 Percutaneous 4 Percutaneous Endoscopic	Z No Device	Z No Qualifier

Section	0	Medical and Surgical
Body System	T	Urinary System
Operation	F	Fragmentation: Breaking solid matter in a body part into pieces

Body Part (4th)	Approach (5th)	Device (6th)	Qualifier (7th)
3 Kidney Pelvis, Right 4 Kidney Pelvis, Left 6 Ureter, Right 7 Ureter, Left B Bladder C Bladder Neck D Urethra	0 Open 3 Percutaneous 4 Percutaneous Endoscopic 7 Via Natural or Artificial Opening 8 Via Natural or Artificial Opening Endoscopic X External	Z No Device	Z No Qualifier

Section	0	Medical and Surgical
Body System	T	Urinary System
Operation	H	Insertion: Putting in a nonbiological appliance that monitors, assists, performs, or prevents a physiological function but does not physically take the place of a body part

Body Part (4th)	Approach (5th)	Device (6th)	Qualifier (7th)
5 Kidney	0 Open 3 Percutaneous 4 Percutaneous Endoscopic 7 Via Natural or Artificial Opening 8 Via Natural or Artificial Opening Endoscopic	1 Radioactive Element 2 Monitoring Device 3 Infusion Device Y Other Device	Z No Qualifier
9 Ureter	0 Open 3 Percutaneous 4 Percutaneous Endoscopic 7 Via Natural or Artificial Opening 8 Via Natural or Artificial Opening Endoscopic	1 Radioactive Element 2 Monitoring Device 3 Infusion Device M Stimulator Lead Y Other Device	Z No Qualifier
B Bladder	0 Open 3 Percutaneous 4 Percutaneous Endoscopic 7 Via Natural or Artificial Opening 8 Via Natural or Artificial Opening Endoscopic	1 Radioactive Element 2 Monitoring Device 3 Infusion Device L Artificial Sphincter M Stimulator Lead Y Other Device	Z No Qualifier
C Bladder Neck	0 Open 3 Percutaneous 4 Percutaneous Endoscopic 7 Via Natural or Artificial Opening 8 Via Natural or Artificial Opening Endoscopic	L Artificial Sphincter	Z No Qualifier
D Urethra	0 Open 3 Percutaneous 4 Percutaneous Endoscopic 7 Via Natural or Artificial Opening 8 Via Natural or Artificial Opening Endoscopic	1 Radioactive Element 2 Monitoring Device 3 Infusion Device L Artificial Sphincter Y Other Device	Z No Qualifier
D Urethra	X External	2 Monitoring Device 3 Infusion Device L Artificial Sphincter	Z No Qualifier

Section   **0**   **Medical and Surgical**
Body System   **T**   **Urinary System**
Operation   **J**   **Inspection:** Visually and/or manually exploring a body part

Body Part (4ᵗʰ)	Approach (5ᵗʰ)	Device (6ᵗʰ)	Qualifier (7ᵗʰ)
5 Kidney 9 Ureter B Bladder D Urethra	0 Open 3 Percutaneous 4 Percutaneous Endoscopic 7 Via Natural or Artificial Opening 8 Via Natural or Artificial Opening Endoscopic X External	Z No Device	Z No Qualifier

Section   **0**   **Medical and Surgical**
Body System   **T**   **Urinary System**
Operation   **L**   **Occlusion:** Completely closing an orifice or the lumen of a tubular body part

Body Part (4ᵗʰ)	Approach (5ᵗʰ)	Device (6ᵗʰ)	Qualifier (7ᵗʰ)
3 Kidney Pelvis, Right 4 Kidney Pelvis, Left 6 Ureter, Right 7 Ureter, Left B Bladder C Bladder Neck	0 Open 3 Percutaneous 4 Percutaneous Endoscopic	C Extraluminal Device D Intraluminal Device Z No Device	Z No Qualifier
3 Kidney Pelvis, Right 4 Kidney Pelvis, Left 6 Ureter, Right 7 Ureter, Left B Bladder C Bladder Neck	7 Via Natural or Artificial Opening 8 Via Natural or Artificial Opening Endoscopic	D Intraluminal Device Z No Device	Z No Qualifier
D Urethra	0 Open 3 Percutaneous 4 Percutaneous Endoscopic X External	C Extraluminal Device D Intraluminal Device Z No Device	Z No Qualifier
D Urethra	7 Via Natural or Artificial Opening 8 Via Natural or Artificial Opening Endoscopic	D Intraluminal Device Z No Device	Z No Qualifier

Section   **0**   **Medical and Surgical**
Body System   **T**   **Urinary System**
Operation   **M**   **Reattachment:** Putting back in or on all or a portion of a separated body part to its normal location or other suitable location

Body Part (4ᵗʰ)	Approach (5ᵗʰ)	Device (6ᵗʰ)	Qualifier (7ᵗʰ)
0 Kidney, Right 1 Kidney, Left 2 Kidneys, Bilateral 3 Kidney Pelvis, Right 4 Kidney Pelvis, Left 6 Ureter, Right 7 Ureter, Left 8 Ureters, Bilateral B Bladder C Bladder Neck D Urethra	0 Open 4 Percutaneous Endoscopic	Z No Device	Z No Qualifier

Section	0	Medical and Surgical
Body System	T	Urinary System
Operation	N	Release: Freeing a body part from an abnormal physical constraint by cutting or by the use of force

Body Part (4th)	Approach (5th)	Device (6th)	Qualifier (7th)
0 Kidney, Right 1 Kidney, Left 3 Kidney Pelvis, Right 4 Kidney Pelvis, Left 6 Ureter, Right 7 Ureter, Left B Bladder C Bladder Neck	0 Open 3 Percutaneous 4 Percutaneous Endoscopic 7 Via Natural or Artificial Opening 8 Via Natural or Artificial Opening Endoscopic	Z No Device	Z No Qualifier
D Urethra	0 Open 3 Percutaneous 4 Percutaneous Endoscopic 7 Via Natural or Artificial Opening 8 Via Natural or Artificial Opening Endoscopic X External	Z No Device	Z No Qualifier

Section	0	Medical and Surgical
Body System	T	Urinary System
Operation	P	Removal: Taking out or off a device from a body part

Body Part (4th)	Approach (5th)	Device (6th)	Qualifier (7th)
5 Kidney	0 Open 3 Percutaneous 4 Percutaneous Endoscopic 7 Via Natural or Artificial Opening 8 Via Natural or Artificial Opening Endoscopic	0 Drainage Device 2 Monitoring Device 3 Infusion Device 7 Autologous Tissue Substitute C Extraluminal Device D Intraluminal Device J Synthetic Substitute K Nonautologous Tissue Substitute Y Other Device	Z No Qualifier
5 Kidney	X External	0 Drainage Device 2 Monitoring Device 3 Infusion Device D Intraluminal Device	Z No Qualifier
9 Ureter	0 Open 3 Percutaneous 4 Percutaneous Endoscopic 7 Via Natural or Artificial Opening 8 Via Natural or Artificial Opening Endoscopic	0 Drainage Device 2 Monitoring Device 3 Infusion Device 7 Autologous Tissue Substitute C Extraluminal Device D Intraluminal Device J Synthetic Substitute K Nonautologous Tissue Substitute M Stimulator Lead Y Other Device	Z No Qualifier
9 Ureter	X External	0 Drainage Device 2 Monitoring Device 3 Infusion Device D Intraluminal Device M Stimulator Lead	Z No Qualifier

Continued →

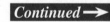

Section 0 Medical and Surgical
Body System T Urinary System
Operation P Removal: Taking out or off a device from a body part

0TP Continued

0TP–0TQ

Body Part (4ᵗʰ)	Approach (5ᵗʰ)	Device (6ᵗʰ)	Qualifier (7ᵗʰ)
B Bladder	**0** Open **3** Percutaneous **4** Percutaneous Endoscopic **7** Via Natural or Artificial Opening **8** Via Natural or Artificial Opening Endoscopic	**0** Drainage Device **2** Monitoring Device **3** Infusion Device **7** Autologous Tissue Substitute **C** Extraluminal Device **D** Intraluminal Device **J** Synthetic Substitute **K** Nonautologous Tissue Substitute **L** Artificial Sphincter **M** Stimulator Lead **Y** Other Device	**Z** No Qualifier
B Bladder	**X** External	**0** Drainage Device **2** Monitoring Device **3** Infusion Device **D** Intraluminal Device **L** Artificial Sphincter **M** Stimulator Lead	**Z** No Qualifier
D Urethra	**0** Open **3** Percutaneous **4** Percutaneous Endoscopic **7** Via Natural or Artificial Opening **8** Via Natural or Artificial Opening Endoscopic	**0** Drainage Device **2** Monitoring Device **3** Infusion Device **7** Autologous Tissue Substitute **C** Extraluminal Device **D** Intraluminal Device **J** Synthetic Substitute **K** Nonautologous Tissue Substitute **L** Artificial Sphincter **Y** Other Device	**Z** No Qualifier
D Urethra	**X** External	**0** Drainage Device **2** Monitoring Device **3** Infusion Device **D** Intraluminal Device **L** Artificial Sphincter	**Z** No Qualifier

Section 0 Medical and Surgical
Body System T Urinary System
Operation Q Repair: Restoring, to the extent possible, a body part to its normal anatomic structure and function

Body Part (4ᵗʰ)	Approach (5ᵗʰ)	Device (6ᵗʰ)	Qualifier (7ᵗʰ)
0 Kidney, Right **1** Kidney, Left **3** Kidney Pelvis, Right **4** Kidney Pelvis, Left **6** Ureter, Right **7** Ureter, Left **B** Bladder **C** Bladder Neck	**0** Open **3** Percutaneous **4** Percutaneous Endoscopic **7** Via Natural or Artificial Opening **8** Via Natural or Artificial Opening Endoscopic	**Z** No Device	**Z** No Qualifier
D Urethra	**0** Open **3** Percutaneous **4** Percutaneous Endoscopic **7** Via Natural or Artificial Opening **8** Via Natural or Artificial Opening Endoscopic **X** External	**Z** No Device	**Z** No Qualifier

Section	0	Medical and Surgical
Body System	T	Urinary System
Operation	R	**Replacement:** Putting in or on biological or synthetic material that physically takes the place and/or function of all or a portion of a body part

Body Part (4th)	Approach (5th)	Device (6th)	Qualifier (7th)
3 Kidney Pelvis, Right 4 Kidney Pelvis, Left 6 Ureter, Right 7 Ureter, Left B Bladder C Bladder Neck	0 Open 4 Percutaneous Endoscopic 7 Via Natural or Artificial Opening 8 Via Natural or Artificial Opening Endoscopic	7 Autologous Tissue Substitute J Synthetic Substitute K Nonautologous Tissue Substitute	Z No Qualifier
D Urethra	0 Open 4 Percutaneous Endoscopic 7 Via Natural or Artificial Opening 8 Via Natural or Artificial Opening Endoscopic X External	7 Autologous Tissue Substitute J Synthetic Substitute K Nonautologous Tissue Substitute	Z No Qualifier

Section	0	Medical and Surgical
Body System	T	Urinary System
Operation	S	**Reposition:** Moving to its normal location, or other suitable location, all or a portion of a body part

Body Part (4th)	Approach (5th)	Device (6th)	Qualifier (7th)
0 Kidney, Right 1 Kidney, Left 2 Kidneys, Bilateral 3 Kidney Pelvis, Right 4 Kidney Pelvis, Left 6 Ureter, Right 7 Ureter, Left 8 Ureters, Bilateral B Bladder C Bladder Neck D Urethra	0 Open 4 Percutaneous Endoscopic	Z No Device	Z No Qualifier

Section	0	Medical and Surgical
Body System	T	Urinary System
Operation	T	**Resection:** Cutting out or off, without replacement, all of a body part

Body Part (4th)	Approach (5th)	Device (6th)	Qualifier (7th)
0 Kidney, Right 1 Kidney, Left 2 Kidneys, Bilateral	0 Open 4 Percutaneous Endoscopic	Z No Device	Z No Qualifier
3 Kidney Pelvis, Right 4 Kidney Pelvis, Left 6 Ureter, Right 7 Ureter, Left B Bladder C Bladder Neck D Urethra	0 Open 4 Percutaneous Endoscopic 7 Via Natural or Artificial Opening 8 Via Natural or Artificial Opening Endoscopic	Z No Device	Z No Qualifier

Section 0 Medical and Surgical
Body System T Urinary System
Operation U Supplement: Putting in or on biological or synthetic material that physically reinforces and/or augments the function of a portion of a body part

Body Part (4th)	Approach (5th)	Device (6th)	Qualifier (7th)
3 Kidney Pelvis, Right 4 Kidney Pelvis, Left 6 Ureter, Right 7 Ureter, Left B Bladder C Bladder Neck	0 Open 4 Percutaneous Endoscopic 7 Via Natural or Artificial Opening 8 Via Natural or Artificial Opening Endoscopic	7 Autologous Tissue Substitute J Synthetic Substitute K Nonautologous Tissue Substitute	Z No Qualifier
D Urethra	0 Open 4 Percutaneous Endoscopic 7 Via Natural or Artificial Opening 8 Via Natural or Artificial Opening Endoscopic X External	7 Autologous Tissue Substitute J Synthetic Substitute K Nonautologous Tissue Substitute	Z No Qualifier

Section 0 Medical and Surgical
Body System T Urinary System
Operation V Restriction: Partially closing an orifice or the lumen of a tubular body part

Body Part (4th)	Approach (5th)	Device (6th)	Qualifier (7th)
3 Kidney Pelvis, Right 4 Kidney Pelvis, Left 6 Ureter, Right 7 Ureter, Left B Bladder C Bladder Neck	0 Open 3 Percutaneous 4 Percutaneous Endoscopic	C Extraluminal Device D Intraluminal Device Z No Device	Z No Qualifier
3 Kidney Pelvis, Right 4 Kidney Pelvis, Left 6 Ureter, Right 7 Ureter, Left B Bladder C Bladder Neck	7 Via Natural or Artificial Opening 8 Via Natural or Artificial Opening Endoscopic	D Intraluminal Device Z No Device	Z No Qualifier
D Urethra	0 Open 3 Percutaneous 4 Percutaneous Endoscopic	C Extraluminal Device D Intraluminal Device Z No Device	Z No Qualifier
D Urethra	7 Via Natural or Artificial Opening 8 Via Natural or Artificial Opening Endoscopic	D Intraluminal Device Z No Device	Z No Qualifier
D Urethra	X External	Z No Device	Z No Qualifier

Section 0 Medical and Surgical
Body System T Urinary System
Operation W Revision: Correcting, to the extent possible, a portion of a malfunctioning device or the position of a displaced device

Body Part (4th)	Approach (5th)	Device (6th)	Qualifier (7th)
5 Kidney	0 Open 3 Percutaneous 4 Percutaneous Endoscopic 7 Via Natural or Artificial Opening 8 Via Natural or Artificial Opening Endoscopic	0 Drainage Device 2 Monitoring Device 3 Infusion Device 7 Autologous Tissue Substitute C Extraluminal Device D Intraluminal Device J Synthetic Substitute K Nonautologous Tissue Substitute Y Other Device	Z No Qualifier

Continued →

Section	0	Medical and Surgical
Body System	T	Urinary System
Operation	W	**Revision:** Correcting, to the extent possible, a portion of a malfunctioning device or the position of a displaced device

Body Part (4th)	Approach (5th)	Device (6th)	Qualifier (7th)
5 Kidney	X External	0 Drainage Device 2 Monitoring Device 3 Infusion Device 7 Autologous Tissue Substitute C Extraluminal Device D Intraluminal Device J Synthetic Substitute K Nonautologous Tissue Substitute	Z No Qualifier
9 Ureter	0 Open 3 Percutaneous 4 Percutaneous Endoscopic 7 Via Natural or Artificial Opening 8 Via Natural or Artificial Opening Endoscopic	0 Drainage Device 2 Monitoring Device 3 Infusion Device 7 Autologous Tissue Substitute C Extraluminal Device D Intraluminal Device J Synthetic Substitute K Nonautologous Tissue Substitute M Stimulator Lead Y Other Device	Z No Qualifier
9 Ureter	X External	0 Drainage Device 2 Monitoring Device 3 Infusion Device 7 Autologous Tissue Substitute C Extraluminal Device D Intraluminal Device J Synthetic Substitute K Nonautologous Tissue Substitute M Stimulator Lead	Z No Qualifier
B Bladder	0 Open 3 Percutaneous 4 Percutaneous Endoscopic 7 Via Natural or Artificial Opening 8 Via Natural or Artificial Opening Endoscopic	0 Drainage Device 2 Monitoring Device 3 Infusion Device 7 Autologous Tissue Substitute C Extraluminal Device D Intraluminal Device J Synthetic Substitute K Nonautologous Tissue Substitute L Artificial Sphincter M Stimulator Lead Y Other Device	Z No Qualifier
B Bladder	X External	0 Drainage Device 2 Monitoring Device 3 Infusion Device 7 Autologous Tissue Substitute C Extraluminal Device D Intraluminal Device J Synthetic Substitute K Nonautologous Tissue Substitute L Artificial Sphincter M Stimulator Lead	Z No Qualifier
D Urethra	0 Open 3 Percutaneous 4 Percutaneous Endoscopic 7 Via Natural or Artificial Opening 8 Via Natural or Artificial Opening Endoscopic	0 Drainage Device 2 Monitoring Device 3 Infusion Device 7 Autologous Tissue Substitute C Extraluminal Device D Intraluminal Device J Synthetic Substitute K Nonautologous Tissue Substitute L Artificial Sphincter Y Other Device	Z No Qualifier

Continued →

Section	0	Medical and Surgical
Body System	T	Urinary System
Operation	W	**Revision:** Correcting, to the extent possible, a portion of a malfunctioning device or the position of a displaced device

Body Part (4ᵗʰ)	Approach (5ᵗʰ)	Device (6ᵗʰ)	Qualifier (7ᵗʰ)
D Urethra	**X** External	**0** Drainage Device **2** Monitoring Device **3** Infusion Device **7** Autologous Tissue Substitute **C** Extraluminal Device **D** Intraluminal Device **J** Synthetic Substitute **K** Nonautologous Tissue Substitute **L** Artificial Sphincter	**Z** No Qualifier

Section	0	Medical and Surgical
Body System	T	Urinary System
Operation	Y	**Transplantation:** Putting in or on all or a portion of a living body part taken from another individual or animal to physically take the place and/or function of all or a portion of a similar body part

Body Part (4ᵗʰ)	Approach (5ᵗʰ)	Device (6ᵗʰ)	Qualifier (7ᵗʰ)
0 Kidney, Right **1** Kidney, Left	**0** Open	**Z** No Device	**0** Allogeneic **1** Syngeneic **2** Zooplastic

AHA Coding Clinic

0T170ZB Bypass Left Ureter to Bladder, Open Approach—AHA CC: 3Q, 2015, 34-35

0T180ZC Bypass Bilateral Ureters to Ileocutaneous, Open Approach—AHA CC: 3Q, 2017, 20-21

0T1B0Z9 Bypass Bladder to Colocutaneous, Open Approach—AHA CC: 3Q, 2017, 21-22

0T768DZ Dilation of Right Ureter with Intraluminal Device, Via Natural or Artificial Opening Endoscopic—AHA CC: 2Q, 2016, 27-28; 4Q, 2017, 111

0T778DZ Dilation of Left Ureter with Intraluminal Device, Via Natural or Artificial Opening Endoscopic—AHA CC: 2Q, 2015, 8-9

0T7D8DZ Dilation of Urethra with Intraluminal Device, Via Natural or Artificial Opening Endoscopic—AHA CC: 4Q, 2013, 123

0T9680Z Drainage of Right Ureter with Drainage Device, Via Natural or Artificial Opening Endoscopic—AHA CC: 3Q, 2017, 19-20

0TBB8ZX Excision of Bladder, Via Natural or Artificial Opening Endoscopic, Diagnostic—AHA CC: 1Q, 2016, 19

0TBB8ZZ Excision of Bladder, Via Natural or Artificial Opening Endoscopic—AHA CC: 2Q, 2014, 8

0TBD8ZZ Excision of Urethra, Via Natural or Artificial Opening Endoscopic—AHA CC: 3Q, 2015, 34

0TC18ZZ Extirpation of Matter from Left Kidney, Via Natural or Artificial Opening Endoscopic—AHA CC: 2Q, 2015, 8-9

0TC48ZZ Extirpation of Matter from Left Kidney Pelvis, Via Natural or Artificial Opening Endoscopic—AHA CC: 2Q, 2015, 7-8

0TC68ZZ Extirpation of Matter from Right Ureter, Via Natural or Artificial Opening Endoscopic—AHA CC: 4Q, 2013, 122-123

0TC78ZZ Extirpation of Matter from Left Ureter, Via Natural or Artificial Opening Endoscopic—AHA CC: 2Q, 2015, 8-9

0TCB8ZZ Extirpation of Matter from Bladder, Via Natural or Artificial Opening Endoscopic—AHA CC: 2Q, 2015, 8-9; 3Q, 2016, 23-24; 3Q, 2019, 4

0TF3XZZ Fragmentation in Right Kidney Pelvis, External Approach—AHA CC: 4Q, 2013, 122

0TP98DZ Removal of Intraluminal Device from Ureter, Via Natural or Artificial Opening Endoscopic—AHA CC: 2Q, 2016, 27-28

0TQD0ZZ Repair Urethra, Open Approach—AHA CC: 1Q, 2017, 37-38

0TRB07Z Replacement of Bladder with Autologous Tissue Substitute, Open Approach—AHA CC: 3Q, 2017, 20-21

0TS60ZZ Reposition Right Ureter, Open Approach—AHA CC: 1Q, 2017, 36-37; 1Q, 2019, 29-30

0TSD0ZZ Reposition Urethra, Open Approach—AHA CC: 1Q, 2016, 15-16

0TT10ZZ Resection of Left Kidney, Open Approach—AHA CC: 3Q, 2014, 16

0TT70ZZ Resection of Left Ureter, Open Approach—AHA CC: 3Q, 2014, 16

0TUB07Z Supplement Bladder with Autologous Tissue Substitute, Open Approach—AHA CC: 3Q, 2017, 21-22

0TUD07Z Supplement Urethra with Autologous Tissue Substitute, Open Approach—AHA CC: 1Q, 2019, 29-30

0TV68ZZ Restriction of Right Ureter, Via Natural or Artificial Opening Endoscopic—AHA CC: 2Q, 2015, 11-12

0TV78ZZ Restriction of Left Ureter, Via Natural or Artificial Opening Endoscopic—AHA CC: 2Q, 2015, 11-12

Female Reproductive System

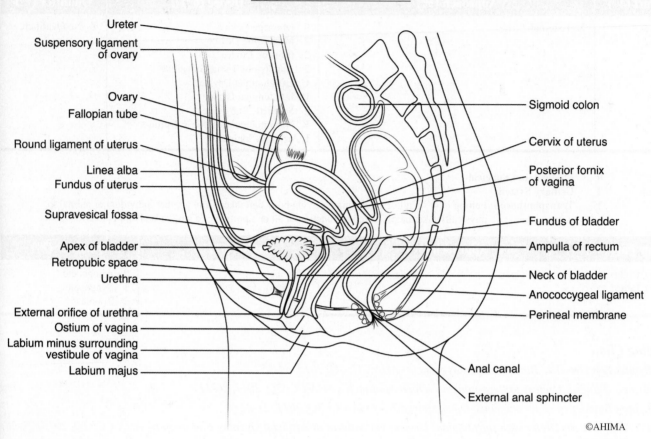

Ureter
Suspensory ligament of ovary
Ovary
Fallopian tube
Round ligament of uterus
Linea alba
Fundus of uterus
Supravesical fossa
Apex of bladder
Retropubic space
Urethra
External orifice of urethra
Ostium of vagina
Labium minus surrounding vestibule of vagina
Labium majus

Sigmoid colon
Cervix of uterus
Posterior fornix of vagina
Fundus of bladder
Ampulla of rectum
Neck of bladder
Anococcygeal ligament
Perineal membrane
Anal canal
External anal sphincter

©AHIMA

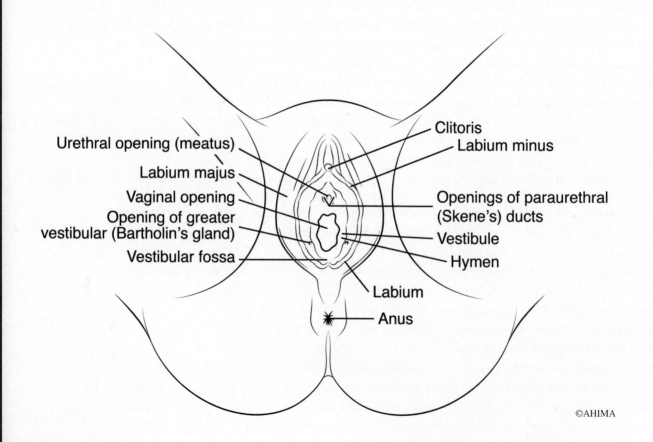

Urethral opening (meatus)
Labium majus
Vaginal opening
Opening of greater vestibular (Bartholin's gland)
Vestibular fossa

Clitoris
Labium minus
Openings of paraurethral (Skene's) ducts
Vestibule
Hymen
Labium
Anus

©AHIMA

Uterus, Ovaries and Uterine Tubes

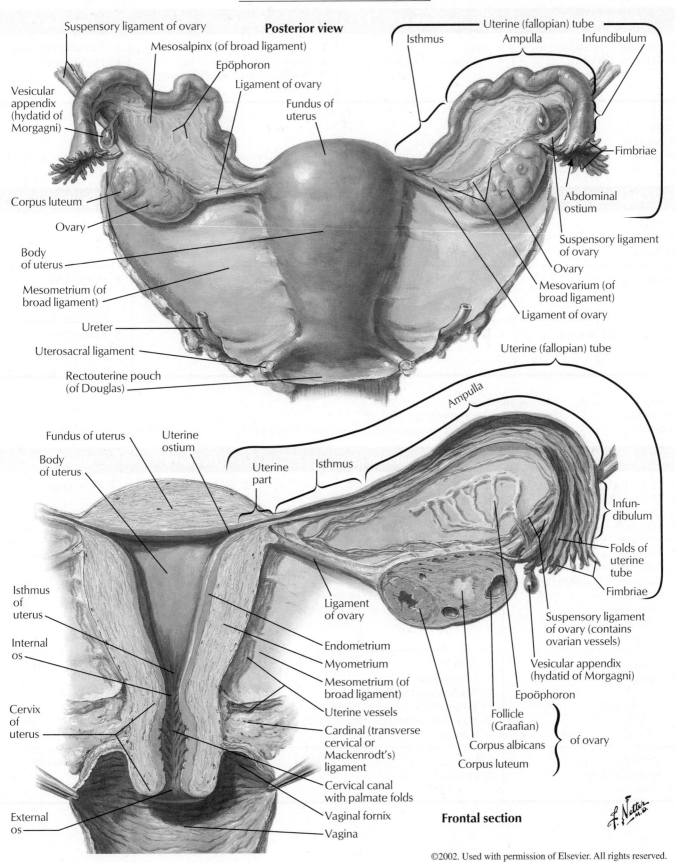

Posterior view

Suspensory ligament of ovary

Mesosalpinx (of broad ligament)

Epöphoron

Ligament of ovary

Fundus of uterus

Vesicular appendix (hydatid of Morgagni)

Corpus luteum

Ovary

Body of uterus

Mesometrium (of broad ligament)

Ureter

Uterosacral ligament

Rectouterine pouch (of Douglas)

Uterine (fallopian) tube

Isthmus

Ampulla

Infundibulum

Fimbriae

Abdominal ostium

Suspensory ligament of ovary

Ovary

Mesovarium (of broad ligament)

Ligament of ovary

Uterine (fallopian) tube

Ampulla

Fundus of uterus

Body of uterus

Uterine ostium

Uterine part

Isthmus

Infundibulum

Folds of uterine tube

Fimbriae

Suspensory ligament of ovary (contains ovarian vessels)

Vesicular appendix (hydatid of Morgagni)

Epoöphoron

Follicle (Graafian)

Corpus albicans

Corpus luteum

of ovary

Isthmus of uterus

Internal os

Cervix of uterus

External os

Ligament of ovary

Endometrium

Myometrium

Mesometrium (of broad ligament)

Uterine vessels

Cardinal (transverse cervical or Mackenrodt's) ligament

Cervical canal with palmate folds

Vaginal fornix

Vagina

Frontal section

f. Netter

Medical and Surgical, Female Reproductive System

Female Reproductive System Tables 0U1–0UY

Section	0	Medical and Surgical
Body System	U	Female Reproductive System
Operation	1	**Bypass:** Altering the route of passage of the contents of a tubular body part

Body Part (4th)	Approach (5th)	Device (6th)	Qualifier (7th)
5 Fallopian Tube, Right 6 Fallopian Tube, Left	0 Open 4 Percutaneous Endoscopic	7 Autologous Tissue Substitute J Synthetic Substitute K Nonautologous Tissue Substitute Z No Device	5 Fallopian Tube, Right 6 Fallopian Tube, Left 9 Uterus

Section	0	Medical and Surgical
Body System	U	Female Reproductive System
Operation	2	**Change:** Taking out or off a device from a body part and putting back an identical or similar device in or on the same body part without cutting or puncturing the skin or a mucous membrane

Body Part (4th)	Approach (5th)	Device (6th)	Qualifier (7th)
3 Ovary 8 Fallopian Tube M Vulva	X External	0 Drainage Device Y Other Device	Z No Qualifier
D Uterus and Cervix	X External	0 Drainage Device H Contraceptive Device Y Other Device	Z No Qualifier
H Vagina and Cul-de-sac	X External	0 Drainage Device G Intraluminal Device, Pessary Y Other Device	Z No Qualifier

Section	0	Medical and Surgical
Body System	U	Female Reproductive System
Operation	5	**Destruction:** Physical eradication of all or a portion of a body part by the direct use of energy, force, or a destructive agent

Body Part (4th)	Approach (5th)	Device (6th)	Qualifier (7th)
0 Ovary, Right 1 Ovary, Left 2 Ovaries, Bilateral 4 Uterine Supporting Structure	0 Open 3 Percutaneous 4 Percutaneous Endoscopic 8 Via Natural or Artificial Opening Endoscopic	Z No Device	Z No Qualifier
5 Fallopian Tube, Right 6 Fallopian Tube, Left 7 Fallopian Tubes, Bilateral 9 Uterus B Endometrium C Cervix F Cul-de-sac	0 Open 3 Percutaneous 4 Percutaneous Endoscopic 7 Via Natural or Artificial Opening 8 Via Natural or Artificial Opening Endoscopic	Z No Device	Z No Qualifier
G Vagina K Hymen	0 Open 3 Percutaneous 4 Percutaneous Endoscopic 7 Via Natural or Artificial Opening 8 Via Natural or Artificial Opening Endoscopic X External	Z No Device	Z No Qualifier
J Clitoris L Vestibular Gland M Vulva	0 Open X External	Z No Device	Z No Qualifier

Section	0	Medical and Surgical
Body System	U	Female Reproductive System
Operation	7	**Dilation:** Expanding an orifice or the lumen of a tubular body part

Body Part (4ᵗʰ)	Approach (5ᵗʰ)	Device (6ᵗʰ)	Qualifier (7ᵗʰ)
5 Fallopian Tube, Right 6 Fallopian Tube, Left 7 Fallopian Tubes, Bilateral 9 Uterus C Cervix G Vagina	0 Open 3 Percutaneous 4 Percutaneous Endoscopic 7 Via Natural or Artificial Opening 8 Via Natural or Artificial Opening Endoscopic	D Intraluminal Device Z No Device	Z No Qualifier
K Hymen	0 Open 3 Percutaneous 4 Percutaneous Endoscopic 7 Via Natural or Artificial Opening 8 Via Natural or Artificial Opening Endoscopic X External	D Intraluminal Device Z No Device	Z No Qualifier

Section	0	Medical and Surgical
Body System	U	Female Reproductive System
Operation	8	**Division:** Cutting into a body part, without draining fluids and/or gases from the body part, in order to separate or transect a body part

Body Part (4ᵗʰ)	Approach (5ᵗʰ)	Device (6ᵗʰ)	Qualifier (7ᵗʰ)
0 Ovary, Right 1 Ovary, Left 2 Ovaries, Bilateral 4 Uterine Supporting Structure	0 Open 3 Percutaneous 4 Percutaneous Endoscopic	Z No Device	Z No Qualifier
K Hymen	7 Via Natural or Artificial Opening 8 Via Natural or Artificial Opening Endoscopic X External	Z No Device	Z No Qualifier

Section	0	Medical and Surgical
Body System	U	Female Reproductive System
Operation	9	**Drainage:** Taking or letting out fluids and/or gases from a body part

Body Part (4ᵗʰ)	Approach (5ᵗʰ)	Device (6ᵗʰ)	Qualifier (7ᵗʰ)
0 Ovary, Right 1 Ovary, Left 2 Ovaries, Bilateral	0 Open 3 Percutaneous 4 Percutaneous Endoscopic 8 Via Natural or Artificial Opening Endoscopic	0 Drainage Device	Z No Qualifier
0 Ovary, Right 1 Ovary, Left 2 Ovaries, Bilateral	0 Open 3 Percutaneous 4 Percutaneous Endoscopic 8 Via Natural or Artificial Opening Endoscopic	Z No Device	X Diagnostic Z No Qualifier
0 Ovary, Right 1 Ovary, Left 2 Ovaries, Bilateral	X External	Z No Device	Z No Qualifier
4 Uterine Supporting Structure	0 Open 3 Percutaneous 4 Percutaneous Endoscopic 8 Via Natural or Artificial Opening Endoscopic	0 Drainage Device	Z No Qualifier
4 Uterine Supporting Structure	0 Open 3 Percutaneous 4 Percutaneous Endoscopic 8 Via Natural or Artificial Opening Endoscopic	Z No Device	X Diagnostic Z No Qualifier

Continued →

Section   **0**   **Medical and Surgical**
Body System   **U**   **Female Reproductive System**
Operation   **9**   **Drainage:** Taking or letting out fluids and/or gases from a body part

Body Part (4th)	Approach (5th)	Device (6th)	Qualifier (7th)
5 Fallopian Tube, Right 6 Fallopian Tube, Left 7 Fallopian Tubes, Bilateral 9 Uterus C Cervix F Cul-de-sac	0 Open 3 Percutaneous 4 Percutaneous Endoscopic 7 Via Natural or Artificial Opening 8 Via Natural or Artificial Opening Endoscopic	0 Drainage Device	Z No Qualifier
5 Fallopian Tube, Right 6 Fallopian Tube, Left 7 Fallopian Tubes, Bilateral 9 Uterus C Cervix F Cul-de-sac	0 Open 3 Percutaneous 4 Percutaneous Endoscopic 7 Via Natural or Artificial Opening 8 Via Natural or Artificial Opening Endoscopic	Z No Device	X Diagnostic Z No Qualifier
G Vagina K Hymen	0 Open 3 Percutaneous 4 Percutaneous Endoscopic 7 Via Natural or Artificial Opening 8 Via Natural or Artificial Opening Endoscopic X External	0 Drainage Device	Z No Qualifier
G Vagina K Hymen	0 Open 3 Percutaneous 4 Percutaneous Endoscopic 7 Via Natural or Artificial Opening 8 Via Natural or Artificial Opening Endoscopic X External	Z No Device	X Diagnostic Z No Qualifier
J Clitoris L Vestibular Gland M Vulva	0 Open X External	0 Drainage Device	Z No Qualifier
J Clitoris L Vestibular Gland M Vulva	0 Open X External	Z No Device	X Diagnostic Z No Qualifier

Section   **0**   **Medical and Surgical**
Body System   **U**   **Female Reproductive System**
Operation   **B**   **Excision:** Cutting out or off, without replacement, a portion of a body part

Body Part (4th)	Approach (5th)	Device (6th)	Qualifier (7th)
0 Ovary, Right 1 Ovary, Left 2 Ovaries, Bilateral 4 Uterine Supporting Structure 5 Fallopian Tube, Right 6 Fallopian Tube, Left 7 Fallopian Tubes, Bilateral 9 Uterus C Cervix F Cul-de-sac	0 Open 3 Percutaneous 4 Percutaneous Endoscopic 7 Via Natural or Artificial Opening 8 Via Natural or Artificial Opening Endoscopic	Z No Device	X Diagnostic Z No Qualifier

Continued →

Section	0	Medical and Surgical
Body System	U	Female Reproductive System
Operation	B	Excision: Cutting out or off, without replacement, a portion of a body part

Body Part (4th)	Approach (5th)	Device (6th)	Qualifier (7th)
G Vagina K Hymen	0 Open 3 Percutaneous 4 Percutaneous Endoscopic 7 Via Natural or Artificial Opening 8 Via Natural or Artificial Opening Endoscopic X External	Z No Device	X Diagnostic Z No Qualifier
J Clitoris L Vestibular Gland M Vulva	0 Open X External	Z No Device	X Diagnostic Z No Qualifier

Section	0	Medical and Surgical
Body System	U	Female Reproductive System
Operation	C	Extirpation: Taking or cutting out solid matter from a body part

Body Part (4th)	Approach (5th)	Device (6th)	Qualifier (7th)
0 Ovary, Right 1 Ovary, Left 2 Ovaries, Bilateral 4 Uterine Supporting Structure	0 Open 3 Percutaneous 4 Percutaneous Endoscopic 8 Via Natural or Artificial Opening Endoscopic	Z No Device	Z No Qualifier
5 Fallopian Tube, Right 6 Fallopian Tube, Left 7 Fallopian Tubes, Bilateral 9 Uterus B Endometrium C Cervix F Cul-de-sac	0 Open 3 Percutaneous 4 Percutaneous Endoscopic 7 Via Natural or Artificial Opening 8 Via Natural or Artificial Opening Endoscopic	Z No Device	Z No Qualifier
G Vagina K Hymen	0 Open 3 Percutaneous 4 Percutaneous Endoscopic 7 Via Natural or Artificial Opening 8 Via Natural or Artificial Opening Endoscopic X External	Z No Device	Z No Qualifier
J Clitoris L Vestibular Gland M Vulva	0 Open X External	Z No Device	Z No Qualifier

Section	0	Medical and Surgical
Body System	U	Female Reproductive System
Operation	D	Extraction: Pulling or stripping out or off all or a portion of a body part by the use of force

Body Part (4th)	Approach (5th)	Device (6th)	Qualifier (7th)
B Endometrium	7 Via Natural or Artificial Opening 8 Via Natural or Artificial Opening Endoscopic	Z No Device	X Diagnostic Z No Qualifier
N Ova	0 Open 3 Percutaneous 4 Percutaneous Endoscopic	Z No Device	Z No Qualifier

Section	0	Medical and Surgical
Body System	U	Female Reproductive System
Operation	F	Fragmentation: Breaking solid matter in a body part into pieces

Body Part (4th)	Approach (5th)	Device (6th)	Qualifier (7th)
5 Fallopian Tube, Right 6 Fallopian Tube, Left 7 Fallopian Tubes, Bilateral 9 Uterus	0 Open 3 Percutaneous 4 Percutaneous Endoscopic 7 Via Natural or Artificial Opening 8 Via Natural or Artificial Opening Endoscopic X External	Z No Device	Z No Qualifier

Section	0	Medical and Surgical
Body System	U	Female Reproductive System
Operation	H	Insertion: Putting in a nonbiological appliance that monitors, assists, performs, or prevents a physiological function but does not physically take the place of a body part

Body Part (4th)	Approach (5th)	Device (6th)	Qualifier (7th)
3 Ovary	0 Open 3 Percutaneous 4 Percutaneous Endoscopic	1 Radioactive Element 3 Infusion Device Y Other Device	Z No Qualifier
3 Ovary	7 Via Natural or Artificial Opening 8 Via Natural or Artificial Opening Endoscopic	1 Radioactive Element Y Other Device	Z No Qualifier
8 Fallopian Tube D Uterus and Cervix H Vagina and Cul-de-sac	0 Open 3 Percutaneous 4 Percutaneous Endoscopic 7 Via Natural or Artificial Opening 8 Via Natural or Artificial Opening Endoscopic	3 Infusion Device Y Other Device	Z No Qualifier
9 Uterus	0 Open 7 Via Natural or Artificial Opening 8 Via Natural or Artificial Opening Endoscopic	1 Radioactive Element H Contraceptive Device	Z No Qualifier
C Cervix	0 Open 3 Percutaneous 4 Percutaneous Endoscopic	1 Radioactive Element	Z No Qualifier
C Cervix	7 Via Natural or Artificial Opening 8 Via Natural or Artificial Opening Endoscopic	1 Radioactive Element H Contraceptive Device	Z No Qualifier
F Cul-de-sac	7 Via Natural or Artificial Opening 8 Via Natural or Artificial Opening Endoscopic	G Intraluminal Device, Pessary	Z No Qualifier
G Vagina	0 Open 3 Percutaneous 4 Percutaneous Endoscopic X External	1 Radioactive Element	Z No Qualifier
G Vagina	7 Via Natural or Artificial Opening 8 Via Natural or Artificial Opening Endoscopic	1 Radioactive Element G Intraluminal Device, Pessary	Z No Qualifier

Section	0	Medical and Surgical
Body System	U	Female Reproductive System
Operation	J	Inspection: Visually and/or manually exploring a body part

Body Part (4th)	Approach (5th)	Device (6th)	Qualifier (7th)
3 Ovary	0 Open 3 Percutaneous 4 Percutaneous Endoscopic 8 Via Natural or Artificial Opening Endoscopic X External	Z No Device	Z No Qualifier

Continued →

Section	0	Medical and Surgical
Body System	U	Female Reproductive System
Operation	J	**Inspection:** Visually and/or manually exploring a body part

Body Part (4ᵗʰ)	Approach (5ᵗʰ)	Device (6ᵗʰ)	Qualifier (7ᵗʰ)
8 Fallopian Tube D Uterus and Cervix H Vagina and Cul-de-sac	0 Open 3 Percutaneous 4 Percutaneous Endoscopic 7 Via Natural or Artificial Opening 8 Via Natural or Artificial Opening Endoscopic X External	Z No Device	Z No Qualifier
M Vulva	0 Open X External	Z No Device	Z No Qualifier

Section	0	Medical and Surgical
Body System	U	Female Reproductive System
Operation	L	**Occlusion:** Completely closing an orifice or the lumen of a tubular body part

Body Part (4ᵗʰ)	Approach (5ᵗʰ)	Device (6ᵗʰ)	Qualifier (7ᵗʰ)
5 Fallopian Tube, Right 6 Fallopian Tube, Left 7 Fallopian Tubes, Bilateral	0 Open 3 Percutaneous 4 Percutaneous Endoscopic	C Extraluminal Device D Intraluminal Device Z No Device	Z No Qualifier
5 Fallopian Tube, Right 6 Fallopian Tube, Left 7 Fallopian Tubes, Bilateral	7 Via Natural or Artificial Opening 8 Via Natural or Artificial Opening Endoscopic	D Intraluminal Device Z No Device	Z No Qualifier
F Cul-de-sac G Vagina	7 Via Natural or Artificial Opening 8 Via Natural or Artificial Opening Endoscopic	D Intraluminal Device Z No Device	Z No Qualifier

Section	0	Medical and Surgical
Body System	U	Female Reproductive System
Operation	M	**Reattachment:** Putting back in or on all or a portion of a separated body part to its normal location or other suitable location

Body Part (4ᵗʰ)	Approach (5ᵗʰ)	Device (6ᵗʰ)	Qualifier (7ᵗʰ)
0 Ovary, Right 1 Ovary, Left 2 Ovaries, Bilateral 4 Uterine Supporting Structure 5 Fallopian Tube, Right 6 Fallopian Tube, Left 7 Fallopian Tubes, Bilateral 9 Uterus C Cervix F Cul-de-sac G Vagina	0 Open 4 Percutaneous Endoscopic	Z No Device	Z No Qualifier
J Clitoris M Vulva	X External	Z No Device	Z No Qualifier
K Hymen	0 Open 4 Percutaneous Endoscopic X External	Z No Device	Z No Qualifier

Section   **0**   **Medical and Surgical**
Body System   **U**   **Female Reproductive System**
Operation   **N**   **Release:** Freeing a body part from an abnormal physical constraint by cutting or by the use of force

Body Part (4th)	Approach (5th)	Device (6th)	Qualifier (7th)
0 Ovary, Right 1 Ovary, Left 2 Ovaries, Bilateral 4 Uterine Supporting Structure	0 Open 3 Percutaneous 4 Percutaneous Endoscopic 8 Via Natural or Artificial Opening Endoscopic	Z No Device	Z No Qualifier
5 Fallopian Tube, Right 6 Fallopian Tube, Left 7 Fallopian Tubes, Bilateral 9 Uterus C Cervix F Cul-de-sac	0 Open 3 Percutaneous 4 Percutaneous Endoscopic 7 Via Natural or Artificial Opening 8 Via Natural or Artificial Opening Endoscopic	Z No Device	Z No Qualifier
G Vagina K Hymen	0 Open 3 Percutaneous 4 Percutaneous Endoscopic 7 Via Natural or Artificial Opening 8 Via Natural or Artificial Opening Endoscopic X External	Z No Device	Z No Qualifier
J Clitoris L Vestibular Gland M Vulva	0 Open X External	Z No Device	Z No Qualifier

Section   **0**   **Medical and Surgical**
Body System   **U**   **Female Reproductive System**
Operation   **P**   **Removal:** Taking out or off a device from a body part

Body Part (4th)	Approach (5th)	Device (6th)	Qualifier (7th)
3 Ovary	0 Open 3 Percutaneous 4 Percutaneous Endoscopic	0 Drainage Device 3 Infusion Device Y Other Device	Z No Qualifier
3 Ovary	7 Via Natural or Artificial Opening 8 Via Natural or Artificial Opening Endoscopic	Y Other Device	Z No Qualifier
3 Ovary	X External	0 Drainage Device 3 Infusion Device	Z No Qualifier
8 Fallopian Tube	0 Open 3 Percutaneous 4 Percutaneous Endoscopic 7 Via Natural or Artificial Opening 8 Via Natural or Artificial Opening Endoscopic	0 Drainage Device 3 Infusion Device 7 Autologous Tissue Substitute C Extraluminal Device D Intraluminal Device J Synthetic Substitute K Nonautologous Tissue Substitute Y Other Device	Z No Qualifier
8 Fallopian Tube	X External	0 Drainage Device 3 Infusion Device D Intraluminal Device	Z No Qualifier
D Uterus and Cervix	0 Open 3 Percutaneous 4 Percutaneous Endoscopic 7 Via Natural or Artificial Opening 8 Via Natural or Artificial Opening Endoscopic	0 Drainage Device 1 Radioactive Element 3 Infusion Device 7 Autologous Tissue Substitute C Extraluminal Device D Intraluminal Device H Contraceptive Device J Synthetic Substitute K Nonautologous Tissue Substitute Y Other Device	Z No Qualifier

Continued →

Section	0	Medical and Surgical
Body System	U	Female Reproductive System
Operation	P	**Removal:** Taking out or off a device from a body part

Body Part (4th)	Approach (5th)	Device (6th)	Qualifier (7th)
D Uterus and Cervix	**X** External	**0** Drainage Device **3** Infusion Device **D** Intraluminal Device **H** Contraceptive Device	**Z** No Qualifier
H Vagina and Cul-de-sac	**0** Open **3** Percutaneous **4** Percutaneous Endoscopic **7** Via Natural or Artificial Opening **8** Via Natural or Artificial Opening Endoscopic	**0** Drainage Device **1** Radioactive Element **3** Infusion Device **7** Autologous Tissue Substitute **D** Intraluminal Device **J** Synthetic Substitute **K** Nonautologous Tissue Substitute **Y** Other Device	**Z** No Qualifier
H Vagina and Cul-de-sac	**X** External	**0** Drainage Device **1** Radioactive Element **3** Infusion Device **D** Intraluminal Device	**Z** No Qualifier
M Vulva	**0** Open	**0** Drainage Device **7** Autologous Tissue Substitute **J** Synthetic Substitute **K** Nonautologous Tissue Substitute	**Z** No Qualifier
M Vulva	**X** External	**0** Drainage Device	**Z** No Qualifier

Section	0	Medical and Surgical
Body System	U	Female Reproductive System
Operation	Q	**Repair:** Restoring, to the extent possible, a body part to its normal anatomic structure and function

Body Part (4th)	Approach (5th)	Device (6th)	Qualifier (7th)
0 Ovary, Right **1** Ovary, Left **2** Ovaries, Bilateral **4** Uterine Supporting Structure	**0** Open **3** Percutaneous **4** Percutaneous Endoscopic **8** Via Natural or Artificial Opening Endoscopic	**Z** No Device	**Z** No Qualifier
5 Fallopian Tube, Right **6** Fallopian Tube, Left **7** Fallopian Tubes, Bilateral **9** Uterus **C** Cervix **F** Cul-de-sac	**0** Open **3** Percutaneous **4** Percutaneous Endoscopic **7** Via Natural or Artificial Opening **8** Via Natural or Artificial Opening Endoscopic	**Z** No Device	**Z** No Qualifier
G Vagina **K** Hymen	**0** Open **3** Percutaneous **4** Percutaneous Endoscopic **7** Via Natural or Artificial Opening **8** Via Natural or Artificial Opening Endoscopic **X** External	**Z** No Device	**Z** No Qualifier
J Clitoris **L** Vestibular Gland **M** Vulva	**0** Open **X** External	**Z** No Device	**Z** No Qualifier

Section	0	Medical and Surgical
Body System	U	Female Reproductive System
Operation	S	Reposition: Moving to its normal location, or other suitable location, all or a portion of a body part

Body Part (4th)	Approach (5th)	Device (6th)	Qualifier (7th)
0 Ovary, Right 1 Ovary, Left 2 Ovaries, Bilateral 4 Uterine Supporting Structure 5 Fallopian Tube, Right 6 Fallopian Tube, Left 7 Fallopian Tubes, Bilateral C Cervix F Cul-de-sac	0 Open 4 Percutaneous Endoscopic 8 Via Natural or Artificial Opening Endoscopic	Z No Device	Z No Qualifier
9 Uterus G Vagina	0 Open 4 Percutaneous Endoscopic 7 Via Natural or Artificial Opening 8 Via Natural or Artificial Opening Endoscopic X External	Z No Device	Z No Qualifier

Section	0	Medical and Surgical
Body System	U	Female Reproductive System
Operation	T	Resection: Cutting out or off, without replacement, all of a body part

Body Part (4th)	Approach (5th)	Device (6th)	Qualifier (7th)
0 Ovary, Right 1 Ovary, Left 2 Ovaries, Bilateral 5 Fallopian Tube, Right 6 Fallopian Tube, Left 7 Fallopian Tubes, Bilateral	0 Open 4 Percutaneous Endoscopic 7 Via Natural or Artificial Opening 8 Via Natural or Artificial Opening Endoscopic F Via Natural or Artificial Opening With Percutaneous Endoscopic Assistance	Z No Device	Z No Qualifier
4 Uterine Supporting Structure C Cervix F Cul-de-sac G Vagina	0 Open 4 Percutaneous Endoscopic 7 Via Natural or Artificial Opening 8 Via Natural or Artificial Opening Endoscopic	Z No Device	Z No Qualifier
9 Uterus	0 Open 4 Percutaneous Endoscopic 7 Via Natural or Artificial Opening 8 Via Natural or Artificial Opening Endoscopic F Via Natural or Artificial Opening with Percutaneous Endoscopic Assistance	Z No Device	L Supracervical Z No Qualifier
J Clitoris L Vestibular Gland M Vulva	0 Open X External	Z No Device	Z No Qualifier
K Hymen	0 Open 4 Percutaneous Endoscopic 7 Via Natural or Artificial Opening 8 Via Natural or Artificial Opening Endoscopic X External	Z No Device	Z No Qualifier

Section	0	Medical and Surgical
Body System	U	Female Reproductive System
Operation	U	Supplement: Putting in or on biological or synthetic material that physically reinforces and/or augments the function of a portion of a body part

Body Part (4th)	Approach (5th)	Device (6th)	Qualifier (7th)
4 Uterine Supporting Structure	**0** Open **4** Percutaneous Endoscopic	**7** Autologous Tissue Substitute **J** Synthetic Substitute **K** Nonautologous Tissue Substitute	**Z** No Qualifier
5 Fallopian Tube, Right **6** Fallopian Tube, Left **7** Fallopian Tubes, Bilateral **F** Cul-de-sac	**0** Open **4** Percutaneous Endoscopic **7** Via Natural or Artificial Opening **8** Via Natural or Artificial Opening Endoscopic	**7** Autologous Tissue Substitute **J** Synthetic Substitute **K** Nonautologous Tissue Substitute	**Z** No Qualifier
G Vagina **K** Hymen	**0** Open **4** Percutaneous Endoscopic **7** Via Natural or Artificial Opening **8** Via Natural or Artificial Opening Endoscopic **X** External	**7** Autologous Tissue Substitute **J** Synthetic Substitute **K** Nonautologous Tissue Substitute	**Z** No Qualifier
J Clitoris **M** Vulva	**0** Open **X** External	**7** Autologous Tissue Substitute **J** Synthetic Substitute **K** Nonautologous Tissue Substitute	**Z** No Qualifier

Section	0	Medical and Surgical
Body System	U	Female Reproductive System
Operation	V	Restriction: Partially closing an orifice or the lumen of a tubular body part

Body Part (4th)	Approach (5th)	Device (6th)	Qualifier (7th)
C Cervix	**0** Open **3** Percutaneous **4** Percutaneous Endoscopic	**C** Extraluminal Device **D** Intraluminal Device **Z** No Device	**Z** No Qualifier
C Cervix	**7** Via Natural or Artificial Opening **8** Via Natural or Artificial Opening Endoscopic	**D** Intraluminal Device **Z** No Device	**Z** No Qualifier

Section	0	Medical and Surgical
Body System	U	Female Reproductive System
Operation	W	Revision: Correcting, to the extent possible, a portion of a malfunctioning device or the position of a displaced device

Body Part (4th)	Approach (5th)	Device (6th)	Qualifier (7th)
3 Ovary	**0** Open **3** Percutaneous **4** Percutaneous Endoscopic	**0** Drainage Device **3** Infusion Device **Y** Other Device	**Z** No Qualifier
3 Ovary	**7** Via Natural or Artificial Opening **8** Via Natural or Artificial Opening Endoscopic	**Y** Other Device	**Z** No Qualifier
3 Ovary	**X** External	**0** Drainage Device **3** Infusion Device	**Z** No Qualifier
8 Fallopian Tube	**0** Open **3** Percutaneous **4** Percutaneous Endoscopic **7** Via Natural or Artificial Opening **8** Via Natural or Artificial Opening Endoscopic **X** External	**0** Drainage Device **3** Infusion Device **7** Autologous Tissue Substitute **C** Extraluminal Device **D** Intraluminal Device **J** Synthetic Substitute **K** Nonautologous Tissue Substitute **Y** Other Device	**Z** No Qualifier

Continued →

Section	0	Medical and Surgical
Body System	U	Female Reproductive System
Operation	W	Revision: Correcting, to the extent possible, a portion of a malfunctioning device or the position of a displaced device

Body Part (4th)	Approach (5th)	Device (6th)	Qualifier (7th)
8 Fallopian Tube	X External	0 Drainage Device 3 Infusion Device 7 Autologous Tissue Substitute C Extraluminal Device D Intraluminal Device J Synthetic Substitute K Nonautologous Tissue Substitute	Z No Qualifier
D Uterus and Cervix	0 Open 3 Percutaneous 4 Percutaneous Endoscopic 7 Via Natural or Artificial Opening 8 Via Natural or Artificial Opening Endoscopic	0 Drainage Device 1 Radioactive Element 3 Infusion Device 7 Autologous Tissue Substitute C Extraluminal Device D Intraluminal Device H Contraceptive Device J Synthetic Substitute K Nonautologous Tissue Substitute Y Other Device	Z No Qualifier
D Uterus and Cervix	X External	0 Drainage Device 3 Infusion Device 7 Autologous Tissue Substitute C Extraluminal Device D Intraluminal Device H Contraceptive Device J Synthetic Substitute K Nonautologous Tissue Substitute	Z No Qualifier
H Vagina and Cul-de-sac	0 Open 3 Percutaneous 4 Percutaneous Endoscopic 7 Via Natural or Artificial Opening 8 Via Natural or Artificial Opening Endoscopic	0 Drainage Device 1 Radioactive Element 3 Infusion Device 7 Autologous Tissue Substitute D Intraluminal Device J Synthetic Substitute K Nonautologous Tissue Substitute Y Other Device	Z No Qualifier
H Vagina and Cul-de-sac	X External	0 Drainage Device 3 Infusion Device 7 Autologous Tissue Substitute D Intraluminal Device J Synthetic Substitute K Nonautologous Tissue Substitute	Z No Qualifier
M Vulva	0 Open X External	0 Drainage Device 7 Autologous Tissue Substitute J Synthetic Substitute K Nonautologous Tissue Substitute	Z No Qualifier

Section	0	Medical and Surgical
Body System	U	Female Reproductive System
Operation	Y	

Transplantation: Putting in or on all or a portion of a living body part taken from another individual or animal to physically take the place and/or function of all or a portion of a similar body part

Body Part (4th)	Approach (5th)	Device (6th)	Qualifier (7th)
0 Ovary, Right 1 Ovary, Left 9 Uterus	0 Open	Z No Device	0 Allogeneic 1 Syngeneic 2 Zooplastic

0U7C7ZZ Dilation of Cervix, Via Natural or Artificial Opening—AHA CC: 2Q, 2020, 30

0U9G7ZZ Drainage of Vagina, Via Natural or Artificial Opening—AHA CC: 4Q, 2016, 58-59

0UB64ZZ Excision of Left Fallopian Tube, Percutaneous Endoscopic Approach—AHA CC: 3Q, 2015, 31-32

0UB70ZZ Excision of Bilateral Fallopian Tubes, Open Approach—AHA CC: 3Q, 2015, 31

0UB90ZZ Excision of Uterus, Open Approach—AHA CC: 4Q, 2014, 16

0UBMXZZ Excision of Vulva, External Approach—AHA CC: 3Q, 2014, 12

0UC97ZZ Extirpation of Matter from Uterus, Via Natural or Artificial Opening—AHA CC: 2Q, 2013, 38

0UCC7ZZ Extirpation of Matter from Cervix, Via Natural or Artificial Opening—AHA CC: 3Q, 2015, 30

0UCC8ZZ Extirpation of Matter from Cervix, Via Natural or Artificial Opening Endoscopic—AHA CC: 3Q, 2015, 30-31

0UH97HZ Insertion of Contraceptive Device into Uterus, Via Natural or Artificial Opening—AHA CC: 2Q, 2013, 34

0UHD7YZ Insertion of Other Device into Uterus and Cervix, Via Natural or Artificial Opening—AHA CC: 4Q, 2017, 104; 1Q, 2018, 25

0UJD4ZZ Inspection of Uterus and Cervix, Percutaneous Endoscopic Approach—AHA CC: 1Q, 2015, 33-34

0UQJXZZ Repair Clitoris, External Approach—AHA CC: 4Q, 2013, 120-121

0UQMXZZ Repair Vulva, External Approach—AHA CC: 4Q, 2014, 18-19

0US9XZZ Reposition Uterus, External Approach—AHA CC: 1Q, 2016, 9

0UT00ZZ Resection of Right Ovary, Open Approach—AHA CC: 1Q, 2013, 24

0UT20ZZ Resection of Bilateral Ovaries, Open Approach—AHA CC: 1Q, 2015, 33-34

0UT70ZZ Resection of Bilateral Fallopian Tubes, Open Approach—AHA CC: 1Q, 2015, 33-34

0UT90ZZ Resection of Uterus, Open Approach—AHA CC: 3Q, 2013, 28; 1Q, 2015, 33-34; 4Q, 2017, 68

0UT97ZL Resection of Uterus, Supracervical, Via Natural or Artificial Opening—AHA CC: 4Q, 2017, 68

0UTC0ZZ Resection of Cervix, Open Approach—AHA CC: 3Q, 2013, 28; 1Q, 2015, 33-34

0UVC7ZZ Restriction of Cervix, Via Natural or Artificial Opening—AHA CC: 3Q, 2015, 30

Male Reproductive System

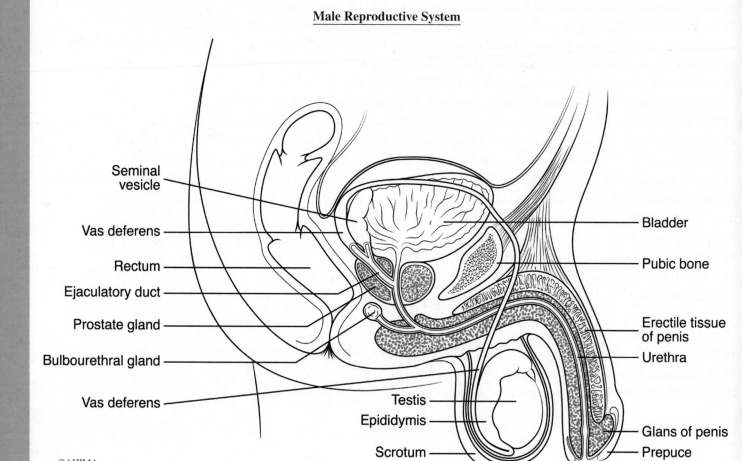

Seminal vesicle

Vas deferens

Rectum

Ejaculatory duct

Prostate gland

Bulbourethral gland

Vas deferens

Bladder

Pubic bone

Erectile tissue of penis

Urethra

Testis

Epididymis

Scrotum

Glans of penis

Prepuce

©AHIMA

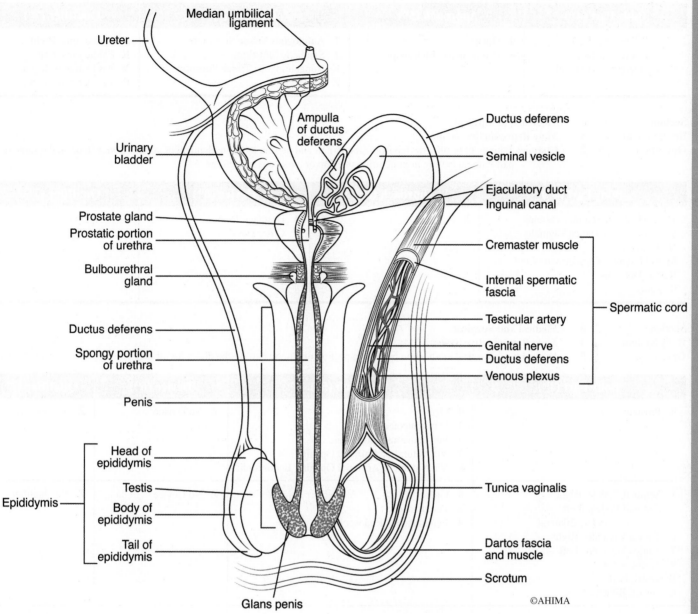

Median umbilical ligament

Ureter

Ampulla of ductus deferens

Ductus deferens

Seminal vesicle

Urinary bladder

Ejaculatory duct

Inguinal canal

Prostate gland

Prostatic portion of urethra

Cremaster muscle

Bulbourethral gland

Internal spermatic fascia

Testicular artery

Ductus deferens

Genital nerve

Spongy portion of urethra

Ductus deferens

Venous plexus

Spermatic cord

Penis

Head of epididymis

Testis

Epididymis

Body of epididymis

Tunica vaginalis

Tail of epididymis

Dartos fascia and muscle

Scrotum

Glans penis

©AHIMA

Male Reproductive System Tables 0V1–0VY

Section   **0**   **Medical and Surgical**
Body System   **V**   **Male Reproductive System**
Operation   **1**   **Bypass:** Altering the route of passage of the contents of a tubular body part

Body Part (4th)	Approach (5th)	Device (6th)	Qualifier (7th)
N Vas Deferens, Right P Vas Deferens, Left Q Vas Deferens, Bilateral	0 Open 4 Percutaneous Endoscopic	7 Autologous Tissue Substitute J Synthetic Substitute K Nonautologous Tissue Substitute Z No Device	J Epididymis, Right K Epididymis, Left N Vas Deferens, Right P Vas Deferens, Left

Section   **0**   **Medical and Surgical**
Body System   **V**   **Male Reproductive System**
Operation   **2**   **Change:** Taking out or off a device from a body part and putting back an identical or similar device in or on the same body part without cutting or puncturing the skin or a mucous membrane

Body Part (4th)	Approach (5th)	Device (6th)	Qualifier (7th)
4 Prostate and Seminal Vesicles 8 Scrotum and Tunica Vaginalis D Testis M Epididymis and Spermatic Cord R Vas Deferens S Penis	X External	0 Drainage Device Y Other Device	Z No Qualifier

Section   **0**   **Medical and Surgical**
Body System   **V**   **Male Reproductive System**
Operation   **5**   **Destruction:** Physical eradication of all or a portion of a body part by the direct use of energy, force, or a destructive agent

Body Part (4th)	Approach (5th)	Device (6th)	Qualifier (7th)
0 Prostate	0 Open 3 Percutaneous 4 Percutaneous Endoscopic 7 Via Natural or Artificial Opening 8 Via Natural or Artificial Opening Endoscopic	Z No Device	Z No Qualifier
1 Seminal Vesicle, Right 2 Seminal Vesicle, Left 3 Seminal Vesicles, Bilateral 6 Tunica Vaginalis, Right 7 Tunica Vaginalis, Left 9 Testis, Right B Testis, Left C Testes, Bilateral	0 Open 3 Percutaneous 4 Percutaneous Endoscopic	Z No Device	Z No Qualifier
5 Scrotum S Penis T Prepuce	0 Open 3 Percutaneous 4 Percutaneous Endoscopic X External	Z No Device	Z No Qualifier
F Spermatic Cord, Right G Spermatic Cord, Left H Spermatic Cords, Bilateral J Epididymis, Right K Epididymis, Left L Epididymis, Bilateral N Vas Deferens, Right P Vas Deferens, Left Q Vas Deferens, Bilateral	0 Open 3 Percutaneous 4 Percutaneous Endoscopic 8 Via Natural or Artificial Opening Endoscopic	Z No Device	Z No Qualifier

Section	0	Medical and Surgical
Body System	V	Male Reproductive System
Operation	7	Dilation: Expanding an orifice or the lumen of a tubular body part

Body Part (4th)	Approach (5th)	Device (6th)	Qualifier (7th)
N Vas Deferens, Right P Vas Deferens, Left Q Vas Deferens, Bilateral	0 Open 3 Percutaneous 4 Percutaneous Endoscopic	D Intraluminal Device Z No Device	Z No Qualifier

Section	0	Medical and Surgical
Body System	V	Male Reproductive System
Operation	9	Drainage: Taking or letting out fluids and/or gases from a body part

Body Part (4th)	Approach (5th)	Device (6th)	Qualifier (7th)
0 Prostate	0 Open 3 Percutaneous 4 Percutaneous Endoscopic 7 Via Natural or Artificial Opening 8 Via Natural or Artificial Opening Endoscopic	0 Drainage Device	Z No Qualifier
0 Prostate	0 Open 3 Percutaneous 4 Percutaneous Endoscopic 7 Via Natural or Artificial Opening 8 Via Natural or Artificial Opening Endoscopic	Z No Device	X Diagnostic Z No Qualifier
1 Seminal Vesicle, Right 2 Seminal Vesicle, Left 3 Seminal Vesicles, Bilateral 6 Tunica Vaginalis, Right 7 Tunica Vaginalis, Left 9 Testis, Right B Testis, Left C Testes, Bilateral F Spermatic Cord, Right G Spermatic Cord, Left H Spermatic Cords, Bilateral J Epididymis, Right K Epididymis, Left L Epididymis, Bilateral N Vas Deferens, Right P Vas Deferens, Left Q Vas Deferens, Bilateral	0 Open 3 Percutaneous 4 Percutaneous Endoscopic	0 Drainage Device	Z No Qualifier
1 Seminal Vesicle, Right 2 Seminal Vesicle, Left 3 Seminal Vesicles, Bilateral 6 Tunica Vaginalis, Right 7 Tunica Vaginalis, Left 9 Testis, Right B Testis, Left C Testes, Bilateral F Spermatic Cord, Right G Spermatic Cord, Left H Spermatic Cords, Bilateral J Epididymis, Right K Epididymis, Left L Epididymis, Bilateral N Vas Deferens, Right P Vas Deferens, Left Q Vas Deferens, Bilateral	0 Open 3 Percutaneous 4 Percutaneous Endoscopic	Z No Device	X Diagnostic Z No Qualifier
5 Scrotum S Penis T Prepuce	0 Open 3 Percutaneous 4 Percutaneous Endoscopic X External	0 Drainage Device	Z No Qualifier

Continued →

Section	0	Medical and Surgical
Body System	V	Male Reproductive System
Operation	9	**Drainage:** Taking or letting out fluids and/or gases from a body part

Body Part (4th)	Approach (5th)	Device (6th)	Qualifier (7th)
5 Scrotum S Penis T Prepuce	0 Open 3 Percutaneous 4 Percutaneous Endoscopic X External	Z No Device	X Diagnostic Z No Qualifier

Section	0	Medical and Surgical
Body System	V	Male Reproductive System
Operation	B	**Excision:** Cutting out or off, without replacement, a portion of a body part

Body Part (4th)	Approach (5th)	Device (6th)	Qualifier (7th)
0 Prostate	0 Open 3 Percutaneous 4 Percutaneous Endoscopic 7 Via Natural or Artificial Opening 8 Via Natural or Artificial Opening Endoscopic	Z No Device	X Diagnostic Z No Qualifier
1 Seminal Vesicle, Right 2 Seminal Vesicle, Left 3 Seminal Vesicles, Bilateral 6 Tunica Vaginalis, Right 7 Tunica Vaginalis, Left 9 Testis, Right B Testis, Left C Testes, Bilateral	0 Open 3 Percutaneous 4 Percutaneous Endoscopic	Z No Device	X Diagnostic Z No Qualifier
5 Scrotum S Penis T Prepuce	0 Open 3 Percutaneous 4 Percutaneous Endoscopic X External	Z No Device	X Diagnostic Z No Qualifier
F Spermatic Cord, Right G Spermatic Cord, Left H Spermatic Cords, Bilateral J Epididymis, Right K Epididymis, Left L Epididymis, Bilateral N Vas Deferens, Right P Vas Deferens, Left Q Vas Deferens, Bilateral	0 Open 3 Percutaneous 4 Percutaneous Endoscopic 8 Via Natural or Artificial Opening Endoscopic	Z No Device	X Diagnostic Z No Qualifier

Section	0	Medical and Surgical
Body System	V	Male Reproductive System
Operation	C	**Extirpation:** Taking or cutting out solid matter from a body part

Body Part (4th)	Approach (5th)	Device (6th)	Qualifier (7th)
0 Prostate	0 Open 3 Percutaneous 4 Percutaneous Endoscopic 7 Via Natural or Artificial Opening 8 Via Natural or Artificial Opening Endoscopic	Z No Device	Z No Qualifier

Continued →

Section   **0**   **Medical and Surgical**
Body System   **V**   **Male Reproductive System**
Operation   **C**   **Extirpation:** Taking or cutting out solid matter from a body part

Body Part (4th)	Approach (5th)	Device (6th)	Qualifier (7th)
1 Seminal Vesicle, Right **2** Seminal Vesicle, Left **3** Seminal Vesicles, Bilateral **6** Tunica Vaginalis, Right **7** Tunica Vaginalis, Left **9** Testis, Right **B** Testis, Left **C** Testes, Bilateral **F** Spermatic Cord, Right **G** Spermatic Cord, Left **H** Spermatic Cords, Bilateral **J** Epididymis, Right **K** Epididymis, Left **L** Epididymis, Bilateral **N** Vas Deferens, Right **P** Vas Deferens, Left **Q** Vas Deferens, Bilateral	**0** Open **3** Percutaneous **4** Percutaneous Endoscopic	**Z** No Device	**Z** No Qualifier
5 Scrotum **S** Penis **T** Prepuce	**0** Open **3** Percutaneous **4** Percutaneous Endoscopic **X** External	**Z** No Device	**Z** No Qualifier

Section   **0**   **Medical and Surgical**
Body System   **V**   **Male Reproductive System**
Operation   **H**   **Insertion:** Putting in a nonbiological appliance that monitors, assists, performs, or prevents a physiological function but does not physically take the place of a body part

Body Part (4th)	Approach (5th)	Device (6th)	Qualifier (7th)
0 Prostate	**0** Open **3** Percutaneous **4** Percutaneous Endoscopic **7** Via Natural or Artificial Opening **8** Via Natural or Artificial Opening Endoscopic	**1** Radioactive Element	**Z** No Qualifier
4 Prostate and Seminal Vesicles **8** Scrotum and Tunica Vaginalis **M** Epididymis and Spermatic Cord **R** Vas Deferens	**0** Open **3** Percutaneous **4** Percutaneous Endoscopic **7** Via Natural or Artificial Opening **8** Via Natural or Artificial Opening Endoscopic	**3** Infusion Device **Y** Other Device	**Z** No Qualifier
D Testis	**0** Open **3** Percutaneous **4** Percutaneous Endoscopic **7** Via Natural or Artificial Opening **8** Via Natural or Artificial Opening Endoscopic	**1** Radioactive Element **3** Infusion Device **Y** Other Device	**Z** No Qualifier
S Penis	**0** Open **3** Percutaneous **4** Percutaneous Endoscopic	**3** Infusion Device **Y** Other Device	**Z** No Qualifier
S Penis	**7** Via Natural or Artificial Opening **8** Via Natural or Artificial Opening Endoscopic	**Y** Other Device	**Z** No Qualifier
S Penis	**X** External	**3** Infusion Device	**Z** No Qualifier

Section	0	Medical and Surgical
Body System	V	Male Reproductive System
Operation	J	**Inspection:** Visually and/or manually exploring a body part

Body Part (4th)	Approach (5th)	Device (6th)	Qualifier (7th)
4 Prostate and Seminal Vesicles 8 Scrotum and Tunica Vaginalis D Testis M Epididymis and Spermatic Cord R Vas Deferens S Penis	0 Open 3 Percutaneous 4 Percutaneous Endoscopic X External	Z No Device	Z No Qualifier

Section	0	Medical and Surgical
Body System	V	Male Reproductive System
Operation	L	**Occlusion:** Completely closing an orifice or the lumen of a tubular body part

Body Part (4th)	Approach (5th)	Device (6th)	Qualifier (7th)
F Spermatic Cord, Right G Spermatic Cord, Left H Spermatic Cords, Bilateral N Vas Deferens, Right P Vas Deferens, Left Q Vas Deferens, Bilateral	0 Open 3 Percutaneous 4 Percutaneous Endoscopic 8 Via Natural or Artificial Opening Endoscopic	C Extraluminal Device D Intraluminal Device Z No Device	Z No Qualifier

Section	0	Medical and Surgical
Body System	V	Male Reproductive System
Operation	M	**Reattachment:** Putting back in or on all or a portion of a separated body part to its normal location or other suitable location

Body Part (4th)	Approach (5th)	Device (6th)	Qualifier (7th)
5 Scrotum S Penis	X External	Z No Device	Z No Qualifier
6 Tunica Vaginalis, Right 7 Tunica Vaginalis, Left 9 Testis, Right B Testis, Left C Testes, Bilateral F Spermatic Cord, Right G Spermatic Cord, Left H Spermatic Cords, Bilateral	0 Open 4 Percutaneous Endoscopic	Z No Device	Z No Qualifier

Section	0	Medical and Surgical
Body System	V	Male Reproductive System
Operation	N	**Release:** Freeing a body part from an abnormal physical constraint by cutting or by the use of force

Body Part (4th)	Approach (5th)	Device (6th)	Qualifier (7th)
0 Prostate	0 Open 3 Percutaneous 4 Percutaneous Endoscopic 7 Via Natural or Artificial Opening 8 Via Natural or Artificial Opening Endoscopic	Z No Device	Z No Qualifier
1 Seminal Vesicle, Right 2 Seminal Vesicle, Left 3 Seminal Vesicles, Bilateral 6 Tunica Vaginalis, Right 7 Tunica Vaginalis, Left 9 Testis, Right B Testis, Left C Testes, Bilateral	0 Open 3 Percutaneous 4 Percutaneous Endoscopic	Z No Device	Z No Qualifier

Continued →

Section 0 Medical and Surgical
Body System V Male Reproductive System
Operation N Release: Freeing a body part from an abnormal physical constraint by cutting or by the use of force

0VN Continued

Body Part (4th)	Approach (5th)	Device (6th)	Qualifier (7th)
5 Scrotum S Penis T Prepuce	0 Open 3 Percutaneous 4 Percutaneous Endoscopic X External	Z No Device	Z No Qualifier
F Spermatic Cord, Right G Spermatic Cord, Left H Spermatic Cords, Bilateral J Epididymis, Right K Epididymis, Left L Epididymis, Bilateral N Vas Deferens, Right P Vas Deferens, Left Q Vas Deferens, Bilateral	0 Open 3 Percutaneous 4 Percutaneous Endoscopic 8 Via Natural or Artificial Opening Endoscopic	Z No Device	Z No Qualifier

Section 0 Medical and Surgical
Body System V Male Reproductive System
Operation P Removal: Taking out or off a device from a body part

Body Part (4th)	Approach (5th)	Device (6th)	Qualifier (7th)
4 Prostate and Seminal Vesicles	0 Open 3 Percutaneous 4 Percutaneous Endoscopic 7 Via Natural or Artificial Opening 8 Via Natural or Artificial Opening Endoscopic	0 Drainage Device 1 Radioactive Element 3 Infusion Device 7 Autologous Tissue Substitute J Synthetic Substitute K Nonautologous Tissue Substitute Y Other Device	Z No Qualifier
4 Prostate and Seminal Vesicles	X External	0 Drainage Device 1 Radioactive Element 3 Infusion Device	Z No Qualifier
8 Scrotum and Tunica Vaginalis D Testis S Penis	0 Open 3 Percutaneous 4 Percutaneous Endoscopic 7 Via Natural or Artificial Opening 8 Via Natural or Artificial Opening Endoscopic	0 Drainage Device 3 Infusion Device 7 Autologous Tissue Substitute J Synthetic Substitute K Nonautologous Tissue Substitute Y Other Device	Z No Qualifier
8 Scrotum and Tunica Vaginalis D Testis S Penis	X External	0 Drainage Device 3 Infusion Device	Z No Qualifier
M Epididymis and Spermatic Cord	0 Open 3 Percutaneous 4 Percutaneous Endoscopic 7 Via Natural or Artificial Opening 8 Via Natural or Artificial Opening Endoscopic	0 Drainage Device 3 Infusion Device 7 Autologous Tissue Substitute C Extraluminal Device J Synthetic Substitute K Nonautologous Tissue Substitute Y Other Device	Z No Qualifier
M Epididymis and Spermatic Cord	X External	0 Drainage Device 3 Infusion Device	Z No Qualifier

Continued →

Section	0	Medical and Surgical
Body System	V	Male Reproductive System
Operation	P	Removal: Taking out or off a device from a body part

Body Part (4th)	Approach (5th)	Device (6th)	Qualifier (7th)
R Vas Deferens	0 Open 3 Percutaneous 4 Percutaneous Endoscopic 7 Via Natural or Artificial Opening 8 Via Natural or Artificial Opening Endoscopic	0 Drainage Device 3 Infusion Device 7 Autologous Tissue Substitute C Extraluminal Device D Intraluminal Device J Synthetic Substitute K Nonautologous Tissue Substitute Y Other Device	Z No Qualifier
R Vas Deferens	X External	0 Drainage Device 3 Infusion Device D Intraluminal Device	Z No Qualifier

Section	0	Medical and Surgical
Body System	V	Male Reproductive System
Operation	Q	Repair: Restoring, to the extent possible, a body part to its normal anatomic structure and function

Body Part (4th)	Approach (5th)	Device (6th)	Qualifier (7th)
0 Prostate	0 Open 3 Percutaneous 4 Percutaneous Endoscopic 7 Via Natural or Artificial Opening 8 Via Natural or Artificial Opening Endoscopic	Z No Device	Z No Qualifier
1 Seminal Vesicle, Right 2 Seminal Vesicle, Left 3 Seminal Vesicles, Bilateral 6 Tunica Vaginalis, Right 7 Tunica Vaginalis, Left 9 Testis, Right B Testis, Left C Testes, Bilateral	0 Open 3 Percutaneous 4 Percutaneous Endoscopic	Z No Device	Z No Qualifier
5 Scrotum S Penis T Prepuce	0 Open 3 Percutaneous 4 Percutaneous Endoscopic X External	Z No Device	Z No Qualifier
F Spermatic Cord, Right G Spermatic Cord, Left H Spermatic Cords, Bilateral J Epididymis, Right K Epididymis, Left L Epididymis, Bilateral N Vas Deferens, Right P Vas Deferens, Left Q Vas Deferens, Bilateral	0 Open 3 Percutaneous 4 Percutaneous Endoscopic 8 Via Natural or Artificial Opening Endoscopic	Z No Device	Z No Qualifier

Section	0	Medical and Surgical
Body System	V	Male Reproductive System
Operation	R	Replacement: Putting in or on biological or synthetic material that physically takes the place and/or function of all or a portion of a body part

Body Part (4th)	Approach (5th)	Device (6th)	Qualifier (7th)
9 Testis, Right B Testis, Left C Testes, Bilateral	0 Open	J Synthetic Substitute	Z No Qualifier

Section	0	Medical and Surgical
Body System	V	Male Reproductive System
Operation	S	Reposition: Moving to its normal location, or other suitable location, all or a portion of a body part

Body Part (4th)	Approach (5th)	Device (6th)	Qualifier (7th)
9 Testis, Right B Testis, Left C Testes, Bilateral F Spermatic Cord, Right G Spermatic Cord, Left H Spermatic Cords, Bilateral	0 Open 3 Percutaneous 4 Percutaneous Endoscopic 8 Via Natural or Artificial Opening Endoscopic	Z No Device	Z No Qualifier

Section	0	Medical and Surgical
Body System	V	Male Reproductive System
Operation	T	Resection: Cutting out or off, without replacement, all of a body part

Body Part (4th)	Approach (5th)	Device (6th)	Qualifier (7th)
0 Prostate	0 Open 4 Percutaneous Endoscopic 7 Via Natural or Artificial Opening 8 Via Natural or Artificial Opening Endoscopic	Z No Device	Z No Qualifier
1 Seminal Vesicle, Right 2 Seminal Vesicle, Left 3 Seminal Vesicles, Bilateral 6 Tunica Vaginalis, Right 7 Tunica Vaginalis, Left 9 Testis, Right B Testis, Left C Testes, Bilateral F Spermatic Cord, Right G Spermatic Cord, Left H Spermatic Cords, Bilateral J Epididymis, Right K Epididymis, Left L Epididymis, Bilateral N Vas Deferens, Right P Vas Deferens, Left Q Vas Deferens, Bilateral	0 Open 4 Percutaneous Endoscopic	Z No Device	Z No Qualifier
5 Scrotum S Penis T Prepuce	0 Open 4 Percutaneous Endoscopic X External	Z No Device	Z No Qualifier

Section	0	Medical and Surgical
Body System	V	Male Reproductive System
Operation	U	Supplement: Putting in or on biological or synthetic material that physically reinforces and/or augments the function of a portion of a body part

Body Part (4th)	Approach (5th)	Device (6th)	Qualifier (7th)
1 Seminal Vesicle, Right 2 Seminal Vesicle, Left 3 Seminal Vesicles, Bilateral 6 Tunica Vaginalis, Right 7 Tunica Vaginalis, Left F Spermatic Cord, Right G Spermatic Cord, Left H Spermatic Cords, Bilateral J Epididymis, Right K Epididymis, Left L Epididymis, Bilateral N Vas Deferens, Right P Vas Deferens, Left Q Vas Deferens, Bilateral	0 Open 4 Percutaneous Endoscopic 8 Via Natural or Artificial Opening Endoscopic	7 Autologous Tissue Substitute J Synthetic Substitute K Nonautologous Tissue Substitute	Z No Qualifier

Continued →

Section	0	Medical and Surgical
Body System	V	Male Reproductive System
Operation	U	Supplement: Putting in or on biological or synthetic material that physically reinforces and/or augments the function of a portion of a body part

Body Part (4th)	Approach (5th)	Device (6th)	Qualifier (7th)
5 Scrotum S Penis T Prepuce	0 Open 4 Percutaneous Endoscopic X External	7 Autologous Tissue Substitute J Synthetic Substitute K Nonautologous Tissue Substitute	Z No Qualifier
9 Testis, Right B Testis, Left C Testes, Bilateral	0 Open	7 Autologous Tissue Substitute J Synthetic Substitute K Nonautologous Tissue Substitute	Z No Qualifier

Section	0	Medical and Surgical
Body System	V	Male Reproductive System
Operation	W	Revision: Correcting, to the extent possible, a portion of a malfunctioning device or the position of a displaced device

Body Part (4th)	Approach (5th)	Device (6th)	Qualifier (7th)
4 Prostate and Seminal Vesicles 8 Scrotum and Tunica Vaginalis D Testis S Penis	0 Open 3 Percutaneous 4 Percutaneous Endoscopic 7 Via Natural or Artificial Opening 8 Via Natural or Artificial Opening Endoscopic	0 Drainage Device 3 Infusion Device 7 Autologous Tissue Substitute J Synthetic Substitute K Nonautologous Tissue Substitute Y Other Device	Z No Qualifier
4 Prostate and Seminal Vesicles 8 Scrotum and Tunica Vaginalis D Testis S Penis	X External	0 Drainage Device 3 Infusion Device 7 Autologous Tissue Substitute J Synthetic Substitute K Nonautologous Tissue Substitute	Z No Qualifier
M Epididymis and Spermatic Cord	0 Open 3 Percutaneous 4 Percutaneous Endoscopic 7 Via Natural or Artificial Opening 8 Via Natural or Artificial Opening Endoscopic	0 Drainage Device 3 Infusion Device 7 Autologous Tissue Substitute C Extraluminal Device J Synthetic Substitute K Nonautologous Tissue Substitute Y Other Device	Z No Qualifier
M Epididymis and Spermatic Cord	X External	0 Drainage Device 3 Infusion Device 7 Autologous Tissue Substitute C Extraluminal Device J Synthetic Substitute K Nonautologous Tissue Substitute	Z No Qualifier
R Vas Deferens	0 Open 3 Percutaneous 4 Percutaneous Endoscopic 7 Via Natural or Artificial Opening 8 Via Natural or Artificial Opening Endoscopic	0 Drainage Device 3 Infusion Device 7 Autologous Tissue Substitute C Extraluminal Device D Intraluminal Device J Synthetic Substitute K Nonautologous Tissue Substitute Y Other Device	Z No Qualifier
R Vas Deferens	X External	0 Drainage Device 3 Infusion Device 7 Autologous Tissue Substitute C Extraluminal Device C Intraluminal Device J Synthetic Substitute K Nonautologous Tissue Substitute	Z No Qualifier

	Section	0	Medical and Surgical
Body System	V	Male Reproductive System
Operation	X	**Transfer:** Moving, without taking out, all or a portion of a body part to another location to take over the function of all or a portion of a body part

Body Part (4ᵗʰ)	Approach (5ᵗʰ)	Device (6ᵗʰ)	Qualifier (7ᵗʰ)
T Prepuce	**0** Open **X** External	**Z** No Device	**D** Urethra **S** Penis

	Section	0	Medical and Surgical
Body System	V	Male Reproductive System
Operation	Y	**Transplantation:** Putting in or on all or a portion of a living body part taken from another individual or animal to physically take the place and/or function of all or a portion of a similar body part

Body Part (4ᵗʰ)	Approach (5ᵗʰ)	Device (6ᵗʰ)	Qualifier (7ᵗʰ)
5 Scrotum **6** Penis	**0** Open	**Z** No Device	**0** Allogeneic **1** Syngeneic **2** Zooplastic

AHA Coding Clinic

0VBQ4ZZ Excision of Bilateral Vas Deferens, Percutaneous Endoscopic Approach—AHA CC: 4Q, 2014, 33-34; 1Q, 2016, 23

0VPS0JZ Removal of Synthetic Substitute from Penis, Open Approach—AHA CC: 2Q, 2016, 28-29

0VQS3ZZ Repair Penis, Percutaneous Approach—AHA CC: 3Q, 2018, 12

0VT04ZZ Resection of Prostate, Percutaneous Endoscopic Approach— AHA CC: 4Q, 2014, 33-34

0VT34ZZ Resection of Bilateral Seminal Vesicles, Percutaneous Endoscopic Approach—AHA CC: 4Q, 2014, 33-34

0VUS07Z Supplement Penis with Autologous Tissue Substitute, Open Approach—AHA CC: 1Q, 2020, 31-32

0VUS0JZ Supplement Penis with Synthetic Substitute, Open Approach—AHA CC: 3Q, 2015, 25; 2Q, 2016, 28-29

Body Cavities

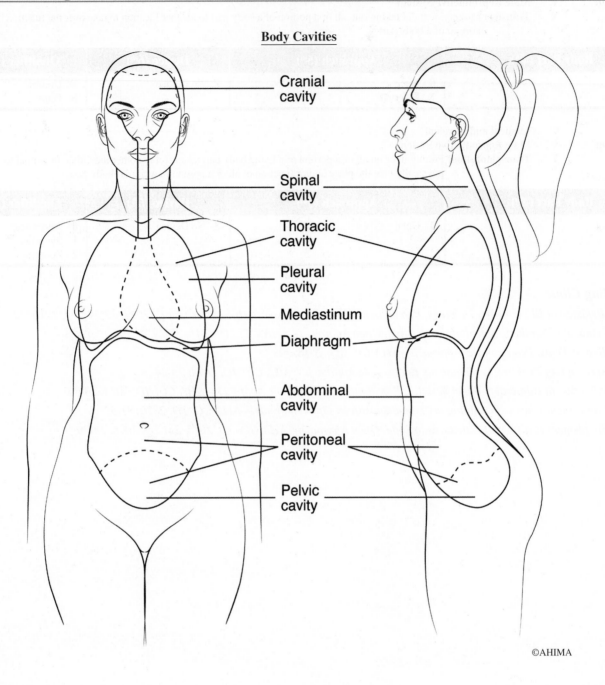

Cranial cavity

Spinal cavity

Thoracic cavity

Pleural cavity

Mediastinum

Diaphragm

Abdominal cavity

Peritoneal cavity

Pelvic cavity

©AHIMA

Body Areas

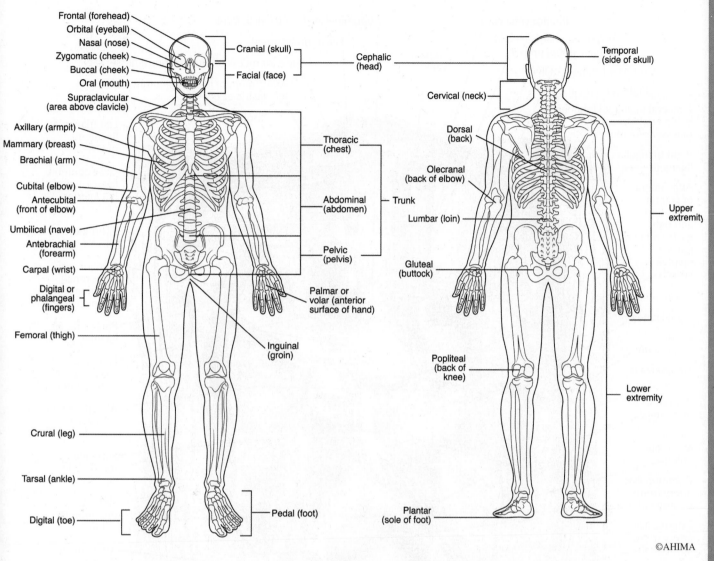

Frontal (forehead)
Orbital (eyeball)
Nasal (nose)
Zygomatic (cheek)
Buccal (cheek)
Oral (mouth)
Supraclavicular
(area above clavicle)
Axillary (armpit)
Mammary (breast)
Brachial (arm)
Cubital (elbow)
Antecubital
(front of elbow)
Umbilical (navel)
Antebrachial
(forearm)
Carpal (wrist)
Digital or
phalangeal
(fingers)
Femoral (thigh)
Crural (leg)
Tarsal (ankle)
Digital (toe)

Cranial (skull)
Facial (face)
Thoracic
(chest)
Abdominal
(abdomen)
Pelvic
(pelvis)
Palmar or
volar (anterior
surface of hand)
Inguinal
(groin)
Pedal (foot)

Cephalic
(head)
Trunk

Temporal
(side of skull)
Cervical (neck)
Dorsal
(back)
Olecranal
(back of elbow)
Lumbar (loin)
Gluteal
(buttock)
Popliteal
(back of
knee)
Plantar
(sole of foot)

Upper
extremity
Lower
extremity

©AHIMA

Peritoneum of Posterior Abdominal Wall

Inferior vena cava

(Common) bile duct and hepatic artery proper

Coronary ligament of liver

Right suprarenal gland

Omental (epiploic) foramen behind right free margin of lesser omentum

Right triangular ligament

Attachment of greater omentum and right gastro-omental (gastro-epiploic) vessels

Duodenum

Right kidney

Parietal peritoneum

Transversalis fascia

Root of mesentery

Site of ascending colon

Common iliac artery (retro-peritoneal)

External iliac artery (retro-peritoneal)

Testicular vessels (retro-peritoneal)

Ureters (retro-peritoneal)

Site of deep inguinal ring

Median umbilical fold (contains urachus)

Hepatic veins

Abdominal aorta and celiac trunk

Falciform ligament

Superior recess of omental bursa (lesser sac)

Attachment of lesser omentum and left gastric artery

Esophagus

Left triangular ligament of liver

Gastrophrenic ligament and left inferior phrenic artery

Short gastric vessels

Splenorenal (lienorenal) ligament and splenic vessels

Phrenicocolic ligament

Pancreas and splenic artery (retroperitoneal)

Attachment of transverse mesocolon

Superior mesenteric vessels

Site of descending colon

Attachment of sigmoid mesocolon and sigmoid vessels

Superior rectal vessels

Sacrogenital fold (ligament)

Lateral umbilical fold (contains inferior epi-gastric vessels)

Medial umbilical fold (contains occluded part of umbilical artery)

Rectum

Urinary bladder

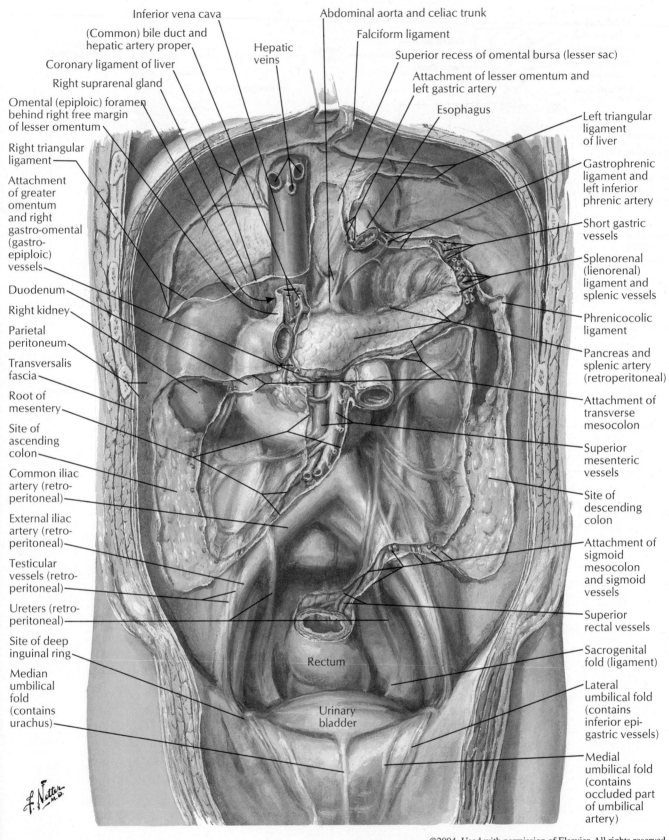

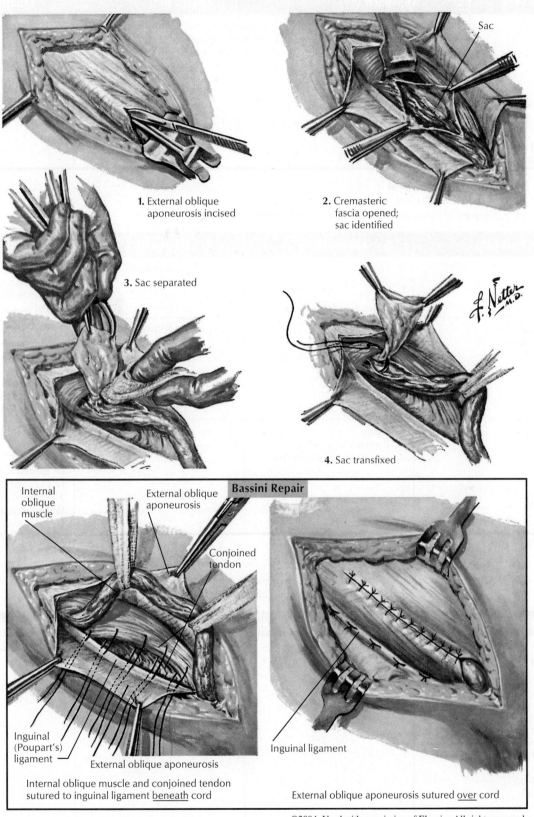

Sac

1. External oblique aponeurosis incised

2. Cremasteric fascia opened; sac identified

3. Sac separated

4. Sac transfixed

Bassini Repair

Internal oblique muscle

External oblique aponeurosis

Conjoined tendon

Inguinal (Poupart's) ligament

External oblique aponeurosis

Internal oblique muscle and conjoined tendon sutured to inguinal ligament <u>beneath</u> cord

Inguinal ligament

External oblique aponeurosis sutured <u>over</u> cord

Medical and Surgical, Anatomical Regions, General

Anatomical Regions, General Tables 0W0–0WY

Section	0	Medical and Surgical
Body System	W	Anatomical Regions, General
Operation	0	**Alteration:** Modifying the anatomic structure of a body part without affecting the function of the body part

Body Part (4th)	Approach (5th)	Device (6th)	Qualifier (7th)
0 Head 2 Face 4 Upper Jaw 5 Lower Jaw 6 Neck 8 Chest Wall F Abdominal Wall K Upper Back L Lower Back M Perineum, Male N Perineum, Female	0 Open 3 Percutaneous 4 Percutaneous Endoscopic	7 Autologous Tissue Substitute J Synthetic Substitute K Nonautologous Tissue Substitute Z No Device	Z No Qualifier

Section	0	Medical and Surgical
Body System	W	Anatomical Regions, General
Operation	1	**Bypass:** Altering the route of passage of the contents of a tubular body part

Body Part (4th)	Approach (5th)	Device (6th)	Qualifier (7th)
1 Cranial Cavity	0 Open	J Synthetic Substitute	9 Pleural Cavity, Right B Pleural Cavity, Left G Peritoneal Cavity J Pelvic Cavity
9 Pleural Cavity, Right B Pleural Cavity, Left J Pelvic Cavity	0 Open 3 Percutaneous 4 Percutaneous Endoscopic	J Synthetic Substitute	4 Cutaneous 9 Pleural Cavity, Right B Pleural Cavity, Left G Peritoneal Cavity J Pelvic Cavity W Upper Vein Y Lower Vein
G Peritoneal Cavity	0 Open 3 Percutaneous 4 Percutaneous Endoscopic	J Synthetic Substitute	4 Cutaneous 6 Bladder 9 Pleural Cavity, Right B Pleural Cavity, Left G Peritoneal Cavity J Pelvic Cavity W Upper Vein Y Lower Vein

Section	0	Medical and Surgical
Body System	W	Anatomical Regions, General
Operation	2	**Change:** Taking out or off a device from a body part and putting back an identical or similar device in or on the same body part without cutting or puncturing the skin or a mucous membrane

Body Part (4th)	Approach (5th)	Device (6th)	Qualifier (7th)
0 Head 1 Cranial Cavity 2 Face 4 Upper Jaw 5 Lower Jaw 6 Neck 8 Chest Wall 9 Pleural Cavity, Right B Pleural Cavity, Left C Mediastinum D Pericardial Cavity F Abdominal Wall G Peritoneal Cavity H Retroperitoneum J Pelvic Cavity K Upper Back L Lower Back M Perineum, Male N Perineum, Female	X External	0 Drainage Device Y Other Device	Z No Qualifier

Section	0	Medical and Surgical
Body System	W	Anatomical Regions, General
Operation	3	Control: Stopping, or attempting to stop, postprocedural or other acute bleeding

Body Part (4th)	Approach (5th)	Device (6th)	Qualifier (7th)
0 Head 1 Cranial Cavity 2 Face 4 Upper Jaw 5 Lower Jaw 6 Neck 8 Chest Wall 9 Pleural Cavity, Right B Pleural Cavity, Left C Mediastinum D Pericardial Cavity F Abdominal Wall G Peritoneal Cavity H Retroperitoneum J Pelvic Cavity K Upper Back L Lower Back M Perineum, Male N Perineum, Female	0 Open 3 Percutaneous 4 Percutaneous Endoscopic	Z No Device	Z No Qualifier
3 Oral Cavity and Throat	0 Open 3 Percutaneous 4 Percutaneous Endoscopic 7 Via Natural or Artificial Opening 8 Via Natural or Artificial Opening Endoscopic X External	Z No Device	Z No Qualifier
P Gastrointestinal Tract Q Respiratory Tract R Genitourinary Tract	0 Open 3 Percutaneous 4 Percutaneous Endoscopic 7 Via Natural or Artificial Opening 8 Via Natural or Artificial Opening Endoscopic	Z No Device	Z No Qualifier

Section	0	Medical and Surgical
Body System	W	Anatomical Regions, General
Operation	4	Creation: Putting in or on biological or synthetic material to form a new body part that to the extent possible replicates the anatomic structure or function of an absent body part

Body Part (4th)	Approach (5th)	Device (6th)	Qualifier (7th)
M Perineum, Male	0 Open	7 Autologous Tissue Substitute J Synthetic Substitute K Nonautologous Tissue Substitute	0 Vagina
N Perineum, Female	0 Open	7 Autologous Tissue Substitute J Synthetic Substitute K Nonautologous Tissue Substitute	1 Penis

Section	0	Medical and Surgical
Body System	W	Anatomical Regions, General
Operation	8	Division: Cutting into a body part, without draining fluids and/or gases from the body part, in order to separate or transect a body part

Body Part (4th)	Approach (5th)	Device (6th)	Qualifier (7th)
N Perineum, Female	X External	Z No Device	Z No Qualifier

Section	0	Medical and Surgical
Body System	W	Anatomical Regions, General
Operation	9	Drainage: Taking or letting out fluids and/or gases from a body part

Body Part (4th)	Approach (5th)	Device (6th)	Qualifier (7th)
0 Head 1 Cranial Cavity 2 Face 3 Oral Cavity and Throat 4 Upper Jaw 5 Lower Jaw 6 Neck 8 Chest Wall 9 Pleural Cavity, Right B Pleural Cavity, Left C Mediastinum D Pericardial Cavity F Abdominal Wall G Peritoneal Cavity H Retroperitoneum K Upper Back L Lower Back M Perineum, Male N Perineum, Female	0 Open 3 Percutaneous 4 Percutaneous Endoscopic	0 Drainage Device	Z No Qualifier
0 Head 1 Cranial Cavity 2 Face 3 Oral Cavity and Throat 4 Upper Jaw 5 Lower Jaw 6 Neck 8 Chest Wall 9 Pleural Cavity, Right B Pleural Cavity, Left C Mediastinum D Pericardial Cavity F Abdominal Wall G Peritoneal Cavity H Retroperitoneum K Upper Back L Lower Back M Perineum, Male N Perineum, Female	0 Open 3 Percutaneous 4 Percutaneous Endoscopic	Z No Device	X Diagnostic Z No Qualifier
J Pelvic Cavity	0 Open 3 Percutaneous 4 Percutaneous Endoscopic 7 Via Natural or Artificial Opening 8 Via Natural or Artificial Opening Endoscopic	0 Drainage Device	Z No Qualifier
J Pelvic Cavity	0 Open 3 Percutaneous 4 Percutaneous Endoscopic 7 Via Natural or Artificial Opening 8 Via Natural or Artificial Opening Endoscopic	Z No Device	X Diagnostic Z No Qualifier

Section	0	Medical and Surgical
Body System	W	Anatomical Regions, General
Operation	B	Excision: Cutting out or off, without replacement, a portion of a body part

Body Part (4th)	Approach (5th)	Device (6th)	Qualifier (7th)
0 Head 2 Face 3 Oral Cavity and Throat 4 Upper Jaw 5 Lower Jaw 8 Chest Wall K Upper Back L Lower Back M Perineum, Male N Perineum, Female	0 Open 3 Percutaneous 4 Percutaneous Endoscopic X External	Z No Device	X Diagnostic Z No Qualifier

Continued →

Body Part (4ᵗʰ)	Approach (5ᵗʰ)	Device (6ᵗʰ)	Qualifier (7ᵗʰ)
6 Neck F Abdominal Wall	0 Open 3 Percutaneous 4 Percutaneous Endoscopic	Z No Device	X Diagnostic Z No Qualifier
6 Neck F Abdominal Wall	X External	Z No Device	2 Stoma X Diagnostic Z No Qualifier
C Mediastinum H Retroperitoneum	0 Open 3 Percutaneous 4 Percutaneous Endoscopic	Z No Device	X Diagnostic Z No Qualifier

Section 0 Medical and Surgical

Body System W Anatomical Regions, General

Operation C Extirpation: Taking or cutting out solid matter from a body part

Body Part (4ᵗʰ)	Approach (5ᵗʰ)	Device (6ᵗʰ)	Qualifier (7ᵗʰ)
1 Cranial Cavity 3 Oral Cavity and Throat 9 Pleural Cavity, Right B Pleural Cavity, Left C Mediastinum D Pericardial Cavity G Peritoneal Cavity H Retroperitoneum J Pelvic Cavity	0 Open 3 Percutaneous 4 Percutaneous Endoscopic X External	Z No Device	Z No Qualifier
4 Upper Jaw 5 Lower Jaw	0 Open 3 Percutaneous 4 Percutaneous Endoscopic	Z No Device	Z No Qualifier
P Gastrointestinal Tract Q Respiratory Tract R Genitourinary Tract	0 Open 3 Percutaneous 4 Percutaneous Endoscopic 7 Via Natural or Artificial Opening 8 Via Natural or Artificial Opening Endoscopic X External	Z No Device	Z No Qualifier

Section 0 Medical and Surgical

Body System W Anatomical Regions, General

Operation F Fragmentation: Breaking solid matter in a body part into pieces

Body Part (4ᵗʰ)	Approach (5ᵗʰ)	Device (6ᵗʰ)	Qualifier (7ᵗʰ)
1 Cranial Cavity 3 Oral Cavity and Throat 9 Pleural Cavity, Right B Pleural Cavity, Left C Mediastinum D Pericardial Cavity G Peritoneal Cavity J Pelvic Cavity	0 Open 3 Percutaneous 4 Percutaneous Endoscopic X External	Z No Device	Z No Qualifier
P Gastrointestinal Tract Q Respiratory Tract R Genitourinary Tract	0 Open 3 Percutaneous 4 Percutaneous Endoscopic 7 Via Natural or Artificial Opening 8 Via Natural or Artificial Opening Endoscopic X External	Z No Device	Z No Qualifier

Section 0 Medical and Surgical
Body System W Anatomical Regions, General
Operation H Insertion: Putting in a nonbiological appliance that monitors, assists, performs, or prevents a physiological function but does not physically take the place of a body part

Body Part (4th)	Approach (5th)	Device (6th)	Qualifier (7th)
0 Head 1 Cranial Cavity 2 Face 3 Oral Cavity and Throat 4 Upper Jaw 5 Lower Jaw 6 Neck 8 Chest Wall 9 Pleural Cavity, Right B Pleural Cavity, Left C Mediastinum D Pericardial Cavity F Abdominal Wall G Peritoneal Cavity H Retroperitoneum J Pelvic Cavity K Upper Back L Lower Back M Perineum, Male N Perineum, Female	0 Open 3 Percutaneous 4 Percutaneous Endoscopic	1 Radioactive Element 3 Infusion Device Y Other Device	Z No Qualifier
P Gastrointestinal Tract Q Respiratory Tract R Genitourinary Tract	0 Open 3 Percutaneous 4 Percutaneous Endoscopic 7 Via Natural or Artificial Opening 8 Via Natural or Artificial Opening Endoscopic	1 Radioactive Element 3 Infusion Device Y Other Device	Z No Qualifier

Section 0 Medical and Surgical
Body System W Anatomical Regions, General
Operation J Inspection: Visually and/or manually exploring a body part

Body Part (4th)	Approach (5th)	Device (6th)	Qualifier (7th)
0 Head 2 Face 3 Oral Cavity and Throat 4 Upper Jaw 5 Lower Jaw 6 Neck 8 Chest Wall F Abdominal Wall K Upper Back L Lower Back M Perineum, Male N Perineum, Female	0 Open 3 Percutaneous 4 Percutaneous Endoscopic X External	Z No Device	Z No Qualifier
1 Cranial Cavity 9 Pleural Cavity, Right B Pleural Cavity, Left C Mediastinum D Pericardial Cavity G Peritoneal Cavity H Retroperitoneum J Pelvic Cavity	0 Open 3 Percutaneous 4 Percutaneous Endoscopic	Z No Device	Z No Qualifier
P Gastrointestinal Tract Q Respiratory Tract R Genitourinary Tract	0 Open 3 Percutaneous 4 Percutaneous Endoscopic 7 Via Natural or Artificial Opening 8 Via Natural or Artificial Opening Endoscopic	Z No Device	Z No Qualifier

Section	0	Medical and Surgical
Body System	W	Anatomical Regions, General
Operation	M	Reattachment: Putting back in or on all or a portion of a separated body part to its normal location or other suitable location

Body Part (4th)	Approach (5th)	Device (6th)	Qualifier (7th)
2 Face 4 Upper Jaw 5 Lower Jaw 6 Neck 8 Chest Wall F Abdominal Wall K Upper Back L Lower Back M Perineum, Male N Perineum, Female	0 Open	Z No Device	Z No Qualifier

Section	0	Medical and Surgical
Body System	W	Anatomical Regions, General
Operation	P	Removal: Taking out or off a device from a body part

Body Part (4th)	Approach (5th)	Device (6th)	Qualifier (7th)
0 Head 2 Face 4 Upper Jaw 5 Lower Jaw 6 Neck 8 Chest Wall C Mediastinum F Abdominal Wall K Upper Back L Lower Back M Perineum, Male N Perineum, Female	0 Open 3 Percutaneous 4 Percutaneous Endoscopic X External	0 Drainage Device 1 Radioactive Element 3 Infusion Device 7 Autologous Tissue Substitute J Synthetic Substitute K Nonautologous Tissue Substitute Y Other Device	Z No Qualifier
1 Cranial Cavity 9 Pleural Cavity, Right B Pleural Cavity, Left G Peritoneal Cavity J Pelvic Cavity	0 Open 3 Percutaneous 4 Percutaneous Endoscopic	0 Drainage Device 1 Radioactive Element 3 Infusion Device J Synthetic Substitute Y Other Device	Z No Qualifier
1 Cranial Cavity 9 Pleural Cavity, Right B Pleural Cavity, Left G Peritoneal Cavity J Pelvic Cavity	X External	0 Drainage Device 1 Radioactive Element 3 Infusion Device	Z No Qualifier
D Pericardial Cavity H Retroperitoneum	0 Open 3 Percutaneous 4 Percutaneous Endoscopic	0 Drainage Device 1 Radioactive Element 3 Infusion Device Y Other Device	Z No Qualifier
D Pericardial Cavity H Retroperitoneum	X External	0 Drainage Device 1 Radioactive Element 3 Infusion Device	Z No Qualifier
P Gastrointestinal Tract Q Respiratory Tract R Genitourinary Tract	0 Open 3 Percutaneous 4 Percutaneous Endoscopic 7 Via Natural or Artificial Opening 8 Via Natural or Artificial Opening Endoscopic X External	1 Radioactive Element 3 Infusion Device Y Other Device	Z No Qualifier

Section	0	Medical and Surgical
Body System	W	Anatomical Regions, General
Operation	Q	Repair: Restoring, to the extent possible, a body part to its normal anatomic structure and function

Body Part (4th)	Approach (5th)	Device (6th)	Qualifier (7th)
0 Head 2 Face 3 Oral Cavity and Throat 4 Upper Jaw 5 Lower Jaw 8 Chest Wall K Upper Back L Lower Back M Perineum, Male N Perineum, Female	0 Open 3 Percutaneous 4 Percutaneous Endoscopic X External	Z No Device	Z No Qualifier
6 Neck F Abdominal Wall	0 Open 3 Percutaneous 4 Percutaneous Endoscopic	Z No Device	Z No Qualifier
6 Neck F Abdominal Wall	X External	Z No Device	2 Stoma Z No Qualifier
C Mediastinum	0 Open 3 Percutaneous 4 Percutaneous Endoscopic	Z No Device	Z No Qualifier

Section	0	Medical and Surgical
Body System	W	Anatomical Regions, General
Operation	U	Supplement: Putting in or on biological or synthetic material that physically reinforces and/or augments the function of a portion of a body part

Body Part (4th)	Approach (5th)	Device (6th)	Qualifier (7th)
0 Head 2 Face 4 Upper Jaw 5 Lower Jaw 6 Neck 8 Chest Wall C Mediastinum F Abdominal Wall K Upper Back L Lower Back M Perineum, Male N Perineum, Female	0 Open 4 Percutaneous Endoscopic	7 Autologous Tissue Substitute J Synthetic Substitute K Nonautologous Tissue Substitute	Z No Qualifier

Section	0	Medical and Surgical
Body System	W	Anatomical Regions, General
Operation	W	Revision: Correcting, to the extent possible, a portion of a malfunctioning device or the position of a displaced device

Body Part (4th)	Approach (5th)	Device (6th)	Qualifier (7th)
0 Head 2 Face 4 Upper Jaw 5 Lower Jaw 6 Neck 8 Chest Wall C Mediastinum F Abdominal Wall K Upper Back L Lower Back M Perineum, Male N Perineum, Female	0 Open 3 Percutaneous 4 Percutaneous Endoscopic X External	0 Drainage Device 1 Radioactive Element 3 Infusion Device 7 Autologous Tissue Substitute J Synthetic Substitute K Nonautologous Tissue Substitute Y Other Device	Z No Qualifier

Continued →

Section	0	Medical and Surgical
Body System	W	Anatomical Regions, General
Operation	W	**Revision:** Correcting, to the extent possible, a portion of a malfunctioning device or the position of a displaced device

Body Part (4ᵗʰ)	Approach (5ᵗʰ)	Device (6ᵗʰ)	Qualifier (7ᵗʰ)
1 Cranial Cavity 9 Pleural Cavity, Right B Pleural Cavity, Left G Peritoneal Cavity J Pelvic Cavity	0 Open 3 Percutaneous 4 Percutaneous Endoscopic X External	0 Drainage Device 1 Radioactive Element 3 Infusion Device J Synthetic Substitute Y Other Device	Z No Qualifier
D Pericardial Cavity H Retroperitoneum	0 Open 3 Percutaneous 4 Percutaneous Endoscopic X External	0 Drainage Device 1 Radioactive Element 3 Infusion Device Y Other Device	Z No Qualifier
P Gastrointestinal Tract Q Respiratory Tract R Genitourinary Tract	0 Open 3 Percutaneous 4 Percutaneous Endoscopic 7 Via Natural or Artificial Opening 8 Via Natural or Artificial Opening Endoscopic X External	1 Radioactive Element 3 Infusion Device Y Other Device	Z No Qualifier

Section	0	Medical and Surgical
Body System	W	Anatomical Regions, General
Operation	Y	**Transplantation:** Putting in or on all or a portion of a living body part taken from another individual or animal to physically take the place and/or function of all or a portion of a similar body part

Body Part (4ᵗʰ)	Approach (5ᵗʰ)	Device (6ᵗʰ)	Qualifier (7th)
2 Face	0 Open	Z No Device	0 Allogeneic 1 Syngeneic

AHA Coding Clinic

0W020ZZ Alteration of Face, Open Approach—AHA CC: 1Q, 2015, 31

0W1G3J4 Bypass Peritoneal Cavity to Cutaneous with Synthetic Substitute, Percutaneous Approach—AHA CC: 4Q, 2013, 126-127

0W1G3JW Bypass Peritoneal Cavity to Upper Vein with Synthetic Substitute, Percutaneous Approach—AHA CC: 4Q, 2018, 42-43

0W310ZZ Control Bleeding in Cranial Cavity, Open Approach—AHA CC: 3Q, 2019, 4-5

0W3F0ZZ Control Bleeding in Abdominal Wall, Open Approach—AHA CC: 4Q, 2016, 100-101

0W3P8ZZ Control Bleeding in Gastrointestinal Tract, Via Natural or Artificial Opening Endoscopic—AHA CC: 4Q, 2016, 99-100; 4Q, 2017, 105; 1Q, 2018, 19

0W3Q7ZZ Control Bleeding in Respiratory Tract, Via Natural or Artificial Opening—AHA CC: 4Q, 2017, 106

0W3Q8ZZ Control Bleeding in Respiratory Tract, Via Natural or Artificial Opening Endoscopic—AHA CC: 1Q, 2018, 19-20

0W3R7ZZ Control Bleeding in Genitourinary Tract, Via Natural or Artificial Opening—AHA CC: 4Q, 2014, 44

0W930ZZ Drainage of Oral Cavity and Throat, Open Approach—AHA CC: 2Q, 2017, 16-17

0W9G3ZZ Drainage of Peritoneal Cavity, Percutaneous Approach—AHA CC: 3Q, 2017, 12-13

0WBF4ZZ Excision of Abdominal Wall, Percutaneous Endoscopic Approach—AHA CC: 1Q, 2016, 21-22

0WBH0ZZ Excision of Retroperitoneum, Open Approach—AHA CC: 1Q, 2019, 27

0WBNXZZ Excision of Female Perineum, External Approach—AHA CC: 4Q, 2013, 119-120

0WC30ZZ Extirpation of Matter from Oral Cavity and Throat, Open Approach—AHA CC: 2Q, 2017, 16

0WHG33Z Insertion of Infusion Device into Peritoneal Cavity, Percutaneous Approach—AHA CC: 2Q, 2015, 36; 2Q, 2016, 14

0WHJ01Z Insertion of Radioactive Element into Pelvic Cavity, Open Approach—AHA CC: 4Q, 2019, 43-44

0WJC0ZZ Inspection of Mediastinum, Open Approach—AHA CC: 3Q, 2018, 29

0WJG4ZZ Inspection of Peritoneal Cavity, Percutaneous Endoscopic Approach—AHA CC: 2Q, 2013, 36-37; 1Q, 2019, 4-5, 25

0WJJ4ZZ Inspection of Pelvic Cavity, Percutaneous Endoscopic Approach—AHA CC: 4Q, 2016, 58-59

0WQF0ZZ Repair Abdominal Wall, Open Approach—AHA CC: 4Q, 2014, 38-39; 3Q, 2014, 28-29; 3Q, 2016, 6; 3Q, 2017, 8-9

0WU80JZ Supplement Chest Wall with Synthetic Substitute, Open Approach—AHA CC: 4Q, 2012, 101-102

0WUF07Z Supplement Abdominal Wall with Autologous Tissue Substitute, Open Approach—AHA CC: 3Q, 2016, 40-41

0WUF0JZ Supplement Abdominal Wall with Synthetic Substitute, Open Approach—AHA CC: 4Q, 2014, 39-40; 3Q, 2017, 8

0WWG4JZ Revision of Synthetic Substitute in Peritoneal Cavity, Percutaneous Endoscopic Approach—AHA CC: 2Q, 2015, 9-10

Anatomical Regions, Upper Extremities

Anatomical Regions, Upper Extremities Tables 0X0–0XY

Section	0	Medical and Surgical
Body System	X	Anatomical Regions, Upper Extremities
Operation	0	**Alteration:** Modifying the anatomic structure of a body part without affecting the function of the body part

Body Part (4th)	Approach (5th)	Device (6th)	Qualifier (7th)
2 Shoulder Region, Right 3 Shoulder Region, Left 4 Axilla, Right 5 Axilla, Left 6 Upper Extremity, Right 7 Upper Extremity, Left 8 Upper Arm, Right 9 Upper Arm, Left B Elbow Region, Right C Elbow Region, Left D Lower Arm, Right F Lower Arm, Left G Wrist Region, Right H Wrist Region, Left	0 Open 3 Percutaneous 4 Percutaneous Endoscopic	7 Autologous Tissue Substitute J Synthetic Substitute K Nonautologous Tissue Substitute Z No Device	Z No Qualifier

Section	0	Medical and Surgical
Body System	X	Anatomical Regions, Upper Extremities
Operation	2	**Change:** Taking out or off a device from a body part and putting back an identical or similar device in or on the same body part without cutting or puncturing the skin or a mucous membrane

Body Part (4th)	Approach (5th)	Device (6th)	Qualifier (7th)
6 Upper Extremity, Right 7 Upper Extremity, Left	X External	0 Drainage Device Y Other Device	Z No Qualifier

Section	0	Medical and Surgical
Body System	X	Anatomical Regions, Upper Extremities
Operation	3	**Control:** Stopping, or attempting to stop, postprocedural or other acute bleeding

Body Part (4th)	Approach (5th)	Device (6th)	Qualifier (7th)
2 Shoulder Region, Right 3 Shoulder Region, Left 4 Axilla, Right 5 Axilla, Left 6 Upper Extremity, Right 7 Upper Extremity, Left 8 Upper Arm, Right 9 Upper Arm, Left B Elbow Region, Right C Elbow Region, Left D Lower Arm, Right F Lower Arm, Left G Wrist Region, Right H Wrist Region, Left J Hand, Right K Hand, Left	0 Open 3 Percutaneous 4 Percutaneous Endoscopic	Z No Device	Z No Qualifier

Section   0   **Medical and Surgical**
Body System   X   **Anatomical Regions, Upper Extremities**
Operation   6   **Detachment:** Cutting off all or a portion of the upper or lower extremities

Body Part (4th)	Approach (5th)	Device (6th)	Qualifier (7th)
0 Forequarter, Right **1** Forequarter, Left **2** Shoulder Region, Right **3** Shoulder Region, Left **B** Elbow Region, Right **C** Elbow Region, Left	**0** Open	**Z** No Device	**Z** No Qualifier
8 Upper Arm, Right **9** Upper Arm, Left **D** Lower Arm, Right **F** Lower Arm, Left	**0** Open	**Z** No Device	**1** High **2** Mid **3** Low
J Hand, Right **K** Hand, Left	**0** Open	**Z** No Device	**0** Complete **4** Complete 1st Ray **5** Complete 2nd Ray **6** Complete 3rd Ray **7** Complete 4th Ray **8** Complete 5th Ray **9** Partial 1st Ray **B** Partial 2nd Ray **C** Partial 3rd Ray **D** Partial 4th Ray **F** Partial 5th Ray
L Thumb, Right **M** Thumb, Left **N** Index Finger, Right **P** Index Finger, Left **Q** Middle Finger, Right **R** Middle Finger, Left **S** Ring Finger, Right **T** Ring Finger, Left **V** Little Finger, Right **W** Little Finger, Left	**0** Open	**Z** No Device	**0** Complete **1** High **2** Mid **3** Low

Section   0   **Medical and Surgical**
Body System   X   **Anatomical Regions, Upper Extremities**
Operation   9   **Drainage:** Taking or letting out fluids and/or gases from a body part

Body Part (4th)	Approach (5th)	Device (6th)	Qualifier (7th)
2 Shoulder Region, Right **3** Shoulder Region, Left **4** Axilla, Right **5** Axilla, Left **6** Upper Extremity, Right **7** Upper Extremity, Left **8** Upper Arm, Right **9** Upper Arm, Left **B** Elbow Region, Right **C** Elbow Region, Left **D** Lower Arm, Right **F** Lower Arm, Left **G** Wrist Region, Right **H** Wrist Region, Left **J** Hand, Right **K** Hand, Left	**0** Open **3** Percutaneous **4** Percutaneous Endoscopic	**0** Drainage Device	**Z** No Qualifier

Continued →

Section	0	Medical and Surgical
Body System	X	Anatomical Regions, Upper Extremities
Operation	9	**Drainage:** Taking or letting out fluids and/or gases from a body part

Body Part (4th)	Approach (5th)	Device (6th)	Qualifier (7th)
2 Shoulder Region, Right **3** Shoulder Region, Left **4** Axilla, Right **5** Axilla, Left **6** Upper Extremity, Right **7** Upper Extremity, Left **8** Upper Arm, Right **9** Upper Arm, Left **B** Elbow Region, Right **C** Elbow Region, Left **D** Lower Arm, Right **F** Lower Arm, Left **G** Wrist Region, Right **H** Wrist Region, Left **J** Hand, Right **K** Hand, Left	**0** Open **3** Percutaneous **4** Percutaneous Endoscopic	**Z** No Device	**X** Diagnostic **Z** No Qualifier

Section	0	Medical and Surgical
Body System	X	Anatomical Regions, Upper Extremities
Operation	B	**Excision:** Cutting out or off, without replacement, a portion of a body part

Body Part (4th)	Approach (5th)	Device (6th)	Qualifier (7th)
2 Shoulder Region, Right **3** Shoulder Region, Left **4** Axilla, Right **5** Axilla, Left **6** Upper Extremity, Right **7** Upper Extremity, Left **8** Upper Arm, Right **9** Upper Arm, Left **B** Elbow Region, Right **C** Elbow Region, Left **D** Lower Arm, Right **F** Lower Arm, Left **G** Wrist Region, Right **H** Wrist Region, Left **J** Hand, Right **K** Hand, Left	**0** Open **3** Percutaneous **4** Percutaneous Endoscopic	**Z** No Device	**X** Diagnostic **Z** No Qualifier

Section	0	Medical and Surgical
Body System	X	Anatomical Regions, Upper Extremities
Operation	H	**Insertion:** Putting in a nonbiological appliance that monitors, assists, performs, or prevents a physiological function but does not physically take the place of a body part

Body Part (4th)	Approach (5th)	Device (6th)	Qualifier (7th)
2 Shoulder Region, Right **3** Shoulder Region, Left **4** Axilla, Right **5** Axilla, Left **6** Upper Extremity, Right **7** Upper Extremity, Left **8** Upper Arm, Right **9** Upper Arm, Left **B** Elbow Region, Right **C** Elbow Region, Left **D** Lower Arm, Right **F** Lower Arm, Left **G** Wrist Region, Right **H** Wrist Region, Left **J** Hand, Right **K** Hand, Left	**0** Open **3** Percutaneous **4** Percutaneous Endoscopic	**1** Radioactive Element **3** Infusion Device **Y** Other Device	**Z** No Qualifier

Section	0	Medical and Surgical
Body System	X	Anatomical Regions, Upper Extremities
Operation	J	**Inspection:** Visually and/or manually exploring a body part

Body Part (4th)	Approach (5th)	Device (6th)	Qualifier (7th)
2 Shoulder Region, Right 3 Shoulder Region, Left 4 Axilla, Right 5 Axilla, Left 6 Upper Extremity, Right 7 Upper Extremity, Left 8 Upper Arm, Right 9 Upper Arm, Left B Elbow Region, Right C Elbow Region, Left D Lower Arm, Right F Lower Arm, Left G Wrist Region, Right H Wrist Region, Left J Hand, Right K Hand, Left	0 Open 3 Percutaneous 4 Percutaneous Endoscopic X External	Z No Device	Z No Qualifier

Section	0	Medical and Surgical
Body System	X	Anatomical Regions, Upper Extremities
Operation	M	**Reattachment:** Putting back in or on all or a portion of a separated body part to its normal location or other suitable location

Body Part (4th)	Approach (5th)	Device (6th)	Qualifier (7th)
0 Forequarter, Right 1 Forequarter, Left 2 Shoulder Region, Right 3 Shoulder Region, Left 4 Axilla, Right 5 Axilla, Left 6 Upper Extremity, Right 7 Upper Extremity, Left 8 Upper Arm, Right 9 Upper Arm, Left B Elbow Region, Right C Elbow Region, Left D Lower Arm, Right F Lower Arm, Left G Wrist Region, Right H Wrist Region, Left J Hand, Right K Hand, Left L Thumb, Right M Thumb, Left N Index Finger, Right P Index Finger, Left Q Middle Finger, Right R Middle Finger, Left S Ring Finger, Right T Ring Finger, Left V Little Finger, Right W Little Finger, Left	0 Open	Z No Device	Z No Qualifier

Section   0   **Medical and Surgical**
Body System   X   **Anatomical Regions, Upper Extremities**
Operation   P   **Removal:** Taking out or off a device from a body part

Body Part (4th)	Approach (5th)	Device (6th)	Qualifier (7th)
6 Upper Extremity, Right 7 Upper Extremity, Left	0 Open 3 Percutaneous 4 Percutaneous Endoscopic X External	0 Drainage Device 1 Radioactive Element 3 Infusion Device 7 Autologous Tissue Substitute J Synthetic Substitute K Nonautologous Tissue Substitute Y Other Device	Z No Qualifier

Section   0   **Medical and Surgical**
Body System   X   **Anatomical Regions, Upper Extremities**
Operation   Q   **Repair:** Restoring, to the extent possible, a body part to its normal anatomic structure and function

Body Part (4th)	Approach (5th)	Device (6th)	Qualifier (7th)
2 Shoulder Region, Right 3 Shoulder Region, Left 4 Axilla, Right 5 Axilla, Left 6 Upper Extremity, Right 7 Upper Extremity, Left 8 Upper Arm, Right 9 Upper Arm, Left B Elbow Region, Right C Elbow Region, Left D Lower Arm, Right F Lower Arm, Left G Wrist Region, Right H Wrist Region, Left J Hand, Right K Hand, Left L Thumb, Right M Thumb, Left N Index Finger, Right P Index Finger, Left Q Middle Finger, Right R Middle Finger, Left S Ring Finger, Right T Ring Finger, Left V Little Finger, Right W Little Finger, Left	0 Open 3 Percutaneous 4 Percutaneous Endoscopic X External	Z No Device	Z No Qualifier

Section   0   **Medical and Surgical**
Body System   X   **Anatomical Regions, Upper Extremities**
Operation   R   **Replacement:** Putting in or on biological or synthetic material that physically takes the place and/or function of all or a portion of a body part

Body Part (4th)	Approach (5th)	Device (6th)	Qualifier (7th)
L Thumb, Right M Thumb, Left	0 Open 4 Percutaneous Endoscopic	7 Autologous Tissue Substitute	N Toe, Right P Toe, Left

Section	0	Medical and Surgical
Body System	X	Anatomical Regions, Upper Extremities
Operation	U	Supplement: Putting in or on biological or synthetic material that physically reinforces and/or augments the function of a portion of a body part

Body Part (4th)	Approach (5th)	Device (6th)	Qualifier (7th)
2 Shoulder Region, Right 3 Shoulder Region, Left 4 Axilla, Right 5 Axilla, Left 6 Upper Extremity, Right 7 Upper Extremity, Left 8 Upper Arm, Right 9 Upper Arm, Left B Elbow Region, Right C Elbow Region, Left D Lower Arm, Right F Lower Arm, Left G Wrist Region, Right H Wrist Region, Left J Hand, Right K Hand, Left L Thumb, Right M Thumb, Left N Index Finger, Right P Index Finger, Left Q Middle Finger, Right R Middle Finger, Left S Ring Finger, Right T Ring Finger, Left V Little Finger, Right W Little Finger, Left	0 Open 4 Percutaneous Endoscopic	7 Autologous Tissue Substitute J Synthetic Substitute K Nonautologous Tissue Substitute	Z No Qualifier

Section	0	Medical and Surgical
Body System	X	Anatomical Regions, Upper Extremities
Operation	W	Revision: Correcting, to the extent possible, a portion of a malfunctioning device or the position of a displaced device

Body Part (4th)	Approach (5th)	Device (6th)	Qualifier (7th)
6 Upper Extremity, Right 7 Upper Extremity, Left	0 Open 3 Percutaneous 4 Percutaneous Endoscopic X External	0 Drainage Device 3 Infusion Device 7 Autologous Tissue Substitute J Synthetic Substitute K Nonautologous Tissue Substitute Y Other Device	Z No Qualifier

Section	0	Medical and Surgical
Body System	X	Anatomical Regions, Upper Extremities
Operation	X	Transfer: Moving, without taking out, all or a portion of a body part to another location to take over the function of all or a portion of a body part

Body Part (4th)	Approach (5th)	Device (6th)	Qualifier (7th)
N Index Finger, Right	0 Open	Z No Device	L Thumb, Right
P Index Finger, Left	0 Open	Z No Device	M Thumb, Left

Section	0	Medical and Surgical
Body System	X	Anatomical Regions, Upper Extremities
Operation	Y	Transplantation: Putting in or on all or a portion of a living body part taken from another individual or animal to physically take the place and/or function of all or a portion of a similar body part

Body Part (4th)	Approach (5th)	Device (6th)	Qualifier (7th)
J Hand, Right K Hand, Left	0 Open	Z No Device	0 Allogeneic 1 Syngeneic

0X370ZZ Control Bleeding in Left Upper Extremity, Open Approach—AHA CC: 1Q, 2015, 35

0X6M0Z3 Detachment at Left Thumb, Low, Open Approach—AHA CC: 3Q, 2016, 33-34; 1Q, 2017, 52

0X6T0Z3 Detachment at Left Ring Finger, Low, Open Approach—AHA CC: 3Q, 2016, 33-34; 1Q, 2017, 52

0X6V0Z0 Detachment at Right Little Finger, Complete, Open Approach—AHA CC: 2Q, 2017, 18-19

0X6W0Z3 Detachment at Left Little Finger, Low, Open Approach—AHA CC: 3Q, 2016, 33-34; 1Q, 2017, 52

0XH90YZ Insertion of Other Device into Left Upper Arm, Open Approach—AHA CC: 2Q, 2017, 20-21

0XP70YZ Removal of Other Device from Left Upper Extremity, Open Approach—AHA CC: 2Q, 2017, 20-21

Anatomical Regions, Lower Extremities

Anatomical Regions, Lower Extremities 0Y0–0YW

Section	0	Medical and Surgical
Body System	Y	Anatomical Regions, Lower Extremities
Operation	0	Alteration: Modifying the anatomic structure of a body part without affecting the function of the body part

Body Part (4th)	Approach (5th)	Device (6th)	Qualifier (7th)
0 Buttock, Right 1 Buttock, Left 9 Lower Extremity, Right B Lower Extremity, Left C Upper Leg, Right D Upper Leg, Left F Knee Region, Right G Knee Region, Left H Lower Leg, Right J Lower Leg, Left K Ankle Region, Right L Ankle Region, Left	0 Open 3 Percutaneous 4 Percutaneous Endoscopic	7 Autologous Tissue Substitute J Synthetic Substitute K Nonautologous Tissue Substitute Z No Device	Z No Qualifier

Section	0	Medical and Surgical
Body System	Y	Anatomical Regions, Lower Extremities
Operation	2	Change: Taking out or off a device from a body part and putting back an identical or similar device in or on the same body part without cutting or puncturing the skin or a mucous membrane

Body Part (4th)	Approach (5th)	Device (6th)	Qualifier (7th)
9 Lower Extremity, Right B Lower Extremity, Left	X External	0 Drainage Device Y Other Device	Z No Qualifier

Section	0	Medical and Surgical
Body System	Y	Anatomical Regions, Lower Extremities
Operation	3	Control: Stopping, or attempting to stop, postprocedural or other acute bleeding

Body Part (4th)	Approach (5th)	Device (6th)	Qualifier (7th)
0 Buttock, Right 1 Buttock, Left 5 Inguinal Region, Right 6 Inguinal Region, Left 7 Femoral Region, Right 8 Femoral Region, Left 9 Lower Extremity, Right B Lower Extremity, Left C Upper Leg, Right D Upper Leg, Left F Knee Region, Right G Knee Region, Left H Lower Leg, Right J Lower Leg, Left K Ankle Region, Right L Ankle Region, Left M Foot, Right N Foot, Left	0 Open 3 Percutaneous 4 Percutaneous Endoscopic	Z No Device	Z No Qualifier

Section	0	Medical and Surgical
Body System	Y	Anatomical Regions, Lower Extremities
Operation	6	Detachment: Cutting off all or a portion of the upper or lower extremities

Body Part (4th)	Approach (5th)	Device (6th)	Qualifier (7th)
2 Hindquarter, Right 3 Hindquarter, Left 4 Hindquarter, Bilateral 7 Femoral Region, Right 8 Femoral Region, Left F Knee Region, Right G Knee Region, Left	0 Open	Z No Device	Z No Qualifier
C Upper Leg, Right D Upper Leg, Left H Lower Leg, Right J Lower Leg, Left	0 Open	Z No Device	1 High 2 Mid 3 Low
M Foot, Right N Foot, Left	0 Open	Z No Device	0 Complete 4 Complete 1st Ray 5 Complete 2nd Ray 6 Complete 3rd Ray 7 Complete 4th Ray 8 Complete 5th Ray 9 Partial 1st Ray B Partial 2nd Ray C Partial 3rd Ray D Partial 4th Ray F Partial 5th Ray
P 1st Toe, Right Q 1st Toe, Left R 2nd Toe, Right S 2nd Toe, Left T 3rd Toe, Right U 3rd Toe, Left V 4th Toe, Right W 4th Toe, Left X 5th Toe, Right Y 5th Toe, Left	0 Open	Z No Device	0 Complete 1 High 2 Mid 3 Low

Section	0	Medical and Surgical
Body System	Y	Anatomical Regions, Lower Extremities
Operation	9	Drainage: Taking or letting out fluids and/or gases from a body part

Body Part (4th)	Approach (5th)	Device (6th)	Qualifier (7th)
0 Buttock, Right 1 Buttock, Left 5 Inguinal Region, Right 6 Inguinal Region, Left 7 Femoral Region, Right 8 Femoral Region, Left 9 Lower Extremity, Right B Lower Extremity, Left C Upper Leg, Right D Upper Leg, Left F Knee Region, Right G Knee Region, Left H Lower Leg, Right J Lower Leg, Left K Ankle Region, Right L Ankle Region, Left M Foot, Right N Foot, Left	0 Open 3 Percutaneous 4 Percutaneous Endoscopic	0 Drainage Device	Z No Qualifier

Continued →

Section	0	Medical and Surgical
Body System	Y	Anatomical Regions, Lower Extremities
Operation	9	Drainage: Taking or letting out fluids and/or gases from a body part

Body Part (4th)	Approach (5th)	Device (6th)	Qualifier (7th)
0 Buttock, Right	0 Open	Z No Device	X Diagnostic
1 Buttock, Left	3 Percutaneous		Z No Qualifier
5 Inguinal Region, Right	4 Percutaneous Endoscopic		
6 Inguinal Region, Left			
7 Femoral Region, Right			
8 Femoral Region, Left			
9 Lower Extremity, Right			
B Lower Extremity, Left			
C Upper Leg, Right			
D Upper Leg, Left			
F Knee Region, Right			
G Knee Region, Left			
H Lower Leg, Right			
J Lower Leg, Left			
K Ankle Region, Right			
L Ankle Region, Left			
M Foot, Right			
N Foot, Left			

Section	0	Medical and Surgical
Body System	Y	Anatomical Regions, Lower Extremities
Operation	B	Excision: Cutting out or off, without replacement, a portion of a body part

Body Part (4th)	Approach (5th)	Device (6th)	Qualifier (7th)
0 Buttock, Right	0 Open	Z No Device	X Diagnostic
1 Buttock, Left	3 Percutaneous		Z No Qualifier
5 Inguinal Region, Right	4 Percutaneous Endoscopic		
6 Inguinal Region, Left			
7 Femoral Region, Right			
8 Femoral Region, Left			
9 Lower Extremity, Right			
B Lower Extremity, Left			
C Upper Leg, Right			
D Upper Leg, Left			
F Knee Region, Right			
G Knee Region, Left			
H Lower Leg, Right			
J Lower Leg, Left			
K Ankle Region, Right			
L Ankle Region, Left			
M Foot, Right			
N Foot, Left			

Section	0	Medical and Surgical
Body System	Y	Anatomical Regions, Lower Extremities
Operation	H	**Insertion:** Putting in a nonbiological appliance that monitors, assists, performs, or prevents a physiological function but does not physically take the place of a body part

Body Part (4th)	Approach (5th)	Device (6th)	Qualifier (7th)
0 Buttock, Right 1 Buttock, Left 5 Inguinal Region, Right 6 Inguinal Region, Left 7 Femoral Region, Right 8 Femoral Region, Left 9 Lower Extremity, Right B Lower Extremity, Left C Upper Leg, Right D Upper Leg, Left F Knee Region, Right G Knee Region, Left H Lower Leg, Right J Lower Leg, Left K Ankle Region, Right L Ankle Region, Left M Foot, Right N Foot, Left	0 Open 3 Percutaneous 4 Percutaneous Endoscopic	1 Radioactive Element 3 Infusion Device Y Other Device	Z No Qualifier

Section	0	Medical and Surgical
Body System	Y	Anatomical Regions, Lower Extremities
Operation	J	**Inspection:** Visually and/or manually exploring a body part

Body Part (4th)	Approach (5th)	Device (6th)	Qualifier (7th)
0 Buttock, Right 1 Buttock, Left 5 Inguinal Region, Right 6 Inguinal Region, Left 7 Femoral Region, Right 8 Femoral Region, Left 9 Lower Extremity, Right A Inguinal Region, Bilateral B Lower Extremity, Left C Upper Leg, Right D Upper Leg, Left E Femoral Region, Bilateral F Knee Region, Right G Knee Region, Left H Lower Leg, Right J Lower Leg, Left K Ankle Region, Right L Ankle Region, Left M Foot, Right N Foot, Left	0 Open 3 Percutaneous 4 Percutaneous Endoscopic X External	Z No Device	Z No Qualifier

Section	0	Medical and Surgical
Body System	Y	Anatomical Regions, Lower Extremities
Operation	M	**Reattachment:** Putting back in or on all or a portion of a separated body part to its normal location or other suitable location

Body Part (4th)	Approach (5th)	Device (6th)	Qualifier (7th)
0 Buttock, Right	0 Open	Z No Device	Z No Qualifier
1 Buttock, Left			
2 Hindquarter, Right			
3 Hindquarter, Left			
4 Hindquarter, Bilateral			
5 Inguinal Region, Right			
6 Inguinal Region, Left			
7 Femoral Region, Right			
8 Femoral Region, Left			
9 Lower Extremity, Right			
B Lower Extremity, Left			
C Upper Leg, Right			
D Upper Leg, Left			
F Knee Region, Right			
G Knee Region, Left			
H Lower Leg, Right			
J Lower Leg, Left			
K Ankle Region, Right			
L Ankle Region, Left			
M Foot, Right			
N Foot, Left			
P 1st Toe, Right			
Q 1st Toe, Left			
R 2nd Toe, Right			
S 2nd Toe, Left			
T 3rd Toe, Right			
U 3rd Toe, Left			
V 4th Toe, Right			
W 4th Toe, Left			
X 5th Toe, Right			
Y 5th Toe, Left			

Section	0	Medical and Surgical
Body System	Y	Anatomical Regions, Lower Extremities
Operation	P	**Removal:** Taking out or off a device from a body part

Body Part (4th)	Approach (5th)	Device (6th)	Qualifier (7th)
9 Lower Extremity, Right	0 Open	0 Drainage Device	Z No Qualifier
B Lower Extremity, Left	3 Percutaneous	1 Radioactive Element	
	4 Percutaneous Endoscopic	3 Infusion Device	
	X External	7 Autologous Tissue Substitute	
		J Synthetic Substitute	
		K Nonautologous Tissue Substitute	
		Y Other Device	

Section	0	Medical and Surgical
Body System	Y	Anatomical Regions, Lower Extremities
Operation	Q	Repair: Restoring, to the extent possible, a body part to its normal anatomic structure and function

Body Part (4th)	Approach (5th)	Device (6th)	Qualifier (7th)
0 Buttock, Right	0 Open	Z No Device	Z No Qualifier
1 Buttock, Left	3 Percutaneous		
5 Inguinal Region, Right	4 Percutaneous Endoscopic		
6 Inguinal Region, Left	X External		
7 Femoral Region, Right			
8 Femoral Region, Left			
9 Lower Extremity, Right			
A Inguinal Region, Bilateral			
B Lower Extremity, Left			
C Upper Leg, Right			
D Upper Leg, Left			
E Femoral Region, Bilateral			
F Knee Region, Right			
G Knee Region, Left			
H Lower Leg, Right			
J Lower Leg, Left			
K Ankle Region, Right			
L Ankle Region, Left			
M Foot, Right			
N Foot, Left			
P 1st Toe, Right			
Q 1st Toe, Left			
R 2nd Toe, Right			
S 2nd Toe, Left			
T 3rd Toe, Right			
U 3rd Toe, Left			
V 4th Toe, Right			
W 4th Toe, Left			
X 5th Toe, Right			
Y 5th Toe, Left			

Section   0   **Medical and Surgical**
Body System   Y   **Anatomical Regions, Lower Extremities**
Operation   U   **Supplement:** Putting in or on biological or synthetic material that physically reinforces and/or augments the function of a portion of a body part

Body Part (4th)	Approach (5th)	Device (6th)	Qualifier (7th)
0 Buttock, Right 1 Buttock, Left 5 Inguinal Region, Right 6 Inguinal Region, Left 7 Femoral Region, Right 8 Femoral Region, Left 9 Lower Extremity, Right A Inguinal Region, Bilateral B Lower Extremity, Left C Upper Leg, Right D Upper Leg, Left E Femoral Region, Bilateral F Knee Region, Right G Knee Region, Left H Lower Leg, Right J Lower Leg, Left K Ankle Region, Right L Ankle Region, Left M Foot, Right N Foot, Left P 1st Toe, Right Q 1st Toe, Left R 2nd Toe, Right S 2nd Toe, Left T 3rd Toe, Right U 3rd Toe, Left V 4th Toe, Right W 4th Toe, Left X 5th Toe, Right Y 5th Toe, Left	0 Open 4 Percutaneous Endoscopic	7 Autologous Tissue Substitute J Synthetic Substitute K Nonautologous Tissue Substitute	Z No Qualifier

Section   0   **Medical and Surgical**
Body System   Y   **Anatomical Regions, Lower Extremities**
Operation   W   **Revision:** Correcting, to the extent possible, a portion of a malfunctioning device or the position of a displaced device

Body Part (4th)	Approach (5th)	Device (6th)	Qualifier (7th)
9 Lower Extremity, Right B Lower Extremity, Left	0 Open 3 Percutaneous 4 Percutaneous Endoscopic X External	0 Drainage Device 3 Infusion Device 7 Autologous Tissue Substitute J Synthetic Substitute K Nonautologous Tissue Substitute Y Other Device	Z No Qualifier

AHA Coding Clinic

0Y6N0Z0 Detachment at Left Foot, Complete, Open Approach—AHA CC: 1Q, 2015, 28; 1Q, 2017, 22-23
0Y6P0Z3 Detachment at Right 1st Toe, Low, Open Approach—AHA CC: 2Q, 2015, 28-29
0Y6Q0Z3 Detachment at Left 1st Toe, Low, Open Approach—AHA CC: 2Q, 2015, 28-29
0Y950ZZ Drainage of Right Inguinal Region, Open Approach—AHA CC: 1Q, 2015, 23
0Y980ZZ Drainage of Left Femoral Region, Open Approach—AHA CC: 1Q, 2015, 22

Within each section of ICD-10-PCS the characters have different meanings. The seven character meanings for the Obstetrics section are illustrated here through the procedure example of *Manually-assisted delivery*.

Section	Body System	Root Operation	Body Part	Approach	Device	Qualifier
Obstetrics	Pregnancy	Delivery	Products of Conception	External	None	None
1	0	E	0	X	Z	Z

Section (Character 1)

All Obstetric procedure codes have a first character value of 1.

Body System (Character 2)

The alphanumeric character for the body system is placed in the second position. The body system applicable to the Obstetrics section is Pregnancy and has a character value of 0.

Root Operations (Character 3)

The alphanumeric character value for root operations is placed in the third position. Listed below are the root operations applicable to the Obstetrics section with their associated meaning.

Character Value	Root Operation	Root Operation Definition
2	Change	Taking out or off a device from a body part and putting back an identical or similar device in or on the same body part without cutting or puncturing the skin or a mucous membrane
9	Drainage	Taking or letting out fluids and/or gases from a body part
A	Abortion	Artificially terminating a pregnancy
D	Extraction	Pulling or stripping out or off all or a portion of a body part by the use of force
E	Delivery	Assisting the passage of the products of conception from the genital canal
H	Insertion	Putting in a nonbiological appliance that monitors, assists, performs, or prevents a physiological function but does not physically take the place of a body part
J	Inspection	Visually and/or manually exploring a body part
P	Removal	Taking out or off a device from a body part, region or orifice
Q	Repair	Restoring, to the extent possible, a body part to its normal anatomic structure and function
S	Reposition	Moving to its normal location, or other suitable location, all or a portion of a body part
T	Resection	Cutting out or off, without replacement, all of a body part
Y	Transplantation	Putting in or on all or a portion of a living body part taken from another individual or animal to physically take the place and/or function of all or a portion of a similar body part

Body Part (Character 4)

For each body system the applicable body part character values will be available for procedure code construction. An example of a body part is Products of Conception.

Approach (Character 5)

The approach is the technique used to reach the procedure site. The following are the approach character values for the Obstetrics section with the associated definitions.

Character Value	Approach	Approach Definition
0	Open	Cutting through the skin or mucous membrane and any other body layers necessary to expose the site of the procedure
3	Percutaneous	Entry, by puncture or minor incision, of instrumentation through the skin or mucous membrane and any other body layers necessary to reach the site of the procedure

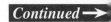
Continued →

Character Value	Approach	Approach Definition
4	Percutaneous Endoscopic	Entry, by puncture or minor incision, of instrumentation through the skin or mucous membrane and any other body layers necessary to reach and visualize the site of the procedure
7	Via Natural or Artificial Opening	Entry of instrumentation through a natural or artificial external opening to reach the site of the procedure
8	Via Natural or Artificial Opening Endoscopic	Entry of instrumentation through a natural or artificial external opening to reach and visualize the site of the procedure
X	External	Procedures performed directly on the skin or mucous membrane and procedures performed indirectly by the application of external force through the skin or mucous membrane

Device (Character 6)

Depending on the procedure performed there may or may not be a device used. There are two types of devices included in the Obstetrics section: monitoring electrode and other device. When a device is not utilized during the procedure, the placeholder Z is the character value that should be reported.

Qualifier (Character 7)

The qualifier represents an additional attribute for the procedure when applicable. For example, drainage procedures in this section include several qualifiers including fetal cerebrospinal fluid that is reported with the character value of A. If there is no qualifier for a procedure, the placeholder Z is the character valve that should be reported.

Obstetric Section Guidelines (section 1)

C. Obstetrics Section

Products of Conception

C1. Procedures performed on the products of conception are coded to the Obstetrics section. Procedures performed on the pregnant female other than the products of conception are coded to the appropriate root operation in the Medical and Surgical section.

Example: Amniocentesis is coded to the products of conception body part in the Obstetrics section. Repair of obstetric urethral laceration is coded to the urethra body part in the Medical and Surgical section.

Procedures following delivery or abortion

C2. Procedures performed following a delivery or abortion for curettage of the endometrium or evacuation of retained products of conception are all coded in the Obstetrics section, to the root operation Extraction and the body part Products of Conception, Retained. Diagnostic or therapeutic dilation and curettage performed during times other than the postpartum or post-abortion period are all coded in the Medical and Surgical section, to the root operation Extraction and the body part Endometrium.

Coding Guidelines References

The table below links ICD-10-PCS coding guidelines to Obstetrics section body system tables. The guidelines identified in the table are provided in order to remind users to reference the coding guidelines prior to code reporting. It is imperative to review the ICD-10-PCS coding guidelines to ensure the procedure code being reported is accurate and complete.

Table References

Table	Root Operation	Coding Guideline(s)
102	Change	C1
10D	Extraction	C2

Obstetrics Section Tables

Obstetrics Tables 102–10Y

Section	1	Obstetrics
Body System	0	Pregnancy
Operation	2	**Change:** Taking out or off a device from a body part and putting back an identical or similar device in or on the same body part without cutting or puncturing the skin or a mucous membrane

Body Part (4th)	Approach (5th)	Device (6th)	Qualifier (7th)
0 Products of Conception	7 Via Natural or Artificial Opening	3 Monitoring Electrode Y Other Device	Z No Qualifier

Section	1	Obstetrics
Body System	0	Pregnancy
Operation	9	**Drainage:** Taking or letting out fluids and/or gases from a body part

Body Part (4th)	Approach (5th)	Device (6th)	Qualifier (7th)
0 Products of Conception	0 Open 3 Percutaneous 4 Percutaneous Endoscopic 7 Via Natural or Artificial Opening 8 Via Natural or Artificial Opening Endoscopic	Z No Device	9 Fetal Blood A Fetal Cerebrospinal Fluid B Fetal Fluid, Other C Amniotic Fluid, Therapeutic D Fluid, Other U Amniotic Fluid, Diagnostic

Section	1	Obstetrics
Body System	0	Pregnancy
Operation	A	**Abortion:** Artificially terminating a pregnancy

Body Part (4th)	Approach (5th)	Device (6th)	Qualifier (7th)
0 Products of Conception	0 Open 3 Percutaneous 4 Percutaneous Endoscopic 8 Via Natural or Artificial Opening Endoscopic	Z No Device	Z No Qualifier
0 Products of Conception	7 Via Natural or Artificial Opening	Z No Device	6 Vacuum W Laminaria X Abortifacient Z No Qualifier

Section	1	Obstetrics
Body System	0	Pregnancy
Operation	D	**Extraction:** Pulling or stripping out or off all or a portion of a body part by the use of force

Body Part (4th)	Approach (5th)	Device (6th)	Qualifier (7th)
0 Products of Conception	0 Open	Z No Device	0 High 1 Low 2 Extraperitoneal
0 Products of Conception	7 Via Natural or Artificial Opening	Z No Device	3 Low Forceps 4 Mid Forceps 5 High Forceps 6 Vacuum 7 Internal Version 8 Other

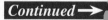

Continued →

Section	1	Obstetrics
Body System	0	Pregnancy
Operation	D	Extraction: Pulling or stripping out or off all or a portion of a body part by the use of force

Body Part (4th)	Approach (5th)	Device (6th)	Qualifier (7th)
1 Products of Conception, Retained	7 Via Natural or Artificial Opening 8 Via Natural or Artificial Opening Endoscopic	Z No Device	9 Manual Z No Qualifier
2 Products of Conception, Ectopic	0 Open 4 Percutaneous Endoscopic 7 Via Natural or Artificial Opening 8 Via Natural or Artificial Opening Endoscopic	Z No Device	Z No Qualifier

Section	1	Obstetrics
Body System	0	Pregnancy
Operation	E	Delivery: Assisting the passage of the products of conception from the genital canal

Body Part (4th)	Approach (5th)	Device (6th)	Qualifier (7th)
0 Products of Conception	X External	Z No Device	Z No Qualifier

Section	1	Obstetrics
Body System	0	Pregnancy
Operation	H	Insertion: Putting in a nonbiological appliance that monitors, assists, performs, or prevents a physiological function but does not physically take the place of a body part

Body Part (4th)	Approach (5th)	Device (6th)	Qualifier (7th)
0 Products of Conception	0 Open 7 Via Natural or Artificial Opening	3 Monitoring Electrode Y Other Device	Z No Qualifier

Section	1	Obstetrics
Body System	0	Pregnancy
Operation	J	Inspection: Visually and/or manually exploring a body part

Body Part (4th)	Approach (5th)	Device (6th)	Qualifier (7th)
0 Products of Conception 1 Products of Conception, Retained 2 Products of Conception, Ectopic	0 Open 3 Percutaneous 4 Percutaneous Endoscopic 7 Via Natural or Artificial Opening 8 Via Natural or Artificial Opening Endoscopic X External	Z No Device	Z No Qualifier

Section	1	Obstetrics
Body System	0	Pregnancy
Operation	P	Removal: Taking out or off a device from a body part, region or orifice

Body Part (4th)	Approach (5th)	Device (6th)	Qualifier (7th)
0 Products of Conception	0 Open 7 Via Natural or Artificial Opening	3 Monitoring Electrode Y Other Device	Z No Qualifier

Section   1   **Obstetrics**
Body System   0   **Pregnancy**
Operation   Q   **Repair:** Restoring, to the extent possible, a body part to its normal anatomic structure and function

Body Part (4th)	Approach (5th)	Device (6th)	Qualifier (7th)
0 Products of Conception	0 Open 3 Percutaneous 4 Percutaneous Endoscopic 7 Via Natural or Artificial Opening 8 Via Natural or Artificial Opening Endoscopic	Y Other Device Z No Device	E Nervous System F Cardiovascular System G Lymphatics and Hemic H Eye J Ear, Nose and Sinus K Respiratory System L Mouth and Throat M Gastrointestinal System N Hepatobiliary and Pancreas P Endocrine System Q Skin R Musculoskeletal System S Urinary System T Female Reproductive System V Male Reproductive System Y Other Body System

Section   1   **Obstetrics**
Body System   0   **Pregnancy**
Operation   S   **Reposition:** Moving to its normal location, or other suitable location, all or a portion of a body part

Body Part (4th)	Approach (5th)	Device (6th)	Qualifier (7th)
0 Products of Conception	7 Via Natural or Artificial Opening X External	Z No Device	Z No Qualifier
2 Products of Conception, Ectopic	0 Open 3 Percutaneous 4 Percutaneous Endoscopic 7 Via Natural or Artificial Opening 8 Via Natural or Artificial Opening Endoscopic	Z No Device	Z No Qualifier

Section   1   **Obstetrics**
Body System   0   **Pregnancy**
Operation   T   **Resection:** Cutting out or off, without replacement, all of a body part

Body Part (4th)	Approach (5th)	Device (6th)	Qualifier (7th)
2 Products of Conception, Ectopic	0 Open 3 Percutaneous 4 Percutaneous Endoscopic 7 Via Natural or Artificial Opening 8 Via Natural or Artificial Opening Endoscopic	Z No Device	Z No Qualifier

Section	1	Obstetrics
Body System	0	Pregnancy
Operation	Y	**Transplantation:** Putting in or on all or a portion of a living body part taken from another individual or animal to physically take the place and/or function of all or a portion of a similar body part

Body Part (4th)	Approach (5th)	Device (6th)	Qualifier (7th)
0 Products of Conception	3 Percutaneous 4 Percutaneous Endoscopic 7 Via Natural or Artificial Opening	Z No Device	E Nervous System F Cardiovascular System G Lymphatics and Hemic H Eye J Ear, Nose and Sinus K Respiratory System L Mouth and Throat M Gastrointestinal System N Hepatobiliary and Pancreas P Endocrine System Q Skin R Musculoskeletal System S Urinary System T Female Reproductive System V Male Reproductive System Y Other Body System

AHA Coding Clinic

10904ZC Drainage of Amniotic Fluid, Therapeutic from Products of Conception, Percutaneous Endoscopic Approach—AHA CC: 3Q, 2014, 12-13

10907ZC Drainage of Amniotic Fluid, Therapeutic from Products of Conception, Via Natural or Artificial Opening—AHA CC: 2Q, 2014, 9-10

10D00Z0 Extraction of Products of Conception, High, Open Approach— AHA CC: 2Q, 2018, 17-18; 4Q, 2018, 51

10D00Z1 Extraction of Products of Conception, Low, Open Approach—AHA CC: 4Q, 2018, 50-51

10D07Z3 Extraction of Products of Conception, Low Forceps, Via Natural or Artificial Opening—AHA CC: 1Q, 2016, 9-10

10D07Z6 Extraction of Products of Conception, Vacuum, Via Natural or Artificial Opening—AHA CC: 4Q, 2014, 43

10E0XZZ Delivery of Products of Conception, External Approach—AHA CC: 2Q, 2014, 9-10; 4Q, 2014, 17-18; 2Q, 2016, 34-35; 3Q, 2017, 5

10H07YZ Insertion of Other Device into Products of Conception, Via Natural or Artificial Opening—AHA CC: 2Q, 2013, 36

10Q04ZY Repair Other Body System in Products of Conception, Percutaneous Endoscopic Approach—AHA CC: 3Q, 2014, 12-13

10T24ZZ Resection of Products of Conception, Ectopic, Percutaneous Endoscopic Approach—AHA CC: 3Q, 2015, 32

Within each section of ICD-10-PCS the characters have different meanings. The seven character meanings for the Placement section are illustrated below through the procedure example of *Placement of pressure dressing on abdominal wall*.

Section	Body System	Root Operation	Body Region	Approach	Device	Qualifier
Placement	Anatomical Regions	Compression	Abdominal Wall	External	Pressure Dressing	None
2	W	1	3	X	6	Z

Section (Character 1)

All Placement procedure codes have a first character value of 2.

Body System (Character 2)

The alphanumeric character for the body system is placed in the second position. There are two character values applicable for the Placement section. The character value of W is reported for anatomical regions. The character value Y is reported for anatomical orifices.

Root Operations (Character 3)

The alphanumeric character value for root operations is placed in the third position. The following are the root operations applicable to the Placement section with their associated meaning.

Character Value	Root Operation	Root Operation Definition
0	Change	Taking out or off a device from a body part and putting back an identical or similar device in or on the same body part without cutting or puncturing the skin or a mucous membrane
1	Compression	Putting pressure on a body region
2	Dressing	Putting material on a body region for protection
3	Immobilization	Limiting or preventing motion of a body region
4	Packing	Putting material in a body region or orifice
5	Removal	Taking out or off a device from a body part
6	Traction	Exerting a pulling force on a body region in a distal direction

Body Region (Character 4)

For each body system the applicable body part character values will be available for procedure code construction. An example of a body region is Chest Wall.

Approach (Character 5)

The only approach technique utilized for the Placement section is External approach and is reported with the character value of X.

Character Value	Approach	Approach Definition
X	External	Procedures performed directly on the skin or mucous membrane and procedures performed indirectly by the application of external force through the skin or mucous membrane

Device (Character 6)

Depending on the procedure performed there may or may not be a device used. There are several types of devices included in the Placement section. Here is a sample list of the devices included in this section:

- Cast
- Packing material
- Pressure dressing
- Traction apparatus

When a device is not utilized during the procedure, the placeholder Z is the character value that should be reported.

Qualifier (Character 7)

The qualifier represents an additional attribute for the procedure when applicable. Currently, there are no qualifiers in the Placement section; therefore, the placeholder character value of Z should be reported.

Coding Guideline References

Before reporting Change and Removal procedures in this section users should review coding guideline B6.1c.

Placement Section Tables

Placement Tables 2W0–2Y5

Section	2	**Placement**
Body System	W	**Anatomical Regions**
Operation	0	**Change:** Taking out or off a device from a body part and putting back an identical or similar device in or on the same body part without cutting or puncturing the skin or a mucous membrane

Body Region (4th)	Approach (5th)	Device (6th)	Qualifier (7th)
0 Head 2 Neck 3 Abdominal Wall 4 Chest Wall 5 Back 6 Inguinal Region, Right 7 Inguinal Region, Left 8 Upper Extremity, Right 9 Upper Extremity, Left A Upper Arm, Right B Upper Arm, Left C Lower Arm, Right D Lower Arm, Left E Hand, Right F Hand, Left G Thumb, Right H Thumb, Left J Finger, Right K Finger, Left L Lower Extremity, Right M Lower Extremity, Left N Upper Leg, Right P Upper Leg, Left Q Lower Leg, Right R Lower Leg, Left S Foot, Right T Foot, Left U Toe, Right V Toe, Left	X External	0 Traction Apparatus 1 Splint 2 Cast 3 Brace 4 Bandage 5 Packing Material 6 Pressure Dressing 7 Intermittent Pressure Device Y Other Device	Z No Qualifier
1 Face	X External	0 Traction Apparatus 1 Splint 2 Cast 3 Brace 4 Bandage 5 Packing Material 6 Pressure Dressing 7 Intermittent Pressure Device 9 Wire Y Other Device	Z No Qualifier

Section	2	Placement
Body System	W	Anatomical Regions
Operation	1	Compression: Putting pressure on a body region

Body Region (4th)	Approach (5th)	Device (6th)	Qualifier (7th)
0 Head 1 Face 2 Neck 3 Abdominal Wall 4 Chest Wall 5 Back 6 Inguinal Region, Right 7 Inguinal Region, Left 8 Upper Extremity, Right 9 Upper Extremity, Left A Upper Arm, Right B Upper Arm, Left C Lower Arm, Right D Lower Arm, Left E Hand, Right F Hand, Left G Thumb, Right H Thumb, Left J Finger, Right K Finger, Left L Lower Extremity, Right M Lower Extremity, Left N Upper Leg, Right P Upper Leg, Left Q Lower Leg, Right R Lower Leg, Left S Foot, Right T Foot, Left U Toe, Right V Toe, Left	X External	6 Pressure Dressing 7 Intermittent Pressure Device	Z No Qualifier

Section	2	Placement
Body System	W	Anatomical Regions
Operation	2	Dressing: Putting material on a body region for protection

Body Region (4th)	Approach (5th)	Device (6th)	Qualifier (7th)
0 Head	X External	4 Bandage	Z No Qualifier
1 Face			
2 Neck			
3 Abdominal Wall			
4 Chest Wall			
5 Back			
6 Inguinal Region, Right			
7 Inguinal Region, Left			
8 Upper Extremity, Right			
9 Upper Extremity, Left			
A Upper Arm, Right			
B Upper Arm, Left			
C Lower Arm, Right			
D Lower Arm, Left			
E Hand, Right			
F Hand, Left			
G Thumb, Right			
H Thumb, Left			
J Finger, Right			
K Finger, Left			
L Lower Extremity, Right			
M Lower Extremity, Left			
N Upper Leg, Right			
P Upper Leg, Left			
Q Lower Leg, Right			
R Lower Leg, Left			
S Foot, Right			
T Foot, Left			
U Toe, Right			
V Toe, Left			

Section	2	Placement
Body System	W	Anatomical Regions
Operation	3	Immobilization: Limiting or preventing motion of a body region

Body Region (4th)	Approach (5th)	Device (6th)	Qualifier (7th)
0 Head 2 Neck 3 Abdominal Wall 4 Chest Wall 5 Back 6 Inguinal Region, Right 7 Inguinal Region, Left 8 Upper Extremity, Right 9 Upper Extremity, Left A Upper Arm, Right B Upper Arm, Left C Lower Arm, Right D Lower Arm, Left E Hand, Right F Hand, Left G Thumb, Right H Thumb, Left J Finger, Right K Finger, Left L Lower Extremity, Right M Lower Extremity, Left N Upper Leg, Right P Upper Leg, Left Q Lower Leg, Right R Lower Leg, Left S Foot, Right T Foot, Left U Toe, Right V Toe, Left	X External	1 Splint 2 Cast 3 Brace Y Other Device	Z No Qualifier
1 Face	X External	1 Splint 2 Cast 3 Brace 9 Wire Y Other Device	Z No Qualifier

	Section	2	Placement
	Body System	W	Anatomical Regions
	Operation	4	Packing: Putting material in a body region or orifice

Body Region (4th)	Approach (5th)	Device (6th)	Qualifier (7th)
0 Head	X External	5 Packing Material	Z No Qualifier
1 Face			
2 Neck			
3 Abdominal Wall			
4 Chest Wall			
5 Back			
6 Inguinal Region, Right			
7 Inguinal Region, Left			
8 Upper Extremity, Right			
9 Upper Extremity, Left			
A Upper Arm, Right			
B Upper Arm, Left			
C Lower Arm, Right			
D Lower Arm, Left			
E Hand, Right			
F Hand, Left			
G Thumb, Right			
H Thumb, Left			
J Finger, Right			
K Finger, Left			
L Lower Extremity, Right			
M Lower Extremity, Left			
N Upper Leg, Right			
P Upper Leg, Left			
Q Lower Leg, Right			
R Lower Leg, Left			
S Foot, Right			
T Foot, Left			
U Toe, Right			
V Toe, Left			

Section   2   **Placement**
Body System   W   **Anatomical Regions**
Operation   5   **Removal:** Taking out or off a device from a body part

Body Region (4ᵗʰ)	Approach (5ᵗʰ)	Device (6ᵗʰ)	Qualifier (7ᵗʰ)
0 Head 2 Neck 3 Abdominal Wall 4 Chest Wall 5 Back 6 Inguinal Region, Right 7 Inguinal Region, Left 8 Upper Extremity, Right 9 Upper Extremity, Left A Upper Arm, Right B Upper Arm, Left C Lower Arm, Right D Lower Arm, Left E Hand, Right F Hand, Left G Thumb, Right H Thumb, Left J Finger, Right K Finger, Left L Lower Extremity, Right M Lower Extremity, Left N Upper Leg, Right P Upper Leg, Left Q Lower Leg, Right R Lower Leg, Left S Foot, Right T Foot, Left U Toe, Right V Toe, Left	X External	0 Traction Apparatus 1 Splint 2 Cast 3 Brace 4 Bandage 5 Packing Material 6 Pressure Dressing 7 Intermittent Pressure Device Y Other Device	Z No Qualifier
1 Face	X External	0 Traction Apparatus 1 Splint 2 Cast 3 Brace 4 Bandage 5 Packing Material 6 Pressure Dressing 7 Intermittent Pressure Device 9 Wire Y Other Device	Z No Qualifier

Section	2	Placement
Body System	W	Anatomical Regions
Operation	6	Traction: Exerting a pulling force on a body region in a distal direction

Body Region (4th)	Approach (5th)	Device (6th)	Qualifier (7th)
0 Head	X External	0 Traction Apparatus	Z No Qualifier
1 Face		Z No Device	
2 Neck			
3 Abdominal Wall			
4 Chest Wall			
5 Back			
6 Inguinal Region, Right			
7 Inguinal Region, Left			
8 Upper Extremity, Right			
9 Upper Extremity, Left			
A Upper Arm, Right			
B Upper Arm, Left			
C Lower Arm, Right			
D Lower Arm, Left			
E Hand, Right			
F Hand, Left			
G Thumb, Right			
H Thumb, Left			
J Finger, Right			
K Finger, Left			
L Lower Extremity, Right			
M Lower Extremity, Left			
N Upper Leg, Right			
P Upper Leg, Left			
Q Lower Leg, Right			
R Lower Leg, Left			
S Foot, Right			
T Foot, Left			
U Toe, Right			
V Toe, Left			

Section	2	Placement
Body System	Y	Anatomical Orifices
Operation	0	Change: Taking out or off a device from a body part and putting back an identical or similar device in or on the same body part without cutting or puncturing the skin or a mucous membrane

Body Region (4th)	Approach (5th)	Device (6th)	Qualifier (7th)
0 Mouth and Pharynx	X External	5 Packing Material	Z No Qualifier
1 Nasal			
2 Ear			
3 Anorectal			
4 Female Genital Tract			
5 Urethra			

Section	2	Placement
Body System	Y	Anatomical Orifices
Operation	4	Packing: Putting material in a body region or orifice

Body Region (4th)	Approach (5th)	Device (6th)	Qualifier (7th)
0 Mouth and Pharynx	X External	5 Packing Material	Z No Qualifier
1 Nasal			
2 Ear			
3 Anorectal			
4 Female Genital Tract			
5 Urethra			

Section	2	Placement
Body System	Y	Anatomical Orifices
Operation	5	**Removal:** Taking out or off a device from a body part

Body Region (4th)	Approach (5th)	Device (6th)	Qualifier (7th)
0 Mouth and Pharynx **1** Nasal **2** Ear **3** Anorectal **4** Female Genital Tract **5** Urethra	**X** External	**5** Packing Material	**Z** No Qualifier

AHA Coding Clinic

2W60X0Z Traction of Head using Traction Apparatus—AHA CC: 2Q, 2013, 39

2W62X0Z Traction of Neck using Traction Apparatus—AHA CC: 2Q, 2015, 35

2Y41X5Z Packing of Nasal Region using Packing Material—AHA CC: 4Q, 2017, 106; 4Q, 2018, 38

Within each section of ICD-10-PCS, the characters have different meanings. The seven character meanings for the Administration section are illustrated here through the procedure example of *Nerve block injection to median nerve*.

Section	Body System	Root Operation	Body System/ Region	Approach	Substance	Qualifier
Administration	Physiological System and Anatomical Region	Introduction	Peripheral Nerves and Plexi	Percutaneous	Regional Anesthetic	None
3	E	0	T	3	C	Z

Section (Character 1)

All Administration procedure codes have a first character value of 3.

Body System (Character 2)

The alphanumeric character for the body system is placed in the second position. There are three character values applicable for the Administration section.

Character Value	Character Value Description
0	Circulatory
C	Indwelling Device
E	Physiological System and Anatomical Region

Root Operations (Character 3)

The alphanumeric character value for root operations is placed in the third position. Listed here are the root operations applicable to the Administration section with their associated meaning.

Character Value	Root Operation	Root Operation Definition
0	Introduction	Putting in or on a therapeutic, diagnostic, nutritional, physiological, or prophylactic substance except blood or blood products
1	Irrigation	Putting in or on a cleansing substance
2	Transfusion	Putting in blood or blood products

Body System/Region (Character 4)

For each body system the applicable body part character values will be available for procedure code construction. An example of a body region is upper GI.

Approach (Character 5)

The approach is the technique used to reach the procedure site. Listed here are the approach character values for the Administration with the associated definitions.

Character Value	Approach	Approach Definition
0	Open	Cutting through the skin or mucous membrane and any other body layers necessary to expose the site of the procedure
3	Percutaneous	Entry, by puncture or minor incision, of instrumentation through the skin or mucous membrane and any other body layers necessary to reach the site of the procedure
4	Percutaneous Endoscopic	Entry, by puncture or minor incision, of instrumentation through the skin or mucous membrane and any other body layers necessary to reach and visualize the site of the procedure
7	Via Natural or Artificial Opening	Entry of instrumentation through a natural or artificial external opening to reach the site of the procedure
8	Via Natural or Artificial Opening Endoscopic	Entry of instrumentation through a natural or artificial external opening to reach and visualize the site of the procedure
X	External	Procedures performed directly on the skin or mucous membrane and procedures performed indirectly by the application of external force through the skin or mucous membrane

Substance (Character 6)

In the Administration section a substance is always utilized. The substance is reported in the sixth character position by the type of substance utilized. The following is a sample list of the substances included in this section:

- Anti-inflammatory
- Antineoplastic
- Bone marrow
- Platelet inhibitor
- Whole blood

Qualifier (Character 7)

The qualifier represents an additional attribute for the procedure when applicable. There are several qualifiers included in the Administration section. For example, transfusion procedures in this section include qualifiers including Autologous and Nonautologous that are reported with the character values of 0 and 1, respectively. If there is no qualifier for a procedure, the placeholder Z is the character value that should be reported.

If a coder is unsure of which option to select for the substance qualifier utilized during the procedure, Appendix F can be used to guide the selection. It is important to note that not all substance qualifier categories are provided by CMS in Appendix F. However, for example, the coding scenario indicates that Clolar was introduced percutaneously via the peripheral vein. The coder references Table 3E0 (Introduction in Physiological Systems and Anatomical Regions) under the peripheral vein, percutaneous approach, anti-neoplastic. Clolar is not a substance qualifier choice. However, the coder can then locate the substance qualifier categories in Appendix F. The category Clofarabine includes Clolar. Therefore, the coder should select P - Clofarabine for the 7th character.

Important Definitions for the Administration Section

Administration Root Operation	Qualifier	Definition
Transfusion (302)	0 - Autologous	Derived or transferred from the same individual's body*
	1 - Nonautologous	Derived or transferred from another individual's body

*Taken from The Free Dictionary by Farlex at www.thefreedictionary.com

Coding Guideline References

Before reporting Transfusion procedures for embryonic stem cells (6th character A), bone marrow (6th character G), cord blood stem cells (6th character X) or hematopoietic stem cells (6th character Y) users should review coding guideline B3.16.

Before reporting Administration codes for all Biliary and Pancreatic Tract (4th character value of J) procedures with a 6th character value of U (Pancreatic Islet Cells), users should review coding guideline B3.16.

Before reporting Irrigation procedures in this section, users should review coding guideline B6.1c.

Administration Section Tables

Administration Tables 302–3E1

Section	3	Administration
Body System	0	Circulatory
Operation	2	**Transfusion:** Putting in blood or blood products

Body System / Region (4th)	Approach (5th)	Substance (6th)	Qualifier (7th)
3 Peripheral Vein 4 Central Vein	0 Open 3 Percutaneous	A Stem Cells, Embryonic	Z No Qualifier
3 Peripheral Vein 4 Central Vein	0 Open 3 Percutaneous	C Hematopoietic Stem/Progenitor Cells, Genetically Modified	0 Autologous
3 Peripheral Vein 4 Central Vein	0 Open 3 Percutaneous	G Bone Marrow X Stem Cells, Cord Blood Y Stem Cells, Hematopoietic	0 Autologous 2 Allogeneic, Related 3 Allogeneic, Unrelated 4 Allogeneic, Unspecified
3 Peripheral Vein 4 Central Vein	0 Open 3 Percutaneous	H Whole Blood J Serum Albumin K Frozen Plasma L Fresh Plasma M Plasma Cryoprecipitate N Red Blood Cells P Frozen Red Cells Q White Cells R Platelets S Globulin T Fibrinogen V Antihemophilic Factors W Factor IX	0 Autologous 1 Nonautologous
3 Peripheral Vein 4 Central Vein	0 Open 3 Percutaneous	U Stem Cells, T-cell Depleted Hematopoietic	2 Allogeneic, Related 3 Allogeneic, Unrelated 4 Allogeneic, Unspecified
7 Products of Conception, Circulatory	3 Percutaneous 7 Via Natural or Artificial Opening	H Whole Blood J Serum Albumin K Frozen Plasma L Fresh Plasma M Plasma Cryoprecipitate N Red Blood Cells P Frozen Red Cells Q White Cells R Platelets S Globulin T Fibrinogen V Antihemophilic Factors W Factor IX	1 Nonautologous
8 Vein	0 Open 3 Percutaneous	B 4-Factor Prothrombin Complex Concentrate	1 Nonautologous

Section	3	Administration
Body System	C	Indwelling Device
Operation	1	**Irrigation:** Putting in or on a cleansing substance

Body System / Region (4th)	Approach (5th)	Substance (6th)	Qualifier (7th)
Z None	X External	8 Irrigating Substance	Z No Qualifier

Section	3	Administration
Body System	E	Physiological Systems and Anatomical Regions
Operation	0	Introduction: Putting in or on a therapeutic, diagnostic, nutritional, physiological, or prophylactic substance except blood or blood products

Body System / Region (4th)	Approach (5th)	Substance (6th)	Qualifier (7th)
0 Skin and Mucous Membranes	X External	0 Antineoplastic	5 Other Antineoplastic M Monoclonal Antibody
0 Skin and Mucous Membranes	X External	2 Anti-infective	8 Oxazolidinones 9 Other Anti-infective
0 Skin and Mucous Membranes	X External	3 Anti-inflammatory B Anesthetic Agent K Other Diagnostic Substance M Pigment N Analgesics, Hypnotics, Sedatives T Destructive Agent	Z No Qualifier
0 Skin and Mucous Membranes	X External	G Other Therapeutic Substance	C Other Substance
1 Subcutaneous Tissue	0 Open	2 Anti-infective	A Anti-Infective Envelope
1 Subcutaneous Tissue	3 Percutaneous	0 Antineoplastic	5 Other Antineoplastic M Monoclonal Antibody
1 Subcutaneous Tissue	3 Percutaneous	2 Anti-infective	8 Oxazolidinones 9 Other Anti-infective A Anti-Infective Envelope
1 Subcutaneous Tissue	3 Percutaneous	3 Anti-inflammatory 6 Nutritional Substance 7 Electrolytic and Water Balance Substance B Anesthetic Agent H Radioactive Substance K Other Diagnostic Substance N Analgesics, Hypnotics, Sedatives T Destructive Agent	Z No Qualifier
1 Subcutaneous Tissue	3 Percutaneous	4 Serum, Toxoid and Vaccine	0 Influenza Vaccine Z No Qualifier
1 Subcutaneous Tissue	3 Percutaneous	G Other Therapeutic Substance	C Other Substance
1 Subcutaneous Tissue	3 Percutaneous	V Hormone	G Insulin J Other Hormone
2 Muscle	3 Percutaneous	0 Antineoplastic	5 Other Antineoplastic M Monoclonal Antibody
2 Muscle	3 Percutaneous	2 Anti-infective	8 Oxazolidinones 9 Other Anti-infective
2 Muscle	3 Percutaneous	3 Anti-inflammatory 6 Nutritional Substance 7 Electrolytic and Water Balance Substance B Anesthetic Agent H Radioactive Substance K Other Diagnostic Substance N Analgesics, Hypnotics, Sedatives T Destructive Agent	Z No Qualifier
2 Muscle	3 Percutaneous	4 Serum, Toxoid and Vaccine	0 Influenza Vaccine Z No Qualifier
2 Muscle	3 Percutaneous	G Other Therapeutic Substance	C Other Substance

Continued →

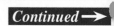

Section 3 Administration
Body System E Physiological Systems and Anatomical Regions
Operation 0 Introduction: Putting in or on a therapeutic, diagnostic, nutritional, physiological, or prophylactic substance except blood or blood products

3E0 Continued

3E0

Body System / Region (4th)	Approach (5th)	Substance (6th)	Qualifier (7th)
3 Peripheral Vein	0 Open	0 Antineoplastic	2 High-dose Interleukin-2 3 Low-dose Interleukin-2 5 Other Antineoplastic M Monoclonal Antibody P Clofarabine
3 Peripheral Vein	0 Open	1 Thrombolytic	6 Recombinant Human-activated Protein C 7 Other Thrombolytic
3 Peripheral Vein	0 Open	2 Anti-infective	8 Oxazolidinones 9 Other Anti-infective
3 Peripheral Vein	0 Open	3 Anti-inflammatory 4 Serum, Toxoid and Vaccine 6 Nutritional Substance 7 Electrolytic and Water Balance Substance F Intracirculatory Anesthetic H Radioactive Substance K Other Diagnostic Substance N Analgesics, Hypnotics, Sedatives P Platelet Inhibitor R Antiarrhythmic T Destructive Agent X Vasopressor	Z No Qualifier
3 Peripheral Vein	0 Open	G Other Therapeutic Substance	C Other Substance N Blood Brain Barrier Disruption
3 Peripheral Vein	0 Open	U Pancreatic Islet Cells	0 Autologous 1 Nonautologous
3 Peripheral Vein	0 Open	V Hormone	G Insulin H Human B-type Natriuretic Peptide J Other Hormone
3 Peripheral Vein	0 Open	W Immunotherapeutic	K Immunostimulator L Immunosuppressive
3 Peripheral Vein	3 Percutaneous	0 Antineoplastic	2 High-dose Interleukin-2 3 Low-dose Interleukin-2 5 Other Antineoplastic M Monoclonal Antibody P Clofarabine
3 Peripheral Vein	3 Percutaneous	1 Thrombolytic	6 Recombinant Human-activated Protein C 7 Other Thrombolytic
3 Peripheral Vein	3 Percutaneous	2 Anti-infective	8 Oxazolidinones 9 Other Anti-infective
3 Peripheral Vein	3 Percutaneous	3 Anti-inflammatory 4 Serum, Toxoid and Vaccine 6 Nutritional Substance 7 Electrolytic and Water Balance Substance F Intracirculatory Anesthetic H Radioactive Substance K Other Diagnostic Substance N Analgesics, Hypnotics, Sedatives P Platelet Inhibitor R Antiarrhythmic T Destructive Agent X Vasopressor	Z No Qualifier

Continued →

Section	3	Administration
Body System	E	**Physiological Systems and Anatomical Regions**
Operation	0	**Introduction:** Putting in or on a therapeutic, diagnostic, nutritional, physiological, or prophylactic substance except blood or blood products

Body System / Region (4ᵗʰ)	Approach (5ᵗʰ)	Substance (6ᵗʰ)	Qualifier (7ᵗʰ)
3 Peripheral Vein	**3** Percutaneous	**G** Other Therapeutic Substance	**C** Other Substance **N** Blood Brain Barrier Disruption **Q** Glucarpidase
3 Peripheral Vein	**3** Percutaneous	**U** Pancreatic Islet Cells	**0** Autologous **1** Nonautologous
3 Peripheral Vein	**3** Percutaneous	**V** Hormone	**G** Insulin **H** Human B-type Natriuretic Peptide **J** Other Hormone
3 Peripheral Vein	**3** Percutaneous	**W** Immunotherapeutic	**K** Immunostimulator **L** Immunosuppressive
4 Central Vein	**0** Open	**0** Antineoplastic	**2** High-dose Interleukin-2 **3** Low-dose Interleukin-2 **5** Other Antineoplastic **M** Monoclonal Antibody **P** Clofarabine
4 Central Vein	**0** Open	**1** Thrombolytic	**6** Recombinant Human-activated Protein C **7** Other Thrombolytic
4 Central Vein	**0** Open	**2** Anti-infective	**8** Oxazolidinones **9** Other Anti-infective
4 Central Vein	**0** Open	**3** Anti-inflammatory **4** Serum, Toxoid and Vaccine **6** Nutritional Substance **7** Electrolytic and Water Balance Substance **F** Intracirculatory Anesthetic **H** Radioactive Substance **K** Other Diagnostic Substance **N** Analgesics, Hypnotics, Sedatives **P** Platelet Inhibitor **R** Antiarrhythmic **T** Destructive Agent **X** Vasopressor	**Z** No Qualifier
4 Central Vein	**0** Open	**G** Other Therapeutic Substance	**C** Other Substance **N** Blood Brain Barrier Disruption
4 Central Vein	**0** Open	**V** Hormone	**G** Insulin **H** Human B-type Natriuretic Peptide **J** Other Hormone
4 Central Vein	**0** Open	**W** Immunotherapeutic	**K** Immunostimulator **L** Immunosuppressive
4 Central Vein	**3** Percutaneous	**0** Antineoplastic	**2** High-dose Interleukin-2 **3** Low-dose Interleukin-2 **5** Other Antineoplastic **M** Monoclonal Antibody **P** Clofarabine
4 Central Vein	**3** Percutaneous	**1** Thrombolytic	**6** Recombinant Human-activated Protein C **7** Other Thrombolytic

Continued →

Section	3	Administration
Body System	E	Physiological Systems and Anatomical Regions
Operation	0	**Introduction:** Putting in or on a therapeutic, diagnostic, nutritional, physiological, or prophylactic substance except blood or blood products

Body System / Region (4th)	Approach (5th)	Substance (6th)	Qualifier (7th)
4 Central Vein	3 Percutaneous	2 Anti-infective	8 Oxazolidinones 9 Other Anti-infective
4 Central Vein	3 Percutaneous	3 Anti-inflammatory 4 Serum, Toxoid and Vaccine 6 Nutritional Substance 7 Electrolytic and Water Balance Substance F Intracirculatory Anesthetic H Radioactive Substance K Other Diagnostic Substance N Analgesics, Hypnotics, Sedatives P Platelet Inhibitor R Antiarrhythmic T Destructive Agent X Vasopressor	Z No Qualifier
4 Central Vein	3 Percutaneous	G Other Therapeutic Substance	C Other Substance N Blood Brain Barrier Disruption Q Glucarpidase
4 Central Vein	3 Percutaneous	V Hormone	G Insulin H Human B-type Natriuretic Peptide J Other Hormone
4 Central Vein	3 Percutaneous	W Immunotherapeutic	K Immunostimulator L Immunosuppressive
5 Peripheral Artery 6 Central Artery	0 Open 3 Percutaneous	0 Antineoplastic	2 High-dose Interleukin-2 3 Low-dose Interleukin-2 5 Other Antineoplastic M Monoclonal Antibody P Clofarabine
5 Peripheral Artery 6 Central Artery	0 Open 3 Percutaneous	1 Thrombolytic	6 Recombinant Human-activated Protein C 7 Other Thrombolytic
5 Peripheral Artery 6 Central Artery	0 Open 3 Percutaneous	2 Anti-infective	8 Oxazolidinones 9 Other Anti-infective
5 Peripheral Artery 6 Central Artery	0 Open 3 Percutaneous	3 Anti-inflammatory 4 Serum, Toxoid and Vaccine 6 Nutritional Substance 7 Electrolytic and Water Balance Substance F Intracirculatory Anesthetic H Radioactive Substance K Other Diagnostic Substance N Analgesics, Hypnotics, Sedatives P Platelet Inhibitor R Antiarrhythmic T Destructive Agent X Vasopressor	Z No Qualifier
5 Peripheral Artery 6 Central Artery	0 Open 3 Percutaneous	G Other Therapeutic Substance	C Other Substance N Blood Brain Barrier Disruption
5 Peripheral Artery 6 Central Artery	0 Open 3 Percutaneous	V Hormone	G Insulin H Human B-type Natriuretic Peptide J Other Hormone

Continued →

3E0

Section   3   **Administration**
Body System   E   **Physiological Systems and Anatomical Regions**
Operation   0   **Introduction:** Putting in or on a therapeutic, diagnostic, nutritional, physiological, or prophylactic substance except blood or blood products

3E0 Continued

Body System / Region (4th)	Approach (5th)	Substance (6th)	Qualifier (7th)
5 Peripheral Artery 6 Central Artery	0 Open 3 Percutaneous	W Immunotherapeutic	K Immunostimulator L Immunosuppressive
7 Coronary Artery 8 Heart	0 Open 3 Percutaneous	1 Thrombolytic	6 Recombinant Human-activated Protein C 7 Other Thrombolytic
7 Coronary Artery 8 Heart	0 Open 3 Percutaneous	G Other Therapeutic Substance	C Other Substance
7 Coronary Artery 8 Heart	0 Open 3 Percutaneous	K Other Diagnostic Substance P Platelet Inhibitor	Z No Qualifier
7 Coronary Artery 8 Heart	4 Percutaneous Endoscopic	G Other Therapeutic Substance	C Other Substance
9 Nose	3 Percutaneous 7 Via Natural or Artificial Opening X External	0 Antineoplastic	5 Other Antineoplastic M Monoclonal Antibody
9 Nose	3 Percutaneous 7 Via Natural or Artificial Opening X External	2 Anti-infective	8 Oxazolidinones 9 Other Anti-infective
9 Nose	3 Percutaneous 7 Via Natural or Artificial Opening X External	3 Anti-inflammatory 4 Serum, Toxoid and Vaccine B Anesthetic Agent H Radioactive Substance K Other Diagnostic Substance N Analgesics, Hypnotics, Sedatives T Destructive Agent	Z No Qualifier
9 Nose	3 Percutaneous 7 Via Natural or Artificial Opening X External	G Other Therapeutic Substance	C Other Substance
A Bone Marrow	3 Percutaneous	0 Antineoplastic	5 Other Antineoplastic M Monoclonal Antibody
A Bone Marrow	3 Percutaneous	G Other Therapeutic Substance	C Other Substance
B Ear	3 Percutaneous 7 Via Natural or Artificial Opening X External	0 Antineoplastic	4 Liquid Brachytherapy Radioisotope 5 Other Antineoplastic M Monoclonal Antibody
B Ear	3 Percutaneous 7 Via Natural or Artificial Opening X External	2 Anti-infective	8 Oxazolidinones 9 Other Anti-infective
B Ear	3 Percutaneous 7 Via Natural or Artificial Opening X External	3 Anti-inflammatory B Anesthetic Agent H Radioactive Substance K Other Diagnostic Substance N Analgesics, Hypnotics, Sedatives T Destructive Agent	Z No Qualifier

Continued →

Section 3 Administration
Body System E Physiological Systems and Anatomical Regions
Operation 0 Introduction: Putting in or on a therapeutic, diagnostic, nutritional, physiological, or prophylactic substance except blood or blood products

3E0 Continued

3E0

Body System / Region (4th)	Approach (5th)	Substance (6th)	Qualifier (7th)
B Ear	3 Percutaneous 7 Via Natural or Artificial Opening X External	G Other Therapeutic Substance	C Other Substance
C Eye	3 Percutaneous 7 Via Natural or Artificial Opening X External	0 Antineoplastic	4 Liquid Brachytherapy Radioisotope 5 Other Antineoplastic M Monoclonal Antibody
C Eye	3 Percutaneous 7 Via Natural or Artificial Opening X External	2 Anti-infective	8 Oxazolidinones 9 Other Anti-infective
C Eye	3 Percutaneous 7 Via Natural or Artificial Opening X External	3 Anti-inflammatory B Anesthetic Agent H Radioactive Substance K Other Diagnostic Substance M Pigment N Analgesics, Hypnotics, Sedatives T Destructive Agent	Z No Qualifier
C Eye	3 Percutaneous 7 Via Natural or Artificial Opening X External	G Other Therapeutic Substance	C Other Substance
C Eye	3 Percutaneous 7 Via Natural or Artificial Opening X External	S Gas	F Other Gas
D Mouth and Pharynx	3 Percutaneous 7 Via Natural or Artificial Opening X External	0 Antineoplastic	4 Liquid Brachytherapy Radioisotope 5 Other Antineoplastic M Monoclonal Antibody
D Mouth and Pharynx	3 Percutaneous 7 Via Natural or Artificial Opening X External	2 Anti-infective	8 Oxazolidinones 9 Other Anti-infective
D Mouth and Pharynx	3 Percutaneous 7 Via Natural or Artificial Opening X External	3 Anti-inflammatory 4 Serum, Toxoid and Vaccine 6 Nutritional Substance 7 Electrolytic and Water Balance Substance B Anesthetic Agent H Radioactive Substance K Other Diagnostic Substance N Analgesics, Hypnotics, Sedatives R Antiarrhythmic T Destructive Agent	Z No Qualifier
D Mouth and Pharynx	3 Percutaneous 7 Via Natural or Artificial Opening X External	G Other Therapeutic Substance	C Other Substance

Continued →

3E0

Section 3 Administration

Body System E Physiological Systems and Anatomical Regions

Operation 0 **Introduction:** Putting in or on a therapeutic, diagnostic, nutritional, physiological, or prophylactic substance except blood or blood products

3E0 Continued

Body System / Region (4th)	Approach (5th)	Substance (6th)	Qualifier (7th)
E Products of Conception G Upper GI H Lower GI K Genitourinary Tract N Male Reproductive	3 Percutaneous 7 Via Natural or Artificial Opening 8 Via Natural or Artificial Opening Endoscopic	0 Antineoplastic	4 Liquid Brachytherapy Radioisotope 5 Other Antineoplastic M Monoclonal Antibody
E Products of Conception G Upper GI H Lower GI K Genitourinary Tract N Male Reproductive	3 Percutaneous 7 Via Natural or Artificial Opening 8 Via Natural or Artificial Opening Endoscopic	2 Anti-infective	8 Oxazolidinones 9 Other Anti-infective
E Products of Conception G Upper GI H Lower GI K Genitourinary Tract N Male Reproductive	3 Percutaneous 7 Via Natural or Artificial Opening 8 Via Natural or Artificial Opening Endoscopic	3 Anti-inflammatory 6 Nutritional Substance 7 Electrolytic and Water Balance Substance B Anesthetic Agent H Radioactive Substance K Other Diagnostic Substance N Analgesics, Hypnotics, Sedatives T Destructive Agent	Z No Qualifier
E Products of Conception G Upper GI H Lower GI K Genitourinary Tract N Male Reproductive	3 Percutaneous 7 Via Natural or Artificial Opening 8 Via Natural or Artificial Opening Endoscopic	G Other Therapeutic Substance	C Other Substance
E Products of Conception G Upper GI H Lower GI K Genitourinary Tract N Male Reproductive	3 Percutaneous 7 Via Natural or Artificial Opening 8 Via Natural or Artificial Opening Endoscopic	S Gas	F Other Gas
E Products of Conception G Upper GI H Lower GI K Genitourinary Tract N Male Reproductive	4 Percutaneous Endoscopic	G Other Therapeutic Substance	C Other Substance
F Respiratory Tract	3 Percutaneous 7 Via Natural or Artificial Opening 8 Via Natural or Artificial Opening Endoscopic	0 Antineoplastic	4 Liquid Brachytherapy Radioisotope 5 Other Antineoplastic M Monoclonal Antibody
F Respiratory Tract	3 Percutaneous 7 Via Natural or Artificial Opening 8 Via Natural or Artificial Opening Endoscopic	2 Anti-infective	8 Oxazolidinones 9 Other Anti-infective
F Respiratory Tract	3 Percutaneous 7 Via Natural or Artificial Opening 8 Via Natural or Artificial Opening Endoscopic	3 Anti-inflammatory 6 Nutritional Substance 7 Electrolytic and Water Balance Substance B Anesthetic Agent H Radioactive Substance K Other Diagnostic Substance N Analgesics, Hypnotics, Sedatives T Destructive Agent	Z No Qualifier

Continued →

Section 3 Administration
Body System E Physiological Systems and Anatomical Regions
Operation 0 Introduction: Putting in or on a therapeutic, diagnostic, nutritional, physiological, or prophylactic substance except blood or blood products

3E0 Continued

3E0

Body System / Region (4th)	Approach (5th)	Substance (6th)	Qualifier (7th)
F Respiratory Tract	3 Percutaneous 7 Via Natural or Artificial Opening 8 Via Natural or Artificial Opening Endoscopic	G Other Therapeutic Substance	C Other Substance
F Respiratory Tract	3 Percutaneous 7 Via Natural or Artificial Opening 8 Via Natural or Artificial Opening Endoscopic	S Gas	D Nitric Oxide F Other Gas
F Respiratory Tract	4 Percutaneous Endoscopic	G Other Therapeutic Substance	C Other Substance
J Biliary and Pancreatic Tract	3 Percutaneous 7 Via Natural or Artificial Opening 8 Via Natural or Artificial Opening Endoscopic	0 Antineoplastic	4 Liquid Brachytherapy Radioisotope 5 Other Antineoplastic M Monoclonal Antibody
J Biliary and Pancreatic Tract	3 Percutaneous 7 Via Natural or Artificial Opening 8 Via Natural or Artificial Opening Endoscopic	2 Anti-infective	8 Oxazolidinones 9 Other Anti-infective
J Biliary and Pancreatic Tract	3 Percutaneous 7 Via Natural or Artificial Opening 8 Via Natural or Artificial Opening Endoscopic	3 Anti-inflammatory 6 Nutritional Substance 7 Electrolytic and Water Balance Substance B Anesthetic Agent H Radioactive Substance K Other Diagnostic Substance N Analgesics, Hypnotics, Sedatives T Destructive Agent	Z No Qualifier
J Biliary and Pancreatic Tract	3 Percutaneous 7 Via Natural or Artificial Opening 8 Via Natural or Artificial Opening Endoscopic	G Other Therapeutic Substance	C Other Substance
J Biliary and Pancreatic Tract	3 Percutaneous 7 Via Natural or Artificial Opening 8 Via Natural or Artificial Opening Endoscopic	S Gas	F Other Gas
J Biliary and Pancreatic Tract	3 Percutaneous 7 Via Natural or Artificial Opening 8 Via Natural or Artificial Opening Endoscopic	U Pancreatic Islet Cells	0 Autologous 1 Nonautologous
J Biliary and Pancreatic Tract	4 Percutaneous Endoscopic	G Other Therapeutic Substance	C Other Substance
L Pleural Cavity	0 Open	5 Adhesion Barrier	Z No Qualifier

Continued →

Section	3	Administration
Body System	E	Physiological Systems and Anatomical Regions
Operation	0	Introduction: Putting in or on a therapeutic, diagnostic, nutritional, physiological, or prophylactic substance except blood or blood products

Body System / Region (4ᵗʰ)	Approach (5ᵗʰ)	Substance (6ᵗʰ)	Qualifier (7ᵗʰ)
L Pleural Cavity	**3** Percutaneous	**0** Antineoplastic	**4** Liquid Brachytherapy Radioisotope **5** Other Antineoplastic **M** Monoclonal Antibody
L Pleural Cavity	**3** Percutaneous	**2** Anti-infective	**8** Oxazolidinones **9** Other Anti-infective
L Pleural Cavity	**3** Percutaneous	**3** Anti-inflammatory **5** Adhesion Barrier **6** Nutritional Substance **7** Electrolytic and Water Balance Substance **B** Anesthetic Agent **H** Radioactive Substance **K** Other Diagnostic Substance **N** Analgesics, Hypnotics, Sedatives **T** Destructive Agent	**Z** No Qualifier
L Pleural Cavity	**3** Percutaneous	**G** Other Therapeutic Substance	**C** Other Substance
L Pleural Cavity	**3** Percutaneous	**S** Gas	**F** Other Gas
L Pleural Cavity	**4** Percutaneous Endoscopic	**5** Adhesion Barrier	**Z** No Qualifier
L Pleural Cavity	**4** Percutaneous Endoscopic	**G** Other Therapeutic Substance	**C** Other Substance
L Pleural Cavity	**7** Via Natural or Artificial Opening	**0** Antineoplastic	**4** Liquid Brachytherapy Radioisotope **5** Other Antineoplastic **M** Monoclonal Antibody
L Pleural Cavity	**7** Via Natural or Artificial Opening	**S** Gas	**F** Other Gas
M Peritoneal Cavity	**0** Open	**5** Adhesion Barrier	**Z** No Qualifier
M Peritoneal Cavity	**3** Percutaneous	**0** Antineoplastic	**4** Liquid Brachytherapy Radioisotope **5** Other Antineoplastic **M** Monoclonal Antibody **Y** Hyperthermic
M Peritoneal Cavity	**3** Percutaneous	**2** Anti-infective	**8** Oxazolidinones **9** Other Anti-infective
M Peritoneal Cavity	**3** Percutaneous	**3** Anti-inflammatory **5** Adhesion Barrier **6** Nutritional Substance **7** Electrolytic and Water Balance Substance **B** Anesthetic Agent **H** Radioactive Substance **K** Other Diagnostic Substance **N** Analgesics, Hypnotics, Sedatives **T** Destructive Agent	**Z** No Qualifier
M Peritoneal Cavity	**3** Percutaneous	**G** Other Therapeutic Substance	**C** Other Substance
M Peritoneal Cavity	**3** Percutaneous	**S** Gas	**F** Other Gas
M Peritoneal Cavity	**4** Percutaneous Endoscopic	**5** Adhesion Barrier	**Z** No Qualifier
M Peritoneal Cavity	**4** Percutaneous Endoscopic	**G** Other Therapeutic Substance	**C** Other Substance

Continued →

Section 3 Administration
Body System E Physiological Systems and Anatomical Regions
Operation 0 Introduction: Putting in or on a therapeutic, diagnostic, nutritional, physiological, or prophylactic substance except blood or blood products

3E0 Continued

3E0

Body System / Region (4th)	Approach (5th)	Substance (6th)	Qualifier (7th)
M Peritoneal Cavity	7 Via Natural or Artificial Opening	0 Antineoplastic	4 Liquid Brachytherapy Radioisotope 5 Other Antineoplastic M Monoclonal Antibody
M Peritoneal Cavity	7 Via Natural or Artificial Opening	S Gas	F Other Gas
P Female Reproductive	0 Open	5 Adhesion Barrier	Z No Qualifier
P Female Reproductive	3 Percutaneous	0 Antineoplastic	4 Liquid Brachytherapy Radioisotope 5 Other Antineoplastic M Monoclonal Antibody
P Female Reproductive	3 Percutaneous	2 Anti-infective	8 Oxazolidinones 9 Other Anti-infective
P Female Reproductive	3 Percutaneous	3 Anti-inflammatory 5 Adhesion Barrier 6 Nutritional Substance 7 Electrolytic and Water Balance Substance B Anesthetic Agent H Radioactive Substance K Other Diagnostic Substance L Sperm N Analgesics, Hypnotics, Sedatives T Destructive Agent V Hormone	Z No Qualifier
P Female Reproductive	3 Percutaneous	G Other Therapeutic Substance	C Other Substance
P Female Reproductive	3 Percutaneous	Q Fertilized Ovum	0 Autologous 1 Nonautologous
P Female Reproductive	3 Percutaneous	S Gas	F Other Gas
P Female Reproductive	4 Percutaneous Endoscopic	5 Adhesion Barrier	Z No Qualifier
P Female Reproductive	4 Percutaneous Endoscopic	G Other Therapeutic Substance	C Other Substance
P Female Reproductive	7 Via Natural or Artificial Opening	0 Antineoplastic	4 Liquid Brachytherapy Radioisotope 5 Other Antineoplastic M Monoclonal Antibody
P Female Reproductive	7 Via Natural or Artificial Opening	2 Anti-infective	8 Oxazolidinones 9 Other Anti-infective
P Female Reproductive	7 Via Natural or Artificial Opening	5 Adhesion Barrier 6 Nutritional Substance 7 Electrolytic and Water Balance Substance B Anesthetic Agent H Radioactive Substance K Other Diagnostic Substance L Sperm N Analgesics, Hypnotics, Sedatives T Destructive Agent V Hormone	Z No Qualifier
P Female Reproductive	7 Via Natural or Artificial Opening	G Other Therapeutic Substance	C Other Substance
P Female Reproductive	7 Via Natural or Artificial Opening	Q Fertilized Ovum	0 Autologous 1 Nonautologous

Continued →

3E0

Section 3 Administration
Body System E Physiological Systems and Anatomical Regions
Operation 0 Introduction: Putting in or on a therapeutic, diagnostic, nutritional, physiological, or prophylactic substance except blood or blood products

3E0 Continued

Body System / Region (4th)	Approach (5th)	Substance (6th)	Qualifier (7th)
P Female Reproductive	**7** Via Natural or Artificial Opening	**S** Gas	**F** Other Gas
P Female Reproductive	**8** Via Natural or Artificial Opening Endoscopic	**0** Antineoplastic	**4** Liquid Brachytherapy Radioisotope **5** Other Antineoplastic **M** Monoclonal Antibody
P Female Reproductive	**8** Via Natural or Artificial Opening Endoscopic	**2** Anti-infective	**8** Oxazolidinones **9** Other Anti-infective
P Female Reproductive	**8** Via Natural or Artificial Opening Endoscopic	**3** Anti-inflammatory **6** Nutritional Substance **7** Electrolytic and Water Balance Substance **B** Anesthetic Agent **H** Radioactive Substance **K** Other Diagnostic Substance **N** Analgesics, Hypnotics, Sedatives **T** Destructive Agent	**Z** No Qualifier
P Female Reproductive	**8** Via Natural or Artificial Opening Endoscopic	**G** Other Therapeutic Substance	**C** Other Substance
P Female Reproductive	**8** Via Natural or Artificial Opening Endoscopic	**S** Gas	**F** Other Gas
Q Cranial Cavity and Brain	**0** Open **3** Percutaneous	**0** Antineoplastic	**4** Liquid Brachytherapy Radioisotope **5** Other Antineoplastic **M** Monoclonal Antibody
Q Cranial Cavity and Brain	**0** Open **3** Percutaneous	**2** Anti-infective	**8** Oxazolidinones **9** Other Anti-infective
Q Cranial Cavity and Brain	**0** Open **3** Percutaneous	**3** Anti-inflammatory **6** Nutritional Substitute **7** Electrolytic and Water Balance Substitute **A** Stem Cells, Embryonic **B** Anesthetic Agent **H** Radioactive Substance **K** Other Diagnostic Substance **N** Analgesics, Hypnotics, Sedatives **T** Destructive Agent	**Z** No Qualifier
Q Cranial Cavity and Brain	**0** Open **3** Percutaneous	**E** Stem Cells, Somatic	**0** Autologous **1** Nonautologous
Q Cranial Cavity and Brain	**0** Open **3** Percutaneous	**G** Other Therapeutic Substance	**C** Other Substance
Q Cranial Cavity and Brain	**0** Open **3** Percutaneous	**S** Gas	**F** Other Gas
Q Cranial Cavity and Brain	**7** Via Natural or Artificial Opening	**0** Antineoplastic	**4** Liquid Brachytherapy Radioisotope **5** Other Antineoplastic **M** Monoclonal Antibody
Q Cranial Cavity and Brain	**7** Via Natural or Artificial Opening	**S** Gas	**F** Other Gas

Continued →

Section 3 Administration
Body System E Physiological Systems and Anatomical Regions
Operation 0 Introduction: Putting in or on a therapeutic, diagnostic, nutritional, physiological, or prophylactic substance except blood or blood products

3E0 Continued

3E0

Body System / Region (4th)	Approach (5th)	Substance (6th)	Qualifier (7th)
R Spinal Canal	**0** Open	**A** Stem Cells, Embryonic	**Z** No Qualifier
R Spinal Canal	**0** Open	**E** Stem Cells, Somatic	**0** Autologous **1** Nonautologous
R Spinal Canal	**3** Percutaneous	**0** Antineoplastic	**2** High-dose Interleukin-2 **3** Low-dose Interleukin-2 **4** Liquid Brachytherapy Radioisotope **5** Other Antineoplastic **M** Monoclonal Antibody
R Spinal Canal	**3** Percutaneous	**2** Anti-infective	**8** Oxazolidinones **9** Other Anti-infective
R Spinal Canal	**3** Percutaneous	**3** Anti-inflammatory **6** Nutritional Substance **7** Electrolytic and Water Balance Substance **A** Stem Cells, Embryonic **B** Anesthetic Agent **H** Radioactive Substance **K** Other Diagnostic Substance **N** Analgesics, Hypnotics, Sedatives **T** Destructive Agent	**Z** No Qualifier
R Spinal Canal	**3** Percutaneous	**E** Stem Cells, Somatic	**0** Autologous **1** Nonautologous
R Spinal Canal	**3** Percutaneous	**G** Other Therapeutic Substance	**C** Other Substance
R Spinal Canal	**3** Percutaneous	**S** Gas	**F** Other Gas
R Spinal Canal	**7** Via Natural or Artificial Opening	**S** Gas	**F** Other Gas
S Epidural Space	**3** Percutaneous	**0** Antineoplastic	**2** High-dose Interleukin-2 **3** Low-dose Interleukin-2 **4** Liquid Brachytherapy Radioisotope **5** Other Antineoplastic **M** Monoclonal Antibody
S Epidural Space	**3** Percutaneous	**2** Anti-infective	**8** Oxazolidinones **9** Other Anti-infective
S Epidural Space	**3** Percutaneous	**3** Anti-inflammatory **6** Nutritional Substance **7** Electrolytic and Water Balance Substance **B** Anesthetic Agent **H** Radioactive Substance **K** Other Diagnostic Substance **N** Analgesics, Hypnotics, Sedatives **T** Destructive Agent	**Z** No Qualifier
S Epidural Space	**3** Percutaneous	**G** Other Therapeutic Substance	**C** Other Substance
S Epidural Space	**3** Percutaneous	**S** Gas	**F** Other Gas
S Epidural Space	**7** Via Natural or Artificial Opening	**S** Gas	**F** Other Gas
T Peripheral Nerves and Plexi **X** Cranial Nerves	**3** Percutaneous	**3** Anti-inflammatory **B** Anesthetic Agent **T** Destructive Agent	**Z** No Qualifier

Continued →

3E0

Section 3 Administration
Body System E Physiological Systems and Anatomical Regions
Operation 0 Introduction: Putting in or on a therapeutic, diagnostic, nutritional, physiological, or prophylactic substance except blood or blood products

3E0 Continued

Body System / Region (4th)	Approach (5th)	Substance (6th)	Qualifier (7th)
T Peripheral Nerves and Plexi **X** Cranial Nerves	**3** Percutaneous	**G** Other Therapeutic Substance	**C** Other Substance
U Joints	**0** Open	**2** Anti-infective	**8** Oxazolidinones **9** Other Anti-infective
U Joints	**0** Open	**G** Other Therapeutic Substance	**B** Recombinant Bone Morphogenetic Protein
U Joints	**3** Percutaneous	**0** Antineoplastic	**4** Liquid Brachytherapy Radioisotope **5** Other Antineoplastic **M** Monoclonal Antibody
U Joints	**3** Percutaneous	**2** Anti-infective	**8** Oxazolidinones **9** Other Anti-infective
U Joints	**3** Percutaneous	**3** Anti-inflammatory **6** Nutritional Substance **7** Electrolytic and Water Balance Substance **B** Anesthetic Agent **H** Radioactive Substance **K** Other Diagnostic Substance **N** Analgesics, Hypnotics, Sedatives **T** Destructive Agent	**Z** No Qualifier
U Joints	**3** Percutaneous	**G** Other Therapeutic Substance	**B** Recombinant Bone Morphogenetic Protein **C** Other Substance
U Joints	**3** Percutaneous	**S** Gas	**F** Other Gas
U Joints	**4** Percutaneous Endoscopic	**G** Other Therapeutic Substance	**C** Other Substance
V Bones	**0** Open	**G** Other Therapeutic Substance	**B** Recombinant Bone Morphogenetic Protein
V Bones	**3** Percutaneous	**0** Antineoplastic	**5** Other Antineoplastic **M** Monoclonal Antibody
V Bones	**3** Percutaneous	**2** Anti-infective	**8** Oxazolidinones **9** Other Anti-infective
V Bones	**3** Percutaneous	**3** Anti-inflammatory **6** Nutritional Substance **7** Electrolytic and Water Balance Substance **B** Anesthetic Agent **H** Radioactive Substance **K** Other Diagnostic Substance **N** Analgesics, Hypnotics, Sedatives **T** Destructive Agent	**Z** No Qualifier
V Bones	**3** Percutaneous	**G** Other Therapeutic Substance	**B** Recombinant Bone Morphogenetic Protein **C** Other Substance
W Lymphatics	**3** Percutaneous	**0** Antineoplastic	**5** Other Antineoplastic **M** Monoclonal Antibody
W Lymphatics	**3** Percutaneous	**2** Anti-infective	**8** Oxazolidinones **9** Other Anti-infective

Continued →

Section	3	Administration
Body System	E	Physiological Systems and Anatomical Regions
Operation	0	Introduction: Putting in or on a therapeutic, diagnostic, nutritional, physiological, or prophylactic substance except blood or blood products

Body System / Region (4th)	Approach (5th)	Substance (6th)	Qualifier (7th)
W Lymphatics	3 Percutaneous	3 Anti-inflammatory 6 Nutritional Substance 7 Electrolytic and Water Balance Substance B Anesthetic Agent H Radioactive Substance K Other Diagnostic Substance N Analgesics, Hypnotics, Sedatives T Destructive Agent	Z No Qualifier
W Lymphatics	3 Percutaneous	G Other Therapeutic Substance	C Other Substance
Y Pericardial Cavity	3 Percutaneous	0 Antineoplastic	4 Liquid Brachytherapy Radioisotope 5 Other Antineoplastic M Monoclonal Antibody
Y Pericardial Cavity	3 Percutaneous	2 Anti-infective	8 Oxazolidinones 9 Other Anti-infective
Y Pericardial Cavity	3 Percutaneous	3 Anti-inflammatory 6 Nutritional Substance 7 Electrolytic and Water Balance Substance B Anesthetic Agent H Radioactive Substance K Other Diagnostic Substance N Analgesics, Hypnotics, Sedatives T Destructive Agent	Z No Qualifier
Y Pericardial Cavity	3 Percutaneous	G Other Therapeutic Substance	C Other Substance
Y Pericardial Cavity	3 Percutaneous	S Gas	F Other Gas
Y Pericardial Cavity	4 Percutaneous Endoscopic	G Other Therapeutic Substance	C Other Substance
Y Pericardial Cavity	7 Via Natural or Artificial Opening	0 Antineoplastic	4 Liquid Brachytherapy Radioisotope 5 Other Antineoplastic M Monoclonal Antibody
Y Pericardial Cavity	7 Via Natural or Artificial Opening	S Gas	F Other Gas

Section	3	Administration
Body System	E	Physiological Systems and Anatomical Regions
Operation	1	Irrigation: Putting in or on a cleansing substance

Body System / Region (4th)	Approach (5th)	Substance (6th)	Qualifier (7th)
0 Skin and Mucous Membranes C Eye	3 Percutaneous X External	8 Irrigating Substance	X Diagnostic Z No Qualifier

Continued →

3E1

Section 3 Administration
Body System E Physiological Systems and Anatomical Regions
Operation 1 Irrigation: Putting in or on a cleansing substance

3E1 Continued

Body System / Region (4th)	Approach (5th)	Substance (6th)	Qualifier (7th)
9 Nose B Ear F Respiratory Tract G Upper GI H Lower GI J Biliary and Pancreatic Tract K Genitourinary Tract N Male Reproductive P Female Reproductive	3 Percutaneous 7 Via Natural or Artificial Opening 8 Via Natural or Artificial Opening Endoscopic	8 Irrigating Substance	X Diagnostic Z No Qualifier
L Pleural Cavity Q Cranial Cavity and Brain R Spinal Canal S Epidural Space Y Pericardial Cavity	3 Percutaneous	8 Irrigating Substance	X Diagnostic Z No Qualifier
M Peritoneal Cavity	3 Percutaneous	8 Irrigating Substance	X Diagnostic Z No Qualifier
M Peritoneal Cavity	3 Percutaneous	9 Dialysate	Z No Qualifier
U Joints	3 Percutaneous 4 Percutaneous Endoscopic	8 Irrigating Substance	X Diagnostic Z No Qualifier

AHA Coding Clinic

3E013GC Introduction of Other Therapeutic Substance into Subcutaneous Tissue, Percutaneous Approach—AHA CC: 2Q, 2014, 10

3E0234Z Introduction of Serum, Toxoid and Vaccine into Muscle, Percutaneous Approach—AHA CC: 4Q, 2014, 16

3E03317 Introduction of Other Thrombolytic into Peripheral Vein, Percutaneous Approach—AHA CC: 4Q, 2013, 124

3E033VJ Introduction of Other Hormone into Peripheral Vein, Percutaneous Approach—AHA CC: 4Q, 2014, 17-18

3E05305 Introduction of Other Antineoplastic into Peripheral Artery, Percutaneous Approach—AHA CC: 1Q, 2015, 38

3E06305 Introduction of Other Antineoplastic into Central Artery, Percutaneous Approach—AHA CC: 3Q, 2014 26-27

3E06317 Introduction of Other Thrombolytic into Central Artery, Percutaneous Approach—AHA CC: 4Q, 2014, 19-20

3E073GC Introduction of Other Therapeutic Substance into Coronary Artery, Percutaneous Approach—AHA CC: 3Q, 2018. 7-8

3E0G76Z Introduction of Nutritional Substance into Upper GI, Via Natural or Artificial Opening—AHA CC: 2Q, 2015, 29

3E0G8GC Introduction of Other Therapeutic Substance into Upper GI, via Natural or Artificial Opening Endoscopic—AHA CC: 3Q, 2015, 24-25

3E0G8TZ Introduction of Destructive Agent into Upper GI, Via Natural or Artificial Opening Endoscopic—AHA CC: 1Q, 2013, 27

3E0H3GC Introduction of Other Therapeutic Substance into Lower GI, Percutaneous Approach—AHA CC: 1Q, 2017, 37

3E0L3GC Introduction of Other Therapeutic Substance into Pleural Cavity, Percutaneous Approach—AHA CC: 2Q, 2015, 31 2Q, 2017, 14-15

3E0M30Y Introduction of Hyperthermic Antineoplastic into Peritoneal Cavity, Percutaneous Approach—AHA CC: 4Q, 2019, 37

3E0M3GC Introduction of Other Therapeutic Substance into Peritoneal Cavity, Percutaneous Approach—AHA CC: 4Q, 2014, 38

3E0P7GC Introduction of Other Therapeutic Substance into Female Reproductive, Via Natural or Artificial Opening—AHA CC: 2Q, 2014, 8-9

3E0Q005 Introduction of Other Antineoplastic into Cranial Cavity and Brain, Open Approach—AHA CC: 4Q, 2016, 114

3E0Q305 Introduction of Other Antineoplastic into Cranial Cavity and Brain, Percutaneous Approach—AHA CC: 4Q, 2014, 34-35

3E0R305 Introduction of Other Antineoplastic into Spinal Canal, Percutaneous Approach—AHA CC: 1Q, 2015, 31

3E0U0GB Introduction of Recombinant Bone Morphogenetic Protein into Joints, Open Approach—AHA CC: 1Q, 2018, 8

3E0V0GB Introduction of Recombinant Bone Morphogenetic Protein into Bones, Open Approach—AHA CC: 3Q, 2016, 29-30

Within each section of ICD-10-PCS the characters have different meanings. The seven character meanings for the Measurement and Monitoring section are illustrated here through the procedure example of *External electrocardiogram (EKG), single reading*.

Section	Body System	Root Operation	Body System	Approach	Function / Device	Qualifier
Measurement and Monitoring	Physiological Systems	Measurement	Cardiac	External	Electrical Activity	None
4	A	0	2	X	4	Z

Section (Character 1)

All Measurement and Monitoring procedure codes have a first character value of 4.

Body System (Character 2)

The alphanumeric character for the body system is placed in the second position. There are two character values applicable for the Measurement and Monitoring section. The character value of A is reported for physiological systems. The character value B is reported for physiological devices.

Root Operations (Character 3)

The alphanumeric character value for root operations is placed in the third position. Listed here are the root operations applicable to the Measurement and Monitoring section with their associated meaning.

Character Value	Root Operation	Root Operation Definition
0	Measurement	Determining the level of a physiological or physical function at a point in time
1	Monitoring	Determining the level of a physiological or physical function repetitively over a period of time

Body System/Region (Character 4)

For each body system the applicable body part character values will be available for procedure code construction. An example of a body region for this section is Respiratory.

Approach (Character 5)

The approach is the technique used to reach the procedure site. The following are the approach character values for the Measurement and Monitoring section with the associated definitions.

Character Value	Approach	Approach Definition
0	Open	Cutting through the skin or mucous membrane and any other body layers necessary to expose the site of the procedure
3	Percutaneous	Entry, by puncture or minor incision, of instrumentation through the skin or mucous membrane and any other body layers necessary to reach the site of the procedure
4	Percutaneous Endoscopic	Entry, by puncture or minor incision, of instrumentation through the skin or mucous membrane and any other body layers necessary to reach and visualize the site of the procedure
7	Via Natural or Artificial Opening	Entry of instrumentation through a natural or artificial external opening to reach the site of the procedure
8	Via Natural or Artificial Opening Endoscopic	Entry of instrumentation through a natural or artificial external opening to reach and visualize the site of the procedure
X	External	Procedures performed directly on the skin or mucous membrane and procedures performed indirectly by the application of external force through the skin or mucous membrane

Function/Device (Character 6)

In the Measurement and Monitoring section a function or device is always utilized. The function or device is reported in the sixth character position by the type of function monitored or measured or by the device utilized. The following is a sample list of the functions and devices included in this section:

- Conductivity
- Flow
- Metabolism
- Pressure
- Sound

Qualifier (Character 7)

The qualifier represents an additional attribute for the procedure when applicable. There are several qualifiers included in the Measurement and Monitoring section. For example, measurement procedures in this section include several qualifiers including stress that is reported with the character value of 4. If there is no qualifier for a procedure, the placeholder Z is the character valve that should be reported.

Measurement and Monitoring Section Tables

Measurement and Monitoring Tables 4A0–4B0

Section	4	Measurement and Monitoring
Body System	A	Physiological Systems
Operation	0	Measurement: Determining the level of a physiological or physical function at a point in time

Body System (4ᵗʰ)	Approach (5ᵗʰ)	Function / Device (6ᵗʰ)	Qualifier (7ᵗʰ)
0 Central Nervous	0 Open	2 Conductivity 4 Electrical Activity B Pressure	Z No Qualifier
0 Central Nervous	3 Percutaneous 7 Via Natural or Artificial Opening 8 Via Natural or Artificial Opening Endoscopic	4 Electrical Activity	Z No Qualifier
0 Central Nervous	3 Percutaneous 7 Via Natural or Artificial Opening 8 Via Natural or Artificial Opening Endoscopic	B Pressure K Temperature R Saturation	D Intracranial
0 Central Nervous	X External	2 Conductivity 4 Electrical Activity	Z No Qualifier
1 Peripheral Nervous	0 Open 3 Percutaneous 7 Via Natural or Artificial Opening 8 Via Natural or Artificial Opening Endoscopic X External	2 Conductivity	9 Sensory B Motor
1 Peripheral Nervous	0 Open 3 Percutaneous 7 Via Natural or Artificial Opening 8 Via Natural or Artificial Opening Endoscopic X External	4 Electrical Activity	Z No Qualifier
2 Cardiac	0 Open 3 Percutaneous 7 Via Natural or Artificial Opening 8 Via Natural or Artificial Opening Endoscopic	4 Electrical Activity 9 Output C Rate F Rhythm H Sound P Action Currents	Z No Qualifier
2 Cardiac	0 Open 3 Percutaneous 7 Via Natural or Artificial Opening 8 Via Natural or Artificial Opening Endoscopic	N Sampling and Pressure	6 Right Heart 7 Left Heart 8 Bilateral
2 Cardiac	X External	4 Electrical Activity	A Guidance Z No Qualifier

Continued →

Section	4	Measurement and Monitoring
Body System	A	Physiological Systems
Operation	0	Measurement: Determining the level of a physiological or physical function at a point in time

Body System (4th)	Approach (5th)	Function / Device (6th)	Qualifier (7th)
2 Cardiac	**X** External	**9** Output **C** Rate **F** Rhythm **H** Sound **P** Action Currents	**Z** No Qualifier
2 Cardiac	**X** External	**M** Total Activity	**4** Stress
3 Arterial	**0** Open **3** Percutaneous	**5** Flow **J** Pulse	**1** Peripheral **3** Pulmonary **C** Coronary
3 Arterial	**0** Open **3** Percutaneous	**B** Pressure	**1** Peripheral **3** Pulmonary **C** Coronary **F** Other Thoracic
3 Arterial	**0** Open **3** Percutaneous	**H** Sound **R** Saturation	**1** Peripheral
3 Arterial	**X** External	**5** Flow	**1** Peripheral **D** Intracranial
3 Arterial	**X** External	**B** Pressure **H** Sound **J** Pulse **R** Saturation	**1** Peripheral
4 Venous	**0** Open **3** Percutaneous	**5** Flow **B** Pressure **J** Pulse	**0** Central **1** Peripheral **2** Portal **3** Pulmonary
4 Venous	**0** Open **3** Percutaneous	**R** Saturation	**1** Peripheral
4 Venous	**4** Percutaneous Endoscopic	**B** Pressure	**2** Portal
4 Venous	**X** External	**5** Flow **B** Pressure **J** Pulse **R** Saturation	**1** Peripheral
5 Circulatory	**X** External	**L** Volume	**Z** No Qualifier
6 Lymphatic	**0** Open **3** Percutaneous **7** Via Natural or Artificial Opening **8** Via Natural or Artificial Opening Endoscopic	**5** Flow **B** Pressure	**Z** No Qualifier
7 Visual	**X** External	**0** Acuity **7** Mobility **B** Pressure	**Z** No Qualifier
8 Olfactory	**X** External	**0** Acuity	**Z** No Qualifier
9 Respiratory	**7** Via Natural or Artificial Opening **8** Via Natural or Artificial Opening Endoscopic **X** External	**1** Capacity **5** Flow **C** Rate **D** Resistance **L** Volume **M** Total Activity	**Z** No Qualifier
B Gastrointestinal	**7** Via Natural or Artificial Opening **8** Via Natural or Artificial Opening Endoscopic	**8** Motility **B** Pressure **G** Secretion	**Z** No Qualifier

Continued →

Section | 4 | **Measurement and Monitoring** | | | | | 4A0 Continued
Body System | A | **Physiological Systems**
Operation | 0 | **Measurement:** Determining the level of a physiological or physical function at a point in time

Body System (4th)	Approach (5th)	Function / Device (6th)	Qualifier (7th)
C Biliary	3 Percutaneous 4 Percutaneous Endoscopic 7 Via Natural or Artificial Opening 8 Via Natural or Artificial Opening Endoscopic	5 Flow B Pressure	Z No Qualifier
D Urinary	7 Via Natural or Artificial Opening 8 Via Natural or Artificial Opening Endoscopic	3 Contractility 5 Flow B Pressure D Resistance L Volume	Z No Qualifier
F Musculoskeletal	3 Percutaneous	3 Contractility	Z No Qualifier
F Musculoskeletal	3 Percutaneous	B Pressure	E Compartment
F Musculoskeletal	X External	3 Contractility	Z No Qualifier
H Products of Conception, Cardiac	7 Via Natural or Artificial Opening 8 Via Natural or Artificial Opening Endoscopic X External	4 Electrical Activity C Rate F Rhythm H Sound	Z No Qualifier
J Products of Conception, Nervous	7 Via Natural or Artificial Opening 8 Via Natural or Artificial Opening Endoscopic X External	2 Conductivity 4 Electrical Activity B Pressure	Z No Qualifier
Z None	7 Via Natural or Artificial Opening	6 Metabolism K Temperature	Z No Qualifier
Z None	X External	6 Metabolism K Temperature Q Sleep	Z No Qualifier

Section | 4 | **Measurement and Monitoring**
Body System | A | **Physiological Systems**
Operation | 1 | **Monitoring:** Determining the level of a physiological or physical function repetitively over a period of time

Body System (4th)	Approach (5th)	Function / Device (6th)	Qualifier (7th)
0 Central Nervous	0 Open	2 Conductivity B Pressure	Z No Qualifier
0 Central Nervous	0 Open	4 Electrical Activity	G Intraoperative Z No Qualifier
0 Central Nervous	3 Percutaneous 7 Via Natural or Artificial Opening 8 Via Natural or Artificial Opening Endoscopic	4 Electrical Activity	G Intraoperative Z No Qualifier
0 Central Nervous	3 Percutaneous 7 Via Natural or Artificial Opening 8 Via Natural or Artificial Opening Endoscopic	B Pressure K Temperature R Saturation	D Intracranial
0 Central Nervous	X External	2 Conductivity	Z No Qualifier
0 Central Nervous	X External	4 Electrical Activity	G Intraoperative Z No Qualifier
1 Peripheral Nervous	0 Open 3 Percutaneous 7 Via Natural or Artificial Opening 8 Via Natural or Artificial Opening Endoscopic X External	2 Conductivity	9 Sensory B Motor

Continued →

Section 4 Measurement and Monitoring
Body System A Physiological Systems
Operation 1 Monitoring: Determining the level of a physiological or physical function repetitively over a period of time

4A1 Continued

4A1

Measurement and Monitoring Section Tables

Body System (4th)	Approach (5th)	Function / Device (6th)	Qualifier (7th)
1 Peripheral Nervous	0 Open 3 Percutaneous 7 Via Natural or Artificial Opening 8 Via Natural or Artificial Opening Endoscopic X External	4 Electrical Activity	G Intraoperative Z No Qualifier
2 Cardiac	0 Open 3 Percutaneous 7 Via Natural or Artificial Opening 8 Via Natural or Artificial Opening Endoscopic	4 Electrical Activity 9 Output C Rate F Rhythm H Sound	Z No Qualifier
2 Cardiac	X External	4 Electrical Activity	5 Ambulatory Z No Qualifier
2 Cardiac	X External	9 Output C Rate F Rhythm H Sound	Z No Qualifier
2 Cardiac	X External	M Total Activity	4 Stress
2 Cardiac	X External	S Vascular Perfusion	H Indocyanine Green Dye
3 Arterial	0 Open 3 Percutaneous	5 Flow B Pressure J Pulse	1 Peripheral 3 Pulmonary C Coronary
3 Arterial	0 Open 3 Percutaneous	H Sound R Saturation	1 Peripheral
3 Arterial	X External	5 Flow B Pressure H Sound J Pulse R Saturation	1 Peripheral
4 Venous	0 Open 3 Percutaneous	5 Flow B Pressure J Pulse	0 Central 1 Peripheral 2 Portal 3 Pulmonary
4 Venous	0 Open 3 Percutaneous	R Saturation	0 Central 2 Portal 3 Pulmonary
4 Venous	X External	5 Flow B Pressure J Pulse	1 Peripheral
6 Lymphatic	0 Open 3 Percutaneous 7 Via Natural or Artificial Opening 8 Via Natural or Artificial Opening Endoscopic	5 Flow	H Indocyanine Green Dye Z No Qualifier
6 Lymphatic	0 Open 3 Percutaneous 7 Via Natural or Artificial Opening 8 Via Natural or Artificial Opening Endoscopic	B Pressure	Z No Qualifier
9 Respiratory	7 Via Natural or Artificial Opening X External	1 Capacity 5 Flow C Rate D Resistance L Volume	Z No Qualifier

Continued →

551

Section	**4**	**Measurement and Monitoring**	
Body System	**A**	**Physiological Systems**	
Operation	**1**	**Monitoring:** Determining the level of a physiological or physical function repetitively over a period of time	*4A1 Continued*

Body System (4th)	Approach (5th)	Function / Device (6th)	Qualifier (7th)
B Gastrointestinal	**7** Via Natural or Artificial Opening **8** Via Natural or Artificial Opening Endoscopic	**8** Motility **B** Pressure **G** Secretion	**Z** No Qualifier
B Gastrointestinal	**X** External	**S** Vascular Perfusion	**H** Indocyanine Green Dye
D Urinary	**7** Via Natural or Artificial Opening **8** Via Natural or Artificial Opening Endoscopic	**3** Contractility **5** Flow **B** Pressure **D** Resistance **L** Volume	**Z** No Qualifier
G Skin and Breast	**X** External	**S** Vascular Perfusion	**H** Indocyanine Green Dye
H Products of Conception, Cardiac	**7** Via Natural or Artificial Opening **8** Via Natural or Artificial Opening Endoscopic **X** External	**4** Electrical Activity **C** Rate **F** Rhythm **H** Sound	**Z** No Qualifier
J Products of Conception, Nervous	**7** Via Natural or Artificial Opening **8** Via Natural or Artificial Opening Endoscopic **X** External	**2** Conductivity **4** Electrical Activity **B** Pressure	**Z** No Qualifier
Z None	**7** Via Natural or Artificial Opening	**K** Temperature	**Z** No Qualifier
Z None	**X** External	**K** Temperature **Q** Sleep	**Z** No Qualifier

Section	**4**	**Measurement and Monitoring**
Body System	**B**	**Physiological Devices**
Operation	**0**	**Measurement:** Determining the level of a physiological or physical function at a point in time

Body System (4th)	Approach (5th)	Function / Device (6th)	Qualifier (7th)
0 Central Nervous **1** Peripheral Nervous **F** Musculoskeletal	**X** External	**V** Stimulator	**Z** No Qualifier
2 Cardiac	**X** External	**S** Pacemaker **T** Defibrillator	**Z** No Qualifier
9 Respiratory	**X** External	**S** Pacemaker	**Z** No Qualifier

AHA Coding Clinic

4A023N6 Measurement of Cardiac Sampling and Pressure, Right Heart, Percutaneous Approach—AHA CC: 3Q, 2019, 32

4A023N8 Measurement of Cardiac Sampling and Pressure, Bilateral, Percutaneous Approach—AHA CC: 1Q, 2018, 12-13

4A02X4Z Measurement of Cardiac Electrical Activity, External Approach—AHA CC: 3Q, 2015, 29

4A033BC Measurement of Arterial Pressure, Coronary, Percutaneous Approach—AHA CC: 3Q, 2016, 37

4A103BD Monitoring of Intracranial Pressure, Percutaneous Approach—AHA CC: 2Q, 2016, 29

4A1134G Monitoring of Peripheral Nervous Electrical Activity, Intraoperative, Percutaneous Approach—AHA CC: 4Q, 2014, 28-29

4A11X4G Monitoring of Peripheral Nervous Electrical Activity, Intraoperative, External Approach—AHA CC: 1Q, 2015, 26; 2Q, 2015, 14

4A1239Z Monitoring of Cardiac Output, Percutaneous Approach—AHA CC: 3Q, 2015, 35

4A133B1 Monitoring of Arterial Pressure, Peripheral, Percutaneous Approach, for Continuous Monitoring of Pressure—AHA CC: 2Q, 2016, 33

4A133B3 Monitoring of Arterial Pressure, Pulmonary, Percutaneous Approach—AHA CC: 3Q, 2015, 35

4A133J1 Monitoring of Arterial Pulse, Peripheral, Percutaneous Approach, for Continuous Monitoring of Pulse—AHA CC: 2Q, 2016, 33

Within each section of ICD-10-PCS the characters have different meanings. The seven character meanings for the Extracorporeal or Systemic Assistance and Performance section are illustrated here through the procedure example of *Hyperbaric oxygenation of wound*.

Section	Body System	Root Operation	Body System	Duration	Function	Qualifier
Extracorporeal or Systemic Assistance and Performance	Physiological Systems	Assistance	Circulatory	Intermittent	Oxygenation	Hyperbaric
5	A	0	5	1	2	1

Section (Character 1)

All Extracorporeal or Systemic Assistance and Performance procedure codes have a first character value of 5.

Body System (Character 2)

The alphanumeric character for the body system is placed in the second position. There is one character value applicable for the Extracorporeal or Systemic Assistance and Performance section. The character value of A is reported for physiological systems.

Root Operations (Character 3)

The alphanumeric character value for root operations is placed in the third position. Listed here are the root operations applicable to the Extracorporeal or Systemic Assistance and Performance section with their associated meaning.

Character Value	Root Operation	Root Operation Definition
0	Assistance	Taking over a portion of a physiological function by extracorporeal means
1	Performance	Completely taking over a physiological function by extracorporeal means
2	Restoration	Returning, or attempting to return, a physiological function to its original state by extracorporeal means

Body System (Character 4)

For each body system, the applicable body part character values will be available for procedure code construction. An example of a body region for this section is respiratory.

Duration (Character 5)

The duration represents the length of time or frequency for which the assistance or performance is utilized. Some examples of duration are Intermittent, Continuous, or Less than 24 consecutive hours.

Function (Character 6)

In the Extracorporeal or Systemic Assistance and Performance section a function is always reported. The function is reported in the sixth character position. The following is a sample list of the functions utilized in this section:

- Output
- Oxygenation
- Pacing
- Ventilation

Qualifier (Character 7)

The qualifier represents an additional attribute for the procedure when applicable. There are several qualifiers included in the Extracorporeal or Systemic Assistance and Performance section. For example, assistance procedures in this section include several qualifiers including Balloon Pump, which is reported with the character value of 0. If there is no qualifier for a procedure, the placeholder Z is the character valve that should be reported.

Extracorporeal or Systemic Assistance and Performance Section Tables

Extracorporeal or Systemic Assistance and Performance Tables 5A0–5A2

Section	5	Extracorporeal or Systemic Assistance and Performance
Body System	A	Physiological Systems
Operation	0	**Assistance:** Taking over a portion of a physiological function by extracorporeal means

Body System (4th)	Duration (5th)	Function (6th)	Qualifier (7th)
2 Cardiac	1 Intermittent 2 Continuous	1 Output	0 Balloon Pump 5 Pulsatile Compression 6 Other Pump D Impeller Pump
5 Circulatory	1 Intermittent 2 Continuous	2 Oxygenation	1 Hyperbaric C Supersaturated
9 Respiratory	2 Continuous	0 Filtration	Z No Qualifier
9 Respiratory	3 Less than 24 Consecutive Hours 4 24-96 Consecutive Hours 5 Greater than 96 Consecutive Hours	5 Ventilation	7 Continuous Positive Airway Pressure 8 Intermittent Positive Airway Pressure 9 Continuous Negative Airway Pressure A High Nasal Flow/Velocity B Intermittent Negative Airway Pressure Z No Qualifier

Section	5	Extracorporeal or Systemic Assistance and Performance
Body System	A	Physiological Systems
Operation	1	**Performance:** Completely taking over a physiological function by extracorporeal means

Body System (4th)	Duration (5th)	Function (6th)	Qualifier (7th)
2 Cardiac	0 Single	1 Output	2 Manual
2 Cardiac	1 Intermittent	3 Pacing	Z No Qualifier
2 Cardiac	2 Continuous	1 Output 3 Pacing	Z No Qualifier
5 Circulatory	2 Continuous A Intraoperative	2 Oxygenation	F Membrane, Central G Membrane, Peripheral Veno-arterial H Membrane, Peripheral Veno-venous
9 Respiratory	0 Single	5 Ventilation	4 Nonmechanical
9 Respiratory	3 Less than 24 Consecutive Hours 4 24-96 Consecutive Hours 5 Greater than 96 Consecutive Hours	5 Ventilation	Z No Qualifier
C Biliary	0 Single 6 Multiple	0 Filtration	Z No Qualifier
D Urinary	7 Intermittent, Less than 6 Hours Per Day 8 Prolonged Intermittent, 6-18 Hours Per Day 9 Continuous, Greater than 18 Hours Per Day	0 Filtration	Z No Qualifier

Section	5	Extracorporeal or Systemic Assistance and Performance
Body System	A	Physiological Systems
Operation	2	**Restoration:** Returning, or attempting to return, a physiological function to its original state by extracorporeal means.

Body System (4th)	Duration (5th)	Function (6th)	Qualifier (7th)
2 Cardiac	0 Single	4 Rhythm	Z No Qualifier

5A02210 Assistance with Cardiac Output using Balloon Pump, Continuous—AHA CC: 3Q, 2013, 18-19; 2Q, 2018, 4-5

5A0221D Assistance with Cardiac Output using Impeller Pump, Continuous—AHA CC: 3Q, 2014, 19; 4Q, 2016, 138-139; 1Q, 2017, 11-12; 4Q, 2017, 43-45

5A09357 Assistance with Respiratory Ventilation, <24 Hrs, CPAP—AHA CC: 4Q, 2014, 9-10; 1Q, 2020, 10-11

5A09457 Assistance with Respiratory Ventilation, 24-96 Hrs, CPAP—AHA CC: 4Q, 2014, 9-10

5A09557 Assistance with Respiratory Ventilation, >96 Hrs, CPAP—AHA CC: 4Q, 2014, 9-10

5A1221Z Performance of Cardiac Output, Continuous—AHA CC: 3Q, 2013, 18-19; 1Q, 2014, 10-11; 3Q, 2014, 16-17, 20-21; 4Q, 2015, 22-25; 1Q, 2016, 27-28; 1Q, 2017, 19-20; 3Q, 2017, 7-8

ECMO, Extracorporeal Oxygenation, Membrane—AHA CC: 3Q, 2019, 19-23; 4Q, 2019, 39-41

5A1223Z Performance of Cardiac Pacing, Continuous—AHA CC: 3Q, 2013, 18-19

5A1522F Extracorporeal Oxygenation, Membrane, Central—AHA CC: 2Q, 2019, 36

5A1522G Extracorporeal Oxygenation, Membrane, Peripheral Veno-arterial—AHA CC: 4Q, 2018, 53-54

5A1522H Extracorporeal Oxygenation, Membrane, Peripheral Veno-venous—AHA CC: 4Q, 2018. 53-54

5A15A2G Extracorporeal Oxygenation, Membrane, Peripheral Veno-arterial, Intraoperative—AHA CC: 4Q, 2019, 39-40

5A1935Z Respiratory Ventilation, Less than 24 Consecutive Hours—AHA CC: 4Q, 2014, 3-15; 1Q, 2018, 13-14

5A1945Z Respiratory Ventilation, 24-96 Consecutive Hours—AHA CC: 4Q, 2014, 3-15

5A1955Z Respiratory Ventilation, Greater than 96 Consecutive Hours—AHA CC: 4Q, 2014, 3-15

5A1C00Z Performance of Biliary Filtration, Single—AHA CC: 1Q, 2016, 28-29

5A1D60Z Performance of Urinary Filtration, Multiple—AHA CC: 1Q, 2016, 29

5A1D70Z Performance of Urinary Filtration, Intermittent, Less than 6 Hours Per Day—AHA CC: 4Q, 2017, 72-73

5A1D80Z Performance of Urinary Filtration, Prolonged Intermittent, 6-18 hours Per Day—AHA CC: 4Q, 2017, 72

5A1D90Z Performance of Urinary Filtration, Continuous, Greater than 18 hours Per Day—AHA CC: 4Q, 2017, 72-73

Within each section of ICD-10-PCS the characters have different meanings. The seven character meanings for the Extracorporeal or Systemic Therapies section are illustrated here through the procedure example of *Ultraviolet light phototherapy, series treatment.*

Section	Body System	Root Operation	Body System	Duration	Qualifier	Qualifier
Extracorporeal or Systemic Therapies	Physiological Systems	UV Light Therapy	Skin	Multiple	None	None
6	A	8	0	1	Z	Z

Section (Character 1)

All Extracorporeal or Systemic Therapies procedure codes have a first character value of 6.

Body System (Character 2)

The alphanumeric character for the body system is placed in the second position. There is one character value applicable for the Extracorporeal or Systemic Therapies section. The character value of A is reported for physiological systems.

Root Operations (Character 3)

The alphanumeric character value for root operations is placed in the third position. Listed below are the root operations applicable to the Extracorporeal or Systemic Therapies section with their associated meaning.

Character Value	Root Operation	Root Operation Definition
0	Atmospheric Control	Extracorporeal control of atmospheric pressure and composition
1	Decompression	Extracorporeal elimination of undissolved gas from body fluids
2	Electromagnetic Therapy	Extracorporeal treatment by electromagnetic rays
3	Hyperthermia	Extracorporeal raising of body temperature
4	Hypothermia	Extracorporeal lowering of body temperature
5	Pheresis	Extracorporeal separation of blood products
6	Phototherapy	Extracorporeal treatment by light rays
7	Ultrasound Therapy	Extracorporeal treatment by ultrasound
8	Ultraviolet Light Therapy	Extracorporeal treatment by ultraviolet light
9	Shock Wave Therapy	Extracorporeal treatment by shock waves
B	Perfusion	Extracorporeal treatment by diffusion of therapeutic fluid

Body System (Character 4)

For each body system the applicable body part character values will be available for procedure code construction. An example of a body region for this section is Skin.

Duration (Character 5)

The duration represents the number of therapy sessions performed. Single is reported with character value 0; Multiple is reported with character value 1.

Qualifier (Character 6)

Character 6 is the first of two qualifier characters for the Extracorporeal or Systemic Therapies section. The qualifier represents an additional attribute for the procedure when applicable. There are currently no qualifier values for the sixth character position, so the character value of Z is always reported.

Qualifier (Character 7)

Character 7 is the second of two qualifier characters for the Extracorporeal or Systemic Therapies section. The qualifier represents an additional attribute for the procedure when applicable. There are some qualifiers included in the Extracorporeal or Systemic Therapies section. For example, pheresis procedures in this section include several qualifiers including Plasma that is reported with the character value of 3. If there is no qualifier for a procedure, the placeholder Z is the character valve that should be reported.

Extracorporeal or Systemic Therapies Tables 6A0–6AB

Section	6	**Extracorporeal or Systemic Therapies**
Body System	A	**Physiological Systems**
Operation	0	**Atmospheric Control:** Extracorporeal control of atmospheric pressure and composition

Body System (4th)	Duration (5th)	Qualifier (6th)	Qualifier (7th)
Z None	0 Single 1 Multiple	Z No Qualifier	Z No Qualifier

Section	6	**Extracorporeal or Systemic Therapies**
Body System	A	**Physiological Systems**
Operation	1	**Decompression:** Extracorporeal elimination of undissolved gas from body fluids

Body System (4th)	Duration (5th)	Qualifier (6th)	Qualifier (7th)
5 Circulatory	0 Single 1 Multiple	Z No Qualifier	Z No Qualifier

Section	6	**Extracorporeal or Systemic Therapies**
Body System	A	**Physiological Systems**
Operation	2	**Electromagnetic Therapy:** Extracorporeal treatment by electromagnetic rays

Body System (4th)	Duration (5th)	Qualifier (6th)	Qualifier (7th)
1 Urinary 2 Central Nervous	0 Single 1 Multiple	Z No Qualifier	Z No Qualifier

Section	6	**Extracorporeal or Systemic Therapies**
Body System	A	**Physiological Systems**
Operation	3	**Hyperthermia:** Extracorporeal raising of body temperature

Body System (4th)	Duration (5th)	Qualifier (6th)	Qualifier (7th)
Z None	0 Single 1 Multiple	Z No Qualifier	Z No Qualifier

Section	6	**Extracorporeal or Systemic Therapies**
Body System	A	**Physiological Systems**
Operation	4	**Hypothermia:** Extracorporeal lowering of body temperature

Body System (4th)	Duration (5th)	Qualifier (6th)	Qualifier (7th)
Z None	0 Single 1 Multiple	Z No Qualifier	Z No Qualifier

Section	6	**Extracorporeal or Systemic Therapies**
Body System	A	**Physiological Systems**
Operation	5	**Pheresis:** Extracorporeal separation of blood products

Body System (4th)	Duration (5th)	Qualifier (6th)	Qualifier (7th)
5 Circulatory	0 Single 1 Multiple	Z No Qualifier	0 Erythrocytes 1 Leukocytes 2 Platelets 3 Plasma T Stem Cells, Cord Blood V Stem Cells, Hematopoietic

Section	6	Extracorporeal or Systemic Therapies
Body System	A	Physiological Systems
Operation	6	**Phototherapy:** Extracorporeal treatment by light rays

Body System (4th)	Duration (5th)	Qualifier (6th)	Qualifier (7th)
0 Skin **5** Circulatory	**0** Single **1** Multiple	**Z** No Qualifier	**Z** No Qualifier

Section	6	Extracorporeal or Systemic Therapies
Body System	A	Physiological Systems
Operation	7	**Ultrasound Therapy:** Extracorporeal treatment by ultrasound

Body System (4th)	Duration (5th)	Qualifier (6th)	Qualifier (7th)
5 Circulatory	**0** Single **1** Multiple	**Z** No Qualifier	**4** Head and Neck Vessels **5** Heart **6** Peripheral Vessels **7** Other Vessels **Z** No Qualifier

Section	6	Extracorporeal or Systemic Therapies
Body System	A	Physiological Systems
Operation	8	**Ultraviolet Light Therapy:** Extracorporeal treatment by ultraviolet light

Body System (4th)	Duration (5th)	Qualifier (6th)	Qualifier (7th)
0 Skin	**0** Single **1** Multiple	**Z** No Qualifier	**Z** No Qualifier

Section	6	Extracorporeal or Systemic Therapies
Body System	A	Physiological Systems
Operation	9	**Shock Wave Therapy:** Extracorporeal treatment by shock waves

Body System (4th)	Duration (5th)	Qualifier (6th)	Qualifier (7th)
3 Musculoskeletal	**0** Single **1** Multiple	**Z** No Qualifier	**Z** No Qualifier

Section	6	Extracorporeal or Systemic Therapies
Body System	A	Physiological Systems
Operation	B	**Perfusion:** Extracorporeal treatment by diffusion of therapeutic fluid

Body System (4th)	Duration (5th)	Qualifier (6th)	Qualifier (7th)
5 Circulatory **B** Respiratory System **F** Hepatobiliary System and Pancreas **T** Urinary System	**0** Single	**B** Donor Organ	**Z** No Qualifier

AHA Coding Clinic

6A4Z0ZZ Hypothermia, Single—AHA CC: 2Q, 2019, 17-18

6A750Z7 Ultrasound Therapy of Other Vessels, Single—AHA CC: 4Q, 2014, 19-20

Within each section of ICD-10-PCS, the characters have different meanings. The seven character meanings for the Osteopathic section are illustrated below through the procedure example of Indirect osteopathic treatment of sacrum.

Section	Body System	Root Operation	Body Region	Approach	Method	Qualifier
Osteopathic	Anatomical Regions	Treatment	Sacrum	External	Indirect	None
7	W	0	4	X	4	Z

Section (Character 1)

All Osteopathic procedure codes have a first character value of 7.

Body System (Character 2)

The alphanumeric character for the body system is placed in the second position. There is one character value applicable for the Osteopathic section. The character value of W is reported for anatomical regions.

Root Operations (Character 3)

The alphanumeric character value for root operations is placed in the third position. Listed here is the root operation applicable to the Osteopathic section with its associated meaning.

Character Value	Root Operation	Root Operation Definition
0	Treatment	Manual treatment to eliminate or alleviate somatic dysfunction and related disorders

Body Region (Character 4)

For each body region the applicable body part character values will be available for procedure code construction. An example of a body region for this section is Head.

Approach (Character 5)

The approach is the technique used to reach the procedure site. The following are the approach character values for the Osteopathic section with the associated definitions.

Character Value	Approach	Approach Definition
X	External	Procedures performed directly on the skin or mucous membrane and procedures performed indirectly by the application of external force through the skin or mucous membrane

Method (Character 6)

The method identifies the treatment method used to complete the osteopathic procedure. The available methods are:

- Articulatory-Raising
- Fascial Release
- General Mobilization
- High Velocity-Low Amplitude
- Indirect
- Low Velocity-High Amplitude
- Lymphatic Pump
- Muscle Energy-Isometric
- Muscle Energy-Isotonic
- Other

Qualifier (Character 7)

The qualifier represents an additional attribute for the procedure when applicable. Currently, there are no qualifiers in the Osteopathic section; therefore, the placeholder character value of Z should be reported.

Osteopathic Section Table

Osteopathic Table 7W0

Section	7	Osteopathic
Body System	W	Anatomical Regions
Operation	0	**Treatment:** Manual treatment to eliminate or alleviate somatic dysfunction and related disorders

Body Region (4th)	Approach (5th)	Method (6th)	Qualifier (7th)
0 Head	X External	0 Articulatory-Raising	Z None
1 Cervical		1 Fascial Release	
2 Thoracic		2 General Mobilization	
3 Lumbar		3 High Velocity-Low Amplitude	
4 Sacrum		4 Indirect	
5 Pelvis		5 Low Velocity-High Amplitude	
6 Lower Extremities		6 Lymphatic Pump	
7 Upper Extremities		7 Muscle Energy-Isometric	
8 Rib Cage		8 Muscle Energy-Isotonic	
9 Abdomen		9 Other Method	

AHA Coding Clinic

No references have been issued for the Osteopathic Section.

Within each section of ICD-10-PCS the characters have different meanings. The seven character meanings for the Other Procedures section are illustrated here through the procedure example of Yoga therapy.

Section	Body System	Root Operation	Body Region	Approach	Method	Qualifier
Other Procedures	Physiological Systems and Anatomical Regions	Other Procedures	None	External	Other Method	Yoga Therapy
8	E	0	Z	X	Y	4

Section (Character 1)

All Other Procedures codes have a first character value of 8.

Body System (Character 2)

The alphanumeric character for the body system is placed in the second position. There are two character values applicable for the Other Procedures section. The character value of C is reported for indwelling device. The character value of E is reported for physiological system and anatomical regions.

Root Operations (Character 3)

The alphanumeric character value for root operations is placed in the third position. Listed here is the root operation applicable to the Other Procedures section with its associated meaning.

Character Value	Root Operation	Root Operation Definition
0	Other Procedures	Methodologies which attempt to remediate or cure a disorder or disease

Body Region (Character 4)

For each body region the applicable body part character values will be available for procedure code construction. An example of a body region for this section is Lower Extremity.

Approach (Character 5)

The approach is the technique used to reach the procedure site. The following are the approach character values for the Other Procedures section with the associated definitions.

Character Value	Approach	Approach Definition
0	Open	Cutting through the skin or mucous membrane and any other body layers necessary to expose the site of the procedure
3	Percutaneous	Entry, by puncture or minor incision, of instrumentation through the skin or mucous membrane and any other body layers necessary to reach the site of the procedure
4	Percutaneous Endoscopic	Entry, by puncture or minor incision, of instrumentation through the skin or mucous membrane and any other body layers necessary to reach and visualize the site of the procedure
7	Via Natural or Artificial Opening	Entry of instrumentation through a natural or artificial external opening to reach the site of the procedure
8	Via Natural or Artificial Opening Endoscopic	Entry of instrumentation through a natural or artificial external opening to reach and visualize the site of the procedure
X	External	Procedures performed directly on the skin or mucous membrane and procedures performed indirectly by the application of external force through the skin or mucous membrane

Method (Character 6)

The method identifies the treatment method used to complete the other procedure. The available methods are:

- Acupuncture
- Collection
- Computer Assisted Procedure
- Near Infrared Spectroscopy
- Robotic Assisted procedure
- Therapeutic Massage
- Other

Qualifier (Character 7)

The qualifier represents an additional attribute for the procedure when applicable. In the preceding example of Yoga therapy, the qualifier of 4 was used to report that the other procedure was Yoga therapy. If there is no qualifier for a procedure, the placeholder Z is the character valve that should be reported.

Other Procedures Section Tables

Other Procedures Tables 8C0–8E0

Section	8	Other Procedures
Body System	C	Indwelling Device
Operation	0	Other Procedures: Methodologies which attempt to remediate or cure a disorder or disease

Body Region (4th)	Approach (5th)	Method (6th)	Qualifier (7th)
1 Nervous System	X External	6 Collection	J Cerebrospinal Fluid L Other Fluid
2 Circulatory System	X External	6 Collection	K Blood L Other Fluid

Section	8	Other Procedures
Body System	E	Physiological Systems and Anatomical Regions
Operation	0	Other Procedures: Methodologies which attempt to remediate or cure a disorder or disease

Body Region (4th)	Approach (5th)	Method (6th)	Qualifier (7th)
1 Nervous System U Female Reproductive System	X External	Y Other Method	7 Examination
2 Circulatory System	3 Percutaneous X External	D Near Infrared Spectroscopy	Z No Qualifier
9 Head and Neck Region	0 Open	C Robotic Assisted Procedure	Z No Qualifier
9 Head and Neck Region	0 Open	E Fluorescence Guided Procedure	M Aminolevulinic Acid Z No Qualifier
9 Head and Neck Region	3 Percutaneous 4 Percutaneous Endoscopic 7 Via Natural or Artificial Opening 8 Via Natural or Artificial Opening Endoscopic	C Robotic Assisted Procedure E Fluorescence Guided Procedure	Z No Qualifier
9 Head and Neck Region	X External	B Computer Assisted Procedure	F With Fluoroscopy G With Computerized Tomography H With Magnetic Resonance Imaging Z No Qualifier
9 Head and Neck Region	X External	C Robotic Assisted Procedure	Z No Qualifier
9 Head and Neck Region	X External	Y Other Method	8 Suture Removal

Continued →

Section	8	Other Procedures					8E0 Continued
Body System	E	Physiological Systems and Anatomical Regions					
Operation	0	Other Procedures: Methodologies which attempt to remediate or cure a disorder or disease					

Body Region (4th)	Approach (5th)	Method (6th)	Qualifier (7th)
H Integumentary System and Breast	**3** Percutaneous	**0** Acupuncture	**0** Anesthesia **Z** No Qualifier
H Integumentary System and Breast	**X** External	**6** Collection	**2** Breast Milk
H Integumentary System and Breast	**X** External	**Y** Other Method	**9** Piercing
K Musculoskeletal System	**X** External	**1** Therapeutic Massage	**Z** No Qualifier
K Musculoskeletal System	**X** External	**Y** Other Method	**7** Examination
V Male Reproductive System	**X** External	**1** Therapeutic Massage	**C** Prostate **D** Rectum
V Male Reproductive System	**X** External	**6** Collection	**3** Sperm
W Trunk Region	**0** Open **3** Percutaneous **4** Percutaneous Endoscopic **7** Via Natural or Artificial Opening **8** Via Natural or Artificial Opening Endoscopic	**C** Robotic Assisted Procedure **E** Fluorescence Guided Procedure	**Z** No Qualifier
W Trunk Region	**X** External	**B** Computer Assisted Procedure	**F** With Fluoroscopy **G** With Computerized Tomography **H** With Magnetic Resonance Imaging **Z** No Qualifier
W Trunk Region	**X** External	**C** Robotic Assisted Procedure	**Z** No Qualifier
W Trunk Region	**X** External	**Y** Other Method	**8** Suture Removal
X Upper Extremity **Y** Lower Extremity	**0** Open **3** Percutaneous **4** Percutaneous Endoscopic	**C** Robotic Assisted Procedure **E** Fluorescence Guided Procedure	**Z** No Qualifier
X Upper Extremity **Y** Lower Extremity	**X** External	**B** Computer Assisted Procedure	**F** With Fluoroscopy **G** With Computerized Tomography **H** With Magnetic Resonance Imaging **Z** No Qualifier
X Upper Extremity **Y** Lower Extremity	**X** External	**C** Robotic Assisted Procedure	**Z** No Qualifier
X Upper Extremity **Y** Lower Extremity	**X** External	**Y** Other Method	**8** Suture Removal
Z None	**X** External	**Y** Other Method	**1** In Vitro Fertilization **4** Yoga Therapy **5** Meditation **6** Isolation

AHA Coding Clinic

8E0W4CZ Robotic Assisted Procedure of Trunk Region, Percutaneous Endoscopic Approach—AHA CC: 4Q, 2014, 33-34; 1Q, 2015, 33-34; 1Q, 2019, 30-31

Chiropractic Section (9WB)

Within each section of ICD-10-PCS the characters have different meanings. The seven character meanings for the Chiropractic section are illustrated here through the procedure example of Chiropractic treatment of cervical spine, short lever specific contact.

Section	Body System	Root Operation	Body Region	Approach	Method	Qualifier
Chiropractic	Anatomical Regions	Manipulation	Cervical	External	Short Lever Specific Contact	None
9	W	B	1	X	H	Z

Section (Character 1)

All Chiropractic procedure codes have a first character value of 9.

Body System (Character 2)

The alphanumeric character for the body system is placed in the second position. There is one character value applicable for the Chiropractic section. The character value of W is reported for anatomical regions.

Root Operations (Character 3)

The alphanumeric character value for root operations is placed in the third position. The following is the root operation applicable to the Chiropractic section with its associated meaning.

Character Value	Root Operation	Root Operation Definition
B	Manipulation	Manual procedure that involves a directed thrust to move a joint past the physiological range of motion, without exceeding the anatomical limit

Body Region (Character 4)

For each body region the applicable body part character values will be available for procedure code construction. An example of a body region for this section is Rib Cage.

Approach (Character 5)

The approach is the technique used to reach the procedure site. The following are the approach character values for the Chiropractic section with the associated definitions.

Character Value	Approach	Approach Definition
X	External	Procedures performed directly on the skin or mucous membrane and procedures performed indirectly by the application of external force through the skin or mucous membrane

Method (Character 6)

The method identifies the treatment method used to complete the chiropractic procedure. The available methods are:

- Non-Manual
- Indirect Visceral
- Extra-Articular
- Direct-Visual
- Long Lever Specific Contact
- Short Lever Specific Contact
- Long and Short Lever Specific Contact
- Mechanically Assisted
- Other

Qualifier (Character 7)

The qualifier represents an additional attribute for the procedure when applicable. Currently, there are no qualifiers in the Chiropractic section; therefore, the placeholder character value of Z should be reported.

Chiropractic Section Table

Chiropractic Table 9WB

Section	9	Chiropractic
Body System	W	Anatomical Regions
Operation	B	**Manipulation:** Manual procedure that involves a directed thrust to move a joint past the physiological range of motion, without exceeding the anatomical limit

Body Region (4th)	Approach (5th)	Method (6th)	Qualifier (7th)
0 Head 1 Cervical 2 Thoracic 3 Lumbar 4 Sacrum 5 Pelvis 6 Lower Extremities 7 Upper Extremities 8 Rib Cage 9 Abdomen	X External	B Non-Manual C Indirect Visceral D Extra-Articular F Direct Visceral G Long Lever Specific Contact H Short Lever Specific Contact J Long and Short Lever Specific Contact K Mechanically Assisted L Other Method	Z None

AHA Coding Clinic

No references have been issued for the Chiropractic Section.

Imaging Section (B00–BY4)

Within each section of ICD-10-PCS the characters have different meanings. The seven character meanings for the Imaging section are illustrated here through the procedure example of X-ray right clavicle, limited study.

Section	Body System	Root Type	Body Part	Contrast	Qualifier	Qualifier
Imaging	Non-Axial Upper Bones	Plain Radiography	Clavicle, right	None	None	None
B	P	0	4	Z	Z	Z

Section (Character 1)

All Imaging procedure codes have a first character value of B.

Body System (Character 2)

The alphanumeric character for the body system is placed in the second position. The following are the body systems applicable to the Imaging section.

Character Value	Character Value Description
0	Central Nervous System
2	Heart
3	Upper Arteries
4	Lower Arteries
5	Veins
7	Lymphatic System
8	Eye
9	Ear, Nose, Mouth and Throat
B	Respiratory System
D	Gastrointestinal System
F	Hepatobiliary System and Pancreas
G	Endocrine System
H	Skin, Subcutaneous Tissue and Breast
L	Connective Tissue
N	Skull and Facial Bones
P	Non-Axial Upper Bones
Q	Non-Axial Lower Bones
R	Axial Skeleton, Except Skull and Facial Bones
T	Urinary System
U	Female Reproductive System
V	Male Reproductive System
W	Anatomical Regions
Y	Fetus and Obstetrical

Root Types (Character 3)

The alphanumeric character value for root types is placed in the third position. Listed here are the root types applicable to the Imaging section with their associated meaning.

Character Value	Root Type	Root Type Definition
0	Plain Radiography	Planar display of an image developed from the capture of external ionizing radiation on photographic or photoconductive plate
1	Fluoroscopy	Single plane or bi-plane real time display of an image developed from the capture of external ionizing radiation on a fluorescent screen. The image may also be stored by either digital or analog means

Continued →

Character Value	Root Type	Root Type Definition
2	Computerized Tomography (CT Scan)	Computer reformatted digital display of multiplanar images developed from the capture of multiple exposures of external ionizing radiation
3	Magnetic Resonance Imaging (MRI)	Computer reformatted digital display of multiplanar images developed from the capture of radiofrequency signals emitted by nuclei in a body site excited within a magnetic field
4	Ultrasonography	Real time display of images of anatomy or flow information developed from the capture of reflected and attenuated high frequency sound waves
5	Other Imaging	Other specified modality for visualizing a body part

Body Part (Character 4)

For each body part the applicable body part character values will be available for procedure code construction. An example of a body part for this section is Spinal Cord.

Contrast (Character 5)

When contrast is utilized during an imaging procedure, the corresponding contrast character value should be reported in the fifth character position. The following are the contrast character values for the Imaging section:

- High Osmolar
- Low Osmolar
- Other Contrast

If contrast is not utilized, the placeholder character value of Z should be reported.

Qualifier (Character 6)

This qualifier character specifies when an image taken without contrast is followed by one with contrast. The character value of 0 is reported for Unenhanced and Enhanced.

Qualifier (Character 7)

The qualifier represents an additional attribute for the procedure when applicable. For example, ultrasonography procedures in this section include the qualifier Densitometry that is reported with the character value of 1 for some body parts. If there is no qualifier for a procedure, the placeholder Z is the character valve that should be reported.

Imaging Section Tables

Imaging Tables B00–BY4

Section	B	Imaging
Body System	0	Central Nervous System
Type	0	**Plain Radiography:** Planar display of an image developed from the capture of external ionizing radiation on photographic or photoconductive plate

Body Part (4th)	Contrast (5th)	Qualifier (6th)	Qualifier (7th)
B Spinal Cord	0 High Osmolar 1 Low Osmolar Y Other Contrast Z None	Z None	Z None

Section	B	Imaging
Body System	0	Central Nervous System
Type	1	**Fluoroscopy:** Single plane or bi-plane real time display of an image developed from the capture of external ionizing radiation on a fluorescent screen. The image may also be stored by either digital or analog means

Body Part (4th)	Contrast (5th)	Qualifier (6th)	Qualifier (7th)
B Spinal Cord	0 High Osmolar 1 Low Osmolar Y Other Contrast Z None	Z None	Z None

Section	B	Imaging
Body System	0	Central Nervous System
Type	2	Computerized Tomography (CT Scan): Computer reformatted digital display of multiplanar images developed from the capture of multiple exposures of external ionizing radiation

Body Part (4th)	Contrast (5th)	Qualifier (6th)	Qualifier (7th)
0 Brain 7 Cisterna 8 Cerebral Ventricle(s) 9 Sella Turcica/Pituitary Gland B Spinal Cord	0 High Osmolar 1 Low Osmolar Y Other Contrast	0 Unenhanced and Enhanced Z None	Z None
0 Brain 7 Cisterna 8 Cerebral Ventricle(s) 9 Sella Turcica/Pituitary Gland B Spinal Cord	Z None	Z None	Z None

Section	B	Imaging
Body System	0	Central Nervous System
Type	3	Magnetic Resonance Imaging (MRI): Computer reformatted digital display of multiplanar images developed from the capture of radiofrequency signals emitted by nuclei in a body site excited within a magnetic field

Body Part (4th)	Contrast (5th)	Qualifier (6th)	Qualifier (7th)
0 Brain 9 Sella Turcica/Pituitary Gland B Spinal Cord C Acoustic Nerves	Y Other Contrast	0 Unenhanced and Enhanced Z None	Z None
0 Brain 9 Sella Turcica/Pituitary Gland B Spinal Cord C Acoustic Nerves	Z None	Z None	Z None

Section	B	Imaging
Body System	0	Central Nervous System
Type	4	Ultrasonography: Real time display of images of anatomy or flow information developed from the capture of reflected and attenuated high frequency sound waves

Body Part (4th)	Contrast (5th)	Qualifier (6th)	Qualifier (7th)
0 Brain B Spinal Cord	Z None	Z None	Z None

Section	B	Imaging
Body System	2	Heart
Type	0	Plain Radiography: Planar display of an image developed from the capture of external ionizing radiation on photographic or photoconductive plate

Body Part (4th)	Contrast (5th)	Qualifier (6th)	Qualifier (7th)
0 Coronary Artery, Single 1 Coronary Arteries, Multiple 2 Coronary Artery Bypass Graft, Single 3 Coronary Artery Bypass Grafts, Multiple 4 Heart, Right 5 Heart, Left 6 Heart, Right and Left 7 Internal Mammary Bypass Graft, Right 8 Internal Mammary Bypass Graft, Left F Bypass Graft, Other	0 High Osmolar 1 Low Osmolar Y Other Contrast	Z None	Z None

Section   **B**   **Imaging**
Body System   **2**   **Heart**
Type   **1**   **Fluoroscopy:** Single plane or bi-plane real time display of an image developed from the capture of external ionizing radiation on a fluorescent screen. The image may also be stored by either digital or analog means

Body Part (4th)	Contrast (5th)	Qualifier (6th)	Qualifier (7th)
0 Coronary Artery, Single 1 Coronary Arteries, Multiple 2 Coronary Artery Bypass Graft, Single 3 Coronary Artery Bypass Grafts, Multiple	0 High Osmolar 1 Low Osmolar Y Other Contrast	1 Laser	0 Intraoperative
0 Coronary Artery, Single 1 Coronary Arteries, Multiple 2 Coronary Artery Bypass Graft, Single 3 Coronary Artery Bypass Grafts, Multiple	0 High Osmolar 1 Low Osmolar Y Other Contrast	Z None	Z None
4 Heart, Right 5 Heart, Left 6 Heart, Right and Left 7 Internal Mammary Bypass Graft, Right 8 Internal Mammary Bypass Graft, Left F Bypass Graft, Other	0 High Osmolar 1 Low Osmolar Y Other Contrast	Z None	Z None

Section   **B**   **Imaging**
Body System   **2**   **Heart**
Type   **2**   **Computerized Tomography (CT Scan):** Computer reformatted digital display of multiplanar images developed from the capture of multiple exposures of external ionizing radiation

Body Part (4th)	Contrast (5th)	Qualifier (6th)	Qualifier (7th)
1 Coronary Arteries, Multiple 3 Coronary Artery Bypass Grafts, Multiple 6 Heart, Right and Left	0 High Osmolar 1 Low Osmolar Y Other Contrast	0 Unenhanced and Enhanced Z None	Z None
1 Coronary Arteries, Multiple 3 Coronary Artery Bypass Grafts, Multiple 6 Heart, Right and Left	Z None	2 Intravascular Optical Coherence Z None	Z None

Section   **B**   **Imaging**
Body System   **2**   **Heart**
Type   **3**   **Magnetic Resonance Imaging (MRI):** Computer reformatted digital display of multiplanar images developed from the capture of radiofrequency signals emitted by nuclei in a body site excited within a magnetic field

Body Part (4th)	Contrast (5th)	Qualifier (6th)	Qualifier (7th)
1 Coronary Arteries, Multiple 3 Coronary Artery Bypass Grafts, Multiple 6 Heart, Right and Left	Y Other Contrast	0 Unenhanced and Enhanced Z None	Z None
1 Coronary Arteries, Multiple 3 Coronary Artery Bypass Grafts, Multiple 6 Heart, Right and Left	Z None	Z None	Z None

Section   **B**   **Imaging**
Body System   **2**   **Heart**
Type   **4**   **Ultrasonography:** Real time display of images of anatomy or flow information developed from the capture of reflected and attenuated high frequency sound waves

Body Part (4th)	Contrast (5th)	Qualifier (6th)	Qualifier (7th)
0 Coronary Artery, Single 1 Coronary Arteries, Multiple 4 Heart, Right 5 Heart, Left 6 Heart, Right and Left B Heart with Aorta C Pericardium D Pediatric Heart	Y Other Contrast	Z None	Z None
0 Coronary Artery, Single 1 Coronary Arteries, Multiple 4 Heart, Right 5 Heart, Left 6 Heart, Right and Left B Heart with Aorta C Pericardium D Pediatric Heart	Z None	Z None	3 Intravascular 4 Transesophageal Z None

Section   **B**   **Imaging**
Body System   **3**   **Upper Arteries**
Type   **0**   **Plain Radiography:** Planar display of an image developed from the capture of external ionizing radiation on photographic or photoconductive plate

Body Part (4th)	Contrast (5th)	Qualifier (6th)	Qualifier (7th)
0 Thoracic Aorta 1 Brachiocephalic-Subclavian Artery, Right 2 Subclavian Artery, Left 3 Common Carotid Artery, Right 4 Common Carotid Artery, Left 5 Common Carotid Arteries, Bilateral 6 Internal Carotid Artery, Right 7 Internal Carotid Artery, Left 8 Internal Carotid Arteries, Bilateral 9 External Carotid Artery, Right B External Carotid Artery, Left C External Carotid Arteries, Bilateral D Vertebral Artery, Right F Vertebral Artery, Left G Vertebral Arteries, Bilateral H Upper Extremity Arteries, Right J Upper Extremity Arteries, Left K Upper Extremity Arteries, Bilateral L Intercostal and Bronchial Arteries M Spinal Arteries N Upper Arteries, Other P Thoraco-Abdominal Aorta Q Cervico-Cerebral Arch R Intracranial Arteries S Pulmonary Artery, Right T Pulmonary Artery, Left	0 High Osmolar 1 Low Osmolar Y Other Contrast Z None	Z None	Z None

Section	B	Imaging
Body System	3	Upper Arteries
Type	1	Fluoroscopy: Single plane or bi-plane real time display of an image developed from the capture of external ionizing radiation on a fluorescent screen. The image may also be stored by either digital or analog means

Body Part (4th)	Contrast (5th)	Qualifier (6th)	Qualifier (7th)
0 Thoracic Aorta 1 Brachiocephalic-Subclavian Artery, Right 2 Subclavian Artery, Left 3 Common Carotid Artery, Right 4 Common Carotid Artery, Left 5 Common Carotid Arteries, Bilateral 6 Internal Carotid Artery, Right 7 Internal Carotid Artery, Left 8 Internal Carotid Arteries, Bilateral 9 External Carotid Artery, Right B External Carotid Artery, Left C External Carotid Arteries, Bilateral D Vertebral Artery, Right F Vertebral Artery, Left G Vertebral Arteries, Bilateral H Upper Extremity Arteries, Right J Upper Extremity Arteries, Left K Upper Extremity Arteries, Bilateral L Intercostal and Bronchial Arteries M Spinal Arteries N Upper Arteries, Other P Thoraco-Abdominal Aorta Q Cervico-Cerebral Arch R Intracranial Arteries S Pulmonary Artery, Right T Pulmonary Artery, Left U Pulmonary Trunk	0 High Osmolar 1 Low Osmolar Y Other Contrast	1 Laser	0 Intraoperative
0 Thoracic Aorta 1 Brachiocephalic-Subclavian Artery, Right 2 Subclavian Artery, Left 3 Common Carotid Artery, Right 4 Common Carotid Artery, Left 5 Common Carotid Arteries, Bilateral 6 Internal Carotid Artery, Right 7 Internal Carotid Artery, Left 8 Internal Carotid Arteries, Bilateral 9 External Carotid Artery, Right B External Carotid Artery, Left C External Carotid Arteries, Bilateral D Vertebral Artery, Right F Vertebral Artery, Left G Vertebral Arteries, Bilateral H Upper Extremity Arteries, Right J Upper Extremity Arteries, Left K Upper Extremity Arteries, Bilateral L Intercostal and Bronchial Arteries M Spinal Arteries N Upper Arteries, Other P Thoraco-Abdominal Aorta Q Cervico-Cerebral Arch R Intracranial Arteries S Pulmonary Artery, Right T Pulmonary Artery, Left U Pulmonary Trunk	0 High Osmolar 1 Low Osmolar Y Other Contrast	Z None	Z None

Continued →

Section	B	Imaging
Body System	3	Upper Arteries
Type	1	**Fluoroscopy:** Single plane or bi-plane real time display of an image developed from the capture of external ionizing radiation on a fluorescent screen. The image may also be stored by either digital or analog means

Body Part (4th)	Contrast (5th)	Qualifier (6th)	Qualifier (7th)
0 Thoracic Aorta	Z None	Z None	Z None
1 Brachiocephalic-Subclavian Artery, Right			
2 Subclavian Artery, Left			
3 Common Carotid Artery, Right			
4 Common Carotid Artery, Left			
5 Common Carotid Arteries, Bilateral			
6 Internal Carotid Artery, Right			
7 Internal Carotid Artery, Left			
8 Internal Carotid Arteries, Bilateral			
9 External Carotid Artery, Right			
B External Carotid Artery, Left			
C External Carotid Arteries, Bilateral			
D Vertebral Artery, Right			
F Vertebral Artery, Left			
G Vertebral Arteries, Bilateral			
H Upper Extremity Arteries, Right			
J Upper Extremity Arteries, Left			
K Upper Extremity Arteries, Bilateral			
L Intercostal and Bronchial Arteries			
M Spinal Arteries			
N Upper Arteries, Other			
P Thoraco-Abdominal Aorta			
Q Cervico-Cerebral Arch			
R Intracranial Arteries			
S Pulmonary Artery, Right			
T Pulmonary Artery, Left			
U Pulmonary Trunk			

Section	B	Imaging
Body System	3	Upper Arteries
Type	2	**Computerized Tomography (CT Scan):** Computer reformatted digital display of multiplanar images developed from the capture of multiple exposures of external ionizing radiation

Body Part (4th)	Contrast (5th)	Qualifier (6th)	Qualifier (7th)
0 Thoracic Aorta	0 High Osmolar	Z None	Z None
5 Common Carotid Arteries, Bilateral	1 Low Osmolar		
8 Internal Carotid Arteries, Bilateral	Y Other Contrast		
G Vertebral Arteries, Bilateral			
R Intracranial Arteries			
S Pulmonary Artery, Right			
T Pulmonary Artery, Left			
0 Thoracic Aorta	Z None	2 Intravascular Optical Coherence	Z None
5 Common Carotid Arteries, Bilateral		Z None	
8 Internal Carotid Arteries, Bilateral			
G Vertebral Arteries, Bilateral			
R Intracranial Arteries			
S Pulmonary Artery, Right			
T Pulmonary Artery, Left			

Section	B	Imaging
Body System	3	Upper Arteries
Type	3	**Magnetic Resonance Imaging (MRI):** Computer reformatted digital display of multiplanar images developed from the capture of radiofrequency signals emitted by nuclei in a body site excited within a magnetic field

Body Part (4th)	Contrast (5th)	Qualifier (6th)	Qualifier (7th)
0 Thoracic Aorta **5** Common Carotid Arteries, Bilateral **8** Internal Carotid Arteries, Bilateral **G** Vertebral Arteries, Bilateral **H** Upper Extremity Arteries, Right **J** Upper Extremity Arteries, Left **K** Upper Extremity Arteries, Bilateral **M** Spinal Arteries **Q** Cervico-Cerebral Arch **R** Intracranial Arteries	**Y** Other Contrast	**0** Unenhanced and Enhanced **Z** None	**Z** None
0 Thoracic Aorta **5** Common Carotid Arteries, Bilateral **8** Internal Carotid Arteries, Bilateral **G** Vertebral Arteries, Bilateral **H** Upper Extremity Arteries, Right **J** Upper Extremity Arteries, Left **K** Upper Extremity Arteries, Bilateral **M** Spinal Arteries **Q** Cervico-Cerebral Arch **R** Intracranial Arteries	**Z** None	**Z** None	**Z** None

Section	B	Imaging
Body System	3	Upper Arteries
Type	4	**Ultrasonography:** Real time display of images of anatomy or flow information developed from the capture of reflected and attenuated high frequency sound waves

Body Part (4th)	Contrast (5th)	Qualifier (6th)	Qualifier (7th)
0 Thoracic Aorta **1** Brachiocephalic-Subclavian Artery, Right **2** Subclavian Artery, Left **3** Common Carotid Artery, Right **4** Common Carotid Artery, Left **5** Common Carotid Arteries, Bilateral **6** Internal Carotid Artery, Right **7** Internal Carotid Artery, Left **8** Internal Carotid Arteries, Bilateral **H** Upper Extremity Arteries, Right **J** Upper Extremity Arteries, Left **K** Upper Extremity Arteries, Bilateral **R** Intracranial Arteries **S** Pulmonary Artery, Right **T** Pulmonary Artery, Left **V** Ophthalmic Arteries	**Z** None	**Z** None	**3** Intravascular **Z** None

Section   **B**   **Imaging**
Body System   **4**   **Lower Arteries**
Type   **0**   **Plain Radiography:** Planar display of an image developed from the capture of external ionizing radiation on photographic or photoconductive plate

Body Part (4th)	Contrast (5th)	Qualifier (6th)	Qualifier (7th)
0 Abdominal Aorta **2** Hepatic Artery **3** Splenic Arteries **4** Superior Mesenteric Artery **5** Inferior Mesenteric Artery **6** Renal Artery, Right **7** Renal Artery, Left **8** Renal Arteries, Bilateral **9** Lumbar Arteries **B** Intra-Abdominal Arteries, Other **C** Pelvic Arteries **D** Aorta and Bilateral Lower Extremity Arteries **F** Lower Extremity Arteries, Right **G** Lower Extremity Arteries, Left **J** Lower Arteries, Other **M** Renal Artery Transplant	**0** High Osmolar **1** Low Osmolar **Y** Other Contrast	**Z** None	**Z** None

Section   **B**   **Imaging**
Body System   **4**   **Lower Arteries**
Type   **1**   **Fluoroscopy:** Single plane or bi-plane real time display of an image developed from the capture of external ionizing radiation on a fluorescent screen. The image may also be stored by either digital or analog means

Body Part (4th)	Contrast (5th)	Qualifier (6th)	Qualifier (7th)
0 Abdominal Aorta **2** Hepatic Artery **3** Splenic Arteries **4** Superior Mesenteric Artery **5** Inferior Mesenteric Artery **6** Renal Artery, Right **7** Renal Artery, Left **8** Renal Arteries, Bilateral **9** Lumbar Arteries **B** Intra-Abdominal Arteries, Other **C** Pelvic Arteries **D** Aorta and Bilateral Lower Extremity Arteries **F** Lower Extremity Arteries, Right **G** Lower Extremity Arteries, Left **J** Lower Arteries, Other	**0** High Osmolar **1** Low Osmolar **Y** Other Contrast	**1** Laser	**0** Intraoperative
0 Abdominal Aorta **2** Hepatic Artery **3** Splenic Arteries **4** Superior Mesenteric Artery **5** Inferior Mesenteric Artery **6** Renal Artery, Right **7** Renal Artery, Left **8** Renal Arteries, Bilateral **9** Lumbar Arteries **B** Intra-Abdominal Arteries, Other **C** Pelvic Arteries **D** Aorta and Bilateral Lower Extremity Arteries **F** Lower Extremity Arteries, Right **G** Lower Extremity Arteries, Left **J** Lower Arteries, Other	**0** High Osmolar **1** Low Osmolar **Y** Other Contrast	**Z** None	**Z** None

Continued →

Section	B	Imaging
Body System	4	Lower Arteries
Type	1	**Fluoroscopy:** Single plane or bi-plane real time display of an image developed from the capture of external ionizing radiation on a fluorescent screen. The image may also be stored by either digital or analog means

Body Part (4ᵗʰ)	Contrast (5ᵗʰ)	Qualifier (6ᵗʰ)	Qualifier (7ᵗʰ)
0 Abdominal Aorta 2 Hepatic Artery 3 Splenic Arteries 4 Superior Mesenteric Artery 5 Inferior Mesenteric Artery 6 Renal Artery, Right 7 Renal Artery, Left 8 Renal Arteries, Bilateral 9 Lumbar Arteries B Intra-Abdominal Arteries, Other C Pelvic Arteries D Aorta and Bilateral Lower Extremity Arteries F Lower Extremity Arteries, Right G Lower Extremity Arteries, Left J Lower Arteries, Other	Z None	Z None	Z None

Section	B	Imaging
Body System	4	Lower Arteries
Type	2	**Computerized Tomography (CT Scan):** Computer reformatted digital display of multiplanar images developed from the capture of multiple exposures of external ionizing radiation

Body Part (4ᵗʰ)	Contrast (5ᵗʰ)	Qualifier (6ᵗʰ)	Qualifier (7ᵗʰ)
0 Abdominal Aorta 1 Celiac Artery 4 Superior Mesenteric Artery 8 Renal Arteries, Bilateral C Pelvic Arteries F Lower Extremity Arteries, Right G Lower Extremity Arteries, Left H Lower Extremity Arteries, Bilateral M Renal Artery Transplant	0 High Osmolar 1 Low Osmolar Y Other Contrast	Z None	Z None
0 Abdominal Aorta 1 Celiac Artery 4 Superior Mesenteric Artery 8 Renal Arteries, Bilateral C Pelvic Arteries F Lower Extremity Arteries, Right G Lower Extremity Arteries, Left H Lower Extremity Arteries, Bilateral M Renal Artery Transplant	Z None	2 Intravascular Optical Coherence Z None	Z None

Section	B	Imaging
Body System	4	Lower Arteries
Type	3	**Magnetic Resonance Imaging (MRI):** Computer reformatted digital display of multiplanar images developed from the capture of radiofrequency signals emitted by nuclei in a body site excited within a magnetic field

Body Part (4ᵗʰ)	Contrast (5ᵗʰ)	Qualifier (6ᵗʰ)	Qualifier (7ᵗʰ)
0 Abdominal Aorta 1 Celiac Artery 4 Superior Mesenteric Artery 8 Renal Arteries, Bilateral C Pelvic Arteries F Lower Extremity Arteries, Right G Lower Extremity Arteries, Left H Lower Extremity Arteries, Bilateral	Y Other Contrast	0 Unenhanced and Enhanced Z None	Z None

Continued →

Section	B	Imaging
Body System	4	Lower Arteries
Type	3	**Magnetic Resonance Imaging (MRI):** Computer reformatted digital display of multiplanar images developed from the capture of radiofrequency signals emitted by nuclei in a body site excited within a magnetic field

Body Part (4th)	Contrast (5th)	Qualifier (6th)	Qualifier (7th)
0 Abdominal Aorta 1 Celiac Artery 4 Superior Mesenteric Artery 8 Renal Arteries, Bilateral C Pelvic Arteries F Lower Extremity Arteries, Right G Lower Extremity Arteries, Left H Lower Extremity Arteries, Bilateral	Z None	Z None	Z None

Section	B	Imaging
Body System	4	Lower Arteries
Type	4	**Ultrasonography:** Real time display of images of anatomy or flow information developed from the capture of reflected and attenuated high frequency sound waves

Body Part (4th)	Contrast (5th)	Qualifier (6th)	Qualifier (7th)
0 Abdominal Aorta 4 Superior Mesenteric Artery 5 Inferior Mesenteric Artery 6 Renal Artery, Right 7 Renal Artery, Left 8 Renal Arteries, Bilateral B Intra-Abdominal Arteries, Other F Lower Extremity Arteries, Right G Lower Extremity Arteries, Left H Lower Extremity Arteries, Bilateral K Celiac and Mesenteric Arteries L Femoral Artery N Penile Arteries	Z None	Z None	3 Intravascular Z None

Section	B	Imaging
Body System	5	Veins
Type	0	**Plain Radiography:** Planar display of an image developed from the capture of external ionizing radiation on photographic or photoconductive plate

Body Part (4th)	Contrast (5th)	Qualifier (6th)	Qualifier (7th)
0 Epidural Veins 1 Cerebral and Cerebellar Veins 2 Intracranial Sinuses 3 Jugular Veins, Right 4 Jugular Veins, Left 5 Jugular Veins, Bilateral 6 Subclavian Vein, Right 7 Subclavian Vein, Left 8 Superior Vena Cava 9 Inferior Vena Cava B Lower Extremity Veins, Right C Lower Extremity Veins, Left D Lower Extremity Veins, Bilateral F Pelvic (Iliac) Veins, Right G Pelvic (Iliac) Veins, Left H Pelvic (Iliac) Veins, Bilateral J Renal Vein, Right K Renal Vein, Left L Renal Veins, Bilateral M Upper Extremity Veins, Right N Upper Extremity Veins, Left P Upper Extremity Veins, Bilateral Q Pulmonary Vein, Right R Pulmonary Vein, Left S Pulmonary Veins, Bilateral T Portal and Splanchnic Veins V Veins, Other W Dialysis Shunt/Fistula	0 High Osmolar 1 Low Osmolar Y Other Contrast	Z None	Z None

Section	B	Imaging
Body System	5	Veins
Type	1	**Fluoroscopy:** Single plane or bi-plane real time display of an image developed from the capture of external ionizing radiation on a fluorescent screen. The image may also be stored by either digital or analog means

Body Part (4th)	Contrast (5th)	Qualifier (6th)	Qualifier (7th)
0 Epidural Veins 1 Cerebral and Cerebellar Veins 2 Intracranial Sinuses 3 Jugular Veins, Right 4 Jugular Veins, Left 5 Jugular Veins, Bilateral 6 Subclavian Vein, Right 7 Subclavian Vein, Left 8 Superior Vena Cava 9 Inferior Vena Cava B Lower Extremity Veins, Right C Lower Extremity Veins, Left D Lower Extremity Veins, Bilateral F Pelvic (Iliac) Veins, Right G Pelvic (Iliac) Veins, Left H Pelvic (Iliac) Veins, Bilateral J Renal Vein, Right K Renal Vein, Left L Renal Veins, Bilateral M Upper Extremity Veins, Right N Upper Extremity Veins, Left P Upper Extremity Veins, Bilateral Q Pulmonary Vein, Right R Pulmonary Vein, Left S Pulmonary Veins, Bilateral T Portal and Splanchnic Veins V Veins, Other W Dialysis Shunt/Fistula	0 High Osmolar 1 Low Osmolar Y Other Contrast Z None	Z None	A Guidance Z None

Section	B	Imaging
Body System	5	Veins
Type	2	**Computerized Tomography (CT Scan):** Computer reformatted digital display of multiplanar images developed from the capture of multiple exposures of external ionizing radiation

Body Part (4th)	Contrast (5th)	Qualifier (6th)	Qualifier (7th)
2 Intracranial Sinuses 8 Superior Vena Cava 9 Inferior Vena Cava F Pelvic (Iliac) Veins, Right G Pelvic (Iliac) Veins, Left H Pelvic (Iliac) Veins, Bilateral J Renal Vein, Right K Renal Vein, Left L Renal Veins, Bilateral Q Pulmonary Vein, Right R Pulmonary Vein, Left S Pulmonary Veins, Bilateral T Portal and Splanchnic Veins	0 High Osmolar 1 Low Osmolar Y Other Contrast	0 Unenhanced and Enhanced Z None	Z None
2 Intracranial Sinuses 8 Superior Vena Cava 9 Inferior Vena Cava F Pelvic (Iliac) Veins, Right G Pelvic (Iliac) Veins, Left H Pelvic (Iliac) Veins, Bilateral J Renal Vein, Right	Z None	2 Intravascular Optical Coherence Z None	Z None
K Renal Vein, Left L Renal Veins, Bilateral Q Pulmonary Vein, Right R Pulmonary Vein, Left S Pulmonary Veins, Bilateral T Portal and Splanchnic Veins			

Section	B	Imaging
Body System	5	Veins
Type	3	**Magnetic Resonance Imaging (MRI):** Computer reformatted digital display of multiplanar images developed from the capture of radiofrequency signals emitted by nuclei in a body site excited within a magnetic field

Body Part (4th)	Contrast (5th)	Qualifier (6th)	Qualifier (7th)
1 Cerebral and Cerebellar Veins 2 Intracranial Sinuses 5 Jugular Veins, Bilateral 8 Superior Vena Cava 9 Inferior Vena Cava B Lower Extremity Veins, Right C Lower Extremity Veins, Left D Lower Extremity Veins, Bilateral H Pelvic (Iliac) Veins, Bilateral L Renal Veins, Bilateral M Upper Extremity Veins, Right N Upper Extremity Veins, Left P Upper Extremity Veins, Bilateral S Pulmonary Veins, Bilateral T Portal and Splanchnic Veins V Veins, Other	Y Other Contrast	0 Unenhanced and Enhanced Z None	Z None

Continued →

Section	B	Imaging
Body System	5	Veins
Type	3	**Magnetic Resonance Imaging (MRI):** Computer reformatted digital display of multiplanar images developed from the capture of radiofrequency signals emitted by nuclei in a body site excited within a magnetic field

Body Part (4th)	Contrast (5th)	Qualifier (6th)	Qualifier (7th)
1 Cerebral and Cerebellar Veins	Z None	Z None	Z None
2 Intracranial Sinuses			
5 Jugular Veins, Bilateral			
8 Superior Vena Cava			
9 Inferior Vena Cava			
B Lower Extremity Veins, Right			
C Lower Extremity Veins, Left			
D Lower Extremity Veins, Bilateral			
H Pelvic (Iliac) Veins, Bilateral			
L Renal Veins, Bilateral			
M Upper Extremity Veins, Right			
N Upper Extremity Veins, Left			
P Upper Extremity Veins, Bilateral			
S Pulmonary Veins, Bilateral			
T Portal and Splanchnic Veins			
V Veins, Other			

Section	B	Imaging
Body System	5	Veins
Type	4	**Ultrasonography:** Real time display of images of anatomy or flow information developed from the capture of reflected and attenuated high frequency sound waves

Body Part (4th)	Contrast (5th)	Qualifier (6th)	Qualifier (7th)
3 Jugular Veins, Right	Z None	Z None	3 Intravascular
4 Jugular Veins, Left			A Guidance
6 Subclavian Vein, Right			Z None
7 Subclavian Vein, Left			
8 Superior Vena Cava			
9 Inferior Vena Cava			
B Lower Extremity Veins, Right			
C Lower Extremity Veins, Left			
D Lower Extremity Veins, Bilateral			
J Renal Vein, Right			
K Renal Vein, Left			
L Renal Veins, Bilateral			
M Upper Extremity Veins, Right			
N Upper Extremity Veins, Left			
P Upper Extremity Veins, Bilateral			
T Portal and Splanchnic Veins			

Section	B	Imaging
Body System	7	Lymphatic System
Type	0	**Plain Radiography:** Planar display of an image developed from the capture of external ionizing radiation on photographic or photoconductive plate

Body Part (4th)	Contrast (5th)	Qualifier (6th)	Qualifier (7th)
0 Abdominal/Retroperitoneal Lymphatics, Unilateral	0 High Osmolar	Z None	Z None
1 Abdominal/Retroperitoneal Lymphatics, Bilateral	1 Low Osmolar		
4 Lymphatics, Head and Neck	Y Other Contrast		
5 Upper Extremity Lymphatics, Right			
6 Upper Extremity Lymphatics, Left			
7 Upper Extremity Lymphatics, Bilateral			
8 Lower Extremity Lymphatics, Right			
9 Lower Extremity Lymphatics, Left			
B Lower Extremity Lymphatics, Bilateral			
C Lymphatics, Pelvic			

Section	B	Imaging
Body System	8	Eye
Type	0	**Plain Radiography:** Planar display of an image developed from the capture of external ionizing radiation on photographic or photoconductive plate

Body Part (4th)	Contrast (5th)	Qualifier (6th)	Qualifier (7th)
0 Lacrimal Duct, Right 1 Lacrimal Duct, Left 2 Lacrimal Ducts, Bilateral	0 High Osmolar 1 Low Osmolar Y Other Contrast	Z None	Z None
3 Optic Foramina, Right 4 Optic Foramina, Left 5 Eye, Right 6 Eye, Left 7 Eyes, Bilateral	Z None	Z None	Z None

Section	B	Imaging
Body System	8	Eye
Type	2	**Computerized Tomography (CT Scan):** Computer reformatted digital display of multiplanar images developed from the capture of multiple exposures of external ionizing radiation

Body Part (4th)	Contrast (5th)	Qualifier (6th)	Qualifier (7th)
5 Eye, Right 6 Eye, Left 7 Eyes, Bilateral	0 High Osmolar 1 Low Osmolar Y Other Contrast	0 Unenhanced and Enhanced Z None	Z None
5 Eye, Right 6 Eye, Left 7 Eyes, Bilateral	Z None	Z None	Z None

Section	B	Imaging
Body System	8	Eye
Type	3	**Magnetic Resonance Imaging (MRI):** Computer reformatted digital display of multiplanar images developed from the capture of radiofrequency signals emitted by nuclei in a body site excited within a magnetic field

Body Part (4th)	Contrast (5th)	Qualifier (6th)	Qualifier (7th)
5 Eye, Right 6 Eye, Left 7 Eyes, Bilateral	Y Other Contrast	0 Unenhanced and Enhanced Z None	Z None
5 Eye, Right 6 Eye, Left 7 Eyes, Bilateral	Z None	Z None	Z None

Section	B	Imaging
Body System	8	Eye
Type	4	**Ultrasonography:** Real time display of images of anatomy or flow information developed from the capture of reflected and attenuated high frequency sound waves

Body Part (4th)	Contrast (5th)	Qualifier (6th)	Qualifier (7th)
5 Eye, Right 6 Eye, Left 7 Eyes, Bilateral	Z None	Z None	Z None

Section	B	Imaging
Body System	9	Ear, Nose, Mouth and Throat
Type	0	**Plain Radiography:** Planar display of an image developed from the capture of external ionizing radiation on photographic or photoconductive plate

Body Part (4th)	Contrast (5th)	Qualifier (6th)	Qualifier (7th)
2 Paranasal Sinuses F Nasopharynx/Oropharynx H Mastoids	Z None	Z None	Z None
4 Parotid Gland, Right 5 Parotid Gland, Left 6 Parotid Glands, Bilateral 7 Submandibular Gland, Right 8 Submandibular Gland, Left 9 Submandibular Glands, Bilateral B Salivary Gland, Right C Salivary Gland, Left D Salivary Glands, Bilateral	0 High Osmolar 1 Low Osmolar Y Other Contrast	Z None	Z None

Section	B	Imaging
Body System	9	Ear, Nose, Mouth and Throat
Type	1	**Fluoroscopy:** Single plane or bi-plane real time display of an image developed from the capture of external ionizing radiation on a fluorescent screen. The image may also be stored by either digital or analog means

Body Part (4th)	Contrast (5th)	Qualifier (6th)	Qualifier (7th)
G Pharynx and Epiglottis J Larynx	Y Other Contrast Z None	Z None	Z None

Section	B	Imaging
Body System	9	Ear, Nose, Mouth and Throat
Type	2	**Computerized Tomography (CT Scan):** Computer reformatted digital display of multiplanar images developed from the capture of multiple exposures of external ionizing radiation

Body Part (4th)	Contrast (5th)	Qualifier (6th)	Qualifier (7th)
0 Ear 2 Paranasal Sinuses 6 Parotid Glands, Bilateral 9 Submandibular Glands, Bilateral D Salivary Glands, Bilateral F Nasopharynx/Oropharynx J Larynx	0 High Osmolar 1 Low Osmolar Y Other Contrast	0 Unenhanced and Enhanced Z None	Z None
0 Ear 2 Paranasal Sinuses 6 Parotid Glands, Bilateral 9 Submandibular Glands, Bilateral D Salivary Glands, Bilateral F Nasopharynx/Oropharynx J Larynx	Z None	Z None	Z None

Section	B	Imaging
Body System	9	Ear, Nose, Mouth and Throat
Type	3	**Magnetic Resonance Imaging (MRI):** Computer reformatted digital display of multiplanar images developed from the capture of radiofrequency signals emitted by nuclei in a body site excited within a magnetic field

Body Part (4th)	Contrast (5th)	Qualifier (6th)	Qualifier (7th)
0 Ear 2 Paranasal Sinuses 6 Parotid Glands, Bilateral 9 Submandibular Glands, Bilateral D Salivary Glands, Bilateral F Nasopharynx/Oropharynx J Larynx	Y Other Contrast	0 Unenhanced and Enhanced Z None	Z None

Continued →

Section	B	Imaging
Body System	9	Ear, Nose, Mouth and Throat
Type	3	**Magnetic Resonance Imaging (MRI):** Computer reformatted digital display of multiplanar images developed from the capture of radiofrequency signals emitted by nuclei in a body site excited within a magnetic field

Body Part (4th)	Contrast (5th)	Qualifier (6th)	Qualifier (7th)
0 Ear 2 Paranasal Sinuses 6 Parotid Glands, Bilateral 9 Submandibular Glands, Bilateral D Salivary Glands, Bilateral F Nasopharynx/Oropharynx J Larynx	Z None	Z None	Z None

Section	B	Imaging
Body System	B	Respiratory System
Type	0	**Plain Radiography:** Planar display of an image developed from the capture of external ionizing radiation on photographic or photoconductive plate

Body Part (4th)	Contrast (5th)	Qualifier (6th)	Qualifier (7th)
7 Tracheobronchial Tree, Right 8 Tracheobronchial Tree, Left 9 Tracheobronchial Trees, Bilateral	Y Other Contrast	Z None	Z None
D Upper Airways	Z None	Z None	Z None

Section	B	Imaging
Body System	B	Respiratory System
Type	1	**Fluoroscopy:** Single plane or bi-plane real time display of an image developed from the capture of external ionizing radiation on a fluorescent screen. The image may also be stored by either digital or analog means

Body Part (4th)	Contrast (5th)	Qualifier (6th)	Qualifier (7th)
2 Lung, Right 3 Lung, Left 4 Lungs, Bilateral 6 Diaphragm C Mediastinum D Upper Airways	Z None	Z None	Z None
7 Tracheobronchial Tree, Right 8 Tracheobronchial Tree, Left 9 Tracheobronchial Trees, Bilateral	Y Other Contrast	Z None	Z None

Section	B	Imaging
Body System	B	Respiratory System
Type	2	**Computerized Tomography (CT Scan):** Computer reformatted digital display of multiplanar images developed from the capture of multiple exposures of external ionizing radiation

Body Part (4th)	Contrast (5th)	Qualifier (6th)	Qualifier (7th)
4 Lungs, Bilateral 7 Tracheobronchial Tree, Right 8 Tracheobronchial Tree, Left 9 Tracheobronchial Trees, Bilateral F Trachea/Airways	0 High Osmolar 1 Low Osmolar Y Other Contrast	0 Unenhanced and Enhanced Z None	Z None
4 Lungs, Bilateral 7 Tracheobronchial Tree, Right 8 Tracheobronchial Tree, Left 9 Tracheobronchial Trees, Bilateral F Trachea/Airways	Z None	Z None	Z None

Section	B	Imaging
Body System	B	Respiratory System
Type	3	**Magnetic Resonance Imaging (MRI):** Computer reformatted digital display of multiplanar images developed from the capture of radiofrequency signals emitted by nuclei in a body site excited within a magnetic field

Body Part (4th)	Contrast (5th)	Qualifier (6th)	Qualifier (7th)
G Lung Apices	**Y** Other Contrast	**0** Unenhanced and Enhanced **Z** None	**Z** None
G Lung Apices	**Z** None	**Z** None	**Z** None

Section	B	Imaging
Body System	B	Respiratory System
Type	4	**Ultrasonography:** Real time display of images of anatomy or flow information developed from the capture of reflected and attenuated high frequency sound waves

Body Part (4th)	Contrast (5th)	Qualifier (6th)	Qualifier (7th)
B Pleura **C** Mediastinum	**Z** None	**Z** None	**Z** None

Section	B	Imaging
Body System	D	Gastrointestinal System
Type	1	**Fluoroscopy:** Single plane or bi-plane real time display of an image developed from the capture of external ionizing radiation on a fluorescent screen. The image may also be stored by either digital or analog means

Body Part (4th)	Contrast (5th)	Qualifier (6th)	Qualifier (7th)
1 Esophagus **2** Stomach **3** Small Bowel **4** Colon **5** Upper GI **6** Upper GI and Small Bowel **9** Duodenum **B** Mouth/Oropharynx	**Y** Other Contrast **Z** None	**Z** None	**Z** None

Section	B	Imaging
Body System	D	Gastrointestinal System
Type	2	**Computerized Tomography (CT Scan):** Computer reformatted digital display of multiplanar images developed from the capture of multiple exposures of external ionizing radiation

Body Part (4th)	Contrast (5th)	Qualifier (6th)	Qualifier (7th)
4 Colon	**0** High Osmolar **1** Low Osmolar **Y** Other Contrast	**0** Unenhanced and Enhanced **Z** None	**Z** None
4 Colon	**Z** None	**Z** None	**Z** None

Section	B	Imaging
Body System	D	Gastrointestinal System
Type	4	**Ultrasonography:** Real time display of images of anatomy or flow information developed from the capture of reflected and attenuated high frequency sound waves

Body Part (4th)	Contrast (5th)	Qualifier (6th)	Qualifier (7th)
1 Esophagus **2** Stomach **7** Gastrointestinal Tract **8** Appendix **9** Duodenum **C** Rectum	**Z** None	**Z** None	**Z** None

Section	B	Imaging
Body System	F	Hepatobiliary System and Pancreas
Type	0	**Plain Radiography:** Planar display of an image developed from the capture of external ionizing radiation on photographic or photoconductive plate

Body Part (4ᵗʰ)	Contrast (5ᵗʰ)	Qualifier (6ᵗʰ)	Qualifier (7ᵗʰ)
0 Bile Ducts 3 Gallbladder and Bile Ducts C Hepatobiliary System, All	0 High Osmolar 1 Low Osmolar Y Other Contrast	Z None	Z None

Section	B	Imaging
Body System	F	Hepatobiliary System and Pancreas
Type	1	**Fluoroscopy:** Single plane or bi-plane real time display of an image developed from the capture of external ionizing radiation on a fluorescent screen. The image may also be stored by either digital or analog means

Body Part (4ᵗʰ)	Contrast (5ᵗʰ)	Qualifier (6ᵗʰ)	Qualifier (7ᵗʰ)
0 Bile Ducts 1 Biliary and Pancreatic Ducts 2 Gallbladder 3 Gallbladder and Bile Ducts 4 Gallbladder, Bile Ducts and Pancreatic Ducts 8 Pancreatic Ducts	0 High Osmolar 1 Low Osmolar Y Other Contrast	Z None	Z None

Section	B	Imaging
Body System	F	Hepatobiliary System and Pancreas
Type	2	**Computerized Tomography (CT Scan):** Computer reformatted digital display of multiplanar images developed from the capture of multiple exposures of external ionizing radiation

Body Part (4ᵗʰ)	Contrast (5ᵗʰ)	Qualifier (6ᵗʰ)	Qualifier (7ᵗʰ)
5 Liver 6 Liver and Spleen 7 Pancreas C Hepatobiliary System, All	0 High Osmolar 1 Low Osmolar Y Other Contrast	0 Unenhanced and Enhanced Z None	Z None
5 Liver 6 Liver and Spleen 7 Pancreas C Hepatobiliary System, All	Z None	Z None	Z None

Section	B	Imaging
Body System	F	Hepatobiliary System and Pancreas
Type	3	**Magnetic Resonance Imaging (MRI):** Computer reformatted digital display of multiplanar images developed from the capture of radiofrequency signals emitted by nuclei in a body site excited within a magnetic field

Body Part (4ᵗʰ)	Contrast (5ᵗʰ)	Qualifier (6ᵗʰ)	Qualifier (7ᵗʰ)
5 Liver 6 Liver and Spleen 7 Pancreas	Y Other Contrast	0 Unenhanced and Enhanced Z None	Z None
5 Liver 6 Liver and Spleen 7 Pancreas	Z None	Z None	Z None

584

Section	B	Imaging
Body System	F	Hepatobiliary System and Pancreas
Type	4	Ultrasonography: Real time display of images of anatomy or flow information developed from the capture of reflected and attenuated high frequency sound waves

Body Part (4th)	Contrast (5th)	Qualifier (6th)	Qualifier (7th)
0 Bile Ducts 2 Gallbladder 3 Gallbladder and Bile Ducts 5 Liver 6 Liver and Spleen 7 Pancreas C Hepatobiliary System, All	Z None	Z None	Z None

Section	B	Imaging
Body System	F	Hepatobiliary System and Pancreas
Type	5	Other Imaging: Other specified modality for visualizing a body part

Body Part (4th)	Contrast (5th)	Qualifier (6th)	Qualifier (7th)
0 Bile Ducts 2 Gallbladder 3 Gallbladder and Bile Ducts 5 Liver 6 Liver and Spleen 7 Pancreas C Hepatobiliary System, All	2 Fluorescing Agent	0 Indocyanine Green Dye Z None	0 Intraoperative Z None

Section	B	Imaging
Body System	G	Endocrine System
Type	2	Computerized Tomography (CT Scan): Computer reformatted digital display of multiplanar images developed from the capture of multiple exposures of external ionizing radiation

Body Part (4th)	Contrast (5th)	Qualifier (6th)	Qualifier (7th)
2 Adrenal Glands, Bilateral 3 Parathyroid Glands 4 Thyroid Gland	0 High Osmolar 1 Low Osmolar Y Other Contrast	0 Unenhanced and Enhanced Z None	Z None
2 Adrenal Glands, Bilateral 3 Parathyroid Glands 4 Thyroid Gland	Z None	Z None	Z None

Section	B	Imaging
Body System	G	Endocrine System
Type	3	Magnetic Resonance Imaging (MRI): Computer reformatted digital display of multiplanar images developed from the capture of radiofrequency signals emitted by nuclei in a body site excited within a magnetic field

Body Part (4th)	Contrast (5th)	Qualifier (6th)	Qualifier (7th)
2 Adrenal Glands, Bilateral 3 Parathyroid Glands 4 Thyroid Gland	Y Other Contrast	0 Unenhanced and Enhanced Z None	Z None
2 Adrenal Glands, Bilateral 3 Parathyroid Glands 4 Thyroid Gland	Z None	Z None	Z None

Section	B	Imaging
Body System	G	Endocrine System
Type	4	**Ultrasonography:** Real time display of images of anatomy or flow information developed from the capture of reflected and attenuated high frequency sound waves

Body Part (4th)	Contrast (5th)	Qualifier (6th)	Qualifier (7th)
0 Adrenal Gland, Right 1 Adrenal Gland, Left 2 Adrenal Glands, Bilateral 3 Parathyroid Glands 4 Thyroid Gland	Z None	Z None	Z None

Section	B	Imaging
Body System	H	Skin, Subcutaneous Tissue and Breast
Type	0	**Plain Radiography:** Planar display of an image developed from the capture of external ionizing radiation on photographic or photoconductive plate

Body Part (4th)	Contrast (5th)	Qualifier (6th)	Qualifier (7th)
0 Breast, Right 1 Breast, Left 2 Breasts, Bilateral	Z None	Z None	Z None
3 Single Mammary Duct, Right 4 Single Mammary Duct, Left 5 Multiple Mammary Ducts, Right 6 Multiple Mammary Ducts, Left	0 High Osmolar 1 Low Osmolar Y Other Contrast Z None	Z None	Z None

Section	B	Imaging
Body System	H	Skin, Subcutaneous Tissue and Breast
Type	3	**Magnetic Resonance Imaging (MRI):** Computer reformatted digital display of multiplanar images developed from the capture of radiofrequency signals emitted by nuclei in a body site excited within a magnetic field

Body Part (4th)	Contrast (5th)	Qualifier (6th)	Qualifier (7th)
0 Breast, Right 1 Breast, Left 2 Breasts, Bilateral D Subcutaneous Tissue, Head/Neck F Subcutaneous Tissue, Upper Extremity G Subcutaneous Tissue, Thorax H Subcutaneous Tissue, Abdomen and Pelvis J Subcutaneous Tissue, Lower Extremity	Y Other Contrast	0 Unenhanced and Enhanced Z None	Z None
0 Breast, Right 1 Breast, Left 2 Breasts, Bilateral D Subcutaneous Tissue, Head/Neck F Subcutaneous Tissue, Upper Extremity G Subcutaneous Tissue, Thorax H Subcutaneous Tissue, Abdomen and Pelvis J Subcutaneous Tissue, Lower Extremity	Z None	Z None	Z None

Section	B	Imaging
Body System	H	Skin, Subcutaneous Tissue and Breast
Type	4	**Ultrasonography:** Real time display of images of anatomy or flow information developed from the capture of reflected and attenuated high frequency sound waves

Body Part (4th)	Contrast (5th)	Qualifier (6th)	Qualifier (7th)
0 Breast, Right 1 Breast, Left 2 Breasts, Bilateral 7 Extremity, Upper 8 Extremity, Lower 9 Abdominal Wall B Chest Wall C Head and Neck	Z None	Z None	Z None

Section	B	Imaging
Body System	L	Connective Tissue
Type	3	**Magnetic Resonance Imaging (MRI):** Computer reformatted digital display of multiplanar images developed from the capture of radiofrequency signals emitted by nuclei in a body site excited within a magnetic field

Body Part (4th)	Contrast (5th)	Qualifier (6th)	Qualifier (7th)
0 Connective Tissue, Upper Extremity 1 Connective Tissue, Lower Extremity 2 Tendons, Upper Extremity 3 Tendons, Lower Extremity	Y Other Contrast	0 Unenhanced and Enhanced Z None	Z None
0 Connective Tissue, Upper Extremity 1 Connective Tissue, Lower Extremity 2 Tendons, Upper Extremity 3 Tendons, Lower Extremity	Z None	Z None	Z None

Section	B	Imaging
Body System	L	Connective Tissue
Type	4	**Ultrasonography:** Real time display of images of anatomy or flow information developed from the capture of reflected and attenuated high frequency sound waves

Body Part (4th)	Contrast (5th)	Qualifier (6th)	Qualifier (7th)
0 Connective Tissue, Upper Extremity 1 Connective Tissue, Lower Extremity 2 Tendons, Upper Extremity 3 Tendons, Lower Extremity	Z None	Z None	Z None

Section	B	Imaging
Body System	N	Skull and Facial Bones
Type	0	**Plain Radiography:** Planar display of an image developed from the capture of external ionizing radiation on photographic or photoconductive plate

Body Part (4th)	Contrast (5th)	Qualifier (6th)	Qualifier (7th)
0 Skull 1 Orbit, Right 2 Orbit, Left 3 Orbits, Bilateral 4 Nasal Bones 5 Facial Bones 6 Mandible B Zygomatic Arch, Right C Zygomatic Arch, Left D Zygomatic Arches, Bilateral G Tooth, Single H Teeth, Multiple J Teeth, All	Z None	Z None	Z None
7 Temporomandibular Joint, Right 8 Temporomandibular Joint, Left 9 Temporomandibular Joints, Bilateral	0 High Osmolar 1 Low Osmolar Y Other Contrast Z None	Z None	Z None

Section	B	Imaging
Body System	N	Skull and Facial Bones
Type	1	**Fluoroscopy:** Single plane or bi-plane real time display of an image developed from the capture of external ionizing radiation on a fluorescent screen. The image may also be stored by either digital or analog means

Body Part (4th)	Contrast (5th)	Qualifier (6th)	Qualifier (7th)
7 Temporomandibular Joint, Right 8 Temporomandibular Joint, Left 9 Temporomandibular Joints, Bilateral	0 High Osmolar 1 Low Osmolar Y Other Contrast Z None	Z None	Z None

Section	B	Imaging
Body System	N	Skull and Facial Bones
Type	2	**Computerized Tomography (CT Scan):** Computer reformatted digital display of multiplanar images developed from the capture of multiple exposures of external ionizing radiation

Body Part (4ᵗʰ)	Contrast (5ᵗʰ)	Qualifier (6ᵗʰ)	Qualifier (7ᵗʰ)
0 Skull 3 Orbits, Bilateral 5 Facial Bones 6 Mandible 9 Temporomandibular Joints, Bilateral F Temporal Bones	0 High Osmolar 1 Low Osmolar Y Other Contrast Z None	Z None	Z None

Section	B	Imaging
Body System	N	Skull and Facial Bones
Type	3	**Magnetic Resonance Imaging (MRI):** Computer reformatted digital display of multiplanar images developed from the capture of radiofrequency signals emitted by nuclei in a body site excited within a magnetic field

Body Part (4ᵗʰ)	Contrast (5ᵗʰ)	Qualifier (6ᵗʰ)	Qualifier (7ᵗʰ)
9 Temporomandibular Joints, Bilateral	Y Other Contrast Z None	Z None	Z None

Section	B	Imaging
Body System	P	Non-Axial Upper Bones
Type	0	**Plain Radiography:** Planar display of an image developed from the capture of external ionizing radiation on photographic or photoconductive plate

Body Part (4ᵗʰ)	Contrast (5ᵗʰ)	Qualifier (6ᵗʰ)	Qualifier (7ᵗʰ)
0 Sternoclavicular Joint, Right 1 Sternoclavicular Joint, Left 2 Sternoclavicular Joints, Bilateral 3 Acromioclavicular Joints, Bilateral 4 Clavicle, Right 5 Clavicle, Left 6 Scapula, Right 7 Scapula, Left A Humerus, Right B Humerus, Left E Upper Arm, Right F Upper Arm, Left J Forearm, Right K Forearm, Left N Hand, Right P Hand, Left R Finger(s), Right S Finger(s), Left X Ribs, Right Y Ribs, Left	Z None	Z None	Z None
8 Shoulder, Right 9 Shoulder, Left C Hand/Finger Joint, Right D Hand/Finger Joint, Left G Elbow, Right H Elbow, Left L Wrist, Right M Wrist, Left	0 High Osmolar 1 Low Osmolar Y Other Contrast Z None	Z None	Z None

Section	B	Imaging
Body System	P	Non-Axial Upper Bones
Type	1	Fluoroscopy: Single plane or bi-plane real time display of an image developed from the capture of external ionizing radiation on a fluorescent screen. The image may also be stored by either digital or analog means

Body Part (4th)	Contrast (5th)	Qualifier (6th)	Qualifier (7th)
0 Sternoclavicular Joint, Right 1 Sternoclavicular Joint, Left 2 Sternoclavicular Joints, Bilateral 3 Acromioclavicular Joints, Bilateral 4 Clavicle, Right 5 Clavicle, Left 6 Scapula, Right 7 Scapula, Left A Humerus, Right B Humerus, Left E Upper Arm, Right F Upper Arm, Left J Forearm, Right K Forearm, Left N Hand, Right P Hand, Left R Finger(s), Right S Finger(s), Left X Ribs, Right Y Ribs, Left	Z None	Z None	Z None
8 Shoulder, Right 9 Shoulder, Left L Wrist, Right M Wrist, Left	0 High Osmolar 1 Low Osmolar Y Other Contrast Z None	Z None	Z None
C Hand/Finger Joint, Right D Hand/Finger Joint, Left G Elbow, Right H Elbow, Left	0 High Osmolar 1 Low Osmolar Y Other Contrast	Z None	Z None

Section	B	Imaging
Body System	P	Non-Axial Upper Bones
Type	2	Computerized Tomography (CT Scan): Computer reformatted digital display of multiplanar images developed from the capture of multiple exposures of external ionizing radiation

Body Part (4th)	Contrast (5th)	Qualifier (6th)	Qualifier (7th)
0 Sternoclavicular Joint, Right 1 Sternoclavicular Joint, Left W Thorax	0 High Osmolar 1 Low Osmolar Y Other Contrast	Z None	Z None

Continued →

Section   **B**   **Imaging**
Body System   **P**   **Non-Axial Upper Bones**
Type   **2**   **Computerized Tomography (CT Scan):** Computer reformatted digital display of multiplanar images developed from the capture of multiple exposures of external ionizing radiation

Body Part (4th)	Contrast (5th)	Qualifier (6th)	Qualifier (7th)
2 Sternoclavicular Joints, Bilateral 3 Acromioclavicular Joints, Bilateral 4 Clavicle, Right 5 Clavicle, Left 6 Scapula, Right 7 Scapula, Left 8 Shoulder, Right 9 Shoulder, Left A Humerus, Right B Humerus, Left E Upper Arm, Right F Upper Arm, Left G Elbow, Right H Elbow, Left J Forearm, Right K Forearm, Left L Wrist, Right M Wrist, Left N Hand, Right P Hand, Left Q Hands and Wrists, Bilateral R Finger(s), Right S Finger(s), Left T Upper Extremity, Right U Upper Extremity, Left V Upper Extremities, Bilateral X Ribs, Right Y Ribs, Left	0 High Osmolar 1 Low Osmolar Y Other Contrast Z None	Z None	Z None
C Hand/Finger Joint, Right D Hand/Finger Joint, Left	Z None	Z None	Z None

Section   **B**   **Imaging**
Body System   **P**   **Non-Axial Upper Bones**
Type   **3**   **Magnetic Resonance Imaging (MRI):** Computer reformatted digital display of multiplanar images developed from the capture of radiofrequency signals emitted by nuclei in a body site excited within a magnetic field

Body Part (4th)	Contrast (5th)	Qualifier (6th)	Qualifier (7th)
8 Shoulder, Right 9 Shoulder, Left C Hand/Finger Joint, Right D Hand/Finger Joint, Left E Upper Arm, Right F Upper Arm, Left G Elbow, Right H Elbow, Left J Forearm, Right K Forearm, Left L Wrist, Right M Wrist, Left	Y Other Contrast	0 Unenhanced and Enhanced Z None	Z None

Continued →

Section	B	Imaging
Body System	P	Non-Axial Upper Bones
Type	3	**Magnetic Resonance Imaging (MRI):** Computer reformatted digital display of multiplanar images developed from the capture of radiofrequency signals emitted by nuclei in a body site excited within a magnetic field

Body Part (4th)	Contrast (5th)	Qualifier (6th)	Qualifier (7th)
8 Shoulder, Right 9 Shoulder, Left C Hand/Finger Joint, Right D Hand/Finger Joint, Left E Upper Arm, Right F Upper Arm, Left G Elbow, Right H Elbow, Left J Forearm, Right K Forearm, Left L Wrist, Right M Wrist, Left	Z None	Z None	Z None

Section	B	Imaging
Body System	P	Non-Axial Upper Bones
Type	4	**Ultrasonography:** Real time display of images of anatomy or flow information developed from the capture of reflected and attenuated high frequency sound waves

Body Part (4th)	Contrast (5th)	Qualifier (6th)	Qualifier (7th)
8 Shoulder, Right 9 Shoulder, Left G Elbow, Right H Elbow, Left L Wrist, Right M Wrist, Left N Hand, Right P Hand, Left	Z None	Z None	1 Densitometry Z None

Section	B	Imaging
Body System	Q	Non-Axial Lower Bones
Type	0	**Plain Radiography:** Planar display of an image developed from the capture of external ionizing radiation on photographic or photoconductive plate

Body Part (4th)	Contrast (5th)	Qualifier (6th)	Qualifier (7th)
0 Hip, Right 1 Hip, Left	0 High Osmolar 1 Low Osmolar Y Other Contrast	Z None	Z None
0 Hip, Right 1 Hip, Left	Z None	Z None	1 Densitometry Z None
3 Femur, Right 4 Femur, Left	Z None	Z None	1 Densitometry Z None
7 Knee, Right 8 Knee, Left G Ankle, Right H Ankle, Left	0 High Osmolar 1 Low Osmolar Y Other Contrast Z None	Z None	Z None
D Lower Leg, Right F Lower Leg, Left J Calcaneus, Right K Calcaneus, Left L Foot, Right M Foot, Left P Toe(s), Right Q Toe(s), Left V Patella, Right W Patella, Left	Z None	Z None	Z None

Continued →

Section	B	Imaging
Body System	Q	Non-Axial Lower Bones
Type	0	**Plain Radiography:** Planar display of an image developed from the capture of external ionizing radiation on photographic or photoconductive plate

Body Part (4th)	Contrast (5th)	Qualifier (6th)	Qualifier (7th)
X Foot/Toe Joint, Right Y Foot/Toe Joint, Left	0 High Osmolar 1 Low Osmolar Y Other Contrast	Z None	Z None

Section	B	Imaging
Body System	Q	Non-Axial Lower Bones
Type	1	**Fluoroscopy:** Single plane or bi-plane real time display of an image developed from the capture of external ionizing radiation on a fluorescent screen. The image may also be stored by either digital or analog means

Body Part (4th)	Contrast (5th)	Qualifier (6th)	Qualifier (7th)
0 Hip, Right 1 Hip, Left 7 Knee, Right 8 Knee, Left G Ankle, Right H Ankle, Left X Foot/Toe Joint, Right Y Foot/Toe Joint, Left	0 High Osmolar 1 Low Osmolar Y Other Contrast Z None	Z None	Z None
3 Femur, Right 4 Femur, Left D Lower Leg, Right F Lower Leg, Left J Calcaneus, Right K Calcaneus, Left L Foot, Right M Foot, Left P Toe(s), Right Q Toe(s), Left V Patella, Right W Patella, Left	Z None	Z None	Z None

Section	B	Imaging
Body System	Q	Non-Axial Lower Bones
Type	2	**Computerized Tomography (CT Scan):** Computer reformatted digital display of multiplanar images developed from the capture of multiple exposures of external ionizing radiation

Body Part (4th)	Contrast (5th)	Qualifier (6th)	Qualifier (7th)
0 Hip, Right 1 Hip, Left 3 Femur, Right 4 Femur, Left 7 Knee, Right 8 Knee, Left D Lower Leg, Right F Lower Leg, Left G Ankle, Right H Ankle, Left J Calcaneus, Right K Calcaneus, Left L Foot, Right M Foot, Left P Toe(s), Right Q Toe(s), Left R Lower Extremity, Right S Lower Extremity, Left V Patella, Right W Patella, Left X Foot/Toe Joint, Right Y Foot/Toe Joint, Left	0 High Osmolar 1 Low Osmolar Y Other Contrast Z None	Z None	Z None

Continued →

Section	B	Imaging
Body System	Q	Non-Axial Lower Bones
Type	2	Computerized Tomography (CT Scan): Computer reformatted digital display of multiplanar images developed from the capture of multiple exposures of external ionizing radiation

Body Part (4th)	Contrast (5th)	Qualifier (6th)	Qualifier (7th)
B Tibia/Fibula, Right C Tibia/Fibula, Left	0 High Osmolar 1 Low Osmolar Y Other Contrast	Z None	Z None

Section	B	Imaging
Body System	Q	Non-Axial Lower Bones
Type	3	Magnetic Resonance Imaging (MRI): Computer reformatted digital display of multiplanar images developed from the capture of radiofrequency signals emitted by nuclei in a body site excited within a magnetic field

Body Part (4th)	Contrast (5th)	Qualifier (6th)	Qualifier (7th)
0 Hip, Right 1 Hip, Left 3 Femur, Right 4 Femur, Left 7 Knee, Right 8 Knee, Left D Lower Leg, Right F Lower Leg, Left G Ankle, Right H Ankle, Left J Calcaneus, Right K Calcaneus, Left L Foot, Right M Foot, Left P Toe(s), Right Q Toe(s), Left V Patella, Right W Patella, Left	Y Other Contrast	0 Unenhanced and Enhanced Z None	Z None
0 Hip, Right 1 Hip, Left 3 Femur, Right 4 Femur, Left 7 Knee, Right 8 Knee, Left D Lower Leg, Right F Lower Leg, Left G Ankle, Right H Ankle, Left J Calcaneus, Right K Calcaneus, Left L Foot, Right M Foot, Left P Toe(s), Right Q Toe(s), Left V Patella, Right W Patella, Left	Z None	Z None	Z None

Section   B   **Imaging**
Body System   Q   **Non-Axial Lower Bones**
Type   4   **Ultrasonography:** Real time display of images of anatomy or flow information developed from the capture of reflected an attenuated high frequency sound waves

Body Part (4ᵗʰ)	Contrast (5ᵗʰ)	Qualifier (6ᵗʰ)	Qualifier (7ᵗʰ)
0 Hip, Right 1 Hip, Left 2 Hips, Bilateral 7 Knee, Right 8 Knee, Left 9 Knees, Bilateral	Z None	Z None	Z None

Section   B   **Imaging**
Body System   R   **Axial Skeleton, Except Skull and Facial Bones**
Type   0   **Plain Radiography:** Planar display of an image developed from the capture of external ionizing radiation on photographic or photoconductive plate

Body Part (4ᵗʰ)	Contrast (5ᵗʰ)	Qualifier (6ᵗʰ)	Qualifier (7ᵗʰ)
0 Cervical Spine 7 Thoracic Spine 9 Lumbar Spine G Whole Spine	Z None	Z None	1 Densitometry Z None
1 Cervical Disc(s) 2 Thoracic Disc(s) 3 Lumbar Disc(s) 4 Cervical Facet Joint(s) 5 Thoracic Facet Joint(s) 6 Lumbar Facet Joint(s) D Sacroiliac Joints	0 High Osmolar 1 Low Osmolar Y Other Contrast Z None	Z None	Z None
8 Thoracolumbar Joint B Lumbosacral Joint C Pelvis F Sacrum and Coccyx H Sternum	Z None	Z None	Z None

Section   B   **Imaging**
Body System   R   **Axial Skeleton, Except Skull and Facial Bones**
Type   1   **Fluoroscopy:** Single plane or bi-plane real time display of an image developed from the capture of external ionizing radiation on a fluorescent screen. The image may also be stored by either digital or analog means

Body Part (4ᵗʰ)	Contrast (5ᵗʰ)	Qualifier (6ᵗʰ)	Qualifier (7ᵗʰ)
0 Cervical Spine 1 Cervical Disc(s) 2 Thoracic Disc(s) 3 Lumbar Disc(s) 4 Cervical Facet Joint(s) 5 Thoracic Facet Joint(s) 6 Lumbar Facet Joint(s) 7 Thoracic Spine 8 Thoracolumbar Joint 9 Lumbar Spine B Lumbosacral Joint C Pelvis D Sacroiliac Joints F Sacrum and Coccyx G Whole Spine H Sternum	0 High Osmolar 1 Low Osmolar Y Other Contrast Z None	Z None	Z None

Section	B	Imaging
Body System	R	Axial Skeleton, Except Skull and Facial Bones
Type	2	**Computerized Tomography (CT Scan):** Computer reformatted digital display of multiplanar images developed from the capture of multiple exposures of external ionizing radiation

Body Part (4th)	Contrast (5th)	Qualifier (6th)	Qualifier (7th)
0 Cervical Spine 7 Thoracic Spine 9 Lumbar Spine C Pelvis D Sacroiliac Joints F Sacrum and Coccyx	0 High Osmolar 1 Low Osmolar Y Other Contrast Z None	Z None	Z None

Section	B	Imaging
Body System	R	Axial Skeleton, Except Skull and Facial Bones
Type	3	**Magnetic Resonance Imaging (MRI):** Computer reformatted digital display of multiplanar images developed from the capture of radiofrequency signals emitted by nuclei in a body site excited within a magnetic field

Body Part (4th)	Contrast (5th)	Qualifier (6th)	Qualifier (7th)
0 Cervical Spine 1 Cervical Disc(s) 2 Thoracic Disc(s) 3 Lumbar Disc(s) 7 Thoracic Spine 9 Lumbar Spine C Pelvis F Sacrum and Coccyx	Y Other Contrast	0 Unenhanced and Enhanced Z None	Z None
0 Cervical Spine 1 Cervical Disc(s) 2 Thoracic Disc(s) 3 Lumbar Disc(s) 7 Thoracic Spine 9 Lumbar Spine C Pelvis F Sacrum and Coccyx	Z None	Z None	Z None

Section	B	Imaging
Body System	R	Axial Skeleton, Except Skull and Facial Bones
Type	4	**Ultrasonography:** Real time display of images of anatomy or flow information developed from the capture of reflected and attenuated high frequency sound waves

Body Part (4th)	Contrast (5th)	Qualifier (6th)	Qualifier (7th)
0 Cervical Spine 7 Thoracic Spine 9 Lumbar Spine F Sacrum and Coccyx	Z None	Z None	Z None

Section	B	Imaging
Body System	T	Urinary System
Type	0	**Plain Radiography:** Planar display of an image developed from the capture of external ionizing radiation on photographic or photoconductive plate

Body Part (4th)	Contrast (5th)	Qualifier (6th)	Qualifier (7th)
0 Bladder 1 Kidney, Right 2 Kidney, Left 3 Kidneys, Bilateral 4 Kidneys, Ureters and Bladder 5 Urethra 6 Ureter, Right 7 Ureter, Left 8 Ureters, Bilateral B Bladder and Urethra C Ileal Diversion Loop	0 High Osmolar 1 Low Osmolar Y Other Contrast Z None	Z None	Z None

Section   **B**   **Imaging**
Body System   **T**   **Urinary System**
Type   **1**   **Fluoroscopy:** Single plane or bi-plane real time display of an image developed from the capture of external ionizing radiation on a fluorescent screen. The image may also be stored by either digital or analog means

Body Part (4th)	Contrast (5th)	Qualifier (6th)	Qualifier (7th)
0 Bladder 1 Kidney, Right 2 Kidney, Left 3 Kidneys, Bilateral 4 Kidneys, Ureters and Bladder 5 Urethra 6 Ureter, Right 7 Ureter, Left B Bladder and Urethra C Ileal Diversion Loop D Kidney, Ureter and Bladder, Right F Kidney, Ureter and Bladder, Left G Ileal Loop, Ureters and Kidneys	0 High Osmolar 1 Low Osmolar Y Other Contrast Z None	Z None	Z None

Section   **B**   **Imaging**
Body System   **T**   **Urinary System**
Type   **2**   **Computerized Tomography (CT Scan):** Computer reformatted digital display of multiplanar images developed from the capture of multiple exposures of external ionizing radiation

Body Part (4th)	Contrast (5th)	Qualifier (6th)	Qualifier (7th)
0 Bladder 1 Kidney, Right 2 Kidney, Left 3 Kidneys, Bilateral 9 Kidney Transplant	0 High Osmolar 1 Low Osmolar Y Other Contrast	0 Unenhanced and Enhanced Z None	Z None
0 Bladder 1 Kidney, Right 2 Kidney, Left 3 Kidneys, Bilateral 9 Kidney Transplant	Z None	Z None	Z None

Section   **B**   **Imaging**
Body System   **T**   **Urinary System**
Type   **3**   **Magnetic Resonance Imaging (MRI):** Computer reformatted digital display of multiplanar images developed from the capture of radiofrequency signals emitted by nuclei in a body site excited within a magnetic field

Body Part (4th)	Contrast (5th)	Qualifier (6th)	Qualifier (7th)
0 Bladder 1 Kidney, Right 2 Kidney, Left 3 Kidneys, Bilateral 9 Kidney Transplant	Y Other Contrast	0 Unenhanced and Enhanced Z None	Z None
0 Bladder 1 Kidney, Right 2 Kidney, Left 3 Kidneys, Bilateral 9 Kidney Transplant	Z None	Z None	Z None

Section	B	Imaging
Body System	T	Urinary System
Type	4	**Ultrasonography:** Real time display of images of anatomy or flow information developed from the capture of reflected and attenuated high frequency sound waves

Body Part (4th)	Contrast (5th)	Qualifier (6th)	Qualifier (7th)
0 Bladder 1 Kidney, Right 2 Kidney, Left 3 Kidneys, Bilateral 5 Urethra 6 Ureter, Right 7 Ureter, Left 8 Ureters, Bilateral 9 Kidney Transplant J Kidneys and Bladder	Z None	Z None	Z None

Section	B	Imaging
Body System	U	Female Reproductive System
Type	0	**Plain Radiography:** Planar display of an image developed from the capture of external ionizing radiation on photographic or photoconductive plate

Body Part (4th)	Contrast (5th)	Qualifier (6th)	Qualifier (7th)
0 Fallopian Tube, Right 1 Fallopian Tube, Left 2 Fallopian Tubes, Bilateral 6 Uterus 8 Uterus and Fallopian Tubes 9 Vagina	0 High Osmolar 1 Low Osmolar Y Other Contrast	Z None	Z None

Section	B	Imaging
Body System	U	Female Reproductive System
Type	1	**Fluoroscopy:** Single plane or bi-plane real time display of an image developed from the capture of external ionizing radiation on a fluorescent screen. The image may also be stored by either digital or analog means

Body Part (4th)	Contrast (5th)	Qualifier (6th)	Qualifier (7th)
0 Fallopian Tube, Right 1 Fallopian Tube, Left 2 Fallopian Tubes, Bilateral 6 Uterus 8 Uterus and Fallopian Tubes 9 Vagina	0 High Osmolar 1 Low Osmolar Y Other Contrast Z None	Z None	Z None

Section	B	Imaging
Body System	U	Female Reproductive System
Type	3	**Magnetic Resonance Imaging (MRI):** Computer reformatted digital display of multiplanar images developed from the capture of radiofrequency signals emitted by nuclei in a body site excited within a magnetic field

Body Part (4th)	Contrast (5th)	Qualifier (6th)	Qualifier (7th)
3 Ovary, Right 4 Ovary, Left 5 Ovaries, Bilateral 6 Uterus 9 Vagina B Pregnant Uterus C Uterus and Ovaries	Y Other Contrast	0 Unenhanced and Enhanced Z None	Z None
3 Ovary, Right 4 Ovary, Left 5 Ovaries, Bilateral 6 Uterus 9 Vagina B Pregnant Uterus C Uterus and Ovaries	Z None	Z None	Z None

Section	B	Imaging
Body System	U	Female Reproductive System
Type	4	**Ultrasonography:** Real time display of images of anatomy or flow information developed from the capture of reflected and attenuated high frequency sound waves

Body Part (4th)	Contrast (5th)	Qualifier (6th)	Qualifier (7th)
0 Fallopian Tube, Right 1 Fallopian Tube, Left 2 Fallopian Tubes, Bilateral 3 Ovary, Right 4 Ovary, Left 5 Ovaries, Bilateral 6 Uterus C Uterus and Ovaries	Y Other Contrast Z None	Z None	Z None

Section	B	Imaging
Body System	V	Male Reproductive System
Type	0	**Plain Radiography:** Planar display of an image developed from the capture of external ionizing radiation on photographic or photoconductive plate

Body Part (4th)	Contrast (5th)	Qualifier (6th)	Qualifier (7th)
0 Corpora Cavernosa 1 Epididymis, Right 2 Epididymis, Left 3 Prostate 5 Testicle, Right 6 Testicle, Left 8 Vasa Vasorum	0 High Osmolar 1 Low Osmolar Y Other Contrast	Z None	Z None

Section	B	Imaging
Body System	V	Male Reproductive System
Type	1	**Fluoroscopy:** Single plane or bi-plane real time display of an image developed from the capture of external ionizing radiation on a fluorescent screen. The image may also be stored by either digital or analog means

Body Part (4th)	Contrast (5th)	Qualifier (6th)	Qualifier (7th)
0 Corpora Cavernosa 8 Vasa Vasorum	0 High Osmolar 1 Low Osmolar Y Other Contrast Z None	Z None	Z None

Section	B	Imaging
Body System	V	Male Reproductive System
Type	2	**Computerized Tomography (CT Scan):** Computer reformatted digital display of multiplanar images developed from the capture of multiple exposures of external ionizing radiation

Body Part (4th)	Contrast (5th)	Qualifier (6th)	Qualifier (7th)
3 Prostate	0 High Osmolar 1 Low Osmolar Y Other Contrast	0 Unenhanced and Enhanced Z None	Z None
3 Prostate	Z None	Z None	Z None

Section	B	Imaging
Body System	V	Male Reproductive System
Type	3	**Magnetic Resonance Imaging (MRI):** Computer reformatted digital display of multiplanar images developed from the capture of radiofrequency signals emitted by nuclei in a body site excited within a magnetic field

Body Part (4th)	Contrast (5th)	Qualifier (6th)	Qualifier (7th)
0 Corpora Cavernosa 3 Prostate 4 Scrotum 5 Testicle, Right 6 Testicle, Left 7 Testicles, Bilateral	Y Other Contrast	0 Unenhanced and Enhanced Z None	Z None
0 Corpora Cavernosa 3 Prostate 4 Scrotum 5 Testicle, Right 6 Testicle, Left 7 Testicles, Bilateral	Z None	Z None	Z None

Section	B	Imaging
Body System	V	Male Reproductive System
Type	4	**Ultrasonography:** Real time display of images of anatomy or flow information developed from the capture of reflected and attenuated high frequency sound waves

Body Part (4th)	Contrast (5th)	Qualifier (6th)	Qualifier (7th)
4 Scrotum 9 Prostate and Seminal Vesicles B Penis	Z None	Z None	Z None

Section	B	Imaging
Body System	W	Anatomical Regions
Type	0	**Plain Radiography:** Planar display of an image developed from the capture of external ionizing radiation on photographic or photoconductive plate

Body Part (4th)	Contrast (5th)	Qualifier (6th)	Qualifier (7th)
0 Abdomen 1 Abdomen and Pelvis 3 Chest B Long Bones, All C Lower Extremity J Upper Extremity K Whole Body L Whole Skeleton M Whole Body, Infant	Z None	Z None	Z None

Section	B	Imaging
Body System	W	Anatomical Regions
Type	1	**Fluoroscopy:** Single plane or bi-plane real time display of an image developed from the capture of external ionizing radiation on a fluorescent screen. The image may also be stored by either digital or analog means

Body Part (4th)	Contrast (5th)	Qualifier (6th)	Qualifier (7th)
1 Abdomen and Pelvis 9 Head and Neck C Lower Extremity J Upper Extremity	0 High Osmolar 1 Low Osmolar Y Other Contrast Z None	Z None	Z None

Section	B	Imaging
Body System	W	Anatomical Regions
Type	2	**Computerized Tomography (CT Scan):** Computer reformatted digital display of multiplanar images developed from the capture of multiple exposures of external ionizing radiation

Body Part (4th)	Contrast (5th)	Qualifier (6th)	Qualifier (7th)
0 Abdomen 1 Abdomen and Pelvis 4 Chest and Abdomen 5 Chest, Abdomen and Pelvis 8 Head 9 Head and Neck F Neck G Pelvic Region	0 High Osmolar 1 Low Osmolar Y Other Contrast	0 Unenhanced and Enhanced Z None	Z None
0 Abdomen 1 Abdomen and Pelvis 4 Chest and Abdomen 5 Chest, Abdomen and Pelvis 8 Head 9 Head and Neck F Neck G Pelvic Region	Z None	Z None	Z None

Section	B	Imaging
Body System	W	Anatomical Regions
Type	3	**Magnetic Resonance Imaging (MRI):** Computer reformatted digital display of multiplanar images developed from the capture of radiofrequency signals emitted by nuclei in a body site excited within a magnetic field

Body Part (4th)	Contrast (5th)	Qualifier (6th)	Qualifier (7th)
0 Abdomen 8 Head F Neck G Pelvic Region H Retroperitoneum P Brachial Plexus	Y Other Contrast	0 Unenhanced and Enhanced Z None	Z None
0 Abdomen 8 Head F Neck G Pelvic Region H Retroperitoneum P Brachial Plexus	Z None	Z None	Z None
3 Chest	Y Other Contrast	0 Unenhanced and Enhanced Z None	Z None

Section	B	Imaging
Body System	W	Anatomical Regions
Type	4	**Ultrasonography:** Real time display of images of anatomy or flow information developed from the capture of reflected and attenuated high frequency sound waves

Body Part (4th)	Contrast (5th)	Qualifier (6th)	Qualifier (7th)
0 Abdomen 1 Abdomen and Pelvis F Neck G Pelvic Region	Z None	Z None	Z None

Section	B	Imaging
Body System	W	Anatomical Regions
Type	5	Other Imaging: Other specified modality for visualizing a body part

Body Part (4th)	Contrast (5th)	Qualifier (6th)	Qualifier (7th)
2 Trunk 9 Head and Neck C Lower Extremity J Upper Extremi	Z None	1 Bacterial Autofluorescence	Z None

Section	B	Imaging
Body System	Y	Fetus and Obstetrical
Type	3	Magnetic Resonance Imaging (MRI): Computer reformatted digital display of multiplanar images developed from the capture of radiofrequency signals emitted by nuclei in a body site excited within a magnetic field

Body Part (4th)	Contrast (5th)	Qualifier (6th)	Qualifier (7th)
0 Fetal Head 1 Fetal Heart 2 Fetal Thorax 3 Fetal Abdomen 4 Fetal Spine 5 Fetal Extremities 6 Whole Fetus	Y Other Contrast	0 Unenhanced and Enhanced Z None	Z None
0 Fetal Head 1 Fetal Heart 2 Fetal Thorax 3 Fetal Abdomen 4 Fetal Spine 5 Fetal Extremities 6 Whole Fetus	Z None	Z None	Z None

Section	B	Imaging
Body System	Y	Fetus and Obstetrical
Type	4	Ultrasonography: Real time display of images of anatomy or flow information developed from the capture of reflected and attenuated high frequency sound waves

Body Part (4th)	Contrast (5th)	Qualifier (6th)	Qualifier (7th)
7 Fetal Umbilical Cord 8 Placenta 9 First Trimester, Single Fetus B First Trimester, Multiple Gestation C Second Trimester, Single Fetus D Second Trimester, Multiple Gestation F Third Trimester, Single Fetus G Third Trimester, Multiple Gestation	Z None	Z None	Z None

AHA Coding Clinic

B2151ZZ Fluoroscopy of Left Heart using Low Osmolar Contrast—AHA CC: 1Q, 2018, 12-13

B518ZZA Fluoroscopy of Superior Vena Cava, Guidance, for Fluoroscopic Guidance used to Place the Renal Dialysis Catheter—AHA CC: 4Q, 2015, 30

Within each section of ICD-10-PCS the characters have different meanings. The seven character meanings for the Nuclear Medicine section are illustrated here through the procedure example of *Technetium tomo scan of liver*.

Section	Body System	Root Type	Body Part	Radionuclide	Qualifier	Qualifier
Nuclear Medicine	Hepatobiliary and Pancreas	Tomographic (Tomo)	Liver	Technetium 99m	None	None
C	F	2	5	1	Z	Z

Section (Character 1)

All Nuclear Medicine procedure codes have a first character value of C.

Body System (Character 2)

The alphanumeric character for the body system is placed in the second position. The following are the body systems applicable to the Nuclear Medicine section.

Character Value	Character Value Description
0	Central Nervous System
2	Heart
5	Veins
7	Lymphatic System
8	Eye
9	Ear, Nose, Mouth and Throat
B	Respiratory System
D	Gastrointestinal System
F	Hepatobiliary System and Pancreas
G	Endocrine System
H	Skin, Subcutaneous Tissue and Breast
P	Musculoskeletal
T	Urinary System
V	Male Reproductive System
W	Anatomical Regions

Root Types (Character 3)

The alphanumeric character value for root types is placed in the third position. The following are the root types applicable to the Nuclear Medicine section with their associated meaning.

Character Value	Root Type	Root Type Definition
1	Planar Nuclear Medicine Imaging	Introduction of radioactive materials into the body for single plane display of images developed from the capture of radioactive emissions
2	Tomographic (Tomo) Nuclear Medicine Imaging	Introduction of radioactive materials into the body for three dimensional display of images developed from the capture of radioactive emissions
3	Positron Emission Tomographic (PET) Imaging	Introduction of radioactive materials into the body for three dimensional display of images developed from the simultaneous capture, 180 degrees apart, of radioactive emissions
4	Nonimaging Nuclear Medicine Uptake	Introduction of radioactive materials into the body for measurements of organ function, from the detection of radioactive emissions
5	Nonimaging Nuclear Medicine Probe	Introduction of radioactive materials into the body for the study of distribution and fate of certain substances by the detection of radioactive emissions; or, alternatively, measurement of absorption of radioactive emissions from an external source

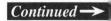

Continued →

Character Value	Root Type	Root Type Definition
6	Nonimaging Nuclear Medicine Assay	Introduction of radioactive materials into the body for the study of body fluids and blood elements, by the detection of radioactive emissions
7	Systemic Nuclear Medicine Therapy	Introduction of unsealed radioactive materials into the body for treatment

Body Part (Character 4)

For each body part the applicable body part character values will be available for procedure code construction. An example of a body part is Cerebrospinal Fluid.

Radionuclide (Character 5)

When radionuclide is utilized during a nuclear medicine procedure, the corresponding radionuclide character value should be reported in the fifth character position. The following are examples of the radionuclide character values available for the Nuclear Medicine section.

- Krypton (Kr-81m)
- Technetium 99m (Tc-99m)
- Xenon 127 (Xe-127)
- Xenon 133 (Xe-133)
- Other Radionuclide

If radionuclide is not utilized, the placeholder character value of Z should be reported.

Qualifier (Character 6)

The qualifier represents an additional attribute for the procedure when applicable. Currently, there are no qualifiers in the Nuclear Medicine section; therefore, the placeholder character value of Z should be reported.

Qualifier (Character 7)

The qualifier represents an additional attribute for the procedure when applicable. Currently, there are no qualifiers in the Nuclear Medicine section; therefore, the placeholder character value of Z should be reported.

Nuclear Medicine Section Tables

Nuclear Medicine Tables C01–CW7

Section	C	**Nuclear Medicine**
Body System	0	**Central Nervous System**
Type	1	**Planar Nuclear Medicine Imaging:** Introduction of radioactive materials into the body for single plane display of images developed from the capture of radioactive emissions

Body Part (4th)	Radionuclide (5th)	Qualifier (6th)	Qualifier (7th)
0 Brain	1 Technetium 99m (Tc-99m) Y Other Radionuclide	Z None	Z None
5 Cerebrospinal Fluid	D Indium 111 (In-111) Y Other Radionuclide	Z None	Z None
Y Central Nervous System	Y Other Radionuclide	Z None	Z None

Section	C	Nuclear Medicine
Body System	0	Central Nervous System
Type	2	**Tomographic (Tomo) Nuclear Medicine Imaging:** Introduction of radioactive materials into the body for three dimensional display of images developed from the capture of radioactive emissions

Body Part (4th)	Radionuclide (5th)	Qualifier (6th)	Qualifier (7th)
0　Brain	1　Technetium 99m (Tc-99m) F　Iodine 123 (I-123) S　Thallium 201 (Tl-201) Y　Other Radionuclide	Z　None	Z　None
5　Cerebrospinal Fluid	D　Indium 111 (In-111) Y　Other Radionuclide	Z　None	Z　None
Y　Central Nervous System	Y　Other Radionuclide	Z　None	Z　None

Section	C	Nuclear Medicine
Body System	0	Central Nervous System
Type	3	**Positron Emission Tomographic (PET) Imaging:** Introduction of radioactive materials into the body for three dimensional display of images developed from the simultaneous capture, 180 degrees apart, of radioactive emissions

Body Part (4th)	Radionuclide (5th)	Qualifier (6th)	Qualifier (7th)
0　Brain	B　Carbon 11 (C-11) K　Fluorine 18 (F-18) M　Oxygen 15 (O-15) Y　Other Radionuclide	Z　None	Z　None
Y　Central Nervous System	Y　Other Radionuclide	Z　None	Z　None

Section	C	Nuclear Medicine
Body System	0	Central Nervous System
Type	5	**Nonimaging Nuclear Medicine Probe:** Introduction of radioactive materials into the body for the study of distribution and fate of certain substances by the detection of radioactive emissions; or, alternatively, measurement of absorption of radioactive emissions from an external source

Body Part (4th)	Radionuclide (5th)	Qualifier (6th)	Qualifier (7th)
0　Brain	V　Xenon 133 (Xe-133) Y　Other Radionuclide	Z　None	Z　None
Y　Central Nervous System	Y　Other Radionuclide	Z　None	Z　None

Section	C	Nuclear Medicine
Body System	2	Heart
Type	1	**Planar Nuclear Medicine Imaging:** Introduction of radioactive materials into the body for single plane display of images developed from the capture of radioactive emissions

Body Part (4th)	Radionuclide (5th)	Qualifier (6th)	Qualifier (7th)
6　Heart, Right and Left	1　Technetium 99m (Tc-99m) Y　Other Radionuclide	Z　None	Z　None
G　Myocardium	1　Technetium 99m (Tc-99m) D　Indium 111 (In-111) S　Thallium 201 (Tl-201) Y　Other Radionuclide Z　None	Z　None	Z　None
Y　Heart	Y　Other Radionuclide	Z　None	Z　None

Section   **C**   **Nuclear Medicine**
Body System   **2**   **Heart**
Type   **2**   **Tomographic (Tomo) Nuclear Medicine Imaging:** Introduction of radioactive materials into the body for three dimensional display of images developed from the capture of radioactive emissions

Body Part (4ᵗʰ)	Radionuclide (5ᵗʰ)	Qualifier (6ᵗʰ)	Qualifier (7ᵗʰ)
6 Heart, Right and Left	**1** Technetium 99m (Tc-99m) **Y** Other Radionuclide	**Z** None	**Z** None
G Myocardium	**1** Technetium 99m (Tc-99m) **D** Indium 111 (In-111) **K** Fluorine 18 (F-18) **S** Thallium 201 (Tl-201) **Y** Other Radionuclide **Z** None	**Z** None	**Z** None
Y Heart	**Y** Other Radionuclide	**Z** None	**Z** None

Section   **C**   **Nuclear Medicine**
Body System   **2**   **Heart**
Type   **3**   **Positron Emission Tomographic (PET) Imaging:** Introduction of radioactive materials into the body for three dimensional display of images developed from the simultaneous capture, 180 degrees apart, of radioactive emissions

Body Part (4ᵗʰ)	Radionuclide (5ᵗʰ)	Qualifier (6ᵗʰ)	Qualifier (7ᵗʰ)
G Myocardium	**K** Fluorine 18 (F-18) **M** Oxygen 15 (O-15) **Q** Rubidium 82 (Rb-82) **R** Nitrogen 13 (N-13) **Y** Other Radionuclide	**Z** None	**Z** None
Y Heart	**Y** Other Radionuclide	**Z** None	**Z** None

Section   **C**   **Nuclear Medicine**
Body System   **2**   **Heart**
Type   **5**   **Nonimaging Nuclear Medicine Probe:** Introduction of radioactive materials into the body for the study of distribution and fate of certain substances by the detection of radioactive emissions; or, alternatively, measurement of absorption of radioactive emissions from an external source

Body Part (4ᵗʰ)	Radionuclide (5ᵗʰ)	Qualifier (6ᵗʰ)	Qualifier (7ᵗʰ)
6 Heart, Right and Left	**1** Technetium 99m (Tc-99m) **Y** Other Radionuclide	**Z** None	**Z** None
Y Heart	**Y** Other Radionuclide	**Z** None	**Z** None

Section   **C**   **Nuclear Medicine**
Body System   **5**   **Veins**
Type   **1**   **Planar Nuclear Medicine Imaging:** Introduction of radioactive materials into the body for single plane display of images developed from the capture of radioactive emissions

Body Part (4ᵗʰ)	Radionuclide (5ᵗʰ)	Qualifier (6ᵗʰ)	Qualifier (7ᵗʰ)
B Lower Extremity Veins, Right **C** Lower Extremity Veins, Left **D** Lower Extremity Veins, Bilateral **N** Upper Extremity Veins, Right **P** Upper Extremity Veins, Left **Q** Upper Extremity Veins, Bilateral **R** Central Veins	**1** Technetium 99m (Tc-99m) **Y** Other Radionuclide	**Z** None	**Z** None
Y Veins	**Y** Other Radionuclide	**Z** None	**Z** None

Section	C	Nuclear Medicine
Body System	7	Lymphatic and Hematologic System
Type	1	**Planar Nuclear Medicine Imaging:** Introduction of radioactive materials into the body for single plane display of images developed from the capture of radioactive emissions

Body Part (4th)	Radionuclide (5th)	Qualifier (6th)	Qualifier (7th)
0 Bone Marrow	1 Technetium 99m (Tc-99m) D Indium 111 (In-111) Y Other Radionuclide	Z None	Z None
2 Spleen 5 Lymphatics, Head and Neck D Lymphatics, Pelvic J Lymphatics, Head K Lymphatics, Neck L Lymphatics, Upper Chest M Lymphatics, Trunk N Lymphatics, Upper Extremity P Lymphatics, Lower Extremity	1 Technetium 99m (Tc-99m) Y Other Radionuclide	Z None	Z None
3 Blood	D Indium 111 (In-111) Y Other Radionuclide	Z None	Z None
Y Lymphatic and Hematologic System	Y Other Radionuclide	Z None	Z None

Section	C	Nuclear Medicine
Body System	7	Lymphatic and Hematologic System
Type	2	**Tomographic (Tomo) Nuclear Medicine Imaging:** Introduction of radioactive materials into the body for three dimensional display of images developed from the capture of radioactive emissions

Body Part (4th)	Radionuclide (5th)	Qualifier (6th)	Qualifier (7th)
2 Spleen	1 Technetium 99m (Tc-99m) Y Other Radionuclide	Z None	Z None
Y Lymphatic and Hematologic System	Y Other Radionuclide	Z None	Z None

Section	C	Nuclear Medicine
Body System	7	Lymphatic and Hematologic System
Type	5	**Nonimaging Nuclear Medicine Probe:** Introduction of radioactive materials into the body for the study of distribution and fate of certain substances by the detection of radioactive emissions; or, alternatively, measurement of absorption of radioactive emissions from an external source

Body Part (4th)	Radionuclide (5th)	Qualifier (6th)	Qualifier (7th)
5 Lymphatics, Head and Neck D Lymphatics, Pelvic J Lymphatics, Head K Lymphatics, Neck L Lymphatics, Upper Chest M Lymphatics, Trunk N Lymphatics, Upper Extremity P Lymphatics, Lower Extremity	1 Technetium 99m (Tc-99m) Y Other Radionuclide	Z None	Z None
Y Lymphatic and Hematologic System	Y Other Radionuclide	Z None	Z None

Section	C	Nuclear Medicine
Body System	7	Lymphatic and Hematologic System
Type	6	**Nonimaging Nuclear Medicine Assay:** Introduction of radioactive materials into the body for the study of body fluids and blood elements, by the detection of radioactive emissions

Body Part (4th)	Radionuclide (5th)	Qualifier (6th)	Qualifier (7th)
3 Blood	1 Technetium 99m (Tc-99m) 7 Cobalt 58 (Co-58) C Cobalt 57 (Co-57) D Indium 111 (In-111) H Iodine 125 (I-125) W Chromium (Cr-51) Y Other Radionuclide	Z None	Z None
Y Lymphatic and Hematologic System	Y Other Radionuclide	Z None	Z None

Section	C	Nuclear Medicine
Body System	8	Eye
Type	1	**Planar Nuclear Medicine Imaging:** Introduction of radioactive materials into the body for single plane display of images developed from the capture of radioactive emissions

Body Part (4th)	Radionuclide (5th)	Qualifier (6th)	Qualifier (7th)
9 Lacrimal Ducts, Bilateral	1 Technetium 99m (Tc-99m) Y Other Radionuclide	Z None	Z None
Y Eye	Y Other Radionuclide	Z None	Z None

Section	C	Nuclear Medicine
Body System	9	Ear, Nose, Mouth and Throat
Type	1	**Planar Nuclear Medicine Imaging:** Introduction of radioactive materials into the body for single plane display of images developed from the capture of radioactive emissions

Body Part (4th)	Radionuclide (5th)	Qualifier (6th)	Qualifier (7th)
B Salivary Glands, Bilateral	1 Technetium 99m (Tc-99m) Y Other Radionuclide	Z None	Z None
Y Ear, Nose, Mouth and Throat	Y Other Radionuclide	Z None	Z None

Section	C	Nuclear Medicine
Body System	B	Respiratory System
Type	1	**Planar Nuclear Medicine Imaging:** Introduction of radioactive materials into the body for single plane display of images developed from the capture of radioactive emissions

Body Part (4th)	Radionuclide (5th)	Qualifier (6th)	Qualifier (7th)
2 Lungs and Bronchi	1 Technetium 99m (Tc-99m) 9 Krypton (Kr-81m) T Xenon 127 (Xe-127) V Xenon 133 (Xe-133) Y Other Radionuclide	Z None	Z None
Y Respiratory System	Y Other Radionuclide	Z None	Z None

Section	C	Nuclear Medicine
Body System	B	Respiratory System
Type	2	**Tomographic (Tomo) Nuclear Medicine Imaging:** Introduction of radioactive materials into the body for three dimensional display of images developed from the capture of radioactive emissions

Body Part (4th)	Radionuclide (5th)	Qualifier (6th)	Qualifier (7th)
2 Lungs and Bronchi	1 Technetium 99m (Tc-99m) 9 Krypton (Kr-81m) Y Other Radionuclide	Z None	Z None
Y Respiratory System	Y Other Radionuclide	Z None	Z None

Section	C	Nuclear Medicine
Body System	B	Respiratory System
Type	3	**Positron Emission Tomographic (PET) Imaging:** Introduction of radioactive materials into the body for three dimensional display of images developed from the simultaneous capture, 180 degrees apart, of radioactive emissions

Body Part (4th)	Radionuclide (5th)	Qualifier (6th)	Qualifier (7th)
2 Lungs and Bronchi	K Fluorine 18 (F-18) Y Other Radionuclide	Z None	Z None
Y Respiratory System	Y Other Radionuclide	Z None	Z None

Section	C	Nuclear Medicine
Body System	D	Gastrointestinal System
Type	1	**Planar Nuclear Medicine Imaging:** Introduction of radioactive materials into the body for single plane display of images developed from the capture of radioactive emissions

Body Part (4th)	Radionuclide (5th)	Qualifier (6th)	Qualifier (7th)
5 Upper Gastrointestinal Tract 7 Gastrointestinal Tract	1 Technetium 99m (Tc-99m) D Indium 111 (In-111) Y Other Radionuclide	Z None	Z None
Y Digestive System	Y Other Radionuclide	Z None	Z None

Section	C	Nuclear Medicine
Body System	D	Gastrointestinal System
Type	2	**Tomographic (Tomo) Nuclear Medicine Imaging:** Introduction of radioactive materials into the body for three dimensional display of images developed from the capture of radioactive emissions

Body Part (4th)	Radionuclide (5th)	Qualifier (6th)	Qualifier (7th)
7 Gastrointestinal Tract	1 Technetium 99m (Tc-99m) D Indium 111 (In-111) Y Other Radionuclide	Z None	Z None
Y Digestive System	Y Other Radionuclide	Z None	Z None

Section	C	Nuclear Medicine
Body System	F	Hepatobiliary System and Pancreas
Type	1	**Planar Nuclear Medicine Imaging:** Introduction of radioactive materials into the body for single plane display of images developed from the capture of radioactive emissions

Body Part (4th)	Radionuclide (5th)	Qualifier (6th)	Qualifier (7th)
4 Gallbladder 5 Liver 6 Liver and Spleen C Hepatobiliary System, All	1 Technetium 99m (Tc-99m) Y Other Radionuclide	Z None	Z None
Y Hepatobiliary System and Pancreas	Y Other Radionuclide	Z None	Z None

Section	C	Nuclear Medicine
Body System	F	Hepatobiliary System and Pancreas
Type	2	Tomographic (Tomo) Nuclear Medicine Imaging: Introduction of radioactive materials into the body for three dimensional display of images developed from the capture of radioactive emissions

Body Part (4th)	Radionuclide (5th)	Qualifier (6th)	Qualifier (7th)
4 Gallbladder 5 Liver 6 Liver and Spleen	1 Technetium 99m (Tc-99m) Y Other Radionuclide	Z None	Z None
Y Hepatobiliary System and Pancreas	Y Other Radionuclide	Z None	Z None

Section	C	Nuclear Medicine
Body System	G	Endocrine System
Type	1	Planar Nuclear Medicine Imaging: Introduction of radioactive materials into the body for single plane display of images developed from the capture of radioactive emissions

Body Part (4th)	Radionuclide (5th)	Qualifier (6th)	Qualifier (7th)
1 Parathyroid Glands	1 Technetium 99m (Tc-99m) S Thallium 201 (Tl-201) Y Other Radionuclide	Z None	Z None
2 Thyroid Gland	1 Technetium 99m (Tc-99m) F Iodine 123 (I-123) G Iodine 131 (I-131) Y Other Radionuclide	Z None	Z None
4 Adrenal Glands, Bilateral	G Iodine 131 (I-131) Y Other Radionuclide	Z None	Z None
Y Endocrine System	Y Other Radionuclide	Z None	Z None

Section	C	Nuclear Medicine
Body System	G	Endocrine System
Type	2	Tomographic (Tomo) Nuclear Medicine Imaging: Introduction of radioactive materials into the body for three dimensional display of images developed from the capture of radioactive emissions

Body Part (4th)	Radionuclide (5th)	Qualifier (6th)	Qualifier (7th)
1 Parathyroid Glands	1 Technetium 99m (Tc-99m) S Thallium 201 (Tl-201) Y Other Radionuclide	Z None	Z None
Y Endocrine System	Y Other Radionuclide	Z None	Z None

Section	C	Nuclear Medicine
Body System	G	Endocrine System
Type	4	Nonimaging Nuclear Medicine Uptake: Introduction of radioactive materials into the body for measurements of organ function, from the detection of radioactive emissions

Body Part (4th)	Radionuclide (5th)	Qualifier (6th)	Qualifier (7th)
2 Thyroid Gland	1 Technetium 99m (Tc-99m) F Iodine 123 (I-123) G Iodine 131 (I-131) Y Other Radionuclide	Z None	Z None
Y Endocrine System	Y Other Radionuclide	Z None	Z None

Section	C	Nuclear Medicine
Body System	H	Skin, Subcutaneous Tissue and Breast
Type	1	**Planar Nuclear Medicine Imaging:** Introduction of radioactive materials into the body for single plane display of images developed from the capture of radioactive emissions

Body Part (4th)	Radionuclide (5th)	Qualifier (6th)	Qualifier (7th)
0 Breast, Right 1 Breast, Left 2 Breasts, Bilateral	1 Technetium 99m (Tc-99m) S Thallium 201 (Tl-201) Y Other Radionuclide	Z None	Z None
Y Skin, Subcutaneous Tissue and Breast	Y Other Radionuclide	Z None	Z None

Section	C	Nuclear Medicine
Body System	H	Skin, Subcutaneous Tissue and Breast
Type	2	**Tomographic (Tomo) Nuclear Medicine Imaging:** Introduction of radioactive materials into the body for three dimensional display of images developed from the capture of radioactive emissions

Body Part (4th)	Radionuclide (5th)	Qualifier (6th)	Qualifier (7th)
0 Breast, Right 1 Breast, Left 2 Breasts, Bilateral	1 Technetium 99m (Tc-99m) S Thallium 201 (Tl-201) Y Other Radionuclide	Z None	Z None
Y Skin, Subcutaneous Tissue and Breast	Y Other Radionuclide	Z None	Z None

Section	C	Nuclear Medicine
Body System	P	Musculoskeletal System
Type	1	**Planar Nuclear Medicine Imaging:** Introduction of radioactive materials into the body for single plane display of images developed from the capture of radioactive emissions

Body Part (4th)	Radionuclide (5th)	Qualifier (6th)	Qualifier (7th)
1 Skull 4 Thorax 5 Spine 6 Pelvis 7 Spine and Pelvis 8 Upper Extremity, Right 9 Upper Extremity, Left B Upper Extremities, Bilateral C Lower Extremity, Right D Lower Extremity, Left F Lower Extremities, Bilateral Z Musculoskeletal System, All	1 Technetium 99m (Tc-99m) Y Other Radionuclide	Z None	Z None
Y Musculoskeletal System, Other	Y Other Radionuclide	Z None	Z None

Section	C	Nuclear Medicine
Body System	P	Musculoskeletal System
Type	2	**Tomographic (Tomo) Nuclear Medicine Imaging:** Introduction of radioactive materials into the body for three dimensional display of images developed from the capture of radioactive emissions

Body Part (4th)	Radionuclide (5th)	Qualifier (6th)	Qualifier (7th)
1 Skull 2 Cervical Spine 3 Skull and Cervical Spine 4 Thorax 6 Pelvis 7 Spine and Pelvis 8 Upper Extremity, Right 9 Upper Extremity, Left B Upper Extremities, Bilateral C Lower Extremity, Right D Lower Extremity, Left F Lower Extremities, Bilateral G Thoracic Spine H Lumbar Spine J Thoracolumbar Spine	1 Technetium 99m (Tc-99m) Y Other Radionuclide	Z None	Z None
Y Musculoskeletal System, Other	Y Other Radionuclide	Z None	Z None

Section	C	Nuclear Medicine
Body System	P	Musculoskeletal System
Type	5	**Nonimaging Nuclear Medicine Probe:** Introduction of radioactive materials into the body for the study of distribution and fate of certain substances by the detection of radioactive emissions; or, alternatively, measurement of absorption of radioactive emissions from an external source

Body Part (4th)	Radionuclide (5th)	Qualifier (6th)	Qualifier (7th)
5 Spine N Upper Extremities P Lower Extremities	Z None	Z None	Z None
Y Musculoskeletal System, Other	Y Other Radionuclide	Z None	Z None

Section	C	Nuclear Medicine
Body System	T	Urinary System
Type	1	**Planar Nuclear Medicine Imaging:** Introduction of radioactive materials into the body for single plane display of images developed from the capture of radioactive emissions

Body Part (4th)	Radionuclide (5th)	Qualifier (6th)	Qualifier (7th)
3 Kidneys, Ureters and Bladder	1 Technetium 99m (Tc-99m) F Iodine 123 (I-123) G Iodine 131 (I-131) Y Other Radionuclide	Z None	Z None
H Bladder and Ureters	1 Technetium 99m (Tc-99m) Y Other Radionuclide	Z None	Z None
Y Urinary System	Y Other Radionuclide	Z None	Z None

Section	C	Nuclear Medicine
Body System	T	Urinary System
Type	2	**Tomographic (Tomo) Nuclear Medicine Imaging:** Introduction of radioactive materials into the body for three dimensional display of images developed from the capture of radioactive emissions

Body Part (4th)	Radionuclide (5th)	Qualifier (6th)	Qualifier (7th)
3 Kidneys, Ureters and Bladder	1 Technetium 99m (Tc-99m) Y Other Radionuclide	Z None	Z None
Y Urinary System	Y Other Radionuclide	Z None	Z None

Section C **Nuclear Medicine**
Body System T **Urinary System**
Type 6 **Nonimaging Nuclear Medicine Assay:** Introduction of radioactive materials into the body for the study of body fluids and blood elements, by the detection of radioactive emissions

Body Part (4th)	Radionuclide (5th)	Qualifier (6th)	Qualifier (7th)
3 Kidneys, Ureters and Bladder	1 Technetium 99m (Tc-99m) F Iodine 123 (I-123) G Iodine 131 (I-131) H Iodine 125 (I-125) Y Other Radionuclide	Z None	Z None
Y Urinary System	Y Other Radionuclide	Z None	Z None

Section C **Nuclear Medicine**
Body System V **Male Reproductive System**
Type 1 **Planar Nuclear Medicine Imaging:** Introduction of radioactive materials into the body for single plane display of images developed from the capture of radioactive emissions

Body Part (4th)	Radionuclide (5th)	Qualifier (6th)	Qualifier (7th)
9 Testicles, Bilateral	1 Technetium 99m (Tc-99m) Y Other Radionuclide	Z None	Z None
Y Male Reproductive System	Y Other Radionuclide	Z None	Z None

Section C **Nuclear Medicine**
Body System W **Anatomical Regions**
Type 1 **Planar Nuclear Medicine Imaging:** Introduction of radioactive materials into the body for single plane display of images developed from the capture of radioactive emissions

Body Part (4th)	Radionuclide (5th)	Qualifier (6th)	Qualifier (7th)
0 Abdomen 1 Abdomen and Pelvis 4 Chest and Abdomen 6 Chest and Neck B Head and Neck D Lower Extremity J Pelvic Region M Upper Extremity N Whole Body	1 Technetium 99m (Tc-99m) D Indium 111 (In-111) F Iodine 123 (I-123) G Iodine 131 (I-131) L Gallium 67 (Ga-67) S Thallium 201 (Tl-201) Y Other Radionuclide	Z None	Z None
3 Chest	1 Technetium 99m (Tc-99m) D Indium 111 (In-111) F Iodine 123 (I-123) G Iodine 131 (I-131) K Fluorine 18 (F-18) L Gallium 67 (Ga-67) S Thallium 201 (Tl-201) Y Other Radionuclide	Z None	Z None
Y Anatomical Regions, Multiple	Y Other Radionuclide	Z None	Z None
Z Anatomical Region, Other	Z None	Z None	Z None

Section	C	Nuclear Medicine
Body System	W	Anatomical Regions
Type	2	**Tomographic (Tomo) Nuclear Medicine Imaging:** Introduction of radioactive materials into the body for three dimensional display of images developed from the capture of radioactive emissions

Body Part (4th)	Radionuclide (5th)	Qualifier (6th)	Qualifier (7th)
0 Abdomen 1 Abdomen and Pelvis 3 Chest 4 Chest and Abdomen 6 Chest and Neck B Head and Neck D Lower Extremity J Pelvic Region M Upper Extremity	1 Technetium 99m (Tc-99m) D Indium 111 (In-111) F Iodine 123 (I-123) G Iodine 131 (I-131) K Fluorine 18 (F-18) L Gallium 67 (Ga-67) S Thallium 201 (Tl-201) Y Other Radionuclide	Z None	Z None
Y Anatomical Regions, Multiple	Y Other Radionuclide	Z None	Z None

Section	C	Nuclear Medicine
Body System	W	Anatomical Regions
Type	3	**Positron Emission Tomographic (PET) Imaging:** Introduction of radioactive materials into the body for three dimensional display of images developed from the simultaneous capture, 180 degrees apart, of radioactive emissions

Body Part (4th)	Radionuclide (5th)	Qualifier (6th)	Qualifier (7th)
N Whole Body	Y Other Radionuclide	Z None	Z None

Section	C	Nuclear Medicine
Body System	W	Anatomical Regions
Type	5	**Nonimaging Nuclear Medicine Probe:** Introduction of radioactive materials into the body for the study of distribution and fate of certain substances by the detection of radioactive emissions; or, alternatively, measurement of absorption of radioactive emissions from an external source

Body Part (4th)	Radionuclide (5th)	Qualifier (6th)	Qualifier (7th)
0 Abdomen 1 Abdomen and Pelvis 3 Chest 4 Chest and Abdomen 6 Chest and Neck B Head and Neck D Lower Extremity J Pelvic Region M Upper Extremity	1 Technetium 99m (Tc-99m) D Indium 111 (In-111) Y Other Radionuclide	Z None	Z None

Section	C	Nuclear Medicine
Body System	W	Anatomical Regions
Type	7	**Systemic Nuclear Medicine Therapy:** Introduction of unsealed radioactive materials into the body for treatment

Body Part (4th)	Radionuclide (5th)	Qualifier (6th)	Qualifier (7th)
0 Abdomen 3 Chest	N Phosphorus 32 (P-32) Y Other Radionuclide	Z None	Z None
G Thyroid	G Iodine 131 (I-131) Y Other Radionuclide	Z None	Z None
N Whole Body	8 Samarium 153 (Sm-153) G Iodine 131 (I-131) N Phosphorus 32 (P-32) P Strontium 89 (Sr-89) Y Other Radionuclide	Z None	Z None
Y Anatomical Regions, Multiple	Y Other Radionuclide	Z None	Z None

AHA Coding Clinic

No references have been issued for the Nuclear Medicine section.

Within each section of ICD-10-PCS the characters have different meanings. The seven character meanings for the Radiation Therapy section are illustrated here through the procedure example of *HDR brachytherapy of prostate using Palladium 103*.

Section	Body System	Modality	Treatment Site	Modality Qualifier	Isotope	Qualifier
Radiation Therapy	Male Reproductive System	Brachytherapy	Prostate	High Dose Rate (HDR)	Palladium 103	None
D	V	1	0	9	B	Z

Section (Character 1)

All Radiation Therapy procedure codes have a first character value of D.

Body System (Character 2)

The alphanumeric character for the body system is placed in the second position. The following are the body systems applicable to the Radiation Therapy section.

Character Value	Character Value Description
0	Central and Peripheral Nervous System
7	Lymphatic and Hematologic System
8	Eye
9	Ear, Nose, Mouth and Throat
B	Respiratory System
D	Gastrointestinal System
F	Hepatobiliary System and Pancreas
G	Endocrine System
H	Skin
M	Breast
P	Musculoskeletal
T	Urinary System
U	Female Reproductive System
V	Male Reproductive System
W	Anatomical Regions

Modality (Character 3)

The alphanumeric character value for root types is placed in the third position. The following are the root types applicable to the Radiation Therapy section with their associated meaning.

Character Value	Modality	Modality Definition
0	Beam Radiation	The external use of high-energy radiation such as x-rays, photons, electrons, or protons
1	Brachytherapy	The use of radioactive sources placed directly into a tumor bearing area to generate local regions of high intensity radiation
2	Stereotactic Radiosurgery	The use of external radiation sources either from a linear accelerator or a special Cobalt-60 irradiator to deliver many beams of radiation directly to an internal structure in a single fraction
Y	Other Radiation	Other types of radiation therapy such as hyperthermia, contact radiation and plaque radiation. *See Modality qualifier, character 5, for specified types of other radiation.*

Source: CSI Navigator for Radiation Oncology, 2010

Treatment Site (Character 4)

For each treatment site the applicable body part character values will be available for procedure code construction. An example of a treatment site for this section is Brain Stem.

Modality Qualifier (Character 5)

The modality qualifier further specifies the treatment modality. The following are examples of the modality qualifier values available for the Radiation Therapy section:

- Photons >10 MeV
- Neutrons
- Electrons
- High Dose Rate
- Hyperthermia

Isotope (Character 6)

When an isotope is utilized during a radiation oncology procedure, the corresponding isotope character value should be reported in the sixth character position. The following are examples of the isotope character values available for the Radiation Therapy section:

- Iridium 192 (Ir-192)
- Iodine 125 (I-125)
- Californium 252 (Cf-252)

Qualifier (Character 7)

The qualifier represents an additional attribute for the procedure when applicable. For example, beam radiation procedures in this section include the qualifier Intraoperative that is reported with the character value of 0 for some body parts. If there is no qualifier for a procedure, the placeholder Z is the character value that should be reported.

Radiation Therapy Section Guidelines (section D)

D. Radiation Therapy Section

Brachytherapy
D1.a

Brachytherapy is coded to the modality Brachytherapy in the Radiation Therapy section. When a radioactive brachytherapy source is left in the body at the end of the procedure, it is coded separately to the root operation Insertion with the device value Radioactive Element.

Example: Brachytherapy with implantation of a low dose rate brachytherapy source left in the body at the end of the procedure is coded to the applicable treatment site in section D, Radiation Therapy, with the modality Brachytherapy, the modality qualifier value, Low Dose Rate, and the applicable isotope value and qualifier value. The implantation of the brachytherapy source is coded separately to the device value Radioactive Element in the appropriate Insertion table of the Medical and Surgical section. The Radiation Therapy section code identifies the specific modality and isotope of the brachytherapy, and the root operation Insertion code identifies the implantation of the brachytherapy source that remain in the body at the end of the procedure.

Exception: Implantation of Cesium-131 brachytherapy seeds embedded in a collagen matrix to the treatment site after resection of brain tumor is coded to the root operation Insertion with the device value Radioactive Element, Cesium-131 Collagen Implant. The procedure is coded to the root operation Insertion only, because the device value identifies both the implantation of the radioactive element and a specific brachytherapy isotope that is not included in the Radiation Therapy section tables.

D1.b

A separate procedure to place a temporary applicator for delivering the brachytherapy is coded to the root operation Insertion and the device value Other Device.

Examples: Intrauterine brachytherapy applicator placed as a separate procedure from the brachytherapy procedure is coded to Insertion of Other Device, and the brachytherapy is coded separately using the modality Brachytherapy in the Radiation Therapy section. Intrauterine brachytherapy applicator placed concomitantly with delivery of the brachytherapy dose is coded with a single code using the modality Brachytherapy in the Radiation Therapy section.

Radiation Therapy Section Tables

Radiation Therapy Tables D00–DWY

Section	D	Radiation Therapy
Body System	0	Central and Peripheral Nervous System
Modality	0	Beam Radiation

Treatment Site (4th)	Modality Qualifier (5th)	Isotope (6th)	Qualifier (7th)
0 Brain 1 Brain Stem 6 Spinal Cord 7 Peripheral Nerve	0 Photons <1 MeV 1 Photons 1 - 10 MeV 2 Photons >10 MeV 4 Heavy Particles (Protons,Ions) 5 Neutrons 6 Neutron Capture	Z None	Z None
0 Brain 1 Brain Stem 6 Spinal Cord 7 Peripheral Nerve	3 Electrons	Z None	0 Intraoperative Z None

Section	D	Radiation Therapy
Body System	0	Central and Peripheral Nervous System
Modality	1	Brachytherapy

Treatment Site (4th)	Modality Qualifier (5th)	Isotope (6th)	Qualifier (7th)
0 Brain 1 Brain Stem 6 Spinal Cord 7 Peripheral Nerve	9 High Dose Rate (HDR)	7 Cesium 137 (Cs-137) 8 Iridium 192 (Ir-192) 9 Iodine 125 (I-125) B Palladium 103 (Pd-103) C Californium 252 (Cf-252) Y Other Isotope	Z None
0 Brain 1 Brain Stem 6 Spinal Cord 7 Peripheral Nerve	B Low Dose Rate (LDR)	6 Cesium 131 (Cs-131) 7 Cesium 137 (Cs-137) 8 Iridium 192 (Ir-192) 9 Iodine 125 (I-125) C Californium 252 (Cf-252) Y Other Isotope	Z None
0 Brain 1 Brain Stem 6 Spinal Cord 7 Peripheral Nerve	B Low Dose Rate (LDR)	B Palladium 103 (Pd-103)	1 Unidirectional Source Z None

Section	D	Radiation Therapy
Body System	0	Central and Peripheral Nervous System
Modality	2	Stereotactic Radiosurgery

Treatment Site (4th)	Modality Qualifier (5th)	Isotope (6th)	Qualifier (7th)
0 Brain 1 Brain Stem 6 Spinal Cord 7 Peripheral Nerve	D Stereotactic Other Photon Radiosurgery H Stereotactic Particulate Radiosurgery J Stereotactic Gamma Beam Radiosurgery	Z None	Z None

Section	D	Radiation Therapy
Body System	0	Central and Peripheral Nervous System
Modality	Y	Other Radiation

Treatment Site (4th)	Modality Qualifier (5th)	Isotope (6th)	Qualifier (7th)
0 Brain 1 Brain Stem 6 Spinal Cord 7 Peripheral Nerve	7 Contact Radiation 8 Hyperthermia C Intraoperative Radiation Therapy (IORT) F Plaque Radiation K Laser Interstitial Thermal Therapy	Z None	Z None

Section   D   Radiation Therapy
Body System   7   Lymphatic and Hematologic System
Modality   0   Beam Radiation

Treatment Site (4th)	Modality Qualifier (5th)	Isotope (6th)	Qualifier (7th)
0 Bone Marrow 1 Thymus 2 Spleen 3 Lymphatics, Neck 4 Lymphatics, Axillary 5 Lymphatics, Thorax 6 Lymphatics, Abdomen 7 Lymphatics, Pelvis 8 Lymphatics, Inguinal	0 Photons <1 MeV 1 Photons 1 - 10 MeV 2 Photons >10 MeV 4 Heavy Particles (Protons,Ions) 5 Neutrons 6 Neutron Capture	Z None	Z None
0 Bone Marrow 1 Thymus 2 Spleen 3 Lymphatics, Neck 4 Lymphatics, Axillary 5 Lymphatics, Thorax 6 Lymphatics, Abdomen 7 Lymphatics, Pelvis 8 Lymphatics, Inguinal	3 Electrons	Z None	0 Intraoperative Z None

Section   D   Radiation Therapy
Body System   7   Lymphatic and Hematologic System
Modality   1   Brachytherapy

Treatment Site (4th)	Modality Qualifier (5th)	Isotope (6th)	Qualifier (7th)
0 Bone Marrow 1 Thymus 2 Spleen 3 Lymphatics, Neck 4 Lymphatics, Axillary 5 Lymphatics, Thorax 6 Lymphatics, Abdomen 7 Lymphatics, Pelvis 8 Lymphatics, Inguinal	9 High Dose Rate (HDR)	7 Cesium 137 (Cs-137) 8 Iridium 192 (Ir-192) 9 Iodine 125 (I-125) B Palladium 103 (Pd-103) C Californium 252 (Cf-252) Y Other Isotope	Z None
0 Bone Marrow 1 Thymus 2 Spleen 3 Lymphatics, Neck 4 Lymphatics, Axillary 5 Lymphatics, Thorax 6 Lymphatics, Abdomen 7 Lymphatics, Pelvis 8 Lymphatics, Inguinal	B Low Dose Rate (LDR)	6 Cesium 131 (Cs-131) 7 Cesium 137 (Cs-137) 8 Iridium 192 (Ir-192) 9 Iodine 125 (I-125) C Californium 252 (Cf-252) Y Other Isotope	Z None
0 Bone Marrow 1 Thymus 2 Spleen 3 Lymphatics, Neck 4 Lymphatics, Axillary 5 Lymphatics, Thorax 6 Lymphatics, Abdomen 7 Lymphatics, Pelvis 8 Lymphatics, Inguinal	B Low Dose Rate (LDR)	B Palladium 103 (Pd-103)	1 Unidirectional Source Z None

Section	D	Radiation Therapy
Body System	7	Lymphatic and Hematologic System
Modality	2	Stereotactic Radiosurgery

Treatment Site (4th)	Modality Qualifier (5th)	Isotope (6th)	Qualifier (7th)
0 Bone Marrow 1 Thymus 2 Spleen 3 Lymphatics, Neck 4 Lymphatics, Axillary 5 Lymphatics, Thorax 6 Lymphatics, Abdomen 7 Lymphatics, Pelvis 8 Lymphatics, Inguinal	D Stereotactic Other Photon Radiosurgery H Stereotactic Particulate Radiosurgery J Stereotactic Gamma Beam Radiosurgery	Z None	Z None

Section	D	Radiation Therapy
Body System	7	Lymphatic and Hematologic System
Modality	Y	Other Radiation

Treatment Site (4th)	Modality Qualifier (5th)	Isotope (6th)	Qualifier (7th)
0 Bone Marrow 1 Thymus 2 Spleen 3 Lymphatics, Neck 4 Lymphatics, Axillary 5 Lymphatics, Thorax 6 Lymphatics, Abdomen 7 Lymphatics, Pelvis 8 Lymphatics, Inguinal	8 Hyperthermia F Plaque Radiation	Z None	Z None

Section	D	Radiation Therapy
Body System	8	Eye
Modality	0	Beam Radiation

Treatment Site (4th)	Modality Qualifier (5th)	Isotope (6th)	Qualifier (7th)
0 Eye	0 Photons <1 MeV 1 Photons 1 - 10 MeV 2 Photons >10 MeV 4 Heavy Particles (Protons,Ions) 5 Neutrons 6 Neutron Capture	Z None	Z None
0 Eye	3 Electrons	Z None	0 Intraoperative Z None

Section	D	Radiation Therapy
Body System	8	Eye
Modality	1	Brachytherapy

Treatment Site (4th)	Modality Qualifier (5th)	Isotope (6th)	Qualifier (7th)
0 Eye	9 High Dose Rate (HDR)	7 Cesium 137 (Cs-137) 8 Iridium 192 (Ir-192) 9 Iodine 125 (I-125) B Palladium 103 (Pd-103) C Californium 252 (Cf-252) Y Other Isotope	Z None
0 Eye	B Low Dose Rate (LDR)	6 Cesium 131 (Cs-131) 7 Cesium 137 (Cs-137) 8 Iridium 192 (Ir-192) 9 Iodine 125 (I-125) C Californium 252 (Cf-252) Y Other Isotope	Z None

Continued →

Section | D | Radiation Therapy
Body System | 8 | Eye
Modality | 1 | Brachytherapy

Treatment Site (4th)	Modality Qualifier (5th)	Isotope (6th)	Qualifier (7th)
0 Eye	**B** Low Dose Rate (LDR)	**B** Palladium 103 (Pd-103)	**1** Unidirectional Source **Z** None

Section | D | Radiation Therapy
Body System | 8 | Eye
Modality | 2 | Stereotactic Radiosurgery

Treatment Site (4th)	Modality Qualifier (5th)	Isotope (6th)	Qualifier (7th)
0 Eye	**D** Stereotactic Other Photon Radiosurgery **H** Stereotactic Particulate Radiosurgery **J** Stereotactic Gamma Beam Radiosurgery	**Z** None	**Z** None

Section | D | Radiation Therapy
Body System | 8 | Eye
Modality | Y | Other Radiation

Treatment Site (4th)	Modality Qualifier (5th)	Isotope (6th)	Qualifier (7th)
0 Eye	**7** Contact Radiation **8** Hyperthermia **F** Plaque Radiation	**Z** None	**Z** None

Section | D | Radiation Therapy
Body System | 9 | Ear, Nose, Mouth and Throat
Modality | 0 | Beam Radiation

Treatment Site (4th)	Modality Qualifier (5th)	Isotope (6th)	Qualifier (7th)
0 Ear **1** Nose **3** Hypopharynx **4** Mouth **5** Tongue **6** Salivary Glands **7** Sinuses **8** Hard Palate **9** Soft Palate **B** Larynx **D** Nasopharynx **F** Oropharynx	**0** Photons <1 MeV **1** Photons 1 - 10 MeV **2** Photons >10 MeV **4** Heavy Particles (Protons,Ions) **5** Neutrons **6** Neutron Capture	**Z** None	**Z** None
0 Ear **1** Nose **3** Hypopharynx **4** Mouth **5** Tongue **6** Salivary Glands **7** Sinuses **8** Hard Palate **9** Soft Palate **B** Larynx **D** Nasopharynx **F** Oropharynx	**3** Electrons	**Z** None	**0** Intraoperative **Z** None

Section	D	Radiation Therapy
Body System	9	Ear, Nose, Mouth and Throat
Modality	1	Brachytherapy

Treatment Site (4th)	Modality Qualifier (5th)	Isotope (6th)	Qualifier (7th)
0 Ear 1 Nose 3 Hypopharynx 4 Mouth 5 Tongue 6 Salivary Glands 7 Sinuses 8 Hard Palate 9 Soft Palate B Larynx D Nasopharynx F Oropharynx	9 High Dose Rate (HDR)	7 Cesium 137 (Cs-137) 8 Iridium 192 (Ir-192) 9 Iodine 125 (I-125) B Palladium 103 (Pd-103) C Californium 252 (Cf-252) Y Other Isotope	Z None
0 Ear 1 Nose 3 Hypopharynx 4 Mouth 5 Tongue 6 Salivary Glands 7 Sinuses 8 Hard Palate 9 Soft Palate B Larynx D Nasopharynx F Oropharynx	B Low Dose Rate (LDR)	6 Cesium 131 (Cs-131) 7 Cesium 137 (Cs-137) 8 Iridium 192 (Ir-192) 9 Iodine 125 (I-125) C Californium 252 (Cf-252) Y Other Isotope	Z None
0 Ear 1 Nose 3 Hypopharynx 4 Mouth 5 Tongue 6 Salivary Glands 7 Sinuses 8 Hard Palate 9 Soft Palate B Larynx D Nasopharynx F Oropharynx	B Low Dose Rate (LDR)	B Palladium 103 (Pd-103)	1 Unidirectional Source Z None

Section	D	Radiation Therapy
Body System	9	Ear, Nose, Mouth and Throat
Modality	2	Stereotactic Radiosurgery

Treatment Site (4th)	Modality Qualifier (5th)	Isotope (6th)	Qualifier (7th)
0 Ear 1 Nose 4 Mouth 5 Tongue 6 Salivary Glands 7 Sinuses 8 Hard Palate 9 Soft Palate B Larynx C Pharynx D Nasopharynx	D Stereotactic Other Photon Radiosurgery H Stereotactic Particulate Radiosurgery J Stereotactic Gamma Beam Radiosurgery	Z None	Z None

Section	D	Radiation Therapy
Body System	9	Ear, Nose, Mouth and Throat
Modality	Y	Other Radiation

Treatment Site (4ᵗʰ)	Modality Qualifier (5ᵗʰ)	Isotope (6ᵗʰ)	Qualifier (7ᵗʰ)
0 Ear 1 Nose 5 Tongue 6 Salivary Glands 7 Sinuses 8 Hard Palate 9 Soft Palate	7 Contact Radiation 8 Hyperthermia F Plaque Radiation	Z None	Z None
3 Hypopharynx F Oropharynx	7 Contact Radiation 8 Hyperthermia	Z None	Z None
4 Mouth B Larynx D Nasopharynx	7 Contact Radiation 8 Hyperthermia C Intraoperative Radiation Therapy (IORT) F Plaque Radiation	Z None	Z None
C Pharynx	C Intraoperative Radiation Therapy (IORT) F Plaque Radiation	Z None	Z None

Section	D	Radiation Therapy
Body System	B	Respiratory System
Modality	0	Beam Radiation

Treatment Site (4ᵗʰ)	Modality Qualifier (5ᵗʰ)	Isotope (6ᵗʰ)	Qualifier (7ᵗʰ)
0 Trachea 1 Bronchus 2 Lung 5 Pleura 6 Mediastinum 7 Chest Wall 8 Diaphragm	0 Photons <1 MeV 1 Photons 1 - 10 MeV 2 Photons >10 MeV 4 Heavy Particles (Protons,Ions) 5 Neutrons 6 Neutron Capture	Z None	Z None
0 Trachea 1 Bronchus 2 Lung 5 Pleura 6 Mediastinum 7 Chest Wall 8 Diaphragm	3 Electrons	Z None	0 Intraoperative Z None

Section	D	Radiation Therapy
Body System	B	Respiratory System
Modality	1	Brachytherapy

Treatment Site (4ᵗʰ)	Modality Qualifier (5ᵗʰ)	Isotope (6ᵗʰ)	Qualifier (7ᵗʰ)
0 Trachea 1 Bronchus 2 Lung 5 Pleura 6 Mediastinum 7 Chest Wall 8 Diaphragm	9 High Dose Rate (HDR)	7 Cesium 137 (Cs-137) 8 Iridium 192 (Ir-192) 9 Iodine 125 (I-125) B Palladium 103 (Pd-103) C Californium 252 (Cf-252) Y Other Isotope	Z None

Continued →

Section	D	Radiation Therapy
Body System	B	Respiratory System
Modality	1	Brachytherapy

Treatment Site (4th)	Modality Qualifier (5th)	Isotope (6th)	Qualifier (7th)
0 Trachea 1 Bronchus 2 Lung 5 Pleura 6 Mediastinum 7 Chest Wall 8 Diaphragm	B Low Dose Rate (LDR)	6 Cesium 131 (Cs-131) 7 Cesium 137 (Cs-137) 8 Iridium 192 (Ir-192) 9 Iodine 125 (I-125) C Californium 252 (Cf-252) Y Other Isotope	Z None
0 Trachea 1 Bronchus 2 Lung 5 Pleura 6 Mediastinum 7 Chest Wall 8 Diaphragm	B Low Dose Rate (LDR)	B Palladium 103 (Pd-103)	1 Unidirectional Source Z None

Section	D	Radiation Therapy
Body System	B	Respiratory System
Modality	2	Stereotactic Radiosurgery

Treatment Site (4th)	Modality Qualifier (5th)	Isotope (6th)	Qualifier (7th)
0 Trachea 1 Bronchus 2 Lung 5 Pleura 6 Mediastinum 7 Chest Wall 8 Diaphragm	D Stereotactic Other Photon Radiosurgery H Stereotactic Particulate Radiosurgery J Stereotactic Gamma Beam Radiosurgery	Z None	Z None

Section	D	Radiation Therapy
Body System	B	Respiratory System
Modality	Y	Other Radiation

Treatment Site (4th)	Modality Qualifier (5th)	Isotope (6th)	Qualifier (7th)
0 Trachea 1 Bronchus 2 Lung 5 Pleura 6 Mediastinum 7 Chest Wall 8 Diaphragm	7 Contact Radiation 8 Hyperthermia F Plaque Radiation K Laser Interstitial Thermal Therapy	Z None	Z None

Section	D	Radiation Therapy
Body System	D	Gastrointestinal System
Modality	0	Beam Radiation

Treatment Site (4th)	Modality Qualifier (5th)	Isotope (6th)	Qualifier (7th)
0 Esophagus 1 Stomach 2 Duodenum 3 Jejunum 4 Ileum 5 Colon 7 Rectum	0 Photons <1 MeV 1 Photons 1 - 10 MeV 2 Photons >10 MeV 4 Heavy Particles (Protons,Ions) 5 Neutrons 6 Neutron Capture	Z None	Z None

Continued →

Section	D	Radiation Therapy
Body System	D	Gastrointestinal System
Modality	0	Beam Radiation

Treatment Site (4th)	Modality Qualifier (5th)	Isotope (6th)	Qualifier (7th)
0 Esophagus 1 Stomach 2 Duodenum 3 Jejunum 4 Ileum 5 Colon 7 Rectum	3 Electrons	Z None	0 Intraoperative Z None

Section	D	Radiation Therapy
Body System	D	Gastrointestinal System
Modality	1	Brachytherapy

Treatment Site (4th)	Modality Qualifier (5th)	Isotope (6th)	Qualifier (7th)
0 Esophagus 1 Stomach 2 Duodenum 3 Jejunum 4 Ileum 5 Colon 7 Rectum	9 High Dose Rate (HDR)	7 Cesium 137 (Cs-137) 8 Iridium 192 (Ir-192) 9 Iodine 125 (I-125) B Palladium 103 (Pd-103) C Californium 252 (Cf-252) Y Other Isotope	Z None
0 Esophagus 1 Stomach 2 Duodenum 3 Jejunum 4 Ileum 5 Colon 7 Rectum	B Low Dose Rate (LDR)	6 Cesium 131 (Cs-131) 7 Cesium 137 (Cs-137) 8 Iridium 192 (Ir-192) 9 Iodine 125 (I-125) C Californium 252 (Cf-252) Y Other Isotope	Z None
0 Esophagus 1 Stomach 2 Duodenum 3 Jejunum 4 Ileum 5 Colon 7 Rectum	B Low Dose Rate (LDR)	B Palladium 103 (Pd-103)	1 Unidirectional Source Z None

Section	D	Radiation Therapy
Body System	D	Gastrointestinal System
Modality	2	Stereotactic Radiosurgery

Treatment Site (4th)	Modality Qualifier (5th)	Isotope (6th)	Qualifier (7th)
0 Esophagus 1 Stomach 2 Duodenum 3 Jejunum 4 Ileum 5 Colon 7 Rectum	D Stereotactic Other Photon Radiosurgery H Stereotactic Particulate Radiosurgery J Stereotactic Gamma Beam Radiosurgery	Z None	Z None

Section	D	Radiation Therapy
Body System	D	Gastrointestinal System
Modality	Y	Other Radiation

Treatment Site (4th)	Modality Qualifier (5th)	Isotope (6th)	Qualifier (7th)
0 Esophagus	7 Contact Radiation 8 Hyperthermia F Plaque Radiation K Laser Interstitial Thermal Therapy	Z None	Z None

Continued →

Section	D	Radiation Therapy
Body System	D	Gastrointestinal System
Modality	Y	Other Radiation

Treatment Site (4th)	Modality Qualifier (5th)	Isotope (6th)	Qualifier (7th)
1 Stomach 2 Duodenum 3 Jejunum 4 Ileum 5 Colon 7 Rectum	7 Contact Radiation 8 Hyperthermia C Intraoperative Radiation Therapy (IORT) F Plaque Radiation K Laser Interstitial Thermal Therapy	Z None	Z None
8 Anus	C Intraoperative Radiation Therapy (IORT) F Plaque Radiation K Laser Interstitial Thermal Therapy	Z None	Z None

Section	D	Radiation Therapy
Body System	F	Hepatobiliary System and Pancreas
Modality	0	Beam Radiation

Treatment Site (4th)	Modality Qualifier (5th)	Isotope (6th)	Qualifier (7th)
0 Liver 1 Gallbladder 2 Bile Ducts 3 Pancreas	0 Photons <1 MeV 1 Photons 1 - 10 MeV 2 Photons >10 MeV 4 Heavy Particles (Protons,Ions) 5 Neutrons 6 Neutron Capture	Z None	Z None
0 Liver 1 Gallbladder 2 Bile Ducts 3 Pancreas	3 Electrons	Z None	0 Intraoperative Z None

Section	D	Radiation Therapy
Body System	F	Hepatobiliary System and Pancreas
Modality	1	Brachytherapy

Treatment Site (4th)	Modality Qualifier (5th)	Isotope (6th)	Qualifier (7th)
0 Liver 1 Gallbladder 2 Bile Ducts 3 Pancreas	9 High Dose Rate (HDR)	7 Cesium 137 (Cs-137) 8 Iridium 192 (Ir-192) 9 Iodine 125 (I-125) B Palladium 103 (Pd-103) C Californium 252 (Cf-252) Y Other Isotope	Z None
0 Liver 1 Gallbladder 2 Bile Ducts 3 Pancreas	B Low Dose Rate (LDR)	6 Cesium 131 (Cs-131) 7 Cesium 137 (Cs-137) 8 Iridium 192 (Ir-192) 9 Iodine 125 (I-125) C Californium 252 (Cf-252) Y Other Isotope	Z None
0 Liver 1 Gallbladder 2 Bile Ducts 3 Pancreas	B Low Dose Rate (LDR)	B Palladium 103 (Pd-103)	1 Unidirectional Source Z None

Section   D   **Radiation Therapy**
Body System   F   **Hepatobiliary System and Pancreas**
Modality   2   **Stereotactic Radiosurgery**

Treatment Site (4th)	Modality Qualifier (5th)	Isotope (6th)	Qualifier (7th)
0 Liver 1 Gallbladder 2 Bile Ducts 3 Pancreas	D Stereotactic Other Photon Radiosurgery H Stereotactic Particulate Radiosurgery J Stereotactic Gamma Beam Radiosurgery	Z None	Z None

Section   D   **Radiation Therapy**
Body System   F   **Hepatobiliary System and Pancreas**
Modality   Y   **Other Radiation**

Treatment Site (4th)	Modality Qualifier (5th)	Isotope (6th)	Qualifier (7th)
0 Liver 1 Gallbladder 2 Bile Ducts 3 Pancreas	7 Contact Radiation 8 Hyperthermia C Intraoperative Radiation Therapy (IORT) F Plaque Radiation K Laser Interstitial Thermal Therapy	Z None	Z None

Section   D   **Radiation Therapy**
Body System   G   **Endocrine System**
Modality   0   **Beam Radiation**

Treatment Site (4th)	Modality Qualifier (5th)	Isotope (6th)	Qualifier (7th)
0 Pituitary Gland 1 Pineal Body 2 Adrenal Glands 4 Parathyroid Glands 5 Thyroid	0 Photons <1 MeV 1 Photons 1 - 10 MeV 2 Photons >10 MeV 5 Neutrons 6 Neutron Capture	Z None	Z None
0 Pituitary Gland 1 Pineal Body 2 Adrenal Glands 4 Parathyroid Glands 5 Thyroid	3 Electrons	Z None	0 Intraoperative Z None

Section   D   **Radiation Therapy**
Body System   G   **Endocrine System**
Modality   1   **Brachytherapy**

Treatment Site (4th)	Modality Qualifier (5th)	Isotope (6th)	Qualifier (7th)
0 Pituitary Gland 1 Pineal Body 2 Adrenal Glands 4 Parathyroid Glands 5 Thyroid	9 High Dose Rate (HDR)	7 Cesium 137 (Cs-137) 8 Iridium 192 (Ir-192) 9 Iodine 125 (I-125) B Palladium 103 (Pd-103) C Californium 252 (Cf-252) Y Other Isotope	Z None
0 Pituitary Gland 1 Pineal Body 2 Adrenal Glands 4 Parathyroid Glands 5 Thyroid	B Low Dose Rate (LDR)	6 Cesium 131 (Cs-131) 7 Cesium 137 (Cs-137) 8 Iridium 192 (Ir-192) 9 Iodine 125 (I-125) C Californium 252 (Cf-252) Y Other Isotope	Z None
0 Pituitary Gland 1 Pineal Body 2 Adrenal Glands 4 Parathyroid Glands 5 Thyroid	B Low Dose Rate (LDR)	B Palladium 103 (Pd-103)	1 Unidirectional Source Z None

Section	D	Radiation Therapy
Body System	G	Endocrine System
Modality	2	Stereotactic Radiosurgery

Treatment Site (4th)	Modality Qualifier (5th)	Isotope (6th)	Qualifier (7th)
0 Pituitary Gland 1 Pineal Body 2 Adrenal Glands 4 Parathyroid Glands 5 Thyroid	D Stereotactic Other Photon Radiosurgery H Stereotactic Particulate Radiosurgery J Stereotactic Gamma Beam Radiosurgery	Z None	Z None

Section	D	Radiation Therapy
Body System	G	Endocrine System
Modality	Y	Other Radiation

Treatment Site (4th)	Modality Qualifier (5th)	Isotope (6th)	Qualifier (7th)
0 Pituitary Gland 1 Pineal Body 2 Adrenal Glands 4 Parathyroid Glands 5 Thyroid	7 Contact Radiation 8 Hyperthermia F Plaque Radiation K Laser Interstitial Thermal Therapy	Z None	Z None

Section	D	Radiation Therapy
Body System	H	Skin
Modality	0	Beam Radiation

Treatment Site (4th)	Modality Qualifier (5th)	Isotope (6th)	Qualifier (7th)
2 Skin, Face 3 Skin, Neck 4 Skin, Arm 6 Skin, Chest 7 Skin, Back 8 Skin, Abdomen 9 Skin, Buttock B Skin, Leg	0 Photons <1 MeV 1 Photons 1 - 10 MeV 2 Photons >10 MeV 4 Heavy Particles (Protons,Ions) 5 Neutrons 6 Neutron Capture	Z None	Z None
2 Skin, Face 3 Skin, Neck 4 Skin, Arm 6 Skin, Chest 7 Skin, Back 8 Skin, Abdomen 9 Skin, Buttock B Skin, Leg	3 Electrons	Z None	0 Intraoperative Z None

Section	D	Radiation Therapy
Body System	H	Skin
Modality	Y	Other Radiation

Treatment Site (4th)	Modality Qualifier (5th)	Isotope (6th)	Qualifier (7th)
2 Skin, Face 3 Skin, Neck 4 Skin, Arm 6 Skin, Chest 7 Skin, Back 8 Skin, Abdomen 9 Skin, Buttock B Skin, Leg	7 Contact Radiation 8 Hyperthermia F Plaque Radiation	Z None	Z None
5 Skin, Hand C Skin, Foot	F Plaque Radiation	Z None	Z None

Section D Radiation Therapy
Body System M Breast
Modality 0 Beam Radiation

Treatment Site (4th)	Modality Qualifier (5th)	Isotope (6th)	Qualifier (7th)
0 Breast, Left 1 Breast, Right	0 Photons <1 MeV 1 Photons 1 - 10 MeV 2 Photons >10 MeV 4 Heavy Particles (Protons,Ions) 5 Neutrons 6 Neutron Capture	Z None	Z None
0 Breast, Left 1 Breast, Right	3 Electrons	Z None	0 Intraoperative Z None

Section D Radiation Therapy
Body System M Breast
Modality 1 Brachytherapy

Treatment Site (4th)	Modality Qualifier (5th)	Isotope (6th)	Qualifier (7th)
0 Breast, Left 1 Breast, Right	9 High Dose Rate (HDR)	7 Cesium 137 (Cs-137) 8 Iridium 192 (Ir-192) 9 Iodine 125 (I-125) B Palladium 103 (Pd-103) C Californium 252 (Cf-252) Y Other Isotope	Z None
0 Breast, Left 1 Breast, Right	B Low Dose Rate (LDR)	6 Cesium 131 (Cs-131) 7 Cesium 137 (Cs-137) 8 Iridium 192 (Ir-192) 9 Iodine 125 (I-125) C Californium 252 (Cf-252) Y Other Isotope	Z None
0 Breast, Left 1 Breast, Right	B Low Dose Rate (LDR)	B Palladium 103 (Pd-103)	1 Unidirectional Source Z None

Section D Radiation Therapy
Body System M Breast
Modality 2 Stereotactic Radiosurgery

Treatment Site (4th)	Modality Qualifier (5th)	Isotope (6th)	Qualifier (7th)
0 Breast, Left 1 Breast, Right	D Stereotactic Other Photon Radiosurgery H Stereotactic Particulate Radiosurgery J Stereotactic Gamma Beam Radiosurgery	Z None	Z None

Section D Radiation Therapy
Body System M Breast
Modality Y Other Radiation

Treatment Site (4th)	Modality Qualifier (5th)	Isotope (6th)	Qualifier (7th)
0 Breast, Left 1 Breast, Right	7 Contact Radiation 8 Hyperthermia F Plaque Radiation K Laser Interstitial Thermal Therapy	Z None	Z None

Section	D	Radiation Therapy
Body System	P	Musculoskeletal System
Modality	0	Beam Radiation

Treatment Site (4th)	Modality Qualifier (5th)	Isotope (6th)	Qualifier (7th)
0 Skull 2 Maxilla 3 Mandible 4 Sternum 5 Rib(s) 6 Humerus 7 Radius/Ulna 8 Pelvic Bones 9 Femur B Tibia/Fibula C Other Bone	0 Photons <1 MeV 1 Photons 1 - 10 MeV 2 Photons >10 MeV 4 Heavy Particles (Protons,Ions) 5 Neutrons 6 Neutron Capture	Z None	Z None
0 Skull 2 Maxilla 3 Mandible 4 Sternum 5 Rib(s) 6 Humerus 7 Radius/Ulna 8 Pelvic Bones 9 Femur B Tibia/Fibula C Other Bone	3 Electrons	Z None	0 Intraoperative Z None

Section	D	Radiation Therapy
Body System	P	Musculoskeletal System
Modality	Y	Other Radiation

Treatment Site (4th)	Modality Qualifier (5th)	Isotope (6th)	Qualifier (7th)
0 Skull 2 Maxilla 3 Mandible 4 Sternum 5 Rib(s) 6 Humerus 7 Radius/Ulna 8 Pelvic Bones 9 Femur B Tibia/Fibula C Other Bone	7 Contact Radiation 8 Hyperthermia F Plaque Radiation	Z None	Z None

Section	D	Radiation Therapy
Body System	T	Urinary System
Modality	0	Beam Radiation

Treatment Site (4th)	Modality Qualifier (5th)	Isotope (6th)	Qualifier (7th)
0 Kidney 1 Ureter 2 Bladder 3 Urethra	0 Photons <1 MeV 1 Photons 1 - 10 MeV 2 Photons >10 MeV 4 Heavy Particles (Protons,Ions) 5 Neutrons 6 Neutron Capture	Z None	Z None
0 Kidney 1 Ureter 2 Bladder 3 Urethra	3 Electrons	Z None	0 Intraoperative Z None

Section   D   **Radiation Therapy**
Body System   T   **Urinary System**
Modality   1   **Brachytherapy**

Treatment Site (4th)	Modality Qualifier (5th)	Isotope (6th)	Qualifier (7th)
0 Kidney 1 Ureter 2 Bladder 3 Urethra	9 High Dose Rate (HDR)	7 Cesium 137 (Cs-137) 8 Iridium 192 (Ir-192) 9 Iodine 125 (I-125) B Palladium 103 (Pd-103) C Californium 252 (Cf-252) Y Other Isotope	Z None
0 Kidney 1 Ureter 2 Bladder 3 Urethra	B Low Dose Rate (LDR)	6 Cesium 131 (Cs-131) 7 Cesium 137 (Cs-137) 8 Iridium 192 (Ir-192) 9 Iodine 125 (I-125) C Californium 252 (Cf-252) Y Other Isotope	Z None
0 Kidney 1 Ureter 2 Bladder 3 Urethra	B Low Dose Rate (LDR)	B Palladium 103 (Pd-103)	1 Unidirectional Source Z None

Section   D   **Radiation Therapy**
Body System   T   **Urinary System**
Modality   2   **Stereotactic Radiosurgery**

Treatment Site (4th)	Modality Qualifier (5th)	Isotope (6th)	Qualifier (7th)
0 Kidney 1 Ureter 2 Bladder 3 Urethra	D Stereotactic Other Photon Radiosurgery H Stereotactic Particulate Radiosurgery J Stereotactic Gamma Beam Radiosurgery	Z None	Z None

Section   D   **Radiation Therapy**
Body System   T   **Urinary System**
Modality   Y   **Other Radiation**

Treatment Site (4th)	Modality Qualifier (5th)	Isotope (6th)	Qualifier (7th)
0 Kidney 1 Ureter 2 Bladder 3 Urethra	7 Contact Radiation 8 Hyperthermia C Intraoperative Radiation Therapy (IORT) F Plaque Radiation	Z None	Z None

Section   D   **Radiation Therapy**
Body System   U   **Female Reproductive System**
Modality   0   **Beam Radiation**

Treatment Site (4th)	Modality Qualifier (5th)	Isotope (6th)	Qualifier (7th)
0 Ovary 1 Cervix 2 Uterus	0 Photons <1 MeV 1 Photons 1 - 10 MeV 2 Photons >10 MeV 4 Heavy Particles (Protons,Ions) 5 Neutrons 6 Neutron Capture	Z None	Z None
0 Ovary 1 Cervix 2 Uterus	3 Electrons	Z None	0 Intraoperative Z None

Section	D	Radiation Therapy
Body System	U	Female Reproductive System
Modality	1	Brachytherapy

Treatment Site (4th)	Modality Qualifier (5th)	Isotope (6th)	Qualifier (7th)
0 Ovary 1 Cervix 2 Uterus	9 High Dose Rate (HDR)	7 Cesium 137 (Cs-137) 8 Iridium 192 (Ir-192) 9 Iodine 125 (I-125) B Palladium 103 (Pd-103) C Californium 252 (Cf-252) Y Other Isotope	Z None
0 Ovary 1 Cervix 2 Uterus	B Low Dose Rate (LDR)	6 Cesium 131 (Cs-131) 7 Cesium 137 (Cs-137) 8 Iridium 192 (Ir-192) 9 Iodine 125 (I-125) C Californium 252 (Cf-252) Y Other Isotope	Z None
0 Ovary 1 Cervix 2 Uterus	B Low Dose Rate (LDR)	B Palladium 103 (Pd-103)	1 Unidirectional Source Z None

Section	D	Radiation Therapy
Body System	U	Female Reproductive System
Modality	2	Stereotactic Radiosurgery

Treatment Site (4th)	Modality Qualifier (5th)	Isotope (6th)	Qualifier (7th)
0 Ovary 1 Cervix 2 Uterus	D Stereotactic Other Photon Radiosurgery H Stereotactic Particulate Radiosurgery J Stereotactic Gamma Beam Radiosurgery	Z None	Z None

Section	D	Radiation Therapy
Body System	U	Female Reproductive System
Modality	Y	Other Radiation

Treatment Site (4th)	Modality Qualifier (5th)	Isotope (6th)	Qualifier (7th)
0 Ovary 1 Cervix 2 Uterus	7 Contact Radiation 8 Hyperthermia C Intraoperative Radiation Therapy (IORT) F Plaque Radiation	Z None	Z None

Section	D	Radiation Therapy
Body System	V	Male Reproductive System
Modality	0	Beam Radiation

Treatment Site (4th)	Modality Qualifier (5th)	Isotope (6th)	Qualifier (7th)
0 Prostate 1 Testis	0 Photons <1 MeV 1 Photons 1 - 10 MeV 2 Photons >10 MeV 4 Heavy Particles (Protons,Ions) 5 Neutrons 6 Neutron Capture	Z None	Z None
0 Prostate 1 Testis	3 Electrons	Z None	0 Intraoperative Z None

Section D Radiation Therapy
Body System V Male Reproductive System
Modality 1 Brachytherapy

Treatment Site (4th)	Modality Qualifier (5th)	Isotope (6th)	Qualifier (7th)
0 Prostate 1 Testis	9 High Dose Rate (HDR)	7 Cesium 137 (Cs-137) 8 Iridium 192 (Ir-192) 9 Iodine 125 (I-125) B Palladium 103 (Pd-103) C Californium 252 (Cf-252) Y Other Isotope	Z None
0 Prostate 1 Testis	B Low Dose Rate (LDR)	6 Cesium 131 (Cs-131) 7 Cesium 137 (Cs-137) 8 Iridium 192 (Ir-192) 9 Iodine 125 (I-125) C Californium 252 (Cf-252) Y Other Isotope	Z None
0 Prostate 1 Testis	B Low Dose Rate (LDR)	B Palladium 103 (Pd-103)	1 Unidirectional Source Z None

Section D Radiation Therapy
Body System V Male Reproductive System
Modality 2 Stereotactic Radiosurgery

Treatment Site (4th)	Modality Qualifier (5th)	Isotope (6th)	Qualifier (7th)
0 Prostate 1 Testis	D Stereotactic Other Photon Radiosurgery H Stereotactic Particulate Radiosurgery J Stereotactic Gamma Beam Radiosurgery	Z None	Z None

Section D Radiation Therapy
Body System V Male Reproductive System
Modality Y Other Radiation

Treatment Site (4th)	Modality Qualifier (5th)	Isotope (6th)	Qualifier (7th)
0 Prostate	7 Contact Radiation 8 Hyperthermia C Intraoperative Radiation Therapy (IORT) F Plaque Radiation K Laser Interstitial Thermal Therapy	Z None	Z None
1 Testis	7 Contact Radiation 8 Hyperthermia F Plaque Radiation	Z None	Z None

Section D Radiation Therapy
Body System W Anatomical Regions
Modality 0 Beam Radiation

Treatment Site (4th)	Modality Qualifier (5th)	Isotope (6th)	Qualifier (7th)
1 Head and Neck 2 Chest 3 Abdomen 4 Hemibody 5 Whole Body 6 Pelvic Region	0 Photons <1 MeV 1 Photons 1 - 10 MeV 2 Photons >10 MeV 4 Heavy Particles (Protons,Ions) 5 Neutrons 6 Neutron Capture	Z None	Z None
1 Head and Neck 2 Chest 3 Abdomen 4 Hemibody 5 Whole Body 6 Pelvic Region	3 Electrons	Z None	0 Intraoperative Z None

Section	D	Radiation Therapy
Body System	W	Anatomical Regions
Modality	1	Brachytherapy

Treatment Site (4th)	Modality Qualifier (5th)	Isotope (6th)	Qualifier (7th)
0 Cranial Cavity K Upper Back L Lower Back P Gastrointestinal Track Q Respiratory Track R Genitourinary Track X Upper Extremity Y Lower Extremity	B Low Dose Rate (LDR)	B Palladium 103 (Pd-103)	1 Unidirectional Source Z None
1 Head and Neck 2 Chest 3 Abdomen 6 Pelvic Region	9 High Dose Rate (HDR)	7 Cesium 137 (Cs-137) 8 Iridium 192 (Ir-192) 9 Iodine 125 (I-125) B Palladium 103 (Pd-103) C Californium 252 (Cf-252) Y Other Isotope	Z None
1 Head and Neck 2 Chest 3 Abdomen 6 Pelvic Region	B Low Dose Rate (LDR)	6 Cesium 131 (Cs-131) 7 Cesium 137 (Cs-137) 8 Iridium 192 (Ir-192) 9 Iodine 125 (I-125) C Californium 252 (Cf-252) Y Other Isotope	Z None
1 Head and Neck 2 Chest 3 Abdomen 6 Pelvic Region	B Low Dose Rate (LDR)	B Palladium 103 (Pd-103)	1 Unidirectional Source Z None

Section	D	Radiation Therapy
Body System	W	Anatomical Regions
Modality	2	Stereotactic Radiosurgery

Treatment Site (4th)	Modality Qualifier (5th)	Isotope (6th)	Qualifier (7th)
1 Head and Neck 2 Chest 3 Abdomen 6 Pelvic Region	D Stereotactic Other Photon Radiosurgery H Stereotactic Particulate Radiosurgery J Stereotactic Gamma Beam Radiosurgery	Z None	Z None

Section	D	Radiation Therapy
Body System	W	Anatomical Regions
Modality	Y	Other Radiation

Treatment Site (4th)	Modality Qualifier (5th)	Isotope (6th)	Qualifier (7th)
1 Head and Neck 2 Chest 3 Abdomen 4 Hemibody 6 Pelvic Region	7 Contact Radiation 8 Hyperthermia F Plaque Radiation	Z None	Z None
5 Whole Body	7 Contact Radiation 8 Hyperthermia F Plaque Radiation	Z None	Z None
5 Whole Body	G Isotope Administration	D Iodine 131 (I-131) F Phosphorus 32 (P-32) G Strontium 89 (Sr-89) H Strontium 90 (Sr-90) Y Other Isotope	Z None

AHA Coding Clinic

DU11B7Z Low Dose Rate (LDR) Brachytherapy of Cervix using Cesium 137 (Cs-137)—AHA CC: 4Q, 2017, 104

DW16BB1 Low Dose Rate (LDR) Brachytherapy of Pelvic Region using Palladium 103 (Pd-103), Unidirectional Source—AHA CC: 4Q, 2019, 43-44

DWY38ZZ Hyperthermia of Abdomen—AHA CC: 4Q, 2019, 37

Within each section of ICD-10-PCS the characters have different meanings. The seven character meanings for the Physical Rehabilitation and Diagnostic Audiology section are illustrated below through the procedure example of *Individual fitting of moveable brace, right knee*.

Section	Section Qualifier	Root Type	Body System/Region	Type Qualifier	Equipment	Qualifier
Physical Rehabilitation and Diagnostic Audiology	Rehabilitation	Device Fitting	None	Dynamic Orthosis	Orthosis	None
F	0	D	Z	6	E	Z

Section (Character 1)

All Physical Rehabilitation and Diagnostic Audiology procedure codes have a first character value of F.

Section Qualifier (Character 2)

The alphanumeric character in the second character position identifies if the procedure is a physical rehabilitation procedure or a diagnostic audiology procedure. Physical rehabilitation is reported with character value 0, and diagnostic audiology is reported with character value 1.

Root Type (Character 3)

The alphanumeric character value for root types is placed in the third position. The following are the root types applicable to the Physical Rehabilitation and Diagnostic Audiology section with their associated meaning.

Character Value	Root Type	Root Type Definition
0	Speech Assessment	Measurement of speech and related functions
1	Motor and/or Nerve Function Assessment	Measurement of motor, nerve, and related functions
2	Activities of Daily Living Assessment	Measurement of functional level for activities of daily living
3	Hearing Assessment	Measurement of hearing and related functions
4	Hearing Aid Assessment	Measurement of the appropriateness and/or effectiveness of a hearing device
5	Vestibular Assessment	Measurement of the vestibular system and related functions
6	Speech Treatment	Application of techniques to improve, augment, or compensate for speech and related functional impairment
7	Motor Treatment	Exercise or activities to increase or facilitate motor function
8	Activities of Daily Living Treatment	Exercise or activities to facilitate functional competence for activities of daily living
9	Hearing Treatment	Application of techniques to improve, augment, or compensate for hearing and related functional impairment
B	Cochlear Implant Treatment	Application of techniques to improve the communication abilities of individuals with cochlear implant
C	Vestibular Treatment	Application of techniques to improve, augment, or compensate for vestibular and related functional impairment
D	Device Fitting	Fitting of a device designed to facilitate or support achievement of a higher level of function
F	Caregiver Training	Training in activities to support patient's optimal level of function

Body System/Region (Character 4)

For each body system/region the applicable body part character values will be available for procedure code construction. An example of a body region for this section is Musculoskeletal System—Lower Back/Lower Extremity.

Type Qualifier (Character 5)

Type qualifier further specifies the root type procedure. For example, the type qualifier of Gait Training/Functional Ambulation is used with Motor Treatment (character value 7) when applicable.

Equipment (Character 6)

If equipment is utilized during the procedure character six is used to report the type. Some examples of equipment are

- Aerobic Endurance and Conditioning
- Electrotherapeutic
- Mechanical
- Orthosis
- Prosthesis

If equipment is not utilized, the placeholder character value of Z should be reported.

Qualifier (Character 7)

The qualifier represents an additional attribute for the procedure when applicable. Currently, there are no qualifiers in the Physical Rehabilitation and Diagnostic Audiology section; therefore, the placeholder character value of Z should be reported.

Physical Rehabilitation and Diagnostic Audiology Section Tables

Physical Rehabilitation and Diagnostic Audiology Tables F00–F15

Section	F	Physical Rehabilitation and Diagnostic Audiology
Section Qualifier	0	Rehabilitation
Type	0	Speech Assessment: Measurement of speech and related functions

Body System / Region (4th)	Type Qualifier (5th)	Equipment (6th)	Qualifier (7th)
3 Neurological System - Whole Body	G Communicative/Cognitive Integration Skills	K Audiovisual M Augmentative / Alternative Communication P Computer Y Other Equipment Z None	Z None
Z None	0 Filtered Speech 3 Staggered Spondaic Word Q Performance Intensity Phonetically Balanced Speech Discrimination R Brief Tone Stimuli S Distorted Speech T Dichotic Stimuli V Temporal Ordering of Stimuli W Masking Patterns	1 Audiometer 2 Sound Field / Booth K Audiovisual Z None	Z None
Z None	1 Speech Threshold 2 Speech/Word Recognition	1 Audiometer 2 Sound Field / Booth 9 Cochlear Implant K Audiovisual Z None	Z None
Z None	4 Sensorineural Acuity Level	1 Audiometer 2 Sound Field / Booth Z None	Z None
Z None	5 Synthetic Sentence Identification	1 Audiometer 2 Sound Field / Booth 9 Cochlear Implant K Audiovisual	Z None
Z None	6 Speech and/or Language Screening 7 Nonspoken Language 8 Receptive/Expressive Language C Aphasia G Communicative/Cognitive Integration Skills L Augmentative/Alternative Communication System	K Audiovisual M Augmentative / Alternative Communication P Computer Y Other Equipment Z None	Z None

Continued →

Section	F	Physical Rehabilitation and Diagnostic Audiology
Section Qualifier	0	Rehabilitation
Type	0	Speech Assessment: Measurement of speech and related functions

Body System / Region (4th)	Type Qualifier (5th)	Equipment (6th)	Qualifier (7th)
Z None	9 Articulation/Phonology	K Audiovisual P Computer Q Speech Analysis Y Other Equipment Z None	Z None
Z None	B Motor Speech	K Audiovisual N Biosensory Feedback P Computer Q Speech Analysis T Aerodynamic Function Y Other Equipment Z None	Z None
Z None	D Fluency	K Audiovisual N Biosensory Feedback P Computer Q Speech Analysis S Voice Analysis T Aerodynamic Function Y Other Equipment Z None	Z None
Z None	F Voice	K Audiovisual N Biosensory Feedback P Computer S Voice Analysis T Aerodynamic Function Y Other Equipment Z None	Z None
Z None	H Bedside Swallowing and Oral Function P Oral Peripheral Mechanism	Y Other Equipment Z None	Z None
Z None	J Instrumental Swallowing and Oral Function	T Aerodynamic Function W Swallowing Y Other Equipment	Z None
Z None	K Orofacial Myofunctional	K Audiovisual P Computer Y Other Equipment Z None	Z None
Z None	M Voice Prosthetic	K Audiovisual P Computer S Voice Analysis V Speech Prosthesis Y Other Equipment Z None	Z None
Z None	N Non-invasive Instrumental Status	N Biosensory Feedback P Computer Q Speech Analysis S Voice Analysis T Aerodynamic Function Y Other Equipment	Z None
Z None	X Other Specified Central Auditory Processing	Z None	Z None

Section	F	Physical Rehabilitation and Diagnostic Audiology
Section Qualifier	0	Rehabilitation
Type	1	Motor and/or Nerve Function Assessment: Measurement of motor, nerve, and related functions

Body System / Region (4th)	Type Qualifier (5th)	Equipment (6th)	Qualifier (7th)
0 Neurological System - Head and Neck 1 Neurological System - Upper Back / Upper Extremity 2 Neurological System - Lower Back / Lower Extremity 3 Neurological System - Whole Body	0 Muscle Performance	E Orthosis F Assistive, Adaptive, Supportive or Protective U Prosthesis Y Other Equipment Z None	Z None
0 Neurological System - Head and Neck 1 Neurological System - Upper Back / Upper Extremity 2 Neurological System - Lower Back / Lower Extremity 3 Neurological System - Whole Body	1 Integumentary Integrity 3 Coordination/Dexterity 4 Motor Function G Reflex Integrity	Z None	Z None
0 Neurological System - Head and Neck 1 Neurological System - Upper Back / Upper Extremity 2 Neurological System - Lower Back / Lower Extremity 3 Neurological System - Whole Body	5 Range of Motion and Joint Integrity 6 Sensory Awareness/ Processing/Integrity	Y Other Equipment Z None	Z None
D Integumentary System - Head and Neck F Integumentary System - Upper Back / Upper Extremity G Integumentary System - Lower Back / Lower Extremity H Integumentary System - Whole Body J Musculoskeletal System - Head and Neck K Musculoskeletal System - Upper Back / Upper Extremity L Musculoskeletal System - Lower Back / Lower Extremity M Musculoskeletal System - Whole Body	0 Muscle Performance	E Orthosis F Assistive, Adaptive, Supportive or Protective U Prosthesis Y Other Equipment Z None	Z None
D Integumentary System - Head and Neck F Integumentary System - Upper Back / Upper Extremity G Integumentary System - Lower Back / Lower Extremity H Integumentary System - Whole Body J Musculoskeletal System - Head and Neck K Musculoskeletal System - Upper Back / Upper Extremity L Musculoskeletal System - Lower Back / Lower Extremity M Musculoskeletal System - Whole Body	1 Integumentary Integrity	Z None	Z None
D Integumentary System - Head and Neck F Integumentary System - Upper Back / Upper Extremity G Integumentary System - Lower Back / Lower Extremity H Integumentary System - Whole Body J Musculoskeletal System - Head and Neck K Musculoskeletal System - Upper Back / Upper Extremity L Musculoskeletal System - Lower Back / Lower Extremity M Musculoskeletal System - Whole Body	5 Range of Motion and Joint Integrity 6 Sensory Awareness/ Processing/Integrity	Y Other Equipment Z None	Z None

Continued →

Section	F	Physical Rehabilitation and Diagnostic Audiology
Section Qualifier	0	Rehabilitation
Type	1	Motor and/or Nerve Function Assessment: Measurement of motor, nerve, and related functions

Body System / Region (4th)	Type Qualifier (5th)	Equipment (6th)	Qualifier (7th)
N Genitourinary System	0 Muscle Performance	E Orthosis F Assistive, Adaptive, Supportive or Protective U Prosthesis Y Other Equipment Z None	Z None
Z None	2 Visual Motor Integration	K Audiovisual M Augmentative / Alternative Communication N Biosensory Feedback P Computer Q Speech Analysis S Voice Analysis Y Other Equipment Z None	Z None
Z None	7 Facial Nerve Function	7 Electrophysiologic	Z None
Z None	9 Somatosensory Evoked Potentials	J Somatosensory	Z None
Z None	B Bed Mobility C Transfer F Wheelchair Mobility	E Orthosis F Assistive, Adaptive, Supportive or Protective U Prosthesis Z None	Z None
Z None	D Gait and/or Balance	E Orthosis F Assistive, Adaptive, Supportive or Protective U Prosthesis Y Other Equipment Z None	Z None

Section	F	Physical Rehabilitation and Diagnostic Audiology
Section Qualifier	0	Rehabilitation
Type	2	Activities of Daily Living Assessment: Measurement of functional level for activities of daily living

Body System / Region (4th)	Type Qualifier (5th)	Equipment (6th)	Qualifier (7th)
0 Neurological System - Head and Neck	9 Cranial Nerve Integrity D Neuromotor Development	Y Other Equipment Z None	Z None
1 Neurological System - Upper Back / Upper Extremity 2 Neurological System - Lower Back / Lower Extremity 3 Neurological System - Whole Body	D Neuromotor Development	Y Other Equipment Z None	Z None
4 Circulatory System - Head and Neck 5 Circulatory System - Upper Back / Upper Extremity 6 Circulatory System - Lower Back / Lower Extremity 8 Respiratory System - Head and Neck 9 Respiratory System - Upper Back / Upper Extremity B Respiratory System - Lower Back / Lower Extremity	G Ventilation, Respiration and Circulation	C Mechanical G Aerobic Endurance and Conditioning Y Other Equipment Z None	Z None

Continued →

Section   F   **Physical Rehabilitation and Diagnostic Audiology**
Section Qualifier   0   **Rehabilitation**
Type   2   **Activities of Daily Living Assessment:** Measurement of functional level for activities of daily living

Body System / Region (4ᵗʰ)	Type Qualifier (5ᵗʰ)	Equipment (6ᵗʰ)	Qualifier (7ᵗʰ)
7 Circulatory System - Whole Body **C** Respiratory System - Whole Body	**7** Aerobic Capacity and Endurance	**E** Orthosis **G** Aerobic Endurance and Conditioning **U** Prosthesis **Y** Other Equipment **Z** None	**Z** None
7 Circulatory System - Whole Body **C** Respiratory System - Whole Body	**G** Ventilation, Respiration and Circulation	**C** Mechanical **G** Aerobic Endurance and Conditioning **Y** Other Equipment **Z** None	**Z** None
Z None	**0** Bathing/Showering **1** Dressing **3** Grooming/Personal Hygiene **4** Home Management	**E** Orthosis **F** Assistive, Adaptive, Supportive or Protective **U** Prosthesis **Z** None	**Z** None
Z None	**2** Feeding/Eating **8** Anthropometric Characteristics **F** Pain	**Y** Other Equipment **Z** None	**Z** None
Z None	**5** Perceptual Processing	**K** Audiovisual **M** Augmentative / Alternative Communication **N** Biosensory Feedback **P** Computer **Q** Speech Analysis **S** Voice Analysis **Y** Other Equipment **Z** None	**Z** None
Z None	**6** Psychosocial Skills	**Z** None	**Z** None
Z None	**B** Environmental, Home and Work Barriers **C** Ergonomics and Body Mechanics	**E** Orthosis **F** Assistive, Adaptive, Supportive or Protective **U** Prosthesis **Y** Other Equipment **Z** None	**Z** None
Z None	**H** Vocational Activities and Functional Community or Work Reintegration Skills	**E** Orthosis **F** Assistive, Adaptive, Supportive or Protective **G** Aerobic Endurance and Conditioning **U** Prosthesis **Y** Other Equipment **Z** None	**Z** None

Section   F   **Physical Rehabilitation and Diagnostic Audiology**
Section Qualifier   0   **Rehabilitation**
Type   6   **Speech Treatment:** Application of techniques to improve, augment, or compensate for speech and related functional impairment

Body System / Region (4ᵗʰ)	Type Qualifier (5ᵗʰ)	Equipment (6ᵗʰ)	Qualifier (7ᵗʰ)
3 Neurological System - Whole Body	**6** Communicative/Cognitive Integration Skills	**K** Audiovisual **M** Augmentative / Alternative Communication **P** Computer **Y** Other Equipment **Z** None	**Z** None

Continued →

Body System / Region (4th)	Type Qualifier (5th)	Equipment (6th)	Qualifier (7th)
Z None	0 Nonspoken Language 3 Aphasia 6 Communicative/Cognitive Integration Skills	K Audiovisual M Augmentative / Alternative Communication P Computer Y Other Equipment Z None	Z None
Z None	1 Speech-Language Pathology and Related Disorders Counseling 2 Speech-Language Pathology and Related Disorders Prevention	K Audiovisual Z None	Z None
Z None	4 Articulation/Phonology	K Audiovisual P Computer Q Speech Analysis T Aerodynamic Function Y Other Equipment Z None	Z None
Z None	5 Aural Rehabilitation	K Audiovisual L Assistive Listening M Augmentative / Alternative Communication N Biosensory Feedback P Computer Q Speech Analysis S Voice Analysis Y Other Equipment Z None	Z None
Z None	7 Fluency	4 Electroacoustic Immitance / Acoustic Reflex K Audiovisual N Biosensory Feedback Q Speech Analysis S Voice Analysis T Aerodynamic Function Y Other Equipment Z None	Z None
Z None	8 Motor Speech	K Audiovisual N Biosensory Feedback P Computer Q Speech Analysis S Voice Analysis T Aerodynamic Function Y Other Equipment Z None	Z None
Z None	9 Orofacial Myofunctional	K Audiovisual P Computer Y Other Equipment Z None	Z None
Z None	B Receptive/Expressive Language	K Audiovisual L Assistive Listening M Augmentative / Alternative Communication P Computer Y Other Equipment Z None	Z None

Continued →

Section F Physical Rehabilitation and Diagnostic Audiology *F06 Continued*
Section Qualifier 0 Rehabilitation
Type 6 **Speech Treatment:** Application of techniques to improve, augment, or compensate for speech and related functional impairment

Body System / Region (4th)	Type Qualifier (5th)	Equipment (6th)	Qualifier (7th)
Z None	C Voice	K Audiovisual N Biosensory Feedback P Computer S Voice Analysis T Aerodynamic Function V Speech Prosthesis Y Other Equipment Z None	Z None
Z None	D Swallowing Dysfunction	M Augmentative / Alternative Communication T Aerodynamic Function V Speech Prosthesis Y Other Equipment Z None	Z None

Section F Physical Rehabilitation and Diagnostic Audiology
Section Qualifier 0 Rehabilitation
Type 7 **Motor Treatment:** Exercise or activities to increase or facilitate motor function

Body System / Region (4th)	Type Qualifier (5th)	Equipment (6th)	Qualifier (7th)
0 Neurological System - Head and Neck 1 Neurological System - Upper Back / Upper Extremity 2 Neurological System - Lower Back / Lower Extremity 3 Neurological System - Whole Body D Integumentary System - Head and Neck F Integumentary System - Upper Back / Upper Extremity G Integumentary System - Lower Back / Lower Extremity H Integumentary System - Whole Body J Musculoskeletal System - Head and Neck K Musculoskeletal System - Upper Back / Upper Extremity L Musculoskeletal System - Lower Back / Lower Extremity M Musculoskeletal System - Whole Body	0 Range of Motion and Joint Mobility 1 Muscle Performance 2 Coordination/Dexterity 3 Motor Function	E Orthosis F Assistive, Adaptive, Supportive or Protective U Prosthesis Y Other Equipment Z None	Z None
0 Neurological System - Head and Neck 1 Neurological System - Upper Back / Upper Extremity 2 Neurological System - Lower Back / Lower Extremity 3 Neurological System - Whole Body D Integumentary System - Head and Neck F Integumentary System - Upper Back / Upper Extremity G Integumentary System - Lower Back / Lower Extremity H Integumentary System - Whole Body J Musculoskeletal System - Head and Neck K Musculoskeletal System - Upper Back / Upper Extremity L Musculoskeletal System - Lower Back / Lower Extremity M Musculoskeletal System - Whole Body	6 Therapeutic Exercise	B Physical Agents C Mechanical D Electrotherapeutic E Orthosis F Assistive, Adaptive, Supportive or Protective G Aerobic Endurance and Conditioning H Mechanical or Electromechanical U Prosthesis Y Other Equipment Z None	Z None

Continued →

	Section	F	Physical Rehabilitation and Diagnostic Audiology
	Section Qualifier	0	Rehabilitation
	Type	7	**Motor Treatment:** Exercise or activities to increase or facilitate motor function

Body System / Region (4th)	Type Qualifier (5th)	Equipment (6th)	Qualifier (7th)
0 Neurological System - Head and Neck 1 Neurological System - Upper Back / Upper Extremity 2 Neurological System - Lower Back / Lower Extremity 3 Neurological System - Whole Body D Integumentary System - Head and Neck F Integumentary System - Upper Back / Upper Extremity G Integumentary System - Lower Back / Lower Extremity H Integumentary System - Whole Body J Musculoskeletal System - Head and Neck K Musculoskeletal System - Upper Back / Upper Extremity L Musculoskeletal System - Lower Back / Lower Extremity M Musculoskeletal System - Whole Body	7 Manual Therapy Techniques	Z None	Z None
4 Circulatory System - Head and Neck 5 Circulatory System - Upper Back / Upper Extremity 6 Circulatory System - Lower Back / Lower Extremity 7 Circulatory System - Whole Body 8 Respiratory System - Head and Neck 9 Respiratory System - Upper Back / Upper Extremity B Respiratory System - Lower Back / Lower Extremity C Respiratory System - Whole Body	6 Therapeutic Exercise	B Physical Agents C Mechanical D Electrotherapeutic E Orthosis F Assistive, Adaptive, Supportive or Protective G Aerobic Endurance and Conditioning H Mechanical or Electromechanical U Prosthesis Y Other Equipment Z None	Z None
N Genitourinary System	1 Muscle Performance	E Orthosis F Assistive, Adaptive, Supportive or Protective U Prosthesis Y Other Equipment Z None	Z None
N Genitourinary System	6 Therapeutic Exercise	B Physical Agents C Mechanical D Electrotherapeutic E Orthosis F Assistive, Adaptive, Supportive or Protective G Aerobic Endurance and Conditioning H Mechanical or Electromechanical U Prosthesis Y Other Equipment Z None	Z None
Z None	4 Wheelchair Mobility	D Electrotherapeutic E Orthosis F Assistive, Adaptive, Supportive or Protective U Prosthesis Y Other Equipment Z None	Z None
Z None	5 Bed Mobility	C Mechanical E Orthosis F Assistive, Adaptive, Supportive or Protective U Prosthesis Y Other Equipment Z None	Z None

Continued →

Section	F	Physical Rehabilitation and Diagnostic Audiology
Section Qualifier	0	Rehabilitation
Type	7	Motor Treatment: Exercise or activities to increase or facilitate motor function

Body System / Region (4th)	Type Qualifier (5th)	Equipment (6th)	Qualifier (7th)
Z None	8 Transfer Training	C Mechanical D Electrotherapeutic E Orthosis F Assistive, Adaptive, Supportive or Protective U Prosthesis Y Other Equipment Z None	Z None
Z None	9 Gait Training/Functional Ambulation	C Mechanical D Electrotherapeutic E Orthosis F Assistive, Adaptive, Supportive or Protective G Aerobic Endurance and Conditioning U Prosthesis Y Other Equipment Z None	Z None

Section	F	Physical Rehabilitation and Diagnostic Audiology
Section Qualifier	0	Rehabilitation
Type	8	Activities of Daily Living Treatment: Exercise or activities to facilitate functional competence for activities of daily living

Body System / Region (4th)	Type Qualifier (5th)	Equipment (6th)	Qualifier (7th)
D Integumentary System - Head and Neck F Integumentary System - Upper Back / Upper Extremity G Integumentary System - Lower Back / Lower Extremity H Integumentary System - Whole Body J Musculoskeletal System - Head and Neck K Musculoskeletal System - Upper Back / Upper Extremity L Musculoskeletal System - Lower Back / Lower Extremity M Musculoskeletal System - Whole Body	5 Wound Management	B Physical Agents C Mechanical D Electrotherapeutic E Orthosis F Assistive, Adaptive, Supportive or Protective U Prosthesis Y Other Equipment Z None	Z None
Z None	0 Bathing/Showering Techniques 1 Dressing Techniques 2 Grooming/Personal Hygiene	E Orthosis F Assistive, Adaptive, Supportive or Protective U Prosthesis Y Other Equipment Z None	Z None
Z None	3 Feeding/Eating	C Mechanical D Electrotherapeutic E Orthosis F Assistive, Adaptive, Supportive or Protective U Prosthesis Y Other Equipment Z None	Z None
Z None	4 Home Management	D Electrotherapeutic E Orthosis F Assistive, Adaptive, Supportive or Protective U Prosthesis Y Other Equipment Z None	Z None

Continued →

Section	F	Physical Rehabilitation and Diagnostic Audiology		*F08 Continued*
Section Qualifier	0	Rehabilitation		
Type	8	Activities of Daily Living Treatment: Exercise or activities to facilitate functional competence for activities of daily living		

Body System / Region (4th)	Type Qualifier (5th)	Equipment (6th)	Qualifier (7th)
Z None	6 Psychosocial Skills	Z None	Z None
Z None	7 Vocational Activities and Functional Community or Work Reintegration Skills	B Physical Agents C Mechanical D Electrotherapeutic E Orthosis F Assistive, Adaptive, Supportive or Protective G Aerobic Endurance and Conditioning U Prosthesis Y Other Equipment Z None	Z None

Section	F	Physical Rehabilitation and Diagnostic Audiology		
Section Qualifier	0	Rehabilitation		
Type	9	Hearing Treatment: Application of techniques to improve, augment, or compensate for hearing and related functional impairment		

Body System / Region (4th)	Type Qualifier (5th)	Equipment (6th)	Qualifier (7th)
Z None	0 Hearing and Related Disorders Counseling 1 Hearing and Related Disorders Prevention	K Audiovisual Z None	Z None
Z None	2 Auditory Processing	K Audiovisual L Assistive Listening P Computer Y Other Equipment Z None	Z None
Z None	3 Cerumen Management	X Cerumen Management Z None	Z None

Section	F	Physical Rehabilitation and Diagnostic Audiology		
Section Qualifier	0	Rehabilitation		
Type	B	Cochlear Implant Treatment: Application of techniques to improve the communication abilities of individuals with cochlear implant		

Body System / Region (4th)	Type Qualifier (5th)	Equipment (6th)	Qualifier (7th)
Z None	0 Cochlear Implant Rehabilitation	1 Audiometer 2 Sound Field / Booth 9 Cochlear Implant K Audiovisual P Computer Y Other Equipment	Z None

Section	F	Physical Rehabilitation and Diagnostic Audiology		
Section Qualifier	0	Rehabilitation		
Type	C	Vestibular Treatment: Application of techniques to improve, augment, or compensate for vestibular and related functional impairment		

Body System / Region (4th)	Type Qualifier (5th)	Equipment (6th)	Qualifier (7th)
3 Neurological System - Whole Body H Integumentary System - Whole Body M Musculoskeletal System - Whole Body	3 Postural Control	E Orthosis F Assistive, Adaptive, Supportive or Protective U Prosthesis Y Other Equipment Z None	Z None

Continued →

Section   **F**   **Physical Rehabilitation and Diagnostic Audiology**
Section Qualifier   **0**   **Rehabilitation**
Type   **C**   **Vestibular Treatment:** Application of techniques to improve, augment, or compensate for vestibular and related functional impairment

Body System / Region (4th)	Type Qualifier (5th)	Equipment (6th)	Qualifier (7th)
Z None	0 Vestibular	8 Vestibular / Balance Z None	Z None
Z None	1 Perceptual Processing 2 Visual Motor Integration	K Audiovisual L Assistive Listening N Biosensory Feedback P Computer Q Speech Analysis S Voice Analysis T Aerodynamic Function Y Other Equipment Z None	Z None

Section   **F**   **Physical Rehabilitation and Diagnostic Audiology**
Section Qualifier   **0**   **Rehabilitation**
Type   **D**   **Device Fitting:** Fitting of a device designed to facilitate or support achievement of a higher level of function

Body System / Region (4th)	Type Qualifier (5th)	Equipment (6th)	Qualifier (7th)
Z None	0 Tinnitus Masker	5 Hearing Aid Selection / Fitting / Test Z None	Z None
Z None	1 Monaural Hearing Aid 2 Binaural Hearing Aid 5 Assistive Listening Device	1 Audiometer 2 Sound Field / Booth 5 Hearing Aid Selection / Fitting / Test K Audiovisual L Assistive Listening Z None	Z None
Z None	3 Augmentative/Alternative Communication System	M Augmentative / Alternative Communication	Z None
Z None	4 Voice Prosthetic	S Voice Analysis V Speech Prosthesis	Z None
Z None	6 Dynamic Orthosis 7 Static Orthosis 8 Prosthesis 9 Assistive, Adaptive, Supportive or Protective Devices	E Orthosis F Assistive, Adaptive, Supportive or Protective U Prosthesis Z None	Z None

Section	F	Physical Rehabilitation and Diagnostic Audiology
Section Qualifier	0	Rehabilitation
Type	F	Caregiver Training: Training in activities to support patient's optimal level of function

Body System / Region (4th)	Type Qualifier (5th)	Equipment (6th)	Qualifier (7th)
Z None	0 Bathing/Showering Technique 1 Dressing 2 Feeding and Eating 3 Grooming/Personal Hygiene 4 Bed Mobility 5 Transfer 6 Wheelchair Mobility 7 Therapeutic Exercise 8 Airway Clearance Techniques 9 Wound Management B Vocational Activities and Functional Community or Work Reintegration Skills C Gait Training/Functional Ambulation D Application, Proper Use and Care of Devices F Application, Proper Use and Care of Orthoses G Application, Proper Use and Care of Prosthesis H Home Management	E Orthosis F Assistive, Adaptive, Supportive or Protective U Prosthesis Z None	Z None
Z None	J Communication Skills	K Audiovisual L Assistive Listening M Augmentative / Alternative Communication P Computer Z None	Z None

Section	F	Physical Rehabilitation and Diagnostic Audiology
Section Qualifier	1	Diagnostic Audiology
Type	3	Hearing Assessment: Measurement of hearing and related functions

Body System / Region (4th)	Type Qualifier (5th)	Equipment (6th)	Qualifier (7th)
Z None	0 Hearing Screening	0 Occupational Hearing 1 Audiometer 2 Sound Field / Booth 3 Tympanometer 8 Vestibular / Balance 9 Cochlear Implant Z None	Z None
Z None	1 Pure Tone Audiometry, Air 2 Pure Tone Audiometry, Air and Bone	0 Occupational Hearing 1 Audiometer 2 Sound Field / Booth Z None	Z None
Z None	3 Bekesy Audiometry 6 Visual Reinforcement Audiometry 9 Short Increment Sensitivity Index B Stenger C Pure Tone Stenger	1 Audiometer 2 Sound Field / Booth Z None	Z None
Z None	4 Conditioned Play Audiometry 5 Select Picture Audiometry	1 Audiometer 2 Sound Field / Booth K Audiovisual Z None	Z None
Z None	7 Alternate Binaural or Monaural Loudness Balance	1 Audiometer K Audiovisual Z None	Z None

Continued →

Section	F	Physical Rehabilitation and Diagnostic Audiology
Section Qualifier	1	Diagnostic Audiology
Type	3	Hearing Assessment: Measurement of hearing and related functions

Body System / Region (4th)	Type Qualifier (5th)	Equipment (6th)	Qualifier (7th)
Z None	8 Tone Decay D Tympanometry F Eustachian Tube Function G Acoustic Reflex Patterns H Acoustic Reflex Threshold J Acoustic Reflex Decay	3 Tympanometer 4 Electroacoustic Immitance / Acoustic Reflex Z None	Z None
Z None	K Electrocochleography L Auditory Evoked Potentials	7 Electrophysiologic Z None	Z None
Z None	M Evoked Otoacoustic Emissions, Screening N Evoked Otoacoustic Emissions, Diagnostic	6 Otoacoustic Emission (OAE) Z None	Z None
Z None	P Aural Rehabilitation Status	1 Audiometer 2 Sound Field / Booth 4 Electroacoustic Immitance / Acoustic Reflex 9 Cochlear Implant K Audiovisual L Assistive Listening P Computer Z None	Z None
Z None	Q Auditory Processing	K Audiovisual P Computer Y Other Equipment Z None	Z None

Section	F	Physical Rehabilitation and Diagnostic Audiology
Section Qualifier	1	Diagnostic Audiology
Type	4	Hearing Aid Assessment: Measurement of the appropriateness and/or effectiveness of a hearing device

Body System / Region (4th)	Type Qualifier (5th)	Equipment (6th)	Qualifier (7th)
Z None	0 Cochlear Implant	1 Audiometer 2 Sound Field / Booth 3 Tympanometer 4 Electroacoustic Immitance / Acoustic Reflex 5 Hearing Aid Selection / Fitting / Test 7 Electrophysiologic 9 Cochlear Implant K Audiovisual L Assistive Listening P Computer Y Other Equipment Z None	Z None
Z None	1 Ear Canal Probe Microphone 6 Binaural Electroacoustic Hearing Aid Check 8 Monaural Electroacoustic Hearing Aid Check	5 Hearing Aid Selection / Fitting / Test Z None	Z None

Continued →

Section Qualifier 1   Diagnostic Audiology
Type   4   **Hearing Aid Assessment:** Measurement of the appropriateness and/or effectiveness of a hearing device

Body System / Region (4th)	Type Qualifier (5th)	Equipment (6th)	Qualifier (7th)
Z None	2 Monaural Hearing Aid 3 Binaural Hearing Aid	1 Audiometer 2 Sound Field / Booth 3 Tympanometer 4 Electroacoustic Immitance / Acoustic Reflex 5 Hearing Aid Selection / Fitting / Test K Audiovisual L Assistive Listening P Computer Z None	Z None
Z None	4 Assistive Listening System/ Device Selection	1 Audiometer 2 Sound Field / Booth 3 Tympanometer 4 Electroacoustic Immitance / Acoustic Reflex K Audiovisual L Assistive Listening Z None	Z None
Z None	5 Sensory Aids	1 Audiometer 2 Sound Field / Booth 3 Tympanometer 4 Electroacoustic Immitance / Acoustic Reflex 5 Hearing Aid Selection / Fitting / Test K Audiovisual L Assistive Listening Z None	Z None
Z None	7 Ear Protector Attentuation	0 Occupational Hearing Z None	Z None

Section   F   **Physical Rehabilitation and Diagnostic Audiology**
Section Qualifier 1   **Diagnostic Audiology**
Type   5   **Vestibular Assessment:** Measurement of the vestibular system and related functions

Body System / Region (4th)	Type Qualifier (5th)	Equipment (6th)	Qualifier (7th)
Z None	0 Bithermal, Binaural Caloric Irrigation 1 Bithermal, Monaural Caloric Irrigation 2 Unithermal Binaural Screen 3 Oscillating Tracking 4 Sinusoidal Vertical Axis Rotational 5 Dix-Hallpike Dynamic 6 Computerized Dynamic Posturography	8 Vestibular / Balance Z None	Z None
Z None	7 Tinnitus Masker	5 Hearing Aid Selection / Fitting / Test Z None	Z None

AHA Coding Clinic

No references have been issued for the Physical Rehabilitation and Diagnostic Audiology section.

Within each section of ICD-10-PCS the characters have different meanings. The seven character meanings for the Mental Health section are illustrated here through the procedure example of *Crisis intervention*.

Section	Body System	Root Type	Qualifier	Qualifier	Qualifier	Qualifier
Mental Health	None	Crisis Intervention	None	None	None	None
G	Z	2	Z	Z	Z	Z

Section (Character 1)

All Mental Health procedure codes have a first character value of G.

Body System (Character 2)

The body system is not specified for mental health; therefore, the placeholder character value of Z is reported in the second character position.

Root Type (Character 3)

The alphanumeric character value for root types is placed in the third position. Listed below are the root types applicable to the Mental Health section with their associated meaning.

Character Value	Root Type	Root Type Definition
1	Psychological Tests	The administration and interpretation of standardized psychological tests and measurement instruments for the assessment of psychological function
2	Crisis Intervention	Treatment of a traumatized, acutely disturbed or distressed individual for the purpose of short-term stabilization
3	Medication Management	Monitoring and adjusting the use of medications for the treatment of a mental health disorder
5	Individual Psychotherapy	Treatment of an individual with a mental health disorder by behavioral, cognitive, psychoanalytic, psychodynamic or psychophysiological means to improve functioning or well-being
6	Counseling	The application of psychological methods to treat an individual with normal developmental issues and psychological problems in order to increase function, improve well-being, alleviate distress, maladjustment or resolve crises
7	Family Psychotherapy	Treatment that includes one or more family members of an individual with a mental health disorder by behavioral, cognitive, psychoanalytic, psychodynamic or psychophysiological means to improve functioning or well-being
B	Electroconvulsive Therapy	The application of controlled electrical voltages to treat a mental health disorder
C	Biofeedback	Provision of information from the monitoring and regulating of physiological processes in conjunction with cognitive-behavioral techniques to improve patient functioning or well-being
F	Hypnosis	Induction of a state of heightened suggestibility by auditory, visual and tactile techniques to elicit an emotional or behavioral response
G	Narcosynthesis	Administration of intravenous barbiturates in order to release suppressed or repressed thoughts
H	Group Psychotherapy	Treatment of two or more individuals with a mental health disorder by behavioral, cognitive, psychoanalytic, psychodynamic or psychophysiological means to improve functioning or well-being
J	Light Therapy	Application of specialized light treatments to improve functioning or well-being

Qualifier (Character 4)

This qualifier further specifies the root type procedure. For example, the qualifier of Development further specifies the type of Psychological Tests.

Qualifier (Character 5)

The qualifier represents an additional attribute for the procedure when applicable. Currently, there are no qualifiers in the Mental Health section; therefore, the placeholder character value of Z should be reported.

Qualifier (Character 6)

The qualifier represents an additional attribute for the procedure when applicable. Currently, there are no qualifiers in the Mental Health section; therefore, the placeholder character value of Z should be reported.

Qualifier (Character 7)

The qualifier represents an additional attribute for the procedure when applicable. Currently, there are no qualifiers in the Mental Health section; therefore, the placeholder character value of Z should be reported.

Mental Health Section Tables

Mental Health Tables GZ1–GZJ

Section	G	Mental Health
Body System	Z	None
Type	1	**Psychological Tests:** The administration and interpretation of standardized psychological tests and measurement instruments for the assessment of psychological function

Qualifier (4th)	Qualifier (5th)	Qualifier (6th)	Qualifier (7th)
0 Developmental 1 Personality and Behavioral 2 Intellectual and Psychoeducational 3 Neuropsychological 4 Neurobehavioral and Cognitive Status	Z None	Z None	Z None

Section	G	Mental Health
Body System	Z	None
Type	2	**Crisis Intervention:** Treatment of a traumatized, acutely disturbed or distressed individual for the purpose of short-term stabilization

Qualifier (4th)	Qualifier (5th)	Qualifier (6th)	Qualifier (7th)
Z None	Z None	Z None	Z None

Section	G	Mental Health
Body System	Z	None
Type	3	**Medication Management:** Monitoring and adjusting the use of medications for the treatment of a mental health disorder

Qualifier (4th)	Qualifier (5th)	Qualifier (6th)	Qualifier (7th)
Z None	Z None	Z None	Z None

Section	G	Mental Health
Body System	Z	None
Type	5	**Individual Psychotherapy:** Treatment of an individual with a mental health disorder by behavioral, cognitive, psychoanalytic, psychodynamic or psychophysiological means to improve functioning or well-being

Qualifier (4th)	Qualifier (5th)	Qualifier (6th)	Qualifier (7th)
0 Interactive 1 Behavioral 2 Cognitive 3 Interpersonal 4 Psychoanalysis 5 Psychodynamic 6 Supportive 8 Cognitive-Behavioral 9 Psychophysiological	Z None	Z None	Z None

Section   **G**   **Mental Health**
Body System   **Z**   **None**
Type   **6**   **Counseling:** The application of psychological methods to treat an individual with normal developmental issues and psychological problems in order to increase function, improve well-being, alleviate distress, maladjustment or resolve crises

Qualifier (4th)	Qualifier (5th)	Qualifier (6th)	Qualifier (7th)
0 Educational 1 Vocational 3 Other Counseling	Z None	Z None	Z None

Section   **G**   **Mental Health**
Body System   **Z**   **None**
Type   **7**   **Family Psychotherapy:** Treatment that includes one or more family members of an individual with a mental health disorder by behavioral, cognitive, psychoanalytic, psychodynamic or psychophysiological means to improve functioning or well-being

Qualifier (4th)	Qualifier (5th)	Qualifier (6th)	Qualifier (7th)
2 Other Family Psychotherapy	Z None	Z None	Z None

Section   **G**   **Mental Health**
Body System   **Z**   **None**
Type   **B**   **Electroconvulsive Therapy:** The application of controlled electrical voltages to treat a mental health disorder

Qualifier (4th)	Qualifier (5th)	Qualifier (6th)	Qualifier (7th)
0 Unilateral-Single Seizure 1 Unilateral-Multiple Seizure 2 Bilateral-Single Seizure 3 Bilateral-Multiple Seizure 4 Other Electroconvulsive Therapy	Z None	Z None	Z None

Section   **G**   **Mental Health**
Body System   **Z**   **None**
Type   **C**   **Biofeedback:** Provision of information from the monitoring and regulating of physiological processes in conjunction with cognitive-behavioral techniques to improve patient functioning or well-being

Qualifier (4th)	Qualifier (5th)	Qualifier (6th)	Qualifier (7th)
9 Other Biofeedback	Z None	Z None	Z None

Section   **G**   **Mental Health**
Body System   **Z**   **None**
Type   **F**   **Hypnosis:** Induction of a state of heightened suggestibility by auditory, visual and tactile techniques to elicit an emotional or behavioral response

Qualifier (4th)	Qualifier (5th)	Qualifier (6th)	Qualifier (7th)
Z None	Z None	Z None	Z None

Section   **G**   **Mental Health**
Body System   **Z**   **None**
Type   **G**   **Narcosynthesis:** Administration of intravenous barbiturates in order to release suppressed or repressed thoughts

Qualifier (4th)	Qualifier (5th)	Qualifier (6th)	Qualifier (7th)
Z None	Z None	Z None	Z None

Section	G	Mental Health
Body System	Z	None
Type	H	**Group Psychotherapy:** Treatment of two or more individuals with a mental health disorder by behavioral, cognitive, psychoanalytic, psychodynamic or psychophysiological means to improve functioning or well-being

Qualifier (4th)	Qualifier (5th)	Qualifier (6th)	Qualifier (7th)
Z None	**Z** None	**Z** None	**Z** None

Section	G	Mental Health
Body System	Z	None
Type	J	**Light Therapy:** Application of specialized light treatments to improve functioning or well-being

Qualifier (4th)	Qualifier (5th)	Qualifier (6th)	Qualifier (7th)
Z None	**Z** None	**Z** None	**Z** None

AHA Coding Clinic

No references have been issued for the Mental Health section.

Within each section of ICD-10-PCS the characters have different meanings. The seven character meanings for the Substance Abuse Treatment section are illustrated below through the procedure example of *Substance abuse family counseling*.

Section	Body System	Root Type	Qualifier	Qualifier	Qualifier	Qualifier
Substance Abuse	None	Family Counseling	Other Family Counseling	None	None	None
H	Z	6	3	Z	Z	Z

Section (Character 1)

All Substance Abuse Treatment procedure codes have a first character value of H.

Body System (Character 2)

The body system is not specified for substance abuse treatment; therefore, the placeholder character value of Z is reported in the second character position.

Root Type (Character 3)

The alphanumeric character value for root types is placed in the third position. The following are the root types applicable to the Substance Abuse Treatment section with their associated meaning.

Character Value	Root Type	Root Type Definition
2	Detoxification Services	Detoxification from alcohol and/or drugs
3	Individual Counseling	The application of psychological methods to treat an individual with addictive behavior
4	Group Counseling	The application of psychological methods to treat two or more individuals with addictive behavior
5	Individual Psychotherapy	Treatment of an individual with addictive behavior by behavioral, cognitive, psychoanalytic, psychodynamic or psychophysiological means
6	Family Counseling	The application of psychological methods that includes one or more family members to treat an individual with addictive behavior
8	Medication Management	Monitoring and adjusting the use of replacement medications for the treatment of addiction
9	Pharmacotherapy	The use of replacement medications for the treatment of addiction

Qualifier (Character 4)

This qualifier further specifies the root type procedure. For example, the qualifier of Cognitive further specifies the type of Individual counseling.

Qualifier (Character 5)

The qualifier represents an additional attribute for the procedure when applicable. Currently, there are no qualifiers in the Substance Abuse Treatment section; therefore, the placeholder character value of Z should be reported.

Qualifier (Character 6)

The qualifier represents an additional attribute for the procedure when applicable. Currently, there are no qualifiers in the Substance Abuse Treatment section; therefore, the placeholder character value of Z should be reported.

Qualifier (Character 7)

The qualifier represents an additional attribute for the procedure when applicable. Currently, there are no qualifiers in the Substance Abuse Treatment section; therefore, the placeholder character value of Z should be reported.

Substance Abuse Treatment Section Tables

Substance Abuse Treatment Tables HZ2–HZ9

Section	H	Substance Abuse Treatment
Body System	Z	None
Type	2	**Detoxification Services:** Detoxification from alcohol and/or drugs

Qualifier (4th)	Qualifier (5th)	Qualifier (6th)	Qualifier (7th)
Z None	**Z** None	**Z** None	**Z** None

Section	H	Substance Abuse Treatment
Body System	Z	None
Type	3	**Individual Counseling:** The application of psychological methods to treat an individual with addictive behavior

Qualifier (4th)	Qualifier (5th)	Qualifier (6th)	Qualifier (7th)
0 Cognitive **1** Behavioral **2** Cognitive-Behavioral **3** 12-Step **4** Interpersonal **5** Vocational **6** Psychoeducation **7** Motivational Enhancement **8** Confrontational **9** Continuing Care **B** Spiritual **C** Pre/Post-Test Infectious Disease	**Z** None	**Z** None	**Z** None

Section	H	Substance Abuse Treatment
Body System	Z	None
Type	4	**Group Counseling:** The application of psychological methods to treat two or more individuals with addictive behavior

Qualifier (4th)	Qualifier (5th)	Qualifier (6th)	Qualifier (7th)
0 Cognitive **1** Behavioral **2** Cognitive-Behavioral **3** 12-Step **4** Interpersonal **5** Vocational **6** Psychoeducation **7** Motivational Enhancement **8** Confrontational **9** Continuing Care **B** Spiritual **C** Pre/Post-Test Infectious Disease	**Z** None	**Z** None	**Z** None

Section	H	Substance Abuse Treatment
Body System	Z	None
Type	5	**Individual Psychotherapy:** Treatment of an individual with addictive behavior by behavioral, cognitive, psychoanalytic, psychodynamic or psychophysiological means

Qualifier (4ᵗʰ)	Qualifier (5ᵗʰ)	Qualifier (6ᵗʰ)	Qualifier (7ᵗʰ)
0 Cognitive	Z None	Z None	Z None
1 Behavioral			
2 Cognitive-Behavioral			
3 12-Step			
4 Interpersonal			
5 Interactive			
6 Psychoeducation			
7 Motivational Enhancement			
8 Confrontational			
9 Supportive			
B Psychoanalysis			
C Psychodynamic			
D Psychophysiological			

Section	H	Substance Abuse Treatment
Body System	Z	None
Type	6	**Family Counseling:** The application of psychological methods that includes one or more family members to treat an individual with addictive behavior

Qualifier (4ᵗʰ)	Qualifier (5ᵗʰ)	Qualifier (6ᵗʰ)	Qualifier (7ᵗʰ)
3 Other Family Counseling	Z None	Z None	Z None

Section	H	Substance Abuse Treatment
Body System	Z	None
Type	8	**Medication Management:** Monitoring and adjusting the use of replacement medications for the treatment of addiction

Qualifier (4ᵗʰ)	Qualifier (5ᵗʰ)	Qualifier (6ᵗʰ)	Qualifier (7ᵗʰ)
0 Nicotine Replacement	Z None	Z None	Z None
1 Methadone Maintenance			
2 Levo-alpha-acetyl-methadol (LAAM)			
3 Antabuse			
4 Naltrexone			
5 Naloxone			
6 Clonidine			
7 Bupropion			
8 Psychiatric Medication			
9 Other Replacement Medication			

Section	H	Substance Abuse Treatment
Body System	Z	None
Type	9	**Pharmacotherapy:** The use of replacement medications for the treatment of addiction

Qualifier (4ᵗʰ)	Qualifier (5ᵗʰ)	Qualifier (6ᵗʰ)	Qualifier (7ᵗʰ)
0 Nicotine Replacement	Z None	Z None	Z None
1 Methadone Maintenance			
2 Levo-alpha-acetyl-methadol (LAAM)			
3 Antabuse			
4 Naltrexone			
5 Naloxone			
6 Clonidine			
7 Bupropion			
8 Psychiatric Medication			
9 Other Replacement Medication			

AHA Coding Clinic

HZ2ZZZZ Detoxification Services for Substance Abuse Treatment—AHA CC: 1Q, 2020, 21-22

HZ98ZZZ Pharmacotherapy for Substance Abuse Treatment, Psychiatric Medication—AHA CC: 1Q, 2020, 21-22

Within each section of ICD-10-PCS the characters have different meanings. The seven character meanings for the New Technology section are illustrated below through the procedure example of *Introduction of ceftazidime-avibactam anti-infective into peripheral vein, percutaneous approach.*

Section	Body System	Root Operation	Body Part	Approach	Device / Substance / Technology	Qualifier
New Technology	Anatomical Regions	Introduction	Peripheral Vein	Percutaneous	Ceftazidime-Avibactam Anti-infective	New Technology Group 1
X	W	0	3	3	2	1

Section (Character 1)

All New Technology procedure codes have a first character value of X.

Body System (Character 2)

For each body system the applicable body part character values will be available for procedure code construction.

Root Operations (Character 3)

The alphanumeric character value for root operations is placed in the third position. Listed below are the root operations applicable to the New Technology section with their associated meaning.

Character Value	Root Operation	Root Operation Definition
A	Assistance	Taking over a portion of a physiological function by extracorporeal means
C	Extirpation	Taking or cutting out solid matter from a body part
E	Measurement	Determining a level of a physiological or physical function at a point in time
G	Fusion	Joining together portions of an articular body part rendering the articular body part immobile
R	Replacement	Putting in or on biological or synthetic material that physically takes the place and/or function of all or a portion of a body part
S	Reposition	Moving to its normal location, or other suitable location, all or a portion of a body part
U	Supplement	Putting in or on biological or synthetic material that physically reinforces and/or augments the function of a portion of a body part
0	Introduction	Putting in or on a therapeutic, diagnostic, nutritional, physiological, or prophylactic substance except blood or blood products
1	Transfusion In Anatomical Regions	Putting in blood or blood products
2	Monitoring In Joints & Urinary System	Determining the level of a physiological or physical function repetitively
2	Transfusion In Anatomical Regions	Putting in blood or blood products
5	Destruction	Physical eradication of all or a portion of a body part by the direct use of energy, force, or a destructive agent
7	Dilation	Expanding an orifice or the lumen of a tubular body part

Body Part (Character 4)

For each body system the applicable body part character values will be available for procedure code construction.

Approach (Character 5)

The approach is the technique used to reach the procedure site. Listed below are the approach character values for the New Technology section with the associated definitions.

Character Value	Approach	Approach Definition
0	Open	Cutting through the skin or mucous membrane and any other body layers necessary to expose the site of the procedure
3	Percutaneous	Entry, by puncture or minor incision, of instrumentation through the skin or mucous membrane and any other body layers necessary to reach the site of the procedure
4	Percutaneous Endoscopic	Entry, by puncture or minor incision, of instrumentation through the skin or mucous membrane and any other body layers necessary to reach and visualize the site of the procedure
7	Via Natural or Artificial Opening	Entry of instrumentation through a natural or artificial external opening to reach the site of the procedure
8	Via Natural or Artificial Opening Endoscopic	Entry of instrumentation through a natural or artificial external opening to reach and visualize the site of the procedure
X	External	Procedures performed directly on the skin or mucous membrane and procedures performed indirectly by the application of external force through the skin or mucous membrane

Device/Substance/Technology (Character 6)

The New Technology section created a place within ICD-10-PCS to include procedure codes for new services that utilize a specific new device, substance, or technology. Procedures in this section may be part of the Inpatient Prospective Payment System (IPPS) new technology add-on payment mechanism. Depending on the procedure performed there is either a device, substance, or new technology utilized.

Qualifier (Character 7)

The qualifier represents the category year in which the new device, substance, or technology was added to the coding system. In federal fiscal year 2016 (October 1, 2015) the first group of device, substance, and technology was added and therefore are labeled as New Technology Group 1.

New Technology Section Guidelines (section X)

E. New Technology Section

General Guidelines

E1.a Section X codes fully represent the specific procedure described in the code title, and do not require any additional codes from other sections of ICD-10-PCS. When section X contains a code title which describes a specific new technology procedure, and it is the only procedure performed, only the X code is reported for the procedure. There is no need to report an additional code in another section of ICD-10-PCS.

Example: XW04321 Introduction of Ceftazidime-Avibactam Anti-infective into Central Vein, Percutaneous Approach, New Technology Group 1 can be coded to indicate that Ceftazidime-Avibactam Anti-infective was administered via a central vein. A separate code from table 3E0 in the Administration section of ICD-10-PCS is not coded in addition to this code.

E1.b When multiple procedures are performed, New Technology section X codes are coded following the multiple procedures guideline.

Examples: Dual filter cerebral embolic filtration used during transcatheter aortic valve replacement (TAVR), X2A5312 Cerebral Embolic Filtration, Dual Filter in Innominate Artery and Left Common Carotid Artery, Percutaneous Approach, New Technology Group 2, is coded for the cerebral embolic filtration, along with an ICD-10-PCS code for the TAVR procedure. Magnetically controlled growth rod (MCGR) placed during a spinal fusion procedure, a code from table XNS, Reposition of the Bones is coded for the MCGR, along with an ICD-10-PCS code for the spinal fusion procedure.

New Technology Tables X27–XY0

Section	X	New Technology
Body System	2	Cardiovascular
Operation	7	**Dilation:** Expanding an orifice or the lumen of a tubular body part

Body Part (4th)	Approach (5th)	Device/Substance/Technology (6th)	Qualifier (7th)
H Femoral Artery, Right J Femoral Artery, Left K Popliteal Artery, Proximal Right L Popliteal Artery, Proximal Left M Popliteal Artery, Distal Right N Popliteal Artery, Distal Left P Anterior Tibial Artery, Right Q Anterior Tibial Artery, Left R Posterior Tibial Artery, Right S Posterior Tibial Artery, Left T Peroneal Tibial Artery, Right U Peroneal Tibial Artery, Left	3 Percutaneous	8 Intraluminal Device, Sustained Release Drug-eluting 9 Intraluminal Device, Sustained Release Drug-eluting, Two B Intraluminal Device, Sustained Release Drug-eluting, Three C Intraluminal Device, Sustained Release Drug-eluting, Four or More	5 New Technology Group 5

Section	X	New Technology
Body System	2	Cardiovascular System
Operation	A	**Assistance:** Taking over a portion of a physiological function by extracorporeal means

Body Part (4th)	Approach (5th)	Device/Substance/Technology (6th)	Qualifier (7th)
5 Innominate Artery and Left Common Carotid Artery	3 Percutaneous	1 Cerebral Embolic Filtration, Dual Filter	2 New Technology Group 2
6 Aortic Arch	3 Percutaneous	2 Cerebral Embolic Filtration, Single Deflection Filter	5 New Technology Group 5
H Common Carotid Artery, Right J Common Carotid Artery, Left	3 Percutaneous	3 Cerebral Embolic Filtration, Extracorporeal Flow Reversal Circuit	6 New Technology Group 6

Section	X	New Technology
Body System	2	Cardiovascular System
Operation	C	**Extirpation:** Taking or cutting out solid matter from a body part

Body Part (4th)	Approach (5th)	Device/Substance/Technology (6th)	Qualifier (7th)
0 Coronary Artery, One Artery 1 Coronary Artery, Two Arteries 2 Coronary Artery, Three Arteries 3 Coronary Artery, Four or More Arteries	3 Percutaneous	6 Orbital Atherectomy Technology	1 New Technology Group 1

Section	X	New Technology
Body System	2	Cardiovascular System
Operation	R	**Replacement:** Putting in or on biological or synthetic material that physically takes the place and/or function of all or a portion of a body part

Body Part (4th)	Approach (5th)	Device/Substance/Technology (6th)	Qualifier (7th)
F Aortic Valve	0 Open 3 Percutaneous 4 Percutaneous Endoscopic	3 Zooplastic Tissue, Rapid Deployment Technique	2 New Technology Group 2

Section   X   New Technology
Body System   H   Skin, Subcutaneous Tissue, Fascia and Breast
Operation   R   **Replacement:** Putting in or on biological or synthetic material that physically takes the place and/or function of all or a portion of a body part

Body Part (4th)	Approach (5th)	Device/Substance/Technology (6th)	Qualifier (7th)
P Skin	X External	L Skin Substitute, Porcine Liver Derived	2 New Technology Group 2

Section   X   New Technology
Body System   K   Muscles, Tendons, Bursae and Ligaments
Operation   0   **Introduction:** Putting in or on a therapeutic, diagnostic, nutritional, physiological, or prophylactic substance except blood or blood products

Body Part (4th)	Approach (5th)	Device/Substance/Technology (6th)	Qualifier (7th)
2 Muscle	3 Percutaneous	0 Concentrated Bone Marrow Aspirate	3 New Technology Group 3

Section   X   New Technology
Body System   N   Bones
Operation   S   **Reposition:** Moving to its normal location, or other suitable location, all or a portion of a body part

Body Part (4th)	Approach (5th)	Device/Substance/Technology (6th)	Qualifier (7th)
0 Lumbar Vertebra 3 Cervical Vertebra 4 Thoracic Vertebra	0 Open 3 Percutaneous	3 Magnetically Controlled Growth Rod(s)	2 New Technology Group 2

Section   X   New Technology
Body System   N   Bones
Operation   U   **Supplement:** Putting in or on biological or synthetic material that physically reinforces and/or augments the function of a portion of a body part

Body Part (4th)	Approach (5th)	Device/Substance/Technology (6th)	Qualifier (7th)
0 Lumbar Vertebra 4 Thoracic Vertebra	3 Percutaneous	5 Synthetic Substitute, Mechanically Expandable (Paired)	6 New Technology Group 6

Section   X   New Technology
Body System   R   Joints
Operation   2   **Monitoring:** Determining the level of a physiological or physical function repetitively over a period of time

Body Part (4th)	Approach (5th)	Device/Substance/Technology (6th)	Qualifier (7th)
G Knee Joint, Right H Knee Joint, Left	0 Open	2 Intraoperative Knee Replacement Sensor	1 New Technology Group 1

Section   X   New Technology
Body System   R   Joints
Operation   G   **Fusion:** Joining together portions of an articular body part rendering the articular body part immobile

Body Part (4th)	Approach (5th)	Device/Substance/Technology (6th)	Qualifier (7th)
0 Occipital-cervical Joint	0 Open	9 Interbody Fusion Device, Nanotextured Surface	2 New Technology Group 2
0 Occipital-cervical Joint	0 Open	F Interbody Fusion Device, Radiolucent Porous	3 New Technology Group 3
1 Cervical Vertebral Joint	0 Open	9 Interbody Fusion Device, Nanotextured Surface	2 New Technology Group 2
1 Cervical Vertebral Joint	0 Open	F Interbody Fusion Device, Radiolucent Porous	3 New Technology Group 3

Continued →

Section	X	New Technology
Body System	R	Joints
Operation	G	**Fusion:** Joining together portions of an articular body part rendering the articular body part immobile

Body Part (4th)	Approach (5th)	Device/Substance/Technology (6th)	Qualifier (7th)
2 Cervical Vertebral Joints, 2 or More	**0** Open	**9** Interbody Fusion Device, Nanotextured Surface	**2** New Technology Group 2
2 Cervical Vertebral Joints, 2 or More	**0** Open	**F** Interbody Fusion Device, Radiolucent Porous	**3** New Technology Group 3
4 Cervicothoracic Vertebral Joint	**0** Open	**9** Interbody Fusion Device, Nanotextured Surface	**2** New Technology Group 2
4 Cervicothoracic Vertebral Joint	**0** Open	**F** Interbody Fusion Device, Radiolucent Porous	**3** New Technology Group 3
6 Thoracic Vertebral Joint	**0** Open	**9** Interbody Fusion Device, Nanotextured Surface	**2** New Technology Group 2
6 Thoracic Vertebral Joint	**0** Open	**F** Interbody Fusion Device, Radiolucent Porous	**3** New Technology Group 3
7 Thoracic Vertebral Joints, 2 to 7	**0** Open	**9** Interbody Fusion Device, Nanotextured Surface	**2** New Technology Group 2
7 Thoracic Vertebral Joints. 2 to 7	**0** Open	**F** Interbody Fusion Device, Radiolucent Porous	**3** New Technology Group 3
8 Thoracic Vertebral Joints, 8 or More	**0** Open	**9** Interbody Fusion Device, Nanotextured Surface	**2** New Technology Group 2
8 Thoracic Vertebral Joints, 8 or More	**0** Open	**F** Interbody Fusion Device, Radiolucent Porous	**3** New Technology Group 3
A Thoracolumbar Vertebral Joint	**0** Open	**9** Interbody Fusion Device, Nanotextured Surface	**2** New Technology Group 2
A Thoracolumbar Vertebral Joint	**0** Open	**F** Interbody Fusion Device, Radiolucent Porous	**3** New Technology Group 3
B Lumbar Vertebral Joint	**0** Open	**9** Interbody Fusion Device, Nanotextured Surface	**2** New Technology Group 2
B Lumbar Vertebral Joint	**0** Open	**F** Interbody Fusion Device, Radiolucent Porous	**3** New Technology Group 3
C Lumbar Vertebral Joints, 2 or More	**0** Open	**9** Interbody Fusion Device, Nanotextured Surface	**2** New Technology Group 2
C Lumbar Vertebral Joints, 2 or More	**0** Open	**F** Interbody Fusion Device, Radiolucent Porous	**3** New Technology Group 3
D Lumbosacral Vertebral Joint	**0** Open	**9** Interbody Fusion Device, Nanotextured Surface	**2** New Technology Group 2
D Lumbosacral Vertebral Joint	**0** Open	**F** Interbody Fusion Device, Radiolucent Porous	**3** New Technology Group 3

Section	X	New Technology
Body System	T	Urinary System
Operation	2	**Monitoring:** Determining the level of a physiological or physical function repetitively over a period of time

Body Part (4th)	Approach (5th)	Device/Substance/Technology (6th)	Qualifier (7th)
5 Kidney	**X** External	**E** Fluorescent Pyrazine	**5** New Technology Group 5

Section	X	New Technology
Body System	V	Male Reproductive System
Operation	5	Destruction: Physical eradication of all or a portion of a body part by the direct use of energy, force, or a destructive agent

Body Part (4th)	Approach (5th)	Device/Substance/Technology (6th)	Qualifier (7th)
0 Prostate	8 Via Natural or Artificial Opening Endoscopic	A Robotic Waterjet Ablation	4 New Technology Group 4

Section	X	New Technology
Body System	W	Anatomical Regions
Operation	0	Introduction: Putting in or on a therapeutic, diagnostic, nutritional, physiological, or prophylactic substance except blood or blood products

Body Part (4th)	Approach (5th)	Device/Substance/Technology (6th)	Qualifier (7th)
1 Subcutaneous Tissue	3 Percutaneous	F Other New Technology Therapeutic Substance W Caplacizumab	5 New Technology Group 5
3 Peripheral Vein	3 Percutaneous	0 Brexanolone	6 New Technology Group 6
3 Peripheral Vein	3 Percutaneous	2 Ceftazidime-Avibactam Anti-infective	1 New Technology Group 1
3 Peripheral Vein	3 Percutaneous	2 Nerinitide	6 New Technology Group 6
3 Peripheral Vein	3 Percutaneous	3 Idarucizumab, Dabigatran Reversal Agent	1 New Technology Group 1
3 Peripheral Vein	3 Percutaneous	3 Durvalumab Antineoplastic	6 New Technology Group 6
3 Peripheral Vein	3 Percutaneous	4 Isavuconazole Anti-infective 5 Blinatumomab Antineoplastic Immunotherapy	1 New Technology Group 1
3 Peripheral Vein	3 Percutaneous	6 Lefamulin Anti-infective	6 New Technology Group 6
3 Peripheral Vein	3 Percutaneous	7 Coagulation Factor Xa, Inactivated 9 Defibrotide Sodium Anticoagulant	2 New Technology Group 2
3 Peripheral Vein	3 Percutaneous	9 Ceftolozane/Tazobactam Anti-infective	6 New Technology Group 6
3 Peripheral Vein	3 Percutaneous	A Bezlotoxumab Monoclonal	3 New Technology Group 3
3 Peripheral Vein	3 Percutaneous	A Cefiderocol Anti-infective	6 New Technology Group 6
3 Peripheral Vein	3 Percutaneous	B Cytarabine and Daunorubicin Liposome Antineoplastic	3 New Technology Group 3
3 Peripheral Vein	3 Percutaneous	B Omadacycline Anti-infective	6 New Technology Group 6
3 Peripheral Vein	3 Percutaneous	C Engineered Autologous Chimeric Antigen Receptor T-cell Immunotherapy	3 New Technology Group 3
3 Peripheral Vein	3 Percutaneous	C Eculizumab D Atezolizumab Antineoplastic	6 New Technology Group 6
3 Peripheral Vein	3 Percutaneous	E Remdesivir Anti-infective	5 New Technology Group 5
3 Peripheral Vein	3 Percutaneous	F Other New Technology Therapeutic Substance	3 New Technology Group 3
3 Peripheral Vein	3 Percutaneous	F Other New Technology Therapeutic Substance	5 New Technology Group 5
3 Peripheral Vein	3 Percutaneous	G Plazomicin Anti-infective	4 New Technology Group 4
3 Peripheral Vein	3 Percutaneous	G Sarilumab	5 New Technology Group 5
3 Peripheral Vein	3 Percutaneous	H Synthetic Human Angiotensin II	4 New Technology Group 4

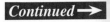

Continued ➡

Section	X	New Technology	*XWO Continued*
Body System	W	Anatomical Regions	
Operation	0	**Introduction:** Putting in or on a therapeutic, diagnostic, nutritional, physiological, or prophylactic substance except blood or blood products	

XW0

Body Part (4th)	Approach (5th)	Device/Substance/Technology (6th)	Qualifier (7th)
3 Peripheral Vein	3 Percutaneous	H Tocilizumab K Fosfomycin Anti-infective N Meropenem-vaborbactam Anti-infective Q Tagraxofusp-erzs Antineoplastic S Iobenguane I-131 Antineoplastic U Imipenem-cilastatin-relebactam Anti-infective W Caplacizumab	5 New Technology Group 5
4 Central Vein	3 Percutaneous	0 Brexanolone	6 New Technology Group 6
4 Central Vein	3 Percutaneous	2 Ceftazidime-Avibactam Anti-infective	1 New Technology Group 1
4 Central Vein	3 Percutaneous	2 Nerinitide	6 New Technology Group 6
4 Central Vein	3 Percutaneous	3 Idarucizumab, Dabigatran Reversal Agent	1 New Technology Group 1
4 Central Vein	3 Percutaneous	3 Durvalumab Antineoplastic	6 New Technology Group 6
4 Central Vein	3 Percutaneous	4 Isavuconazole Anti-infective 5 Blinatumomab Antineoplastic Immunotherapy	1 New Technology Group 1
4 Central Vein	3 Percutaneous	6 Lefamulin Anti-infective	6 New Technology Group 6
4 Central Vein	3 Percutaneous	7 Coagulation Factor Xa, Inactivated 9 Defibrotide Sodium Anticoagulant	2 New Technology Group 2
4 Central Vein	3 Percutaneous	9 Ceftolozane/Tazobactam Anti-infective	6 New Technology Group 6
4 Central Vein	3 Percutaneous	A Bezlotoxumab Monoclonal	3 New Technology Group 3
4 Central Vein	3 Percutaneous	A Cefiderocol Anti-infective	6 New Technology Group 6
4 Central Vein	3 Percutaneous	B Cytarabine and Daunorubicin Liposome Antineoplastic	3 New Technology Group 3
4 Central Vein	3 Percutaneous	B Omadacycline Anti-infective	6 New Technology Group 6
4 Central Vein	3 Percutaneous	C Engineered Autologous Chimeric Antigen Receptor T-cell Immunotherapy	3 New Technology Group 3
4 Central Vein	3 Percutaneous	C Eculizumab D Atezolizumab Antineoplastic	6 New Technology Group 6
4 Central Vein	3 Percutaneous	E Remdesivir Anti-infective	5 New Technology Group 5
4 Central Vein	3 Percutaneous	F Other New Technology Therapeutic Substance	3 New Technology Group 3
4 Central Vein	3 Percutaneous	F Other New Technology Therapeutic Substance	5 New Technology Group 5
4 Central Vein	3 Percutaneous	G Plazomicin Anti-infective	4 New Technology Group 4
4 Central Vein	3 Percutaneous	G Sarilumab	5 New Technology Group 5
4 Central Vein	3 Percutaneous	H Synthetic Human Angiotensin II	4 New Technology Group 4
4 Central Vein	3 Percutaneous	H Tocilizumab K Fosfomycin Anti-infective N Meropenem-vaborbactam Anti-infective Q Tagraxofusp-erzs Antineoplastic S Iobenguane I-131 Antineoplastic U Imipenem-cilastatin-relebactam Anti-infective W Caplacizumab	5 New Technology Group 5

Continued →

Section	X	New Technology
Body System	W	Anatomical Regions
Operation	0	Introduction: Putting in or on a therapeutic, diagnostic, nutritional, physiological, or prophylactic substance except blood or blood products

Body Part (4th)	Approach (5th)	Device/Substance/Technology (6th)	Qualifier (7th)
9 Nose	7 Via Natural or Artificial Opening	M Esketamine Hydrochloride	5 New Technology Group 5
D Mouth and Pharynx	X External	6 Lefamulin Anti-infective	6 New Technology Group 6
D Mouth and Pharynx	X External	8 Uridine Triacetate	2 New Technology Group 2
D Mouth and Pharynx	X External	F Other New Technology Therapeutic Substance J Apalutamide Antienoplastic L Erdafitinib Antineoplastic R Venetoclax Antineoplastic T Ruxolitnib V Gilteritinib Antineoplastic	5 New Technology Group 5
G Upper GI H Lower GI	8 Via Natural or Artificial Opening Endoscopic	8 Mineral-based Topical Hemostatic Agent	6 New Technology Group 6
Q Cranial Cavity and Brain	3 Percutaneous	1 Eladocagene exuparvovec	6 New Technology Group 6

Section	X	New Technology
Body System	W	Anatomical Regions
Operation	1	Transfusion: Putting in blood or blood products

Body Part (4th)	Approach (5th)	Device/Substance/Technology (6th)	Qualifier (7th)
3 Peripheral Vein 4 Central Vein	3 Percutaneous	2 Plasma, Convalescent (Nonautologous)	5 New Technology Group 5

Section	X	New Technology
Body System	W	Anatomical Regions
Operation	2	Transfusion: Putting in blood or blood products

Body Part (4th)	Approach (5th)	Device/Substance/Technology (6th)	Qualifier (7th)
3 Peripheral Vein 4 Central Vein	3 Percutaneous	4 Brexucabtagene Autoleucel Immunotherapy 7 Lisocabtagene Maraleucel Immunotherapy	6 New Technology Group 6

Section	X	New Technology
Body System	X	Physiological Systems
Operation	E	Measurement: Determining the level of a physiological or physical function at a point in time

Body Part (4th)	Approach (5th)	Device/Substance/Technology (6th)	Qualifier (7th)
5 Circulatory	X External	M Infection, Whole Blood Nucleic Acid-base Microbial Detection	5 New Technology Group 5
5 Circulatory	X External	N Infection, Positive Blood Culture Fluorescence Hybridization for Organism Identification, Concentration and Susceptibility	6 New Technology Group 6
B Respiratory	X External	Q Infection, Lower Respiratory Fluid Nucleic Acid-base Microbial Detection	6 New Technology Group 6

Section	X	New Technology
Body System	Y	Extracorporeal
Operation	0	**Introduction:** Putting in or on a therapeutic, diagnostic, nutritional, physiological, or prophylactic substance except blood or blood products

Body Part (4th)	Approach (5th)	Device/Substance/Technology (6th)	Qualifier (7th)
V Vein Graft	X External	8 Endothelial Damage Inhibitor	3 New Technology Group 3

AHA Coding Clinic

X2C0361 Extirpation of Matter from Coronary Artery, One Site Using Orbital Atherectomy Technology, Percutaneous Approach, New Technology Group 1—AHA CC: 4Q, 2015, 13-14

XNS0032 Reposition of Lumbar Vertebra using Magnetically Controlled Growth Rod(s), Open Approach, New Technology Group 2—AHA CC: 4Q, 2017, 75

XRGB0F3 Fusion of Lumbar Vertebral Joint using Radiolucent Porous Interbody Fusion Device, Open Approach, New Technology Group 3—AHA CC: 4Q, 2017, 76-77

XRGD0F3 Fusion of Lumbosacral Joint using Radiolucent Porous Interbody Fusion Device, Open Approach, New Technology Group 3—AHA CC: 4Q, 2017, 76-77

XV508A4 Destruction of Prostate using Robotic Waterjet Ablation, Via Natural or Artificial Opening Endoscopic, New Technology Group 4—AHA CC: 4Q, 2018, 55

XW04331 Introduction of Idarucizumab, Dabigatran Reversal Agent into Central Vein, Percutaneous Approach, New Technology Group 1—AHA CC: 4Q, 2015, 13

XW04351 Introduction of Blinatumomab Antineoplastic into Central Vein, Percutaneous Approach, New Technology Group 1—AHA CC: 4Q, 2015, 14-15

Appendix A: Root Operations Definitions

Section 0 - Medical and Surgical — Character 3 - Root Operation

Alteration (0)	**Definition:** Modifying the anatomic structure of a body part without affecting the function of the body part **Explanation:** Principal purpose is to improve appearance **Includes/Examples:** Face lift, breast augmentation
Bypass (1)	**Definition:** Altering the route of passage of the contents of a tubular body part **Explanation:** Rerouting contents of a body part to a downstream area of the normal route, to a similar route and body part, or to an abnormal route and dissimilar body part. Includes one or more anastomoses, with or without the use of a device **Includes/Examples:** Coronary artery bypass, colostomy formation
Change (2)	**Definition:** Taking out or off a device from a body part and putting back an identical or similar device in or on the same body part without cutting or puncturing the skin or a mucous membrane **Explanation:** All CHANGE procedures are coded using the approach EXTERNAL **Includes/Examples:** Urinary catheter change, gastrostomy tube change
Control (3)	**Definition:** Stopping, or attempting to stop, postprocedural or other acute bleeding **Includes/Examples:** Control of post-prostatectomy hemorrhage, control of intracranial subdural hemorrhage, control of bleeding duodenal ulcer, control of retroperitoneal hemorrhage
Creation (4)	**Definition:** Putting in or on biological or synthetic material to form a new body part that to the extent possible replicates the anatomic structure or function of an absent body part **Explanation:** Used for gender reassignment surgery and corrective procedures in individuals with congenital anomalies **Includes/Examples:** Creation of vagina in a male, creation of right and left atrioventricular valve from common atrioventricular valve
Destruction (5)	**Definition:** Physical eradication of all or a portion of a body part by the direct use of energy, force, or a destructive agent **Explanation:** None of the body part is physically taken out **Includes/Examples:** Fulguration of rectal polyp, cautery of skin lesion
Detachment (6)	**Definition:** Cutting off all or a portion of the upper or lower extremities **Explanation:** The body part value is the site of the detachment, with a qualifier if applicable to further specify the level where the extremity was detached **Includes/Examples:** Below knee amputation, disarticulation of shoulder
Dilation (7)	**Definition:** Expanding an orifice or the lumen of a tubular body part **Explanation:** The orifice can be a natural orifice or an artificially created orifice. Accomplished by stretching a tubular body part using intraluminal pressure or by cutting part of the orifice or wall of the tubular body part **Includes/Examples:** Percutaneous transluminal angioplasty, internal urethrotomy
Division (8)	**Definition:** Cutting into a body part, without draining fluids and/or gases from the body part, in order to separate or transect a body part **Explanation:** All or a portion of the body part is separated into two or more portions **Includes/Examples:** Spinal cordotomy, osteotomy
Drainage (9)	**Definition:** Taking or letting out fluids and/or gases from a body part **Explanation:** The qualifier DIAGNOSTIC is used to identify drainage procedures that are biopsies **Includes/Examples:** Thoracentesis, incision and drainage
Excision (B)	**Definition:** Cutting out or off, without replacement, a portion of a body part **Explanation:** The qualifier DIAGNOSTIC is used to identify excision procedures that are biopsies **Includes/Examples:** Partial nephrectomy, liver biopsy
Extirpation (C)	**Definition:** Taking or cutting out solid matter from a body part **Explanation:** The solid matter may be an abnormal byproduct of a biological function or a foreign body; it may be imbedded in a body part or in the lumen of a tubular body part. The solid matter may or may not have been previously broken into pieces **Includes/Examples:** Thrombectomy, choledocholithotomy
Extraction (D)	**Definition:** Pulling or stripping out or off all or a portion of a body part by the use of force **Explanation:** The qualifier DIAGNOSTIC is used to identify extraction procedures that are biopsies **Includes/Examples:** Dilation and curettage, vein stripping
Fragmentation (F)	**Definition:** Breaking solid matter in a body part into pieces **Explanation:** Physical force (e.g., manual, ultrasonic) applied directly or indirectly is used to break the solid matter into pieces. The solid matter may be an abnormal byproduct of a biological function or a foreign body. The pieces of solid matter are not taken out **Includes/Examples:** Extracorporeal shockwave lithotripsy, transurethral lithotripsy
Fusion (G)	**Definition:** Joining together portions of an articular body part rendering the articular body part immobile **Explanation:** The body part is joined together by fixation device, bone graft, or other means **Includes/Examples:** Spinal fusion, ankle arthrodesis
Insertion (H)	**Definition:** Putting in a nonbiological appliance that monitors, assists, performs, or prevents a physiological function but does not physically take the place of a body part **Includes/Examples:** Insertion of radioactive implant, insertion of central venous catheter

Continued →

Inspection (J)	**Definition:** Visually and/or manually exploring a body part **Explanation:** Visual exploration may be performed with or without optical instrumentation. Manual exploration may be performed directly or through intervening body layers **Includes/Examples:** Diagnostic arthroscopy, exploratory laparotomy
Map (K)	**Definition:** Locating the route of passage of electrical impulses and/or locating functional areas in a body part **Explanation:** Applicable only to the cardiac conduction mechanism and the central nervous system **Includes/Examples:** Cardiac mapping, cortical mapping
Occlusion (L)	**Definition:** Completely closing an orifice or the lumen of a tubular body part **Explanation:** The orifice can be a natural orifice or an artificially created orifice **Includes/Examples:** Fallopian tube ligation, ligation of inferior vena cava
Reattachment (M)	**Definition:** Putting back in or on all or a portion of a separated body part to its normal location or other suitable location **Explanation:** Vascular circulation and nervous pathways may or may not be reestablished **Includes/Examples:** Reattachment of hand, reattachment of avulsed kidney
Release (N)	**Definition:** Freeing a body part from an abnormal physical constraint by cutting or by the use of force **Explanation:** Some of the restraining tissue may be taken out but none of the body part is taken out **Includes/Examples:** Adhesiolysis, carpal tunnel release
Removal (P)	**Definition:** Taking out or off a device from a body part **Explanation:** If a device is taken out and a similar device put in without cutting or puncturing the skin or mucous membrane, the procedure is coded to the root operation CHANGE. Otherwise, the procedure for taking out a device is coded to the root operation REMOVAL **Includes/Examples:** Drainage tube removal, cardiac pacemaker removal
Repair (Q)	**Definition:** Restoring, to the extent possible, a body part to its normal anatomic structure and function **Explanation:** Used only when the method to accomplish the repair is not one of the other root operations **Includes/Examples:** Colostomy takedown, suture of laceration
Replacement (R)	**Definition:** Putting in or on biological or synthetic material that physically takes the place and/or function of all or a portion of a body part **Explanation:** The body part may have been taken out or replaced, or may be taken out, physically eradicated, or rendered nonfunctional during the Replacement procedure. A Removal procedure is coded for taking out the device used in a previous replacement procedure **Includes/Examples:** Total hip replacement, bone graft, free skin graft
Reposition (S)	**Definition:** Moving to its normal location, or other suitable location, all or a portion of a body part **Explanation:** The body part is moved to a new location from an abnormal location, or from a normal location where it is not functioning correctly. The body part may or may not be cut out or off to be moved to the new location **Includes/Examples:** Reposition of undescended testicle, fracture reduction
Resection (T)	**Definition:** Cutting out or off, without replacement, all of a body part **Includes/Examples:** Total nephrectomy, total lobectomy of lung
Restriction (V)	**Definition:** Partially closing an orifice or the lumen of a tubular body part **Explanation:** The orifice can be a natural orifice or an artificially created orifice **Includes/Examples:** Esophagogastric fundoplication, cervical cerclage
Revision (W)	**Definition:** Correcting, to the extent possible, a portion of a malfunctioning device or the position of a displaced device **Explanation:** Revision can include correcting a malfunctioning or displaced device by taking out or putting in components of the device such as a screw or pin **Includes/Examples:** Adjustment of position of pacemaker lead, recementing of hip prosthesis
Supplement (U)	**Definition:** Putting in or on biological or synthetic material that physically reinforces and/or augments the function of a portion of a body part **Explanation:** The biological material is non-living, or is living and from the same individual. The body part may have been previously replaced, and the Supplement procedure is performed to physically reinforce and/or augment the function of the replaced body part **Includes/Examples:** Herniorrhaphy using mesh, mitral valve ring annuloplasty, put a new acetabular liner in a previous hip replacement
Transfer (X)	**Definition:** Moving, without taking out, all or a portion of a body part to another location to take over the function of all or a portion of a body part **Explanation:** The body part transferred remains connected to its vascular and nervous supply **Includes/Examples:** Tendon transfer, skin pedicle flap transfer
Transplantation (Y)	**Definition:** Putting in or on all or a portion of a living body part taken from another individual or animal to physically take the place and/or function of all or a portion of a similar body part **Explanation:** The native body part may or may not be taken out, and the transplanted body part may take over all or a portion of its function **Includes/Examples:** Kidney transplant, heart transplant

Section 1 - Obstetrics — Character 3 - Root Operations Unique to Obstetrics

Abortion (A)	**Definition:** Artificially terminating a pregnancy **Explanation:** Subdivided according to whether an additional device such as a laminaria or abortifacient is used, or whether the abortion was performed by mechanical means **Includes/Example:** Transvaginal abortion using vacuum aspiration technique

Continued ⟶

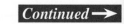

Appendix A

Section 1 - Obstetrics — Character 3 - Root Operations Unique to Obstetrics

Delivery (E)	**Definition:** Assisting the passage of the products of conception from the genital canal **Explanation:** Applies only to manually-assisted, vaginal delivery **Includes/Example:** Manually-assisted delivery

Section 2 - Placement — Character 3 - Root Operation

Change (0)	**Definition:** Taking out or off a device from a body part and putting back an identical or similar device in or on the same body part without cutting or puncturing the skin or a mucous membrane **Includes/Example:** Change of vaginal packing
Compression (1)	**Definition:** Putting pressure on a body region **Includes/Example:** Placement of pressure dressing on abdominal wall
Dressing (2)	**Definition:** Putting material on a body region for protection **Includes/Example:** Application of sterile dressing to head wound
Immobilization (3)	**Definition:** Limiting or preventing motion of a body region **Includes/Example:** Placement of splint on left finger
Packing (4)	**Definition:** Putting material in a body region or orifice **Includes/Example:** Placement of nasal packing
Removal (5)	**Definition:** Taking out or off a device from a body part **Includes/Example:** Removal of cast from right lower leg
Traction (6)	**Definition:** Exerting a pulling force on a body region in a distal direction **Includes/Example:** Lumbar traction using motorized split-traction table

Section 3 - Administration — Character 3 - Root Operation

Introduction (0)	**Definition:** Putting in or on a therapeutic, diagnostic, nutritional, physiological, or prophylactic substance except blood or blood products **Includes/Example:** Nerve block injection to median nerve
Irrigation (1)	**Definition:** Putting in or on a cleansing substance **Includes/Example:** Flushing of eye
Transfusion (2)	**Definition:** Putting in blood or blood products **Includes/Example:** Transfusion of cell saver red cells into central venous line

Section 4 - Measurement and Monitoring — Character 3 - Root Operation

Measurement (0)	**Definition:** Determining the level of a physiological or physical function at a point in time **Includes/Example:** External electrocardiogram (EKG), single reading
Monitoring (1)	**Definition:** Determining the level of a physiological or physical function repetitively over a period of time **Includes/Example:** Urinary pressure monitoring

Section 5 - Extracorporeal Assistance and Performance — Character 3 - Root Operation

Assistance (0)	**Definition:** Taking over a portion of a physiological function by extracorporeal means **Includes/Example:** Hyperbaric oxygenation of wound
Performance (1)	**Definition:** Completely taking over a physiological function by extracorporeal means **Includes/Example:** Cardiopulmonary bypass in conjunction with CABG
Restoration (2)	**Definition:** Returning, or attempting to return, a physiological function to its original state by extracorporeal means. **Includes/Example:** Attempted cardiac defibrillation, unsuccessful

Section 6 - Extracorporeal Therapies — Character 3 - Root Operation

Atmospheric Control (0)	**Definition:** Extracorporeal control of atmospheric pressure and composition **Includes/Example:** Atmospheric control, single treatment
Decompression (1)	**Definition:** Extracorporeal elimination of undissolved gas from body fluids **Includes/Example:** Hyperbaric decompression treatment, single
Electromagnetic Therapy (2)	**Definition:** Extracorporeal treatment by electromagnetic rays **Includes/Example:** Electromagnetic therapy, central nervous, multiple treatments
Hyperthermia (3)	**Definition:** Extracorporeal raising of body temperature **Includes/Example:** Hyperthermia, single treatment

Continued →

Section 6 - Extracorporeal Therapies — Character 3 - Root Operation

Hypothermia (4)	**Definition:** Extracorporeal lowering of body temperature **Includes/Example:** Whole body hypothermia treatment for temperature imbalances, series treatment
Perfusion (B)	**Definition:** Extracorporeal treatment by diffusion of therapeutic fluid
Pheresis (5)	**Definition:** Extracorporeal separation of blood products **Includes/Example:** Therapeutic leukopheresis, single treatment
Phototherapy (6)	**Definition:** Extracorporeal treatment by light rays **Includes/Example:** Phototherapy of circulatory system, series treatment
Shock Wave Therapy (7)	**Definition:** Extracorporeal treatment by shock waves **Includes/Example:** Shock wave therapy, musculoskeletal, single treatment
Ultrasound Therapy (8)	**Definition:** Extracorporeal treatment by ultrasound **Includes/Example:** Ultrasound therapy of the heart, single treatment
Ultraviolet Light Therapy (9)	**Definition:** Extracorporeal treatment by ultraviolet light **Includes/Example:** Ultraviolet light phototherapy, series treatment

Section 7 - Osteopathic — Character 3 - Root Operation

Treatment (0)	**Definition:** Manual treatment to eliminate or alleviate somatic dysfunction and related disorders **Includes/Example:** Fascial release of abdomen, osteopathic treatment

Section 8 - Other Procedures — Character 3 - Root Operation

Other Procedures (0)	**Definition:** Methodologies which attempt to remediate or cure a disorder or disease **Includes/Example:** Acupuncture

Section 9 - Chiropractic — Character 3 - Root Operation

Manipulation (B)	**Definition:** Manual procedure that involves a directed thrust to move a joint past the physiological range of motion, without exceeding the anatomical limit **Includes/Example:** Chiropractic treatment of cervical spine, short lever specific contact

Section X - New Technology — Character 3 - Root Operation

Assistance (A)	**Definition:** Taking over a portion of a physiological function by extracorporeal means
Destruction (5)	**Definition:** Physical eradication of all or a portion of a body part by the direct use of energy, force, or a destructive agent **Explanation:** None of the body part is physically taken out **Includes/Examples:** Fulguration of rectal polyp, cautery of skin lesion
Dilation (7)	**Definition:** Expanding an orifice or the lumen of a tubular body part **Explanation:** The orifice can be a natural orifice or an artificially created orifice. Accomplished by stretching a tubular body part using intraluminal pressure or by cutting part of the orifice or wall of the tubular body part
Extirpation (C)	**Definition:** Taking or cutting out solid matter from a body part **Explanation:** The solid matter may be an abnormal by product of a biological function or a foreign body; it may be imbedded in a body part or in the lumen of a tubular body part. The solid matter may or may not have been previously broken into pieces **Includes/Example:** Thrombectomy, choledocholithotomy
Fusion (G)	**Definition:** Joining together portions of an articular body part rendering the articular body part immobile **Explanation:** The body part is joined together by fixation device, bone graft, or other means **Includes/Examples:** Spinal fusion, ankle arthrodesis
Introduction (0)	**Definition:** Putting in or on a therapeutic, diagnostic, nutritional, physiological, or prophylactic substance except blood or blood products
Measurement (E)	**Definition:** Determining the level of a physiological or physical function at a point in time
Monitoring (2)	**Definition:** Determining the level of a physiological or physical function repetitively over a period of time
Replacement (R)	**Definition:** Putting in or on biological or synthetic material that physically takes the place and/or function of all or a portion of a body part **Explanation:** The body part may have been taken out or replaced, or may be taken out, physically eradicated, or rendered nonfunctional during the Replacement procedure. A Removal procedure is coded for taking out the device used in a previous replacement procedure. **Includes/Examples:** Total hip replacement, bone graft, free skin graft
Reposition (S)	**Definition:** Moving to its normal location, or other suitable location, all or a portion of a body part **Explanation:** The body part is moved to a new location from an abnormal location, or from a normal location where it is not functioning correctly. The body part may or may not be cut out or off to be moved to the new location. **Includes/Examples:** Reposition of undescended testicle, fracture reduction
Supplement (U)	**Definition:** Putting in or on biological or synthetic material that physically reinforces and/or augments the function of a portion of a body part
Transfusion (1&2)	**Definition:** Putting in blood or blood products

Appendix B: Type and Qualifier Definitions

Section B - Imaging — Character 3 - Root Type

Computerized Tomography (CT Scan) (2)	**Definition:** Computer reformatted digital display of multiplanar images developed from the capture of multiple exposures of external ionizing radiation
Fluoroscopy (1)	**Definition:** Single plane or bi-plane real time display of an image developed from the capture of external ionizing radiation on a fluorescent screen. The image may also be stored by either digital or analog means
Magnetic Resonance Imaging (MRI) (3)	**Definition:** Computer reformatted digital display of multiplanar images developed from the capture of radiofrequency signals emitted by nuclei in a body site excited within a magnetic field
Other Imaging (5)	**Definition:** Other specified modality for visualizing a body part
Plain Radiography (0)	**Definition:** Planar display of an image developed from the capture of external ionizing radiation on photographic or photoconductive plate
Ultrasonography (4)	**Definition:** Real time display of images of anatomy or flow information developed from the capture of reflected and attenuated high frequency sound waves

Section C - Nuclear Medicine — Character 3 - Root Type

Nonimaging Nuclear Medicine Assay (6)	**Definition:** Introduction of radioactive materials into the body for the study of body fluids and blood elements, by the detection of radioactive emissions
Nonimaging Nuclear Medicine Probe (5)	**Definition:** Introduction of radioactive materials into the body for the study of distribution and fate of certain substances by the detection of radioactive emissions; or, alternatively, measurement of absorption of radioactive emissions from an external source
Nonimaging Nuclear Medicine Uptake (4)	**Definition:** Introduction of radioactive materials into the body for measurements of organ function, from the detection of radioactive emissions
Planar Nuclear Medicine Imaging (1)	**Definition:** Introduction of radioactive materials into the body for single plane display of images developed from the capture of radioactive emissions
Positron Emission Tomographic (PET) Imaging (3)	**Definition:** Introduction of radioactive materials into the body for three dimensional display of images developed from the simultaneous capture, 180 degrees apart, of radioactive emissions
Systemic Nuclear Medicine Therapy (7)	**Definition:** Introduction of unsealed radioactive materials into the body for treatment
Tomographic (Tomo) Nuclear Medicine Imaging (2)	**Definition:** Introduction of radioactive materials into the body for three dimensional display of images developed from the capture of radioactive emissions

Section F - Physical Rehabilitation and Diagnostic Audiology — Character 3 - Root Type

Activities of Daily Living Assessment	**Definition:** Measurement of functional level for activities of daily living
Activities of Daily Living Treatment	**Definition:** Exercise or activities to facilitate functional competence for activities of daily living
Caregiver Training	**Definition:** Training in activities to support patient's optimal level of function
Cochlear Implant Treatment	**Definition:** Application of techniques to improve the communication abilities of individuals with cochlear implant
Device Fitting	**Definition:** Fitting of a device designed to facilitate or support achievement of a higher level of function
Hearing Aid Assessment	**Definition:** Measurement of the appropriateness and/or effectiveness of a hearing device
Hearing Assessment	**Definition:** Measurement of hearing and related functions
Hearing Treatment	**Definition:** Application of techniques to improve, augment, or compensate for hearing and related functional impairment
Motor and/or Nerve Function Assessment	**Definition:** Measurement of motor, nerve, and related functions
Motor Treatment	**Definition:** Exercise or activities to increase or facilitate motor function
Speech Assessment	**Definition:** Measurement of speech and related functions
Speech Treatment	**Definition:** Application of techniques to improve, augment, or compensate for speech and related functional impairment
Vestibular Assessment	**Definition:** Measurement of the vestibular system and related functions
Vestibular Treatment	**Definition:** Application of techniques to improve, augment, or compensate for vestibular and related functional impairment

Acoustic Reflex Decay	**Definition:** Measures reduction in size/strength of acoustic reflex over time **Includes/Examples:** Includes site of lesion test
Acoustic Reflex Patterns	**Definition:** Defines site of lesion based upon presence/absence of acoustic reflexes with ipsilateral vs. contralateral stimulation
Acoustic Reflex Threshold	**Definition:** Determines minimal intensity that acoustic reflex occurs with ipsilateral and/or contralateral stimulation
Aerobic Capacity and Endurance	**Definition:** Measures autonomic responses to positional changes; perceived exertion, dyspnea or angina during activity; performance during exercise protocols; standard vital signs; and blood gas analysis or oxygen consumption
Alternate Binaural or Monaural Loudness Balance	**Definition:** Determines auditory stimulus parameter that yields the same objective sensation **Includes/Examples:** Sound intensities that yield same loudness perception
Anthropometric Characteristics	**Definition:** Measures edema, body fat composition, height, weight, length and girth
Aphasia (Assessment)	**Definition:** Measures expressive and receptive speech and language function including reading and writing
Aphasia (Treatment)	**Definition:** Applying techniques to improve, augment, or compensate for receptive/expressive language impairments
Articulation/Phonology (Assessment)	**Definition:** Measures speech production
Articulation/Phonology (Treatment)	**Definition:** Applying techniques to correct, improve, or compensate for speech productive impairment
Assistive Listening Device	**Definition:** Assists in use of effective and appropriate assistive listening device/system
Assistive Listening System/Device Selection	**Definition:** Measures the effectiveness and appropriateness of assistive listening systems/devices
Assistive, Adaptive, Supportive or Protective Devices	**Explanation:** Devices to facilitate or support achievement of a higher level of function in wheelchair mobility; bed mobility; transfer or ambulation ability; bath and showering ability; dressing; grooming; personal hygiene; play or leisure
Auditory Evoked Potentials	**Definition:** Measures electric responses produced by the VIIIth cranial nerve and brainstem following auditory stimulation
Auditory Processing (Assessment)	**Definition:** Evaluates ability to receive and process auditory information and comprehension of spoken language
Auditory Processing (Treatment)	**Definition:** Applying techniques to improve the receiving and processing of auditory information and comprehension of spoken language
Augmentative/Alternative Communication System (Assessment)	**Definition:** Determines the appropriateness of aids, techniques, symbols, and/or strategies to augment or replace speech and enhance communication **Includes/Examples:** Includes the use of telephones, writing equipment, emergency equipment, and TDD
Augmentative/Alternative Communication System (Treatment)	**Includes/Examples:** Includes augmentative communication devices and aids
Aural Rehabilitation	**Definition:** Applying techniques to improve the communication abilities associated with hearing loss
Aural Rehabilitation Status	**Definition:** Measures impact of a hearing loss including evaluation of receptive and expressive communication skills
Bathing/Showering	**Includes/Examples:** Includes obtaining and using supplies; soaping, rinsing, and drying body parts; maintaining bathing position; and transferring to and from bathing positions
Bathing/Showering Techniques	**Definition:** Activities to facilitate obtaining and using supplies, soaping, rinsing and drying body parts, maintaining bathing position, and transferring to and from bathing positions
Bed Mobility (Assessment)	**Definition:** Transitional movement within bed
Bed Mobility (Treatment)	**Definition:** Exercise or activities to facilitate transitional movements within bed
Bedside Swallowing and Oral Function	**Includes/Examples:** Bedside swallowing includes assessment of sucking, masticating, coughing, and swallowing. Oral function includes assessment of musculature for controlled movements, structures and functions to determine coordination and phonation
Bekesy Audiometry	**Definition:** Uses an instrument that provides a choice of discrete or continuously varying pure tones; choice of pulsed or continuous signal
Binaural Electroacoustic Hearing Aid Check	**Definition:** Determines mechanical and electroacoustic function of bilateral hearing aids using hearing aid test box
Binaural Hearing Aid (Assessment)	**Definition:** Measures the candidacy, effectiveness, and appropriateness of a hearing aids **Explanation:** Measures bilateral fit

Continued →

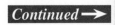

Binaural Hearing Aid (Treatment)	**Explanation:** Assists in achieving maximum understanding and performance
Bithermal, Binaural Caloric Irrigation	**Definition:** Measures the rhythmic eye movements stimulated by changing the temperature of the vestibular system
Bithermal, Monaural Caloric Irrigation	**Definition:** Measures the rhythmic eye movements stimulated by changing the temperature of the vestibular system in one ear
Brief Tone Stimuli	**Definition:** Measures specific central auditory process
Cerumen Management	**Definition:** Includes examination of external auditory canal and tympanic membrane and removal of cerumen from external ear canal
Cochlear Implant	**Definition:** Measures candidacy for cochlear implant
Cochlear Implant Rehabilitation	**Definition:** Applying techniques to improve the communication abilities of individuals with cochlear implant; includes programming the device, providing patients/families with information
Communicative/Cognitive Integration Skills (Assessment)	**Definition:** Measures ability to use higher cortical functions **Includes/Examples:** Includes orientation, recognition, attention span, initiation and termination of activity, memory, sequencing, categorizing, concept formation, spatial operations, judgment, problem solving, generalization and pragmatic communication
Communicative/Cognitive Integration Skills (Treatment)	**Definition:** Activities to facilitate the use of higher cortical functions **Includes/Examples:** Includes level of arousal, orientation, recognition, attention span, initiation and termination of activity, memory sequencing, judgment and problem solving, learning and generalization, and pragmatic communication
Computerized Dynamic Posturography	**Definition:** Measures the status of the peripheral and central vestibular system and the sensory/motor component of balance; evaluates the efficacy of vestibular rehabilitation
Conditioned Play Audiometry	**Definition:** Behavioral measures using nonspeech and speech stimuli to obtain frequency-specific and ear-specific information on auditory status from the patient **Explanation:** Obtains speech reception threshold by having patient point to pictures of spondaic words
Coordination/Dexterity (Assessment)	**Definition:** Measures large and small muscle groups for controlled goal-directed movements **Explanation:** Dexterity includes object manipulation
Coordination/Dexterity (Treatment)	**Definition:** Exercise or activities to facilitate gross coordination and fine coordination
Cranial Nerve Integrity	**Definition:** Measures cranial nerve sensory and motor functions, including tastes, smell and facial expression
Dichotic Stimuli	**Definition:** Measures specific central auditory process
Distorted Speech	**Definition:** Measures specific central auditory process
Dix-Hallpike Dynamic	**Definition:** Measures nystagmus following Dix-Hallpike maneuver
Dressing	**Includes/Examples:** Includes selecting clothing and accessories, obtaining clothing from storage, dressing, fastening and adjusting clothing and shoes, and applying and removing personal devices, prosthesis or orthosis
Dressing Techniques	**Definition:** Activities to facilitate selecting clothing and accessories, dressing and undressing, adjusting clothing and shoes, applying and removing devices, prostheses or orthoses
Dynamic Orthosis	**Includes/Examples:** Includes customized and prefabricated splints, inhibitory casts, spinal and other braces, and protective devices; allows motion through transfer of movement from other body parts or by use of outside forces
Ear Canal Probe Microphone	**Definition:** Real ear measures
Ear Protector Attentuation	**Definition:** Measures ear protector fit and effectiveness
Electrocochleography	**Definition:** Measures the VIIIth cranial nerve action potential
Environmental, Home and Work Barriers	**Definition:** Measures current and potential barriers to optimal function, including safety hazards, access problems and home or office design
Ergonomics and Body Mechanics	**Definition:** Ergonomic measurement of job tasks, work hardening or work conditioning needs; functional capacity; and body mechanics
Eustachian Tube Function	**Definition:** Measures eustachian tube function and patency of eustachian tube
Evoked Otoacoustic Emissions, Diagnostic	**Definition:** Measures auditory evoked potentials in a diagnostic format
Evoked Otoacoustic Emissions, Screening	**Definition:** Measures auditory evoked potentials in a screening format
Facial Nerve Function	**Definition:** Measures electrical activity of the VIIth cranial nerve (facial nerve)
Feeding/Eating (Assessment)	**Includes/Examples:** Includes setting up food, selecting and using utensils and tableware, bringing food or drink to mouth, cleaning face, hands, and clothing, and management of alternative methods of nourishment

Continued →

Feeding/Eating (Treatment)	**Definition:** Exercise or activities to facilitate setting up food, selecting and using utensils and tableware, bringing food or drink to mouth, cleaning face, hands, and clothing, and management of alternative methods of nourishment
Filtered Speech	**Definition:** Uses high or low pass filtered speech stimuli to assess central auditory processing disorders, site of lesion testing
Fluency (Assessment)	**Definition:** Measures speech fluency or stuttering
Fluency (Treatment)	**Definition:** Applying techniques to improve and augment fluent speech
Gait and/or Balance	**Definition:** Measures biomechanical, arthrokinematic and other spatial and temporal characteristics of gait and balance
Gait Training/Functional Ambulation	**Definition:** Exercise or activities to facilitate ambulation on a variety of surfaces and in a variety of environments
Grooming/Personal Hygiene (Assessment)	**Includes/Examples:** Includes ability to obtain and use supplies in a sequential fashion, general grooming, oral hygiene, toilet hygiene, personal care devices, including care for artificial airways
Grooming/Personal Hygiene (Treatment)	**Definition:** Activities to facilitate obtaining and using supplies in a sequential fashion: general grooming, oral hygiene, toilet hygiene, cleaning body, and personal care devices, including artificial airways
Hearing and Related Disorders Counseling	**Definition:** Provides patients/families/caregivers with information, support, referrals to facilitate recovery from a communication disorder **Includes/Examples:** Includes strategies for psychosocial adjustment to hearing loss for clients and families/caregivers
Hearing and Related Disorders Prevention	**Definition:** Provides patients/families/caregivers with information and support to prevent communication disorders
Hearing Screening	**Definition:** Pass/refer measures designed to identify need for further audiologic assessment
Home Management (Assessment)	**Definition:** Obtaining and maintaining personal and household possessions and environment **Includes/Examples:** Includes clothing care, cleaning, meal preparation and cleanup, shopping, money management, household maintenance, safety procedures, and childcare/parenting
Home Management (Treatment)	**Definition:** Activities to facilitate obtaining and maintaining personal household possessions and environment **Includes/Examples:** Includes clothing care, cleaning, meal preparation and clean-up, shopping, money management, household maintenance, safety procedures, childcare/parenting
Instrumental Swallowing and Oral Function	**Definition:** Measures swallowing function using instrumental diagnostic procedures **Explanation:** Methods include videofluoroscopy, ultrasound, manometry, endoscopy
Integumentary Integrity	**Includes/Examples:** Includes burns, skin conditions, ecchymosis, bleeding, blisters, scar tissue, wounds and other traumas, tissue mobility, turgor and texture
Manual Therapy Techniques	**Definition:** Techniques in which the therapist uses his/her hands to administer skilled movements **Includes/Examples:** Includes connective tissue massage, joint mobilization and manipulation, manual lymph drainage, manual traction, soft tissue mobilization and manipulation
Masking Patterns	**Definition:** Measures central auditory processing status
Monaural Electroacoustic Hearing Aid Check	**Definition:** Determines mechanical and electroacoustic function of one hearing aid using hearing aid test box
Monaural Hearing Aid (Assessment)	**Definition:** Measures the candidacy, effectiveness, and appropriateness of a hearing aid **Explanation:** Measures unilateral fit
Monaural Hearing Aid (Treatment)	**Explanation:** Assists in achieving maximum understanding and performance
Motor Function (Assessment)	**Definition:** Measures the body's functional and versatile movement patterns **Includes/Examples:** Includes motor assessment scales, analysis of head, trunk and limb movement, and assessment of motor learning
Motor Function (Treatment)	**Definition:** Exercise or activities to facilitate crossing midline, laterality, bilateral integration, praxis, neuromuscular relaxation, inhibition, facilitation, motor function and motor learning
Motor Speech (Assessment)	**Definition:** Measures neurological motor aspects of speech production
Motor Speech (Treatment)	**Definition:** Applying techniques to improve and augment the impaired neurological motor aspects of speech production
Muscle Performance (Assessment)	**Definition:** Measures muscle strength, power and endurance using manual testing, dynamometry or computer-assisted electromechanical muscle test; functional muscle strength, power and endurance; muscle pain, tone, or soreness; or pelvic-floor musculature **Explanation:** Muscle endurance refers to the ability to contract a muscle repeatedly over time

Continued →

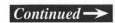

Appendix B

Muscle Performance (Treatment)	**Definition:** Exercise or activities to increase the capacity of a muscle to do work in terms of strength, power, and/or endurance **Explanation:** Muscle strength is the force exerted to overcome resistance in one maximal effort. Muscle power is work produced per unit of time, or the product of strength and speed. Muscle endurance is the ability to contract a muscle repeatedly over time
Neuromotor Development	**Definition:** Measures motor development, righting and equilibrium reactions, and reflex and equilibrium reactions
Non-invasive Instrumental Status	**Definition:** Instrumental measures of oral, nasal, vocal, and velopharyngeal functions as they pertain to speech production
Nonspoken Language (Assessment)	**Definition:** Measures nonspoken language (print, sign, symbols) for communication
Nonspoken Language (Treatment)	**Definition:** Applying techniques that improve, augment, or compensate spoken communication
Oral Peripheral Mechanism	**Definition:** Structural measures of face, jaw, lips, tongue, teeth, hard and soft palate, pharynx as related to speech production
Orofacial Myofunctional (Assessment)	**Definition:** Measures orofacial myofunctional patterns for speech and related functions
Orofacial Myofunctional (Treatment)	**Definition:** Applying techniques to improve, alter, or augment impaired orofacial myofunctional patterns and related speech production errors
Oscillating Tracking	**Definition:** Measures ability to visually track
Pain	**Definition:** Measures muscle soreness, pain and soreness with joint movement, and pain perception **Includes/Examples:** Includes questionnaires, graphs, symptom magnification scales or visual analog scales
Perceptual Processing (Assessment)	**Definition:** Measures stereognosis, kinesthesia, body schema, right-left discrimination, form constancy, position in space, visual closure, figure-ground, depth perception, spatial relations and topographical orientation
Perceptual Processing (Treatment)	**Definition:** Exercise and activities to facilitate perceptual processing **Explanation:** Includes stereognosis, kinesthesia, body schema, right-left discrimination, form constancy, position in space, visual closure, figure-ground, depth perception, spatial relations, and topographical orientation **Includes/Examples:** Includes stereognosis, kinesthesia, body schema, right-left discrimination, form constancy, position in space, visual closure, figure-ground, depth perception, spatial relations, and topographical orientation
Performance Intensity Phonetically Balanced Speech Discrimination	**Definition:** Measures word recognition over varying intensity levels
Postural Control	**Definition:** Exercise or activities to increase postural alignment and control
Prosthesis	**Definition:** Artificial substitutes for missing body parts that augment performance or function **Includes/Examples:** Limb prosthesis, ocular prosthesis
Psychosocial Skills (Assessment)	**Definition:** The ability to interact in society and to process emotions **Includes/Examples:** Includes psychological (values, interests, self-concept); social (role performance, social conduct, interpersonal skills, self expression); self-management (coping skills, time management, self-control)
Psychosocial Skills (Treatment)	**Definition:** The ability to interact in society and to process emotions **Includes/Examples:** Includes psychological (values, interests, self-concept); social (role performance, social conduct, interpersonal skills, self expression); self-management (coping skills, time management, self-control)
Pure Tone Audiometry, Air	**Definition:** Air-conduction pure tone threshold measures with appropriate masking
Pure Tone Audiometry, Air and Bone	**Definition:** Air-conduction and bone-conduction pure tone threshold measures with appropriate masking
Pure Tone Stenger	**Definition:** Measures unilateral nonorganic hearing loss based on simultaneous presentation of pure tones of differing volume
Range of Motion and Joint Integrity	**Definition:** Measures quantity, quality, grade, and classification of joint movement and/or mobility **Explanation:** Range of Motion is the space, distance or angle through which movement occurs at a joint or series of joints. Joint integrity is the conformance of joints to expected anatomic, biomechanical and kinematic norms
Range of Motion and Joint Mobility	**Definition:** Exercise or activities to increase muscle length and joint mobility
Receptive/Expressive Language (Assessment)	**Definition:** Measures receptive and expressive language
Receptive/Expressive Language (Treatment)	**Definition:** Applying techniques to improve and augment receptive/expressive language

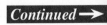

Continued →

Reflex Integrity	**Definition:** Measures the presence, absence, or exaggeration of developmentally appropriate, pathologic or normal reflexes
Select Picture Audiometry	**Definition:** Establishes hearing threshold levels for speech using pictures
Sensorineural Acuity Level	**Definition:** Measures sensorineural acuity masking presented via bone conduction
Sensory Aids	**Definition:** Determines the appropriateness of a sensory prosthetic device, other than a hearing aid or assistive listening system/device
Sensory Awareness/Processing/Integrity	**Includes/Examples:** Includes light touch, pressure, temperature, pain, sharp/dull, proprioception, vestibular, visual, auditory, gustatory, and olfactory
Short Increment Sensitivity Index	**Definition:** Measures the ear's ability to detect small intensity changes; site of lesion test requiring a behavioral response
Sinusoidal Vertical Axis Rotational	**Definition:** Measures nystagmus following rotation
Somatosensory Evoked Potentials	**Definition:** Measures neural activity from sites throughout the body
Speech and/or Language Screening	**Definition:** Identifies need for further speech and/or language evaluation
Speech Threshold	**Definition:** Measures minimal intensity needed to repeat spondaic words
Speech-Language Pathology and Related Disorders Counseling	**Definition:** Provides patients/families with information, support, referrals to facilitate recovery from a communication disorder
Speech-Language Pathology and Related Disorders Prevention	**Definition:** Applying techniques to avoid or minimize onset and/or development of a communication disorder
Speech/Word Recognition	**Definition:** Measures ability to repeat/identify single syllable words; scores given as a percentage; includes word recognition/speech discrimination
Staggered Spondaic Word	**Definition:** Measures central auditory processing site of lesion based upon dichotic presentation of spondaic words
Static Orthosis	**Includes/Examples:** Includes customized and prefabricated splints, inhibitory casts, spinal and other braces, and protective devices; has no moving parts, maintains joint(s) in desired position
Stenger	**Definition:** Measures unilateral nonorganic hearing loss based on simultaneous presentation of signals of differing volume
Swallowing Dysfunction	**Definition:** Activities to improve swallowing function in coordination with respiratory function **Includes/Examples:** Includes function and coordination of sucking, mastication, coughing, swallowing
Synthetic Sentence Identification	**Definition:** Measures central auditory dysfunction using identification of third order approximations of sentences and competing messages
Temporal Ordering of Stimuli	**Definition:** Measures specific central auditory process
Therapeutic Exercise	**Definition:** Exercise or activities to facilitate sensory awareness, sensory processing, sensory integration, balance training, conditioning, reconditioning **Includes/Examples:** Includes developmental activities, breathing exercises, aerobic endurance activities, aquatic exercises, stretching and ventilatory muscle training
Tinnitus Masker (Assessment)	**Definition:** Determines candidacy for tinnitus masker
Tinnitus Masker (Treatment)	**Explanation:** Used to verify physical fit, acoustic appropriateness, and benefit; assists in achieving maximum benefit
Tone Decay	**Definition:** Measures decrease in hearing sensitivity to a tone; site of lesion test requiring a behavioral response
Transfer	**Definition:** Transitional movement from one surface to another
Transfer Training	**Definition:** Exercise or activities to facilitate movement from one surface to another
Tympanometry	**Definition:** Measures the integrity of the middle ear; measures ease at which sound flows through the tympanic membrane while air pressure against the membrane is varied
Unithermal Binaural Screen	**Definition:** Measures the rhythmic eye movements stimulated by changing the temperature of the vestibular system in both ears using warm water, screening format
Ventilation, Respiration and Circulation	**Definition:** Measures ventilatory muscle strength, power and endurance, pulmonary function and ventilatory mechanics **Includes/Examples:** Includes ability to clear airway, activities that aggravate or relieve edema, pain, dyspnea or other symptoms, chest wall mobility, cardiopulmonary response to performance of ADL and IAD, cough and sputum, standard vital signs
Vestibular	**Definition:** Applying techniques to compensate for balance disorders; includes habituation, exercise therapy, and balance retraining

Continued →

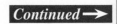

Appendix B

Section F - Physical Rehabilitation and Diagnostic Audiology — Character 5 - Type Qualifier

Visual Motor Integration (Assessment)	**Definition:** Coordinating the interaction of information from the eyes with body movement during activity
Visual Motor Integration (Treatment)	**Definition:** Exercise or activities to facilitate coordinating the interaction of information from eyes with body movement during activity
Visual Reinforcement Audiometry	**Definition:** Behavioral measures using nonspeech and speech stimuli to obtain frequency/ear-specific information on auditory status **Includes/Examples:** Includes a conditioned response of looking toward a visual reinforcer (e.g., lights, animated toy) every time auditory stimuli are heard
Vocational Activities and Functional Community or Work Reintegration Skills (Assessment)	**Definition:** Measures environmental, home, work (job/school/play) barriers that keep patients from functioning optimally in their environment **Includes/Examples:** Includes assessment of vocational skill and interests, environment of work (job/school/play), injury potential and injury prevention or reduction, ergonomic stressors, transportation skills, and ability to access and use community resources
Vocational Activities and Functional Community or Work Reintegration Skills (Treatment)	**Definition:** Activities to facilitate vocational exploration, body mechanics training, job acquisition, and environmental or work (job/school/play) task adaptation **Includes/Examples:** Includes injury prevention and reduction, ergonomic stressor reduction, job coaching and simulation, work hardening and conditioning, driving training, transportation skills, and use of community resources
Voice (Assessment)	**Definition:** Measures vocal structure, function and production
Voice (Treatment)	**Definition:** Applying techniques to improve voice and vocal function
Voice Prosthetic (Assessment)	**Definition:** Determines the appropriateness of voice prosthetic/adaptive device to enhance or facilitate communication
Voice Prosthetic (Treatment)	**Includes/Examples:** Includes electrolarynx, and other assistive, adaptive, supportive devices
Wheelchair Mobility (Assessment)	**Definition:** Measures fit and functional abilities within wheelchair in a variety of environments
Wheelchair Mobility (Treatment)	**Definition:** Management, maintenance and controlled operation of a wheelchair, scooter or other device, in and on a variety of surfaces and environments
Wound Management	**Includes/Examples:** Includes non-selective and selective debridement (enzymes, autolysis, sharp debridement), dressings (wound coverings, hydrogel, vacuum-assisted closure), topical agents, etc.

Section G - Mental Health — Character 3 - Root Type

Biofeedback	**Definition:** Provision of information from the monitoring and regulating of physiological processes in conjunction with cognitive-behavioral techniques to improve patient functioning or well-being **Includes/Examples:** Includes EEG, blood pressure, skin temperature or peripheral blood flow, ECG, electrooculogram, EMG, respirometry or capnometry, GSR/EDR, perineometry to monitor/regulate bowel/bladder activity, electrogastrogram to monitor/regulate gastric motility
Counseling	**Definition:** The application of psychological methods to treat an individual with normal developmental issues and psychological problems in order to increase function, improve well-being, alleviate distress, maladjustment or resolve crises
Crisis Intervention	**Definition:** Treatment of a traumatized, acutely disturbed or distressed individual for the purpose of short-term stabilization **Includes/Examples:** Includes defusing, debriefing, counseling, psychotherapy and/or coordination of care with other providers or agencies
Electroconvulsive Therapy	**Definition:** The application of controlled electrical voltages to treat a mental health disorder **Includes/Examples:** Includes appropriate sedation and other preparation of the individual
Family Psychotherapy	**Definition:** Treatment that includes one or more family members of an individual with a mental health disorder by behavioral, cognitive, psychoanalytic, psychodynamic or psychophysiological means to improve functioning or well-being **Explanation:** Remediation of emotional or behavioral problems presented by one or more family members in cases where psychotherapy with more than one family member is indicated
Group Psychotherapy	**Definition:** Treatment of two or more individuals with a mental health disorder by behavioral, cognitive, psychoanalytic, psychodynamic or psychophysiological means to improve functioning or well-being
Hypnosis	**Definition:** Induction of a state of heightened suggestibility by auditory, visual and tactile techniques to elicit an emotional or behavioral response
Individual Psychotherapy	**Definition:** Treatment of an individual with a mental health disorder by behavioral, cognitive, psychoanalytic, psychodynamic or psychophysiological means to improve functioning or well-being
Light Therapy	**Definition:** Application of specialized light treatments to improve functioning or well-being

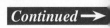

Continued →

Section G - Mental Health — Character 3 - Root Type

Medication Management	**Definition:** Monitoring and adjusting the use of medications for the treatment of a mental health disorder
Narcosynthesis	**Definition:** Administration of intravenous barbiturates in order to release suppressed or repressed thoughts
Psychological Tests	**Definition:** The administration and interpretation of standardized psychological tests and measurement instruments for the assessment of psychological function

Section G - Mental Health — Character 4 - Type Qualifier

Behavioral	**Definition:** Primarily to modify behavior **Includes/Examples:** Includes modeling and role playing, positive reinforcement of target behaviors, response cost, and training of self-management skills
Cognitive	**Definition:** Primarily to correct cognitive distortions and errors
Cognitive-Behavioral	**Definition:** Combining cognitive and behavioral treatment strategies to improve functioning **Explanation:** Maladaptive responses are examined to determine how cognitions relate to behavior patterns in response to an event. Uses learning principles and information-processing models
Developmental	**Definition:** Age-normed developmental status of cognitive, social and adaptive behavior skills
Intellectual and Psychoeducational	**Definition:** Intellectual abilities, academic achievement and learning capabilities (including behaviors and emotional factors affecting learning)
Interactive	**Definition:** Uses primarily physical aids and other forms of non-oral interaction with a patient who is physically, psychologically or developmentally unable to use ordinary language for communication **Includes/Examples:** Includes the use of toys in symbolic play
Interpersonal	**Definition:** Helps an individual make changes in interpersonal behaviors to reduce psychological dysfunction **Includes/Examples:** Includes exploratory techniques, encouragement of affective expression, clarification of patient statements, analysis of communication patterns, use of therapy relationship and behavior change techniques
Neurobehavioral and Cognitive Status	**Definition:** Includes neurobehavioral status exam, interview(s), and observation for the clinical assessment of thinking, reasoning and judgment, acquired knowledge, attention, memory, visual spatial abilities, language functions, and planning
Neuropsychological	**Definition:** Thinking, reasoning and judgment, acquired knowledge, attention, memory, visual spatial abilities, language functions, planning
Personality and Behavioral	**Definition:** Mood, emotion, behavior, social functioning, psychopathological conditions, personality traits and characteristics
Psychoanalysis	**Definition:** Methods of obtaining a detailed account of past and present mental and emotional experiences to determine the source and eliminate or diminish the undesirable effects of unconscious conflicts **Explanation:** Accomplished by making the individual aware of their existence, origin, and inappropriate expression in emotions and behavior
Psychodynamic	**Definition:** Exploration of past and present emotional experiences to understand motives and drives using insight-oriented techniques to reduce the undesirable effects of internal conflicts on emotions and behavior **Explanation:** Techniques include empathetic listening, clarifying self-defeating behavior patterns, and exploring adaptive alternatives
Psychophysiological	**Definition:** Monitoring and alteration of physiological processes to help the individual associate physiological reactions combined with cognitive and behavioral strategies to gain improved control of these processes to help the individual cope more effectively
Supportive	**Definition:** Formation of therapeutic relationship primarily for providing emotional support to prevent further deterioration in functioning during periods of particular stress **Explanation:** Often used in conjunction with other therapeutic approaches
Vocational	**Definition:** Exploration of vocational interests, aptitudes and required adaptive behavior skills to develop and carry out a plan for achieving a successful vocational placement **Includes/Examples:** Includes enhancing work related adjustment and/or pursuing viable options in training education or preparation

Section H - Substance Abuse Treatment — Character 3 - Root Type

Detoxification Services	**Definition:** Detoxification from alcohol and/or drugs **Explanation:** Not a treatment modality, but helps the patient stabilize physically and psychologically until the body becomes free of drugs and the effects of alcohol
Family Counseling	**Definition:** The application of psychological methods that includes one or more family members to treat an individual with addictive behavior **Explanation:** Provides support and education for family members of addicted individuals. Family member participation is seen as a critical area of substance abuse treatment

Continued →

Section H - Substance Abuse Treatment — Character 3 - Root Type

Group Counseling	**Definition:** The application of psychological methods to treat two or more individuals with addictive behavior **Explanation:** Provides structured group counseling sessions and healing power through the connection with others
Individual Counseling	**Definition:** The application of psychological methods to treat an individual with addictive behavior **Explanation:** Comprised of several different techniques, which apply various strategies to address drug addiction
Individual Psychotherapy	**Definition:** Treatment of an individual with addictive behavior by behavioral, cognitive, psychoanalytic, psychodynamic or psychophysiological means
Medication Management	**Definition:** Monitoring and adjusting the use of replacement medications for the treatment of addiction
Pharmacotherapy	**Definition:** The use of replacement medications for the treatment of addiction

Appendix C: Approach Definitions

Section 0 - Medical and Surgical — Character 5 - Approach

External (X)	**Definition:** Procedures performed directly on the skin or mucous membrane and procedures performed indirectly by the application of external force through the skin or mucous membrane
Open (0)	**Definition:** Cutting through the skin or mucous membrane and any other body layers necessary to expose the site of the procedure
Percutaneous (3)	**Definition:** Entry, by puncture or minor incision, of instrumentation through the skin or mucous membrane and any other body layers necessary to reach the site of the procedure
Percutaneous Endoscopic (4)	**Definition:** Entry, by puncture or minor incision, of instrumentation through the skin or mucous membrane and any other body layers necessary to reach and visualize the site of the procedure
Via Natural or Artificial Opening (7)	**Definition:** Entry of instrumentation through a natural or artificial external opening to reach the site of the procedure
Via Natural or Artificial Opening Endoscopic (8)	**Definition:** Entry of instrumentation through a natural or artificial external opening to reach and visualize the site of the procedure
Via Natural or Artificial Opening With Percutaneous Endoscopic Assistance (F)	**Definition:** Entry of instrumentation through a natural or artificial external opening and entry, by puncture or minor incision, of instrumentation through the skin or mucous membrane and any other body layers necessary to aid in the performance of the procedure

Section 1 - Obstetrics — Character 5 - Approach

External (X)	**Definition:** Procedures performed directly on the skin or mucous membrane and procedures performed indirectly by the application of external force through the skin or mucous membrane
Open (0)	**Definition:** Cutting through the skin or mucous membrane and any other body layers necessary to expose the site of the procedure
Percutaneous (3)	**Definition:** Entry, by puncture or minor incision, of instrumentation through the skin or mucous membrane and any other body layers necessary to reach the site of the procedure
Percutaneous Endoscopic (4)	**Definition:** Entry, by puncture or minor incision, of instrumentation through the skin or mucous membrane and any other body layers necessary to reach and visualize the site of the procedure
Via Natural or Artificial Opening (7)	**Definition:** Entry of instrumentation through a natural or artificial external opening to reach the site of the procedure
Via Natural or Artificial Opening Endoscopic (8)	**Definition:** Entry of instrumentation through a natural or artificial external opening to reach and visualize the site of the procedure

Section 2 - Placement — Character 5 - Approach

External (X)	**Definition:** Procedures performed directly on the skin or mucous membrane and procedures performed indirectly by the application of external force through the skin or mucous membrane

Section 3 - Administration — Character 5 - Approach

External (X)	**Definition:** Procedures performed directly on the skin or mucous membrane and procedures performed indirectly by the application of external force through the skin or mucous membrane
Open (0)	**Definition:** Cutting through the skin or mucous membrane and any other body layers necessary to expose the site of the procedure

Continued →

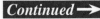

Section 3 - Administration — Character 5 - Approach

Percutaneous (3)	**Definition:** Entry, by puncture or minor incision, of instrumentation through the skin or mucous membrane and any other body layers necessary to reach the site of the procedure
Percutaneous Endoscopic (4)	**Definition:** Entry, by puncture or minor incision, of instrumentation through the skin or mucous membrane and any other body layers necessary to reach and visualize the site of the procedure
Via Natural or Artificial Opening (7)	**Definition:** Entry of instrumentation through a natural or artificial external opening to reach the site of the procedure
Via Natural or Artificial Opening Endoscopic (8)	**Definition:** Entry of instrumentation through a natural or artificial external opening to reach and visualize the site of the procedure

Section 4 - Measurement and Monitoring — Character 5 - Approach

External (X)	**Definition:** Procedures performed directly on the skin or mucous membrane and procedures performed indirectly by the application of external force through the skin or mucous membrane
Open (0)	**Definition:** Cutting through the skin or mucous membrane and any other body layers necessary to expose the site of the procedure
Percutaneous (3)	**Definition:** Entry, by puncture or minor incision, of instrumentation through the skin or mucous membrane and any other body layers necessary to reach the site of the procedure
Percutaneous Endoscopic (4)	**Definition:** Entry, by puncture or minor incision, of instrumentation through the skin or mucous membrane and any other body layers necessary to reach and visualize the site of the procedure
Via Natural or Artificial Opening (7)	**Definition:** Entry of instrumentation through a natural or artificial external opening to reach the site of the procedure
Via Natural or Artificial Opening Endoscopic (8)	**Definition:** Entry of instrumentation through a natural or artificial external opening to reach and visualize the site of the procedure

Section 7 - Osteopathic — Character 5 - Approach

External (X)	**Definition:** Procedures performed directly on the skin or mucous membrane and procedures performed indirectly by the application of external force through the skin or mucous membrane

Section 8 - Other Procedures — Character 5 - Approach

External (X)	**Definition:** Procedures performed directly on the skin or mucous membrane and procedures performed indirectly by the application of external force through the skin or mucous membrane
Open (0)	**Definition:** Cutting through the skin or mucous membrane and any other body layers necessary to expose the site of the procedure
Percutaneous (3)	**Definition:** Entry, by puncture or minor incision, of instrumentation through the skin or mucous membrane and any other body layers necessary to reach the site of the procedure
Percutaneous Endoscopic (4)	**Definition:** Entry, by puncture or minor incision, of instrumentation through the skin or mucous membrane and any other body layers necessary to reach and visualize the site of the procedure
Via Natural or Artificial Opening (7)	**Definition:** Entry of instrumentation through a natural or artificial external opening to reach the site of the procedure
Via Natural or Artificial Opening Endoscopic (8)	**Definition:** Entry of instrumentation through a natural or artificial external opening to reach and visualize the site of the procedure

Section 9 - Chiropractic — Character 5 - Approach

External (X)	**Definition:** Procedures performed directly on the skin or mucous membrane and procedures performed indirectly by the application of external force through the skin or mucous membrane

Section X - New Technology — Character 5 - Approach

External (X)	**Definition:** Procedures performed directly on the skin or mucous membrane and procedures performed indirectly by the application of external force through the skin or mucous membrane
Open (0)	**Definition:** Cutting through the skin or mucous membrane and any other body layers necessary to expose the site of the procedure
Percutaneous (3)	**Definition:** Entry, by puncture or minor incision, of instrumentation through the skin or mucous membrane and any other body layers necessary to reach the site of the procedure
Percutaneous Endoscopic (4)	**Definition:** Entry, by puncture or minor incision, of instrumentation through the skin or mucous membrane and any other body layers necessary to reach and visualize the site of the procedure
Via Natural or Artificial Opening (7)	**Definition:** Entry of instrumentation through a natural or artificial external opening to reach the site of the procedure
Via Natural or Artificial Opening Endoscopic (8)	**Definition:** Entry of instrumentation through a natural or artificial external opening to reach and visualize the site of the procedure

Appendices D–F are structured to assist coders with confirming character selections within the Tables. For example, if the coder is considering the body part of Abdomen Muscle, appendix D can be referenced to identify all of the muscles that are included in the body part Abdomen Muscle (see row 2 in the table below). After reviewing the information, the coder can determine if the body part under consideration is correct or if another body part should be reviewed. The same process can be followed for devices which are included in appendix E and substances which are included in appendix F.

Section 0 - Medical and Surgical — Character 4 - Body Part

1st Toe, Left **1st** Toe, Right	**Includes:** Hallux
Abdomen Muscle, Left **Abdomen** Muscle, Right	**Includes:** External oblique muscle Internal oblique muscle Pyramidalis muscle Rectus abdominis muscle Transversus abdominis muscle
Abdominal Aorta	**Includes:** Inferior phrenic artery Lumbar artery Median sacral artery Middle suprarenal artery Ovarian artery Testicular artery
Abdominal Sympathetic Nerve	**Includes:** Abdominal aortic plexus Auerbach's (myenteric) plexus Celiac (solar) plexus Celiac ganglion Gastric plexus Hepatic plexus Inferior hypogastric plexus Inferior mesenteric ganglion Inferior mesenteric plexus Meissner's (submucous) plexus Myenteric (Auerbach's) plexus Pancreatic plexus Pelvic splanchnic nerve Renal nerve Renal plexus Solar (celiac) plexus Splenic plexus Submucous (Meissner's) plexus Superior hypogastric plexus Superior mesenteric ganglion Superior mesenteric plexus Suprarenal plexus
Abducens Nerve	**Includes:** Sixth cranial nerve
Accessory Nerve	**Includes:** Eleventh cranial nerve
Acoustic Nerve	**Includes:** Cochlear nerve Eighth cranial nerve Scarpa's (vestibular) ganglion Spiral ganglion Vestibular (Scarpa's) ganglion Vestibular nerve Vestibulocochlear nerve
Adenoids	**Includes:** Pharyngeal tonsil

Section 0 - Medical and Surgical — Character 4 - Body Part

Body Part	Includes
Adrenal Gland **Adrenal** Gland, Left **Adrenal** Gland, Right **Adrenal** Glands, Bilateral	**Includes:** Suprarenal gland
Ampulla of Vater	**Includes:** Duodenal ampulla Hepatopancreatic ampulla
Anal Sphincter	**Includes:** External anal sphincter Internal anal sphincter
Ankle Bursa and Ligament, Left **Ankle** Bursa and Ligament, Right	**Includes:** Calcaneofibular ligament Deltoid ligament Ligament of the lateral malleolus Talofibular ligament
Ankle Joint, Left **Ankle** Joint, Right	**Includes:** Inferior tibiofibular joint Talocrural joint
Anterior Chamber, Left **Anterior** Chamber, Right	**Includes:** Aqueous humour
Anterior Tibial Artery, Left **Anterior** Tibial Artery, Right	**Includes:** Anterior lateral malleolar artery Anterior medial malleolar artery Anterior tibial recurrent artery Dorsalis pedis artery Posterior tibial recurrent artery
Anus	**Includes:** Anal orifice
Aortic Valve	**Includes:** Aortic annulus
Appendix	**Includes:** Vermiform appendix
Atrial Septum	**Includes:** Interatrial septum
Atrium, Left	**Includes:** Atrium pulmonale Left auricular appendix
Atrium, Right	**Includes:** Atrium dextrum cordis Right auricular appendix Sinus venosus
Auditory Ossicle, Left **Auditory** Ossicle, Right	**Includes:** Incus Malleus Stapes

Continued →

	Includes:
Axillary Artery, Left **Axillary** Artery, Right	Anterior circumflex humeral artery Lateral thoracic artery Posterior circumflex humeral artery Subscapular artery Superior thoracic artery Thoracoacromial artery
Azygos Vein	Includes: Right ascending lumbar vein Right subcostal vein
Basal Ganglia	Includes: Basal nuclei Claustrum Corpus striatum Globus pallidus Substantia nigra Subthalamic nucleus
Basilic Vein, Left **Basilic** Vein, Right	Includes: Median antebrachial vein Median cubital vein
Bladder	Includes: Trigone of bladder
Brachial Artery, Left **Brachial** Artery, Right	Includes: Inferior ulnar collateral artery Profunda brachii Superior ulnar collateral artery
Brachial Plexus	Includes: Axillary nerve Dorsal scapular nerve First intercostal nerve Long thoracic nerve Musculocutaneous nerve Subclavius nerve Suprascapular nerve
Brachial Vein, Left **Brachial** Vein, Right	Includes: Radial vein Ulnar vein
Brain	Includes: Cerebrum Corpus callosum Encephalon
Breast, Bilateral **Breast,** Left **Breast,** Right	Includes: Mammary duct Mammary gland
Buccal Mucosa	Includes: Buccal gland Molar gland Palatine gland
Carotid Bodies, Bilateral **Carotid** Body, Left **Carotid** Body, Right	Includes: Carotid glomus
Carpal Joint, Left **Carpal** Joint, Right	Includes: Intercarpal joint Midcarpal joint

	Includes:
Carpal, Left **Carpal,** Right	Capitate bone Hamate bone Lunate bone Pisiform bone Scaphoid bone Trapezium bone Trapezoid bone Triquetral bone
Celiac Artery	Includes: Celiac trunk
Cephalic Vein, Left **Cephalic** Vein, Right	Includes: Accessory cephalic vein
Cerebellum	Includes: Culmen
Cerebral Hemisphere	Includes: Frontal lobe Occipital lobe Parietal lobe Temporal lobe
Cerebral Meninges	Includes: Arachnoid mater, intracranial Leptomeninges, intracranial Pia mater, intracranial
Cerebral Ventricle	Includes: Aqueduct of Sylvius Cerebral aqueduct (Sylvius) Choroid plexus Ependyma Foramen of Monro (intraventricular) Fourth ventricle Interventricular foramen (Monro) Left lateral ventricle Right lateral ventricle Third ventricle
Cervical Nerve	Includes: Greater occipital nerve Spinal nerve, cervical Suboccipital nerve Third occipital nerve
Cervical Plexus	Includes: Ansa cervicalis Cutaneous (transverse) cervical nerve Great auricular nerve Lesser occipital nerve Supraclavicular nerve Transverse (cutaneous) cervical nerve
Cervical Vertebra	Includes: Dens Odontoid process Spinous process Transverse foramen Transverse process Vertebral arch Vertebral body Vertebral foramen Vertebral lamina Vertebral pedicle

Continued →

Cervical Vertebral Joint	**Includes:** Atlantoaxial joint Cervical facet joint
Cervical Vertebral Joints, 2 or more	**Includes:** Cervical facet joint
Cervicothoracic Vertebral Joint	**Includes:** Cervicothoracic facet joint
Cisterna Chyli	**Includes:** Intestinal lymphatic trunk Lumbar lymphatic trunk
Coccygeal Glomus	**Includes:** Coccygeal body
Colic Vein	**Includes:** Ileocolic vein Left colic vein Middle colic vein Right colic vein
Conduction Mechanism	**Includes:** Atrioventricular node Bundle of His Bundle of Kent Sinoatrial node
Conjunctiva, Left **Conjunctiva,** Right	**Includes:** Plica semilunaris
Dura Mater	**Includes:** Diaphragma sellae Dura mater, intracranial Falx cerebri Tentorium cerebelli
Elbow Bursa and Ligament, Left **Elbow** Bursa and Ligament, Right	**Includes:** Annular ligament Olecranon bursa Radial collateral ligament Ulnar collateral ligament
Elbow Joint, Left **Elbow** Joint, Right	**Includes:** Distal humerus, involving joint Humeroradial joint Humeroulnar joint Proximal radioulnar joint
Epidural Space, Intracranial	**Includes:** Extradural space, intracranial
Epiglottis	**Includes:** Glossoepiglottic fold
Esophagogastric Junction	**Includes:** Cardia Cardioesophageal junction Gastroesophageal (GE) junction
Esophagus, Lower	**Includes:** Abdominal esophagus
Esophagus, Middle	**Includes:** Thoracic esophagus
Esophagus, Upper	**Includes:** Cervical esophagus
Ethmoid Bone, Left **Ethmoid** Bone, Right	**Includes:** Cribriform plate
Ethmoid Sinus, Left **Ethmoid** Sinus, Right	**Includes:** Ethmoidal air cell

Eustachian Tube, Left **Eustachian** Tube, Right	**Includes:** Auditory tube Pharyngotympanic tube
External Auditory Canal, Left **External** Auditory Canal, Right	**Includes:** External auditory meatus
External Carotid Artery, Left **External** Carotid Artery, Right	**Includes:** Ascending pharyngeal artery Internal maxillary artery Lingual artery Maxillary artery Occipital artery Posterior auricular artery Superior thyroid artery
External Ear, Bilateral **External** Ear, Left **External** Ear, Right	**Includes:** Antihelix Antitragus Auricle Earlobe Helix Pinna Tragus
External Iliac Artery, Left **External** Iliac Artery, Right	**Includes:** Deep circumflex iliac artery Inferior epigastric artery
External Jugular Vein, Left **External** Jugular Vein, Right	**Includes:** Posterior auricular vein
Extraocular Muscle, Left **Extraocular** Muscle, Right	**Includes:** Inferior oblique muscle Inferior rectus muscle Lateral rectus muscle Medial rectus muscle Superior oblique muscle Superior rectus muscle
Eye, Left **Eye,** Right	**Includes:** Ciliary body Posterior chamber
Face Artery	**Includes:** Angular artery Ascending palatine artery External maxillary artery Facial artery Inferior labial artery Submental artery Superior labial artery
Face Vein, Left **Face** Vein, Right	**Includes:** Angular vein Anterior facial vein Common facial vein Deep facial vein Frontal vein Posterior facial (retromandibular) vein Supraorbital vein
Facial Muscle	**Includes:** Buccinator muscle Corrugator supercilii muscle Depressor anguli oris muscle Depressor labii inferioris muscle

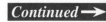

Continued →

	Includes:
	Depressor septi nasi muscle
	Depressor supercilii muscle
	Levator anguli oris muscle
	Levator labii superioris alaeque nasi
	Levator labii superioris alaeque nasi
	Levator labii superioris alaeque nasi
	Levator labii superioris muscle
	Mentalis muscle
	Nasalis muscle
	Occipitofrontalis muscle
	Orbicularis oris muscle
	Procerus muscle
	Risorius muscle
	Zygomaticus muscle
Facial Nerve	**Includes:** Chorda tympani Geniculate ganglion Greater superficial petrosal nerve Nerve to the stapedius Parotid plexus Posterior auricular nerve Seventh cranial nerve Submandibular ganglion
Fallopian Tube, Left **Fallopian** Tube, Right	**Includes:** Oviduct Salpinx Uterine tube
Femoral Artery, Left **Femoral** Artery, Right	**Includes:** Circumflex iliac artery Deep femoral artery Descending genicular artery External pudendal artery Superficial epigastric artery
Femoral Nerve	**Includes:** Anterior crural nerve Saphenous nerve
Femoral Shaft, Left **Femoral** Shaft, Right	**Includes:** Body of femur
Femoral Vein, Left **Femoral** Vein, Right	**Includes:** Deep femoral (profunda femoris) vein Popliteal vein Profunda femoris (deep femoral) vein
Fibula, Left **Fibula,** Right	**Includes:** Body of fibula Head of fibula Lateral malleolus
Finger Nail	**Includes:** Nail bed Nail plate
Finger Phalangeal Joint, Left **Finger** Phalangeal Joint, Right	**Includes:** Interphalangeal (IP) joint
Foot Artery, Left **Foot** Artery, Right	**Includes:** Arcuate artery Dorsal metatarsal artery Lateral plantar artery Lateral tarsal artery Medial plantar artery

	Includes:
Foot Bursa and Ligament, Left **Foot** Bursa and Ligament, Right	**Includes:** Calcaneocuboid ligament Cuneonavicular ligament Intercuneiform ligament Interphalangeal ligament Metatarsal ligament Metatarsophalangeal ligament Subtalar ligament Talocalcaneal ligament Talocalcaneonavicular ligament Tarsometatarsal ligament
Foot Muscle, Left **Foot** Muscle, Right	**Includes:** Abductor hallucis muscle Adductor hallucis muscle Extensor digitorum brevis muscle Extensor hallucis brevis muscle Flexor digitorum brevis muscle Flexor hallucis brevis muscle Quadratus plantae muscle
Foot Vein, Left **Foot** Vein, Right	**Includes:** Common digital vein Dorsal metatarsal vein Dorsal venous arch Plantar digital vein Plantar metatarsal vein Plantar venous arch
Frontal Bone	**Includes:** Zygomatic process of frontal bone
Gastric Artery	**Includes:** Left gastric artery Right gastric artery
Glenoid Cavity, Left **Glenoid** Cavity, Right	**Includes:** Glenoid fossa (of scapula)
Glomus Jugulare	**Includes:** Jugular body
Glossopharyngeal Nerve	**Includes:** Carotid sinus nerve Ninth cranial nerve Tympanic nerve
Hand Artery, Left **Hand** Artery, Right	**Includes:** Deep palmar arch Princeps pollicis artery Radialis indicis Superficial palmar arch
Hand Bursa and Ligament, Left **Hand** Bursa and Ligament, Right	**Includes:** Carpometacarpal ligament Intercarpal ligament Interphalangeal ligament Lunotriquetral ligament Metacarpal ligament Metacarpophalangeal ligament Pisohamate ligament Pisometacarpal ligament Scaphotrapezium ligament
Hand Muscle, Left **Hand** Muscle, Right	**Includes:** Hypothenar muscle Palmar interosseous muscle Thenar muscle

Continued →

Hand Vein, Left **Hand** Vein, Right	**Includes:** Dorsal metacarpal vein Palmar (volar) digital vein Palmar (volar) metacarpal vein Superficial palmar venous arch Volar (palmar) digital vein Volar (palmar) metacarpal vein
Head and Neck Bursa and Ligament	**Includes:** Alar ligament of axis Cervical interspinous ligament Cervical intertransverse ligament Cervical ligamentum flavum Interspinous ligament cervical Intertransverse ligament, cervical Lateral temporomandibular ligament Ligamentum flavum, cervical Sphenomandibular ligament Stylomandibular ligament Transverse ligament of atlas
Head and Neck Sympathetic Nerve	**Includes:** Cavernous plexus Cervical ganglion Ciliary ganglion Internal carotid plexus Otic ganglion Pterygopalatine (sphenopalatine) ganglion Sphenopalatine (pterygopalatine) ganglion Stellate ganglion Submandibular ganglion Submaxillary ganglion
Head Muscle	**Includes:** Auricularis muscle Masseter muscle Pterygoid muscle Splenius capitis muscle Temporalis muscle Temporoparietalis muscle
Heart, Left	**Includes:** Left coronary sulcus Obtuse margin
Heart, Right	**Includes:** Right coronary sulcus
Hemiazygos Vein	**Includes:** Left ascending lumbar vein Left subcostal vein
Hepatic Artery	**Includes:** Common hepatic artery Gastroduodenal artery Hepatic artery proper
Hip Bursa and Ligament, Left **Hip** Bursa and Ligament, Right	**Includes:** Iliofemoral ligament Ischiofemoral ligament Pubofemoral ligament Transverse acetabular ligament Trochanteric bursa
Hip Joint, Left **Hip** Joint, Right	**Includes:** Acetabulofemoral joint

Hip Muscle, Left **Hip** Muscle, Right	**Includes:** Gemellus muscle Gluteus maximus muscle Gluteus medius muscle Gluteus minimus muscle Iliacus muscle Obturator muscle Piriformis muscle Psoas muscle Quadratus femoris muscle Tensor fasciae latae muscle
Humeral Head, Left **Humeral** Head, Right	**Includes:** Greater tuberosity Lesser tuberosity Neck of humerus (anatomical) (surgical)
Humeral Shaft, Left **Humeral** Shaft, Right	**Includes:** Distal humerus Humerus, distal Lateral epicondyle of humerus Medial epicondyle of humerus
Hypogastric Vein, Left **Hypogastric** Vein, Right	**Includes:** Gluteal vein Internal iliac vein Internal pudendal vein Lateral sacral vein Middle hemorrhoidal vein Obturator vein Uterine vein Vaginal vein Vesical vein
Hypoglossal Nerve	**Includes:** Twelfth cranial nerve
Hypothalamus	**Includes:** Mammillary body
Inferior Mesenteric Artery	**Includes:** Sigmoid artery Superior rectal artery
Inferior Mesenteric Vein	**Includes:** Sigmoid vein Superior rectal vein
Inferior Vena Cava	**Includes:** Postcava Right inferior phrenic vein Right ovarian vein Right second lumbar vein Right suprarenal vein Right testicular vein
Inguinal Region, Bilateral **Inguinal** Region, Left **Inguinal** Region, Right	**Includes:** Inguinal canal Inguinal triangle
Inner Ear, Left **Inner** Ear, Right	**Includes:** Bony labyrinth Bony vestibule Cochlea Round window Semicircular canal

Continued →

Innominate Artery	**Includes:** Brachiocephalic artery Brachiocephalic trunk
Innominate Vein, Left **Innominate** Vein, Right	**Includes:** Brachiocephalic vein Inferior thyroid vein
Internal Carotid Artery, Left **Internal** Carotid Artery, Right	**Includes:** Caroticotympanic artery Carotid sinus
Internal Iliac Artery, Left **Internal** Iliac Artery, Right	**Includes:** Deferential artery Hypogastric artery Iliolumbar artery Inferior gluteal artery Inferior vesical artery Internal pudendal artery Lateral sacral artery Middle rectal artery Obturator artery Superior gluteal artery Umbilical artery Uterine artery Vaginal artery
Internal Mammary Artery, Left **Internal** Mammary Artery, Right	**Includes:** Anterior intercostal artery Internal thoracic artery Musculophrenic artery Pericardiophrenic artery Superior epigastric artery
Intracranial Artery	**Includes:** Anterior cerebral artery Anterior choroidal artery Anterior communicating artery Basilar artery Circle of Willis Internal carotid artery, intracranial portion Middle cerebral artery Ophthalmic artery Posterior cerebral artery Posterior communicating artery Posterior inferior cerebellar artery (PICA)
Intracranial Vein	**Includes:** Anterior cerebral vein Basal (internal) cerebral vein Dural venous sinus Great cerebral vein Inferior cerebellar vein Inferior cerebral vein Internal (basal) cerebral vein Middle cerebral vein Ophthalmic vein Superior cerebellar vein Superior cerebral vein
Jejunum	**Includes:** Duodenojejunal flexure

Kidney	**Includes:** Renal calyx Renal capsule Renal cortex Renal segment
Kidney Pelvis, Left **Kidney** Pelvis, Right	**Includes:** Ureteropelvic junction (UPJ)
Kidney, Left **Kidney,** Right **Kidneys,** Bilateral	**Includes:** Renal calyx Renal capsule Renal cortex Renal segment
Knee Bursa and Ligament, Left **Knee** Bursa and Ligament, Right	**Includes:** Anterior cruciate ligament (ACL) Lateral collateral ligament (LCL) Ligament of head of fibula Medial collateral ligament (MCL) Patellar ligament Popliteal ligament Posterior cruciate ligament (PCL) Prepatellar bursa
Knee Joint, Femoral Surface, Left **Knee** Joint, Femoral Surface, Right	**Includes:** Femoropatellar joint Patellofemoral joint
Knee Joint, Left **Knee** Joint, Right	**Includes:** Femoropatellar joint Femorotibial joint Lateral meniscus Medial meniscus Patellofemoral joint Tibiofemoral joint
Knee Joint, Tibial Surface, Left **Knee** Joint, Tibial Surface, Right	**Includes:** Femorotibial joint Tibiofemoral joint
Knee Tendon, Left **Knee** Tendon, Right	**Includes:** Patellar tendon
Lacrimal Duct, Left **Lacrimal** Duct, Right	**Includes:** Lacrimal canaliculus Lacrimal punctum Lacrimal sac Nasolacrimal duct
Larynx	**Includes:** Aryepiglottic fold Arytenoid cartilage Corniculate cartilage Cuneiform cartilage False vocal cord Glottis Rima glottidis Thyroid cartilage Ventricular fold
Lens, Left **Lens,** Right	**Includes:** Zonule of Zinn
Liver	**Includes:** Quadrate lobe

Continued →

Lower Arm and Wrist Muscle, Left **Lower** Arm and Wrist Muscle, Right	**Includes:** Anatomical snuffbox Brachioradialis muscle Extensor carpi radialis muscle Extensor carpi ulnaris muscle Flexor carpi radialis muscle Flexor carpi ulnaris muscle Flexor pollicis longus muscle Palmaris longus muscle Pronator quadratus muscle Pronator teres muscle
Lower Artery	Umbilical artery
Lower Eyelid, Left **Lower** Eyelid, Right	**Includes:** Inferior tarsal plate Medial canthus
Lower Femur, Left **Lower** Femur, Right	**Includes:** Lateral condyle of femur Lateral epicondyle of femur Medial condyle of femur Medial epicondyle of femur
Lower Leg Muscle, Left **Lower** Leg Muscle, Right	**Includes:** Extensor digitorum longus muscle Extensor hallucis longus muscle Fibularis brevis muscle Fibularis longus muscle Flexor digitorum longus muscle Flexor hallucis longus muscle Gastrocnemius muscle Peroneus brevis muscle Peroneus longus muscle Popliteus muscle Soleus muscle Tibialis anterior muscle Tibialis posterior muscle
Lower Leg Tendon, Left **Lower** Leg Tendon, Right	**Includes:** Achilles tendon
Lower Lip	**Includes:** Frenulum labii inferioris Labial gland Vermilion border
Lower Spine Bursa and Ligament	Iliolumbar ligament Interspinous ligament, lumbar Intertransverse ligament, lumbar Ligamentum flavum, lumbar Sacrococcygeal ligament Sacroiliac ligament Sacrospinous ligament Sacrotuberous ligament Supraspinous ligament
Lumbar Nerve	**Includes:** Lumbosacral trunk Spinal nerve, lumbar Superior clunic (cluneal) nerve
Lumbar Plexus	**Includes:** Accessory obturator nerve Genitofemoral nerve Iliohypogastric nerve Ilioinguinal nerve Lateral femoral cutaneous nerve Obturator nerve Superior gluteal nerve

Lumbar Spinal Cord	**Includes:** Cauda equina Conus medullaris
Lumbar Sympathetic Nerve	**Includes:** Lumbar ganglion Lumbar splanchnic nerve
Lumbar Vertebra	**Includes:** Spinous process Transverse process Vertebral arch Vertebral body Vertebral foramen Vertebral lamina Vertebral pedicle
Lumbar Vertebral Joint	**Includes:** Lumbar facet joint
Lumbosacral Joint	**Includes:** Lumbosacral facet joint
Lymphatic, Aortic	**Includes:** Celiac lymph node Gastric lymph node Hepatic lymph node Lumbar lymph node Pancreaticosplenic lymph node Paraaortic lymph node Retroperitoneal lymph node
Lymphatic, Head	**Includes:** Buccinator lymph node Infraauricular lymph node Infraparotid lymph node Parotid lymph node Preauricular lymph node Submandibular lymph node Submaxillary lymph node Submental lymph node Subparotid lymph node Suprahyoid lymph node
Lymphatic, Left Axillary	**Includes:** Anterior (pectoral) lymph node Apical (subclavicular) lymph node Brachial (lateral) lymph node Central axillary lymph node Lateral (brachial) lymph node Pectoral (anterior) lymph node Posterior (subscapular) lymph node Subclavicular (apical) lymph node Subscapular (posterior) lymph node
Lymphatic, Left Lower Extremity	**Includes:** Femoral lymph node Popliteal lymph node

Lymphatic, Left Neck	**Includes:**
	Cervical lymph node
	Jugular lymph node
	Mastoid (postauricular) lymph node
	Occipital lymph node
	Postauricular (mastoid) lymph node
	Retropharyngeal lymph node
	Supraclavicular (Virchow's)
	    lymph node
	Virchow's (supraclavicular)
	    lymph node

Continued →

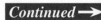

Body Part	Includes
Lymphatic, Left Upper Extremity	**Includes:** Cubital lymph node Deltopectoral (infraclavicular) lymph node Epitrochlear lymph node Infraclavicular (deltopectoral) lymph node Supratrochlear lymph node
Lymphatic, Mesenteric	**Includes:** Inferior mesenteric lymph node Pararectal lymph node Superior mesenteric lymph node
Lymphatic, Pelvis	**Includes:** Common iliac (subaortic) lymph node Gluteal lymph node Iliac lymph node Inferior epigastric lymph node Obturator lymph node Sacral lymph node Subaortic (common iliac) lymph node Suprainguinal lymph node
Lymphatic, Right Axillary	**Includes:** Anterior (pectoral) lymph node Apical (subclavicular) lymph node Brachial (lateral) lymph node Central axillary lymph node Lateral (brachial) lymph node Pectoral (anterior) lymph node Posterior (subscapular) lymph node Subclavicular (apical) lymph node Subscapular (posterior) lymph node
Lymphatic, Right Lower Extremity	**Includes:** Femoral lymph node Popliteal lymph node
Lymphatic, Right Neck	**Includes:** Cervical lymph node Jugular lymph node Mastoid (postauricular) lymph node Occipital lymph node Postauricular (mastoid) lymph node Retropharyngeal lymph node Right jugular trunk Right lymphatic duct Right subclavian trunk Supraclavicular (Virchow's) lymph node Virchow's (supraclavicular) lymph node
Lymphatic, Right Upper Extremity	**Includes:** Cubital lymph node Deltopectoral (infraclavicular) lymph node Epitrochlear lymph node Infraclavicular (deltopectoral) lymph node Supratrochlear lymph node
Lymphatic, Thorax	**Includes:** Intercostal lymph node Mediastinal lymph node Parasternal lymph node Paratracheal lymph node Tracheobronchial lymph node

Body Part	Includes
Main Bronchus, Right	**Includes:** Bronchus Intermedius Intermediate bronchus
Mandible, Left **Mandible,** Right	**Includes:** Alveolar process of mandible Condyloid process Mandibular notch Mental foramen
Mastoid Sinus, Left **Mastoid** Sinus, Right	**Includes:** Mastoid air cells
Maxilla	**Includes:** Alveolar process of maxilla
Maxillary Sinus, Left **Maxillary** Sinus, Right	**Includes:** Antrum of Highmore
Median Nerve	**Includes:** Anterior interosseous nerve Palmar cutaneous nerve
Mediastinum	Mediastinal cavity Mediastinal space
Medulla Oblongata	**Includes:** Myelencephalon
Mesentery	**Includes:** Mesoappendix Mesocolon
Metatarsal-Phalangeal Joint, Left **Metatarsal-Phalangeal** Joint, Right	**Includes:** Metatarsophalangeal (MTP) joint
Middle Ear, Left **Middle** Ear, Right	**Includes:** Oval window Tympanic cavity
Minor Salivary Gland	**Includes:** Anterior lingual gland
Mitral Valve	**Includes:** Bicuspid valve Left atrioventricular valve Mitral annulus
Nasal Bone	**Includes:** Vomer of nasal septum
Nasal Mucosa and Soft Tissue	Columella External naris Greater alar cartilage Internal naris Lateral nasal cartilage Lesser alar cartilage Nasal cavity Nostril
Nasal Septum	**Includes:** Quadrangular cartilage Septal cartilage Vomer bone
Nasal Turbinate	**Includes:** Inferior turbinate Middle turbinate Nasal concha Superior turbinate

Continued →

Nasopharynx	**Includes:** Choana Fossa of Rosenmuller Pharyngeal recess Rhinopharynx
Neck Muscle, Left **Neck** Muscle, Right	**Includes:** Anterior vertebral muscle Arytenoid muscle Cricothyroid muscle Infrahyoid muscle Levator scapulae muscle Platysma muscle Scalene muscle Splenius cervicis muscle Sternocleidomastoid muscle Suprahyoid muscle Thyroarytenoid muscle
Nipple, Left **Nipple,** Right	**Includes:** Areola
Occipital Bone	**Includes:** Foramen magnum
Oculomotor Nerve	**Includes:** Third cranial nerve
Olfactory Nerve	**Includes:** First cranial nerve Olfactory bulb
Omentum	Gastrocolic ligament Gastrocolic omentum Gastrohepatic omentum Gastrophrenic ligament Gastrosplenic ligament Greater Omentum Hepatogastric liagment Lesser Omentum
Optic Nerve	**Includes:** Optic chiasma Second cranial nerve
Orbit, Left **Orbit,** Right	**Includes:** Bony orbit Orbital portion of ethmoid bone Orbital portion of frontal bone Orbital portion of lacrimal bone Orbital portion of maxilla Orbital portion of palatine bone Orbital portion of sphenoid bone Orbital portion of zygomatic bone
Pancreatic Duct	**Includes:** Duct of Wirsung
Pancreatic Duct, Accessory	**Includes:** Duct of Santorini
Parotid Duct, Left **Parotid** Duct, Right	**Includes:** Stensen's duct
Pelvic Bone, Left **Pelvic** Bone, Right	**Includes:** Iliac crest Ilium Ischium Pubis
Pelvic Cavity	**Includes:** Retropubic space

Penis	**Includes:** Corpus cavernosum Corpus spongiosum
Perineum Muscle	**Includes:** Bulbospongiosus muscle Cremaster muscle Deep transverse perineal muscle Ischiocavernosus muscle Levator ani muscle Superficial transverse perineal muscle
Peritoneum	**Includes:** Epiploic foramen
Peroneal Artery, Left **Peroneal** Artery, Right	**Includes:** Fibular artery
Peroneal Nerve	**Includes:** Common fibular nerve Common peroneal nerve External popliteal nerve Lateral sural cutaneous nerve
Pharynx	**Includes:** Base of Tongue Hypopharynx Laryngopharynx Lignual tonsil Oropharynx Piriform recess (sinus) Tongue, base of
Phrenic Nerve	**Includes:** Accessory phrenic nerve
Pituitary Gland	**Includes:** Adenohypophysis Hypophysis Neurohypophysis
Pons	**Includes:** Apneustic center Basis pontis Locus ceruleus Pneumotaxic center Pontine tegmentum Superior olivary nucleus
Popliteal Artery, Left **Popliteal** Artery, Right	**Includes:** Inferior genicular artery Middle genicular artery Superior genicular artery Sural artery Tibioperoneal trunk
Portal Vein	**Includes:** Hepatic portal vein
Prepuce	**Includes:** Foreskin Glans penis
Pudendal Nerve	**Includes:** Posterior labial nerve Posterior scrotal nerve
Pulmonary Artery, Left	**Includes:** Arterial canal (duct) Botallo's duct Pulmoaortic canal
Pulmonary Valve	**Includes:** Pulmonary annulus Pulmonic valve

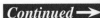

Pulmonary Vein, Left	**Includes:** Left inferior pulmonary vein Left superior pulmonary vein
Pulmonary Vein, Right	**Includes:** Right inferior pulmonary vein Right superior pulmonary vein
Radial Artery, Left **Radial** Artery, Right	**Includes:** Radial recurrent artery
Radial Nerve	**Includes:** Dorsal digital nerve Musculospiral nerve Palmar cutaneous nerve Posterior interosseous nerve
Radius, Left **Radius,** Right	**Includes:** Ulnar notch
Rectum	**Includes:** Anorectal junction
Renal Artery, Left **Renal** Artery, Right	**Includes:** Inferior suprarenal artery Renal segmental artery
Renal Vein, Left	**Includes:** Left inferior phrenic vein Left ovarian vein Left second lumbar vein Left suprarenal vein Left testicular vein
Retina, Left **Retina,** Right	**Includes:** Fovea Macula Optic disc
Retroperitoneum	**Includes:** Retroperitoneal cavity Retroperitoneal space
Rib(s) Bursa and Ligament	Costotransverse ligament
Sacral Nerve	**Includes:** Spinal nerve, sacral
Sacral Plexus	**Includes:** Inferior gluteal nerve Posterior femoral cutaneous nerve Pudendal nerve
Sacral Sympathetic Nerve	**Includes:** Ganglion impar (ganglion of Walther) Pelvic splanchnic nerve Sacral ganglion Sacral splanchnic nerve
Sacrococcygeal Joint	**Includes:** Sacrococcygeal symphysis
Saphenous Vein, Left **Saphenous** Vein, Right	External pudendal vein Great(er) saphenous vein Lesser saphenous vein Small saphenous vein Superficial circumflex iliac vein Superficial epigastric vein
Scapula, Left **Scapula,** Right	**Includes:** Acromion (process) Coracoid process
Sciatic Nerve	**Includes:** Ischiatic nerve

Shoulder Bursa and Ligament, Left **Shoulder** Bursa and Ligament, Right	**Includes:** Acromioclavicular ligament Coracoacromial ligament Coracoclavicular ligament Coracohumeral ligament
	Costoclavicular ligament Glenohumeral ligament Interclavicular ligament Sternoclavicular ligament Subacromial bursa Transverse humeral ligament Transverse scapular ligament
Shoulder Joint, Left **Shoulder** Joint, Right	**Includes:** Glenohumeral joint Glenoid ligament (labrum)
Shoulder Muscle, Left **Shoulder** Muscle, Right	**Includes:** Deltoid muscle Infraspinatus muscle Subscapularis muscle Supraspinatus muscle Teres major muscle Teres minor muscle
Sigmoid Colon	**Includes:** Rectosigmoid junction Sigmoid flexure
Skin	**Includes:** Dermis Epidermis Sebaceous gland Sweat gland
Skin, Chest	Breast procedures, skin only
Sphenoid Bone	**Includes:** Greater wing Lesser wing Optic foramen Pterygoid process Sella turcica
Spinal Canal	**Includes:** Epidural space, spinal Extradural space, spinal Subarachnoid space, spinal Subdural space, spinal Vertebral canal
Spinal Meninges	**Includes:** Arachnoid mater, spinal Denticulate (dentate) ligament Dura mater, spinal Filum terminale Leptomeninges, spinal Pia mater, spinal
Spleen	**Includes:** Accessory spleen
Splenic Artery	**Includes:** Left gastroepiploic artery Pancreatic artery Short gastric artery
Splenic Vein	**Includes:** Left gastroepiploic vein Pancreatic vein

Continued →

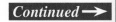

Sternum	**Includes:** Manubrium Suprasternal notch Xiphoid process
Sternum Bursa and Ligament	Costotransverse ligament Costoxiphoid ligament Sternocostal ligament
Stomach, Pylorus	**Includes:** Pyloric antrum Pyloric canal Pyloric sphincter
Subclavian Artery, Left **Subclavian** Artery, Right	**Includes:** Costocervical trunk Dorsal scapular artery Internal thoracic artery
Subcutaneous Tissue and Fascia, Chest	**Includes:** Pectoral fascia
Subcutaneous Tissue and Fascia, Face	**Includes:** Masseteric fascia Orbital fascia Submandibular space
Subcutaneous Tissue and Fascia, Left Foot	**Includes:** Plantar fascia (aponeurosis)
Subcutaneous Tissue and Fascia, Left Hand	**Includes:** Palmar fascia (aponeurosis)
Subcutaneous Tissue and Fascia, Left Lower Arm	**Includes:** Antebrachial fascia Bicipital aponeurosis
Subcutaneous Tissue and Fascia, Left Neck	Deep cervical fascia Pretracheal fascia Prevertebral fascia
Subcutaneous Tissue and Fascia, Left Upper Arm	**Includes:** Axillary fascia Deltoid fascia Infraspinatus fascia Subscapular aponeurosis Supraspinatus fascia
Subcutaneous Tissue and Fascia, Left Upper Leg	**Includes:** Crural fascia Fascia lata Iliac fascia Iliotibial tract (band)
Subcutaneous Tissue and Fascia, Right Foot	**Includes:** Plantar fascia (aponeurosis)
Subcutaneous Tissue and Fascia, Right Hand	**Includes:** Palmar fascia (aponeurosis)
Subcutaneous Tissue and Fascia, Right Lower Arm	**Includes:** Antebrachial fascia Bicipital aponeurosis
Subcutaneous Tissue and Fascia, Right Neck	Deep cervical fascia Pretracheal fascia Prevertebral fascia
Subcutaneous Tissue and Fascia, Right Upper Arm	**Includes:** Axillary fascia Deltoid fascia Infraspinatus fascia Subscapular aponeurosis Supraspinatus fascia

Subcutaneous Tissue and Fascia, Right Upper Leg	**Includes:** Crural fascia Fascia lata Iliac fascia Iliotibial tract (band)
Subcutaneous Tissue and Fascia, Scalp	**Includes:** Galea aponeurotica
Subcutaneous Tissue and Fascia, Trunk	**Includes:** External oblique aponeurosis Transversalis fascia
Submaxillary Gland, Left **Submaxillary** Gland, Right	**Includes:** Submandibular gland
Superior Mesenteric Artery	**Includes:** Ileal artery Ileocolic artery Inferior pancreaticoduodenal artery Jejunal artery
Superior Mesenteric Vein	**Includes:** Right gastroepiploic vein
Superior Vena Cava	**Includes:** Precava
Tarsal Joint, Left **Tarsal** Joint, Right	**Includes:** Calcaneocuboid joint Cuboideonavicular joint Cuneonavicular joint Intercuneiform joint Subtalar (talocalcaneal) joint Talocalcaneal (subtalar) joint Talocalcaneonavicular joint
Tarsal, Left **Tarsal,** Right	**Includes:** Calcaneus Cuboid bone Intermediate cuneiform bone Lateral cuneiform bone Medial cuneiform bone Navicular bone Talus bone
Temporal Artery, Left **Temporal** Artery, Right	**Includes:** Middle temporal artery Superficial temporal artery Transverse facial artery
Temporal Bone, Left **Temporal** Bone, Right	**Includes:** Mastoid process Petrous part of temoporal bone Tympanic part of temoporal bone Zygomatic process of temporal bone
Thalamus	**Includes:** Epithalamus Geniculate nucleus Metathalamus Pulvinar
Thoracic Aorta Ascending/ Arch	**Includes:** Aortic arch Ascending aorta

Continued →

Thoracic Duct	**Includes:** Left jugular trunk Left subclavian trunk
Thoracic Nerve	**Includes:** Intercostal nerve Intercostobrachial nerve Spinal nerve, thoracic Subcostal nerve
Thoracic Sympathetic Nerve	**Includes:** Cardiac plexus Esophageal plexus Greater splanchnic nerve Inferior cardiac nerve Least splanchnic nerve Lesser splanchnic nerve Middle cardiac nerve Pulmonary plexus Superior cardiac nerve Thoracic aortic plexus Thoracic ganglion
Thoracic Vertebra	**Includes:** Spinous process Transverse process Vertebral arch Vertebral body Vertebral foramen Vertebral lamina Vertebral pedicle
Thoracic Vertebral Joint	**Includes:** Costotransverse joint Costovertebral joint Thoracic facet joint
Thoracolumbar Vertebral Joint	**Includes:** Thoracolumbar facet joint
Thorax Muscle, Left **Thorax** Muscle, Right	**Includes:** Intercostal muscle Levatores costarum muscle Pectoralis major muscle Pectoralis minor muscle Serratus anterior muscle Subclavius muscle Subcostal muscle Transverse thoracis muscle
Thymus	**Includes:** Thymus gland
Thyroid Artery, Left **Thyroid** Artery, Right	**Includes:** Cricothyroid artery Hyoid artery Sternocleidomastoid artery Superior laryngeal artery Superior thyroid artery Thyrocervical trunk
Tibia, Left **Tibia,** Right	**Includes:** Lateral condyle of tibia Medial condyle of tibia Medial malleolus
Tibial Nerve	**Includes:** Lateral plantar nerve Medial plantar nerve Medial popliteal nerve Medial sural cutaneous nerve

Toe Nail	**Includes:** Nail bed Nail plate
Toe Phalangeal Joint, Left **Toe** Phalangeal Joint, Right	**Includes:** Interphalangeal (IP) joint
Tongue	**Includes:** Frenulum linguae
Tongue, Palate, Pharynx Muscle	**Includes:** Chondroglossus muscle Genioglossus muscle Hyoglossus muscle Inferior longitudinal muscle Levator veli palatini muscle Palatoglossal muscle Palatopharyngeal muscle Pharyngeal constrictor muscle Salpingopharyngeus muscle Styloglossus muscle Stylopharyngeus muscle Superior longitudinal muscle Tensor veli palatini muscle
Tonsils	**Includes:** Palatine tonsil
Trachea	**Includes:** Cricoid cartilage
Transverse Colon	**Includes:** Hepatic flexure Splenic flexure
Tricuspid Valve	**Includes:** Right atrioventricular valve Tricuspid annulus
Trigeminal Nerve	**Includes:** Fifth cranial nerve Gasserian ganglion Mandibular nerve Maxillary nerve Ophthalmic nerve Trifacial nerve
Trochlear Nerve	**Includes:** Fourth cranial nerve
Trunk Muscle, Left **Trunk** Muscle, Right	**Includes:** Coccygeus muscle Erector spinae muscle Interspinalis muscle Intertransversarius muscle Latissimus dorsi muscle Quadratus lumborum muscle Rhomboid major muscle Rhomboid minor muscle Serratus posterior muscle Transversospinalis muscle Trapezius muscle
Tympanic Membrane, Left **Tympanic** Membrane, Right	**Includes:** Pars flaccida
Ulna, Left **Ulna,** Right	**Includes:** Olecranon process Radial notch

Continued ➝

Ulnar Artery, Left **Ulnar** Artery, Right	**Includes:** Anterior ulnar recurrent artery Common interosseous artery Posterior ulnar recurrent artery
Ulnar Nerve	**Includes:** Cubital nerve
Upper Arm Muscle, Left **Upper** Arm Muscle, Right	**Includes:** Biceps brachii muscle Brachialis muscle Coracobrachialis muscle Triceps brachii muscle
Upper Artery	**Includes:** Aortic intercostal artery Bronchial artery Esophageal artery Subcostal artery
Upper Eyelid, Left **Upper** Eyelid, Right	**Includes:** Lateral canthus Levator palpebrae superioris muscle Orbicularis oculi muscle Superior tarsal plate
Upper Femur, Left **Upper** Femur, Right	**Includes:** Femoral head Greater trochanter Lesser trochanter Neck of femur
Upper Leg Muscle, Left **Upper** Leg Muscle, Right	**Includes:** Adductor brevis muscle Adductor longus muscle Adductor magnus muscle Biceps femoris muscle Gracilis muscle Pectineus muscle Quadriceps (femoris) Rectus femoris muscle Sartorius muscle Semimembranosus muscle Semitendinosus muscle Vastus intermedius muscle Vastus lateralis muscle Vastus medialis muscle
Upper Lip	**Includes:** Frenulum labii superioris Labial gland Vermilion border
Upper Spine Bursa and Ligament	Interspinous ligament, thoracic Intertransverse ligament, thoracic Ligamentum flavum, thoracic Supraspinous ligament
Ureter **Ureter,** Left **Ureter,** Right **Ureters,** Bilateral	**Includes:** Ureteral orifice Ureterovesical orifice
Urethra	**Includes:** Bulbourethral (Cowper's) gland Cowper's (bulbourethral) gland External urethral sphincter Internal urethral sphincter Membranous urethra Penile urethra Prostatic urethra

Uterine Supporting Structure	**Includes:** Broad ligament Infundibulopelvic ligament Ovarian ligament Round ligament of uterus
Uterus	**Includes:** Fundus uteri Myometrium Perimetrium Uterine cornu
Uvula	**Includes:** Palatine uvula
Vagus Nerve	**Includes:** Anterior vagal trunk Pharyngeal plexus Pneumogastric nerve Posterior vagal trunk Pulmonary plexus Recurrent laryngeal nerve Superior laryngeal nerve Tenth cranial nerve
Vas Deferens **Vas** Deferens, Bilateral **Vas** Deferens, Left **Vas** Deferens, Right	**Includes:** Ductus deferens Ejaculatory duct
Ventricle, Right	**Includes:** Conus arteriosus
Ventricular Septum	**Includes:** Interventricular septum
Vertebral Artery, Left **Vertebral** Artery, Right	**Includes:** Anterior spinal artery Posterior spinal artery
Vertebral Vein, Left **Vertebral** Vein, Right	**Includes:** Deep cervical vein Suboccipital venous plexus
Vestibular Gland	**Includes:** Bartholin's (greater vestibular) gland Greater vestibular (Bartholin's) gland Paraurethral (Skene's) gland Skene's (paraurethral) gland
Vitreous, Left **Vitreous,** Right	**Includes:** Vitreous body
Vocal Cord, Left **Vocal** Cord, Right	**Includes:** Vocal fold
Vulva	**Includes:** Labia majora Labia minora
Wrist Bursa and Ligament, Left **Wrist** Bursa and Ligament, Right	**Includes:** Palmar ulnocarpal ligament Radial collateral carpal ligament Radiocarpal ligament Radioulnar ligament Scapholunate ligament Ulnar collateral carpal ligament
Wrist Joint, Left **Wrist** Joint, Right	**Includes:** Distal radioulnar joint Radiocarpal joint

Appendix D

Section 0 - Medical and Surgical — Character 6 - Device

Articulating Spacer in Lower Joints	**Includes:** Articulating Spacer (Antibiotic) Spacer, Articulating (Antibiotic)
Artificial Sphincter in Gastrointestinal System	**Includes:** Artificial anal sphincter (AAS) Artificial bowel sphincter (neosphincter)
Artificial Sphincter in Urinary System	**Includes:** AMS 800® Urinary Control System Artificial urinary sphincter (AUS)
Autologous Arterial Tissue in Heart and Great Vessels	**Includes:** Autologous artery graft
Autologous Arterial Tissue in Lower Arteries	**Includes:** Autologous artery graft
Autologous Arterial Tissue in Lower Veins	**Includes:** Autologous artery graft
Autologous Arterial Tissue in Upper Arteries	**Includes:** Autologous artery graft
Autologous Arterial Tissue in Upper Veins	**Includes:** Autologous artery graft
Autologous Tissue Substitute	**Includes:** Autograft Cultured epidermal cell autograft Epicel® cultured epidermal autograft
Autologous Venous Tissue in Heart and Great Vessels	**Includes:** Autologous vein graft
Autologous Venous Tissue in Lower Arteries	**Includes:** Autologous vein graft
Autologous Venous Tissue in Lower Veins	**Includes:** Autologous vein graft
Autologous Venous Tissue in Upper Arteries	**Includes:** Autologous vein graft
Autologous Venous Tissue in Upper Veins	**Includes:** Autologous vein graft
Bone Growth Stimulator in Head and Facial Bones	**Includes:** Electrical bone growth stimulator (EBGS) Ultrasonic osteogenic stimulator Ultrasound bone healing system
Bone Growth Stimulator in Lower Bones	**Includes:** Electrical bone growth stimulator (EBGS) Ultrasonic osteogenic stimulator Ultrasound bone healing system
Bone Growth Stimulator in Upper Bones	**Includes:** Electrical bone growth stimulator (EBGS) Ultrasonic osteogenic stimulator Ultrasound bone healing system
Cardiac Lead in Heart and Great Vessels	**Includes:** Cardiac contractility modulation lead
Cardiac Lead, Defibrillator for Insertion in Heart and Great Vessels	**Includes:** ACUITY™ Steerable Lead Attain Ability® lead Attain StarFix® (OTW) lead

Section 0 - Medical and Surgical — Character 6 - Device

	Cardiac resynchronization therapy (CRT) lead Corox (OTW) Bipolar Lead Durata® Defibrillation Lead ENDOTAK RELIANCE® (G) Defibrillation Lead
Cardiac Lead, Pacemaker for Insertion in Heart and Great Vessels	**Includes:** ACUITY™ Steerable Lead Attain Ability® lead Attain StarFix® (OTW) lead Cardiac resynchronization therapy (CRT) lead Corox (OTW) Bipolar Lead
Cardiac Resynchronization Defibrillator Pulse Generator for Insertion in Subcutaneous Tissue and Fascia	**Includes:** COGNIS® CRT-D Concerto II CRT-D Consulta CRT-D CONTAK RENEWAL® 3 RF (HE) CRT-D LIVIAN™ CRT-D Maximo II DR CRT-D Ovatio™ CRT-D Protecta XT CRT-D Viva (XT)(S)
Cardiac Resynchronization Pacemaker Pulse Generator for Insertion in Subcutaneous Tissue and Fascia	**Includes:** Consulta CRT-P Stratos LV Synchra CRT-P
Contraceptive Device in Female Reproductive System	**Includes:** Intrauterine device (IUD)
Contraceptive Device in Subcutaneous Tissue and Fascia	**Includes:** Subdermal progesterone implant
Contractility Modulation Device for Insertion in Subcutaneous Tissue and Fascia	**Includes:** Optimizer™ III implantable pulse generator
Defibrillator Generator for Insertion in Subcutaneous Tissue and Fascia	**Includes:** Evera (XT)(S)(DR/VR) Implantable cardioverter-defibrillator (ICD) Maximo II DR (VR) Protecta XT DR (XT VR) Secura (DR) (VR) Virtuoso (II) (DR) (VR)
Diaphragmatic Pacemaker Lead in Respiratory System	**Includes:** Phrenic nerve stimulator lead
Drainage Device	**Includes:** Cystostomy tube Foley catheter Percutaneous nephrostomy catheter Thoracostomy tube

Continued →

External Fixation Device in Head and Facial Bones	**Includes:** External fixator
External Fixation Device in Lower Bones	**Includes:** External fixator
External Fixation Device in Lower Joints	**Includes:** External fixator
External Fixation Device in Upper Bones	**Includes:** External fixator
External Fixation Device in Upper Joints	**Includes:** External fixator
External Fixation Device, Hybrid for Insertion in Upper Bones	**Includes:** Delta frame external fixator Sheffield hybrid external fixator
External Fixation Device, Hybrid for Insertion in Lower Bones	**Includes:** Delta frame external fixator Sheffield hybrid external fixator
External Fixation Device, Hybrid for Reposition in Upper Bones	**Includes:** Delta frame external fixator Sheffield hybrid external fixator
External Fixation Device, Hybrid for Reposition in Lower Bones	**Includes:** Delta frame external fixator Sheffield hybrid external fixator
External Fixation Device, Limb Lengthening for Insertion in Upper Bones	**Includes:** Ilizarov-Vecklich device
External Fixation Device, Limb Lengthening for Insertion in Lower Bones	**Includes:** Ilizarov-Vecklich device
External Fixation Device, Monoplanar for Insertion in Upper Bones	**Includes:** Uniplanar external fixator
External Fixation Device, Monoplanar for Insertion in Lower Bones	**Includes:** Uniplanar external fixator
External Fixation Device, Monoplanar for Reposition in Upper Bones	**Includes:** Uniplanar external fixator
External Fixation Device, Monoplanar for Reposition in Lower Bones	**Includes:** Uniplanar external fixator
External Fixation Device, Ring for Insertion in Upper Bones	**Includes:** Ilizarov external fixator Sheffield ring external fixator
External Fixation Device, Ring for Insertion in Lower Bones	**Includes:** Ilizarov external fixator Sheffield ring external fixator
External Fixation Device, Ring for Reposition in Upper Bones	**Includes:** Ilizarov external fixator Sheffield ring external fixator
External Fixation Device, Ring for Reposition in Lower Bones	**Includes:** Ilizarov external fixator Sheffield ring external fixator

Extraluminal Device	**Includes:** AtriClip LAA Exclusion System LAP-BAND® adjustable gastric banding system REALIZE® Adjustable Gastric Band
Feeding Device in Gastrointestinal System	**Includes:** Percutaneous endoscopic gastrojejunostomy (PEG/J) tube Percutaneous endoscopic gastrostomy (PEG) tube
Hearing Device in Ear, Nose, Sinus	**Includes:** Esteem® implantable hearing system
Hearing Device in Head and Facial Bones	**Includes:** Bone anchored hearing device
Hearing Device, Bone Conduction for Insertion in Ear, Nose, Sinus	**Includes:** Bone anchored hearing device
Hearing Device, Multiple Channel Cochlear Prosthesis for Insertion in Ear, Nose, Sinus	**Includes:** Cochlear implant (CI), multiple channel (electrode)
Hearing Device, Single Channel Cochlear Prosthesis for Insertion in Ear, Nose, Sinus	**Includes:** Cochlear implant (CI), single channel (electrode)
Implantable Heart Assist System in Heart and Great Vessels	**Includes:** Berlin Heart Ventricular Assist Device DeBakey Left Ventricular Assist Device DuraHeart Left Ventricular Assist System HeartMate II® Left Ventricular Assist Device (LVAD) HeartMate 3® LVAS HeartMate XVE® Left Ventricular Assist Device (LVAD) MicroMed HeartAssist Novacor Left Ventricular Assist Device Thoratec IVAD (Implantable Ventricular Assist Device)
Infusion Device	**Includes:** Ascenda Intrathecal Catheter InDura, intrathecal catheter (1P) (spinal) Non-tunneled central venous catheter Peripherally inserted central catheter (PICC) Tunneled spinal (intrathecal) catheter
Infusion Device, Pump in Subcutaneous Tissue and Fascia	**Includes:** Implantable drug infusion pump (anti-spasmodic)(chemotherapy)(pain) Injection reservoir, pump Pump reservoir Subcutaneous injection reservoir, pump SynchroMed pump
Interbody Fusion Device in Lower Joints	**Includes:** Axial Lumbar Interbody Fusion System AxiaLIF® System CoRoent® XL Direct Lateral Interbody Fusion (DLIF) device EXtreme Lateral Interbody Fusion (XLIF) device Interbody fusion (spine) cage XLIF® System

Continued →

Interbody Fusion Device in Upper Joints	**Includes:** BAK/C® Interbody Cervical Fusion System Interbody fusion (spine) cage
Internal Fixation Device in Head and Facial Bones	**Includes:** Bone screw (interlocking)(lag)(pedicle) (recessed) Kirschner wire (K-wire) Neutralization plate
Internal Fixation Device in Lower Bones	**Includes:** Bone screw (interlocking)(lag)(pedicle) (recessed) Clamp and rod internal fixation system (CRIF) Kirschner wire (K-wire) Neutralization plate
Internal Fixation Device in Lower Joints	**Includes:** Fusion screw (compression)(lag) (locking) Joint fixation plate Kirschner wire (K-wire)
Internal Fixation Device in Upper Bones	**Includes:** Bone screw (interlocking)(lag)(pedicle) (recessed) Clamp and rod internal fixation system (CRIF) Kirschner wire (K-wire) Neutralization plate
Internal Fixation Device in Upper Joints	**Includes:** Fusion screw (compression)(lag) (locking) Joint fixation plate Kirschner wire (K-wire)
Internal Fixation Device, Intramedullary in Lower Bones	**Includes:** Intramedullary (IM) rod (nail) Intramedullary skeletal kinetic distractor (ISKD) Kuntscher nail
Internal Fixation Device, Intramedullary in Upper Bones	**Includes:** Intramedullary (IM) rod (nail) Intramedullary skeletal kinetic distractor (ISKD) Kuntscher nail
Internal Fixation Device, Intramedullary Limb Lengthening for Insertion in Lower Bones	**Includes:** PRECICE intramedullary limb lengthening system
Internal Fixation Device, Intramedullary Limb Lengthening for Insertion in Upper Bones	**Includes:** PRECICE intramedullary limb lengthening system
Internal Fixation Device, Rigid Plate for Insertion in Upper Bones	**Includes:** Titanium Sternal Fixation System (TSFS)
Internal Fixation Device, Rigid Plate for Reposition in Upper Bones	**Includes:** Titanium Sternal Fixation System (TSFS)
Internal Fixation Device, Sustained Compression for Fusion in Lower Joints	**Includes:** DynaNail® DynaNail Mini®

Internal Fixation Device, Sustained Compression for Fusion in Upper Joints	**Includes:** DynaNail® DynaNail Mini®
Intraluminal Device	**Includes:** Absolute Pro Vascular (OTW) Self-Expanding Stent System Acculink (RX) Carotid Stent System AFX® Endovascular AAA System AneuRx® AAA Advantage® Assurant (Cobalt) stent Carotid WALLSTENT® Monorail® Endoprosthesis CoAxia NeuroFlo catheter Colonic Z-Stent® Complete (SE) stent Cook Zenith AAA Endovascular Graft Driver stent (RX) (OTW) E-Luminexx™ (Biliary)(Vascular) Stent Embolization coil(s) Endologix AFX® Endovascular AAA System Endurant® II AAA stent graft system Endurant® Endovascular Stent Graft EXCLUDER® AAA Endoprosthesis Express® (LD) Premounted Stent System Express® Biliary SD Monorail® Premounted Stent System Express® SD Renal Monorail® Premounted Stent System FLAIR® Endovascular Stent Graft Formula™ Balloon-Expandable Renal Stent System GORE EXCLUDER® AAA Endoprosthesis GORE TAG® Thoracic Endoprosthesis Herculink (RX) Elite Renal Stent System LifeStent® (Flexstar)(XL) Vascular Stent System Medtronic Endurant® II AAA stent graft system Micro-Driver stent (RX) (OTW) MULTI-LINK (VISION)(MINI-VISION) (ULTRA) Coronary Stent System Omnilink Elite Vascular Balloon Expandable Stent System Protégé® RX Carotid Stent System Stent, intraluminal (cardiovascular) (gastrointestinal)(hepatobiliary)(urinary) Talent® Converter Talent® Occluder Talent® Stent Graft (abdominal)(thoracic) Therapeutic occlusion coil(s) Ultraflex™ Precision Colonic Stent System Valiant Thoracic Stent Graft WALLSTENT® Endoprosthesis Xact Carotid Stent System Zenith AAA Endovascular Graft Zenith Flex® AAA Endovascular Graft Zenith® Renu™ AAA Ancillary Graft Zenith TX2® TAA Endovascular Graft
Intraluminal Device, Airway in Ear, Nose, Sinus	**Includes:** Nasopharyngeal airway (NPA)

Continued →

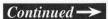

Intraluminal Device, Airway in Gastrointestinal System	**Includes:** Esophageal obturator airway (EOA)
Intraluminal Device, Airway in Mouth and Throat	**Includes:** Guedel airway Oropharyngeal airway (OPA)
Intraluminal Device, Bioactive in Upper Arteries	**Includes:** Bioactive embolization coil(s) Micrus CERECYTE microcoil

Intraluminal Device, Branched or Fenestrated, One or Two Arteries for Restriction in Lower Arteries	**Includes:**
	Cook Zenith® Fenestrated AAA
	    Endovascular Graft
	EXCLUDER® AAA Endoprosthesis
	EXCLUDER® IBE Endoprosthesis
	GORE EXCLUDER® AAA
	    Endoprosthesis
	GORE EXCLUDER® IBE Endoprosthesis
	Zenith® Fenestrated AAA Endovascular
	    Graft

Intraluminal Device, Branched or Fenestrated, Three or More Arteries for Restriction in Lower Arteries	**Includes:**
	Cook Zenith® Fenestrated AAA
	    Endovascular Graft
	EXCLUDER® AAA Endoprosthesis
	GORE EXCLUDER® AAA Endoprosthesis
	Zenith® Fenestrated AAA Endovascular
	    Graft

Intraluminal Device, Drug-eluting in Heart and Great Vessels	**Includes:**
	CYPHER® Stent
	Endeavor® (III)(IV) (Sprint) Zotarolimus-
	    eluting Coronary Stent System
	Everolimus-eluting coronary stent
	Paclitaxel-eluting coronary stent
	Sirolimus-eluting coronary stent
	TAXUS® Liberté® Paclitaxel-eluting
	    Coronary Stent System
	XIENCE Everolimus Eluting Coronary
	    Stent System
	Zotarolimus-eluting coronary stent

Intraluminal Device, Drug-eluting in Lower Arteries	**Includes:** Paclitaxel-eluting peripheral stent Zilver® PTX® (paclitaxel) Drug-Eluting Peripheral Stent
Intraluminal Device, Drug-eluting in Upper Arteries	**Includes:** Paclitaxel-eluting peripheral stent Zilver® PTX® (paclitaxel) Drug-Eluting Peripheral Stent
Intraluminal Device, Endobronchial Valve in Respiratory System	**Includes:** Spiration IBV™ Valve System
Intraluminal Device, Flow Diverter for Restriction in Upper Arteries	**Includes:** Flow Diverter embolization device Pipeline™ (Flex) embolization device Surpass Streamline™ Flow Diverter
Intraluminal Device, Pessary in Female Reproductive System	**Includes:** Pessary ring Vaginal pessary
Intraluminal Device, Endotracheal Airway in Respiratory System	**Includes:** Endotracheal tube (cuffed)(double-lumen)

Liner in Lower Joints	**Includes:** Acetabular cup Hip (joint) liner Joint liner (insert) Knee (implant) insert Tibial insert
Monitoring Device	**Includes:** Blood glucose monitoring system Cardiac event recorder Continuous Glucose Monitoring (CGM) device Implantable glucose monitoring device Loop recorder, implantable Reveal (LINQ)(DX)(XT)
Monitoring Device, Hemodynamic for Insertion in Subcutaneous Tissue and Fascia	**Includes:** Implantable hemodynamic monitor (IHM) Implantable hemodynamic monitoring system (IHMS)
Monitoring Device, Pressure Sensor for Insertion in Heart and Great Vessels	**Includes:** CardioMEMS® pressure sensor EndoSure® sensor
Neurostimulator Lead in Central Nervous System and Cranial Nerves	**Includes:** Cortical strip neurostimulator lead DBS lead Deep brain neurostimulator lead RNS System lead Spinal cord neurostimulator lead
Neurostimulator Lead in Peripheral Nervous System	**Includes:** InterStim® Therapy lead
Neurostimulator Generator in Head and Facial Bones	**Includes:** RNS system neurostimulator generator
Nonautologous Tissue Substitute	**Includes:** Acellular Hydrated Dermis Bone bank bone graft Cook Biodesign® Fistula Plug(s) Cook Biodesign® Hernia Graft(s) Cook Biodesign® Layered Graft(s) Cook Zenapro™ Layered Grafts(s) Tissue bank graft
Pacemaker, Dual Chamber for Insertion in Subcutaneous Tissue and Fascia	**Includes:** Advisa (MRI) EnRhythm Kappa Revo MRI™ SureScan® pacemaker Two lead pacemaker Versa
Pacemaker, Single Chamber for Insertion in Subcutaneous Tissue and Fascia	**Includes:** Single lead pacemaker (atrium)(ventricle)
Pacemaker, Single Chamber Rate Responsive for Insertion in Subcutaneous Tissue and Fascia	**Includes:** Single lead rate responsive pacemaker (atrium)(ventricle)
Radioactive Element	**Includes:** Brachytherapy seeds CivaSheet®

Continued →

Radioactive Element, Cesium-131 Collagen Implant for Insertion in Central Nervous System and Cranial Nerves	Cesium-131 Collagen Implant GammaTile™
Resurfacing Device in Lower Joints	**Includes:** CONSERVE® PLUS Total Resurfacing Hip System Cormet Hip Resurfacing System
Short-term External Heart Assist System in Heart and Great Vessels	Biventricular external heart assist system BVS 5000 Ventricular Assist Device Centrimag® Blood Pump Impella® heart pump TandemHeart® System Thoratec Paracorporeal Ventricular Assist Device
Spacer in Lower Joints	**Includes:** Joint spacer (antibiotic) Spacer, Static (Antibiotic) Static Spacer (Antibiotic)
Spacer in Upper Joints	**Includes:** Joint spacer (antibiotic)
Spinal Stabilization Device, Facet Replacement for Insertion in Upper Joints	**Includes:** Facet replacement spinal stabilization device
Spinal Stabilization Device, Facet Replacement for Insertion in Lower Joints	**Includes:** Facet replacement spinal stabilization device
Spinal Stabilization Device, Interspinous Process for Insertion in Upper Joints	**Includes:** Interspinous process spinal stabilization device X-STOP® Spacer
Spinal Stabilization Device, Interspinous Process for Insertion in Lower Joints	**Includes:** Interspinous process spinal stabilization device X-STOP® Spacer
Spinal Stabilization Device, Pedicle-Based for Insertion in Upper Joints	**Includes:** Dynesys® Dynamic Stabilization System Pedicle-based dynamic stabilization device
Spinal Stabilization Device, Pedicle-Based for Insertion in Lower Joints	**Includes:** Dynesys® Dynamic Stabilization System Pedicle-based dynamic stabilization device
Stimulator Generator in Subcutaneous Tissue and Fascia	**Includes:** Baroreflex Activation Therapy® (BAT®) Diaphragmatic pacemaker generator Mark IV Breathing Pacemaker System Phrenic nerve stimulator generator Rheos® System device
Stimulator Generator, Multiple Array for Insertion in Subcutaneous Tissue and Fascia	**Includes:** Activa PC neurostimulator Enterra gastric neurostimulator Neurostimulator generator, multiple channel PrimeAdvanced neurostimulator (SureScan)(MRI Safe)

Stimulator Generator, Multiple Array Rechargeable for Insertion in Subcutaneous Tissue and Fascia	**Includes:** Activa RC neurostimulator Neurostimulator generator, multiple channel rechargeable RestoreAdvanced neurostimulator (SureScan)(MRI Safe) RestoreSensor neurostimulator (SureScan)(MRI Safe) RestoreUltra neurostimulator (SureScan) (MRI Safe)
Stimulator Generator, Single Array for Insertion in Subcutaneous Tissue and Fascia	**Includes:** Activa SC neurostimulator InterStim® Therapy neurostimulator Itrel (3)(4) neurostimulator Neurostimulator generator, single channel
Stimulator Generator, Single Array Rechargeable for Insertion in Subcutaneous Tissue and Fascia	**Includes:** Neurostimulator generator, single channel rechargeable
Stimulator Lead in Gastrointestinal System	**Includes:** Gastric electrical stimulation (GES) lead Gastric pacemaker lead
Stimulator Lead in Muscles	**Includes:** Electrical muscle stimulation (EMS) lead Electronic muscle stimulator lead Neuromuscular electrical stimulation (NEMS) lead
Stimulator Lead in Upper Arteries	**Includes:** Baroreflex Activation Therapy® (BAT®) Carotid (artery) sinus (baroreceptor) lead Rheos® System lead
Stimulator Lead in Urinary System	**Includes:** Sacral nerve modulation (SNM) lead Sacral neuromodulation lead Urinary incontinence stimulator lead
Subcutaneous Defibrillator Lead in Subcutaneous Tissue and Fascia	**Includes:** S-ICD™ lead

Continued →

Synthetic Substitute	**Includes:** AbioCor® Total Replacement Heart AMPLATZER® Muscular VSD Occluder Annuloplasty ring Bard® Composix® (E/X)(LP) mesh Bard® Composix® Kugel® patch Bard® Dulex™ mesh Bard® Ventralex™ hernia patch Barricaid® Annular Closure Device (ACD) BRYAN® Cervical Disc System Corvia IASD® Ex-PRESS™ mini glaucoma shunt Flexible Composite Mesh GORE® DUALMESH® Holter valve ventricular shunt IASD® (InterAtrial Shunt Device), Corvia InterAtrial Shunt Device IASD®, Corvia MitraClip valve repair system Nitinol framed polymer mesh Open Pivot Aortic Valve Graft (AVG) Open Pivot (mechanical) valve Partially absorbable mesh PHYSIOMESH™ Flexible Composite Mesh Polymethylmethacrylate (PMMA) Polypropylene mesh PRESTIGE® Cervical Disc PROCEED™ Ventral Patch Prodisc-C Prodisc-L PROLENE Polypropylene Hernia System (PHS) Rebound HRD® (Hernia Repair Device) SynCardia Total Artificial Heart Total artificial (replacement) heart ULTRAPRO Hernia System (UHS) ULTRAPRO Partially Absorbable Lightweight Mesh ULTRAPRO Plug V-WAVE Interatrial Shunt System Ventrio™ Hernia Patch Zimmer® NexGen® LPS Mobile Bearing Knee Zimmer® NexGen® LPS-Flex Mobile Knee
Synthetic Substitute, Ceramic for Replacement in Lower Joints	**Includes:** Ceramic on ceramic bearing surface Novation® Ceramic AHS® (Articulation Hip System)
Synthetic Substitute, Intraocular Telescope for Replacement in Eye	**Includes:** Implantable Miniature Telescope™ (IMT)
Synthetic Substitute, Metal for Replacement in Lower Joints	**Includes:** Cobalt/chromium head and socket Metal on metal bearing surface

Synthetic Substitute, Metal on Polyethylene for Replacement in Lower Joints	**Includes:** Cobalt/chromium head and polyethylene socket
Synthetic Substitute, Oxidized Zirconium on Polyethylene for Replacement in Lower Joints	OXINIUM
Synthetic Substitute, Polyethylene for Replacement in Lower Joints	**Includes:** Polyethylene socket
Synthetic Substitute, Reverse Ball and Socket for Replacement in Upper Joints	**Includes:** Delta III Reverse shoulder prosthesis Reverse® Shoulder Prosthesis
Tissue Expander in Skin and Breast	**Includes:** Tissue expander (inflatable)(injectable)
Tissue Expander in Subcutaneous Tissue and Fascia	**Includes:** Tissue expander (inflatable)(injectable)
Tracheostomy Device in Respiratory System	**Includes:** Tracheostomy tube
Vascular Access Device, Totally Implantable in Subcutaneous Tissue and Fascia	**Includes:** Implanted (venous)(access) port Injection reservoir, port Subcutaneous injection reservoir, port
Vascular Access Device, Tunneled in Subcutaneous Tissue and Fascia	Tunneled central venous catheter Vectra® Vascular Access Graft
Zooplastic Tissue in Heart and Great Vessels	**Includes:** 3f (Aortic) Bioprosthesis valve Bovine pericardial valve Bovine pericardium graft Contegra Pulmonary Valved Conduit CoreValve transcatheter aortic valve Epic™ Stented Tissue Valve (aortic) Freestyle (Stentless) Aortic Root Bioprosthesis Hancock Bioprosthesis (aortic) (mitral) valve Hancock Bioprosthetic Valved Conduit Melody® transcatheter pulmonary valve Mitroflow® Aortic Pericardial Heart Valve Mosaic Bioprosthesis (aortic) (mitral) valve Porcine (bioprosthetic) valve SAPIEN transcatheter aortic valve SJM Biocor® Stented Valve System Stented tissue valve Trifecta™ Valve (aortic) Xenograft

Device Aggregation Table

Specific Device	for Operation	in Body System	General Device	
Autologous Arterial Tissue	All applicable	Heart and Great Vessels Lower Arteries Lower Veins Upper Arteries Upper Veins	7	Autologous Tissue Substitute
Autologous Venous Tissue	All applicable	Heart and Great Vessels Lower Arteries Lower Veins Upper Arteries Upper Veins	7	Autologous Tissue Substitute
Cardiac Lead, Defibrillator	Insertion	Heart and Great Vessels	M	Cardiac Lead
Cardiac Lead, Pacemaker	Insertion	Heart and Great Vessels	M	Cardiac Lead
Cardiac Resynchronization Defibrillator Pulse Generator	Insertion	Subcutaneous Tissue and Fascia	P	Cardiac Rhythm Related Device
Cardiac Resynchronization Pacemaker Pulse Generator	Insertion	Subcutaneous Tissue and Fascia	P	Cardiac Rhythm Related Device
Contractility Modulation Device	Insertion	Subcutaneous Tissue and Fascia	P	Cardiac Rhythm Related Device
Defibrillator Generator	Insertion	Subcutaneous Tissue and Fascia	P	Cardiac Rhythm Related Device
Epiretinal Visual Prosthesis	All applicable	Eye	J	Synthetic Substitute
External Fixation Device, Hybrid	Insertion	Lower Bones Upper Bones	5	External Fixation Device
External Fixation Device, Hybrid	Reposition	Lower Bones Upper Bones	5	External Fixation Device
External Fixation Device, Limb Lengthening	Insertion	Lower Bones Upper Bones	5	External Fixation Device
External Fixation Device, Monoplanar	Insertion	Lower Bones Upper Bones	5	External Fixation Device
External Fixation Device, Monoplanar	Reposition	Lower Bones Upper Bones	5	External Fixation Device
External Fixation Device, Ring	Insertion	Lower Bones Upper Bones	5	External Fixation Device
External Fixation Device, Ring	Reposition	Lower Bones Upper Bones	5	External Fixation Device
Hearing Device, Bone Conduction	Insertion	Ear, Nose, Sinus	S	Hearing Device
Hearing Device, Multiple Channel Cochlear Prosthesis	Insertion	Ear, Nose, Sinus	S	Hearing Device
Hearing Device, Single Channel Cochlear Prosthesis	Insertion	Ear, Nose, Sinus	S	Hearing Device
Internal Fixation Device, Intramedullary	All applicable	Lower Bones Upper Bones	4	Internal Fixation Device
Internal Fixation Device, Intramedullary Limb Lengthening	Insertion	Lower Bones Upper Bones	6	Internal Fixation Device Intramedullary
Internal Fixation Device, Rigid Plate	Insertion	Upper Bones	4	Internal Fixation Device
Internal Fixation Device, Rigid Plate	Reposition	Upper Bones	4	Internal Fixation Device

Continued →

Specific Device	for Operation	in Body System	General Device	
Intraluminal Device, Airway	All applicable	Ear, Nose, Sinus Gastrointestinal System Mouth and Throat	**D**	Intraluminal Device
Intraluminal Device, Bioactive	All applicable	Upper Arteries	**D**	Intraluminal Device
Intraluminal Device, Branched or Fenestrated, One or Two Arteries	Restriction	Heart and Great Vessels Lower Arteries	**D**	Intraluminal Device
Intraluminal Device, Branched or Fenestrated, Three or More Arteries	Restriction	Heart and Great Vessels Lower Arteries	**D**	Intraluminal Device
Intraluminal Device, Drug-eluting	All applicable	Heart and Great Vessels Lower Arteries Upper Arteries	**D**	Intraluminal Device
Intraluminal Device, Drug-eluting, Four or More	All applicable	Heart and Great Vessels Lower Arteries Upper Arteries	**D**	Intraluminal Device
Intraluminal Device, Drug-eluting, Three	All applicable	Heart and Great Vessels Lower Arteries Upper Arteries	**D**	Intraluminal Device
Intraluminal Device, Drug-eluting, Two	All applicable	Heart and Great Vessels Lower Arteries Upper Arteries	**D**	Intraluminal Device
Intraluminal Device, Endobronchial Valve	All applicable	Respiratory System	**D**	Intraluminal Device
Intraluminal Device, Endotracheal Airway	All applicable	Respiratory System	**D**	Intraluminal Device
Intraluminal Device, Flow Diverter	Restriction	Upper Arteries	**D**	Intraluminal Device
Intraluminal Device, Four or More	All applicable	Heart and Great Vessels Lower Arteries Upper Arteries	**D**	Intraluminal Device
Intraluminal Device, Pessary	All applicable	Female Reproductive System	**D**	Intraluminal Device
Intraluminal Device, Radioactive	All applicable	Heart and Great Vessels	**D**	Intraluminal Device
Intraluminal Device, Three	All applicable	Heart and Great Vessels Lower Arteries Upper Arteries	**D**	Intraluminal Device
Intraluminal Device, Two	All applicable	Heart and Great Vessels Lower Arteries Upper Arteries	**D**	Intraluminal Device
Monitoring Device, Hemodynamic	Insertion	Subcutaneous Tissue and Fascia	**2**	Monitoring Device
Monitoring Device, Pressure Sensor	Insertion	Heart and Great Vessels	**2**	Monitoring Device
Pacemaker, Dual Chamber	Insertion	Subcutaneous Tissue and Fascia	**P**	Cardiac Rhythm Related Device
Pacemaker, Single Chamber	Insertion	Subcutaneous Tissue and Fascia	**P**	Cardiac Rhythm Related Device
Pacemaker, Single Chamber Rate Responsive	Insertion	Subcutaneous Tissue and Fascia	**P**	Cardiac Rhythm Related Device
Spinal Stabilization Device, Facet Replacement	Insertion	Lower Joints Upper Joints	**4**	Internal Fixation Device
Spinal Stabilization Device, Interspinous Process	Insertion	Lower Joints Upper Joints	**4**	Internal Fixation Device

Continued →

Specific Device	for Operation	in Body System	General Device	
Spinal Stabilization Device, Pedicle-Based	Insertion	Lower Joints Upper Joints	4	Internal Fixation Device
Stimulator Generator, Multiple Array	Insertion	Subcutaneous Tissue and Fascia	M	Stimulator Generator
Stimulator Generator, Multiple Array Rechargeable	Insertion	Subcutaneous Tissue and Fascia	M	Stimulator Generator
Stimulator Generator, Single Array	Insertion	Subcutaneous Tissue and Fascia	M	Stimulator Generator
Stimulator Generator, Single Array Rechargeable	Insertion	Subcutaneous Tissue and Fascia	M	Stimulator Generator
Synthetic Substitute, Ceramic	Replacement	Lower Joints	J	Synthetic Substitute
Synthetic Substitute, Ceramic on Polyethylene	Replacement	Lower Joints	J	Synthetic Substitute
Synthetic Substitute, Intraocular Telescope	Replacement	Eye	J	Synthetic Substitute
Synthetic Substitute, Metal	Replacement	Lower Joints	J	Synthetic Substitute
Synthetic Substitute, Metal on Polyethylene	Replacement	Lower Joints	J	Synthetic Substitute
Synthetic Substitute, Oxidized Zirconium on Polyethylene	Replacement	Lower Joints	J	Synthetic Substitute
Synthetic Substitute, Polyethylene	Replacement	Lower Joints	J	Synthetic Substitute
Synthetic Substitute, Reverse Ball and Socket	Replacement	Upper Joints	J	Synthetic Substitute

Section 3 – Administration Character 6 – Substance

4-Factor Prothrombin Complex Concentrate	**Includes:** Kcentra
Adhesion Barrier	**Includes:** Seprafilm
Anti-Infective Envelope	**Includes:** AIGISRx Antibacterial Envelope Antibacterial Envelope (TYRX) (AIGISRx) Antimicrobial envelope TYRX Antibacterial Envelope
Clofarabine	**Includes:** Clolar
Glucarpidase	**Includes:** Voraxaze
Hematopoietic Stem/ Progenitor Cells, Genetically Modified	**Includes:** OTL-101
Human B-type Natriuretic Peptide	**Includes:** Nesiritide
Other Thrombolytic	**Includes:** Tissue Plasinogen Activator (tPA)(r-tPA)
Oxazolidinones	**Includes:** Zyvox
Recombinant Bone Morphogenetic Protein	**Includes:** Bone morphogenetic protein 2 (BMP 2) rhBMP-2

Section X - New Technology - Character 6 - Device/ Substance/Technology

Apalutamide Antineoplastic	ERLEADA™
Atezolizumab Antineoplastic	TECENTRIQ®
Bezlotoxumab Monoclonal Antibody	ZINPLAVA™
Brexanolone	ZULRESSO™
Brexucabtagene Autoleucel Immunotherapy	Brexucabtagene Autoleucel
Cefiderocol Anti-infective	FETROJA®
Ceftolozane/Tazobactam Anti-infective	ZERBAXA®
Coagulation Factor Xa, Inactivated	Andexanet Alfa, Factor Xa Inhibitor Reversal Agent Andexxa Coagulation Factor Xa, (Recombinant) Inactivated Factor Xa Inhibitor Reversal Agent, Andexanet Alfa
Concentrated Bone Marrow Aspirate	CBMA (Concentrated Bone Marrow Aspirate)
Cytarabine and Daunorubicin Liposome Antineoplastic	VYXEOS™
Defibrotide Sodium Anticoagulant	Defitelio
Durvalumab Antineoplastic	IMFINZI®
Eculizumab	Soliris®
Endothelial Damage Inhibitor	DuraGraft® Endothelial Damage Inhibitor
Engineered Autologous Chimeric Antigent Receptor T-cell Immunotherapy	Axicabtagene Ciloeucel KYMRIAH Tisagenlecleucel
Esketamine Hydrochloride	SPRAVATO™
Fosfomycin Anti-infective	CONTEPO™ Fosfomycin injection
Gilteritinib Antineoplastic	XOSPATA®
Imipenem-cilastatin-relebactam Anti-infective	IMI/REL
Interbody Fusion Device, Nanotextured Surface in New Technology	nanoLOCK™ interbody fusion device
Interbody Fusion Device, Radiolucent Porous in New Technology	COALESCE® radiolucent interbody fusion device COHERE® radiolucent interbody fusion device
Intraluminal Device, Sustained Release Drug-eluting in New Technology	Eluvia™ Drug-Eluting Vascular Stent System SAVAL below-the-knee (BTK) drug-eluting stent system
Intraluminal Device, Sustained Release Drug-eluting, Four or more in New Technology	Eluvia™ Drug-Eluting Vascular Stent System SAVAL below-the-knee (BTK) drug-eluting stent system

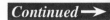

Continued →

Intraluminal Device, Sustained Release Drug-eluting, Three in New Technology	Eluvia™ Drug-Eluting Vascular Stent System SAVAL below-the-knee (BTK) drug-eluting stent system
Intraluminal Device, Sustained Release Drug-eluting, Two in New Technology	Eluvia™ Drug-Eluting Vascular Stent System SAVAL below-the-knee (BTK) drug-eluting stent system
Iobenguane I-131 Antineoplastic	AZEDRA® Iobenguane I-131, High Specific Activity (HSA)
Lefamulin Anti-Infective	XENLETA™
Lisocabtagene Maraleucel Immunotherapy	Lisocabtagene Maraleucel
Magnetically Controlled Growth Rod(s) in New Technology	MAGEC® Spinal Bracing and Distraction System Spinal growth rods, magnetically controlled
Meropenem-vaborbactam Anti-infective	Vabomere™
Mineral-based Topical Hemostatic Agent	Hemospray® Endoscopic Hemostat
Nerinitide	NA-1 (Nerinitide)
Omadacycline Anti-infective	NUZYRA™
Other New Technology Therapeutic Substance	STELARA® Ustekinumab

Remdesivir Anti-infective	GS-5734 Veklury
Ruxolitinib	Jakafi®
Sarilumab	KEVZARA®
Skin Substitute, Porcine Liver Derived in New Technology	MIRODERM™ Biologic Wound Matrix
Synthetic Human Angiotensin II	Angiotensin II GIAPREZA™ Human angiotensin II, synthetic
Synthetic Substitute, Mechanically Expandable (Paired) in New Technology	SpineJack® system
Tagraxofusp-erzs Antineoplastic	ELZONRIS™
Tocilizumab	ACTEMRA®
Uridine Triacetate	Vistogard®
Venetoclax Antineoplastic	Venclexta®
Zooplastic Tissue, Rapid Deployment Technique in New Technology	EDWARDS INTUITY Elite valve system INTUITY elite valve system, EDWARDS Perceval sutureless valve Sutureless valve, Perceval

Appendix G is provided online in a format suitable for spreadsheet and/or database use. Go to http://ahimapress.org/casto8130, click the "Online Resources" link, and enter case sensitive password AHIMA7Dc3w2021 to download files.

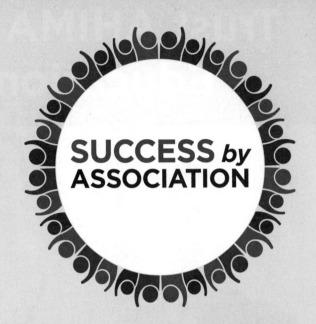
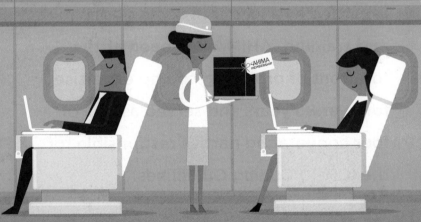
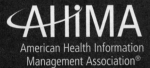

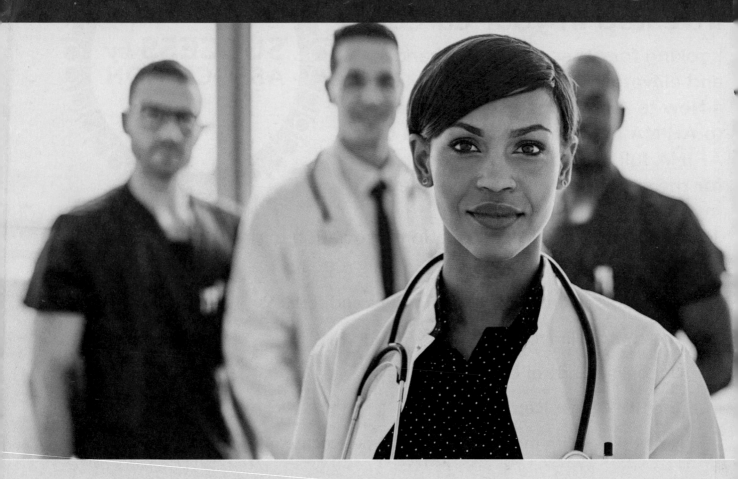
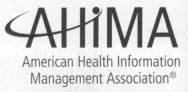